Handbook of

Healthcare Delivery Systems

Industrial and Systems Engineering

Series Editor

Gavriel Salvendy

Professor Emeritus
School of Industrial Engineering
Purdue University

Chair Professor & Head
Department of Industrial Engineering
Tsinghua University
Beijing, People's Republic of China

Published Titles

Handbook of Healthcare Delivery Systems, *edited by Yuehwern Yih*

Forthcoming Titles

Cultural Factors in Systems Design: Decision Making and Action, *Robert W. Proctor, Shimon Y. Nof, and Yuehwern Yih*

Data Mining Techniques: Concepts and Methodologies of Discovering and Modeling Data Patterns, *Nong Ye*

Design and Management of RFID-Enabled Enterprises, *edited by Sangtae Kim and Nagabhushana Prabhu*

Managing Professional Services Delivery: Nine Rules for Success, *Barry Mundt and Francis J. Smith*

Handbook of Healthcare Delivery Systems

Edited by
Yuehwern Yih

CRC Press
Taylor & Francis Group
Boca Raton London New York

CRC Press is an imprint of the
Taylor & Francis Group, an **informa** business

CRC Press
Taylor & Francis Group
6000 Broken Sound Parkway NW, Suite 300
Boca Raton, FL 33487-2742

Printed in the United States of America on acid-free paper
10 9 8 7 6 5 4 3 2 1

International Standard Book Number: 978-1-4398-0333-2 (Hardback)

Library of Congress Cataloging-in-Publication Data

Handbook of healthcare delivery systems / edited by Yuehwern Yih.
p. ; cm. -- (Industrial and systems engineering series)
Includes bibliographical references and index.
Summary: "A resource covering the delivery of all healthcare services, this handbook provides the collective source to promote and facilitate integrated system solutions for healthcare. Written from a systems engineering perspective, it provides theoretical foundations, methodologies, and case studies in each main sector of healthcare delivery systems for designing, assessing, optimizing, and managing each healthcare outcome. It covers the state-of-the-art in modern technologies and offers a comprehensive description of the healthcare delivery system from the macro level (e.g. hospitals) to the micro level (e.g. operation room)"--Provided by publisher.
ISBN 978-1-4398-0333-2 (hardcover : alkaline paper)
1. Integrated delivery of health care--Handbooks, manuals, etc. I. Yih, Yuehwern, editor. II. Series: Industrial and systems engineering series.
[DNLM: 1. Delivery of Health Care, Integrated. 2. Outcome and Process Assessment (Health Care) 3. Systems Analysis. W 84.1]

RA971.H277 2011
362.1068--dc22 2010043718

Visit the Taylor & Francis Web site at
http://www.taylorandfrancis.com

and the CRC Press Web site at
http://www.crcpress.com

Contents

Foreword xi

Preface xiii

Editor xv

Contributors xvii

PART I Healthcare Delivery System Overview

1 Healthcare: How Did We Get Here and Where Are We Going? 1-1
David M. Lawrence

2 Engineering and the Healthcare Delivery System 2-1
Proctor P. Reid and W. Dale Compton

3 The VA Healthcare Delivery System 3-1
Elizabeth M. Yano

4 Outpatient Clinics: Primary and Specialty Care 4-1
Deanna R. Willis

5 Designing a Nurse-Managed Healthcare Delivery System 5-1
Julie Cowan Novak

6 Long-Term Care 6-1
Kathleen Abrahamson and Karis Pressler

7 Healthcare Insurance: An Introduction 7-1
Vinod K. Sahney and Ann Tousignant

8 An Integrated Model of Healthcare Delivery 8-1
Steven M. Witz and Kenneth J. Musselman

PART II Performance Assessment and Process Improvement Management

9 Performance Assessment for Healthcare Organizations 9-1
Peter Arthur Woodbridge and George Oscar Allen

10 Managing Physician Panels in Primary Care 10-1
Hari Balasubramanian, Brian T. Denton, and Qi Ming Lin

11 Lean in Healthcare 11-1
Philip C. Jones and Barrett W. Thomas

12 Patient Safety and Proactive Risk Assessment 12-1
Pascale Carayon, Hélène Faye, Ann Schoofs Hundt, Ben-Tzion Karsh, and Tosha B. Wetterneck

13 Toward More Effective Implementation of Evidence-Based Practice: Relational and Contextual Considerations 13-1
Priscilla A. Arling, Rebekah L. Fox, and Bradley N. Doebbeling

PART III System Engineering: Technologies and Methodologies

14 Computer Simulation in Healthcare 14-1
Sean Carr and Stephen D. Roberts

15 An Introduction to Optimization Models and Applications in Healthcare Delivery Systems 15-1
Wenhua Cao and Gino J. Lim

16 Queueing Theory and Modeling 16-1
Linda V. Green

17 Markov Decision Processes and Its Applications in Healthcare 17-1
Jonathan Patrick and Mehmet A. Begen

18 Statistical Analysis and Modeling 18-1
Min Zhang and Mark E. Cowen

19 Analyzing Decisions Using Datasets with Multiple Attributes: A Machine Learning Approach 19-1
Janusz Wojtusiak and Farrokh Alemi

20 The Shaping of Inventory Systems in Health Services 20-1
Jan de Vries and Karen Spens

21 Facility Planning and Design 21-1
Richard L. Miller

22 Work Design, Task Analysis, and Value Stream Mapping 22-1
Cindy Jimmerson

23 Scheduling and Sequencing 23-1
Edmund K. Burke, Timothy Curtois, Tomas Eric Nordlander, and Atle Riise

24 Data Mining 24-1
Niels Peek

25 Applications to HIV Prevention Strategies 25-1
Paul G. Farnham and Arielle Lasry

26 Causal Risk Analysis: Revisiting the Vioxx Study 26-1
Farrokh Alemi and Manaf Zargoush

PART IV Design, Planning, Control, and Management of Healthcare Systems

IV.A Preventive Care

27 Vaccine Production 27-1
Karen M. Polizzi and Cleo Kontoravdi

28 Economic Implications of Preventive Care 28-1
George H. Avery, Kara E. Leonard, and Steve P. McKenzie

IV.B Telemedicine

29 Interactive Medicine 29-1
Pamela Whitten, Samantha A. Nazione, and Jennifer Cornacchione

IV.C Transplant Services

30 The U.S. Organ Transplant Network: History, Structure, and Functions 30-1
Timothy L. Pruett and Joel D. Newman

IV.D Pharmacy Operation

31 Pharmacoeconomics and the Drug Development Process 31-1
Stephanie R. Earnshaw, Thomas N. Taylor, and Cheryl McDade

IV.E ED/ICU Operation

32 Emergency Department Crowding 32-1
Joshua A. Hilton and Jesse M. Pines

33 Emergency Department Throughput from a Healthcare Leader's Perspective 33-1
Airica Steed

IV.F OR Management

34 Capacity Planning in Operating Rooms 34-1
John T. Blake

35 Managing Critical Resources through an Improved Surgery Scheduling Process 35-1
Erik Demeulemeester, Jeroen Beliën, and Brecht Cardoen

36 Anesthesia Group Management and Strategies 36-1
William H. Hass, Alex Macario, and Randal G. Garner

IV.G Decontamination Service

37 Turnovers and Turnarounds in the Healthcare System 37-1
June M. Worley and Toni L. Doolen

38 Decontamination Service 38-1
Peter F. Hooper

IV.H Laboratories

39 Quality Control in Hospital Clinical Laboratories: A System Approach.... 39-1
George G. Klee

IV.I Emergency Response and Pandemics Planning

40 Emergency Planning Model for Pandemics 40-1
J. Eric Dietz, David R. Black, Julia E. Drifmeyer, and Jennifer A. Smock

41 Public Health and Medical Preparedness 41-1
Eva K. Lee, Anna Yang Yang, Ferdinand Pietz, and Bernard Benecke

IV.J Mental Health

42 Mental Health Allocation and Planning Simulation Model 42-1
H. Stephen Leff, David R. Hughes, Clifton M. Chow, Steven Noyes, and Laysha Ostrow

43 Correlation with Social and Medical Factors 43-1
Kathleen Abrahamson, Karis Pressler, and Melissa Grabner-Hagen

IV.K Food and Supplies

44 Healthcare Foodservice 44-1
L. Charnette Norton

45 Healthcare-Product Supply Chains: Medical–Surgical Supplies, Pharmaceuticals, and Orthopedic Devices: Flows of Product, Information, and Dollars 45-1
Leroy B. Schwarz

IV.L Tracking and Information Systems

46 Wireless Sensor Network 46-1
James A.C. Patterson, Raza Ali, and Guang-Zhong Yang

47 Bar Coding in Medication Administration 47-1
Ben-Tzion Karsh, Tosha B. Wetterneck, Richard J. Holden, A. Joy Rivera-Rodriguez, Hélène Faye, Matthew C. Scanlon, Pascale Carayon, and Samuel J. Alper

48 Clinical Decision Support Systems **48**-1
Sze-jung Sandra Wu, Mark Lehto, and Yuehwern Yih

49 Health Informatics: Systems and Design Considerations **49**-1
Jose Antonio Valdez and Rupa Sheth Valdez

50 Privacy/Security/Personal Health Record Service **50**-1
Jeff Donnell

Index **Index**-1

Foreword

Th [illegible] blished at a very opportune time. According to [illegible] thcare delivery in the Middle East and Africa ac [illegible] rn Europe and Russia it accounts for 5.9%, in La [illegible] nd in North America for a whopping 15.5%. C [illegible] 65 worldwide. As this number continues to in [illegible] st of healthcare in terms of percentage of the gr [illegible] turn, will drive up costs and raise the old age de [illegible] o fund healthcare systems everywhere.

This handbook presents the latest and best methods and tools of systems engineering aimed at improving the design, planning, control, and management of healthcare delivery. Experience in a variety of other industries suggests that when these known industrial engineering tools were applied to the design, operation, and management of enterprise, costs were typically reduced by 25% or more. In addition to the concern about the rising cost of healthcare delivery, there is also a major concern about the quality of healthcare delivery and the reduction of errors, which impact costs and the well-being of the patient. If industrial engineering tools and methods such as total quality management, Six Sigma, and other process improvement and methods are effectively applied, they will improve quality and reduce the error rate by 40% or higher.

With this in mind, the utilization of the information presented in this handbook will have a major impact on reducing costs and improving the quality of healthcare worldwide. This information is presented in 50 chapters authored by 106 contributors from 8 countries. The handbook consists of 41 useful tables and 132 figures that visually illustrate the utilization of tools and methods; it also provides over 2000 references for those who would like to pursue an in-depth study of the subject matter. The handbook should be of special value to administrators of healthcare delivery systems, including those working in hospitals, clinics, insurance companies, and to those involved in the consultancy and research of healthcare delivery systems.

Gavriel Salvendy
Series Editor

Preface

Today we are facing many challenges in healthcare, ranging from patient access, safety, care quality, and cost effectiveness. The rapidly rising cost of healthcare has a direct impact on the economy as well as on our standard of living. The Committee on the Quality of Health Care in America released two reports, *To Err Is Human* (1999) and *Crossing the Quality Chasm* (2001), to address issues of patient safety and overall healthcare delivery systems. The six main areas of concern include safety, effectiveness, patient-centeredness, timeliness, efficiency, and equity. To develop strategies to address these areas requires a holistic approach by understanding the processes, patients, families, providers, payers, governments, and organizations in the healthcare delivery system, and their dependencies and interactions. Furthermore, due to specialization in medicine and advances in science and technology, the healthcare delivery system intersects with the disciplines of medicine, engineering, management, science, technology, and sociology.

This handbook aims to document the healthcare delivery system from a system engineering perspective to provide theoretical foundations, methodologies, and case studies in each sector of the system. In particular, it covers the system engineering methodologies and their applications in designing, evaluating, and optimizing the operations of the healthcare system to improve patient outcomes and cost effectiveness. The handbook consists of 50 chapters divided into four parts. The four broad parts are as follows: Healthcare Delivery System Overview; Performance Assessment and Process Improvement Management; System Engineering: Technologies and Methodologies; and Design, Planning, Control, and Management of Healthcare Systems.

Part I presents an overview of the history and current challenges of the healthcare system, and the potential impact of system engineering on healthcare and healthcare-related networks and organizations, such as VA systems, outpatient clinics, nurse-managed clinics, long-term care, and third-party payers. The last chapter in this part (Chapter 8) describes an integrated framework for the delivery system. Part II describes the tools and methodologies used, such as lean concept, evidence-based practice, and risk assessment, for performance assessment and process improvement in healthcare systems. Part III reviews system engineering methodologies and technologies and their applications in healthcare. Each chapter in this part introduces a system engineering method with a case study in healthcare application. The methods discussed include simulation, optimization, queuing theory, Markov decision processes, statistical analysis and modeling, machine learning, inventory model, facility planning, value stream mapping, scheduling, data mining, economic analysis, and causal risk analysis.

Part IV is devoted to the design, planning, control, and management of healthcare systems. The chapters in this part are divided into 12 service sectors: preventive care, telemedicine, transplant services, pharmacy operation, ED/ICU operation, OR management, decontamination service, laboratories, emergency response and pandemics planning, mental health, food and supplies, and tracking and information systems. This part presents the state-of-the-art operations and the challenges in each service unit. It is clear that system engineering concepts have been broadly applied in healthcare systems. However, most of the improvements have focused on a specific segment or unit of the delivery system.

For example, in a hospital, there are process improvement projects within individual units, such as ED, OR, Lab, and Radiology. However, each unit has a strong interaction with the other units and any significant improvement is more likely to be sustained over time by integrating the process and reevaluating the system design from a holistic point of view. Redesigning the delivery system with an integrated approach will transform the operations of the healthcare system, improving patient safety, care quality, patient access, system efficiency, and overall cost effectiveness. By providing an overview of individual operational sectors in the extremely complex healthcare system and introducing a wide array of engineering methods and tools, this handbook establishes the foundation to facilitate integrated system thinking to redesign the next-generation healthcare system.

I would like to express my sincere gratitude and appreciation to over 100 authors who took the time and effort to share their scientific insights and invaluable experiences in healthcare research and practices. I am particularly touched by the fact that all the authors contributed to this book with their jam-packed schedules and some despite personal tragedies. I would also like to thank the Advisory Board of this handbook, Dr. W. Dale Compton, Dr. Steven M. Witz, and Dr. James P. Bagian, who helped define and shape the scope of this book. My personal thanks go to Sanmit Ambedkar, Vishal Chandrasekar, Tze Chao Chiam, Vikram Chitnis, Imran Hasan, Sangbok Lee, Haocheng (Vincent) Liu, Daiki Min, Sally Perng, Varun Ramamohan, Benjavan (Den) Upatising, and Sue Wongweragiat for their assistance, and Dr. Gavriel Salvendy for his continuous support and encouragement. Lastly, I would like to thank my husband, Daniel, for his patience and understanding that made this project possible.

Yuehwern Yih
Regenstrief Center for Healthcare Engineering Faculty Scholar
School of Industrial Engineering
Purdue University
West Lafayette, Indiana

Editor

Dr. Yuehwern Yih is a professor in the School of Industrial Engineering and the director of the Smart Systems and Operations Laboratory at Purdue University, West Lafayette, Indiana. She is the faculty scholar of the Regenstrief Center for Healthcare Engineering. Dr. Yih received her BS from the National Tsing Hua University in Taiwan and her PhD in industrial engineering from the University of Wisconsin–Madison, Madison, Wisconsin. She specializes in system and process designing, monitoring, and controlling to improve its quality and efficiency. Her research work has been focused on dynamic process control and decision making for operations in complex systems (or systems in systems), such as healthcare delivery systems, manufacturing systems, supply chains, and advanced life support systems for missions to Mars.

Dr. Yih has published over 100 journal papers, conference proceedings, and book chapters on system and operation control, and her contributions in this area have been recognized through national awards and fellowships. She is an IIE Fellow and a member of the Institute for Operations Research and Management Science, the Society of Automobile Engineers, and the Omega Rho Honor Society.

Contributors

Kathleen Abrahamson
Department of Public Health
Western Kentucky University
Bowling Green, Kentucky

Farrokh Alemi
Health Systems Administration
Georgetown University
Washington, District of Columbia

Raza Ali
Royal Society/Wolfson MIC Laboratory
Department of Computing
Imperial College London
London, United Kingdom

George Oscar Allen
Department of Veterans Affairs
Nebraska-Western Iowa Health Care System
Omaha, Nebraska

Samuel J. Alper
Exponent
Chicago, Illinois

Priscilla A. Arling
College of Business
Butler University
Indianapolis, Indiana

George H. Avery
Department of Health and Kinesiology
Purdue University
West Lafayette, Indiana

Hari Balasubramanian
Department of Mechanical and Industrial Engineering
University of Massachusetts at Amherst
Amherst, Massachusetts

Mehmet A. Begen
Richard Ivey School of Business
University of Western Ontario
London, Ontario, Canada

Jeroen Beliën
Center for Modeling and Simulation
Hogeschool Universiteit Brussel
Brussels, Belgium

Bernard Benecke
Strategic National Stockpile
Centers for Disease Control and Prevention
Atlanta, Georgia

David R. Black
College of Health and Human Services
Purdue University
West Lafayette, Indiana

John T. Blake
Department of Industrial Engineering
Dalhousie University
Halifax, Nova Scotia, Canada

Edmund K. Burke
School of Computer Science
University of Nottingham
Nottingham, United Kingdom

Wenhua Cao
Department of Industrial Engineering
University of Houston
Houston, Texas

Pascale Carayon
Center for Quality and Productivity Improvement
Department of Industrial and Systems Engineering
University of Wisconsin–Madison
Madison, Wisconsin

Brecht Cardoen
Operations and Technology Management Center
Vlerick Leuven Gent Management School
Gent, Belgium

Sean Carr
Edward P. Fitts Department of Industrial and Systems Engineering
North Carolina State University
Raleigh, North Carolina

Clifton M. Chow
Human Services Research Institute
Cambridge, Massachusetts

W. Dale Compton
School of Industrial Engineering
Purdue University
West Lafayette, Indiana

Jennifer Cornacchione
College of Communication Arts and Sciences
Michigan State University
East Lansing, Michigan

Mark E. Cowen
St. Joseph Mercy Health System
Ypsilanti, Michigan

Timothy Curtois
School of Computer Science
University of Nottingham
Nottingham, United Kingdom

Erik Demeulemeester
Department of Decision Sciences and Information Management
Research Center for Operations Management
Katholieke Universiteit Leuven
Leuven, Belgium

Brian T. Denton
Edward P. Fitts Department of Industrial and Systems Engineering
North Carolina State University
Raleigh, North Carolina

J. Eric Dietz
Purdue Homeland Security Institute
and
Computer and Information Technology
Purdue University
West Lafayette, Indiana

Bradley N. Doebbeling
Veterans Affairs Health Services Research & Development Center on Implementing Evidence-Based Practice
and
Regenstrief Institute, Inc.
and
Indiana Transforming Healthcare Research Initiative
Indiana University School of Medicine
Indianapolis, Indiana

Jeff Donnell
NoMoreClipboard.com
Indianapolis, Indiana

Toni L. Doolen
School of Mechanical, Industrial, and Manufacturing Engineering
Oregon State University
Corvallis, Oregon

Julia E. Drifmeyer
Purdue Homeland Security Institute
Purdue University
West Lafayette, Indiana

Stephanie R. Earnshaw
RTI Health Solutions
RTI International
Research Triangle Park, North Carolina

Paul G. Farnham
Division of HIV/AIDS Prevention
Centers for Disease Control and Prevention
Atlanta, Georgia

Hélène Faye
Institut de Radioprotection et de Sûreté Nucléaire
Fontenay-aux-Roses, France

Rebekah L. Fox
Department of Communication Studies
Texas State University
San Marcos, Texas

Randal G. Garner
Medical Practice & Management Partners, Inc.
Grayson, Georgia

Melissa Grabner-Hagen
Department of Educational Psychology
Indiana University
Kokomo, Indiana

Linda V. Green
Decision, Risk and Operations Division
Columbia Business School
Columbia University
New York, New York

William H. Hass
Anesthesia Cooperative of the Panhandle
Pensacola, Florida

Joshua A. Hilton
Department of Emergency Medicine
University of Pennsylvania
Philadelphia, Pennsylvania

Richard J. Holden
School of Medicine and Public Health
University of Wisconsin–Madison
Madison, Wisconsin

Peter F. Hooper
Central Sterilising Club
Banbury, United Kingdom

David R. Hughes
Human Services Research Institute
Cambridge, Massachusetts

Ann Schoofs Hundt
Center for Quality and Productivity Improvement
University of Wisconsin–Madison
Madison, Wisconsin

Cindy Jimmerson
Lean Healthcare West
Missoula, Montana

Philip C. Jones
Department of Management Sciences
Tippie College of Business
University of Iowa
Iowa City, Iowa

Ben-Tzion Karsh
Department of Industrial and Systems Engineering
University of Wisconsin–Madison
Madison, Wisconsin

George G. Klee
Department of Laboratory Medicine and Pathology
Mayo Clinic
Rochester, Minnesota

Cleo Kontoravdi
Department of Chemical Engineering
Imperial College London
London, United Kingdom

Arielle Lasry
Division of HIV/AIDS Prevention
Centers for Disease Control and Prevention
Atlanta, Georgia

David M. Lawrence
Kaiser Foundation Health Plan and Hospitals
Healdsburg, California

Eva K. Lee
School of Industrial and Systems Engineering
Georgia Institute of Technology
Atlanta, Georgia

H. Stephen Leff
Human Services Research Institute
Cambridge, Massachusetts

Mark Lehto
School of Industrial Engineering
Purdue University
West Lafayette, Indiana

Kara E. Leonard
Division of Management, Policy, and Community Health School of Public Health
University of Texas Medical Branch
Houston, Texas

Gino J. Lim
Department of Industrial Engineering
University of Houston
Houston, Texas

Qi Ming Lin
EInk Corporation
Cambridge, Massachusetts

Alex Macario
Stanford University Medical Center
Stanford University School of Medicine
Stanford, California

Cheryl McDade
RTI Health Solutions
RTI International
Research Triangle Park, North Carolina

Steve P. McKenzie
Department of Health and Kinesiology
and
Department of Foods and Nutrition
Purdue University
West Lafayette, Indiana

Richard L. Miller
Earl Swensson Associates, Inc. (ESa)
Nashville, Tennessee

Kenneth J. Musselman
Regenstrief Center for Healthcare Engineering
Purdue University
West Lafayette, Indiana

Samantha A. Nazione
College of Communication Arts and Sciences
Michigan State University
East Lansing, Michigan

Joel D. Newman
UNOS Communications
Richmond, Virginia

Tomas Eric Nordlander
Department of Applied Mathematics
SINTEF Information and Communication Technology
Trondheim, Norway

L. Charnette Norton
DM & A
Chula Vista, California
and
The Norton Group, Inc.
Missouri City, Texas

Julie Cowan Novak
School of Nursing
University of Texas Health Science Center at San Antonio
San Antonio, Texas

Steven Noyes
Human Services Research Institute
Cambridge, Massachusetts

Laysha Ostrow
Human Services Research Institute
Cambridge, Massachusetts

Jonathan Patrick
Telfer School of Management
University of Ottawa
Ottawa, Ontario, Canada

James A.C. Patterson
Royal Society/Wolfson MIC Laboratory
Department of Computing
Imperial College London
London, United Kingdom

Niels Peek
Department of Medical Informatics
Academic Medical Center
University of Amsterdam
Amsterdam, the Netherlands

Ferdinand Pietz
Strategic National Stockpile
Centers for Disease Control and Prevention
Atlanta, Georgia

Jesse M. Pines
Department of Emergency Medicine and Health Policy
George Washington University
Washington, District of Columbia

Karen M. Polizzi
Division of Molecular Biosciences
Department of Life Sciences and Department of Chemical Engineering
Imperial College London
London, United Kingdom

Karis Pressler
Department of Sociology
Purdue University
West Lafayette, Indiana

Timothy L. Pruett
Division of Transplantation
University of Minnesota
Minneapolis, Minnesota

Proctor P. Reid
National Academy of Engineering
Washington, District of Columbia

Atle Riise
Department of Applied Mathematics
SINTEF Information and Communication Technology
Trondheim, Norway

A. Joy Rivera-Rodriguez
Department of Industrial and Systems Engineering
University of Wisconsin–Madison
Madison, Wisconsin

Stephen D. Roberts
Edward P. Fitts Department of Industrial and Systems Engineering
North Carolina State University
Raleigh, North Carolina

Vinod K. Sahney
Blue Cross Blue Shield of Massachusetts
Boston, Massachusetts

Matthew C. Scanlon
Department of Pediatrics
Medical College of Wisconsin
Milwaukee, Wisconsin

Leroy B. Schwarz
Krannert Graduate School of Management
Purdue University
West Lafayette, Indiana

Jennifer A. Smock
National Association of County and City Health Officials (NACCHO)
Washington, District of Columbia

Karen Spens
Department of Marketing
Hanken School of Economics
Helsinki, Finland

Airica Steed
Advocate Health Care
Libertyville, Illinois

Thomas N. Taylor
Department of Pharmacy Practice
Wayne State University
Detroit, Michigan

Barrett W. Thomas
Department of Management Sciences
Tippie College of Business
University of Iowa
Iowa City, Iowa

Ann Tousignant
Blue Cross Blue Shield of Massachusetts
Boston, Massachusetts

Jose Antonio Valdez
Quality Resources Department
University of Wisconsin Hospital and Clinics
Madison, Wisconsin

Rupa Sheth Valdez
Department of Industrial and Systems Engineering
University of Wisconsin–Madison
Madison, Wisconsin

Jan de Vries
Faculty of Economics and Business
University of Groningen
Groningen, the Netherlands

Tosha B. Wetterneck
School of Medicine and Public Health
University of Wisconsin–Madison
Madison, Wisconsin

Pamela Whitten
College of Communication Arts and Sciences
Michigan State University
East Lansing, Michigan

Deanna R. Willis
Department of Family Medicine
Indiana University School of Medicine
Indianapolis, Indiana

Steven M. Witz
Regenstrief Center for Healthcare Engineering
Purdue University
West Lafayette, Indiana

Janusz Wojtusiak
Department of Health Administration and Policy
George Mason University
Fairfax, Virginia

Peter Arthur Woodbridge
College of Public Health
University of Nebraska Medical Center
and
Department of Veterans Affairs
Mid-West Mountain Veterans Engineering Resource Center
and
Department of Veterans Affairs
Nebraska-Western Iowa Health Care System
Omaha, Nebraska

June M. Worley
School of Mechanical, Industrial, and Manufacturing Engineering
Oregon State University
Corvallis, Oregon

Sze-jung Sandra Wu
Risk Department
JP Morgan Chase
Wilmington, Delaware

Anna Yang Yang
School of Industrial and Systems Engineering
Georgia Institute of Technology
Atlanta, Georgia

Guang-Zhong Yang
Royal Society/Wolfson MIC Laboratory
Department of Computing
Imperial College London
London, United Kingdom

Elizabeth M. Yano
Veterans Affairs Greater Los Angeles Health Services Research & Development Center of Excellence
Sepulveda, California
and
School of Public Health
University of California, Los Angeles
Los Angeles, California

Yuehwern Yih
Regenstrief Center for Healthcare Engineering
School of Industrial Engineering
Purdue University
West Lafayette, Indiana

Manaf Zargoush
ESSEC Business School
Paris, France

Min Zhang
Department of Statistics
Purdue University
West Lafayette, Indiana

I

Healthcare Delivery System Overview

1 **Healthcare: How Did We Get Here and Where Are We Going?** *David M. Lawrence* **1**-1
Introduction • What Does This Mean for the Future? • Final Thoughts • References

2 **Engineering and the Healthcare Delivery System** *Proctor P. Reid and W. Dale Compton* **2**-1
Engineering Systems • Quality of Healthcare • System Tools • Challenges • Barriers to Cooperation • Needs and Opportunities • Conclusion • References

3 **The VA Healthcare Delivery System** *Elizabeth M. Yano* **3**-1
Historical Evolution of the VA Healthcare Delivery System • VA's Quality Transformation • Veterans and the VA Healthcare Systems • Leadership and Organizational Structure • VA Healthcare Budget and Financing Mechanisms • VA Healthcare Delivery • Health and Healthcare Utilization among Veterans • Quality Improvement in the VA Healthcare System • Special Populations in VA Healthcare Settings • Future Perspectives • References

4 **Outpatient Clinics: Primary and Specialty Care** *Deanna R. Willis* **4**-1
Background • Size and Scope • Structure • Practice Expenses and Overhead • Revenue and Payment for Services • Quality • Medical Home • Care Coordination • Primary Care Shortage • References

5 **Designing a Nurse-Managed Healthcare Delivery System** *Julie Cowan Novak* **5**-1
Introduction • Direct Practice • Program Costs • Challenges to Nurse-Managed Clinics and Faculty Practice • DNP Development: Implications for Faculty Practice • References

6 **Long-Term Care** *Kathleen Abrahamson and Karis Pressler* **6**-1
Role of Families in the Provision of Long-Term Care • Nursing Home Decision • Nursing Homes • Family Caregiver Involvement in Long-Term Care Facilities • Assisted Living Facilities • Financing Long-Term Care • Long-Term Care Culture • Conclusion • References

7 Healthcare Insurance: An Introduction *Vinod K. Sahney and Ann Tousignant* 7-1
Introduction • Third-Party Payers • Healthcare Financing • Roots of Employer-Sponsored Healthcare Coverage • Issues Raised by Third-Party Payment • Private Healthcare Insurance • Healthcare Insurance Products • Regulation of Private Health Insurance • Healthcare Reimbursement Systems • Discussion • References

8 An Integrated Model of Healthcare Delivery *Steven M. Witz and Kenneth J. Musselman* **8**-1
Background • Integrated Healthcare Delivery Model • Research Opportunities • Conclusion • References

1

Healthcare: How Did We Get Here and Where Are We Going?

David M. Lawrence
Kaiser Foundation Health Plan and Hospitals

Introduction 1-1
How Did We Get Here? • Physician Culture • Growth of Medical Science • Changing Demographics and Demand
What Does This Mean for the Future? 1-9
Balanced Healthcare • Four Battlefronts • Sick Care Delivery System • Consumer-Health Ecosystem • New Personalized Medicine Paradigm • Accountable Organizations
Final Thoughts 1-14
References 1-14

Between the health care we have and the care we could have lies not just a gap, but a chasm.

Institute of Medicine (2001)

Introduction

Healthcare delivery is in transition. A new administration pledges to overhaul the "broken" system as part of a comprehensive economic stimulus package; the recent report of the Medicare Trust Fund indicates that Medicare will be insolvent in less than a decade; a national comparative effectiveness program will determine which treatments are most useful; and the innovations in care delivery continue to come. To understand where these changes could lead requires an understanding of the starting point.

This chapter provides a short overview of the growth of the healthcare system during the twentieth century and the significant forces that will shape it going forward. Based on these observations, I suggest four areas where important battles are most likely in the future: inside the sick care system; between the sick care system and the emerging consumer-health ecosystem; over-personalized or predictive medicine; and in the so-called accountable healthcare organizations. In each instance the battles will revolve around critical questions: What is included in care? Who is in charge? And what do doctors do? The outcomes of these battles will determine, in large measure, the future of heath care in the United States.

How Did We Get Here?

Prior to World War II, medical care in the United States was provided by generalist physicians who wielded limited diagnostic and therapeutic technologies in their solo practices and community hospitals staffed by nonacademically prepared nurses. In just over half a century since, care has become a maze of nearly unfathomable complexity: well over 600,000 physicians practice in one or more of nearly 130 specialties (U.S. Department of Labor, 2009), supported by more than 200 distinct categories of support personnel, in a wide variety of clinical settings where uncertain accountabilities and competing professional and economic imperatives abound. The care that results is superb for some, but its costs are unsustainable, its quality and safety unpredictable, and the value it delivers (health/dollar invested) markedly lower than that found in other developed countries (Arnold and Carrie, 2009).[*,†] Accessing and navigating through this maze is a challenge, especially for those with limited financial means, for minorities, and those for whom English is a second language.[‡] As a consequence, the benefits of outstanding individual physicians and world-leading clinical science and technology are often lost in impersonal, confusing, and fragmented care, while the threat of personal bankruptcy grows as medical expenses exceed the ability of patients and their families to pay.[§]

In its 2001 study, "Crossing the Quality Chasm: A New System for the 21st Century," the Institute of Medicine decried the absence of "real progress towards solving these problems" because care delivery continues to rely on "...outmoded systems of work. Poor designs set the workforce up to fail, regardless of how hard they try. If we want safer, higher-quality care, we will need to have redesigned systems of care" (Institute of Medicine, 2001).

Little has changed since the report was written nearly a decade ago. Why? Why are systems of work outmoded? Why is care, so rich in talent and resources, an expensive "nightmare to navigate" for many patients.[¶] Why has it proven so difficult to build integrated care organizations after more than half a century of recommendations to do just that?[**] Why is there a chasm between "...the care we have and the care we could have"?

The performance of the care system, I suggest, is a predictable outcome of a rapidly growing scientific enterprise and fundamental shifts in consumer demands that are incompatible with the organizing assumptions and practices of a dominant physician culture. A deeply challenged U.S. economy adds further urgency to the need to find better ways to organize and deliver care in the future. The fee for service payment system reinforces the problems, and little improvement in care can be expected until this changes. But the payment system is not a primary cause. It is, after all, the result of decades of effort by doctors and hospitals to be paid for what they have been prepared to do.[††] Nor is the managed care movement of the late 1980s and early 1990s the culprit, though the aftereffects of

---

[*] The study reports a 23% "value gap" between the United States and the G-5 (Canada, Japan, Germany, United Kingdom, and France), and a 46% value gap with emerging competitors Brazil, India, and China (Arnold and Carrie, 2009).

[†] Elizabeth McGlynn and colleagues at the RAND Corporation have pioneered studies that explore the consistency with which patients receive scientifically "appropriate" medical care. See, for example, McGlynn et al. (2003).

[‡] The issue of access, and in particular access for minorities and those for whom English is a second language, has been of concern to policy makers for at least two decades. The IOM has published several reports on the subject.

[§] This is a controversial issue. The organization "Fact Check" concludes that there is a relationship, but that the extent to which medical expenses "cause" bankruptcy remains unclear. http://www.factcheck.org/askfactcheck/what_is_the_percentage_of_total_personal.html (last accessed on March 20, 2010).

[¶] The "nightmare to navigate" description is found in the joint publication of the Picker Institute with the American Hospital Association (1996). The Picker Institute assesses the interactions of patients, families with the care system "through the eyes of the patient." (http://www.pickerinstitute.org/)

[**] The modern Mayo Clinic traces its origins to the mid-1880s. In the report of the independent "Committee on Cost Containment" 1927–1932, a key recommendation was to form multi-specialty groups to offset fragmentation and cost pressures. The HMO act in 1973 was designed to foster organized systems of care. And the IOM series on quality of care in the United States, published over the period 1999–2002, argued for the formation of organized, integrated systems of care.

[††] Health insurance, which began in the 1920s, grew rapidly in the 1930s as doctors and hospitals sought ways to ensure steady incomes during the Depression. The boards of the Blues plans were dominated by physicians and hospital administrators until the rise of the for-profit health insurers, including the conversion of a number of Blues plans from not-for-profit to for-profit companies.

that experiment remain (Ludmerer, 1999). The movement opened the black box of clinical decision-making and care organization that until then had been largely under the control of physicians, in effect weakening their sovereignty over the medical care enterprise and introducing scarcity and the need for choices into the public debate. These are important shifts. But the failure of the movement to control costs and improve care over the longer term says as much about the power that physicians are still able to wield when their sovereignty is threatened as it does about the many flaws in the movement itself.

Physician Culture

Autonomy

Not until the 1930s, after decades of struggle to emerge from a hodgepodge of charlatans, quacks, and self-trained healers, did physicians assume leadership of American medicine and establish the unique physician culture as the bedrock for today's care system.* Central to that culture is the concept of professional autonomy. The doctor is his own judge, responsible to himself and his profession to make decisions in the interest of his patients based on the best combination of science, experience, and judgment that he can bring together.† A trained skeptic of the work of others, gathering his own information by carrying out an independent assessment of each patient, he prefers to work alone surrounded by his support staff, interacting with his patients on his terms. Only when he reaches the limits of his largely self-defined competence (or his tolerance for legal risk), does he refer the patient to another doctor, who repeats the same process. He is responsible for staying current with the latest treatments and procedures throughout his professional career, and is accountable to himself and his physician peers for his decisions and judgments.‡

This is not surprising. A profession is "...a calling requiring specialized knowledge and often long and intensive academic preparation" (Webster, 2009). For the physician, the educational process is particularly extended; the knowledge to master and the judgments and skills to develop require intensive study and supervised practice. What most distinguishes the physician culture from other professionals, though, is the extent to which autonomy is its defining feature. The reinforcement for autonomy finds its way into every nook and cranny of the physician's early development, encouraged by senior physicians and medical school curricula that provide few opportunities to learn the skills of shared decision-making or to work in teams of physicians or other health professionals (Lawrence, 2002).§ The doctor is socialized, then, over long years of medical school and residency training to function highly independently within the tightly protected world of his profession.

Doctors practice this way when their formal training ends. Although there has been a slow but growing trend among younger physicians to practice in small groups, the majority of physicians still practice in single-specialty groups of 10 physicians or less, and a third of all physicians work alone (Liebhaber and Grossman, 2007). Beyond practice choice, autonomy expresses itself in the profession's battles

* Starr argues that the physicians became sovereign in medical care, establishing their leadership of the hierarchy within the care system, the laws and regulations surrounding the practice of medicine, the control of the hospitals where they practice, and the development of reimbursement and federal and state support models. The sovereign physician model is the prototype for medical delivery systems throughout the world. Only where there is insufficient physician manpower are nonphysician alternatives encouraged from a policy point of view. Of course, many cultures have extensive networks of nonphysician local healers, but even these exist side by side with the physician-centric solutions of "modern" medicine (Starr, 1982).

† For ease of reading, I refer to physicians in the masculine form, recognizing that within the past 20 years, the proportion of women entering the profession is roughly equal to men.

‡ Of course, he is accountable to the legal system, although typically most court cases include dueling physician expert witnesses.

§ In its first roundtable, the Lucian Leape Institute of the National Patient Safety Foundation focused on the preparation of physicians, and the lack of emphasis on collaborative learning and care.

with administrators and managed care companies over the control of the clinical workplace, and in the 50-year fight to limit the roles that nurse practitioners, physician's assistants, and, more recently, pharmacists, play in providing care to patients. It contributes to the wide variation in physician practice patterns observed from one community to the next,* and is one important reason why doctors have resisted the transparency that shared information technology introduces into the care-delivery process. It produces a fragmented "job shop" organization of care in which each independent doctor-cum-small-businessman customizes his practice to his preference and his interpretation of what his patients need and expect.

As one might anticipate, autonomy is the major stumbling block to the formation of effective care organizations.† Group decision-making, transparency, and accountability that organizations require to be effective are in conflict with the expectation for clinical autonomy that guides physicians. This can lead to profound discomfort and suspicion. Doctors have limited exposure to the tools required to address the complex problems that organizations must resolve, where the wisdom of the collective and the deliberative process itself is critical to successful problem resolution and decision implementation. Even the process of clinical decision-making is different from organizational decision-making;‡ as a result physicians are ill-prepared to deal with the ambiguities, trade-offs, and workforce engagement challenges that drive organizational strategy and operational effectiveness.

Physician Exceptionalism

As central as autonomy is to the physician culture, it is not the only element that shapes the care system. The physician is trained to employ his long training, deep knowledge, well-honed judgment, and advanced skills—his professional insights—to distinguish the common problem from the serious illness in disguise, then customize the care he provides to meet the unique needs of each patient. He seeks the uncommon behind the apparently simple clinical presentation (Groopman, 2007). And he is trained to believe that only a doctor is capable of these insights. The *sine qua non* of care excellence is the doctor–patient relationship, to be protected at all costs from anything that threatens it; and above all, the doctor must be in the lead in the care process. As a result, physicians have been slow to accept practices and clinical approaches that differ from their own experiences; have resisted efforts to codify clinical decision-making using "best practices" or evidence-based medicine; and have fought the introduction of nonphysician clinicians into daily practice unless they are under their direct supervision and control.

Intuition versus Prediction

The resistance to organizations, especially those not controlled by physicians; the dismissing of clinical pathways and guidelines as "cookbook medicine"; the unwillingness to accept transparency and accountability; and the belief in physician exceptionalism—these are the direct outgrowth of the physician culture that has shaped the care system into what we see today. In their recent book, *The Innovator's Prescription*, Christensen, Grossman, and Hwang provide a useful framework to help understand how this culture affects the organization of care (Christensen et al., 2009). The authors describe care as a continuum of problem-solving challenges from intuition to predictive precision, with empiricism

* Wennberg, Elliot, and their colleagues at Dartmouth have documented these "small area variations" in medical practice since the early 1970s.

† In the interest of simplicity, I use the term "effective" to cover the six goals for care systems of the future articulated in the Crossing the Quality Chasm report: effectiveness, safety, timeliness, responsiveness, affordability, and equity.

‡ In clinical practice one utilizes two frameworks. First is a pattern-recognition skill in which a problem is "slotted" into a diagnosis and treatment based on its similarity to previously encountered "patterns" of illness presentation and treatment. Second is a heuristic in which the physician makes judgments based on the likelihood that a given collection of objective and subjective information is disease x, y, or z.

somewhere in the middle, the result of the developments in the science of medicine. The expectations of the physician, however, are that most medicine is intuitive. The arduous training to develop the physician's clinical acumen guides this view, colors his assessment of efforts to introduce empiricism into care ("best practices; evidence-based medicine"), and lies at the heart of his resistance to the precision of predictive care. As a consequence, the doctor's professional identity and the systems of work that result conflict with the care that medical science now makes possible, as well as the care that health consumers increasingly demand and need.

Growth of Medical Science

Biological Science

In parallel with the development of the modern care system, in fact fueling many of the advances that have been introduced over the past half century, is the creation of a powerful medical scientific enterprise. The National Institutes of Health (NIH) is the primary engine of discovery for the biological sciences in the nation. Created by Congress in 1946 to expand the scientific, primarily biological base of medicine, its budget grew from $8 million in 1947 to more than $1 billion in 1966, $13.7 billion by 1997, and $29 billion in 2008. It now supports over 200,000 scientists in 3100 research centers around the country, in addition to its intramural scientists and programs located at the NIH home, and includes 27 centers and institutes covering a broad range of clinical conditions.*

Other sources have played significant roles in biomedical research and development. Pharmaceutical company investments in research and development ("R&D") overtook federal support for the NIH in 1980 and have continued at a higher level since then. In 1970 the industry invested approximately $8B in R&D; by 2008 that number had grown to $50.3B. In addition, the publicly listed biotech drug industry invested $14.6B in 2008, bringing the total private sector investment in basic science and bio-pharma to $65B ($64.9B) (Burrill & Company, 2009).† Added to this are the estimated 6000 medical device companies that build on advances in engineering, microcircuitry, imaging, computing, and wireless communications to produce a wide assortment of diagnostic and therapeutic devices. According to the group "Research!America," investments in medical science and technology from all these sources reached $111B by 2005.‡

Today, advanced bio-computational capabilities join with deepening understanding of how individual human molecules operate to enable investigators to explore complex biological pathways and clinical correlations for relationships that escape notice with less sophisticated tools. As the capacity to identify and read information related to genes and proteins grows, so too does the ability to analyze millions of bits of information using complex computer algorithms to identify patterns (so-called signatures) correlated to the presence of disease or pre-disease. Already this has led to advances in cancer and heart disease diagnosis and treatment.§

---

* See History of the National Institutes of Health; Wikipedia.

† Available from Burrill and Company, San Francisco, California. The numbers are inconsistent because some reports are only for publicly listed companies; others include venture funding for early-stage companies. A figure of around $65B in 2008 is as accurate an estimate as can be found.

‡ Some controversy exists over this total related to the estimates of private sector investments in R&D. Research!America errs on the high side of the estimates. Ralph Snyderman, MD, Chancellor Emeritus of Duke University Health Sciences Center, once estimated that between 1950 and 2000, the United States invested $1 trillion in public and privately financed medical R&D. Based on current estimates, the same amount will be invested between 2000 and 2010. (personal communications) (Research!America, 2005).

§ Perhaps the best example of this can be found in a graph developed by David Altshuler for the IOM meeting of October 8, 2007. Altshuler illustrates the rapid growth in the identification of gene variants associated with common diseases. The graph is found in Learning Healthcare System Concepts v. 2008 (Institute of Medicine, 2009). A recent series of articles in the *New England Journal of Medicine* sound a cautionary note about how quickly these advances are occurring (see e.g., Kraft and Hunter, 2009).

Population Science

Increasingly powerful computational technologies and biostatistical and epidemiological techniques support large-scale population studies that provide insights into the ways populations are affected by disease. The 60-year-old Framingham Heart Study, for example, is an investigation into the risks, causes, and presentations for heart disease across three generations in the community of Framingham, Massachusetts.* Another multi-decade study involves nurses, followed for more than 30 years.† Two recent studies on the value of screening for prostate cancer in men employ similar tools.‡ Common to these approaches is the ability to identify and follow the clinical course of large populations, often across different geographies, over a long-enough period of time to understand how diseases present and change.

Social Science

Each major health profession has added further research to the knowledge pool, distributed as for physicians through a network of professional journals, so-called gray literature,§ blogs, and a variety of profession-specific meetings. They have contributed significantly to the understanding of the relationships between social context and illness, and the ability of alternative delivery models to improve patient compliance, safety, and quality using different combinations of care professionals.

New Organizational Tools

Innovative delivery solutions have also begun to emerge from decades-long advances in wireless communications, microcircuitry applied to monitoring devices, Internet search and networking systems, computing power, and the like, as new players enter the care-delivery field. For example, Qualcomm and Johnson & Johnson sponsor the Wireless Life-Sciences Alliance, focused on the discovery of wireless-based tools to monitor health or illnesses, that enable providers and consumers to communicate quickly and efficiently using wireless technologies.¶ A recently announced partnership between Intel and GE brings their expertise and financial resources to the development of home-based monitoring solutions for patients with chronic illnesses; they will compete directly with Philips, long a leader in consumer electronics and large imaging solutions and more recently a major provider of home-based care solutions (Clark and Glader, 2009). Companies like these, joined by myriad start-up companies and a growing venture community, are creating a "consumer-health ecosystem," a parallel delivery capability to the sick care system that provides the consumer with the tools and support required to enable him or her to get care outside the more expensive, often less accessible sick care system of today.

What Do These Advances Mean?

The investment in medical science over the last six decades has provided the nation with access to therapeutic and diagnostic advances that have the potential to reduce morbidity and mortality and improve quality of life far beyond what was possible half a century ago. It also has enabled much of medicine

---

* The Framingham Heart Study is one of the oldest of this genre, and has produced an extraordinary series of insights on cardiac risk factors, disease prevalence, etc. For more information, see: http://www.framinghamheartstudy.org/

† The Nurses' Health Study was started in 1976 and covers a population of 289,000 registered nurses. For more details, see http://www.channing.harvard.edu/nhs/ (last accessed on March 20, 2010).

‡ Both studies appeared in a recent issue of the *New England Journal of Medicine*. The first covered 76,693 men followed for 9 years in 10 centers in the United States. The second involved 162,243 men drawn from registries in seven European countries and followed for about a decade (Andriole et al., 2009; Schroder et al., 2009).

§ These are the articles in non-juried magazines and newsletters apprising the readers of new studies, or new approaches to diagnosis and treatment. The distinction is that these are not screened by a "jury" of peers and researchers to ensure scientific validity, absence of professional conflicts, etc.

¶ Information about the meetings can be found at www.wirelesslifesciences.org

to move from the realm of sophisticated intuition to empirical and predictive problem solving.* The deepening understanding of human biology and disease, together with advances in computing, communications technologies, miniaturization, and integrated microcircuitry, form the backbone for new delivery models that provide more solutions and greater ease of use for consumers, improve the productivity and reliability of the formal care system, and provide opportunities to substitute less expensive care providers for the most expensive of them all—the physician.

But these advances create a basic conflict. Inherent in the physician culture, as noted, is the belief that clinical uncertainty is high and only a doctor has the preparation and judgment to resolve these diagnostic and therapeutic problems. When medical science was less robust and the understanding of disease less well-developed, this approach provided needed protections for the patient. But now that we have greater understanding and certainty for many, though certainly not all, medical conditions, the physician no longer has to be central to the care process. Other health professionals can perform the histories, order the diagnostic tests, and determine and manage the treatments without jeopardizing safety or effectiveness. And they can do so less expensively, even more responsively than physicians. Technology, especially more accurate diagnostic tests and computer-aided decision support tools, add precision and safety to the care process, further reducing costs. As science continues to advance, more conflicts will arise between the traditional physician culture and the emerging models that are able to use different combinations of nonphysician caregivers and technology to meet the demands from consumers for solutions that respond to their needs and their pockets.

Importantly, our understanding of illness and wellness in humans is broader than that of molecular biology. While deep insights into human biology remain the cornerstone for appropriate diagnosis and effective treatment of specific illnesses, we also know more today about the factors that influence care seeking and care compliance patterns among patients and their families. We know more about how illnesses occur in communities; how communities foster healthy lifestyles; how behaviors can be modified. We have learned to find illnesses through population screening before they become symptomatic. And we understand more about how to lower the risks to keep them from becoming serious. Our knowledge is not perfect, of course. Far from it. But it far exceeds what we knew a half century ago. This knowledge, and the organization and management of the interventions that bring it to patients and communities, resides with many different care professionals and managers in addition to doctors. And in fact, the doctor may not even be best suited to deliver them.

These scientific advances are exciting, but the understanding and tools they support outpace the ability of the care system to use them appropriately and safely. As a result, they often add expense and create more complexity in the already fragmented and confusing medical care process. The tsunami of discovery continues unabated, though, stimulated by new federal allocations and continued private sector investment. As a result, while the future for health-related science has never looked brighter, the implications for doctors and consumers are profound.

Changing Demographics and Demand

Growth, Diversity, and Aging

The last major force that influences the care system is the dramatically changed demand for care in the United States, the result of unprecedented demographic shifts in population growth, diversity, and aging. Birth rates in minority groups, especially the Latino and African-American populations, have contributed to a U.S. population projected to reach 439,010,253 by 2050 (Demographics of the United States, 2008). The population is growing at nearly 1% per year, among the highest in the developed world (Demographics of the United States, 2008), and the proportion of the U.S. population born outside

* Of course, part of medicine remains ambiguous, requiring sophisticated judgments by physician specialists. This is unlikely to change in our lifetimes, though the specific conditions might shift over time.

the United States is the largest since the large immigrant waves of the early 1900s (Demographics of the United States, 2008), resulting in a dizzying array of languages and dialects spoken in the major urban centers of the United States. The linguistic scholar, Professor Vyacheslav Ivanov, discovered 224 languages spoken in Los Angeles, not including dialects, and 180 language-specific publications in the city.* Just over 50% of children born since 2000 in the United States are nonwhite; looking ahead, over half the population is projected to be of nonwhite origin by 2050 at current birth and replacement rates (Demographics of the United States, 2008; Passel and Cohn, 2008). Four states are so-called minority–majority states already; based on the Y2000 U.S. census, in Hawaii, California, Texas, and New Mexico, the nonwhite population outnumbers the white-non-Hispanic population.

The age distribution of the population is changing as well. Driven primarily by the aging of the "baby boom" generation, the proportion of the population over 65 years of age will increase from 13% today to 20% by 2025. The fastest growing subpopulation in the United States is the over-85-year-olds, and the number of centenarians reached approximately 80,000 in 2008 (Demographics of the United States, 2008).

Implications

Together these trends have serious implications for care delivery. Not only are the nation's medical and nursing schools incapable of producing enough physicians and nurses to meet the changing and growing demands, but the gap between the linguistic, cultural, and racial make up of the country and the diversity of the physician and nursing workforce continues to grow (Bodenheimer et al., 2009).

Beyond this challenge lies another—the disparity between the care that physicians are trained to provide and the care the U.S. population now requires (Bodenheimer et al., 2009). In 1950, 4 of the 10 leading causes of death in the United States, occupying the fifth, sixth, seventh, and ninth positions, were acute illnesses. By the beginning of the twenty-first century, only two of these remained in the top 10; the others were chronic illnesses. The Centers for Disease Control estimate that approximately 75% of the dollars spent on healthcare in the United States are for chronic diseases and their complications.† A recent issue of the policy journal, *Health Affairs* was devoted to the subject of the "crisis" in chronic disease care. Contributors described emerging trends in the organization of chronic care, noting that the requirements for effective chronic disease care are different from acute sick care, and the resources are lacking to deliver these services effectively or efficiently (The Crisis in Chronic Disease, 2009).‡

Chronic disease care begins with screening for early signs of disease or the risk factors associated with those illnesses, and proceeds to help consumers make the behavioral changes and incorporate the preventive treatments into their daily lives. This requires the support of caregivers who can work across cultures and languages, as these influence compliance and downstream costs, quality of life, and worker productivity. The care most patients get instead is designed to help them if they are seriously and acutely ill, not when they want to minimize the consequences of their illnesses. Doctors are not trained or organized to do these things—to work in teams, to collaborate with their peers or other professionals to decide what the best combination of treatments is. They are not trained to work with the patient and family as partners. Their culture stands in the way, engendering distrust of the very practices and organizational models that can provide the patients and the population with the care required.

---

* Professor Ivanov, a Russian scholar of language and culture, divides his time between Moscow and Los Angeles, where he teaches at the UCLA (U.S. Census Bureau, 2000).

† http://www.cdc.gov/nccdphp/overview.htm (last accessed on October 1, 2009).

‡ I distinguish between "acute sick care," "chronic care," and "health care" as follows: sick care is the traditional way medicine is practiced, focused on treating acutely ill patients suffering life-threatening, or potentially life-threatening illnesses. Chronic disease care is directed to the detection and management of any one of many chronic illnesses for which effective treatment control can be achieved. Healthcare is the larger array of services that includes wellness and prevention, triage, navigation support, chronic disease management, end-of-life care, and sick care per se.

Prevention and Wellness

The physician culture is also in conflict with efforts to bring broader prevention and wellness services directly to consumers. Effective prevention and wellness care requires more than assuring that appropriate care is provided when patients seek out the doctor. It involves dealing with both population and patient, reaching out to people where they live and work, educating them about the things they do in their daily lives that increase their risks of illness, providing them with effective, low-cost screening to determine what their risks are. It involves education and counseling, and, in all probability, incentives to promote needed behavior changes. And importantly, it involves doing these things in a culturally sophisticated and sensitive way. Doctors cannot be expected to do these things. There is already plenty of work for them; no one can replace their skills and judgments for problems that are uncertain, ambiguous; no one is better able to balance the competing diagnostic and therapeutic options when a patient suffers from complex, multisystem problems. But an ever-increasing part of care is no longer about such clinical ambiguities, and requires new delivery and payment solutions instead (Bohmer and Lawrence, 2008). This is the benefit, and the irony, of the nation's commitment to advancing medical science, and the consequence of a growing, diverse, and aging population with new and different demands.

What Does This Mean for the Future?

We are at a crossroad. The traditional physician culture and the outmoded physician-dominated delivery model it has built are under growing pressure from rapidly changing science and shifting consumer demands. New delivery solutions offer the potential for different pricing and effectiveness for consumers. At the same time significant efforts are necessary to improve the performance of the sick care system itself, using the experiences and tools of other industries. These also hold considerable promise but require changes in the sick care model that, as observed by the Institute of Medicine, have been so slow to occur.

As physicians struggle to respond to these challenges, they will be forced to redefine their roles—where their unique perspectives and judgments still apply, where the new balance of power lies within the care systems, and what their role is in leading the emerging institutions. Science will move ahead with an inexorability driven by powerful momentum and significant public and private sector funding. And the dynamic changes in consumer demand will force the system to change, creating opportunities for still more alternatives to emerge. And all of this will take place under the storm clouds of a distorted economy.

Balanced Healthcare

We are moving slowly and painfully toward a more balanced care system, one that builds more robust capabilities around the traditional, "sick care" system that dominates today. For example, the need for more effective wellness and prevention services is well understood. So too are the requirements for better, more accessible triage care that can help the individual consumer make wise decisions about when and how to use the "sick care" system. Once inside the sick care system, individuals need help making their way: where to go, whom to seek care from, what questions to ask, how to choose among competing of conflicting recommendations, how to obtain the best solutions within one's healthcare budget and coverage, etc. As more patients suffer from chronic illnesses, the value of effective chronic disease care management is indisputable in reducing overall human and economic costs to patients and society. Finally, pathways are required to help terminally ill patients move out of the sick care system into a palliative care system that preserves their dignity and respects their individual choices. When these pieces are in place, together with a strong sick care system, healthcare is "balanced" and the health of the population is likely to be most positive as a result.

Four Battlefronts

The "balanced" care system enables consumers to get the care and services they need most effectively. Getting there from where we are now will involve four major "fronts" in what promises to be an epic battle for the future of healthcare delivery as traditional roles and models collide with the emerging ones driven by the forces discussed throughout this chapter. The most immediate and difficult of these fronts is in the sick care system itself.

Sick Care Delivery System

Most of the attention, investments, hopes, and policy interventions focus on driving the sick care system to higher levels of performance. The working assumptions are straightforward: (1) the sick care system is wasteful and "broken"; (2) it will work better if the doctors are encouraged to do the right things and coordinate their care more effectively, especially for chronic disease care; (3) this will happen if the reimbursement system is redesigned; and (4) if integrated organizations are created to knit together the disparate pieces into a more coherent and patient-centered care; using (5) a combination of health-related information technologies and industrial organizational.

Major improvements in the effectiveness of the sick care system are possible and most likely will come from the creation of new organizations where accountability for performance can be assigned, the resources for supporting the needed changes can be produced, and patients can find the integrated solutions to their medical problems that require sophisticated, often highly expensive diagnostic and therapeutic tools and skills. But this solution is a leap of faith for the nation's physicians steeped in their culture of autonomy.

The logic for integrating care is impeccable. The potential for healthcare information technology and industrial tools to transform sick care is indisputable. But getting there is a major battle. There are examples of organizations in which physicians have joined together to practice integrated care and provide collective leadership to the enterprise—Mayo Clinic, Kaiser Permanente, and Virginia Mason come to mind. But most physicians do not practice in organizations at all, let alone in integrated ones.

The key to the improved performance of the sick care system lies in how effectively the physicians can organize care-delivery models integrated for the benefit of the patient and the cost-effectiveness that our society requires. Tools will help; this is the reason for this book. But the outcome of the struggle depends largely on the extent to which a different, more supportive physician culture emerges.

This new professional culture must be built on the principle of collaboration: with physician peers, with other professionals, and with the patient and family. Successful care, we know, depends on how well the perspectives and training of each professional, as well as the willingness and capabilities of the patient and family, are combined to develop a coherent approach to ensuring the patient that he or she receives the best possible outcome, given the clinical problems at hand. Physician autonomy still has a place—every physician must maintain his skills and employ his capabilities in the best interest of the patient. But the complexity of the science and the demands of the consumer require that this occurs in the larger context of organized teams of caregivers—a collaboration for which the physicians are ill-prepared.* The transformative potential of industrial engineering approaches and the power of a health information technology system that links the disparate elements of the care "production" process together are greatest within a culture of collaboration, where providers, support personnel, suppliers, patients and families, can work together.

Major improvements in performance have been possible in industries outside healthcare, even in those already operating at levels of reliability and efficiency well beyond that of healthcare.† According

* I develop this argument more fully in Lawrence (2002).

† Six Sigma is a popular name for an approach to industrial improvement that drives out errors or defects. The target of six sigma reliability means that for every one million "products" produced, no more than 3.4 are defective. For more information see http://www.isixsigma.com/sixsigma/six_sigma.asp (last accessed on March 20, 2010).

to Donald Berwick, the founder and president of the Institute for Healthcare Improvement, levels of one to two sigma are the norm in sick care delivery instead of the six sigma levels seen in many high-performing companies.* This means that a defect or error occurs about once every 10 times something is done for a patient, and at best once every 100 times care is given, instead of once or twice in every 1,000,000 times something is done. The opportunities for improvement are substantial; the techniques of industrial engineering can drive large improvements in efficiency and quality and safety when applied within the right context (National Academy of Engineering and Institute of Medicine, 2005).

This, then, is the first front in the struggle to build a more effective care system: the conflict between the imperative to create integrated organizations that can use the well-tested tools of information technology and industrial engineering to drive unprecedented performance, on the one hand, and a physician culture built on the principle of autonomy, customization for each patient, and physician control over the care system on the other.

Consumer-Health Ecosystem

Meanwhile, new solutions are emerging around the edges of the sick care system. These are the second "front" in the battle for the future of healthcare: solutions for consumers built on sound science, the increasingly powerful and ubiquitous information management and communications technologies, and the breakthroughs in miniaturization and microcircuitry in electrical and image engineering. They take advantage of distortions in the care market created by a sick care system that is slow to change, a resistant but still dominant physician culture, changing consumer requirements, and the availability of innovation capital to develop "disruptive" new solutions for consumers.

This is a major threat to the sick care system, especially doctors. The solutions often compete with the physician-based delivery model, and shift work done previously in hospitals, outpatient clinics, and doctors' offices to homes and shopping malls, to cell phones and home-monitoring devices, to call centers and computer-aided diagnostic and treatment libraries. Because they leverage technology, standardization, algorithms, reduced variation, and lower-cost care personnel (nurses instead of doctors, health educators instead of nurses, etc.) the way the sick care has not, these solutions can be more personalized, less expensive, and more reliable than the sick care system in which physicians continue to place limits on the pace and scope of change based on traditional assumptions and practices.

The advances in the consumer-health ecosystem are likely to occur in several areas. Most obvious is primary care, the entry point for health consumers into the sick care system. And within the general area of primary care the most appealing target is wellness and prevention. As noted earlier, neither the sick care system nor the doctors are prepared, rewarded, or organized to provide effective wellness and prevention services. U.S. Preventive Medicine and RedBrick Health are early-stage companies that deliver prevention and wellness services in new ways through employers. Physic Ventures, a young San Francisco-based venture fund, is devoted to building companies that provide these services in innovative ways directly to consumers.†

A second area is triage, the process of helping patients determine whether or not their illnesses are serious enough to merit going into the "sick" care system for further treatment; and how to navigate through that system most effectively once there. Here, too, the sick care system does a poor job at a high price. Too few physicians are in primary care and those who are often charge dearly for their services. The data reflect the failure: the growing use of emergency rooms for "routine" care, "triage" care, and the emergence of triage alternatives such as the "doc in the box," the nurse-clinics in shopping malls and pharmacies, the advice companies that use well-developed technologies to provide help in navigating through the system, etc. Again, since most illnesses are routine and non-life-threatening,

* Berwick provided this analysis during the hearings of the "Improving Community Cancer Care" Committee, sponsored by the National Cancer Institute.

† The author is an advisor to Physic Ventures.

nonphysician professionals can provide care that previously only doctors could. Technology helps, especially computer-based decision support tools and information libraries for consumers, and ubiquitous connectivity for purposes of telecommunications and computer-aided consultations. Companies like MedExpert have built their franchises around the principle that the information about which doctor is recognized as best and safest, which hospital is the "best," which care system provides the best outcomes for a given illness, is publicly available and can be delivered to patients and medical consumers inexpensively and effectively using a combination of expert educators, telecommunications, and computer-aided search systems.*

Yet another potential area for disruption concerns routine chronic disease management. Here too care teams using advanced monitoring and communications tools can help people with chronic illnesses avoid or delay complications, maintain quality of life, and prevent premature (avoidable) deaths. They can do this more efficiently than a doctor working alone or several physician specialists working in their individual private clinics. This is possible, once again, because the advances in science and supporting technologies enable more precise and earlier diagnosis, more refined treatments, and clearer understanding of disease progression, complications, and their recognition and prevention through effective therapeutic control and education.†

An additional aspect of chronic illness management is the role patient- and family-based peer groups play in helping support one another by sharing "tricks" for achieving control and complying with therapeutic regimens, dealing with the emotional ups and downs, finding appropriate providers, etc. Building on the success of network models like FaceBook or Linkedin, for example, innovators are experimenting with online communities for patients and families who must deal with chronic illnesses.

Though it is a less likely candidate for a technology-driven disruption than those just mentioned, the End-of-Life Care system is ripe for change as well. A large number of people remain in the "sick care" system after there is no hope for cure. Robert Martensen writes movingly of this problem in his book, *A Life Worth Living: A Doctor's Reflections on Illness in a High-Tech Era* (Rosen, 2009). Of course it is difficult, if not impossible, to know when cure is no longer possible. It is also profoundly difficult to deal with the deeply personal decision that a patient and family make to accept the inevitability of death. Not surprisingly, in spite of efforts to promote death with dignity and advanced directives, many people still die in hospitals in the vain hope that the unlikely will happen.

Creating a solution is difficult; technology is not the answer as the process itself is so intensely personal. A variety of people may be required to help a patient and family reach a decision: a clergyman, a nurse, a peer, a family member, a doctor, and sometimes all of the above. The disruption, if it is to occur, may be more psychological and cultural than organizational or technological.

The emerging consumer-health ecosystem, then, is the second major battlefront in the future. It challenges many aspects of the sick care system by delivering less expensive, more responsive care directly to consumers, a classic "disruption." It divides the sick care system into piece parts, repackaged into solutions for consumers. It is made possible by unmet demands, new technologies, simpler solutions, and the difficulty the sick care system has in changing itself fast enough to keep up with the forces that are driving the changes.

New Personalized Medicine Paradigm

A third front in the battle will occur in the field of personalized medicine, sometimes called "predictive" or "prospective" medicine. As described by many (President's Council of Advisors on Science and Technology, 2008), this is the growing capacity to understand illness at the level of the human molecule

* For more information, see www.medexpert.com. The author is an advisor to MedExpert.

† Diabetes care is the classic example in which careful blood sugar control through continuous monitoring by the patient and adjusting of insulin as required has revolutionized diabetes care. The same is true in asthma care (see, for example, Lawrence, 2002).

and genome, enabling the recognition of illnesses before they produce symptoms and complications. It is the knowledge base required to establish individual risk and understand what therapies are most likely to work for an individual patient based on genetic predilections and molecular pathways.

This is a sea change from the way patients have been cared for up to now. Physicians assume that science is unpredictable and each patient requires a custom solution. To solve problems they focus on phenotype: what is seen, felt, and heard when the patient is in front of them. Personalized medicine is molecular and submolecular, predictive, precise, and based on explicit probabilities. Not only is the physician delivery model poorly designed for this kind of care, but the established diagnostic and therapeutic technologies are becoming obsolete as the tools of molecular and genetic diagnostics continue to develop.

Several conflicts will occur as this new science rolls out. The most obvious is the one waged by physicians and hospitals for control of the science and accompanying technology, as the traditional delivery models (and the regulatory and legal systems that reinforce them) seek to incorporate these capabilities into their institutions and practices. At the same time, efforts to build alternative platforms to deliver these services are emerging, funded with venture capital.* These propose to deliver these reliable and personalized solutions directly to consumers. The battle, once again, is over disintermediation.

Within the traditional care system further conflicts can be expected. Which specialists will control the knowledge, technologies, and patient flows? Will "focused factories" develop within the traditional care system, still built on the central role of physicians but using different business models such as Shouldice Clinic (Herzlinger, 1997; Porter and Teisberg, 2006; Christensen et al., 2009)? How will payment for these services and technologies occur? Under whose control? How will they be regulated? Paid?

As in the other battlefronts, the emerging science and supporting technologies, coupled with strong and changing consumer demands, represent a unique opportunity to develop new delivery models. If successful, they will break the control of the sick care system, and change the way these technologies are rolled out. Instead of the traditional approach in which older technologies are used alongside new ones, adding not lowering costs, these new approaches can work better for consumers and deliver greater value for every healthcare dollar spent.

Accountable Organizations

If medical care is badly fragmented now, will not the addition of the new delivery models create another form of the same disease? It is a valid and important concern that underscores the need for new forms of care organizations to bring the pieces together. This is the fourth and final front in the battle. "Accountable healthcare organizations," as they are called in the current health reform debates, would take responsibility for the health and well-being of the consumers who choose to join them. They would ensure that both the medical care and the wellness and prevention care are delivered in the most effective manner possible. The accountable healthcare organization, then, assumes accountability for assuring that the healthcare spend creates the highest value return for the buyers and payers alike.†

One can readily anticipate the conflicts that will arise as these organizations evolve. How will they be structured and governed? What will be the role of the doctors in their leadership? How will competing clinical and population health requirements be balanced? How will conflicts between clinicians and managers be resolved?

In addition, battles over disputed territory are likely—will accountable care organizations be expected to integrate all aspects of care to create the "balanced care system" described earlier, or will they focus on

* Physic Ventures is dedicated to building companies in this space, for example.

† This idea is not new. Under the leadership of Mark McClellan, Director of CMS (in the Federal Department of Health and Human Services), considerable work was done to define and advance this concept into practice. It is part of the current health reform debate in Washington, District of Columbia, especially as new forms of bundled payments are considered to accelerate innovation within the traditional system.

improving performance and value within the sick care system? If their scope is to include the elements of the balanced care system, how will they integrate the rapidly innovating solutions without stifling them as often happens in many large organizations when innovation clashes with the status quo?

Final Thoughts

We can predict where the battlefronts are most likely to be going forward but not how they will play out. History provides little help, for the situation is without precedent. One thing is clear: if health reform places significant controls on the care system in terms of what is paid for and how, how care is to be delivered and who should deliver it, etc., the traditional physicians and institutions of medical care will be the winners in the short term. This, after all, is where the power lies; consumers lack the lobbying "heft" to force the system to open up through public policy interventions, and the fragmented efforts of the venture community are no match for the entrenched powers in the traditional care system. If, on the other hand, care reform protects and even promotes the sea changes underway, then the changes underway will occur more rapidly.

Whatever the outcome of the current national reform debate, the expanding science and dramatic shifts in consumer demands are unlikely to be stopped in the longer term; the physicians cannot hope to contain these forces as hard as they may try. The traditional system and its sovereign physicians will have to adapt as the alternatives emerge if they hope to keep pace with the rapidly changing and expanding science of care and the growing and changing demands from consumers.

But it is difficult to overstate the significant battles that lie ahead. Within the sick care system physicians will struggle to retain control of the organizations formed to drive greater efficiency, quality, and safety. The sick care system and the emerging consumer-health ecosystem will battle over who provides the care and where. Further downstream will be battles over the influence of accountable healthcare organizations charged with knitting together the fragments into an integrated array of services and accountability for the care consumer. Here too the conflicts will be for control of the formation, operation, and scope of these entities.

There are too many unknowns at this point, too many moving parts, to predict how these struggles will play out. In the meantime, it is critical to focus on improving the performance of the sick care system by applying the tools and perspectives that other industries have used with great success. The sick care system has become a collection of complex production processes, but efforts to improve performance have largely failed because of the overriding need to preserve an obsolete organizing model. The application of the tools of industrial design can help change this. As we improve performance, innovations will continue around the sick care system, forcing it to change more rapidly, in turn enabling the tools of industrial design to have their greatest impact. This is the pathway to the balanced care system that can provide consumers the care they need and want in the future at a price the nation can afford.

References

Andriole, G.L., E.D. Crawford, R.L. Grubb III, S.S. Buys, D. Chia, T.R. Church, M.N. Fouad, E.P. Gelmann, P.A. Kvale, and D.J. Reding. 2009. Mortality results from a randomized prostate-cancer screening trial. *The New England Journal of Medicine* 360(13): 1310–1319.

Arnold, M. and H.C. Carrie. 2009. Health care value comparability study. Washington, DC: Business Roundtable. www.businessroundtable.org (accessed March 18, 2010).

Burrill & Company. 2009. Biotech 2009—Life sciences: Navigating the sea changes. Available at: www.burrillandco.com

Bodenheimer, T., E. Chen, and H.D. Bennett. 2009. Confronting the growing burden of chronic disease: Can the US health care workforce do the job? *Health Affairs* 28(1): 64–74.

Bohmer, R.M.J. and D.M. Lawrence. 2008. Care platforms: A basic building block for care delivery. *Health Affairs* 27(5): 1336–1340.

Christensen, C.M., J.H. Grossman, C. Clayton, and J. Hwang. 2009. *The Innovator's Prescription: A Disruptive Solution for Health Care*. New York: McGraw Hill Professional.

Clark, D. and P. Glader. 2009. Intel, GE form health-care alliance. *Wall Street Journal*, http://online.wsj.com/article/SB123861157569679175.html (accessed March 20, 2010).

Demographics of the United States. 2008. Wikipedia. http://en.wikipedia.org/wiki/Demographics_of_the_United_States (accessed March 20, 2010).

Groopman, J. 2007. *How Doctors Think*. New York: Houghton Mifflin Co.

Herzlinger, R.E. 1997. *Market-Driven Health Care: Who Wins, Who Loses in the Transformation of America's Largest Service Industry*. New York: Perseus Books.

Institute of Medicine. 2001. Crossing the quality chasm: A new health system for the 21st century. Washington, DC.

Institute of Medicine. 2009. Learning health care system concepts v. 2008. Oakland, CA: California Healthcare Foundations.

Kraft, P. and D.J. Hunter. 2009, April 23. Generic risk prediction—Are we there yet? *The New England Journal of Medicine* 360(17): 1701–1703.

Lawrence, D. 2002. *From Chaos to Care: The Promise of Team-Based Medicine*. New York: Perseus Press.

Liebhaber, A. and J. Grossman. 2007. Physicians moving to mid-sized, single-specialty practices. http://www.hschange.org/CONTENT/941/ (accessed March 12, 2010).

Ludmerer, K.M. 1999. *Time to Heal: American Medical Education from the Turn of the Century to the Era of Managed Care*. New York: Oxford University Press.

McGlynn, E.A., S.M. Asch, J. Adams, J. Keesey, J. Hicks, A. DeCristofaro, and E.A. Kerr. 2003. The quality of health care delivered to adults in the United States. *The New England Journal of Medicine* 348(26): 2635.

National Academy of Engineering and Institute of Medicine. 2005. Building a better delivery system: A new engineering/health care partnership. Washington, DC: National Academies Press.

Passel, J. and D. Cohn. 2008. Immigration to Play Lead Role In Future U.S. Growth: U.S. Population Projections: 2005–2050. Washington, DC: Pew Research Center.

Porter, M.E. and E.O. Teisberg. 2006. *Redefining Health Care: Creating Value-Based Competition on Results*. Boston, MA: Harvard Business School Press.

President's Council of Advisors on Science and Technology. 2008. Priorities for Personalized Medicine.

Research!America. 2005. Investment in U.S. health research. www.researchamerica.org/app/webroot/uploads/healthdollar2005.pdf (accessed March 19, 2010).

Rosen, D. 2009. A life worth living: A doctor's reflections on illness in a high-tech era. *JAMA* 302(6): 693–695.

Schroder, F.H., J. Hugosson, M.J. Roobol, T.L.J. Tammela, S. Ciatto, V. Nelen, M. Kwiatkowski, M. Lujan, H. Lilja, and M. Zappa. 2009. Screening and prostate-cancer mortality in a randomized European study. *New England Journal of Medicine* 360(13): 1320–1328.

Starr, P. 1982. *The Social Transformation of American Medicine*. New York, NY: Basic Books.

The Crisis in Chronic Disease. 2009. *Health Affairs* 28(1).

U.S. Census Bureau. 2000. Language spoken at home—persons 5 years of age and older. http://www.laalmanac.com/population/po47.htm (accessed March 20, 2010).

U.S. Department of Labor. 2009. Physicians and surgeons. In *Occupational Outlook Handbook*, 2010–2011 edition. http://www.bls.gov/oco/ocos074.htm (accessed December 2009).

2

Engineering and the Healthcare Delivery System

Proctor P. Reid
National Academy of Engineering

W. Dale Compton
Purdue University

Engineering Systems 2-1
Quality of Healthcare 2-1
System Tools 2-2
Challenges 2-3
Barriers to Cooperation 2-4
Needs and Opportunities 2-5
Short-Term Projects • Long-Term Opportunities
Conclusion 2-7
References 2-8

Engineering Systems

Large numbers of entities that operate collectively to meet a set of objectives are commonly referred to as "systems"; examples are telecommunications systems, trucking systems, energy systems, and manufacturing systems. A well-designed, efficient operating system requires that the overall objectives be clearly understood by all elements of the system, that feedback loops be supported by good communications and controls, and that some entity be in charge of the system and responsible for ensuring that its performance meets its stated goals. The reason we seldom hear about a healthcare delivery "system" is that healthcare delivery was never designed as a system and does not operate as one. Rather, as David Lawrence notes in the previous chapter, healthcare delivery as a whole is fragmented, disorganized, and unaccountably variable.

American medicine has defined the cutting edge in most fields of clinical research, training, and practice, and engineers have made many important contributions to improvements in medical devices, new sensors, new diagnostic devices, and new materials. Ongoing changes in bioengineering and genomics and the promise of quantum advances in diagnostic tools and therapies testify to the continued vitality of the partnership between medicine and engineering. Nevertheless, in stark contrast to these successes, there has been relatively little technical talent or material resources devoted to improving or optimizing operations or measuring the quality and productivity of the overall healthcare system. In fact, engineers have contributed only marginally to improvements in the operations of healthcare delivery.

Quality of Healthcare

Statistics clearly indicate the magnitude of the task of improving the quality of U.S. healthcare delivery. Every year, more than 98,000 Americans die and more than one million patients are injured as a result of broken healthcare processes and system failures (IOM, 2000; Starfield, 2000). The gulf between a rapidly advancing medical knowledge base and its application to patient care is growing. Little more than half of U.S. patients are treated with known "best practices" for their illnesses (Casalino et al., 2003; McGlynn et al., 2003). According to one survey, 75% of patients consider the healthcare system fragmented and fractured, a "nightmare" to navigate, and plagued by duplication of effort, lack of communication, conflicting advice regarding treatment, and tenuous links to the evolving medical evidence base (Picker Institute, 2000).

Poor quality is costly. Lawrence estimates that \$.30 to \$.40 of every dollar spent on healthcare, more than a half trillion dollars per year, is spent on costs associated with "overuse, underuse, misuse, duplication, system failures, unnecessary repetition, poor communication, and inefficiency" (Lawrence, 2005). Meanwhile, healthcare costs have been rising by double digits since the late 1990s—roughly three times the rate of inflation—claiming a growing share of each American's income, inflicting economic hardship on many, and decreasing access to care. In 2007, the nation's uninsured population stood at nearly 46 million, more than 15% of the U.S. population under the age of 65 (DeNavas-Walt et al., 2008).

In *Crossing the Chasm: A New Health System for the 21st Century*, a 2001 study by the Institute of Medicine (IOM), a committee of experts identified six interrelated characteristics of a healthcare system that should guide efforts to improve the quality of care. The twenty-first-century healthcare system must be safe, effective, patient-centered, timely, efficient, and equitable (IOM, 2001):

- Safe—avoiding injuries to patients from the care that is intended to help them
- Effective—providing services based on scientific knowledge to all who could benefit and refraining from providing service to those not likely to benefit (avoiding underuse and overuse, respectively)
- Patient-centered—providing care that is respectful of and responsive to individual patient preferences, needs, and values and ensuring that patient values guide all clinical decisions
- Timely—reducing waiting times and sometimes harmful delays for those who receive and those who give care
- Efficient—avoiding waste, including waste of equipment, supplies, ideas, and energy
- Equitable—providing care that does not vary in quality because of personal characteristics, such as gender, ethnicity, geographic location, and socioeconomic status

The IOM committee identified "patient-centeredness" as the unifying principle.

In that same report, the committee urged the engineering community to assist in transforming the healthcare delivery system to meet these six objectives, each of which includes many aspects that are relevant to engineering. For example, the meaning of efficiency can be broadened to include the optimization of operations, the reduction of costs, and the avoidance of errors; and "timely" healthcare delivery might include better scheduling of facilities and personnel.

System Tools

The principles, tools, and techniques developed in engineering disciplines associated with the analysis, design, and control of complex systems (e.g., systems engineering, industrial engineering, operations research, human-factors engineering, financial engineering/risk analysis, materials/microelectromechanical systems engineering) have been integral to improving, and sometimes transforming many manufacturing and services industries. However, these tools and techniques are largely unknown in the clinical operations of healthcare delivery.

Alan Pritzker, the author of many treatises on large-scale modeling and simulation, has defined the system approach as "a methodology that seeks to ensure that changes in any part of the system will result in significant improvements in total system performance" (Pritzker, 1990). System analyses, which include possible trade-offs and/or synergies among objectives, can be used to improve the overall performance of systems with multiple, potentially conflicting objectives (e.g., cost containment and patient-centeredness). They can also reveal how individual goals can be adjusted to support the overall goals of the entire system.

Engineers have developed systems analyses that can show how complex systems operate, how well systems meet overall goals and objectives, and how they can be improved. Analyses can work on many levels. For example, they may focus on a single unit in a large system (e.g., the flow of patients through a facility or the scheduling of personnel). The results of these analyses can be used to evaluate how changes in procedures might lead to better, more efficient performance. On a higher level, a system analysis may take in the overall operation of a hospital, including its ambulatory clinic and pharmacy.

For a system analysis to reflect the actual performance of a system, the model must include all of the participants and components, representations of their functions, and descriptions of how each participant or part interacts with other participants and parts. Obviously, as the size and complexity of the system increases, the complexity of the model also increases. Mathematical tools have been developed that enable systems engineers to develop models that can investigate "what if" questions, such as, what would happen if the scheduling for laboratory personnel were changed to this? Or to that? Or, what if the inventory of items A, B, and C were reduced by 10%? Or, what would the likely cost savings be if hospitals X and Y, in two different systems, combined their ambulance fleets?

System tools can also be used to design new systems. The usual starting point is an existing system that is similar in structure and operation to the projected new system. Just as "what if" questions can be asked to investigate changes in performance of an existing system, the same type of questions can be asked about the performance of the new system. The questions can be modified to fit within the framework of constraints on the operation of the new system (e.g., budget constraints, fixed personnel costs, space limitations). As radically new or innovative changes to the system are examined, it may be necessary to use data from systems unrelated to healthcare delivery or to construct data sets using first "principles." Obviously, conclusions based on systems analyses must be carefully evaluated.

Finally, system tools can be used to control a system and inform workers and management when the system is about to become unstable or when the operations of the system have moved from a desirable operating point. Key system attributes can be easily identified and performance data can be collected and represented in such a way that performance is easy to understand. These types of controls provide "trend data" that enable management and workers to take corrective action before a change becomes catastrophic. Sections II, III, and IV of this handbook provide more thorough discussions of the current uses and opportunities for engineering tools to improve the delivery of healthcare.

Challenges

Understanding the factors that affect the performance of a system begins with an examination of the data on all aspects of performance. Data relating to the financial performance of healthcare delivery are usually available, but data on the variables that determine the operational performance of the system are often sparse, or even nonexistent. Thus, an engineer prepared to attempt to improve performance must usually begin with laboriously collecting necessary data. In many instances, this task is hampered by an information technology system that does not interface with the operating system in terms of physical variables, so collecting data can lead to time delays and substantial costs. Even more frustrating, once data have been collected and analyzed the same tasks must be repeated to ascertain whether changes in operations have the desired outcome.

A major barrier to the widespread use of the above identified systems-engineering tools is the variability in operating procedures in various healthcare provider facilities. Improvements at one facility turn out to be not directly amenable to another facility. A major research effort is required to create analytic systems that, in connection with information technology systems, can be used to analyze many different operating systems.

As the severe quality and cost challenges to U.S. healthcare suggest, the current care delivery "system" is poorly aligned with the healthcare needs of the American population. In the past half-century, in response to an explosive increase in medical knowledge, the number of medical specialties has increased from fewer than 10 to more than 100 (Lawrence, 2005). This increase has contributed to the "cottage industry" structure of healthcare, helping to create a delivery system characterized by myriad disconnected silos of function and specialization. There are approximately 700,000 clinicians in the United States, representing more than 100 different clinical specialties, and more than 80% of them practice medicine in groups of 10 or less (Lawrence, 2005).

This highly specialized, fragmented, independent practitioner-driven system of healthcare delivery has not kept pace with rapid advances in medical knowledge, nor has it been adapted to address the growing burden of chronic care. Even as more and more clinicians embrace the concept of "evidence-based medicine" (the notion that there is a fundamentally right way to diagnose and treat patients with a given condition) and understand that an individual clinician cannot possibly keep up with, let alone deliver, evidence-based care on his or her own, most of them do not have the tools or infrastructure to access and apply the medical evidence base in a timely way.

Thanks to advances in acute care, and improvements in diet and other lifestyle factors, many Americans are living longer, but with a higher incidence of chronic disease. As in other developed countries, about 125 million people—half of the U.S. population—have a chronic condition; and of these, about 60 million have more than one (Partnership for Solutions, 2002). Three-quarters of our healthcare dollars are spent on patients with chronic conditions (Halvorson, 2007), yet most chronic-care patients do not receive the integrated, longitudinal care they need; longitudinal care can be defined as continuity of care that requires connectivity among diverse, distributed care providers (e.g., patient, family members, physicians, nurses, pharmacists, et al.) and the coordination of multiple functions and specialized knowledge and skill sets over time.

A major challenge is to deliver healthcare to this diverse population in a way that is not only responsive to their needs and well coordinated, but that also reduces the need for frequent trips to care providers. Meeting this challenge will require distance communication between patient and provider(s), both in terms of providers receiving information about a patient's condition and of patients being able to interface with providers. Advances in telemedicine and supporting information technologies (the Internet, communications systems, sensors, etc.) have the potential to improve patient access to convenient/timely, better-coordinated, cost-effective, high-quality healthcare regardless of location. Realizing this promise, however, will require changes in the way healthcare services are priced and reimbursed (i.e., services delivered remotely must be compensated just as services delivered in face-to-face visits are compensated).

Engineering will be crucial for tapping into the potential of advanced telemedicine, but this will require overcoming significant challenges. Advanced telemedicine must confront significant barriers in information technology, sensors, and communication systems, as well as changes in work processes that will be necessary for patients to communicate effectively with their care providers and for providers to remotely assess the status of their patients, coordinate their care, and engage them in self-care.

Barriers to Cooperation*

In a joint National Academy of Engineering (NAE)/IOM report, *Building a Better Delivery System: A New Engineering/Health Care Partnership*, the study committee noted that the "recent history of multiple, interrelated crises of quality, access, and cost in the healthcare system testifies to [its] inherent complexity … and a desperate need for systems-engineering tools and information/communications technology" (NAE/IOM, 2005). The report included discussions of many ways systems engineering might be applied to improve the performance of healthcare processes, units, and departments at the tactical level. It also included discussions of a number of serious barriers to more extensive cooperation between engineers and health professionals.

The way healthcare delivery is currently organized, managed, and regulated provides few incentives for providers to turn to systems engineers for help. Current reimbursement practices, regulatory

* Reprinted from National Academy of Sciences. 2005. *Building a Better Delivery System: A New Engineering/Health Care Partnership*, National Academy Press, Washington, DC, 2005. With permission. © 2005 by the National Academy of Sciences.

frameworks, and the absence of support for research have discouraged the development, adaptation, and use of systems-engineering tools. Moreover, cultural, organizational, and policy-related factors (e.g., regulation, licensing) have contributed to a rigid division of labor in many areas of healthcare that has impeded the widespread use of system tools.

Underlying all of these structural, organizational, cultural, and policy-related barriers is a fundamental lack of understanding and trust between healthcare professionals and engineers, two professions with distinct epistemologies, vocabularies, analytical tools, approaches to problem solving (double-blind trials vs. prototyping), and ethics/values backed by two distinct, highly specialized, relatively insular professional education and training systems. Relatively few healthcare professionals or administrators have learned to think analytically about healthcare delivery as a system or to appreciate the relevance of systems-engineering tools. Few healthcare professionals know what questions to ask system engineers or what to do with the answers that they might receive.

On the other side of the divide, very few engineers are knowledgeable of the complex socio-technical fabric of healthcare processes and systems. The lack of exposure to the rudimentary concepts and ethics of each other's disciplines has tended to inhibit communication between engineers and healthcare professionals and to generate distrust in the other's methods and approaches.

Needs and Opportunities

Short-Term Projects

As engineers begin to address the problems in healthcare delivery, they must also establish their credibility with healthcare professionals. One way that has proved successful in accomplishing this is to work with healthcare professionals on choosing a short-term problem that is acknowledged by everyone to limit performance (e.g., the scheduling of appointments in a facility with a high rate of "no show" patients). By working with medical personnel to solve their problem, engineers can demonstrate their capacity and willingness to help. In addition, addressing a short-term practical problem is a good way to introduce engineering students to the medical environment.

Efforts to improve operational performance in healthcare delivery are most effective if undertaken in the medical environment—sometimes called the "living laboratory." Once a receptive location has been found, engineers can immediately begin to identify and help open up bottlenecks in the operation, at the same time providing their students with "real-world" experience in a healthcare facility. Additionally, it is not uncommon for longer-term research projects to evolve from efforts to solve near-term problems.

Long-Term Opportunities

Information and Communication

Information and information exchange are crucial to the delivery of care at all levels of the healthcare system—the patient, the care team, the healthcare organization, and the encompassing political–economic environment. But integrating information streams that arise at each of these levels will require training/education, decision support, information management, and new communication tools.

Unfortunately, the healthcare sector has historically been far behind most other sectors in investing in information/communication technologies and has only recently undertaken significant measures to establish a National Health Information Infrastructure (NHII). These measures include interrelated efforts to develop (1) healthcare standards and technical infrastructure; (2) core clinical applications, including electronic health records (EHRs), computerized physician order entry (CPOE) systems, digital sources of medical knowledge, and decision-support tools; and (3) information/communication systems.

In early 2009, with the passage of the American Recovery and Reinvestment Act (ARRA), which provided $19 billion for the development of health information technology (HIT) and associated infrastructure, the Obama administration and Congress committed the nation to a significant, sustained investment in improving healthcare delivery (U.S. Congress, 2009). ARRA required the Office of the National Coordinator for HIT to develop FY2009 guidelines for the investment of these foundational funds in an operating plan that described how expenditures would be aligned with the specific objectives, milestones, and metrics of the Federal Health Information Technology Strategic Plan.

The remainder of the investment ($34 billion for 2011–2016) will be in the form of entitlement incentives that build on the foundational work. By December 2009, the U.S. Department of Health and Human Services was required to adopt initial standards, implementation specifications, and certification criteria related to these incentives including technologies to protect the privacy of health information and ensure security in EHRs; the development of NHII; the creation of a certified EHR for each person in the United States by 2014; the use of certified EHRs to improve the quality of healthcare; technologies that protect the privacy of individually identifiable health information; the use of electronic systems to collect patient demographic data; and technologies that address the needs of children and other vulnerable populations. The administration is holding itself accountable for investing these funds in ways that result in a significant reduction in healthcare costs.

The engineering community can provide important, timely information and experience in helping government and the healthcare sector achieve the aims set forth in ARRA to advance the broader objectives of NHII. In a recent National Research Council report, *Computational Technology for Effective Health Care*, a committee of experts identified five principles to guide the nationwide deployment of HIT in the near term and specified a number of specific targets for engineering involvement. The five principles are (1) focus on improvements in care rather than technology; (2) seek incremental improvements from incremental efforts; (3) record available data so that current biomedical knowledge can be used to interpret data to support care, process improvement, and research; (4) design for human and organizational factors; and (5) provide support for the cognitive functions of all caregivers (NRC, 2009).

Multidisciplinary Centers

Earlier in this chapter, difficulties of communication between healthcare professionals and engineers were described. The lack of a vocabulary common to both disciplines contributes to this. Many believe that this strategic limitation can only be overcome by creating environments where professionals from both disciplines can work together on common problems.

In *Building A Better Delivery System: A New Engineering/Healthcare Partnership*, the NAE/IOM study committee recommended that multidisciplinary centers be established, modeled after similar centers that have been established in other domains; the research at these centers will involve both healthcare professionals and engineers. The committee noted that the experiences of government agencies with such centers had yielded two lessons. First, the centers have contributed to solving important research problems and to broadening the education of students. Focused on a multidisciplinary area (e.g., tissue engineering, earthquake engineering, surgical technology), each center necessarily addressed system problems. Second, the centers have identified cross-disciplinary research topics that might not have been undertaken by researchers in a single discipline; this has led to the development of new curricular offerings and materials.

Based on these experiences and the communication problems identified above, the committee made the following recommendations (NAE/IOM, 2005, p. 85):

- **Recommendation A.** The federal government, in partnership with the private sector, universities, federal laboratories, and state governments, should establish multidisciplinary centers at institutions of higher learning throughout the country capable of bringing together researchers, practitioners, educators, and students from appropriate fields of engineering, health sciences, management, social and behavioral sciences, and other disciplines to address the quality and productivity challenges facing the nation's healthcare delivery system. To ensure that the centers have a nationwide impact, they should be geographically distributed. The committee estimated that 30–50 centers would be necessary to accomplish these goals.

- **Recommendation B.** These multidisciplinary research centers should have a three-fold mission: (1) to conduct basic and applied research on the system challenges to healthcare delivery and on the development and use of systems-engineering tools, information/communications technologies, and complementary knowledge from other fields to address them; (2) to demonstrate and diffuse the use of these tools, technologies, and knowledge throughout the healthcare delivery system (technology transfer); and (3) to educate and train a large cadre of current and future healthcare, engineering, and management professionals and researchers in the science, practices, and challenges of systems engineering for healthcare delivery.

Making systems-engineering tools, information technologies, and complementary social-science, cognitive-science, and business/management knowledge available and training individuals to use them will require commitment and cooperation by healthcare and engineering professionals. It will also require long-term changes in the cultures of both professions. These changes must begin in the formative years of professional education and will require that students in both professions have opportunities to participate in learning and research environments in which they can contribute to a new approach to healthcare delivery.

The interdisciplinary centers recommended in the NAE/IOM report are not intended to produce healthcare professionals who can individually apply systems-engineering tools or engineers who can deliver healthcare. They are intended to provide an environment in which engineers and health professionals can work together and share experiences, thus breaking down disciplinary, cultural, and linguistic barriers and building mutual trust and a shared understanding of the problems facing healthcare and the systems-engineering tools and information/communications technologies that can help address them.

Challenge for Educators of Health Professionals

Recognizing and exploiting the potential contributions of systems engineering to healthcare delivery will be an enormous challenge, especially for the educators of health professionals. The current concept of professional excellence accepted by healthcare providers will have to be expanded to encompass public health and the structure, processes, and systems of healthcare delivery. Physicians, nurses, and other health professionals will need new skills to work effectively with engineering and management professionals to change the design, implementation, and understanding of the structures and processes of healthcare to ensure that care is ultimately safe, effective, timely, efficient, patient-centered, and equitable.

Thus, the training of health professionals will have to be changed. The curriculum will have to include systems-engineering concepts and skills, both directly in dedicated courses and indirectly through integrated material in other courses and units of study and practice. This will require that faculty with expertise in healthcare delivery be identified or recruited and that educational and research links be established among clinical professionals and engineers.

Challenges for Schools of Engineering, Management, and Public Health

To encourage engineering and management students to be prepared to participate in helping solve these many problems, curricula in schools of engineering, management, and public health will have to be expanded to encompass problems, concepts, and topics in healthcare delivery. These changes will have to be incorporated into formal classroom education, applied training, and continuing education. Thus, new models of education and training will have to be designed, implemented, and evaluated.

Conclusion

The main argument of this chapter is that the engineering profession can make important contributions to ongoing efforts to make healthcare delivery safe, efficient, patient-centered, timely, and equitable.

Accomplishing these objectives will require the commitment of leaders in the healthcare community and leaders in the engineering community. Working together, we believe they can make great progress and ultimately vastly improve the delivery of healthcare in the United States.

References

Casalino, L., R.R. Gillies, S.M. Shortell, J.A. Schmittdiel, T. Bodenheimer, J.C. Robinson, T. Rundall, N. Oswald, H. Schauffler, and M.C. Wang. 2003. External incentives, information technology, and organized processes to improve health care quality for patients with chronic diseases. *Journal of the American Medical Association* 289(4): 434–441.

DeNavas-Walt, C., B.D. Proctor, and J.C. Smith. 2008. U.S. Census Bureau, Current Population Reports, P60–235, *Income, Poverty, and Health Insurance Coverage in the United States, 2007*. Washington, DC, U.S. Government Printing Office.

Halvorson, G. 2007. *Health Care Reform Now!: A Prescription for Change*. San Francisco, CA, Jossey Bass.

IOM (Institute of Medicine). 2000. *To Err Is Human: Building a Safer Health System*, edited by L.T. Kohn, J.M. Corrigan, and M.S. Donaldson. Washington, DC, National Academy Press.

IOM. 2001. *Crossing the Quality Chasm: A New Health System for the 21st Century*. Washington, DC, National Academy Press.

Lawrence, D. 2005. Bridging the quality chasm. pp. 99–101 in *Building a Better Delivery System: A New Engineering/Health Care Partnership*. Washington, DC, National Academies Press.

McGlynn, E.A., S.M. Asch, J. Adams, J. Keesey, J. Hicks, A. DeCristofaro, and E.A. Kerr. 2003. The quality of health care delivered to adults in the United States. *New England Journal of Medicine* 348(26): 2635–2645.

NAE (National Academy of Engineering)/IOM. 2005. *Building a Better Delivery System: A New Engineering/Health Care Partnership*. Washington, DC, National Academies Press.

NRC (National Research Council). 2009. *Computational Technology for Effective Health Care: Immediate Steps and Strategic Directions*. Washington, DC, National Academies Press.

Partnership for Solutions. 2002. *Chronic Conditions: Making the Case for Ongoing Care*. Prepared for the Robert Wood Johnson Foundation. Baltimore, MD, Johns Hopkins University Press.

Picker Institute. 2000. *Eye on Patients*. A report by the Picker Institute for the American Hospital Association. Boston, MA, Picker Institute.

Starfield, B. 2000. Is U.S. health really the best in the world? *Journal of the American Medical Association* 284(4): 483–485.

U.S. Congress. 2009. American Recovery and Reinvestment Act of 2009. Washington, DC, U.S. Government Printing Office. Available online at: http://frwebgate.access.gpo.gov/cgi-bin/getdoc.cgi?dbname=111_cong_bills&docid=f:h1enr.pdf

3

The VA Healthcare Delivery System

Historical Evolution of the VA Healthcare Delivery System 3-1
VA's Quality Transformation 3-3
Veterans and the VA Healthcare Systems 3-4
Whom Does the VA Healthcare System Serve? • Mission and Goals of the VA Healthcare System
Leadership and Organizational Structure 3-6
Veterans Health Administration • Veterans Integrated Service Networks (VISNs) • VA Medical Centers • VA Community-Based Outpatient Clinics
VA Healthcare Budget and Financing Mechanisms 3-9
VA Appropriations • Veterans Equitable Resource Allocation System • Fee Basis and Contract Care • Medical Care Cost Recovery
VA Healthcare Delivery 3-10
Scope of Patient Care Services in VA Facilities • VA's Computerized Patient Record System
Health and Healthcare Utilization among Veterans 3-11
Health Status of Veteran Users of the VA Healthcare System • Veterans' Healthcare Utilization
Quality Improvement in the VA Healthcare System 3-13
VA Performance Measurement System • National VA Patient Safety Registry • Using Research–Clinical Partnerships to Systematically Improve Care
Special Populations in VA Healthcare Settings 3-14
Veterans with Mental Health and/or Substance Abuse Problems • Veterans with Spinal Cord Injuries • Women Veterans • Operation Enduring Freedom and Operation Iraqi Freedom Veterans
Future Perspectives 3-16
References 3-17

Elizabeth M. Yano
Veterans Affairs Greater Los Angeles Health Services Research & Development Center of Excellence
and
University of California

Historical Evolution of the VA Healthcare Delivery System

Care for veterans has spanned centuries in America, with the notion of the first benefits system tracing back to 1636, when the Pilgrims of the Plymouth Colony were at war with the Pequot Indians and colonists subsequently passed a law that assured that soldiers disabled in the war were to be supported by the colony thereafter (Kizer et al., 1997). By 1776, the Continental Congress extended these beginnings by promising pensions for disabled soldiers, though some historians suggest this was chiefly a mechanism to encourage enlistments during the Revolutionary War, as direct medical and hospital care were actually provided by the states and local communities. It was not until 1811 that the first formal domiciliary and medical facility for veterans was authorized by the federal government. After the Civil War, states also established veterans' homes (Kizer et al., 2000).

By 1917, Congress established a new system of veteran benefits when the United States entered World War I. This new system included domiciliary care, as well as incidental medical and hospital treatment for injuries and diseases among veterans. The system also assured service for indigent and disabled veterans. By the 1920s, three federal agencies that addressed veterans' needs were created: the Veterans' Bureau, the Bureau of Pensions of the Interior Department, and the National Home for Disabled Volunteer Soldiers. These agencies added disability compensation, insurance for military service persons and veterans, and vocational rehabilitation services for disabled veterans. Throughout the nineteenth century, veterans' benefits were also expanded to include their widows and dependents. Care for dependents became a long-term commitment of such programs. For example, the last dependent of the Revolutionary War died in 1911, the last dependent of the War of 1812 died in 1946, and the last of the Mexican War died in 1962. Indeed, there are widows and/or children of veterans of the Civil War, Indian Wars, and Spanish–American War who still draw Veterans Administration (VA) compensation or pension benefits. Originally established to treat combat-related injuries and to rehabilitate veterans with service-connected disabilities, in 1924, the safety net mission was created as Congress gave access to wartime veterans with non-service-connected conditions.

By the time of the Great Depression, the system of veterans' benefits was consolidated as the VA in the face of unprecedented demand. President Roosevelt later authorized construction of additional VA hospital beds in 1937 to meet the demand for neuropsychiatric care, tuberculosis, respiratory illness, and other health concerns, as well as to increase equitable geographic access to care. Casualties from World War II sparked greater VA expansion, with a huge increase in the number of veterans seeking services (26,000 were wait listed), followed by a large array of new benefits, including the GI Bill, signed into law by Congress in 1944 (DeLuca, 2000).

Despite the return and discharge of military veterans after World War II, even by 1946, the initial high demand for VA care waned and many VA hospitals faced an excess of beds, in part because of the Hill–Burton Act, which served to increase the supply of community hospital beds. By the 1950s, veterans of the Korean War soaked up the excess beds, adding a new cohort of veterans seeking use of VA services, followed by the increased volume of veterans and VA demand caused by the Vietnam War during the 1960s and 1970s. By 1980, the veteran population had increased to 28.6 million. Admissions also doubled from 1963 to 1980, from 585,000 to 1.2 million, with admission rates escalating from 24 to 41 per 1000. Consistent with cost increases in U.S. healthcare from the 1950s onward, the costs of VA healthcare also continued to climb. In the 1970s, the Institute of Medicine convened a panel of national experts to debate the fate of the VA healthcare system, with nontrivial suggestions that perhaps closing the VA would provide better benefits to our nation's veterans than trying to fix what was considered an irreparably broken system.

The drivers of the VA's subsequent reorganization began to accelerate in the 1980s. Despite a history of ever-increasing demand (and higher costs), by the 1980s, VA hospital demand began to decline, as did the number of veterans eligible to use VA care. However, while community hospitals reduced their bed size (from a peak of >1 million in the 1980s to 873,000 by 1995) and faced closures (the number of U.S. hospitals declined by 12% between 1975 and 1995), there was virtually no comparable action among VA hospitals to reduce beds or close facilities. The VA also retained a hospital-centric and specialty-oriented system of care, such that while the private sector was shifting to ambulatory care, VA facilities were relatively slow to take advantage of changes in medical technology that enabled outpatient management of conditions and procedures once only cared for in acute care facilities. Demand for VA care was also largely unaffected by changes in the insurance industry. Financial incentives and utilization control mechanisms to reduce hospital admissions and length of stay through the prospective payment system (PPS), capitation, and other payment reforms did not touch the VA healthcare system. While demand for VA care continued to decline through the 1980s, elderly veterans' use of VA hospitals dropped by 50% between 1975 and 1996, as VA hospitals faced competition with Medicare's reimbursement of veterans' care at other public and private hospitals. These shifts occurred at the same time that managed care organizations through health maintenance organizations (HMOs) and health plans were on the rise, with little or no cost sharing, which may have added to the decline in VA demand for services. In 1989, in the midst of these changes and challenges, President Bush elevated the status of the VA benefits system to that of a Cabinet-level agency, thus creating the Department of Veterans Affairs (P.L. No. 100–527). The Department, then and now, is comprised of the Veterans Health Administration (VHA)—which houses the VA healthcare delivery system, the Veterans Benefits Administration (VBA), and the Veterans Cemetery Service.

By 1993, the Clinton Administration's efforts to reform healthcare—with its potential end game of giving every American a national healthcare card, extending private insurance to 50% of VA users—had a transformative effect on the VA healthcare system (Young, 2000). With 172 VA hospitals suffering from waning demand and perceptions of poor quality and customer service, the VA established a Healthcare Reform Task Force to assess the implications of Clinton's reform efforts for veterans. The Task Force aimed to determine system readiness for the adoption of managed care-type arrangements that might support organizational change and also oversaw internal market research efforts to determine where veterans might go if given greater choice. The results revealed a system heavily focused on inpatient and specialty care (with a roughly 70% specialists to 30% generalist physician split) and a virtual absence of primary care delivery arrangements (i.e., walk-in care was the national norm). In addition, three out of four veterans indicated that they would "vote with their feet" and leave the VA if given the opportunity. This threat to survival served as a call to action.

VA's Quality Transformation

For the VA healthcare system, the ensuing decade was a period of unprecedented change. One of the first reactions to the results of the VA's national assessment of the systems' readiness for managed care, armed with results from a regional VA primary care program demonstration project, was the development of the VA Primary Care Directive (1994). The Directive mandated the development of VA primary care programs in every facility nationwide, with an emphasis on team-based models, by the end of 1996. Within 2 short years, VA medical centers (VAMCs) had nearly universal adoption of primary care teams (57%–94%), with substantial increases in primary care physician, nurse, and administrative staffing. The sufficiency of primary care resources increased dramatically between 1993 and 1996 (i.e., computer workstations quadrupled; space for administrative offices, exam rooms, and patient education doubled). The early implementation of electronic medical records may have also supported the two- to sixfold increases in primary care notification systems, alerting primary care providers of their patients' admissions, emergency room visits, and specialty consult results. By 1996, over 80% of VA facilities reported that they served the majority of veterans in their primary care practices, up from about half in 1993.

With primary care internal restructuring and expansion serving as a critical substrate for the changes ahead, a new Under Secretary for Health (USH), Dr. Kenneth Kizer, took the helm and proceeded to shepherd the largest U.S. healthcare delivery system through an unusual depth and breadth of practice and policy changes to transition the VA from being a loosely coupled set of specialty-oriented hospitals to an integrated delivery system rooted in ambulatory care. Not unlike current calls for the transformation of primary care practices into patient-centered medical homes, the vision for the "new VA" in the mid-1990s was focused on putting patients first, organizing primary care services to achieve "first contact care, continuity, comprehensiveness, and coordination," reducing distance to care by bringing services to veterans' communities through community-based outpatient clinics (CBOCs), and creating a seamless continuum of care across the rest of VA healthcare services.

VA's subsequent policy guidance and strategic plans called for (and achieved) substantive changes in network restructuring (i.e., from 172 independent VAMCs into 22 Veterans' Integrated Service Networks or VISNs), implementation of a Computerized Patient Record System (CPRS) (with substantial decision support capabilities), an overhaul of VA healthcare financing to a capitated system, and a performance measurement system that incentivized the achievement of administration and clinical quality targets. The new VISN leadership had budget control and accountable performance agreements across an average of 5–7 VA hospitals, 25–30 outpatient clinics, 4–7 nursing homes, and 1–2 domiciliaries. Primary care enrollments grew from 38% in 1993 to 45% in 1996 and then more than doubled to 95% by 1999. Increased access to nonphysician providers was another hallmark of VA's primary care expansion, demonstrated chiefly by a doubling of the number of nurse practitioners and more modest increase in the number of physician assistants in VA practices. Primary care-based quality improvement programs also expanded rapidly, likely mapped to the many performance measures (e.g., flu shots, colorectal cancer screening) sensitive to the organizational supports for and attention of primary care providers. In 1996, the Veterans' Health Care Eligibility Reform Act (P.L. 104–262) was also passed, which expanded eligibility for comprehensive outpatient services to all veterans, limited only by Congressional appropriations and local VA facilities' capacities. The Act enabled VA's fundamental transition into a health plan with veterans as enrollees, while maintaining priority care for veterans with disabilities (service-connected over non-service-connected) and those unable to defray the costs of medical care before other groups.

Between 1994 and 1998, VA hospital bed-day rates declined by 50%, urgent care visit rates fell by 35%, with only moderate increases in outpatient clinic visits (Ashton et al., 2003). The decline in VA hospital use did not result in increased non-VA hospital use, increased mortality, or declines in access (Ashton et al., 2003). While only 10% of patients were enrolled in primary care in 1994, 80% could identify their primary care provider by 1998. Annual inpatient admissions decreased by 24%, while outpatient visits increased by 30%. Ambulatory surgery rates also increased (35%–75%). System-wide staffing was also reduced by 11% during this period, even while the volume of patients served increased by 10% (including increases among veterans with special needs, with 8% increases among veterans with psychiatric illness or substance abuse problems, 19% more homeless veterans, and 21% more blind rehabilitation patients).

By 2000, the VA healthcare system had achieved its now widely lauded "quality transformation" (Greenfield and Kaplan, 2004). Before VA's reorganization (1994–1995), chronic disease and prevention performance were poor for nearly all areas measured (e.g., only about a quarter of patients eligible for vaccination for pneumococcal pneumonia were immunized). By 2000, VA performance increased in 12 of 13 measures, demonstrating substantial changes in processes of care over time, while the VA healthcare system outperformed Medicare fee-for-service on all 11 measures for which comparable data were available (Jha et al., 2003). Subsequent work demonstrated that VA's quality of care achievements outweighed other sectors as well, earning veterans 67% of recommended care vs. 55% for a nationally representative sample of all Americans (Asch et al., 2004). Kerr et al. also found that quality of diabetes care was better in VA compared to commercially managed care organizations (Kerr et al., 2004). These and other advances in VA care have spurred hopes that the VA could serve as a model delivery system for the United States (Oliver, 2007, 2008).

Veterans and the VA Healthcare Systems

Whom Does the VA Healthcare System Serve?

Veterans represent adult men and women (18 years of age or older) who have been discharged from military service. As of September 30, 2007, the estimated U.S. veteran population was approximately 23.8 million, with the largest period of service group represented by Vietnam Era veterans (nearly 7.9 million) and the second largest group represented by Gulf War era veterans (nearly 5.0 million). All veterans' median age was 60 years, with veterans under 45 representing about 20%, those 45–64 years old representing 41%, and those 65 years and older representing 39% of the total. Women veterans represent about 7.5% of the total veteran population (nearly 1.8 million). Veterans, on average, have a higher percent of high school completion or some college compared to nonveterans, but a lower percent of bachelors and advanced degrees. Nationally, veterans have higher personal income than nonveterans.

Not all veterans are eligible to use the VA healthcare system. Concurrent with the launch of VA's reorganization in the mid-1990s, Congress enacted eligibility reform legislation (P.L. 104–262, 1996) to expand eligibility for comprehensive services to all veterans (limited only by Congressional appropriations, i.e., how far those dollars can go) and to establish an enrollment process to help manage demand. Top enrollment categories reflect veterans with the greatest needs (e.g., service-connected disabilities, former prisoners of war, and catastrophically disabled and housebound regardless of service connection), followed by veterans unable to defray the cost of medical care (low income), other selected groups, and then all other veterans. Distributed into seven priority groups, in 2002, Congress split Priority 7 (all other veterans, about 32% of the total) into two categories, distinguishing between higher- and lower-income levels among veterans without service-connected conditions and later approved the suspension of VA enrollment for the higher-income group because of the growth in the number of veterans seeking care (Sprague, 2004).

Mission and Goals of the VA Healthcare System

The mission of the VHA focuses on ensuring access to veterans' needed healthcare services, providing education and training to healthcare professionals, supporting research of relevance to veterans and the VA healthcare system, and contributing to public health and emergency management needs.

Medical Care

The primary mission of VHA is to provide healthcare to eligible veterans. The medical care mission focuses on improving the health and functioning of veterans, and reducing the impact and burden of their illnesses and injury-related disabilities. Increased emphasis has also been on ensuring smooth transitions for veterans from active military service to civilian life. There are VA healthcare facilities in all 50 states and the District of Columbia, as well as Puerto Rico, Guam, the Philippines, and the U.S. Virgin Islands.

Education and Training

As part of its statutory mission, the VA has a strong education and training mission, realized through affiliations with over 1,200 educational institutions (including 107 of the nation's 128 medical schools), training over 100,000 students, residents, and fellows in over 40 disciplines per year. The VA healthcare system is central to the development and training of the U.S. physician workforce with about one-third of residents and half of all medical students receiving all or part of their clinical training in VA. Over 65% of all U.S. physicians have trained at one time or another in the VA healthcare system. Reflecting VA's educational mission, the majority of VA hospitals are academically affiliated with one or more healthcare professional schools, including schools of medicine, dentistry, nursing, social welfare, among others. VA is the third largest source of funding for graduate medical education in the United States after Medicare and Medicaid.

Research

The VA has a long tradition of fostering healthcare-related research as part of its third statutory mission. VA research spans biomedical/laboratory, clinical sciences, rehabilitation, and health services research, and represents substantial intramural and extramural funding (e.g., NIH, foundation, and other sources). In addition to clinical breakthroughs relevant to all Americans (e.g., pacemakers, MRIs, CT scanners, and the nicotine patch), VA researchers also specialize in the development of new treatments and devices for conditions more commonly seen among veterans (e.g., posttraumatic stress disorder [PTSD], traumatic brain injury [TBI], prosthetics, polytrauma). In addition to basic science discoveries and translation into clinical applications, VA has invested in health services research for over 25 years, contributing to advances in evidence-based practice and policy. VA health service researchers commonly partner with management and operations leaders to critically evaluate VA care for purposes of improvement. These efforts are supported in part by VA's Quality Enhancement Research Initiative (QUERI), aimed at implementing research into practice.

Contingency Support and Emergency Management

Not often as recognized as VA's other mission foci, the VA is designed to provide a source of federal contingency support in two main ways. First, the VA serves as a primary contingency backup to the U.S. Department of Defense (DoD) during times of war. For example, VA providers and staff may sign on to provide direct medical care and administrative support during military conflicts, leaving their VA posts to serve alongside military providers and staff. Also, if war casualties exceed the capacity of the military's healthcare system (which is entirely distinct from the VA healthcare system), the VA may provide assistance and support as needed. Second, the VA assists the U.S. Public Health Service (PHS) and other U.S. agencies and departments during regional or national emergencies (e.g., earthquakes, hurricanes). Unlike other healthcare systems, the VA is capable of airlifting VA personnel and mobile clinics into affected areas within 24–48 hours, helping to operationalize federal disaster plans. The VA is also the largest provider of services to homeless patients, given veterans' disproportionate representation among their ranks. Therefore, the VA serves as a critical public health safety net, capitalizing on the VA as a national healthcare system in the context of its capabilities of mobilizing significant healthcare and administrative support resources to areas of need.

Leadership and Organizational Structure

Veterans Health Administration

With the U.S. Department of Veterans Affairs as a Cabinet-level agency, and thus led by a Secretary appointed by the U.S. President and confirmed by Congress, the VHA is led by a USH. Appointed and confirmed through similar procedures as the Secretary, the USH is the official responsible for the strategic planning and implementation of VHA's mission and vision through effective oversight and deployment of over 230,000 employees in the context of a \$110 billion budget (FY10).

Accountable to the Secretary and Congress, as well as to the veterans and their families, the USH manages the U.S.'s largest healthcare system through a combination of Deputy Under Secretaries and Offices based in VA Central Office (VACO) in Washington, District of Columbia. While the very top leadership of VHA changes with each Administration (unless a new President elects to retain one or more of the prior Administration's selections), leadership of program offices remains relatively consistent over time, as incumbents are government employees rather than political appointees. However, with changes in top leadership, the types and organizational structure of individual offices may change as well.

Currently, VHA is led by a USH, with a Principal Deputy Under Secretary for Health (PDUSH) responsible for oversight of other Deputy Under Secretaries (e.g., Deputy Under Secretary for Operations and Management or DUSHOM) and Chief Officers (e.g., Chief Quality and Performance Officer, Chief Research and Development Officer). Each office may have one or more Strategic Healthcare Programs, run by Chief Consultants (though they are regular VA employees, not "consultants" in the business sense). Mapped to the VHA's mission, main offices include the Office of Patient Care Services (PCS), the Office of Quality and Performance (OQP) (now overseen by an Assistant Deputy Under Secretary for Health for Safety and Quality), the Office of Policy and Planning, the Office of Research and Development (ORD), the Office of Public Health and Environmental Hazards (OPHEH), the Office of Academic Affiliations (OAA), and the Office of Nursing Services, among others (e.g., Information Technology, Readjustment Counseling, Finance, Employee Education, Ethics) (Figure 3.1).

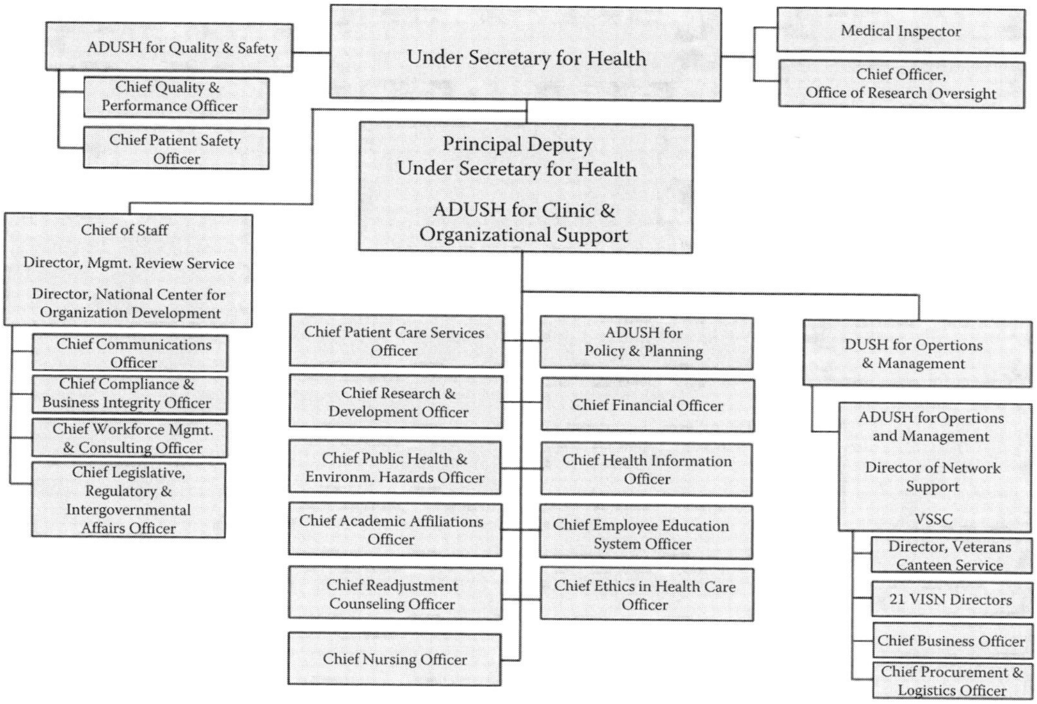

FIGURE 3.1 Organizational chart of the VHA. (Adapted from Veterans Health Administration, Washington, DC, http://www4.va.gov/ofcadmin/docs/vaorgbb.pdf)

Veterans Integrated Service Networks (VISNs)

Central to the restructuring of the VA healthcare system started in the mid-1990s was the move from loosely organized regional offices (e.g., the Western Region) generally supporting large geographic areas of the United States to the development of 22 (now 21) VISNs (Oliver, 2007). The DUSHOM in VACO oversees the VISNs in the field. The DUSHOM and VISN Directors are members of a National Leadership Board (NLB), which in turn has a series of Committees that focus on key strategic areas (e.g., Health Systems Committee). Committee membership commonly represents combinations of VHA Central Office and VISN field-based leaders, as well as selected experts and leaders in the field from individual VA facilities.

Unlike the previous regional offices, which had no direct authority over local VA facilities, VISNs are accountable for the clinical and financial performance of the facilities they oversee in their respective geographic service areas. For example, VHA sets the bar for performance targets and integrates them into executive performance agreements with VISN leaders rather than with VA facilities directly. VISN leaders, in turn, decide how to oversee, manage, coordinate, incentivize, or otherwise enact comparable agreements and performance improvement actions at individual facilities through their respective leaders. Similarly, funding runs from VHA to the VISNs, not to the individual VA facilities as had been the case prior to VA's major reorganization in the mid-1990s. The VISNs, therefore, had new decision-making authority regarding how individual facilities would receive both their core annual budgets, as well as special allocations or project funding based on need during each fiscal year. These changes represented a fundamental reworking of relationships, expectations, and processes, with substantive cultural changes in lines of authority and accountability on all levels (i.e., VHA, VISN, and VA facility).

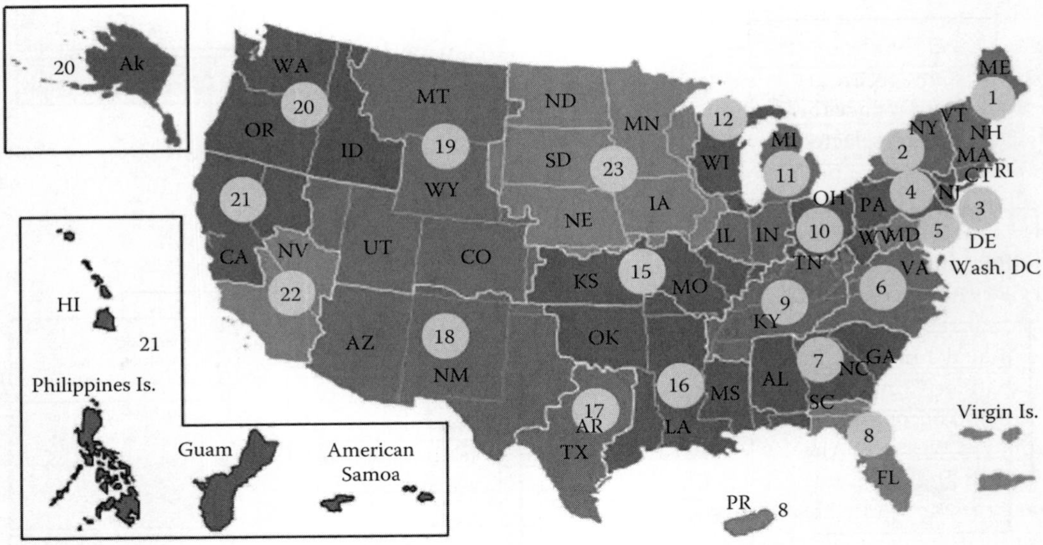

FIGURE 3.2 Map of VISNs. (Adapted from Veterans Health Administration, Washington, DC.)

Each VISN is led by a VISN Director and Chief Medical Officer (CMO) and retains a relatively small staff, despite being the conduit for the budget for all healthcare facilities under their respective purviews. VISN staffing is not proscribed, and thus each VISN Director and CMO may structure and staff VISN operational and management functions somewhat differently (e.g., they may have a Quality Management Officer, a Chief Information Officer, or other functions at the VISN level). VISNs commonly leverage this relatively small core by incorporating supports from their member facilities through task forces, work groups, or, in some cases, VISN-wide restructuring along service lines (e.g., designating a VISN primary care service line chief, overseeing policy and practice issues across all primary care practices in the VISN) or other approaches.

Each VISN is comprised of multiple VA facilities that report to the VISN director through a facility director. A typical VISN may include 5–7 VAMCs, 5–10 CBOCs, multiple nursing home care units, Vet Centers, domiciliaries, and other units (described below in more detail). The geographic service areas for each VISN vary, and commonly span multiple states (e.g., VISN 22 covers Southern California and parts of Nevada) (Figure 3.2).

VISN directors commonly lead the strategic planning and management of administrative operations and clinical care delivery across member VA facilities through VISN-level executive leadership councils. Such councils (or boards) may include combinations of facility-level directors, chiefs of staff (i.e., medical directors), chief nurses, chiefs of medicine, or other service chiefs or representatives (i.e., va facilities have historically been structured around services—such as medical service or research service, rather than departments, but variation in local terminology and structure exists).

VA Medical Centers

VAMCs are the main clinical care hubs of the national VA healthcare system. VAMCs are hospitals that typically include a broad range of acute care, long-term care, rehabilitation, and ambulatory care services (both specialty and primary care), in addition to urgent and emergency care. The specific scope of services and complexity of care available at any given VAMC may vary, requiring care arrangements that may require veterans to travel to another VA facility (e.g., to obtain specialized surgical services from a larger volume hospital or ambulatory surgery center) or to have care obtained in non-VA hospitals or other healthcare organizations in the community. The VA may pay for these services through fee basis or contract care arrangements or other mechanisms (see "Fee Basis and Contract Care" section).

In order to reduce the duplication of services and shift healthcare delivery infrastructure to match delivery needs, selected VAMCs have also undergone facility integrations. In facility integrations, two hospitals have been typically merged under a single, common leadership structure, with the individual hospitals becoming divisions within a newly integrated VA healthcare system. An example is the VA Greater Los Angeles Healthcare System (GLA) in Southern California. While many facility integrations have occurred as a result of a systematic, strategic planning process based on reviews of market penetration, caseload/workload, and overlapping service areas, the GLA integration was the result of the loss of the Sepulveda VAMC's hospital as a consequence of the Northridge Earthquake in 1994. Initially, the Sepulveda VAMC merged with other area CBOCs (Los Angeles Outpatient Clinic, Bakersfield Satellite Outpatient Clinic and Santa Barbara Satellite Outpatient Clinic) to become the VA Southern California System of Clinics (SCSC), which obtained acute care from the West Los Angeles VAMC (and for Bakersfield patients, selected admissions in the Fresno VAMC). The SCSC was subsequently merged with the West Los Angeles VAMC to become one of the largest integrated healthcare systems within VHA. The resulting facility integration has a single facility director, single chief of staff, etc., and integrated almost all other services into multicampus programs under a single service chief. Other VAMCs with single hospitals but with an array of community-based satellite clinics and programs have also renamed themselves as VA healthcare systems.

VA Community-Based Outpatient Clinics

In order to bring VA healthcare services closer to veterans where they live, the VA healthcare system has a long history of developing "satellite" clinics that are affiliated with a "parent" VAMC but may range anywhere from 10 to over 100 miles or more from the main facility. These satellites were renamed CBOCs (called "see-box"), and were part of VHA's efforts to improve the accessibility of VA healthcare services to veterans whose residences were beyond a 30-minute commute to the main VAMCs. Since 1995, more than 600 new CBOCs have been established (including 118 additional CBOCs since 2008). While not an explicit aim of CBOC expansion, the placement of new access points in communities where significant volumes of veterans resided had the concomitant impact of increasing the number of veterans who enrolled in and used VA health services. CBOCs are typically primary care clinics, but have worked to integrate mental healthcare in all satellite locations given the mental health needs of veterans. To enable such expansion, the VA has both leased clinic space (but staffed them with VA providers) and also contracted with non-VA clinics.

VA Healthcare Budget and Financing Mechanisms

VA Appropriations

Congress appropriates medical care funds to the VA healthcare system on an annual basis to cover the costs of patient care, research, education, equipment, and maintenance expenses. As a fixed sum, VA's annual appropriation must cover VHA and VISN wide budget needs and expenditures. In fiscal year 2009, the national U.S. Department of Veterans Affairs' budget was approximately $96.9 billion. Nearly half of this budget goes to veterans and their families in the form of disability payments, income support, and other needs. The majority of the remainder supports the VA healthcare system ($43.5 billion), and includes medical services, medical support and compliance, medical facilities, and medical and prosthetic research. The budget for fiscal year 2010 recommends a significant boost to VA healthcare spending to support returning veterans from Iraq and Afghanistan, as well as a new transformational agenda (see "Future perspectives" section).

Veterans Equitable Resource Allocation System

In 1997, VHA adopted the Veterans Equitable Resource Allocation (VERA) system to transition to a capitated system. Under VERA, federal budget dollars followed where veterans went for their care and considered how they were focusing healthcare spending on veterans of highest priority—namely, those whose conditions were service connected and those with special healthcare needs (e.g., blind or spinal cord injured veterans). The initial deployment of VERA produced profound shifts in the locus of funding in many parts of the country. These included shifts from commonly well-resourced areas in Chicago, Boston, and New York, that had seen 17%–20% losses from 1990 to 2000, to areas of rapid growth of veterans (e.g., Phoenix, Tampa, Las Vegas), that had seen 20%–30% increases. Veteran casemix adjustments were refined over time based on a RAND appraisal of the VERA model (Wasserman et al., 2004). VA healthcare delivery costs also reflect the aging of the physical infrastructure of VA buildings, some 40% of which are more than 50 years old and roughly one-third of which have historical significance (Wasserman et al., 2001).

Fee Basis and Contract Care

For services that local VA facilities cannot deliver (e.g., due to lack of an available or accessible specialist), VA managers and providers may utilize fee basis providers (i.e., providers paid fees to deliver specific services to eligible veterans) or contract care (e.g., mammograms or specific procedures) in the community. For example, women veterans are commonly referred to community providers on a fee basis if their local VA facility lacks providers experienced and credentialed in specialty reproductive health services (e.g., obstetrical care).

Medical Care Cost Recovery

In addition to Congressional appropriations, the VA has established mechanisms for recovering the costs of medical care that VA providers deliver from veterans' insurance plans. Historically not a major focus, VA collections from health insurance companies topped $100 million per month. These funds used to be retained by the U.S. Treasury, but are now retained and used by the VA for patient care needs.

While efforts to recover medical care costs from veterans' other insurance has been successful, efforts to recover costs from Medicare for the large volume of veterans dually eligible for VA and Medicare coverage (i.e., called Medicare subvention) failed (Oliver, 2007). The VA, therefore, delivers services to Medicare-covered veterans without reimbursement.

VA Healthcare Delivery

The VA operates the largest direct healthcare delivery system in the United States, with VA healthcare facilities in all 50 states, the District of Columbia, Puerto Rico, and U.S. territories. As of June 2009, VHA operated 153 hospitals and 995 outpatient clinics (including both hospital- and community-based), in addition to 135 community-living centers, and 49 domiciliary residential rehabilitation treatment programs. VA also staffs 232 Vet Centers, which provide readjustment counseling, outreach and links to community services, and 88 comprehensive home-care programs. With over 235,000 employees, VHA employs over 14,500 physicians and dentists, and about 58,000 nurses, making VA the largest employer of nurses in the United States (Perlin et al., 2004).

Scope of Patient Care Services in VA Facilities

VAMCs and healthcare systems typically provide a full spectrum of acute care hospital-based services, surgical care, specialty care, primary care, geriatrics and extended care, as well as dental care, with special programs and capabilities in mental healthcare (including substance abuse care), rehabilitation, prosthetics, vision/hearing care, and spinal cord injury care. VA's medical benefits package also includes prescription drugs, over-the-counter medications, medical supplies, and durable medical equipment. Most VA hospitals have 365/24/7 emergency rooms (ERs), while CBOCs must refer emergent cases to nearby VA hospitals or community ERs. VA's also deliver care through telemedicine (e.g., telepsychiatry), in addition to providing occupational and environmental health services. The goal of VA PCS is to deliver the full continuum of care from health promotion/disease prevention (including health education and immunizations), diagnostic, therapeutic, and rehabilitative care through to home health, palliative care, and hospice services.

VA CBOCs provide chiefly primary care services, with integration of mental health services over the past several years. Larger CBOCs may also include selected specialty ambulatory care services, depending on service needs and availability. Otherwise, veterans must either travel to the nearest VAMC or obtain services in the community as arranged by VA staff.

Over time, Congress has continued to expand veterans' benefits, including healthcare benefits. The Veterans Millennium Healthcare and Benefits Act of 2001 focused on long-term care expansions, requiring that the VA provide or pay for nursing home care for all veterans who are rated 70% or more disabled and those needing nursing home care because of a service-connected disability. The Act also required VA to provide adult day healthcare and home care as alternatives to institutionalization for elderly and disabled veterans (Sprague, 2004).

VA's Computerized Patient Record System

The VA's CPRS has been noted as one of the best electronic medical record systems in the world. Designed in a partnership among both VA information technology (IT) specialists and VA providers, CPRS has decision support functions, including reminders and specialized templates that help guide providers through care decisions, links patients to consults online, and provides population management capabilities (Evans et al., 2006). Clinician order entry has also been integral to VA clinical care for decades before CPRS was implemented.

CPRS data are specific to each VA healthcare facility, but have been rolled up into VISN data warehouses in many VISNs nationwide. Regional and corporate (national) data warehouses now enable tracking of patient care activities across systems for the purposes of care coordination, and also support analysis for quality improvement, utilization management, and research. The VA has also invested in the development of an online patient portal, called MyHealth*e*Vet, which provides patient education and other information for veterans, and will become a tool for patient online scheduling and secure messaging (Nazi et al., 2010).

Health and Healthcare Utilization among Veterans

The health status and healthcare utilization among veterans who use the VA healthcare system differs from veteran nonusers as well as from nonveterans.

Health Status of Veteran Users of the VA Healthcare System

Historically, veteran users of the VA healthcare system have been older, with lower income, less likely to have private insurance, in poor or fair health, and/or unable to work for pay due to their having limits on their activities of daily living (Wilson and Kizer, 1997). About 45% of VA enrollees are 65 years or older, with another approximately 40% between the ages of 45 and 64. Conditions such as hypertension and diabetes are prevalent.

Because of the prioritization of veterans with service-connected disabilities, VA facilities must be prepared to meet their special healthcare needs. Environmental exposures are of special concern, and may include exposure to radiation fallout (e.g., nuclear, weapons testing, and fire), biological and chemical weapons, Agent Orange, infectious disease agents (e.g., exotic and tropical), as well as iatrogenic exposures (e.g., vaccine "cocktails"), and Gulf War Syndrome. Congress has also legislated care for Special Emphasis Programs, including targeted resources for veterans with spinal cord injury, blindness, PTSD, and homeless veterans. The impacts of military service also include military trauma and violence exposure, requiring services for veterans with combat exposure (i.e., physical assault and trauma, stress-related illness and injury, emotional trauma, and military sexual trauma), support for transitions back to civilian life, and transitions to care programs following military discharge.

Comorbid psychiatric illness is also common among VA users, with substantial rates of depression, anxiety, substance abuse, and PTSD. Veterans who use the VA have average physical and mental health functional status that is substantially lower than the general population, akin to having about two additional chronic conditions (Rogers et al., 2004). Despite this, veterans' risk-adjusted mortality is lower than male seniors under Medicare Advantage (Selim et al., 2009).

Veterans' Healthcare Utilization

The determinants of VA utilization include service-connected disability, insurance status (i.e., uninsured veterans typically rely on VA services), employment (i.e., related to age, disability status, and availability of employer-based insurance), perceptions of VA quality of care, and proximity to VA facilities (Payne et al., 2005; Washington et al., 2006). In 2005, VHA served 5.3 million veterans, roughly 75% of the 7.7 million enrolled. VA providers delivered 57.5 million outpatient visits (in addition to paying for 2.4 million visits through fee-basis providers) and cared for veterans in over 587,000 inpatient stays (approximately 60% acute, 14% psychiatric, and 12% nursing home). Unlike most other U.S. healthcare systems, health plans, and payors, VA has not capped veterans' healthcare utilization, especially in areas of mental healthcare, making it relatively unique among other systems. VA formulary management has increasingly used cost-effectiveness analysis to help guide rational pharmacy benefits policy (Aspinall et al., 2005; Sales et al., 2005).

Over time, the proportion of veterans using the VA healthcare system has continued to increase (Liu et al., 2005). Between 1995 and 2005, veteran enrollment increased from 2.5 million to 5.3 million patients (Perlin, 2005). By 2008, nearly 8 million veterans had enrolled in VA's healthcare system (Congressional Budget Office, 2009). Veterans more likely to use the VA are in poorer health, and have more comorbid medical conditions and higher medical resource use than the general population (Agha et al., 2000; Hynes et al., 2007). However, veterans' resource use is comparable to that outside the VA, when adjusting for their sociodemographic and health status characteristics. Veteran users also tend to be older, less educated, predominantly male, and more likely to be uninsured and unemployed, compared to civilians and to veterans who do not use the VA, reflecting VA's safety net mission (Liu et al., 2005). Nonetheless, a majority of veterans who use VA healthcare services also have alternative healthcare coverage, including over half with Medicare coverage (i.e., among elderly and disabled veterans) (Fleming et al., 1992; Wright et al., 1997), nearly 20% having other private insurance without Medicare coverage, and about 5% having Medicaid coverage (with or without Medicare) (Shen et al., 2003). In a given year, over 90% of VA enrollees have used healthcare, with about 38% using the VA only, 36% using both VA and non-VA healthcare (so nearly three-quarters used VA to some degree), and about 19% using non-VA providers only (Shen et al., 2003).

Quality Improvement in the VA Healthcare System

VA's historical problems with quality of care have been the subject of substantial concern in policy arenas (e.g., Institute of Medicine) and in the public's eye (e.g., the movie, *Born on the Fourth of July*, released in 1989) for decades. A transformative shift to a quality-focused culture was central to Kizer's reorganization of the VA beginning in 1995. Currently, leadership of VA quality improvement activities chiefly comes from the VA OQP, as well as partnered programs in Systems Redesign, a National Surgical Quality Improvement Program (NSQIP), and Inpatient Evaluation Center, all with support from, for example, a national VA Healthcare Analysis and Information Group and a highly active health services research program. OQP oversees accreditation, credentialing and privileging, performance measurement, utilization management, and risk management activities. Institution of a nationwide VA performance measurement system and a national patient safety registry, among other tools and programs, started over 10 years ago, continue to support VA quality improvement (Perlin et al., 2004).

VA Performance Measurement System

Central to the VA reorganization was the development of a national performance measurement system comprised of administrative, patient ratings of care and clinical quality targets. These targets were expressed through executive performance agreements with VISN directors, who, in turn, established performance agreements with facility directors under their oversight. Routine publication of VISN-by-VISN comparison charts became the norm, with VISNs that remained among low performers facing significant scrutiny, in addition to support for improving their management strategies.

The VA performance measurement system has relied on primary data collection and secondary analyses of VA's substantial data resources. For patient ratings of care, random samples of clinic visitors and inpatients at each VA are surveyed using validated survey measures of patient satisfaction, continuity, coordination, and accessibility, among others. The Survey of Healthcare Experiences for Patients (SHEPs) has been the primary survey tool for several years, with a recent shift toward CAHPS to facilitate benchmarking with other providers and health plans. For clinical quality measures, the VA launched the External Peer Review Program (EPRP), wherein an external contractor trains nurse abstractors who review random samples of patients' charts based on clinical guideline-based processes of care (e.g., diabetic foot sensation exam, provision of flu shots for eligible veterans) and intermediate outcomes (e.g., HbA1c, blood pressure control). For administrative data (e.g., tracking utilization patterns), the VA capitalizes on its national data repositories (setting-specific datasets, such as the Outpatient Clinic file), which represent all VA clinical encounters.

VA performance measures are overseen by a national work group that reviews and agrees upon new measures over time to reflect changing priorities. Some measures have been retained since the mid-1990s (e.g., colorectal cancer screening), but have been augmented with other measures and monitors to continue to push the field to higher quality standards. For example, the VA used to measure detection of smokers, later measured smoking cessation counseling, and has added measures of smoking cessation treatment (e.g., referral to smoking cessation clinics and prescription of nicotine replacement therapy) more recently.

National VA Patient Safety Registry

Before the Institute of Medicine published *To Err is Human*, the VA had established a national VA patient safety registry. Unique and forward thinking at the time, the registry was a database that represented information on adverse events and their root causes across the entire VA healthcare system, enabling systematic appraisal not only of individual events but patterns of safety problems. The VA also founded the VHA National Center for Patient Safety, in addition to establishing a patient safety improvement awards program to incentivize reporting and problem solving, rather than punitive strategies.

Using Research–Clinical Partnerships to Systematically Improve Care

VHA has also invested in programs in health services research and quality improvement/implementation research through an intramural program that funds scientifically meritorious research proposals that study veterans' health and healthcare issues and interventions. For example, health services researchers have also been instrumental in systematically improving VA's health IT capabilities (e.g., decision support systems) (Hynes et al., 2010).

The VA QUERI is a key example of VA's work to improve care by implementing research into routine clinical practice. QUERI investigators study mechanisms by which healthcare organizations (i.e., teams, clinics, hospitals, and networks) adopt, implement, and sustain evidence-based practice (Demakis et al., 2000; Atkins, 2009).

Special Populations in VA Healthcare Settings

The VA delivers healthcare to a large population of veterans, many of whom have special healthcare needs. As a result, the VA has developed a number of special programs to meet those needs, with the concomitant development of specialized expertise in key clinical areas. The following section describes the challenges of VA care delivery for several of these special populations.

Veterans with Mental Health and/or Substance Abuse Problems

Because of the prevalence of mental health conditions (e.g., major depression, anxiety, PTSD, bipolar disorder, schizophrenia) and substance abuse disorders, the VA Office of Mental Health Services oversees the provision of virtually uncapped mental health and substance abuse services to eligible veterans. VA mental healthcare supports recovery, aiming to provide treatment and achieve optimal function and potential through a wide array of specialty inpatient and outpatient mental health services, in addition to integrated mental health services in VA primary care clinics, nursing homes, and residential care facilities. Specialized programs also include intensive case management units, day centers, work programs, and psychosocial rehabilitation for seriously mentally ill veterans, as well as programs focused on the needs of veterans who are homeless or incarcerated. The VA also provides specialized PTSD services, in addition to supporting clinical research and program evaluation services through the National Center for PTSD (www.ptsd.va.gov). Screening and counseling for veterans with exposure to military sexual trauma (MST), ranging from harassment to rape, are also available as part of a nationally mandated program for both women and men, in addition to violence prevention. Given the mental health burden among veterans who use the VA for care, the VA has also established suicide prevention programs, including a national hotline call and suicide prevention coordinators at each VA facility. Consistent with the VA's public health mission, the VA also oversees mental health disaster response, as well as post-deployment activities. The VA has established several program evaluation centers (e.g., the North East Program Evaluation Center in West Haven, the Program Evaluation and Resource Center in Palo Alto) and has funded a VA Mental Health QUERI Center (www.queri.research.va.gov/mh/) to study and implement evidence-based practice for prevalent mental health conditions (initially, major depression and schizophrenia).

Veterans with Spinal Cord Injuries

About 42,000 of the approximately 250,000 Americans with serious spinal cord injuries (SCI) and disorders are veterans who are eligible for VA healthcare services either because their injuries were sustained as a result of military service or because the nature of their non-service-connected injuries have resulted in catastrophic disability or low income eligibility. Veterans with SCI may receive monthly disability compensation from the VBA, in addition to direct healthcare services. The VA has the largest network of SCI care in the United States, integrating healthcare, vocational, psychological, and social services throughout their lives. VA SCI services are delivered through a "hub and spoke" model, relying on 24 regional SCI centers ("hubs") offering primary and specialty care by multidisciplinary SCI teams and 134 SCI primary care teams or support clinics ("spokes") (Department of Veteran Affairs, January 2009).

The VA leads research in rehabilitation and engineering for improving the care and quality of life of spinal cord injured veterans, including functional electrical stimulation, wheelchair and other adaptive technologies, cell transplantation, treatment of SCI-related medical complications, among other research areas. The VA has also funded a Spinal Cord Injury QUERI Center to identify and develop interventions to improve the quality of SCI care.

Women Veterans

Women veterans are among one of the fastest growing segments of new users of VA healthcare services. Breaking through the 2% cap historically placed on their participation in the military, women now comprise as much as 20% of new recruits, changing the demographics of the military and of the veterans seen by the VA healthcare system. Intermittent U.S. Government Accounting Service (GAO) reports over the past 25 years have continued to bring issues of privacy, access to gender-specific services, and quality of care to the fore, yielding policy and legislative advances designed to ensure women veterans' access to equitable, high-quality, and comprehensive services. Responsible for overseeing women veterans' health policy and practice, the Women Veterans Health Strategic Healthcare Group (within the VA OPHEH, as a special population) oversees deputy field directors, who, in turn, oversee fulltime Women Veteran Program managers (WVPMs) placed at every VAMC nationwide. The roles of WVPMs have evolved over time, but chiefly focus on ensuring the delivery of needed services, outreach/education, and coordination of care for women.

Focused outreach and education among all veterans returning from Iraq and Afghanistan has had particular impacts among women veterans, yielding a greater than 40% VA market penetration among a new generation of young women. Projections suggest that the absolute numbers of women veterans being seen in VHA will double in a few short years, forcing local VA facilities to rapidly reconsider the scope and practice of gender-specific care, including new primary care models, gender-sensitive mental healthcare, and reproductive services (Frayne et al., 2007). Over two-thirds of VAMCs and larger CBOCs have developed women's health clinics to accommodate the special needs of women (Yano et al., 2006).

Operation Enduring Freedom and Operation Iraqi Freedom Veterans

U.S. wars in Iraq and Afghanistan have produced a generation of chiefly young veterans with high rates of physical and mental health problems. Many of those suffering physical traumas have survived injuries that would have killed service members in prior wars, thanks to advances in battlefield medicine and the infrastructure for transporting the injured and ill out of combat zones to military medical installations. Exposure to blast injuries, for example, from IEDs have created a large cohort of young men and women with mild to severe TBI, now named the "signature" injury among Operation Enduring Freedom and Operation Iraqi Freedom (OEF/OIF) veterans (Hoge et al., 2008). Chronic widespread pain is also common and related to poor role functioning post-discharge (Helmer et al., 2009). Rates of major depression, anxiety, and PTSD ranged from about 15% to 18% after duty in Iraq, with veterans' problems being exacerbated by perceptions of stigma and barriers to mental healthcare (Hoge et al., 2004), with substantial TBI and PTSD comorbidity (Hoge et al., 2008). Among those OEF/OIF veterans who enroll in VA care, about 25% received mental health diagnoses (Seal et al., 2007). The VA healthcare system has responded with the development of multidisciplinary post-deployment health clinics and other programs to integrate services for OEF/OIF veterans.

The wars in Iraq and Afghanistan also have an important distinction insofar as they represent conflicts with high use of Reserve and National Guard members, who have not typically been afforded access to the VA healthcare system. Effective in 2008, Reservists and National Guard members who were discharged from active duty now establish veteran status and may be eligible for VA care for up to five years post-discharge, with variations depending on service-connected disability and combat service.

Future Perspectives

The VA is on the verge of yet another transformation into what VA leaders are calling a "21st Century organization that is Veteran-centric, results-driven and forwarding-looking." Goals for medical care include gradual expansion of healthcare eligibility to provide access to more than 500,000 previously ineligible veterans by 2013; increased funding for the expansion of VA inpatient residential care, outpatient mental health programs, institutional and noninstitutional long-term care, and homeless programs, as well as improved access in rural areas and programs to meet the specific needs of women veterans. Modernization of VA's IT infrastructure is also included, with funds set aside to bring veterans' online access to their electronic health records to full implementation.

At the same time, outside the VA, U.S. primary care delivery is at a crossroads. An ever increasing proportion of medical trainees are moving on to specialty careers (i.e., only 2% of trainees are considering primary care careers in contrast to the 50+% needed), while current primary care providers are leaving practice at an increased rate in the face of dwindling reimbursements (O'Reilly et al., 2008). Pundits point to a "perfect storm" of increased work with decreased rewards, and predict the impending "collapse of primary care" (Ornish, 2008). Recent national surveys demonstrate that VA primary care challenges are consistent with those outside VA, with over 30% of VA practices reporting moderate to a great deal of stress, over half reporting the pace of primary care practice as overly busy to hectic/chaotic, with substantial numbers of unfilled primary care clinician vacancies (Yano et al., 2008). Preliminary evidence also suggests that VAs in nationally recognized primary care shortage areas have significantly lower quality of care compared to areas where primary care staffing remains stable. Two fundamental initiatives are also underway to transform VA's primary care programs into patient-centered medical homes and to recapture and extend VA's cultural shifts to focus on veteran-centered care. These efforts build on special initiatives in recent years to better integrate VA primary care and mental healthcare services (i.e., the National Primary Care–Mental Health Integration Initiative), placing mental health personnel in every primary care clinic nationwide, and a history of building primary care infrastructure to achieve the tenets of the Institute of Medicine's *Crossing the Quality Chasm* report (Institute of Medicine, 2001; Yano et al., 2007).

Meeting the needs of returning veterans from Iraq and Afghanistan has also been a challenge, especially given the complexities inherent in these wars' signature injuries (e.g., TBI). With an initially limited evidence base for delivering care to many of these veterans, especially around mild TBI, the Departments of Veterans Affairs and Defense focused efforts to develop appropriate clinical guidelines (VA/DoD Clinical Practice Guideline for Management of Concussion/Mild Traumatic Brain Injury, 2009). Just as VA has invested significant resources in developing the technologies and treatments for veterans from previous wars (e.g., prosthetics, SCI, rehabilitation, mental health treatments), the VA is currently focused on developing new care models (e.g., polytrauma programs, post-deployment health clinics) and funding intramural research to develop better screening tools and treatments (Sayer et al., 2009).

Similarly, the VA is implementing strategies to provide optimal care for different segments of the population it serves. Women veterans have been a special challenge given their extreme numerical minority and a history of limited experience among VA providers with gender-specific services. The VA's structure has enabled top policymakers to develop comprehensive women's healthcare models that are being planned for and implemented through VISNs and their respective VAMCs and CBOCs in response to research evidence (Yano et al., 2010). Few other systems have established the capabilities and expectations for this approach to promoting evidence-based management and practice (Whittle and Segal, 2010).

Efforts to reform U.S. healthcare delivery under the Obama Administration are faced with substantial challenges. Yet, the VA healthcare system as a public sector turnaround, with its ongoing efforts to continually improve the delivery of high-quality care for a complex population of patients, remains a strong reminder of the potential of a national healthcare system in the United States. At the heart of current healthcare debates are economic arguments about whether we can afford such a system. While methodological challenges abound (Hendricks et al., 1999; Nugent and Hendricks, 2003; Roselle et al., 2003), economic analyses suggest that the costs of VA care are about 20% lower than what VA care would cost at Medicare prices (Nugent et al., 2004). In sharp contrast, using more recent data and different methods, others argue that the VA costs 33% more, questioning VA's "inpatient advantage" and raising concerns about VA surgical care outcomes (Weeks et al., 2009). One thing is for certain: as the U.S. government's only national healthcare system, the VA healthcare system will continue to operate under substantial scrutiny, for both its problems and its promise.

References

Agha, Z., R.P. Lofgren, J.V. VanRuiswyk, and P.M. Layde. 2000. Are patients at Veterans Affairs Medical Centers sicker?: A comparative analysis of health status and medical resource use. *Archives of Internal Medicine* 160(21):3252–3257.

Asch, S.M., E.A. McGlynn, M.M. Hogan, R.A. Hayward, P. Shekelle, L. Rubenstein, J. Keesey, J. Adams, and E.A. Kerr. 2004. Comparison of quality of care for patients in the Veterans Health Administration and patients in a national sample. *Annals of Internal Medicine* 141(12):938–945.

Ashton, C.M., J. Souchek, N.J. Petersen, T.J. Menke, T.C. Collins, K.W. Kizer, S.M. Wright, and N.P. Wray. 2003. Hospital use and survival among Veterans Affairs Beneficiaries. *The New England Journal of Medicine* 349(17):1637–1646.

Aspinall, S.L., C.B. Good, P.A. Glassman, and M.A. Valentino. 2005. The evolving use of cost-effectiveness analysis in formulary management within the Department of Veterans Affairs. *Medical care* 43(7):II20–I126.

Atkins, D. 2009. QUERI and implementation research: Emerging from adolescence into adulthood: QUERI Series. *Implementation Science* 4(1):12.

Congressional Budget Office. August 2009. Quality initiatives undertaken by the Veterans Health Administration, Washington, DC.

DeLuca, M.A. 2000. Trans-Atlantic experiences in health reform: The United Kingdom's National Health Service and the United States Veterans Health Administration. *IBM Center for the Business of Government*, Arlington, VA: PricewaterhouseCoopers Endowment for the Business of Government.

Department of Veterans Affairs. January 2009. VA and Spinal Cord Injury, Fact Sheet, Washington, DC. http://www1.va.gov/opa/publications/fs_spinalcord_injury.pdf (accessed January 10, 2010).

Demakis, J.G., L. McQueen, K.W. Kizer, and J.R. Feussner. 2000. Quality Enhancement Research Initiative (QUERI): A collaboration between research and clinical practice. *Medical Care* 38(6):17–25.

Evans, D.C., W.P. Nichol, and J.B. Perlin. 2006. Effect of the implementation of an enterprise-wide Electronic Health Record on productivity in the Veterans Health Administration. *Health Economics, Policy and Law* 1(02):163–169.

Fleming, C., E.S. Fisher, C.H. Chang, T.A. Bubolz, and D.J. Malenka. 1992. Studying outcomes and hospital utilization in the elderly: The advantages of a merged data base for Medicare and Veterans Affairs hospitals. *Medical care* 30(5):377–391.

Frayne, S.M., W. Yu, E.M. Yano, L. Ananth, S. Iqbal, A. Thrailkill, and C.S. Phibbs. 2007. Gender and use of care: Planning for tomorrow's Veterans Health Administration. *Journal of Women's Health* 16(8):1188–1199.

Greenfield, S. and S.H. Kaplan. 2004. Creating a culture of quality: The remarkable transformation of the department of Veterans Affairs health care system. *Annals of Internal Medicine* 141(4):316–318.

Helmer, D.A., H.K. Chandler, K.S. Quigley, M. Blatt, R. Teichman, and G. Lange. 2009. Chronic widespread pain, mental health, and physical role function in OEF/OIF veterans. *Pain Medicine* 10(7):1174–1182.

Hendricks, A.M., D.K. Remler, and M.J. Prashker. 1999. More or less?: Methods to compare VA and non-VA health care costs. *Medical Care* 37(4):AS54–AS62.

Hoge, C.W., C.A. Castro, S.C. Messer, D. McGurk, D.I. Cotting, and R.L. Koffman. 2004. Combat duty in Iraq and Afghanistan, mental health problems, and barriers to care. *The New England Journal of Medicine* 351(1):13–22.

Hoge, C.W., D. McGurk, J.L. Thomas, A.L. Cox, C.C. Engel, and C.A. Castro. 2008. Mild traumatic brain injury in US soldiers returning from Iraq. *The New England Journal of Medicine* 358(5):453–463.

Hynes, D.M., K. Koelling, K. Stroupe, N. Arnold, K. Mallin, M.W. Sohn, F.M. Weaver, L. Manheim, and L. Kok. 2007. Veterans' access to and use of Medicare and Veterans Affairs health care. *Medical Care* 45(3):214–222.

Hynes, D.M., T. Weddle, N. Smith, E. Whittier, D. Atkins, and J. Francis. 2010. Use of Health information technology to advance evidence-based care: Lessons from the VA QUERI program. *Journal of General Internal Medicine* 25:44–49.

Institute of Medicine. 2000. *To Err Is Human: Building a Safer Health System*, Washington, DC: National Academy Press.

Institute of Medicine. 2001. *Crossing the Quality Chasm: A New Health System for the 21st Century*, Washington, DC: National Academy Press.

Jha, A.K., J.B. Perlin, K.W. Kizer, and R.A. Dudley. 2003. Effect of the transformation of the Veterans Affairs Health Care System on the quality of care. *The New England Journal of Medicine* 348(22):2218–2227.

Kerr, E.A., R.B. Gerzoff, S.L. Krein, J.V. Selby, J.D. Piette, J.D. Curb, W.H. Herman, D.G. Marrero, K.M. Narayan, and M.M. Safford. 2004. Diabetes care quality in the Veterans Affairs Health Care System and commercial managed care: The TRIAD study. *Annals of Internal Medicine* 141(4):272–281.

Kizer, K.W., J.G. Demakis, and J.R. Feussner. 2000. Reinventing VA health care: Systematizing quality improvement and quality innovation. *Medical Care* 38(6):7–16.

Kizer, K.W., M.L. Fonseca, and L.M. Long. 1997. The veterans healthcare system: Preparing for the twenty-first century. *Hospital & Health Services Administration* 42(3):283–298.

Liu, C.F., M.L. Maciejewski, and A.E.B. Sales. 2005. Changes in characteristics of veterans using the VHA health care system between 1996 and 1999. *Health Research Policy and Systems* 3(1):5.

Nazi, K.M., T.P. Hogan, T.H. Wagner, D.K. McInnes, B.M. Smith, D. Haggstrom, N.R. Chumbler, A.L. Gifford, K.G. Charters, and J.J. Saleem. 2010. Embracing a health services research perspective on personal health records: Lessons learned from the VA My HealtheVet System. *Journal of General Internal Medicine* 25:62–67.

Nugent, G. and A. Hendricks. 2003. Estimating private sector values for VA health care: An overview. *Medical Care* 41(6):II2–II10.

Nugent, G.N., A. Hendricks, L. Nugent, and M.L. Render. 2004. Value for taxpayers' dollars: What VA care would cost at medicare prices. *Medical Care Research and Review* 61(4):495–508.

Oliver, A. 2007. The Veterans Health Administration: An American success story? *The Milbank Quarterly* 85(1):5–35.

Oliver, A. 2008. Public-sector health-care reforms that work? A case study of the US Veterans Health Administration. *The Lancet* 371(9619):1211–1213.

O'Reilly, K.B. and B. Hedger. 2008. Doctors urge: Rescue primary care or work force shortage will mount. AMNews. http://www.ama-assn.org/amednews/2008/12/08/prl111208.htm (accessed December 1, 2008).

Ornish, D. 2008. The collapse of primary care. *Newsweek*, September 11, 2008.

Payne, S., A. Lee, J.A. Clark, W.H. Rogers, D.R. Miller, K.M. Skinner, X.S. Ren, and L.E. Kazis. 2005. Utilization of medical services by Veterans Health Study (VHS) respondents. *The Journal of Ambulatory Care Management* 28(2):125–140.

Perlin, J.B. 2005. Under Secretary for Health's Information Letter. VHA mission, core values, vision, domains of value and planning strategies, Washington, DC: Veterans Health Administration.

Perlin, J.B., R.M. Kolodner, and R.H. Roswell. 2004. The Veterans Health Administration: Quality, value, accountability, and information as transforming strategies for patient-centered care. *American Journal of Managed Care* 10(2):828–836.

Rogers, W.H., L.E. Kazis, D.R. Miller, K.M. Skinner, J.A. Clark, A. Spiro III, and B.G. Fincke. 2004. Comparing the health status of VA and non-VA ambulatory patients: The veterans' health and medical outcomes studies. *The Journal of Ambulatory Care Management* 27(3):249–262.

Roselle, G., M.L. Render, N.B. Nugent, and G.N. Nugent. 2003. Estimating private sector professional fees for VA providers. *Medical Care* 41(6 Suppl):I123–I132.

Sales, M.M., F.E. Cunningham, P.A. Glassman, M.A. Valentino, and C.B. Good. 2005. Pharmacy benefits management in the Veterans Health Administration: 1995 to 2003. *American Journal of Managed Care* 11(2):104–112.

Sayer, N.A., D.X. Cifu, S. McNamee, C.E. Chiros, B.J. Sigford, S. Scott, and H.L. Lew. 2009. Rehabilitation needs of combat-injured service members admitted to the VA polytrauma rehabilitation centers: The role of PM&R in the care of wounded warriors. *Physical Medicine and Rehabilitation* 1(1):23–28.

Seal, K., D. Berenthal, C. Miner, S. Sen, and C. Marmar. 2007. Bringing the war back home. *Archives of Internal Medicine* 167(5):476–482.

Selim, A.J., D. Berlowitz, L.E. Kazis, W. Rogers, S.M. Wright, S.X. Qian, J.A. Rothendler, A. Spiro III, D. Miller, and B.J. Selim. 2010. Comparison of health outcomes for male seniors in the Veterans Health Administration and Medicare advantage plans. *Health Services Research* 45(2):379–396.

Shen, Y., A. Hendricks, S. Zhang, and L.E. Kazis. 2003. VHA enrollees' health care coverage and use of care. *Medical Care Research and Review* 60(2):253–267.

Sprague, L. 2004. Veterans' health care: Balancing resources and responsibilities. *Issue brief (George Washington University. National Health Policy Forum)* 796:1–20.

U.S. Department of Veterans Affairs. *VA Organizational Briefing Book*, Washington, DC. http://www4.va.gov/ofcadmin/docs/vaorgbb.pdf (accessed October 1, 2009).

Washington, D.L., E.M. Yano, B. Simon, and S. Sun. 2006. To use or not to use: What influences why women veterans choose VA health care. *Journal of General Internal Medicine* 21(S3):S11–S18.

Wasserman, J., J. Ringel, K. Ricci, J. Malkin, B. Wynn, J. Zwanziger, S. Newberry, M. Suttorp, and A. Rastegar 2004. *Understanding Potential Changes to the Veterans Equitable Resource Allocation (VERA) System: A Regression-Based Approach*, Pittsburgh, PA: RAND Corporation.

Wasserman, J., J. Ringel, B. Wynn, J. Zwanziger, K. Ricci, S. Newberry, B. Genovese, and M. Schoenbaum. 2001. *An Analysis of the Veterans Equitable Resource Allocation (VERA) System*, Pittsburgh, PA: RAND Corporation.

Weeks, W.B., A.E. Wallace, T.A. Wallace, and D.J. Gottlieb. 2009. Does the VA offer good health care value? *Journal of Health Care Finance* 35(4):1–12.

Whittle, J. and J.B. Segal. 2010. What can the VA teach us about implementing proven advances into routine clinical practice? *Journal of General Internal Medicine* 25:77–78.

Wilson, N.J. and K.W. Kizer. 1997. The VA health care system: An unrecognized national safety net. *Health Affairs (Project Hope)* 16(4):200–204.

Wright, S.M., J. Daley, E.S. Fisher, and G.E. Thibault. 1997. Where do elderly veterans obtain care for acute myocardial infarction: Department of Veterans Affairs or Medicare? *Health Services Research* 31(6):739–754.

Yano E.M., B. Fleming, I. Canelo et al. 2008. VHA clinical practice organizational survey: National results for the PC director module, Sepulveda, CA: VA HSR&D Report No. MRC 05-093.

Yano, E.M., C. Goldzweig, I. Canelo, and D.L. Washington. 2006. Diffusion of innovation in women's health care delivery: The Department of Veterans Affairs' adoption of women's health clinics. *Women's Health Issues* 16(5):226–235.

Yano, E.M., P. Hayes, S.M. Wright, P.P. Schnurr, L. Lipson, B. Bean-Mayberry, and D.L. Washington. 2010. Integration of women veterans into VA quality improvement research efforts: What researchers need to know. *Journal of General Internal Medicine* 25:56–61.

Yano, E.M., B.F. Simon, A.B. Lanto, and L.V. Rubenstein. 2007. The evolution of changes in primary care delivery underlying the veterans health administration's quality transformation. *American Journal of Public Health* 97(12):2151–2159.

Young, G.J. 2000. Transforming government: The revitalization of the Veterans Health Administration, Arlington, VA: The PricewaterhouseCoopers Endowment for the Business of Government.

4

Outpatient Clinics: Primary and Specialty Care

Deanna R. Willis
Indiana University School of Medicine

Background 4-1
Size and Scope 4-1
Structure 4-2
Practice Expenses and Overhead 4-3
Revenue and Payment for Services 4-4
Quality 4-5
Medical Home 4-7
Care Coordination 4-7
Primary Care Shortage 4-8
References 4-8

Background

Outpatient clinics provide an important and essential part of the U.S. healthcare system. Being less costly than more intensive parts of the healthcare delivery system, such as inpatient hospital units, outpatient clinics serve as an efficient location for large volumes of patients to receive care from physicians and other healthcare professionals. By providing coordination with other parts of the healthcare system, outpatient clinics can serve as a hub or home location for the medical care of individual patients. Reimbursement mechanisms create unique challenges in the outpatient clinic setting, most notably by not providing funding for this coordination of care across the care continuum. Revenues are generated by face-to-face encounters between patients and providers and office procedures. This payment methodology promotes high volume–low margin activity. The high volume–low margin concept is central to many issues that provide challenges and opportunities in the outpatient clinic setting.

Size and Scope

In the United States, outpatient clinics are one of the most common places for patients to receive healthcare services. The National Center for Health Statistics (Cherry et al., 2007) estimates that in 2005, approximately 963.6 million visits were made to office-based physicians. This is an average of about 3.31 office visits per person in that calendar year. Sixty percent of those office visits were to primary care physicians, a group that is generally thought to include family medicine, general internal medicine, general pediatrics, and obstetrics and gynecology. While general practitioners in other countries are often fully trained in a primary care specialty, in the United States, general practice typically refers to a provider who did not complete a full residency training program. General practice physicians are becoming rare in the United States, mostly a remnant of those training prior to the growth of family medicine, which was recognized as a distinct discipline in 1969. Med-peds, or combined internal medicine-pediatrics, is another primary care medical specialty, however, it is typically difficult to elicit separately in national level statistics. The remaining 40% of office visits is relatively evenly split between medical and surgical subspecialties. Orthopedic surgery and ophthalmology, two surgical specialties, had the most office visits of any of the specialty care clinics, at 4.8% and 6.1%, respectively.

Eighty-seven percent of all outpatient clinic visits occurred to physicians in metropolitan service areas, while only 80% of clinics are in those areas. This discrepancy could be for a number of reasons, such as

- Rural physicians are able to provide more services in one visit. This occurs because more nonmetropolitan physicians are practicing full scope medicine across the healthcare continuum than their urban counterparts (i.e., more rural physicians doing inpatient and outpatient medicine than those in metropolitan areas) (Jones, 2004).
- Patients in nonmetropolitan areas going to metropolitan areas for outpatient clinic appointments (e.g., nonmetropolitan areas may not have as many subspecialists and, thus, patients in those areas have to travel to metropolitan areas to see subspecialists) (The American Psychological Association, 2001).
- Patients in rural areas may culturally be less likely to go to the doctor, and thus have fewer visits per patient per year than patients in urban areas (Friedson, 1961).

Fifty-three percent of office visits occurred for the primary purpose of treating a chronic health condition. The most common chronic health condition was hypertension that accounted for 23% of outpatient office visits. Hypertension has been the leading cause for office visits since 1995, when it accounted for 19% of outpatient clinic visits. The 4% increase could be attributed to several reasons, such as improvement in the rate at which patients are diagnosed for hypertension, intensification of treatment for hypertension (i.e., patients coming in more often once they have a diagnosis of hypertension), or an increase in the prevalence of hypertension in the American population. Routine child health check was the most common diagnosis for infants, children, and adolescents up to the age of 21 years.

Nearly one in ten office visits had diagnostic or screening services ordered or provided. Women were more likely to have a depression screening ordered or provided, and were also more likely to have some type of body imaging ordered or provided. This difference in the rate of body imaging between women and men is mostly attributable to mammography and ultrasound (Cherry et al., 2007).

Structure

In the United States, outpatient clinics typically fall under one of two designation categories from the Centers for Medicare and Medicaid Services (CMS). These two categories are office based and hospital based.

In a typical office-based setting, the physician group owns the practice, employs the support staff of front and back office workers (such as scheduling personnel, medical assistants, and nurses), owns the equipment, and either owns or leases the building. The benefit of this type of structure is that the physician group maintains autonomy from other organizations in the healthcare system and can make its own strategic decisions and have greater flexibility in issues such as incentive compensation for staff members. Additionally, the physician group can collect both the professional and technical components for procedures or ancillary testing performed in the clinic. For example, if the practice owns radiology equipment and performs x-rays, the practice can collect fees for both the performance of the x-ray itself (the technical component) as well as for the reading of the x-ray by the physician (the professional component).

The biggest downside to office-based clinics is that there are often services that are provided in a clinic for which there is no billable revenue and that the costs of operating the clinic cannot be offset by the downstream revenues to the greater healthcare system. An example of lost revenue might be a patient who comes in for a blood pressure check and the blood pressure is checked by a licensed practical nurse (LPN) rather than a registered nurse (RN). Generally, this service could not be billed by the clinic unless the physician also saw the patient. Downstream revenues are created in a healthcare system when patients come into a clinic and then require further services at a hospital or other part of the healthcare system. For example, if a patient sees a surgeon in the clinic and is deemed to need a complex surgery that is performed at the hospital, then that clinic visit generates the downstream revenues that the hospital will receive for providing that surgery. Thus, it is generally considered difficult, in today's healthcare market to have an independent office-based practice that is financially successful unless a significant number of procedures or ancillary testing are performed at the clinic.

Hospital-based clinics, by comparison, are owned by and closely affiliated with the hospital. The hospital employs the support staff of front and back office workers (such as scheduling personnel, medical assistants, and nurses), owns the equipment, and either owns or leases the building.

In this category of clinic, the hospital is able to charge for the services of its support staff through a fee called the facility fee. The facility fee is charged, in addition to the professional fee charged by the physicians, on every patient encounter. The professional fees of the physicians are generally around 85% lower than in office-based settings, but the physicians no longer have to pay wages and benefits to support staff or pay rent for the clinic space (Keagy and Thomas, 2004). The total amount of revenue received for a visit (facility fee plus professional fee) is usually greater than the total amount of revenue received for a visit in an office-based clinic (which just bills the professional fee).

Clinics can be designated by the CMS as hospital based if they are closely affiliated with the hospital, as demonstrated by activities such as use of the hospital's information systems and provision of unique services that could only be provided by the larger hospital system (such as a multidisciplinary clinic). In addition to the greater potential revenue for encounters, this type of clinic can benefit from the close alignment to the bigger hospital system through economies of scale and other collaborative activities.

One downside to a hospital-based clinic is that there is less local autonomy since the clinic is owned and controlled by the bigger hospital system. Another downside to this type of clinic has arisen as part of the increased consumerism of the American healthcare industry. As health plans have shifted an increasing amount of cost into the control of the patient-consumer, patients are increasingly cost sensitive and concerned about the additional facility fee in hospital-based clinics.

Practice Expenses and Overhead

As a service industry, the greatest expense for outpatient clinics is the cost of providers and support staff. Provider compensation models can vary greatly and vary significantly based on the degree of ownership and the type of employment model.

The number and distribution of support staff is the primary driver of support staff expense. Benchmarks based on the type of clinic and specialties present are available for purchase from vendors such as Medical Group Management Association (MGMA). Management of this expense is generally accomplished by monitoring the number of support staff per physician full-time equivalent (FTE), support staff expense per visit, or other management measures.

When support staff are absent from work, most outpatient clinics require the use of temporary support staff from an agency, because the high volume–low margin situation of most outpatient clinics results in a lack of excess workforce capacity. Not only do temporary support staff come at a premium cost, it can sometimes be difficult to hire a temporary worker with only the minimum skill set needed. For example, if a regularly employed medical assistant is not at work under the Family Medical Leave Act (FMLA), it can be difficult in some regions of the country to find a medical assistant to hire through a temporary support staff agency. In this situation, outpatient clinics are often left with no choice but to lease a licensed nurse through the agency, thus driving the premium paid for the skill set needed up even further. Across a large, multisite outpatient clinic system, the cost can be substantial. Thus, many outpatient clinics monitor the use of temporary support staff and/or have processes or guidelines in place about when and where temporary support staff can be utilized.

In years past, the remainder of variable overhead expense was spread across a number of categories. More recently, outpatient clinics that perform or administer injectable medications (such as childhood immunizations or therapeutic medications) find the expense of acquisition of those injectables to be the second largest variable practice expense. With acquisition costs for several vaccinations over $800 per vial, developing and implementing effective management practices in this area can be imperative.

Revenue and Payment for Services

Increased consumerism in the United States has led discussions about the need for pricing transparency on healthcare services. With the high volume of outpatient clinic visits, outpatient clinics have been one area of focus in these discussions. The challenge to the healthcare delivery system in meeting this need for transparency is significant.

A large amount of private health insurance in the United States is provided by third-party payors. In the third-party system, the private insurance company sells a health insurance product to an employer or group of employers. Based on the negotiations, products, and pricing options purchased by the employer, the policy may be based on a standard contract or a nonstandard contract with the insurer. In addition, large employers often become self-insured, where the employer uses actuarial and insurance information to estimate the amount needed in a pool of money to set aside to compensate for future potential healthcare costs of its employees. Self-insured employers often contract with a private insurance company to manage the membership, claims, medical management, quality management, reinsurance, and other typical services of an insurance company. The insurance company does these services for a fee, but uses the pool of money set aside by the self-insured employer to pay the claims of that employer's employees, and dependents, healthcare, and pays according to the rules of coverage developed by the self-insured employer.

Understanding the nature of these employer-driven options is important to understanding the challenge of transparency for outpatient clinics. In other parts of the healthcare delivery system, care is either delivered emergently, with billing occurring retrospectively, or care is delivered on a scheduled basis, with billing approval occurring prospectively. In outpatient clinics, care is often delivered with little advance scheduling, and most patients have a billing component that needs to be collected at the time of service. The information about the patient's third-party insurance is communicated to the outpatient clinic using an insurance card. The insurance card tells the outpatient clinic how much of a copayment should be collected at the time of service or if the patient owes a percent of the charges. Because of the number of different types of policies or insurance products offered by each private insurance company, outpatient clinics often do not know whether or not the insurance coverage for each particular patient covers a particular service until the time the claim for the service is adjudicated, a process where the insurance coverage is applied to the claim. For example, some employers do not purchase preventative care service coverage for their employees. Unless the patient is aware of this exclusion and notifies the outpatient clinic, the outpatient clinic does not readily have a way to know that the payment from the private insurance company will be denied and the money will need to be collected from the patient for the services provided.

Even if a particular outpatient clinic service is reliably covered by the majority of insurance products on the market, the outpatient clinic still may not have a readily available way to know the fee agreed upon between the contracting entity for the provider and the private insurer. Each private insurer contracts separately with the provider group, and thus, the negotiated price for each service varies from insurer to insurer.

This concept of individual insurer pricing, carries over into the financial management of the practice. Each outpatient clinic generally sets its fee schedule or a list of the prices it will charge for each service it provides, and updates it yearly. In addition, each insurer generally sets a standard fee schedule or a list of the prices it will pay for each service it provides, and updates it yearly. Negotiations between the private insurance company and the provider group occur based on the difference between the fee schedule of the provider and the standard fee schedule of the private insurance company. This negotiated rate is formalized in a contract and providers then adjust their financial management reports to reflect those contractual rates by insurer.

One important financial indicator for outpatient clinics is the payor mix, or the percent of services provided to patients with each type of insurance because of the mixed basket of rates of pay for each service. Monitoring the payor mix is important to make sure that the practice is not becoming too heavily predominated by services with low reimbursement (including reimbursement that is below the cost of providing the service), but also to make sure that no one particular private insurer is too predominant such that a shift in their negotiated contractual fees could jeopardize the financial viability of the practice.

Most outpatient clinics need to carefully manage their cash flow because of the low margins. In addition, the earlier money is collected in the revenue cycle, the process from when the financial information to provide the service is collected until the payment for the service is received, the greater the percent of total revenue that is collected. Thus, aging of accounts receivables is another financial management report that is important to outpatient clinics. By looking at the amount of receivables in typical categories of length of time outstanding by payor, outpatient clinics can benchmark their revenue cycle performance and monitor the rapidity with which each payor pays for services.

Managing the productivity, or the number and type of services provided by each provider, is important for outpatient clinics. Determining how to measure productivity depends on the distribution of payment methodologies in the practice. Capitation-based managed care, or the payment of a monthly fee for the entirety of services provided to a population of patients, as a payment methodology in the United States has become less common. Discounted fee-for-service, where contractually negotiated payments are paid on the basis of the services provided, is once again becoming more common. In a fee-for-service or discounted fee-for-service predominated market, outpatient clinics often use work Relative Value Units (wRVUs) to measure productivity.

Relative Value Units (RVUs) are standardized weights assigned to each medical procedure or service that uses a Current Procedural Terminology (CPT) code. Each RVU is built to incorporate the work provided by the physician, the practice expense, and the malpractice expense. The part of the RVU that recognizes the work provided by the physician is the wRVU. By benchmarking wRVUs with other similar specialty physicians, the clinic can develop a more targeted approach to improving operations.

Quality

Pay-for-performance (P4P) has become a common mechanism for value-based purchasing in healthcare. Most P4P programs are developed and implemented by individual payors to help increase the payor's relative quality performance in the marketplace. While significant progress has been made over the years at standardizing the measures that are incentivized in P4P programs, there is still significant fragmentation between providers on the structure and financing of the different programs, and little overlap on the populations of patients covered in the P4P incentive. This compartmentalization can lead to inefficient use of resources for outpatient clinic providers and staff while trying to optimize performance under various programs.

Most P4P programs are payor based, and thus, the measures are generally derived from administrative claims data. The benefit of this type of measure design is that the reports are directly related to the services provided to or utilized by a patient. In addition, little additional work is necessary to use the data since the billing data is already submitted for most services. The greatest downside to the administrative claims quality measures is that they do not capture the clinical aspects of the care particularly well, for example, they do not capture the degree of control for many chronic illnesses. An administrative claims quality measures can tell a payor that a hemoglobin A1c was performed on a diabetic patient in the last 6 months, but it cannot tell the payor what the clinical value of that hemoglobin A1c was. In order to combat this challenge, some measures allow the use of hybrid methodology, or the combination of administrative claims data and clinical data to build the quality measure. The downside to this methodology is that because of the resource burden required to collect hybrid measure data, hybrid measures are most often done on a sample of the patient population of interest. By comparison, administrative claims quality measures are most often performed on a full population basis for those patients of interest.

One nationwide P4P program is the CMS Physician Quality Reporting Initiative (PQRI). The PQRI program uses a unique methodology to collect quality data for the payor, in this case, Medicare. CMS is using a special set of CPT codes, called CPT2 codes. These CPT2 codes are specially designed to communicate clinical information related to quality of care, in this case, on Medicare beneficiaries. There is no associated fee for the CPT2 codes, but, in the PQRI program, they must be submitted along with the usual CPT codes that are used to bill for face-to-face services between a physician and a Medicare beneficiary. By meeting reporting requirements, providers can earn up to 1.5% additional revenue on the Medicare services they provide.

Mixed reception by physician groups has led to reports that penetration of the program has been less than intended. One of the challenges reported by physician groups is that the program has a high degree of complexity. CMS published a report in April of 2009 showing the number of valid Quality-Data Codes submitted nationwide in the 2008 PQRI program. This report shows that the error rates of submissions vary depending on the measure. The measures with the highest percent of valid codes submitted had rates as high as 94.7% valid, while other measures had zero percent validity. The overall validity of submissions was 68.29%, which demonstrates room for reduction in complexities, and other related challenges in reporting, which could tremendously benefit quality reporting expectations for outpatient clinics (Centers for Medicare and Medicaid Services, 2009).

One of the perceived benefits of the PQRI is that it offers an opportunity to consolidate quality reporting efforts. Other payors generally develop and implement their own P4P programs. These programs vary tremendously both on the infrastructure and payment methodology, but also on the number and types of measures reported. Additionally, few P4P programs offer physicians the ability to view their patient level data in a real-time manner. Most often, reports come from the payors after a claims run-out, or waiting period for claims to be submitted, has occurred. If PQRI can be implemented effectively, it may offer a standard solution for capturing and reporting physician-based quality measures.

In June 2009, the University Health System Consortium and the American Association of Medical Colleges' Faculty Practice Solutions compiled a review of how seven academic practices implemented and sustained PQRI reporting. The issue brief reports that for most practices, money was not the primary motivator for participating. More commonly, the leadership of the physician practice chose to do PQRI reporting because they expected the program, which is currently pay-for-reporting, to mature into a true P4P program. All of the practices reported that they wanted to learn how to report on the PQRI measures successfully and consolidate the reporting programs from different payors. The brief goes on to further report that each of the physician groups implemented strategies to select specific PQRI measures and collect and report the data efficiently because they did not want to adversely impact productivity or cash flow. Because of the cross-functional nature of PQRI reporting within a practice (including care delivery, billing, and compliance), each group had a strong physician leader and some also designated a PQRI team with leaders from different parts of the practice (University Health System Consortium, 2009).

Another opportunity for outpatient clinics to consolidate quality reporting expectations is physician recognition programs. Some payors are allowing providers to forgo the payors' individual P4P program criteria if the provider has achieved recognition by the National Committee for Quality Assurance (NCQA) through one of their designated physician recognition programs (National Commission for Quality Assurance, 2007). Many of these recognition programs are focused on the presence of infrastructure that supports high-quality care and demonstration or documentation of processes of care that lead to quality outcomes. Thus, for the high-volume outpatient clinic environment, being recognized for an environment that reduces missed opportunities of care is a much more efficient mechanism of demonstrating high quality than focusing on cleaning and reporting individual patient data that is retrospective to the delivery of the care.

Medical Home

One of the NCQA physician recognition programs is the Patient-Centered Medical Home (PC-MH). Medical home has emerged as a central concept to outpatient care in the United States. The American Academy of Pediatrics, the American Academy of Family Physicians, the American College of Physicians, and the American Osteopathic Association, which jointly represent approximately 330,000 physicians in the United States, released a document in 2007 called the Joint Principles of the Patient Centered-Medical Home (American Academy of Pediatrics et al., 2007). According to the Joint Principles document, PC-MH is an approach to providing comprehensive primary care for children, youth and adults, which is a healthcare setting that facilitates partnerships between individual patients, and their personal physicians, and when appropriate, the patient's family. The central concepts to PC-MH are

- Every patient has a personal physician.
- The medical practice is physician directed.
- Care is oriented to the whole person.
- Care is coordinated and/or integrated.
- The environment promotes quality and safety.
- Patients have enhanced access to their medical home care.
- Presence of payment recognition for systems designed according to these principles.

A variety of not-for-profit and commercial organizations are completing demonstration projects to assess the financial and operational viability of the medical home model in outpatient practices at national and state levels.

Care Coordination

One of the central concepts to the medical home initiative is care coordination. Care coordination takes many forms in outpatient clinics. While there is no standard definition of care coordination, it is generally thought to be a program that provides the patient with assistance in navigating and understanding the healthcare system by helping the patient obtain needed services for their health, social, and psychosocial needs. Patients with complex and/or chronic medical conditions most commonly benefit from care coordination services.

Integrated and/or coordinated care across the healthcare delivery system is increasingly important in the complex healthcare environment. Even as medical homes are being created across the country, payors and hospital systems are also developing mechanisms of integrating the care they deliver. Outpatient clinics are at the front of the care coordination effort since it is the most common place for patients to have repeated encounters over time. In primary care clinics, there has been little margin to provide care coordination services over the years unless the clinic is hospital based and the hospital sees the financial benefit of the coordination of services. The medical home effort will have a tremendous impact on this aspect if financing changes, which are being sought as part of the medical home movement, are put into place that pay for care coordination.

Specialty clinics offer care coordination more commonly in the present environment, typically in the form of a clinical nurse specialist or a nurse practitioner. Not only is the margin higher in specialty services, compared to primary care, but the pay differential is also greater between the physician and the clinical nurse specialist or nurse practitioner. When the pay differential is greater, the financial justification is greater to shift more care to the lower-paid provider so that the higher-paid provider can generate a higher volume of higher-margin care. Thus, specialty clinics are more likely to find a business case for care coordination in the current marketplace.

Care coordination is thought of as a continuum of services that includes a variety of more focused education and system navigation assistance. Two of the more common types of services, along this spectrum, in outpatient settings, include case management and disease management.

Case management services are commonly provided by insurance companies. The focus in case management is typically centered on the patient's medical needs. Since the insurance company is the organization providing the service, case management usually focuses on coordination of covered services, or services that are included as part of the benefits of the insurance policy. Physicians in outpatient clinics are occasionally contacted by case managers to approve or order services that are deemed to be beneficial for the patient as part of the case management program.

Disease management services are often limited to the coordination of care for one particular disease or condition. For patients with chronic illness, the degree to which they understand and engage proactively in the care of their illness is directly related to many health outcomes. Education and training in self management skills are usually included in the repertoire of services in these programs. Outpatient physicians are contacted by disease manager when additional services or supplies are needed for the patient. The outpatient clinic may interact more closely with the disease management program, since some of the services needed by the patient may be delivered on-site at the outpatient clinic.

Community health centers, including Federally Qualified Health Centers (FQHCs) and Rural Health Centers (RHCs), are designed to promote care coordination for medically underserved areas and populations. By co-locating a variety of health and social agencies on-site, employing social workers and other ancillary medical personnel, and hosting community services, these clinics facilitate meeting the broad needs of patients. FQHCs and RHCs receive special designation from the federal government and are eligible for enhanced revenue. As the role of care coordination expands across the United States, these clinics may serve as a model for implementation.

Primary Care Shortage

One last, but important, area of relevance to outpatient clinics is the primary care shortage. Experts predict that by the year 2020, the United States will face a shortage of 40,000 family physicians (Lloyd, 2009). Medical student interest in primary care has dropped to 51.8% since 1997. In addition, 78 million Baby Boomers born from 1946 to 1964 will begin to turn 65 in the year 2011, thus requiring increasing medical care. With 60% of outpatient clinic visits occurring in primary care offices (Cherry et al., 2007), the current and impending shortage of primary care physicians will have a growing impact on the delivery of healthcare in outpatient clinics in the United States. The outcome of this impact is largely dependent on the design and implementation of healthcare reform measures.

References

American Academy of Pediatrics, American Academy of Family Physicians, American College of Physicians, and American Osteopathic Association. March 2007. Joint principles of patient centered-medical home. http://www.medicalhomeinfo.org/joint%20Statement.pdf (accessed September 1, 2009).

Centers for Medicare and Medicaid Services. April 2009. Quality-data code submission error report: 2008 physician quality reporting initiative. http://www.cms.hhs.gov/PQRI/Downloads/2008QualityDataCodeSubmissionErrorReportFinal04-03-09.pdf (accessed March 12, 2010).

Cherry, D.K., D.A. Woodwell, and E.A. Rechtsteiner. 2007. *National Ambulatory Medical Care Survey: 2005 Summary—Advance Data from Vital and Health Statistics; No. 387*. National Center for Health Statistics, Hyattsville, MD.

Friedson, E. 1961. *Patients' Views of Medical Practice.* Russell Sage Foundation, New York.

Jones, R. 2004. *Oxford Textbook of Primary Medical Care*, Vol. 1, eds. N. Britten, L. Culpepper et al. Oxford University Press, Oxford, U.K., p. 34.

Keagy, B.A. and M.S. Thomas. 2004. *Essentials of Physician Practice Management.* John Wiley and Sons, San Francisco, CA, p. 448.

Lloyd, J. 2009. Doctor shortage looms as primary care loses its pull, *USA Today*, August 18, 2009, p. 1.

National Commission for Quality Assurance. 2007. Washington, DC. http://www.ncqa.org/tabid/58/Default.aspx (accessed September 1, 2009).

The American Psychological Association. 2001. Executive summary of the behavioral health care needs of rural women: The report of the rural women's work group and the committee on rural health of the American Psychological Association. http://www.apa.org/pubs/info/reports/rural-women-summary.pdf (accessed September 13, 2009).

University HealthSystem Consortium. June 2009. *Faculty Practice Solutions Center® Issue Brief. Physician Quality Reporting Initiative: How 7 Faculty Practice Plans Implemented and Maintained Reporting*, Oak Brook, IL.

5

Designing a Nurse-Managed Healthcare Delivery System

Julie Cowan Novak
University of Texas Health Science Center at San Antonio

Introduction 5-1
Direct Practice 5-2
Program Costs 5-3
Challenges to Nurse-Managed Clinics and Faculty Practice 5-7
DNP Development: Implications for Faculty Practice 5-7
References 5-9

Introduction

For over 40 years, schools of nursing have developed nurse-managed clinics for the purpose of integrating their discovery, learning, and engagement mission. Most early models were grant-supported and often did not survive beyond the 3 to 5 years of foundation, state, or federal grant support. Over the past decade, with a growing emphasis on systems approaches, sustainability, business models, electronic health records, development of nursing center coalitions/data warehouses, fewer barriers to nurse practitioner practice, and healthcare reform, nurse-managed clinics are increasingly viewed as an important solution to the healthcare crisis. The model has evolved from a single source support to a mosaic of support, acquiring and generating multiple sources of revenue.

Faculty practice models underpin nurse-managed clinic successes and challenges. Models vary by definition, mission, philosophy, values, and region of the country. For the purpose of this chapter, faculty practice elements will include direct practice, indirect practice, and consultation. These models provide opportunities for an integration of the mission, provide a revenue stream, and increase access to high quality, efficient, and effective care.

Potash and Taylor (1993) described three major categories of faculty practice plans (FPP) including the unification model, the collaborative model, and the entrepreneurial model. In this chapter, exemplars will be provided that incorporate elements of each of these models as featured in the FPP of three well-established nurse-managed clinic models including: the North Central Nursing Clinics (NCNC), an affiliate of the Purdue University School of Nursing, the University of Texas Health Science Center–Houston and the University of Texas Health Science Center at San Antonio. Texas Tech University, Purdue, and Vanderbilt University have been designated as Federally Qualified Health Clinics (FQHCs) funded by the Department of Health and Human Services, the Health Resources Services Administration (DHHS/HRSA), and the 2009 Americans for Relief and Recovery Act (ARRA) (Novak, 2008). Other schools of nursing that have developed nurse-managed clinic models and established FPP include: the University of Wisconsin, Milwaukee, Arizona State University, the University of California, San Francisco, Michigan State University, the University of Michigan, the University of Minnesota, the

University of Pennsylvania, and the University of South Carolina. This list is not all inclusive. Due to space constraints for this chapter, please refer to each of their web sites for additional information.

Furthermore, with the development of the doctor of nursing practice (DNP), FPP/nurse-managed clinic models will become more prevalent and more sophisticated. In less than a decade, 130 schools have developed DNP programs and admitted and graduated students; over 200 programs are in the developmental stages. Thus, the evolution of the DNP in nursing education and its effect on nurse-managed clinics and faculty practice will also be addressed.

Direct Practice

Direct practice may include provision of care to individuals and families across a variety of settings. Direct practice models may be fee-for-service or capitated. Models may include nurse-managed clinics supported by federal, state and foundation grants, patient revenues, Medicaid, Medicare, private insurers, and/or private donors. Faculty full time equivalent (FTE) may also be purchased by private or community clinics, health maintenance organizations, hospitals, or industry. Advanced practice nurses including nurse practitioners, clinical nurse specialists, nurse anesthetists and nurse midwives often find this integrated model of teaching and practice most satisfactory as clinical expertise is maintained while accruing hours for recertification. If well designed, this can be beneficial to the School of Nursing as education and practice have the potential to be more relevant and more evidence-based. Faculty practice also can increase the financial viability of the school through revenue production while creating additional preceptorship sites for graduate students and capstone placements for baccalaureate students. These sites provide horizontal and vertical integration models of education. Horizontal integration includes the opportunity for a variety of faculty to serve as role models in a single site. This allows students to compare and contrast practice styles and to be mentored by a variety of faculty who possess different expertise and areas of specialization. Vertical integration is created through settings that may include a range of novice interdisciplinary students to graduate students with varying levels of expertise (Novak, 2007).

Exemplar 1: The University of Texas–Houston (UT Houston) School of Nursing

One of the most sophisticated School of Nursing faculty practice models was developed and implemented at the University of Texas–Houston under the leadership of Dr. Tom Mackey. The faculty practice program links The University of Texas Health Science Center–Houston School of Nursing with community agencies to provide clinical and/or research services on a fee-for-service or contractual basis. UT Houston is a national leader and trendsetter in this concept of joining consultation with healthcare agencies.

Examples of these linked services include employee health, nurse practitioner prenatal clinics, cardiovascular rehabilitation services, group therapy for bipolar disorders, and emergency nurse practitioners for triage and urgent care, and industry partnerships. Benefits include the provision of a nursing expert in the clinical site without the cost of a full-time salary and benefits. Thus, the arrangement contributes to the growth and the development of the agency. The program offers not only a selected faculty member, but also other RNs enrolled at the School of Nursing who are seeking professional learning experiences through various clinical projects. The program enhances capabilities to document clinical, cost and quality outcomes, and affords the opportunity to recruit students following graduation.

An agency or industry expresses a need for a certain service or set of services and determines how much time it will require. The School of Nursing matches the need with faculty expertise and arranges for the two parties to meet to discuss mutual interest. When an agreement has been reached, fees are calculated, the agreement contract is signed, and the services are initiated. Faculty members interview with the agency before the final selection. A match between philosophies and working styles are very important for a successful outcome (http://son.uth.tmc.edu/).

Program Costs

Fees are calculated based on the level of expertise, taking into account the degree held and advance practice certification. Faculty members are ranked as Consultants I, II, or III. Since the School of Nursing is a not-for-profit state agency, fees are used to cover only expenses, keeping costs for the agencies at a reasonable level and far below other means of obtaining these services. The contract is for a 12-month period and is renewable by mutual consent. Every agreement has an escape clause where either party, at any time, may give a 60-day notice of intent to cancel the contract. In case of emergencies, shorter notices are negotiated on an individual basis.

Revenues are dispersed according to a formula: 50% toward the Teaching Support Fund/replacement cost, 20% to the participating faculty member, 20% to the department or center, and 10% to the Dean's office (http://son.uth.tmc.edu/).

Exemplar 2: North Central Nursing Clinics, an Affiliate of Purdue University School of Nursing

Established in 1995 and 2006, respectively, the Family Health Clinic of Carroll County (FHCCC) and the Family Health Clinic of Monon (FHC-M) are supported by the Indiana State Department of Health, the university, the State of Indiana Tobacco Control Trust Fund, patient revenues, foundations, private donors/gifts, and Medicaid and Medicare billing. As with many clinics and businesses in general, it took years to reach revenue neutral status. With the worsening economy; however, a budget neutral status became more and more challenging. In February 2009, a $1.3 million DHHS/HRSA/ARRA grant was secured for operating costs relieving financial pressures significantly (Novak and Richards, 2009). In addition, the two rural NCNC clinics partnered with the Institute for Nursing Centers (INC) housed at the Michigan Institute for Public Health. This partnership led to funding from WK Kellogg and the Agency for Health Care Research and Quality (AHRQ) to support the integration of electronic health record software for patient management, electronic record keeping, evidence-based practice and data collection, pooling, analysis, and dissemination.

The NCNC incorporates both vertical and horizontal learning integration models. The FHCCC and the FHC-M, located in the rural communities of Delphi and Monon, Indiana, provide appropriate, affordable, and accessible primary healthcare to individuals and families. The focus of the services is directed to a growing Medicaid and Medicare population and uninsured or underinsured families living primarily in rural Carroll, White, and 10 other surrounding counties. The staff is comprised of three family nurse practitioners, an adult nurse practitioner, one pediatric nurse practitioner, an office manager, a biller, and a secretary. Of the five NPs, four have primary teaching responsibilities and participate in a rudimentary faculty practice plan. Since obtaining FQHC designation and HRSA funding, an executive director and chief financial officer were also hired. Senior nursing students have public health and capstone experiences in the clinics and graduate students have preceptorships, cognate residencies, and clinical research projects. Faculty, staff, and students study and analyze healthcare costs, aspects of sustainability, simulation, systems design, staffing, and patient flow.

Since their inception, the clinics have grown and expanded their services; client visits have grown 300%. The NCNC maintains an open door policy; no one is denied services because of inability to pay. Objectives include meeting the healthcare needs of individuals, families, and communities across the life span. The clinic focuses on health promotion, health maintenance, and management of acute and stable chronic health problems with specific state funding sources for chronic disease management of diabetes, asthma, cardiovascular disease, and cancer. This value-added service is reducing healthcare costs in the participating counties (Novak, 2007).

Child and adolescent health services include immunizations, health promotion, health supervision, developmental assessment, anticipatory guidance, diagnosis and treatment of acute illnesses, management of stable chronic conditions, basic diagnostic laboratory testing, and integrated mental health services. Women's health services include health promotion, annual pap and pelvic exams, breast health, mammogram referral, birth control, pregnancy testing, and pregnancy care while men's health services include general health promotion, prostate and testicular cancer screening, and education. Counseling/coaching related to nutrition/exercise, obesity prevention/intervention, stress management, tobacco use prevention/cessation, STD prevention and treatment, and screening and diagnostic laboratory testing are also key components.

The clinic meets the needs of the growing Latino/Hispanic population, currently 27%–50% of the patient population in Delphi and Monon, respectively. Faculty and staff members each have some degree of Spanish fluency ranging from high school to Spanish for Healthcare Professionals (an elective in the School of Nursing) to full fluency. The clinic RN and nurse practitioners also provide case management, health system navigation, and serve as an information resource for the community.

Limited space had been a barrier to the expansion of the FHCCC programs with the number of annual client visits at 3000. With private foundation support, a new building was designed, built, and dedicated in 2008. Over a 3-year period, the clinic director met with leaders of other community service agencies who ultimately decided to share space. In addition to public health nursing and advanced practice students, community partners include: WIC, Area Four Aging, Work One, and CDC Developmental Services. This integration of public health nursing students and their professors further strengthen community outreach, in-home care management, and continuity. A community room is used by the NCNC Board, other nonprofit agencies, and the staff for monthly meetings and educational programs (Novak, 2007).

Faculty nurse practitioners who provide care at the NCNC consistently report that the opportunity to teach, practice, and conduct research in an integrated model, while maintaining their clinical expertise and certification, are the reasons that they maintain their faculty role. The added incentive of full-time or part-time summer employment, additional merit salary supplements, and travel support increases their satisfaction. In an era of lucrative opportunities in private practice, the healthcare system, and industry, maintaining faculty satisfaction, growth, and development is critical. The community need for this nurse-managed system of care was documented through a United Way survey noting the lack of access to healthcare as the number one community concern. The high cost of healthcare, physician refusal to accept Medicaid patients, lack of transportation to larger communities for increased healthcare options, the use of costly ERs for primary healthcare, the highest rates of child abuse and neglect in the state, and a waiting list of >300 clients and families at the local Head Start, were reasons to launch and sustain the clinics. The child health component provides health and developmental assessment, immunizations, management of minor acute and stable chronic illnesses, and educational programs based upon a needs assessment. The Braselton Touchpoints model provides a framework for the care of children and their parents. Evaluation of the NCNC model and parent/patient satisfaction is measured quarterly, presented to the Board, and provided to HRSA.

Exemplar 3: Indirect Care Contracts

Indirect care is exemplified through population-based models. For example, public health and community health faculty provide expertise to departments of health in areas, such as county and statewide immunization programs, natural disaster preparedness, chronic disease management models, homeland security, and public health department accreditation. In this model, a portion of the faculty member's contract is purchased for research projects, community assessment and planning, program design, implementation, evaluation, and health policy development. Contracts range from 10% to 40% of the faculty member's salary.

Exemplar 4: Consultation

Consultation models overlap with indirect practice models. Consultation may include the provision of faculty experts for hospitals in the areas of better patient flow/scheduling models, operating room or critical care unit design, patient safety, cost containment, or organizational design. Since hospitals are challenged by the increasingly competitive healthcare market and realize they must improve their processes, share best practices, and improve efficiencies, a healthcare technical assistance program (HTAP) was created by Purdue University. Through the Faculty Practice Plan, a nursing faculty member was subcontracted for 0.4 to 0.5 FTEs during the academic year and full-time during the summer to lead projects with individual hospitals focusing on productivity, quality, safety, design, and cost. Supply management, pharmacy processes, data management, organization of equipment for repetitive tasks in admissions, nursing stations, maintenance, patient rooms, and medical procedure rooms have been addressed.

These seed projects are evolving into longer term projects involving additional nursing faculty practice contracts and DNP projects.

Exemplar 5: Payment Models

In addition to direct purchase of faculty time based upon the faculty member's base salary, time may be purchased at a higher rate based upon hospital or agency salaries. If X is the faculty member's base salary and Y reflects grants and contracts, and clinical revenues that the faculty member brings to the school, then Z can be shared with the faculty in a salary bonus or placed in an enhancement account accessed by the faculty member for approved university purchases, e.g., travel, supplies and equipment, a research assistant, and/or a teaching assistant.

For faculty practice to realize optimal financial benefit, advanced practice nurses must be named to provider panels. Being on a provider panel increases the billing opportunities to private insurers, as well as federally funded programs. This will not only allow increased access and freedom of choice for patients, but also added revenue options that will lead to additional incentive payments to faculty. A cost analysis confirms that nurse-managed clinics can provide high-quality, safe, efficient, and effective care for 30%–50% of the cost of standard medical model care.

Exemplar 6: UT Nursing Clinical Enterprise

The Office of Practice and Engagement (OPE) of the UT Health Science Center San Antonio (UTHSCSA) School of Nursing was created in September 2009 with hiring the first Associate Dean for Practice and Engagement. The practice initiatives for this Office evolved into the UT Nursing Clinical Enterprise which emphasizes financial aspects and sustainability related to nurse-managed clinic development and enhancement and other practice opportunities (see Figure 5.1). The OPE creates or enhances practice settings where faculty and students integrate discovery, learning, and engagement. The OPE offer students and faculty a unique opportunity to increase cultural awareness, acquire cultural knowledge, and become culturally proficient in providing healthcare to diverse populations. Undergraduate and graduate nursing students, under faculty supervision, participate in a broad range of clinical learning experiences. Students are prepared to help reduce health disparities in at-risk populations. Typical learning experiences include health promotion/disease prevention, education and screenings, primary care across the life span, immunization clinics, school-based health services, employment physicals, and chronic disease management.

Internally, within the UT System, the Clinical Enterprise includes the Student Health Center (SHC) run by the School of Nursing since 2007. In September 2009, the SHC expanded from 2 to 4 exam rooms and 2 to 7 faculty nurse practitioners to improve the system of care for 3600 Health Science Center students (nursing, medicine, dentistry, physical therapy, occupational therapy, physician assistant, and basic science), and to expand clinical sites and faculty practice opportunities. Collaboration with the Behavioral Health Department for UTHSCSA students has also increased with the integration of behavioral health services into the Student Health Center primary care model. Over the past year, the SHC has moved from breaking even to billing 15 insurance companies, securing reimbursements and student fees of $20,000 monthly—a 25% increase over the preceding 3 months. This learning laboratory allows students and faculty to understand the business of healthcare while creating an effective, safe, high-quality nurse-managed system of care.

Due to the success of the SHC, documented need, faculty expertise, and access to research populations, the OPE/UT Nursing Clinical Enterprise was invited and agreed to submit a proposal to create

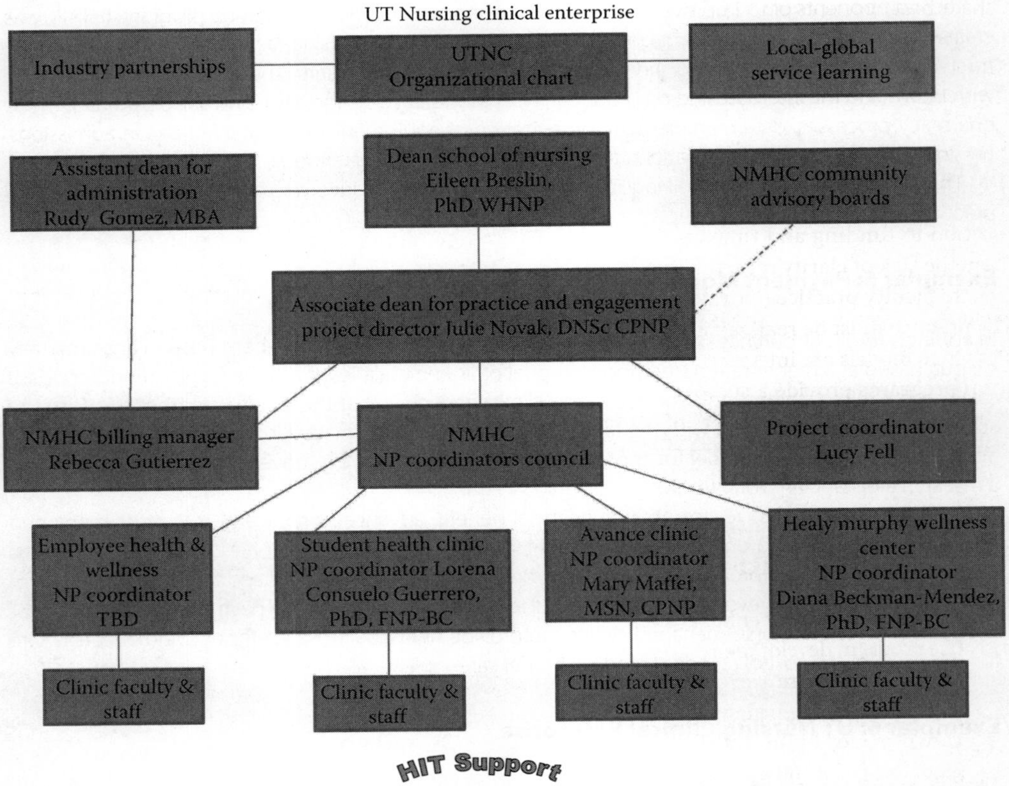

FIGURE 5.1 UT Nursing Clinical Enterprise, Julie Cowan Novak, August 2010.

an Employee Health and Wellness/Occupational Health Clinic. The Associate Dean created a rendering in collaboration with facilities management/university architects. The proposal was approved and "fast tracked"; completion of the new clinic is projected to be October 2010. Over 7000 UTHSCSA employees will have the opportunity to obtain healthcare on campus in the new clinic. The partnerships that have been developed over the past year will culminate in a campus-wide health fair and fun run/walk in conjunction with the dedication of the new clinic and new campus perimeter walking trail. This inaugural student, faculty, staff event will launch a series of health promotion and disease prevention initiatives.

Engagement activities external to the university have occurred in several areas. The Avance Community Partnership Clinic is part of the Early Head Start program. A UTHSCSA faculty pediatric nurse practitioner is the care provider. She also directs the pediatric nurse practitioner (PNP) program; thus Avance is a learning laboratory for PNP students. The success of this program has led to a request from Head Start to expand the model to other San Antonio Head Start facilities. Five Health Homes are being created by the UT Nursing Clinical Enterprise in partnership with Head Start. The San Antonio Independent School District (SAISD) requested Health Home model development for the district; thus the UT Nursing Clinical Enterprise team submitted a $7 million proposal at the request of the state. If funded, the model will provide a nurse-managed clinic health home at each of the eight SAISD high schools.

The second established community site was the Healy Murphy Alternative High School and Day Care Center. Two faculty APNs developed faculty practice sites in the setting and expanded operations to create a nurse-managed Health Home and clinical learning sites as a component of the Office of Practice and Engagement/UT Nursing Clinical Enterprise. Electronic health records adoption will "go live" in December 2010. The EHR system will link the Avance and Healy Murphy Clinics with the Student Health Center. Each of these NMCs provides care for designated medically underserved populations (MUPs).

Other components of the Clinical Enterprise include private practice contracts, industry partnerships and local to global service learning projects. From disaster response to program development for global HIV/AIDS prevention and treatment initiatives, nurse-managed clinics provide effective community-based interventions and the integration of service learning (Richards et al., 2009; Richards and Novak, 2010).

Challenges to Nurse-Managed Clinics and Faculty Practice

In addition to funding and time constraints, inconsistent administrative support and business expertise, and the lack of clarity regarding academic rewards (promotion and tenure), are the most significant barriers to faculty practice (Novak, 2007). These issues must be addressed and a shared commitment to faculty practice must be realized in order to mitigate these challenges.

If practice models are integrated and unified, if business expertise is provided or nursing masters and doctoral programs provide a subspecialization in business practices, and if practice/service/community engagement is clarified and valued in the promotion and tenure process, then these challenges are not insurmountable. Nurse-managed health and wellness centers work because they are focused at the community level where national and state health policies and social realities meet (Hansen-Turton et al., 2009).

DNP Development: Implications for Faculty Practice

The development of the DNP enhances systems approaches to the design of nurse-managed clinics and faculty practice program development. In the past decade, 130 DNP programs have been established across the United States and 200 more are in various stages of development. DNP educational models range from the application of engineering principles to healthcare to executive healthcare leadership, to the highest level of direct care provided by advanced practice nurses. Nurse-managed clinics provide learning laboratories and the opportunity for integration of the mission. DNP students and their faculty create innovative program designs for healthcare delivery, systems analysis, evidence-based practice, informatics and electronic health records, quality and safety analysis, and health policy development. A series of Institute of Medicine Reports were tipping points in patient safety. These reports were a catalyst for the development of the doctor of nursing practice and the expansion of the nurse-managed clinic model (Rapala and Novak, 2007a,b).

The practice doctorate prepares individuals at the highest level of practice and is the terminal practice degree. The DNP program is designed to fill the growing need for expert clinicians who can strengthen healthcare delivery systems. Direct faculty practice in nurse-managed settings, indirect practice with populations of patients, and consultation with a variety of healthcare agencies, serve as models for DNP students in their cognate residencies and for graduates who will be prepared to change the face of healthcare (Novak, 2006). Graduates of the DNP program will ultimately affect the entire healthcare delivery system due to the unique focus on healthcare systems, leadership, and evidence-based practice.

The degree represents the highest level of practice in nursing and incorporates the most independent and advanced nursing skills. The program is structured to prepare the students for cutting edge roles in a changing healthcare system, knowing that the system will demand ever-higher levels of clinical skills and knowledge. Graduates will be experts in designing, implementing, managing, and evaluating healthcare delivery systems. At the same time, they will be prepared to provide leadership in maintaining the complex balance between quality of care, access, and fiscal responsibilities (Wall et al., 2005).

Advanced practice nursing faculty who are masters-prepared have the option to complete the DNP program and its cognate residencies in nurse-managed clinics and other faculty practice sites. Transforming healthcare delivery recognizes the need for clinicians to design, evaluate, and continuously improve the context within which care is delivered. Removing barriers to advanced nursing practice is critical to finding solutions to the problems of a fragmented healthcare delivery system. Cost-effective nurse-managed clinic delivery systems and sophisticated faculty practice initiatives provide excellent alternatives to a healthcare delivery system in the United States that is in turmoil and has been described as "broken." Nursing leaders at the highest levels have determined that a practice doctorate as the terminal degree is the best response to this crisis (Wall et al., 2005).

Due to the information explosion and complexity of the healthcare delivery system, many masters programs in nursing now exceed 55 credits in order to prepare graduates. Over the next decade, it is projected that although bedside nurses still may come from a variety of educational programs leading to baccalaureate degrees and RN licensure, nurses in leadership positions and advanced practice roles must be prepared at the doctoral level. Nurses who currently hold master's degrees will have the option of obtaining a practice doctorate or they may choose to remain in their current clinical positions. These practice doctorates must have a skill and a knowledge set that provides clear value-added service; faculty must be engaged in integrated models of practice, research, and education for these graduates to reach their full potential. A clear understanding of the science and the application of systems engineering, finance, and policy is critical to the effectiveness and maximal impact of the role.

Nursing has many of the answers to the predominant healthcare dilemmas of the future, including: (1) problems associated with normal human development, particularly aging; (2) chronic illness management across the life span; (3) health disparities associated with socioeconomic dislocations, such as global migration, classism and sexism; and (4) the need for health promotion and disease prevention (American Association of Colleges of Nursing, 2004).

Over the past decade, an upswing of interest in developing a viable alternative to the research-focused degrees—Doctor of Philosophy (PhD) and Doctor of Nursing Science (DNS, DNSc, DSN)—has occurred. In 2002, the American Association of Colleges of Nursing (AACN) charged a task force to examine the current status of clinical or practice doctoral development. It recommended that the practice-focused doctoral program be a distinct model of doctoral education that provides an additional option for attaining a terminal degree in nursing.

Informational shifts, demographic changes, growing disparities in healthcare delivery and access, and stakeholder expectations are all creating new demands on the nursing profession. The practice doctorate, with a focus on direct practice, healthcare leadership, and delivery systems offers nursing an exciting opportunity to meet these demands (Wall et al., 2005). The DNP presents a clinical practice-oriented leadership development opportunity that allows the nurse to focus on evidence-based practice, defined as "the conscientious use of current best evidence in making decisions about patient care" and "a problem-solving approach to clinical practice that integrates (1) a systematic search for and a critical appraisal of the most relevant evidence to answer a clinical question; (2) one's own clinical expertise; and (3) patient preferences and values" (Sackett et al., 2000). The nurse also focuses on research utilization for the improvement of clinical care delivery, patient outcomes, and systems management. Such credibility is essential for securing funding from federal or private sources.

With growing emphasis on evidence-based practice, healthcare facilities are desperately looking for nurses with doctorates who can integrate systems approaches, provide leadership in interdisciplinary settings, bring "best practice" to patient care, insure a safe passage through the systems, and understand the importance of ongoing outcomes evaluation and the efficacy of nursing practice. Nurse scientists need to be "linked" with nurses, other healthcare providers, and engineers to aid the translation of research into practice. Joint academic-clinical appointments are feasible and rewarding routes for faculty to connect research and practice through the facilitation of EBP efforts. In fact, facilitation is critical to the success of translation efforts (Hopp, 2005). Integrated nurse-managed clinic models of faculty practice provide settings for this translation to occur.

The growth of advanced practice nursing and the DNP, the knowledge and information explosion, and the increasing complexity of healthcare support the need for interdisciplinary solutions that apply systems engineering concepts. In order for practice and education to be evidenced-based and relevant, nursing and other healthcare disciplines must steer away from ivory tower, siloed models of the past. With the severe faculty shortage, professors who are encouraged to maintain their clinical expertise will experience greater role satisfaction. Finally, nurse-managed clinics and faculty practice facilitate access to research populations, innovations, and policy makers. If nursing is to play a significant role in reengineering healthcare, then faculty members must be less insular and more collaborative with a broad range of healthcare professionals fully engaged in their communities.

References

American Association of Colleges of Nursing. 2004. *White Paper on the Doctor of Nursing Practice.* Washington, DC: AACN.

Hansen-Turton, T., M. E. Miller, and P. A. Greiner. 2009. *Nurse-Managed Wellness Centers.* New York: Springer.

Hopp, L. 2005. Minding the gap: Evidence-based practice brings the academy to clinical practice, editorial. *Clinical Nurse Specialist* 19: 190–192.

Novak, J. C. 2005. *School of Nursing Faculty Survey.* West Lafayette, IN: Purdue University.

Novak, J. C. 2006. Faculty practice. In *Business and Legal Essentials for Nurse Practitioners,* S. Reel and I. Abraham. (Eds.). Philadelphia, PA: Mosby Elsevier.

Novak, J. and R. Richards. 2009. *North Central Nursing Clinics: Care for Rural Underserved Populations.* Washington, DC: DHHS/HRSA/ARRA.

Potash, M. and D. Taylor. 1993. *Nursing Faculty Practice: Models and Methods.* Washington, DC: National Organization of Nurse Practitioner Faculties.

Rapala, K. and J. Novak. 2007a. *Integrating Patient Safety into Curriculum: The Doctor of Nursing Practice.* Marietta, GA: Patient Safety & Quality Healthcare, March/April, pp. 16–23.

Rapala, K. and J. Novak. 2007b. Clinical patient safety: Achieving high reliability in a complex environment. In *Digital Human Modeling,* V. Duffy (Ed.). Springer, Berlin, Germany, pp. 710–716.

Richards, E. and J. Novak. 2010. From Biloxi to Capetown: Curricular integration of service learning. *Journal of Community health Nursing* 27(1): 46–50.

Richards, E., J. C. Novak, and L. Davis. 2009. Disaster response after Hurricane Katrina: A model for academic–community partnership in Mississippi. *Journal of Community Health Nursing* 26(1): 3.

Sackett, D. L., S. E. Straus, W. S. Richardson, W. Rosenberg, and R. B. Haynes. 2000. Evidence-based medicine: How to practice and teach EBM. *The Journal of the American Medical Association* 284(18): 2382–2383.

Wall, B. M., J. C. Novak, and S. A. Wilkerson. 2005. The doctor of nursing practice: Reengineering health care. *Journal of Nursing Education* 44(9): 396–403.

6

Long-Term Care

Kathleen Abrahamson
Western Kentucky University

Karis Pressler
Purdue University

Role of Families in the Provision of Long-Term Care 6-1
Nursing Home Decision 6-2
Nursing Homes 6-3
Family Caregiver Involvement in Long-Term Care Facilities 6-4
Assisted Living Facilities 6-5
Financing Long-Term Care 6-6
Long-Term Care Culture 6-7
Conclusion 6-9
References 6-9

Long-term care is an umbrella term describing "a variety of services and supports to meet health or personal care needs over an extended period of time" (U.S. Department of Health and Human Services 2009). Long-term care is focused upon maintaining safety, mobility, and functional ability in terms of activities of daily living (ADL), such as bathing, eating, toileting, and dressing, and is delivered in a variety of settings, notably home care, assisted living facilities, and nursing homes. At over $135 billion annually, long-term care is a significant area of expenditure in the United States' healthcare system (Brown and Finkelstein 2006). Though long-term care encompasses a wide variety of settings and recipient needs, this chapter will focus upon care provided to the aged population, both informally by family members and within residential institutions.

Role of Families in the Provision of Long-Term Care

Family members provide the greater portion of long-term care to the frail and aged (Pyke and Bengtson 1996). Most primary caregivers are women, with a prevalent caregiving dyad being an adult daughter caring for a dependent mother (Walker et al. 1990b, Walker and Pratt 1991, Walker et al. 1995). Demographic trends, such as increased longevity and improved medical management of chronic conditions are expected to increase the prevalence of family caregiving to the frail and elderly. Smaller family sizes increase the likelihood that an individual will experience the caregiver role (Marks 1996, Pyke and Bengtson 1996).

Obtaining a clear definition of family caregiving can be difficult as the exchange of assistance between family members is a common, nearly defining feature of family. Most caregiving tasks completed by the family are instrumental in nature (shopping, paying bills, running errands), as opposed to the provision of physical care (Walker et al. 1995). Reports of caregiving activity are dependent upon the caregivers' perception of tasks as "caring" and divergent from the normal routine. Especially given that the majority of caregivers are women, the exchange of assistance between family members may be underestimated during assessment by healthcare providers. For example, a man may feel that making breakfast for his wife is a caregiving task, whereas a woman may perceive this work to be part of her routine responsibilities (Walker et al. 1995). Those receiving care may also underestimate the work of their caregiver. Zweibel and Lydens (1990) find that 70% of care recipients perceive themselves to be less dependent then they are perceived to be by their caregivers.

Caregiving norms vary greatly between families (Keith 1995, Walker et al. 1995, Pyke and Bengtson 1996). Much caregiving research focuses upon the existence of a sole caregiver who takes on the majority of caregiving tasks, a caregiving model that may not reflect the experiences of many families (Kleban et al. 1989). Both practitioners and researchers are likely to ask, "Who is the primary caregiver?" in order to ascertain information, compelling a response which may not accurately reflect a family's caregiving system (Keith 1995).

A majority of previous caregiving research focuses upon the burden of caring for an aged family member. Caregivers tend to report poorer health and lower life satisfaction than non-caregivers (Hoyert and Seltzer 1992, Pavalko and Woodbury 2000). Poor or declining caregiver health is the strongest predictor of an increase in caregiver burden (Mui 1995). The intragenerational caregiving experience of wives tends to be less burdensome than the intergenerational caregiving experience of daughters (Hoyert and Seltzer 1992, Mui 1995, Walker et al. 1995, Dorfman et al. 1996). African American caregivers report less overall burden than White caregivers, though African Americans with high incomes have a burden level similar to that of White caregivers (Walker et al. 1995).

Caregiver burden is influenced by gender as well, as many women take on caregiving as an additional role, whereas males, who are frequently aged husbands of dependent wives, are likely to take on caregiving as a replacement for past roles, such as that of employee or family breadwinner (Mui 1995). Caregiving daughters who have minor children are more likely to express burden (Walker et al. 1990). Employed women are equally as likely as women who do not work outside the home to become caregivers, perhaps reflecting the predominance of adult daughters as caregivers for the aged (Kleban et al. 1989, Walker et al. 1995, Pavalko and Woodbury 2000). However, Pavalko and Woodbury (2000) find caregivers are less likely to be employed and more likely to report adverse health after years of caregiving, indicating possible effects of caregiver burden combined with the progressive aging of caregivers themselves.

Research addressing the relationship between duration of caregiving and burden has yielded mixed results. There is evidence that burden is cumulative, increasing as duration of care increases, but also adaptive, decreasing as the caregiver becomes accustomed to negotiating the caregiver role (Hoyert and Seltzer 1992, Pavalko and Woodbury 2000). The issue of coresidence with the care recipient is unclear as well. Caregivers who live with the care recipient may benefit from the convenience of close proximity, yet may also feel the heavy burden of a caregiving situation that is essentially never ending (Hoyert and Seltzer 1992). Consistent with the concept of life course consistency, previous emotional well-being is highly correlated with the perception that the caregiver experience is emotionally rewarding (Moen et al. 1995).

Burden is mediated, and may be almost eliminated in situations where the caregiver perceives high self-efficacy and a supportive social network (Dorfman et al. 1996). Walker et al. (1990), in an examination of mother/adult daughter caregiving dyads, find that almost half of caregiving daughters report positive changes in the relationship with their mothers as a result of caregiving. Caregivers may receive reciprocal aid in exchange for caring. Walker et al. (1992) find that 90% of caregiving daughters report receiving love from mothers in exchange for care, 75% report receiving information, and 87% indicate that the aid they receive from care-receiving mothers is valuable.

Nursing Home Decision

It is frequently the family caregiver, not the care recipient, who makes the decision to discontinue caregiving in the home and to commit the care recipient into a long-term care facility. This decision is often rushed, many times related to a medical crisis or hospitalization, and frequently based upon inadequate information (Castle 2003). Miller and Weinstein (2007), using a sample of working age patients, found that 27.9% of nursing home residents had no involvement in the decision to enter a facility. Previous research has shown that younger residents report greater input to the admission decision; studies using aged samples have shown that up to 50% of residents have little or no input into the admission decision (Miller and Weinstein 2007).

Reasons given by caregivers for nursing home admission include, the need for more skilled care, difficulty managing recipient behaviors, need for the caregiver to have more help, and a decline in caregiver health (Buhr et al. 2006). The level of caregiver burden predicts nursing home placement, as do resident need for continuous supervision, caregiver sleep disruption, and a lack of caregiver leisure time. Older caregivers tend to report higher levels of physical burden prior to institutionalization, while younger caregivers report higher levels of emotion-based stress (Chenier 1997). Conversely, caregivers who report positive aspects of the caregiving experience are less likely to select nursing home placement (Schultz et al. 2004).

Nursing Homes

One and a half million Americans live in long-term nursing institutions, or nursing homes. The number of persons over age 65, who require institutional care is expected to double by 2030. Nursing homes employ 1.5 million full-time caregiving staff, primarily licensed nurses and certified nursing assistants. Thus, millions of residents, family members, and employees are affected by the interpersonal environment of nursing homes (Feder et al. 2000, Jones 2002).

Long-term care facilities in the United States vary in terms of size, location, profit status, and reimbursement structure. A majority of long-term care facilities are located in the Midwest (33.3%) and in the South (33.2%). Over 60% of facilities are located within metropolitan areas. Long-term care facilities with under one hundred beds represent just over half (50.2%) of the United States' nursing homes, while 41.8% have 100–199 beds, and only 8% of facilities have accommodations for 200 or more residents (Jones 2002).

Nursing homes receive less attention than hospitals from researchers and agents of economic development. The system of healthcare delivery in the United States takes an acute care focus, distributing the majority of resources toward short term, technological intervention (Feder et al. 2000). Institutional care has a poor reputation. Admitting a loved one to a nursing home is frequently a care choice of the last resort, representing a time of crisis for residents and families. Long-term care facilities are challenging environments for staff as well, who grapple with low pay, stressful working conditions, and high staff turnover (Abrahamson 2008) rates.

Unique in comparison to long-term care delivery in other industrialized nations, the majority of long-term care facilities in the United States (67%), are proprietary or for-profit organizations (Jones 2002). There is evidence that quality of care is lower in nursing homes with for-profit status, perhaps because of differences in staffing patterns (Hillmer et al. 2005). Proprietary facilities offer nursing staff significantly higher wages yet staff nursing units with fewer nurses and nursing assistants per resident than nonprofit facilities. Despite offering higher wages, for-profit facilities experience higher levels of nursing staff turnover for both licensed nurses and certified nursing assistants (Banaszak-Holl and Hines 1996, Kash et al. 2006, Donoghue and Castle 2009).

Physical care in nursing homes is primarily delivered by unlicensed nursing assistants. Nursing assistants have less than six months of technical training and are certified by the state in which they practice. They provide the majority of hands-on care, such as feeding, bathing, dressing, and toileting. Nursing assistants are supervised by Licensed Practical/Vocational Nurses (LPN/LVN) and Registered Nurses (RN). Licensed Practical/Vocational Nurses have approximately one year of technical training. In the long-term care setting LPN/LVN's participate in both patient care and supervisory tasks. The long-term care setting differs from the acute care setting in that LPN/LVN's are frequently given the charge nurse role, a role that is differentiated very little from that of the Registered Nurse. Registered Nurses have at minimum, two years of post-high school education. Registered Nurses working in long-term care function as charge nurses and perform primarily supervisory duties and technical tasks, such as management of intravenous medications (United States Department of Labor 2007). Both LPN/LVN's and RN's are licensed by the state in which they work.

Staff turnover is a significant problem in nursing homes, with turnover estimates as high as 100% for direct care providers (Anderson et al. 2004, Pillemer et al. 2008). The turnover of nursing staff is lower in facilities that maintain adequate staffing levels and have a stable leadership (Anderson et al. 2004). Management styles influence turnover rate as well. Donoghue and Castle (2009) find nursing home administrators who lead in a consensus style, encouraging input from all staff levels, have the least staff turnover. This is consistent with the work of Anderson et al. (2004), who found lower turnover in facilities that have administrative climates that promote open, accurate communication. There is a correlation between registered nurse turnover and administrative turnover; both seem to influence the other (Anderson et al. 2004, Castle et al. 2007). In a randomized, controlled trial, Pillemer et al. (2008) found that facilities that used the services of a staff retention specialist within the nursing home setting had reduced turnover when compared with facilities that did not use a retention specialist. Thus, concentrated resources and management efforts may be necessary to improve the retention of caregiving staff.

Nursing home residents are largely of advanced age (90% over age 65, 46% over age 85), females (72%), and Caucasians (86%). Long-term care residents and their families present staff with a wide variety of needs (Jones 2002). An aged population brings to the institution well-established lifestyle patterns that vary greatly among individuals (Wellin and Jaffe 2004). Due to the long-term and the all encompassing nature of nursing home care, nursing home staff are expected to manage these individual differences and to provide the type of care normally ascribed to families, and at the same time adhere to organizational guidelines; a situation that is challenging for nursing home staff (Pillemer et al. 2003).

The work of nursing home staff is unique from that of care staff in acute care settings. While acute care facilities, primarily hospitals, focus upon care that is curative, disease focused, and generally technological in nature, long-term care facilities focus their efforts toward maintenance of functional status, management of chronic illness, and assistance with ADL, such as bathing, toileting, and feeding of residents (Feder et al. 2000). Until the early twentieth century, the type of ADL-based care provided by long-term care facilities was managed by families and their private employees. The institutional provision of long-term care represents not only a transition in the physical location of care but a transition in the social relationships between caregivers as well. Once considered experts in the care of their aged relatives, input from family members is now often secondary to that of credentialed professionals working within organizational structures (Levine and Zuckerman 2000, Levine and Murray 2004).

Family Caregiver Involvement in Long-Term Care Facilities

Contrary to the "myth of abandonment", admission to a long-term care facility does not mean the end of family caregiving (Duncan and Morgan 1994, Dupuis and Norris 1997). Most family caregivers maintain frequent contact with the care recipient post-institutionalization (Port et al. 2001). Family caregivers who report high levels of involvement prior to nursing home admission, who live close to the facility, and who care for a recently admitted resident, are the most likely to remain involved in resident care (Hook et al. 1982, Port et al. 2001, Port 2004).

Though physical exertion and demands on caregiver leisure time decrease with nursing home admission, other types of stress increase resulting in a level of caregiver burden that is essentially unchanged (Dellasega 1991, Keefe and Fancey 2000). Instrumental responsibilities, such as financial management, legal assistance, and emotional burden often increase upon nursing home admission (Dellasega 1991). Family members take on new roles of advocate and monitor, roles that can be ambiguous and emotionally draining (Stull et al. 1997, Zarit and Whitlatch 1992).

Caregiver exhaustion or decline in caregiver health is frequently the catalyst for institutionalization (Bauer and Nay 2003). Transition from caregiving in the community to caregiving within an institution involves negotiation of new role expectations with the care receiver, family members, and facility staff. The addition of facility staff to the caregiver's role involves particularly stressful negations, as clear role expectations of family within long-term care facilities are rarely established (Krause et al. 1999, Whitlach et al. 2001, Bauer 2005). Relocation from familiar surroundings can have negative health effects on the patient as well. Planning, preparation, emphasis on the similarities between the home and the facility environment can enhance resident and family member coping (Castle 2001).

There is abundant evidence that family members tend to focus upon care tasks that preserve the care recipient's self-worth, personal identity, and dignity post institutionalization. Family caregivers sense a tendency toward uniformity of caregiving within an institution and strive to differentiate their relative as a unique individual, distinct from other nursing home residents (Bauer and Nay 2003). Bartlett (1994) finds that wives of institutionalized husbands seek to provide care that is personal and affective in nature; care they feel is missing from the work of facility staff. Bowers (1987) describes the family focus on personalization of care as "protective caregiving," meaning care meant to protect the resident's self and identity as they are threatened by a task-oriented institution. Family members tend to evaluate the quality of nursing care more in terms of staff ability to maintain positive relationships and support a resident's self-esteem than by technical competence, often resulting in role conflict for staff members who face demands for improved efficiency and technical competence from employers (Friedeman et al. 1997).

Family members are an important, often underutilized resource to nursing home staff (Schwartz and Vogel 1990, Dupuis and Norris 1997, Ryan and Scullion, 2000). Family members act as resident advocates, system "watchdogs," decision makers, and often provide at least minimal direct care within long-term care facilities (Levine and Zuckerman 2000). Family caregivers bring to the facility, knowledge of resident history and care preferences often inaccessible to staff, especially in situations where a resident is cognitively impaired (Rowles and High 1996). Harvath et al. (1994) describe the knowledge of families as "local," meaning specific to the resident, and the knowledge of staff as "cosmopolitan," meaning generalized and oriented toward scientific principles. Using the analogy of a ship captain's need for both the cosmopolitan knowledge of ship commandeering and the local knowledge of maps created by those most familiar with the landscape to safely enter a harbor, Harvath et al. (1994) note the importance of combining family knowledge of the personal with nursing knowledge of the technical, to provide quality long-term care.

Assisted Living Facilities

Traditional nursing facilities are autonomy-restricted environments; choices for residents, such as when and what to eat, when to rise from bed, and room furnishings are frequently limited or highly regulated. Dependence upon staff is often fostered through the structured nature of institutionalization (Funk 2004). Though there has been a culture change movement in long-term care resulting in a number of patient-centered nursing home models such as the Green House, the Wellspring, and the Eden Alternative, most nursing homes remain highly institutionalized environments (Yeatts and Cready 2007).

Perhaps, because of their more flexible structures, assisted living facilities have become the fastest growing residential alternative to nursing home care for the aged (Golant 2004). The definition of assisted living is highly variable. There is no federal standard for assisted living facilities; regulation, licensure, and definition of assisted living vary from state to state. Even within states, there is great variation in what is considered assisted living. Some assisted living facilities are luxurious and offer a wide variety of services and amenities; others differ little from nursing homes or offer very limited staffing and services. The majority of the assisted living population are aged, white, female and unmarried. Currently only 10%–20% of assisted living residents are not elderly (Golant 2004, Mollica 2008, Street et al. 2009).

What staffing and services are offered by assisted living facilities is driven by both the market and the state regulation (Golant 2004; Kane 2008). Though assisted living is generally not funded through either Medicare or Medicaid dollars, states that allow for Medicaid waivers to cover the cost of assisted living services for those who cannot pay privately, significantly increase the size and the diversity of the population served by assisted living facilities. Regulation of the care recipients served varies between states as well. Some states separate assisted living residences for the aged from those serving younger, chronically disabled, or mentally ill populations; other states allow for a heterogeneous population within a single facility (Kane 2008).

Because assisted living facilities are generally without 24 hour skilled nursing services, admission criteria may limit the acuity of persons entering assisted living environments. There are however, in states with more flexible regulations, some very ill or complex patients residing in assisted living environments (Golant 2004). There is concern that flexible admission standards allow high-acuity residents to be admitted to assisted living facilities that do not have the staff or resources to care for their needs (Street et al. 2009). For example, Sloane et al. (2005) find that while assisted living facilities are able to meet the social and the functional needs of dementia residents, they are often unable to manage complex medical conditions resulting in increased hospitalization rates.

However, admission and acuity standards that are more stringent create situations where residents who are declining in functional or medical status must relocate to receive adequate care (Golant 2004). It is the preference of many aged individuals to "age in place," or remain in their current location if their status declines. Relocation is most difficult when it is forced by policy as opposed to resident choice (Shippee 2009). As the assisted living marketplace continues to expand, clarification is needed as to the amount of regulation necessary to provide safe care while still providing an individualized, homelike setting that adapts to the changing medical needs of individual residents (Mollica 2008).

Financing Long-Term Care

Ninety-eight percent of United States long-term care facilities, both proprietary and non-profit, are certified to accept government reimbursement through Medicare, Medicaid, or both (Jones 2002). Government reimbursement in long-term care is based upon a case mix system that links level of care and facility certification to the amount of payment received (Abrams et al. 1995). The mix of reimbursement sources within an individual facility varies between facilities. Medicare reimburses only for short-term recovery from acute illness or specific skilled nursing/rehabilitation needs (Brown and Finkelstein 2006). Medicare per diem payment is higher and carries more stringent care criteria than Medicaid, ($166 average per diem Medicare bed charge, $116 average per diem Medicaid bed charge). Thus, facilities and units that are designated as Medicare tend to provide more income. The result is a hierarchy of reimbursement sources, both within and between facilities, that influences staffing patterns, average length of stay, and patient acuity (Kash et al. 2006).

Very little—only 4%—of long-term care is paid for through private insurance. The largest payment source apart from individual funds, at 35%, is Medicaid (Brown and Finkelstein 2006). Medicaid funds are administered through 50% federal funds and 50% state funds, allowing states to have control over how long-term care reimbursement is administered. Though the federal government maintains broad regulatory power, key decisions regarding institutional versus noninstitutional reimbursement via waiver programs, funding of ancillary services, such as transportation, and emphasis on quality improvement and innovation are made at the state level. The result is a long-term care delivery system that varies greatly in terms of quality, organization and priority from state to state (Kane 2008). The population of elders requiring institution-based long-term care is expected to rise substantially (Feder et al. 2000, Jones 2002). As demand for services increases, it may become necessary to change the current system of long-term care reimbursement to assure equitable access to quality care across state and socioeconomic boundaries.

Long-Term Care Culture

Older adults move into long-term care settings for a variety of reasons, including but not limited to health conditions, functional decline, difficulty managing the home, and inability to drive (Young 1998, Krout et al. 2002). Long-term care facilities offer a unique venue where aspects of the institution coalesce and interplay with individual personalities, relationships, health trajectories, and life events. Research within these facilities has documented the textured lives of residents and the struggle of staff to optimize and preserve resident autonomy and dignity while simultaneously providing care to residents in a group setting. Although these settings are considered age homogenous, the older adults living within the walls of long-term care facilities are anything but similar. A myriad of personal histories, personalities, and needs comprise long-term care facilities, creating a culture that is unique to that setting, yet similarities across facilities persist. The following descriptions and anecdotes provide a brief overview of the some of the similarities observed within the culture of long-term care across settings.

Research based on Assisted Living facilities and Continuing Care Retirement Communities (CCRC) present a unique opportunity to explore the colorful and complex culture in long-term care settings. The CCRC is a slowly expanding model of retirement home living that caters largely to white, highly educated individuals who move into a CCRC facility while still independent, and generally progress through different levels of care from independent living, to assisted living, and then to nursing home care or dementia care as their health needs accumulate (Binstock et al. 1996, Shippee 2009). The setting is unique because admittance is generally accompanied by a large fee in addition to monthly payments. In one CCRC study setting, the entry fee was $100,000, while monthly fees ranged from $1,500 to $2,000 (Krout et al. 2002). While the demographics of the CCRC population limit the generalizability of research findings to other long-term care settings, the structure of the environment makes for a fascinating case study of culture within a setting where residents usually enter the setting in good health and age-in-place with the guarantee of always being cared for (Sherwood et al. 1997, Heisler et al. 2004). On the other hand, Assisted Living facilities offer a more affordable yet similar age-in-place approach compared to CCRCs. However, residents who become more dependent and require specialized care may have to move outside of the facility to a nursing home that can meet their needs (Eckert et al. 2009). The structure of both of these settings compliment research using the life course perspective because residents generally move into these settings while they can still perform some ADL and expect to stay in the long-term care setting until death (Elder 1994, Moen et al. 2000).

Preserving autonomy is one way to maintain or to improve quality of life among Assisted Living residents (Ball et al. 2000). In a study that asked residents what they look "forward to every day, a male Assisted Living resident responded, 'Being *able* to get up and go to the bathroom'" (Ball et al. 2000, p. 314, emphasis added) with "able" having a double entendre. Not only did this resident have the functional ability to go to the bathroom, but he was allowed to exercise this ability and act independently. The authors observed that residents were only able to achieve autonomy in a limited number of circumstances—for instance, while residents chose which tasks and activities they wanted to attend, autonomy was limited for residents with respect to what they ate and when they ate. Also, the majority of residents expressed that the decision to move into the facility was not their own. Social interaction with friends and family outside the facility was limited for some, with 33% of residents saying they lost contact with friends after moving into the facility. Some residents viewed other fellow-residents as "friendly" but noted that the caliber of friendship among residents could never reach that of relationships formed prior to moving into the facility. However, those who lost contact with outside friends valued the bond they formed with fellow-residents, and the bonds formed with the staff who cared for them (Ball et al. 2000).

Health and the appearance of being healthy is a pervasive theme in long-term care cultures, where residents feel the need to display their independence. Small (2000) documented how female residents, in what she described a communal retirement home setting with independent living apartments, strived to keep their minds and bodies active to maintain an independent appearance. Keeping the mind active included placing physical reminders, such as the pill box in a certain place to remind a resident to take pills at a certain time. Mental activity also included making social comparisons and articulating observations of the setting and its residents. Several female residents reported abandoning use of a knee or back brace in public places within the facility in order to maintain their healthy appearance because the meaning attached to these braces was indicative of physical decline. "I will give into vanity" reported one resident who refused to wear her knee brace in the dining room and endured unnecessary pain in order to appear independent (Small 2000, p. 580). Research illustrates the importance of appearing independent. In Eckert et al. (2009)'s study, assisted living residents who observed other residents experiencing health decline thought that these residents "don't belong" in the setting, despite the fact that assisted living is structured to accommodate a certain amount of health decline (p. 157).

The importance of meal time to residents in long-term care settings is undisputed in long-term care literature. Within Small (2000)'s ethnography, female residents spoke of the importance of dressing up, while Shippee (2009) found this finding echoed in her research where CCRC residents felt that clothing such as shorts were unacceptable in the dining room. Meal time is an important ritual to those in long-term care settings where food is associated with familiar memories and special occasions. Meal time in these settings provide an opportunity for residents to gather, socialize, see and be seen, discuss, observe, and eat (Small 2000, Eckert et al. 2009, Shippee 2009).

Transitions between levels of care can be difficult for residents. In her richly detailed study of transitions within a CCRC, Shippee (2009) observed that residents, despite buying into the CCRC model, were well aware that declining health precipitated transitions within the facility, and transitions were associated with greater dependence, sickness, and imminent death. Residents who lived in cottages associated with the facility but located outside the main facility called the main building "The Big House," referring to the prison-like grip the institutional aspects of retirement home living had on residents (Shippee 2009, p. 422). Despite the best efforts of long-term care to shift away from a medical model and focus on a more social and individualized model of care, older adults in retirement home settings still encounter a structured environment that is impossible to escape in a congregate setting (Eckert et al. 2009).

Identities do not disappear in institutionalized settings. Moen et al. (2000) studied the personal identities of new CCRC residents prior to and following their move into the setting, to better understand how social roles and identities change. Among the most popular and pervasive identities identified by residents was that of spouse. Research suggests that couples who move into a CCRC together do so to ensure that when one spouse passes, the other will be taken care of (Cohen et al. 1988, Krout et al. 2002). How do the newly widowed fare in the CCRC settings?

Several studies have documented the stigmatization widows and widowers experience in retirement settings. Goffman (1963) associated stigma with a spoiled identity and research has illustrated the stigma experienced by widows and widowers and the relevance of presentation of self in retirement home settings (Goffman 1959). Van den Hoonard (1994, 2002) interviewed residents within a retirement community and learned that widow/ers were among several groups of people who lived on the community's social periphery. Interestingly, 10 years prior, the majority of residents were married, but with time widowhood became more prevalent. Despite its increasing prevalence, "It seemed to me that members of couples would probably have been happier if the widowed were not around and reminding them that they might be next" noted Van den Hoonard (1994, p. 125). One resident observed that the widows were dropped "like a hot potato" by their married friends following their husbands' deaths (Van den Hoonard 2002, p. 60).

Complex, and at times unspoken rules, norms, and expectations were ascribed to widow/ers in this community (Van den Hoonard 1994, 2002). Widows would not invite couples out to dinner, but rather wait to be invited and would act as followers and not leaders, letting the couples decide where to eat. Couples who invited a widow/er to dinner viewed this action as a favor, and the male of the couple would usually insist on *appearing* to pay for the widow, yet the widow would quietly pay the male for her portion either before or after the meal. Couples generally perceived widow/ers as wanting to stick around each other.

Residents also revealed the symbols inherent in the setting—if a widow removed her wedding band, this symbolized her willingness to be in a relationship with a man. Timing of the ring removal was also observed by residents. Women who removed their wedding bands too soon were frowned upon as there was an expected standard of when it is acceptable for a woman to explore romantic relationships following her conjugal loss (Van den Hoonard 1994).

The ratio of widow/ers to nonwidow/ers within retirement communities has been shown to affect the widow/er's life satisfaction and well-being. Hong and Duff (1994) studied how the ratio of widows to widowers in seven retirement communities influenced life satisfaction scores. Widow/ers in retirement communities where the number of couples outnumbered the number of widow/ers, had lower satisfaction scores compared to retirement communities where there were more widow/ers than married individuals. Widow/ers, in majority married communities, were less likely than those in widowed majority communities to participate in group activities.

Although long-term care settings are designed and organized to assist older adults in maintaining a quality of life and to continue to find meaning in life, the settings often house an array of spoken and unspoken norms, customs, and rules. Rules at times serve to preserve the appearance of independence and autonomy that encourage residents to appear healthy (Small 2000), but rules may also cause undue strain and hardship for those experiencing physical decline and loss (Van den Hoonard 1994, 2002, Shippee 2009). These cultures evolve and revolve around residents, and future research should continue to unveil the long-term care experience from the viewpoint of residents who strive to call these settings "home."

Conclusion

As the number of individuals living into later life increases, so does the need for long-term care (Feder et al. 2000, Spillman and Lubitz 2000). Long-term care comes in a variety of forms, including care provided by family members in the community, or in institutionalized settings including nursing homes, assisted living facilities, and CCRCs. Despite the pressing need for long-term care, relatively little is known about life inside the walls of these facilities from residents' perspectives. This chapter provides a brief overview of the trends in long-term care facilities, the types of settings, the payment for long-term care, as well as a snapshot of life within long-term care settings.

References

Abrahamson, K. 2008. Role expectations, conflict and burnout among nursing staff in the long-term care setting. PhD dissertation, Purdue University, West Lafayette, IN.

Abrams, W. B., M. H. Beers, and R. Berkow. 1995. *The Merck Manual of Geriatrics,* 2nd ed. Whitehouse Station, NJ: Merck Research Laboratories.

Anderson, R. A., K. N. Corazzini, and R. R. McDaniel. 2004. Complexity science and the dynamics of climate and communication: Reducing nursing home turnover. *The Gerontologist* 44(3): 378–388.

Ball, M. M., F. J. Whittington, M. M. Perkins, V. L. Patterson, C. Hollingsworth, S. V. King, and B. L. Combs. 2000. Quality of life in assisted living facilities: Viewpoints of residents. *The Journal of Applied Gerontology* 19(3): 304–325.

Banaszak-Holl, J. and M. A. Hines. 1996. Factors associated with nursing home staff turnover. *The Gerontologist* 36(4): 512–517.

Bartlett, M. 1994. Married widows: The wives of men in long term care. *Journal of Women and Aging* 6(1): 91–106.

Bauer, M. 2005. Collaboration and control: Nurses' constructions of the role of family in nursing home care. *Journal of Advanced Nursing* 54(1): 45–52.

Bauer, M. and R. Nay. 2003. Family and staff partnerships in long-term care: A review of the literature. *Journal of Gerontological Nursing* 29(10): 46–53.

Binstock, R. H., L. E. Cluff, and O. von Mering. 1996. Issues affecting the future of long-term care. In *The Future of Long-Term Care*, eds. R. H. Binstock, L. E. Cluff, and O. Von Mering, pp. 3–18. Baltimore, MD: Johns Hopkins University Press.

Bowers, B. J. 1987. Intergenerational caregiving: Adult caregivers and their aging parents. *Advanced Nursing Science* 9(2): 20–31.

Brown, J. R. and A. Finkelstein. 2006. The interaction of public and private insurance: Medicaid and the long-term care insurance market. In *Proceedings of the CESIFO Area Conference on Public Sector Economics*, Munich, Germany.

Buhr, G. T., M. Kuchibhatla, and E. C. Clipp. 2006. Caregivers' reasons for nursing home placement: Clues for improving discussions with families prior to the transition. *The Gerontologist* 46(1): 52–61.

Castle, N. G. 2001. Relocation of the elderly. *Medical Care Research and Review* 58(3): 291–333.

Castle, N. G. 2003. Searching for and selecting a nursing facility. *Medical Care Research and Review* 60(2): 223–247.

Castle, N. G., J. Engberg, and R. A. Anderson. 2007. Job satisfaction of nursing home administrators and turnover. *Medical Care Research and Review* 64(2): 191–211.

Chenier, M. C. 1997. Review and analysis of caregiver burden and nursing home placement. *Geriatric Nursing* 18(3): 121–126.

Cohen, M. A., E. J. Tell, H. L. Batten, and M. J. Larson. 1988. Attitudes toward joining continuing care retirement communities. *The Gerontologist* 28(5): 637–643.

Dellasega, C. 1991. Caregiving stress among community caregivers for the elderly: Does institutionalization make a difference? *Journal of Community Health Nursing* 8(4): 197–205.

Donoghue, C. and N. G. Castle. 2009. Leadership styles of nursing home administrators and their association with staff turnover. *The Gerontologist* 49(2): 166–174.

Dorfman, L. T., C. A., Holmes, and K. L. Berlin. 1996. Wife caregivers of frail elderly veterans: Correlates of caregiver satisfaction and caregiver strain. *Family Relations* 45(1): 46–55.

Duncan, M. T. and D. L. Morgan. 1994. Sharing the caring: Family caregivers' views of their relationships with nursing home staff. *The Gerontologist* 34(2): 235–244.

Dupuis, S. L. and J. E. Norris. 1997. A multidimensional and contextual framework for understanding diverse family members' roles in long-term care facilities. *Journal of Aging Studies* 11(4): 297–325.

Eckert, J. K., P. C. Carder, L. A. Morgan, A. C. Frankowski, and E. G. Roth. 2009. *Inside Assisted Living: The Search for Home*. Baltimore, MD: Johns Hopkins University Press.

Elder, G. H. 1994. Time, human agency, and social change: Perspective on the life course. *Social Psychology Quarterly* 57(1): 4–15.

Feder, J., H. L. Komisar, and M. Niefeld. 2000. Long-term care in the united states: An overview. *Health Affairs* 19(3): 40–56.

Friedeman, M. L., R. J. Montgomery, B. Maiberger, and A. A. Smith. 1997. Family involvement in the nursing home: Family-oriented practices and staff-family relationships. *Research in Nursing and Health* 20(6): 527–537.

Funk, L. M. 2004. Who wants to be involved? Decision-making preferences among residents of long-term care facilities. *Canadian Journal on Aging* 23(1): 47–58.

Goffman, E. 1959. *The Presentation of Self in Everyday Life*. New York: Doubleday.

Goffman, E. 1963. *Stigma: Notes on the Management of Spoiled Identity*. New York: Simon and Schuster, Inc.

Golant, S. M. 2004. Do impaired older persons with health care needs occupy U.S. assisted living facilities? An analysis of six national studies. *Journal of Gerontology: Social Sciences* 59B(2): S68–S79.

Harvath, T. A., P. G. Archbold, B. J. Stewart, S. Gadow, J. M. Kirschling, L. Miller, J. Hagan, K. Brody, and J. Schook. 1994. Establishing partnerships with family caregivers: Local and cosmopolitan knowledge. *Journal of Gerontological Nursing* 20(2): 29–35.

Heisler, E., G. W. Evans, and P. Moen. 2004. Health and social outcomes of moving to a continuing care retirement community. *Journal of Housing for the Elderly* 18(1): 5–23.

Hillmer, M. P., W. P. Wodchis, S. S. Gill, G. M. Anderson, and P. A. Rochon. 2005. Nursing home profit status and quality of care: Is there any evidence of an association? *Medical Care Research and Review* 62(2): 139–166.

Hong, L. K. and R. W. Duff. 1994. Widows in retirement communities: the social context of subjective well-being. *The Gerontologist* 34(3): 347–352.

Hook, W. F., J. Sobal, and J. C. Oak. 1982. Frequency of visitation in nursing homes: Patterns of contact across boundaries of total institutions. *The Gerontologist* 22(4): 424–428.

Hoyert, D. L. and M. M. Seltzer. 1992. Factors related to the well-being and life activities of family caregivers. *Family Relations* 41(1): 74–81.

Jones, A. 2002. The national nursing home survey: 1999 summary. *Vital and Health Statistics* 13(152): 1–116.

Kane, R. A. 2008. States as architects and drivers of long-term-care reform for older people. *Generations* 32(3): 47–52.

Kash, B. A., N. G. Castle, G. S. Naufal, and C. Hawes. 2006. Effect of staff turnover on staffing: A closer look at registered nurses, licensed vocational nurses, and certified nursing assistants. *The Gerontologist* 46(4): 609–619.

Keefe, J. and P. Fancey. 2000. The care continues: responsibility for elderly relatives before and after admission to a long term care facility. *Family Relations* 49(3): 235–244.

Keith, C. 1995. Family caregiving systems: Models, resources, and values. *Journal of Marriage and the Family* 57(1): 179–189.

Kleban, M. H., E. M. Brody, C. B. Schoonover, and C. Hoffman. 1989. Family help to the elderly: Perceptions of sons-in-law regarding parent care. *Journal of Marriage and Family* 51(2): 303–312.

Krause, A. M., L. D. Grant, and B. C. Long. 1999. Sources of stress reported by daughters of nursing home residents. *Journal of Aging Studies* 13(3): 349–364.

Krout, J. A., P. Moen, H. H. Holmes, J. Oggins, and N. Bowen. 2002. Reasons for relocation to a continuing care retirement community. *Journal of Applied Gerontology* 21(2): 236–256.

Levine, C. and H. Murray. 2004. *The Cultures of Caregiving: Conflict and Common Ground Among Families, Health Professionals, and Policy Makers*. Baltimore, MD: Johns Hopkins University Press.

Levine, C. and C. Zuckerman. 2000. Hands on/hands off: Why health care professionals depend on families but keep them at arm's length. *The Journal of Law, Medicine and Ethics* 28(1): 5–18.

Marks, N. F. 1996. Caregiving across the lifespan: National prevalence and predictors. *Family Relations* 45(1): 27–36.

Miller, N. and M. Weinstein. 2007. Participation and knowledge related to a nursing home admission decision among a working age population. *Social Science and Medicine* 64(2): 303–313.

Moen, P., M. A. Erickson, and D. Dempster-McClain. 2000. Social role identities among older adults in a continuing care retirement community. *Research on Aging* 22(5): 559–579.

Moen, P., J. Robison, and D. Dempster-McClain. 1995. Caregiving and women's well-being: A life course approach. *Journal of Health and Social Behavior* 36(3): 259–273.

Mollica, R. L. 2008. Trends in state regulation of assisted living. *Generations* 32(3): 67–70.

Mui, A. C. 1995. Multidimensional predictors of caregiving strain among older persons caring for frail spouses. *Journal of Marriage and Family* 57(3): 733–740.

Pavalko, E. K., and S. Woodbury. 2000. Social roles as process: Caregiving careers and women's health. *Journal of Health and Social Behavior* 41(1): 91–105.

Pillemer, K., R. Meador, C. Henderson, J. Robison, C. Hegeman, E. Graham, and L. Schultz. 2008. A facility specialist model for improving retention of nursing home staff: Results from a randomized, controlled study. *The Gerontologist* 48(S1): 80–89.

Pillemer, K., J. J. Suitor, C. R. Henderson, R. Meador, L. Schultz, J. Robison, and C. Hegeman. 2003. A cooperative communication intervention for nursing home staff and family members of residents. *The Gerontologist* 43(S2): 96–106.

Port, C. L. 2004. Identifying changeable barriers to family involvement in the nursing home for cognitively impaired residents. *The Gerontologist* 44(6): 770–778.

Port, C. L., A. L. Gruber-Baldini, L. Burton, M. Baumgarten, J. R. Hebel, S. I. Zimmerman, and J. Magaziner. 2001. Resident contact with family and friends following nursing home admission. *The Gerontologist* 41(5): 589–596.

Pyke, K. D. and V. L. Bengtson. 1996. Caring more or less: Individualistic and collectivist systems of family eldercare. *Journal of Marriage and Family* 58(2): 379–392.

Rowles, G. D. and D. M. High. 1996. Individualizing care: Family roles in nursing home decision-making. *Journal of Gerontological Nursing* 22(3): 20–25.

Ryan, A. A. and H. F. Scullion. 2000. Family and staff perceptions of the role of families in nursing homes. *Journal of Advanced Nursing* 32(3): 626–634.

Schultz, R., S. H. Belle, S. J. Czaja, K. A. McGinnis, A. Stevens, and S. Zhang. 2004. Long term care placement of dementia patients and caregiver health and wellbeing. *Journal of the American Medical Association* 292: 961–967.

Schwartz, A. N. and M. E. Vogel. 1990. Nursing home staff and residents' families role expectations. *The Gerontologist* 30(1): 49–53.

Sherwood, S., H. S. Ruchlin, C. C. Sherwood, and S. A. Morris. 1997. *Continuing Care Retirement Communities*. Baltimore, MD: Johns Hopkins University Press.

Shippee, T. P. 2009. "But I am not moving": Resident's perspective on transitions within a continuing care retirement community. *The Gerontologist* 49(3): 418–427.

Sloane, P. D., S. Zimmerman, A. L. Gruber-Baldini, J. R. Hebel, J. Magaziner, and T. R. Konrad. 2005. Health and functional outcomes and health care utilization of persons with dementia in residential care and assisted living facilities: Comparison with nursing homes. *The Gerontologist* 45(S1): 124–132.

Small, L. M. 2000. Material memories ethnography: Women's purposeful use of popular cultural anachronisms in quasi-communal retirement. *Journal of Contemporary Ethnography* 29(5): 563–592.

Spillman, B. C. and J. Lubitz. 2000. The effect of longevity on spending for acute and long-term care. *The New England Journal of Medicine* 342(19): 1409–1415.

Street, D., S. Burge, and J. Quadagno. 2009. The effect of licensure type on the policies, practices, and resident composition of Florida assisted living facilities. *The Gerontologist* 49(2): 211–223.

Stull, D. E., J. Cosbey, K. Bowman, and W. McNutt. 1997. Institutionalization: A continuation of family care. *Journal of Applied Gerontology* 16(4): 379–401.

United States Department of Labor. 2007. Statistics on professional and related occupations. http://www.bls.gov/oco/ocos083.htm (accessed July 13, 2009).

U.S. Department of Health and Human Services. 2009. National clearinghouse for long-term care information. http://www.longtermcare.gov/LTC/Main_Site/Understanding_Long_Term_Care/Basics/Basics.aspx (accessed July 13, 2009).

Van den Hoonard, D. K. 1994. Paradise lost: Widowhood in a Florida retirement community. *Journal of Aging Studies* 8(2): 121–132.

Van den Hoonard, D. K. 2002. Life on the margins of a Florida retirement community: The experience of snowbirds, newcomers, and widowed persons. *Research on Aging* 24(1): 50–66.

Walker, A. J., and C. C. Pratt. 1991. Daughters' help to mothers: Intergenerational aid versus caregiving. *Journal of Marriage and the Family* 53(1): 3–12.

Walker, A. J., C. C. Pratt, and L. Eddy. 1995. Informal caregiving to aging family members: A critical review. *Family Relations* 44(4): 402–411.

Walker, A. J., C. C. Pratt, and N. C. Oppy. 1992. Perceived reciprocity in family caregiving. *Family Relations* 41(1): 82–85.

Walker, A. J., C. C. Pratt, H. Y. Shin, and L. L. Jones. 1990b. Motives for parental caregiving and relationship quality. *Family Relations* 39(1): 51–56.

Walker, A. J., H. Y. Shin, and D. N. Bird. 1990a. Perceptions of relationship change and caregiver satisfaction. *Family Relations* 39(2): 147–152.

Wellin, C. and D. J. Jaffe. 2004. In search of "personal care": Challenges to identity support in residential care for elders with cognitive illness. *Journal of Aging Studies* 18(3): 275–295.

Whitlach, C. J., D. Schur, L. S. Noelker, F. K. Ejaz, and W. J. Loorman. 2001. The stress process of family caregiving in institutional settings. *The Gerontologist* 41(4): 462–473.

Yeatts, D. E. and C. M. Cready. 2007. Consequences of empowered CNA teams in nursing home settings: A longitudinal assessment. *The Gerontologist* 47(3): 323–339.

Young, H. M. 1998. Moving to congregate housing: The last chosen home. *Journal of Aging Studies* 12(2): 149–165.

Zarit, S. H. and C. J. Whitlatch. 1992. Institutional placement: Phases of the transition. *The Gerontologist* 32(5): 665–672.

Zweibel, N. and L. A. Lydens. 1990. Incongruent perceptions of older adult/caregiver dyads. *Family Relations* 39(1): 63–67.

7

Healthcare Insurance: An Introduction

Vinod K. Sahney
Blue Cross Blue Shield of Massachusetts

Ann Tousignant
Blue Cross Blue Shield of Massachusetts

Introduction 7-1
Third-Party Payers 7-1
Healthcare Financing 7-2
Roots of Employer-Sponsored Healthcare Coverage 7-3
Issues Raised by Third-Party Payment 7-4
Private Healthcare Insurance 7-5
State-Licensed Insurance Companies/Organizations • Self-Funded Employer Health Benefit Plans
Healthcare Insurance Products 7-5
Regulation of Private Health Insurance 7-6
Healthcare Reimbursement Systems 7-6
Discussion 7-7
References 7-7

Introduction

There are many parallels between 1929 and 2009. Most obvious are the economic crisis, rising levels of unemployment, and the rippling global impact of these occurrences. Another parallel exists related to healthcare financing, which in 2009 was a critical topic and a top priority on the U.S. political agenda. As healthcare expenditures continue to grow and currently consume more than 16%–17% of the U.S. gross domestic product (GDP), health expenditures are viewed as a contributor to the economic crisis, and/or health reform is viewed as an essential component of achieving fiscal solvency.

Ironically, events that occurred in 1929 formed the structure and conceptual basis for financing the U.S. healthcare system. As Starr (1982, p. 20) notes, "1929 marked the emergence of commercial health insurance" or third-party reimbursement. One event that marked the start of managed care took place in California at the Roos-Loos Clinic. Nearly simultaneously at Baylor Hospital in Texas, the foundations that eventually formed the basis of the Blue Cross system were laid (http://www.futureofchildren.org/, Palo Alto Medical Foundation, a Sutter Health Affiliate 2010, Thomasson 2003).

Third-Party Payers

In contrast to many other industrialized countries, the U.S. healthcare system is characterized by the role of "third-party payers." In essence, it is an arrangement in which the flow of funds between providers and patients flows through a "third-party payer" on the commercial side. It is an arrangement where an individual or employer pays insurance premiums to a third party (or insurer). Typically, the insurer develops a network of providers, negotiates terms of payment, handles administrative functions such as paying claims, collecting premiums, certifying eligibility, and, depending on the arrangement, may assume some financial risk. With regard to public programs (e.g., Medicare and Medicaid), third parties function as fiscal intermediaries performing similar administrative functions on behalf of government programs. The overall profile of the U.S. healthcare financing system is thus a mixed public–private structure—the foundation being employer-sponsored insurance (Gould 2008, Kaiser Family Foundation 2008).

Today, more than 200 million people in the United States have health insurance covered through employers and government-sponsored programs or by directly purchasing private health insurance (Kaiser Family Foundation 2008). Approximately 45 million residents of the United States do not have any health insurance coverage.

Healthcare Financing

Healthcare is financed in the United States through a collection of disjointed programs provided in both the private and government sector. In the private sector, health insurance for the most part is provided to individuals and their families as part of employee benefits by each individual's employer. Most employers contract with a third-party healthcare insurance company who then administers the program on behalf of the employer. Most employers offer different policies with various levels of cost sharing to their employees. Some employers even offer multiple insurance companies, each with varying healthcare policies. Almost all employers allow their employees to choose their healthcare options once a year for their families. Table 7.1 lists the top 10 private healthcare insurance companies and their enrollment in 2008. In 2007, private healthcare insurance covered 67.5% of the population—59.3% were covered by employer-based programs and 8.9% by individual plans (Blue Cross Blue Shield Association 2009, p. 8). In 2008, 63% of the employers offered some form of health insurance to their employees, 99% of employers with more than 200 employees offered health insurance, and only 78% of employers with less than 25 employees offered health insurance (Blue Cross Blue Shield Association 2009, p. 9).

The public healthcare insurance programs cover different segments of the population including

- Federal Employees Health Benefits Program open to federal employees and their dependents.
- Medicare—This program covers citizens above the age of 65 years. Part A of the program provides hospital insurance coverage. Part B of the program covers outpatient and physician costs. A more recent program called Part D provides pharmacy and drug coverage for seniors. The Medicare program is a federal program and the benefit package is uniform throughout the country. Under some limited conditions, people under the age of 65 can also be covered by the program. In 2007, Medicare A, B, and D covered 43.5 million, 40.0 million, and 17.4 million enrollees (Blue Cross Blue Shield Association 2009, p. 11).
- Medicaid—This program is a federal and state partnership and covers the poor. Each state defines the benefits and the income level below which individuals are covered under this program. Eligibility for coverage can vary from annual income of $5,000 to as high as $30,000 in different states. The cost of the program is shared equally by the state and the federal government. In 2007, Medicaid programs covered 48.1 million Americans (Blue Cross Blue Shield Association 2009, p. 11).
- State Children's Health Insurance Program (SCHIP)—This program provides health insurance to children under the age of 18

TABLE 7.1 Top 10 Healthcare Insurance Companies and Enrollment

Company	Membership (Millions)
United Health Group	32.7
Wellpoint	30.6
Aetna	16.9
HCSC	12.2
Cigna	9.9
Kaiser	8.5
Humana	8.5
Health Net	6.2
Highmark	5.2
BCBSMI	5.0
Total	135.7

Source: Copeland, W. et al., Survival of the fittest: How independent health plans can survive in today's economy, Deloitte, New York City, pp. 1–20, 2008.

years and is a state/federal health insurance program. In 2007, the SCHIP program covered 7.2 million enrollees (Blue Cross Blue Shield Association 2009, p. 12).

- Military Health System—For active members of the U.S. military and their dependents, healthcare is provided in hospitals managed by the various branches of the military. In addition, the military contracts with private healthcare insurance companies to provide coverage through a program called TRICARE.
- Veteran's Health Administration (VHA)—This program provides care to Americans who have served in the military and have healthcare needs related to their service. VHA runs hospitals and outpatient clinics throughout the country.
- Indian Health Service—This is a healthcare program that provides care to the Native American community through specialized healthcare facilities located in tribal communities.

In spite of the complex patch work of government and private healthcare insurance programs, approximately 15% or 45 million Americans are not covered by healthcare insurance (U.S. Census Bureau 2008). Another 20 million Americans are underinsured for the medical costs they may incur if they get sick (Families U.S.A. 2009). The United States spends more per capita in healthcare than any other nation and still not all citizens are covered (WHO 2009). Medical debt is the principal cause of personal bankruptcies in the United States (Anonymous 2009).

In 2008, national healthcare expenditures were $2.4 trillion, 16.6% of GDP, and are projected to reach $3.8 trillion or 18.8% of GDP (Blue Cross Blue Shield Association 2009, p. 19). In 2008, the United States spent $7868 per capita on healthcare (Blue Cross Blue Shield Association 2009, p. 19). National healthcare expenditures are increasing at three times the consumer price index for the past 5 years. Table 7.2 shows the national healthcare expenditures and the source of the money. Table 7.3 shows the percentage of the expenditures in each of the healthcare sectors.

TABLE 7.2 National Healthcare Expenditures: Sources

Source	Percentage (%)
Private insurance	34
Medicare	19
Medicaid/SCHIP	15
Other public	12
Out of pocket	12
Other/private	7

Source: Blue Cross Blue Shield Association, Chicago, IL, http://www.bcbs.com/, 2009.

TABLE 7.3 National Healthcare Expenditures: Sectors

Sector	Percentage (%)
Hospital care	31
Other spending—dental, DME, medical products	22
Physician/clinical services	21
Prescription drugs	10
Administration	7
Nursing homes	6
Home health	3

Source: Blue Cross Blue Shield Association, Chicago, IL, http://www.bcbs.com/, 2009.

According to the Institute of Medicine of the National Academy of Science, the United States is the only developed country without health coverage for all of its citizens (Institute of Medicine 2004). In another report, it was estimated that more than 100,000 Americans die each year due to a lack of health insurance (Himmelstein and Woolhandeller 1997).

Roots of Employer-Sponsored Healthcare Coverage

The roots for employer-sponsored healthcare insurance began in the 1920s. Initially, private companies covered care for injuries, but eventually these services expanded to include sickness care (Starr 1982). As previously mentioned, in 1929, managed care and commercial health insurance began in the United States. Employees of the Louisiana Department of Water and Power contracted with two physicians, Ross and Loos, "to provide comprehensive services for 2000 workers and their families" (Palo Alto Medical Foundation, a Sutter Health Affiliate 2010). The plan was unusual in that it provided for hospital stays as well as office-based medical care (Starr 1982). By 1935, the Ross–Loos Clinic had more than 12,000 workers and 25,000 dependents. (On average, subscribers paid $2.69 per month.) In 1933, Dr. Sidney Garfield started providing medical care on a prepaid basis to workers in Los Angeles. By

1938, Garfield began providing similar services on behalf of the Henry J. Kaiser Company for workers building the Grand Coulee Dam—a prominent part of the economic stimulus on the part of FDR. This initial contract became the basis of the Kaiser Permanente Health Plans (http://www.futureofchildren.org/ and Palo Alto Medical Foundation, a Sutter Health Affiliate 2010).

Midway across the country, the roots of Blue Cross were founded, also in 1929. Baylor University agreed to provide school teachers with up to 21 days of hospital care for a per capita fee ($6 per person). Just as this and other health insurance plans were emerging, the impact of the Great Depression struck. It helped transform these medical cooperatives into broad-based health insurance plans. The American Hospital Association endorsed hospital insurance as a "practicable solution to the problem of fiscal instability of hospitals during the depression" (http://www.futureofchildren.org/; Palo Alto Medical Foundation, a Sutter Health Affiliate 2010).

Issues Raised by Third-Party Payment

Just as in 1929, the current debate around healthcare reform is framed by the perspectives of free-market advocates vs. the supporters' public and private systems (Dr. Stuart Altman). Many economists argue that the traditional market dynamics between suppliers and consumers do not work in healthcare. For example, patients or their employers "purchase insurance, not a product." At the time of purchase of insurance covering healthcare, the decision is made on the basis of premium price; there is a lack of transparency, both about the true costs of services and dimensions of quality. The buyer and seller are not functioning as independent agents; in fact, the buyer (i.e., the patient) may be totally dependent on the supplier for access to information and referrals. Consumers lack information and the complex nature of health information may exacerbate the need to rely on providers. Faced with finding healthcare providers, often for urgent or emergent situations, consumers lack the ability, motivation, and time to identify the best price, quality, or overall "value" (Goodman et al. 2004, p. 235, Orszag 2008, p. 7).

In a recent article in *The New Yorker*, Atul Gawande argues for an incremental approach to healthcare reform in the United States—and provides a cogent historical perspective on why the healthcare systems in selected countries have evolved in very different ways. Most healthcare reform can be traced to the impact of World War II.

- England anticipated that air raids would be focused on disrupting large cities. In response, the national government encouraged people to relocate to the countryside. The exodus of 3.5 million people required building hospitals in areas where none existed before to provide care for them, as well as to make sure that there was sufficient capacity to handle the anticipated surge of wounded civilians and troops. The government provided free treatment for war-related injuries—both hospital and physician costs. This emergency medical service was intended to last only for the duration of the war, but it was so successful in gaining support from patients and providers that it was retained and became the basis for the National Health Service (Gawande 2010).
- After the war, France faced shortages of food, housing, and medical care. The only "system" in place was one established by some employers through a payroll tax. This system was expanded to include all employers and eventually the self-employed, and now the Securite Sociale is still financed through a payroll tax system administered by local health funds (Gawande 2010).
- When Switzerland looked to provide universal health coverage, it had no public programs to build upon; it required all citizens to buy private health insurance, with subsidies for low income residents.

Gawande (2010) points out that in the United States, we have employer-based health insurance, public financing through Medicare and Medicaid, the Veteran's Administration system of physicians and hospitals, and employer-sponsored healthcare insurance for many. He suggests we build on these systems to create a more comprehensive system that may not be elegant in design but that will work in practice.

Private Healthcare Insurance

Private healthcare insurance is provided by two different types of organizations. These organizations are either state-licensed insurance companies/organizations or self-funded employee health benefit plans.

State-Licensed Insurance Companies/Organizations

These are organizations that are under state law and usually fall under the following three categories:

- Blue Cross Blue Shield Plans—These plans were formed as not-for-profit organizations under special state laws for hospital care (Blue Cross) and medical care (Blue Shield). At one time, there were more than 100 such plans. In most states, the Blue Cross plans and Blue Shield plans have merged to form Blue Cross Blue Shield plans. In 12 states, Blue Cross Blue Shield plans have converted from not-for-profit to for-profit status and merged into a national plan which is known as Wellpoint. Four other plans covering Illinois, Texas, Oklahoma, and New Mexico have converted to a mutual member-owned plan and merged to form Health Care Services Corporation (HCSC).
- Commercial Health Insurers—These insurance companies are organized as stock companies owned by stockholders and offer insurance policies on a nationwide basis. United Healthcare, Aetna, Cigna, and Humana are four of the largest commercial healthcare companies in the United States.
- Health Maintenance Organizations (HMOs)—HMOs are licensed in each state as a combination of health insurance and providers. The largest such plan is the Kaiser Foundation health plan with more than 8.5 million members. The plan also owns many hospitals, ambulatory care facilities, and medical groups in different geographical areas.

Self-Funded Employer Health Benefit Plans

These plans operate under federal laws and are usually sponsored by employers or employee organizations. These plans contract with a private healthcare insurance company to administer their healthcare plan but retain the risks themselves. The organizations administering the plans are called "Third-Party Administrators."

Healthcare Insurance Products

Whether it is state-licensed insurance plans or the self-funded employee health benefit plans, they can offer a variety of healthcare insurance products as outlined below. Healthcare insurance products include preferred provider organizations (PPOs), HMOs, point of service plans (POS), high deductible health plans (HDHPs) including health savings accounts (HSAs), health reimbursement accounts (HRAs), and traditional insurance plans. Table 7.4 shows the distribution of employer-sponsored health plan enrollment in 2007.

TABLE 7.4 Healthcare Insurance Plans

Plan	Percentage (%)
PPO	57
HMO	21
POS	13
HDHP	5
Traditional	3

Source: Kaiser Family Foundation, Menlo Park, CA, http://www.kff.org/insurance/7766.cfm, 2008.

- HMO—The original concept of HMOs was to provide care to enrollees for a fixed price per month. Early HMOs were staff model HMOs. The organization employed physicians and either had their own hospitals or contracted with hospitals for the care of their enrollees. Examples are the Group Health Cooperative of Puget Sound and Kaiser Permanente of California.
- PPO—Preferred provider organizations are networks that include physicians and hospitals that agree to provide their services on a

discounted basis to a healthcare insurance plan. Most commonly, members are given incentives to use network providers.

- POS—The Point of Service insurance product is a hybrid of fee-for-service and HMO concepts. Under the HMO concept, members are restricted to a defined network. Under the fee-for-service concept, enrollees can get services from a wider network of physicians and hospitals. The POS product allows members to go outside their network but requires a member to pay higher copays or deductibles if they use this option.
- HSAs/HRAs—Under new federal laws, HSAs and health reimbursement accounts (HRAs) are set up tax free to pay for healthcare expenditures for members of such plans. These plans require that a member enroll in high deductible health insurance plans and also offer a HSA. The money left over in an HSA account can be rolled over to be used in following years.

Regulation of Private Health Insurance

Most health insurance policies offered in this country are regulated by a complex set of rules enacted by the states and the federal government. The most important federal law is called ERISA (Employee Retirement Income Security Act of 1974). This act established standards for employee benefit plans in terms of coverage. Similarly, each state regulates insurance policies and insurance companies under state laws. These laws may cover such issues as minimum required coverage under policies issued in the state, financial standards, reserve requirements, etc. Most states also regulate rate bands. Rate bands are the differences between the lowest and highest premium that can be charged to individuals for the same coverage.

Healthcare Reimbursement Systems

Healthcare insurance companies pay the providers in a number of different ways which are called reimbursement systems. The objective of these payment systems are to pay providers for time and resources used to provide services to patients, but at the same time provide providers with incentives to become more efficient and effective. Some of the common reimbursement systems are described below.

- Fee-for-Service—This is the most common system for paying healthcare providers including physicians, hospitals, clinical laboratories, physical therapists, etc. Each provider sets a fee for each of the services they provide. The insurance company sets a maximum fee for each of the services. The providers bill the insurance company for their services. The insurance company pays the provider the lower of their billed fees or the maximum set by the insurance company. Under fee-for-service, providers have the incentive to prescribe more and more services, even when there is little justification or need for them. This sets up an interesting conflict between the provider and the insurance company. Providers argue that a particular service is needed or they are prescribing it to practice defensive medicine in case they get sued. Insurance companies periodically deny services when they believe there is no justification for them. Since most Americans believe that more care is better, they almost always side with their physician and accuse insurers of denying them needed services. In a recent report published by the New England Healthcare Institute (2008), more than 400 peer-reviewed papers were cited listing studies in the last 10 years documenting unneeded care exceeding 30% of all care provided or $700 billion of waste.
- DRGs—Diagnostic-related groups were developed by Dr. Robert Fetter and researchers at Yale University as a means of paying hospitals for inpatient care on a bundled payment instead of using the fee-for-service system. Hospitals were paid by insurance companies for each service provided to a patient on a fee-for-service basis or in some cases based on costs incurred by the hospitals. In 1985, Medicare changed its payment method to DRGs. All hospital care was grouped into approximately 500 groups and a fixed payment was set for each group. Immediately after this

implementation by Medicare, most healthcare insurance companies began paying for care on a DRG basis. Hospitals immediately embarked on an effort to make inpatient care more efficient. Length of stay for hospitalizations dropped from an average of 10 days to less than 5 days.
- Capitation—Capitation programs are a fixed payment per patient to a healthcare provider to deliver all medical services for one calendar year. Capitation programs were initially established as a basis for HMOs. The concept was that healthcare organizations could provide preventive care on an ongoing basis and thus reduce the need for costly inpatient care. Capitation programs rapidly grew from 1980 to 2000 but fell out of favor because of a few providers and insurance companies denying needed services to patients. In addition, consumers demanded greater freedom of choice in selecting physicians. Recently, capitation programs have been staging a comeback with modifications that include quality indicators under which providers are rewarded to prevent denial of care. Blue Cross Blue Shield of Massachusetts has pioneered such a program and signed more than 10 large healthcare systems to 5-year contracts called Alternative Quality Contracts.
- Pay for Performance—Many insurance companies are rewarding their providers for achieving improvement in quality for various services. Pay for Performance (also know as P4P) varies by individual contracts negotiated by insurance companies and providers including physicians and hospitals. In general, these indicators have only an upside for providers achieving quality goals in well-defined areas. More recently, insurance companies have announced events termed "never events" for which providers will not be paid. An example of a "never event" is a surgeon operating on the wrong site, for example, left knee when the right knee was the correct site.

Discussion

The U.S. healthcare insurance systems are a patchwork with a confusing array of organizations providing coverage to defined groups of individuals and families. Because of this patchwork, there are a number of problems. One key issue is that when an individual loses his/her job, they lose their healthcare coverage as well. There are federal laws that require an organization to allow departing employees to continue their healthcare coverage for a limited period of time by paying premiums out of pocket. When the individual finds a new job, the new employer provides coverage. If the period between leaving one job and finding another job is too long, individuals and families end up not having coverage. In addition, the new insurance company may deny insurance for preexisting health conditions. A second problem is that each insurance company has their own approved network of doctors and hospitals. A change of job may require changing doctors and hospitals.

Healthcare insurance reform is all about correcting these problems. The problem is that without universal coverage, it is very difficult to fix these problems.

References

Anonymous. 2009. Medical debt huge bankruptcy culprit—study: It's behind six in ten personal filings. http://www.cbsnews.com/stories/2009/06/05/earlyshow/health/main5064981.shtml (accessed March 17, 2010).

Blue Cross Blue Shield Association. 2009. Healthcare trends in America: A reference guide. Chicago, IL, http://www.bcbs.com/

Copeland, W., D. Davies, S. Birchard, and F. Irwin. 2008. Survival of the fittest: How independent health plans can survive in today's economy. Deloitte, New York City, pp. 1–20.

Families U.S.A. 2009. Press release summarizing at Lewin Corp Study, "New report finds 86.7 million Americans were uninsured at some point in 2007–2008." http://www.familiesusa.org/

Gawande, A. 2009. Getting there from here. *The New Yorker*. http://www.newyorker.com/reporting/2009/01/26/090126fa_fact_gawande (accessed January 14, 2010).

Goodman J. C., G. L. Musgrave, and D. M. Herrick (Eds.). 2004. Designing ideal health insurance. In *Lives at Risk: Single Payer National Health Insurance Around the World*. Lanham, MD: Rowman and Littlefield Publishers, Inc.

Gould, E. 2008. The erosion of employer-sponsored health insurance: Declines continue for seven years running. Briefing paper no. 223, Economic Policy Institute, Washington, DC.

Himmelstein, D. and S. Woolhandeller. 1997. The inhuman state of U.S. health care. *NEJM* 11: 336.

Institute of Medicine. 2004. *Insuring America's Health: Principles and Recommendations*. Washington, DC: National Academies Press.

Kaiser Family Foundation. 2008. How private health coverage works: A primer—2008 update. Menlo Park, CA, http://www.kff.org/insurance/7766.cfm

New England Healthcare Institute. 2008. How many more studies will it take? http://www.nehi.net/publications/30/how_many_more_studies_will_it_take

Orszag, P. 2008. Opportunities to increase efficiency in health care. Congressional Budget Office, Washington, DC. http://www.cbo.gov/doc.cfm?index=9384 (accessed March 19, 2010).

Palo Alto Medical Foundation, a Sutter Health Affiliate. 2010. Early experiments with managed care. Palo Alto, CA. http://www.pamf.org/about/pamfhistory/managedcare.html

Starr, P. 1982. *The Social Transformation of American Medicine: The Rise of a Sovereign Profession and the Making of a Vast Industry*. New York: Basic Books.

Thomasson, M. 2003. Health insurance in the United States. In R. Whaples (Ed.), *EH.Net Encyclopedia*, http://eh.net/encyclopedia/article/thomasson.insurance.health.us (accessed March 17, 2010).

U.S. Census Bureau. 2008. Income, poverty and health insurance coverage in the United States: 2007. Washington, DC. http://www.census.gov/

WHO. 2009. World health statistics 2009. Geneva, Switzerland. http://www.who.int/en/

8

An Integrated Model of Healthcare Delivery

Steven M. Witz
Purdue University

Kenneth J. Musselman
Purdue University

Background 8-1
Complexity • Fragmentation • Acute to Chronic Care • Healthcare Information and Communications Technology • Linking System Performance and Goals
Integrated Healthcare Delivery Model 8-4
Provider Levels • Healthcare Delivery • Outcomes • Population Extension
Research Opportunities 8-8
Complexity • Fragmentation • Acute to Chronic Care • Healthcare Information and Communications Technology • Multidimensional Metrics • Individual in the Integrated Healthcare Delivery Model • Healthcare System in the Integrated Healthcare Delivery Model
Conclusion 8-11
References 8-11

The application of engineering science in clinical research, medical technology, and public health has a long and robust tradition of enabling important innovations. Healthcare engineering builds on this tradition and offers opportunities for the application of systems engineering to improve healthcare delivery (Reid et al., 2005). These opportunities are extremely relevant to the increasingly urgent need for healthcare reform and to bolster enthusiasm for this area of engineering practice.

Healthcare engineering is the transdisciplinary application of engineering, science, management, and information technologies to improve healthcare delivery. The application seeks to provide a systems perspective in an effort to achieve significant improvements in the delivery of care, both on an individual level and on a population level.

The practice of healthcare engineering is evolving as a result of collaborations and methodology developments across multiple disciplines. The fundamental premise of this chapter is that there is a need for a model of healthcare delivery to guide continued development of healthcare engineering, to assimilate multidisciplinary knowledge in this area, and to encourage the synergistic application of this knowledge. Such a model will help to: (1) easily recognize the components of the delivery system, (2) appropriately represent their functional relationships, (3) creatively link processes and subsystems for improved healthcare value and population health status, and (4) constructively categorize areas for further research and methodology development.

Background

The need for improved healthcare delivery has generated new evaluations and performance assessments of the delivery system itself. In doing so, attention is being paid to fundamental barriers in the system, such as (1) complexity, (2) fragmentation, (3) shift from acute to chronic care needs, (4) a deficit of investment in and development of healthcare information and communications technology, and (5) failure to link performance to goal attainment. An integrated model of healthcare delivery should be informed by this work and provide a conceptual framework for how healthcare delivery systems can overcome the limitations imposed by these barriers.

Complexity

Complexity in the healthcare delivery system is a deterrent to improving performance. Applying high-performance organizational structures from other industries has been proposed as a means to reduce this complexity. For example, microsystems have been suggested as a fundamental building block for higher performance (Nelson et al., 2001). These systems, defined as "a small group of people who regularly work together to provide care to a patient subpopulation," (Nelson et al., 2001) are characterized as "minimum replicable units" (Quinn, 1992) of service delivery. They have both clinical and business aims, linked processes, a shared information environment, and performance-based outcomes. Larger healthcare delivery organizations are often composed of these microsystems, and an organization's performance is dependent on the performance of its embedded microsystems.

Care platforms have also been suggested as an organizing structure to reduce system complexity (Bohmer and Lawrence, 2008). They are defined as fundamental units of service distinguished by the provision of care offered patients with similar medical conditions. Care platforms attempt to integrate patient care by identifying groups of interventions or medical conditions, standardizing requirements per group, designing clinical production systems specific to these groups, creating mechanisms for dealing with exceptions, and establishing accountability for providers (Bohmer and Lawrence, 2008).

Both microsystems and care platforms suggest a hierarchical organizational structure for healthcare delivery. They start with basic production units and then integrate these basic units to provide expanded scopes of care. This organizational structure reduces system complexity by concentrating the care processes and their durations.

Fragmentation

The need to integrate care delivery, or reduce fragmentation of healthcare services, underlies the concept of another approach to organizing care delivery, namely care episodes. "Episode-based approaches are viewed as a means to drive improvements in the quality and efficiency of healthcare delivery. Under an episode approach, some or all of the services related to the management of a patient's chronic condition or acute medical condition would be grouped together" (Hussey et al., 2009). Another view of care episodes is that they are composed of services such as those provided by hospitals and physicians utilized in the treatment of either acute conditions or a chronic condition for a limited period of the total required care (Davis, 2007). This care concept recognizes that healthcare outcomes are dependent on the appropriate integration and delivery of healthcare services. Moreover, it provides the next hierarchical level in organizing healthcare delivery by combining the products of microsystems and care platforms.

There is neither a generally accepted definition for nor a fully implemented application of care episodes. Several demonstration projects are currently underway and may assist in the development of a consensus definition (Gosfield, 2008; Paulus et al., 2008; Trisolini et al., 2008). The scope of services provided, the number of providers involved, and the length of time over which the care is delivered are primary variables differentiating the various definitions (Hussey et al., 2009).

Reducing fragmentation in healthcare delivery requires the ability to effectively link and coordinate related units of care to achieve the desired patient outcomes. Care episodes represent one conceptual approach to improving care coordination. This concept introduces two additional and important considerations. First, while operational complexity may be reduced by viewing delivery processes at an elemental level, improving care outcomes requires functional integration. "If episodes are being used for performance measurement, it may be more appropriate to define episodes to include multiple, interrelated conditions that are often treated concurrently. Such a definition would provide a broader perspective on the clinical management of complex patients" (Hussey et al., 2009). The second consideration is that when the delivery system is viewed in terms of its outcomes, the focus of the process changes from an emphasis on production to the individual and the family.

Acute to Chronic Care

The healthcare delivery system is shifting its attention from acute to chronic care to accommodate the care requirements of an aging population and an increasing prevalence of risk factors for chronic illnesses. To address this expanded view, the concept of a care cycle has been advanced. Care cycles define the provision of a broader scope of care than care episodes (Porter and Teisberg, 2004). Care cycles have been defined as including: (1) prevention, wellness, screening, and routine health maintenance services; (2) a focus on a medical condition; (3) services required for coexisting conditions and complications; and (4) an extended scope of care and time for a chronic illness (Porter, 2009). The organization of healthcare into care cycles may be most applicable for chronic illnesses and other conditions requiring continuous care.

Healthcare Information and Communications Technology

Amidst the growing complexity of care delivery, the value of information and the ability to communicate it among those delivering and receiving care are of increasing importance. Yet, the vast majority of clinical records used in the care delivery system remain paper based. Paper-based medical records restrict access to information to one person at a time, require logistics to route and track the information so it is available where and when needed, and tend to be restricted to the organization producing the records. Multiorganizational involvement in an individual's care often results in multiple medical records; none of which are comprehensive, resulting in the promulgation of fragmentation. In addition, information in paper-based records hinders the aggregation of data and the ability to analyze it for purposes of care improvement.

Healthcare information systems have been developed and implemented to address specific functions. The independent development of systems addressing different functionalities has lead to difficulties in linking critical information necessary for complex decision making. One example of this is the historical separation between clinical and administrative data in healthcare organizations. The inability to link data from these two systems has been a barrier in situations such as the determination of relative cost-effectiveness across alternate care protocols.

Linking System Performance and Goals

Healthcare system performance must be focused on definable goals. Unfortunately, many goals are used in evaluating the performance of the healthcare system. Without a consensus on goals, a means to classify these goals into groups, and an agreement on their priorities, evaluations are difficult to interpret and often fail to establish critical agreement on the highest needs for system improvement.

The Institute of Medicine's critique of the U.S. healthcare system provided "Six Aims for the 21st Century Healthcare System" (Institute of Medicine, 2001). These aims call for healthcare to be safe, effective, patient centered, timely, efficient, and equitable. An integrated model of healthcare delivery needs to link system performance to the achievement of these goals.

Integrated Healthcare Delivery Model

The integrated healthcare delivery model shown in Figure 8.1 provides a framework that identifies the components of the healthcare delivery system and their functional relationships with each other. The model represents a process-driven rather than event-based view of healthcare.

Provider Levels

Four levels of change—individual provider, care team, organization, and environment—have been identified as necessary to effect and sustain improvements in healthcare delivery (Ferlie and Shortell, 2001). This multilevel approach is advocated to assure the inclusion of essential participants and their interactive effect on healthcare. The integrated healthcare delivery model borrows these four levels and portrays them as a basic component of the healthcare delivery system. It also extends this systems view by adding a critically important component, namely the individual/family.

The integrated healthcare delivery model is individual- and family-centric, emphasizing healthcare as a patient-centered process (Berwick, 2009). Although alternate terms for the individual may be used in this model (e.g., patient, consumer, service recipient), there are several important characteristics associated with this component. First, the individual is an essential and active participant in the delivery process. Without individual/family engagement in healthcare and their collaboration with the delivery system, desired outcomes cannot be achieved. Second, delivery processes should be customized to accommodate individual differences to facilitate effective engagement. The delivery of care needs to be tailored to the individual/family to accommodate socioeconomic, cultural, ethnic, and other factors that influence their expectations, engagement in effective self-care, and overall satisfaction with their healthcare providers. Finally, the model recognizes that healthcare delivery must seek a balance between outcomes measured in terms of the individual and those measured for a population.

Although both disease and system issues strongly influence healthcare delivery, they are not, in and of themselves, the central focus of the delivery process, as described here. The model portrays improvement of healthcare delivery as the result of consumer-focused innovations.

The family influences individual decisions and in some cases may serve as a proxy decision maker for the individual. The family can support adherence to care protocols and also shares in the responsibility for and impact of care outcomes. This focus on the individual and family applies throughout the life course—prenatal care, infancy, childhood, adolescence, adulthood, and advanced aging. It is this longitudinal need for integrated healthcare that forms the basis of the healthcare delivery model.

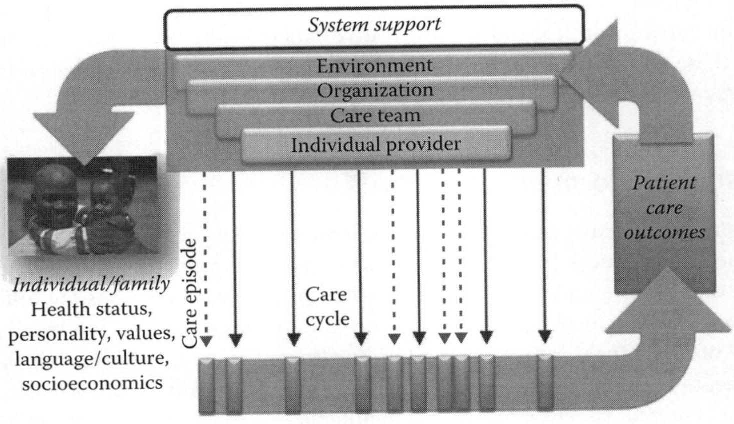

FIGURE 8.1 Integrated healthcare delivery model.

Working in collaboration with the individual/family are the integrated levels of healthcare providers. At the basic level are the individual providers. They perform the explicit tasks required to deliver healthcare. Next, the care team refers to the collective and coordinated efforts of these providers. Care can also be provided at the organizational level, meaning a business unit composed of healthcare professionals or teams working to produce coordinated services. Examples include a hospital or a pharmacy. As the levels of providers expand from individual providers, to care teams, and finally organizations, the scope and comprehensiveness of services also expand. Finally, the environment refers to a variety of care resources, including, but not limited to, state healthcare agencies, technology providers, financiers, policy makers, and regulators. The environment represents entities that finance healthcare, regulate care delivery, provide labor, and supply consumable goods, services, and technology. Although frequently not directly involved in delivering services to the individual and family, entities at the environment level enable service delivery.

Healthcare Delivery

The integrated healthcare delivery model represents care delivery as inclusive of four fundamental activities: (1) the provision of explicit services (e.g., diagnostic test, pharmaceutical dispensation, evaluation, and management services in a medical office setting); (2) care episodes (a complete, self-contained medical interaction between an individual and healthcare provider with a defined clinical objective); (3) care cycles (a series of care episodes required for the prevention, diagnosis, and treatment of a medical condition); and (4) system support (e.g., healthcare information and communications technology, scheduling systems, management information systems). Each of these is covered in greater detail below.

Explicit Services

The application of healthcare engineering in the delivery of explicit services may have the greatest commonality with engineering applications in other industries. The general focus of engineering at this level is to improve service processes. Outcomes typically relate to efficiency gains and safer operations. Efficiencies generally result from improved service methods and more effective resource consumption, whereas safety is often enriched through improved production quality and administration.

Some services may be required by providers or healthcare organizations at the time of use by the patient, such as an x-ray. Other services may be provided in off-site locations, such as clinical laboratory tests provided by a reference lab, and may necessitate additional logistical considerations, such as associated specimen transport and timely results reporting. When services are not able to be produced and stored in advance of their use, service capacity and demand characteristics (e.g., rate, variance) tend to become additional considerations.

Care Episodes

A care episode, as introduced earlier, represents a discrete healthcare event involving the delivery of a service or combination of services over a relatively short time period. Outcomes measured by efficiency and effectiveness are dependent on the quality of the service, the appropriate amount and type of service used, and the effective delivery and administration of that service. Effective delivery is intended to be inclusive of individual considerations such as allergies, concurrent contraindicated therapies, and individualized response to a therapeutic course.

Care episodes place additional demands on healthcare engineering over and above those considerations associated with explicit services. Greater complexity in clinical decision making due to the use of multiple services and the probability of multiple providers are representative of these additional considerations. Work design and task assignments can be critical, as is the information exchange necessary to properly coordinate multiple providers. The timing and sequencing of service delivery may add yet another level of complexity.

Although care episodes are critically important to the delivery process, it is interesting to note the seemingly divergent definitional points of view from the medical and engineering fields. The medical community would likely define a care episode in terms of a medical interaction between a patient and a healthcare provider. This emphasizes the care side of the event and is more person oriented in its description, for the medical profession generally looks to improve healthcare delivery by advancing individual care. The engineering community, on the other hand, would likely view a care episode as a point in time when the state of the delivery system (including the person's health status) may change (Pritsker, 1974; Pritsker and O'Reilly, 1999). As an example, when a person enters the hospital with a broken arm, the number of people in the emergency room is increased by one. Thus, the state of the system or, more precisely, the set of variable values used to describe the system has changed. This view is more system oriented, for engineers look to improve care to the individual by improving the process of care. This engineering perspective facilitates the application of engineering methods such as modeling. Both viewpoints have their place when seeking improvement in the delivery of care.

Care episodes occur in the delivery of care for individuals with either acute care or chronic care conditions. Acute care episodes (represented by the dashed arrows in Figure 8.1) capture the infrequent nature of care and represent the majority of care required to resolve the acute health problem. Chronic care episodes (represented by the solid arrows) depict separate care events that are likely to be repetitive in nature and associated with a longer duration of care. Individuals with diabetes, asthma, congestive heart failure, cancer, or depression may have chronic care episodes. Chronic care can last many years (if not a lifetime), encompasses a variety of care episodes, and may require an assortment of providers.

Care Cycles

People can experience both acute and chronic care episodes. Regardless of the type, though, a person's series of care episodes forms, what was mentioned earlier, a care cycle. This cycle provides a longitudinal, cumulative view of the person's care, in which review of and changes in his or her medical condition and treatment are represented.

A care cycle is defined relative to a medical condition (Porter and Teisberg, 2004). Principally, a cycle differs from a care episode only in scope, for a cycle is more comprehensive. It is inclusive of all the care necessary to create value for the patient. The value proposition is dependent on extending care to include: (1) assessment and reduction of risk through prevention and disease management, (2) treatment and associated rehabilitation, and (3) longitudinal care management involving multiple providers. This value is further enhanced when delivered in an integrated manner, enabling care coordination.

The contribution of care cycles to the integrated healthcare delivery model is to emphasize the value and importance of integrated care. In particular, care cycles provide a conceptual integration of services to help reduce the consequences of medical conditions.

Given the medical condition basis for defining care cycles, it follows that individuals may receive care for multiple conditions simultaneously and thus experience overlapping care cycles. In some situations, these cycles may be easily differentiated (e.g., a simultaneous acute episode for an individual with a chronic disease). In others, cycles may be difficult to distinguish from one another (e.g., an individual with multiple chronic conditions).

The resulting pattern of care episodes defines a frequency curve, represented by the cyclical arrows in Figure 8.2. This care frequency curve captures the increase and decrease in the number of episodes over a given time interval. It also highlights the variability in provider interaction with the patient—another challenge in healthcare delivery. More frequent and consistent monitoring and treatment should increase the span of time one is free of chronic disease and reduce the likelihood of that person's premature morbidity, disability, and death. Also impacting this care frequency curve is age. As people age, the frequency of medical care use usually increases, reflecting the uptrend in morbidity rates with this older population.

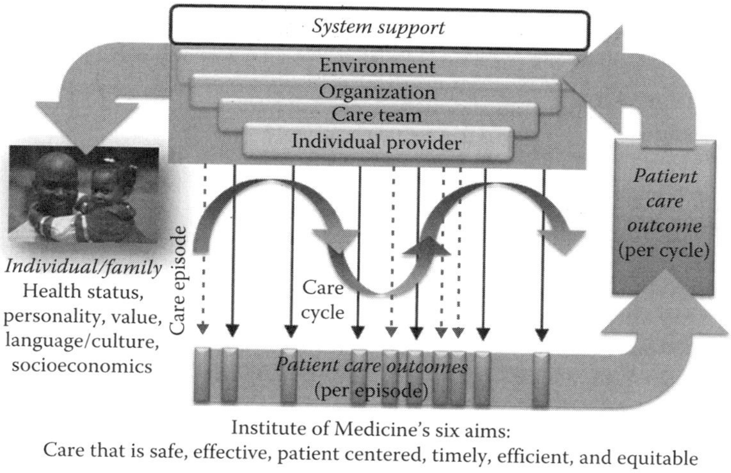

FIGURE 8.2 Care frequency curve and outcome aims.

System Support

The provision of healthcare by a complex delivery system requires significant support. System support, as the name implies, refers to the supplies and services that support the care delivery process. Examples of supplies include labor, consumables, information, technology, and capital. Services, on the other hand, cover things such as IT support and back-office operations like scheduling and financial reporting. Supply chains extend this support service concept beyond the organization. They refer to the iterative flow of money, information, and material from supplier to customer to satisfy the requisite needs of pharmacies and hospitals, for example.

Outcomes

For each care episode, there is an associated outcome, and the management of a person's care over time is based, in part, on the outcomes of previous care episodes. These outcomes provide feedback to inform both the provider and the individual on how to improve care delivery. For each care cycle, there is also an associated outcome that is partially dependent on the combination of episode outcomes, but is also dependent on the appropriate number, type, and timing of episodes relative to treatment of the medical condition. The care cycle outcome assessment then is a reflection of the level of care coordination in a person's treatment.

The development of metrics to measure outcomes and the application of this information for continuous improvement are essential aspects of the integrated healthcare delivery model. The delivery model utilizes the Institute of Medicine's six aims, stated earlier, as a statement of the general attributes of outcomes. Healthcare engineering can join research and development efforts of organizations like the Agency for Healthcare Research and Quality (www.ahrq.gov) and the National Quality Forum (www.qualityforum.org) to establish metrics to measure these attributes and create evaluative feedback loops for continued improvement in healthcare delivery.

Population Extension

As mentioned earlier, the integrated healthcare delivery model, in its base representation, centers on the individual. When considering population health, however, the model changes in dimension. In Figure 8.3, numerous delivery sequences are shown, representing healthcare use by a population. Simultaneous

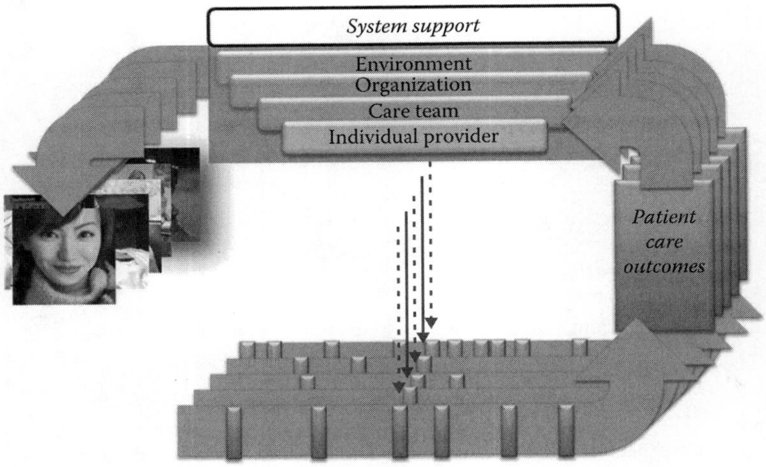

FIGURE 8.3 Population extension.

demand on the healthcare system is displayed by the series of arrows in the same time period. An example of this would be an immunization program. The actual act of immunizing an individual would be an example of an episode that seeks to provide an appropriate outcome relative to that person's needs. The population health perspective, on the other hand, addresses how the population's health outcomes would be best achieved. These outcomes may, in fact, be most effectively accomplished by not providing vaccination to all individuals at the time they request this explicit service, but by allocating the vaccine to individuals in the population based on their risk or potential to transmit infection. Investigations of this cross-section of care are germane to the study of healthcare delivery as is the orthogonal view of a person's care sequence, which has been emphasized to this point. It is the confluence of these two demand streams that captures another healthcare delivery challenge: honoring the requests of individuals while simultaneously serving the needs of the general public.

Research Opportunities

Healthcare engineering is replete with research opportunities. Areas of need are presented below using the concepts presented earlier as a framework for discussion.

Complexity

Microsystem and care platform concepts emphasize delivery system structure as an important aspect in a model of healthcare delivery and suggest that an elemental production view is useful in reducing complexity and enabling process reengineering. This structure provides a useful context in which to improve delivery efficiency and effectiveness. Engineering tools used to improve production in other industries can be adapted for application in the delivery of healthcare services.

Fragmentation

Organizing care in episodes is intended to promote efficient, effective, and timely integration of care services, thus reducing fragmentation and improving care coordination. An open question is how best to do this. Additional research opportunities exist in reconciling inconsistencies in simultaneously addressing system complexity and fragmentation. The imposition of a hierarchical structure for organizing care delivery includes the formation of small production units, whereas the reduction of fragmentation is accomplished through the integration of these units into a system of coordinated delivery. Healthcare engineering research can contribute to enhanced models of delivery efficiency and effectiveness that can be functionally integrated into higher performance systems. Implicit in this work is the need to evolve definitions of work product at the service and episodic levels, with associated determinants of required resources at each of these levels.

Acute to Chronic Care

Several research opportunities exist in the application of care cycles. First of all, some patients may have multiple coexisting conditions and/or multiple chronic illnesses. Clinical guidelines for many of these patients have not been sufficiently developed to determine when appropriate care is being delivered. Thus, in these situations, the ability to organize and evaluate care delivery using care cycles is limited by not having an ability to assign a distinct common medical condition with an associated consensus on appropriate care. Research into evidence-based treatment guidelines and the subsequent translation of these guidelines into cycle-managed care procedures could significantly improve patient care outcomes.

With the expansion of scope and duration of care associated with a cycle, the number of providers involved in the delivery process usually increases. The involvement of multiple providers has been linked to increased complexity in the delivery of care (Pham et al., 2007; Hussey et al., 2009). Research is required to develop and evaluate models for improving care coordination and reducing fragmentation that accompanies this type of complex longitudinal care. The Patient-Centered Medical Home is an example of a model that stresses the benefits of medical management provided in primary care practices (Kellerman and Kirk, 2007). Also, bundled reimbursement models provide financial incentives for provider self-organization to improve care coordination and reduce fragmentation (Hackbarth et al., 2008). Accountable Care Organizations represent yet another type of model with purported benefits for care coordination and efficiencies associated with more comprehensive healthcare delivery organizations (Fisher et al., 2007). Research evaluating the benefits associated with each of these models is critical. Healthcare delivery reengineering efforts need to be informed by these evaluations.

Increasing care coordination and reducing fragmentation through accountable care delivery models such as the Patient-Centered Medical Home and Accountable Care Organizations have a common prerequisite. They require reengineered care delivery processes with an emphasis on improving practice support systems. Research on the development and evaluation of effective practice support systems would fill an important operational gap in the fight to reduce fragmentation and improve care coordination.

A final concern with organizing healthcare delivery as an integrated model is that providers may not be able to assume complete responsibility for care outcomes. Individual and family involvement is particularly important, especially in relationship to chronic disease outcomes. The individual assumes critical responsibility for prevention, behavioral risk modification to avoid disease complications, and adherence to treatment plans. Research is required to improve care delivery systems that enable effective and consistent interfaces with patients and their families.

Healthcare Information and Communications Technology

Research on the development of healthcare information and communications technology is required as a corollary activity for most healthcare engineering. Research opportunities include resolving problems in the development of comprehensive, electronic patient care information systems and developing new ways to use this information to improve care delivery.

One fundamental problem in the development of information systems is resolving barriers to interoperability, that is, how information is exchanged and used across information systems to enable sufficiently comprehensive knowledge transfer. Interoperability can be an issue both within a healthcare organization and in sharing information among organizations. The previously mentioned need for integration of administrative data with clinical data is an example of the former. An example of the latter is the support for meaningful use of information accumulated across multiple organizations. Models for how this may be accomplished include Community Health Information Networks (Zinn, 1994), Regional Health Information Organizations (Lawrence, 2007), and Health Information Exchanges (Vreeman et al., 2008).

Another area of research in health information pertains to mitigating issues surrounding organizations adopting information technology. This research can be broadly grouped into three areas: (1) accommodating changing workflows as a result of new information system adoption, (2) improving factors associated with the use of this technology, and (3) designing and developing information systems that are affordable to the organizations purchasing these systems.

Ultimately, health information systems seek to improve the delivery of care, both to the individual and to the population. This requires research to identify the areas where new information may be applied for greatest benefit in diagnosing illnesses and executing coordinated care delivery.

Multidimensional Metrics

Measuring performance is critical for systems engineering to be effective in healthcare. Particularly important are the development of metrics for each of the attributes of healthcare outcomes and the design of monitoring systems to modify healthcare delivery to attain maximum safety, effectiveness, patient centeredness, and equitability. Most of the engineering methods that currently contribute to the improvement of healthcare delivery presume a single objective function. By adopting more than one attribute for healthcare outcomes, multiple objective analysis becomes a necessary consequence and the trade-offs among these objectives evolve into a central and interesting area of research.

Individual in the Integrated Healthcare Delivery Model

The integrated healthcare delivery model identifies patient-centered care as an attribute of outcome assessment. It furthermore recognizes the pertinent characteristics which require customization of care delivery to meet individual requirements. Additional work is required in healthcare engineering to achieve patient-centered care delivery tailored to these individual expectations and in a manner that achieves equitable and cost-effective care to a population.

Healthcare System in the Integrated Healthcare Delivery Model

Research on the interactions among members of the healthcare system can provide insights into how to improve care. To this end, effective use of healthcare information and communications technology is an important strategy, but significant work remains in determining: (1) what information is critical at various care stages, (2) how that information should be collected and presented to decision makers, (3) how to best interact with these information systems, and (4) how to exchange information across multiple members of the healthcare system to enable safe and efficient care delivery and longitudinal care coordination.

An area of particularly promising research is the use of information as feedback to the individual in support of effective self-care. This information may be presented to the individual in several forms. Personal health records, for example, may provide individuals with feedback on their efforts to reduce risk factors and serve to reinforce positive behavior change. When the personal health record is integrated with the provider's electronic health record, better coordination of individual and provider care may occur, resulting in improved health outcomes. For another direction for research, consider devices, for example, that remind individuals of the appropriate time to self-administer a pharmaceutical. If this feedback is presented in an efficient manner that is adjusted to the cultural and literacy needs of the patient and his or her family, care effectiveness can be significantly improved.

Care Episodes

Care episode effectiveness is likely a function of the degree to which provider services are congruent with evidenced-based guidelines. The implicit assumption is that when care is provided in a manner that adheres to these guidelines, health outcomes are better. Research is required to develop methods that can be used across multiple patient populations to determine whether the care actually delivered is consistent with these guidelines and what amount of deviation affects outcomes. Armed with this information, healthcare engineers would be able to measure the deviation between actual and evidenced-based care, determine system factors influencing these gaps, and redesign care systems accordingly.

Care Cycles

A fundamental question of interest is how to treat patients with multiple chronic illnesses. Should each condition be cared for independently? Are there contraindications for some of the care and where in the care cycle does this occur? Does the presence of multiple chronic conditions actually define a unique medical condition that requires exclusive treatment? Healthcare engineering can contribute to the development of this knowledge by measuring current approaches and correlating them to treatment outcomes.

System Support

Engineering can contribute significantly to improving the healthcare delivery system by focusing on factors associated with the organization and work of healthcare providers. Efforts directed to aiding effective self-care, such as appropriately timed screenings and adherence to jointly established treatment plans, are extremely important in disease prevention and maintenance. Process design to enable useful patient engagement also represents significant opportunities to improve health outcomes. In addition, opportunities to reengineer provider support systems (e.g., scheduling and warehouse management) and increase organizational effectiveness are plentiful. Increasing pressures for cost management in healthcare will continue to represent the need for work analyses and reduction of operating costs. The existing and projected shortages in critical professional categories will provide engineering challenges in work redesign and technology development to increase labor productivity. Other important opportunities exist for reengineering relationships among healthcare providers and other entities in the healthcare environment. Examples include redesigning healthcare supply chains and implementing e-commerce systems to streamline billing and payment between healthcare providers and payers.

Conclusion

The need for improvement in the U.S. healthcare system is now, as is the opportunity for significant impact. This chapter provides a brief overview of some of the fundamental barriers in the healthcare system, concepts of how to describe care delivery in an effort to overcome these barriers, and an integrated view of the healthcare process to highlight the need for a systems approach. Numerous healthcare engineering research opportunities were also advanced. The hope is that this will bring added attention to the healthcare engineering field and inspire continued advances in healthcare delivery.

References

Berwick, D. M. 2009. What 'patient-centered' should mean: Confessions of an extremist. *Health Aff.* 28(4): 555–565.

Bohmer, R. M. and D. M. Lawrence. 2008. Care platforms: A basic building block for care delivery. *Health Aff. (Millwood)* 27(5): 1336–1340.

Davis, K. 2007. Paying for care episodes and care coordination. *N. Engl. J. Med.* 356(11): 1166–1168.

Ferlie, E. B. and S. M. Shortell. 2001. Improving the quality of healthcare in the United Kingdom and the United States: A framework for change. *Milbank Q.* 79(2): 281–325.

Fisher, E. S., D. O. Staiger, J. P. Bynum, and D. J. Gottlieb. 2007. Creating accountable care organizations: The extended hospital medical staff. *Health Aff.* (*Millwood*) 26(1): w44–w57.

Gosfield, A. G. 2008. *PROMETHEUS Newsletter*. Issue 1 (December). http://www.rwjf.org/files/research/prometheus2008issue1.pdf

Hackbarth, G., R. Reischauer, and A. Mutti. 2008. Collective accountability for medical care—Toward bundled Medicare payments. *N. Engl. J. Med.* 359(1): 3–5.

Hussey, P. S., M. E. Sorbero, A. Mehrotra, H. Liu, and C. L. Damberg. 2009. Episode-based performance measurement and payment: Making it a reality. *Health Aff.* (*Millwood*) 28(5): 1406–1417.

Institute of Medicine. 2001. Crossing the Quality Chasm: A New Health System for the 21st Century (No. 0-309-07280-8). Washington, DC: National Academy Press.

Kellerman, R. and L. Kirk. 2007. Principles of the patient-centered medical home. *Am. Fam. Physician* 76(6): 774–775.

Lawrence, D. 2007. Doing it right. While the key to the perfect RHIO may still be a mystery, a number of them are off and running. *Healthc. Inform.* 24(9): 38–40.

Nelson, E., P. Batalden, T. Huber et al. 2001. *Microsystems in Health Care: The Essential Building Blocks of High Performing Systems*. Princeton, NJ: Robert Wood Johnson Foundation.

Paulus, R. A., K. Davis, and G. D. Steele. 2008. Continuous innovation in health care: Implications of the Geisinger experience. *Health Aff.* (*Millwood*) 27(5): 1235–1245.

Pham, H. H., D. Schrag, A. S. O'Malley, B. Wu, and P. B. Bach. 2007. Care patterns in medicare and their implications for pay for performance. *N. Engl. J. Med.* 356(11): 1130–1139.

Porter, M. E. 2009. A strategy for health care reform—Toward a value-based system. *N. Engl. J. Med.* 361(2): 109–112.

Porter, M. E. and E. O. Teisberg. 2004. Redefining competition in health care. *Harv. Bus. Rev.* 82(6): 65–76.

Pritsker, A. A. 1974. *The GASP IV Simulation Language*. New York: John Wiley & Sons.

Pritsker, A. A. and J. J. O'Reilly. 1999. *Simulation with Visual SLAM and AweSim*. New York: John Wiley & Sons.

Quinn, J. B. 1992. *Intelligent Enterprise: A Knowledge and Service Based Paradigm for Industry*. New York: The Free Press.

Reid, P. P., W. D. Compton, J. H. Grossman, and G. Fanjiang (eds.). 2005. *Building a Better Delivery System: A New Engineering/Health Care Partnership*. Washington, DC: National Academy Press.

Trisolini, M., J. Aggarwal, M. Leung, G. Pope, and J. Kautter. 2008. *The Medicare Physician Group Practice Demonstration: Lessons Learned on Improving Quality and Efficiency in Health Care*. New York: The Commonwealth Fund.

Vreeman, D. J., M. Stark, G. L. Tomashefski, D. R. Phillips, and P. R. Dexter. 2008. Embracing change in a health information exchange. *AMIA Annu. Symp. Proc.* 2008: 768–772.

Zinn, T. K. February 1994. A CHIN primer. *Health Manag. Technol.* 15(2): 28–32.

II

Performance Assessment and Process Improvement Management

9 **Performance Assessment for Healthcare Organizations** *Peter Arthur Woodbridge and George Oscar Allen* 9-1
Performance Measures Rationale • Healthcare Performance Measurement • Healthcare Performance Measurement Systems • Performance Assessment in the Veterans Health Administration • Healthcare Performance Measure Barrier • The Future • Summary • References

10 **Managing Physician Panels in Primary Care** *Hari Balasubramanian, Brian T. Denton, and Qi Ming Lin* 10-1
Introduction • Background and Literature • Patient Classifications • Managing Physician Panels • Emerging Trends in Primary Care • Summary and Conclusions • References

11 **Lean in Healthcare** *Philip C. Jones and Barrett W. Thomas* 11-1
Introduction • Lean Overview • Historical Perspective • Does Lean Work in Healthcare? • Analysis and Discussion • Conclusion • References

12 **Patient Safety and Proactive Risk Assessment** *Pascale Carayon, Hélène Faye, Ann Schoofs Hundt, Ben-Tzion Karsh, and Tosha B. Wetterneck* 12-1
Patient Safety and the Need for Proactive Risk Assessment • Proactive Risk Assessment • Practical Considerations of Proactive Risk Assessment • Case Studies • Conclusion • References

13 Toward More Effective Implementation of Evidence-Based Practice: Relational and Contextual Considerations *Priscilla A. Arling, Rebekah L. Fox, and Bradley N. Doebbeling* **13**-1
Evidence-Based Practice • Social Capital Theory • Conclusions • References

9

Performance Assessment for Healthcare Organizations

Peter Arthur Woodbridge
University of Nebraska Medical Center
and
Mid-West Mountain Veterans Engineering Resource Center
and
Nebraska-Western Iowa Healthcare System

George Oscar Allen
Nebraska-Western Iowa Healthcare System

Performance Measures Rationale 9-1
Healthcare Performance Measurement 9-3
Healthcare Performance Measurement Systems 9-5
Performance Assessment in the Veterans Health Administration 9-6
OQP and EPRP • IPEC
Healthcare Performance Measure Barrier 9-7
Establishing Performance Measures • Obtaining Performance Measure Data • Performance Measure Proliferation • Effectiveness of Individual Measures • Performance Measure Aggregation
The Future 9-9
Natural Language Processing • Operational Business Intelligence
Summary 9-11
References 9-12

Performance Measures Rationale

Performance measures "motivate, illuminate, and communicate" (Metzenbaum, 2006, p. 22). Performance measures motivate by enabling tangible goal-setting and factual feedback, which in turn clarifies expectations, promotes accountability, and shapes behavior. Performance measures illuminate by establishing objectivity and consistency, leading to enhanced problem solving, modeling, decision making, and progress tracking. Performance measures communicate by increasing the visibility of goal attainment and performance gaps, thereby focusing on organizational attention, understanding, and organizational alignment.

Performance measures motivate when linked to performance goals (Behn, 2003; Latham, 2004). Differences in goals account for differences in performance (Latham, 2004). Under circumstances of equal ability, individuals with difficult but specific goals outperform individuals with easy goals (Latham, 2004). Specific, difficult, goals lead to higher performance while general exhortations to "do better" do not (Locke and Latham, 2002). Goals have these effects without linkage to incentives or penalties (Latham, 2004).

The likelihood of achieving difficult performance goals increases with individual commitment (Klein et al., 1999). Commitment and effort directed to achieving specific goals rests on self-efficacy (Bandura, 2004) and the perceived importance of the goals (Locke and Latham, 2002). Self-efficacy in this context is the belief that one can attain a specific goal. The effort that an individual puts into achieving a performance goal increases with task difficulty up to the point of limits in ability or commitment (Locke and Latham, 2002).

Performance does not depend on who sets the goal (Latham, 2004). Goal commitment and performance is equal whether goal setting was participatory (the individual participated in deciding the goal) or assigned (someone in authority assigned the goal) (Latham, 2004). However, there are two exceptions: (1) assigned goals are less effective if the person assigning the goal is terse and does not take time to explain the logic or rationale for the goal and (2) assigned goals are more sensitive to the impact of self-efficacy (Locke and Latham, 2002).

Once specific measurable goals have been set, regular reporting of summary (feedback) data motivates and sustains performance (Locke and Latham, 2002). Individuals adjust their effort and strategies when they receive data that tracks their progress toward goal attainment (Locke and Latham, 2002). With complex goals or goals that rest on discovery to uncover solutions, setting proximal (intermediate) goals, seeking and receiving frequent quantitative performance measure feedback, and reacting to that feedback accelerates goal attainment (Dorner, 1991; Frese and Zapf, 1994; Latham and Seijts, 1999).

Performance measures may also contribute to organizational dysfunction (Spitzer, 2007). In particular, performance measurement drives dysfunctional behavior when used for both positive reinforcement (rewards) and negative reinforcement (punishment) (Spitzer, 2007). Measurement dysfunction manifests itself in many forms: "studying to the test" (doing only what is needed to attain a high score regardless of impact on actual service or quality); "gaming the system" (e.g., selecting the clinics "that count" while ignoring those that are not included in the measure); and "cheating" (engaging in dishonest behavior to the point of breaking laws and policies). Pay for performance in particular can lead to dysfunctional behavior (Hayward and Kent, 2008).

The degree to which individuals engage in performance measurement-driven dysfunctional behavior is a function of the individual and organizational context (Spitzer, 2007). Some individuals so fear performance measures that they will engage in dysfunctional behaviors (Metzenbaum, 2006). Performance measurement fear-driven behaviors include: data manipulation; accountability avoidance (e.g., "I cannot be held accountable for this measure—I do not control the entire system"); attempts to dismantle or discredit measurement systems (e.g., prolonged discussions on the statistical validity of the system of metrics); and attempts to negotiate watered-down measures (Metzenbaum, 2006). Watered-down performance measures can take several forms (Metzenbaum, 2006, p. 40)—e.g., a goal that is incremental rather than transformative, process or output measures rather than outcome measures. Key contextual elements that determine how individuals in an organization respond to performance measures include: organizational climate (e.g., learning organization or coercive bureaucracy), organizational values (e.g., quarterly profitability or "doing the right thing"), leadership attitudes to measurement (e.g., data or relationship driven), past experiences with measurement (e.g., positive or punitive), method of communication (e.g., terse or explanatory), and availability of resources to measure and improve (Spitzer, 2007).

Using peer performance measure comparisons yields mixed results (Bandura and Cervone, 1983). Individuals respond differently to comparison and competition (Metzenbaum, 2006, p. 22). Some individuals treat publication of highest performance scores as a de facto goal; for others, it acts as an inhibitor (Tauer and Harackiewicz, 1999). An individual's reaction to comparison is tempered by organizational culture, the perceived fairness of the comparison (Greenburg, 2004), and links to rewards and penalties (Metzenbaum, 2006, p. 22). Inaccurate measures used for ranking are particularly disaffecting (Metzenbaum, 2006, p. 25). Ranking tends to discourage performance by diminishing self-efficacy for the 50% of individuals below the mean (Bandura, 2004).

The method of presenting peer comparative data impacts its acceptance and the reaction of individuals (Metzenbaum, 2006, p. 22). Publishing comparisons in rank order can be particularly alienating while allowing individuals to opt-in or opt-out of the comparison improves acceptance (Metzenbaum, 2006, p. 23). Opting in and out enables individuals that thrive on competition to self-select for comparisons (Metzenbaum, 2006, p. 22). Informing individuals of their scores privately (but not rank), of the group median, and of the score of the leader seems to be effective (Metzenbaum, 2006, p. 24). Multidimensional comparisons add to complexity and are only useful if they support drill-down to individual measures that contribute to the performance gap (Metzenbaum, 2006, p. 24).

While comparative ranking of individuals as a motivational tool yields mixed results, comparative ranking does improve performance as a tool for illumination (Metzenbaum, 2006, p. 25). Identifying performance leaders enables others to learn and emulate (Metzenbaum, 2006).

Performance measures serve to illuminate in a number of ways (Metzenbaum, 2006; Spitzer, 2007). Performance measures illuminate by creating objectivity (Spitzer, 2007). Discussions and decision making are driven by data rather than opinion. Unexpected findings (anomalies and outliers) signal a need for deeper investigation (Metzenbaum, 2006). Performance measure fallout clusters suggest patterns that require analysis and investigation (Metzenbaum, 2006). Uniformly measured and applied performance measures, particularly in large corporate environment, create consistency and support informed decision making (Spitzer, 2007). Comparative performance measurement facilitates problem solving (Spitzer, 2007). Identifying performance leaders serves to identify better practices and systems that can inform others. Identifying performance laggards serves to focus attention on systems or groups that need assistance. Trending performance measures enables prediction and forecasting (Spitzer, 2007).

Performance measures serve as a communication tool within organizations (Metzenbaum, 2006; Spitzer, 2007). They increase visibility of performance. In doing so, they create a climate of transparency (Metzenbaum, 2006). By highlighting specific elements of performance, they help focus organizational attention, build organizational alignment, and clarify expectations (Spitzer, 2007). As such, they serve as a shorthand method to communicate status, thereby enhancing understanding (Metzenbaum, 2006; Spitzer, 2007). Trending communicates direction both by predicting movement toward success and by providing early warning of emerging performance gaps (Metzenbaum, 2006; Spitzer, 2007).

Healthcare Performance Measurement

Since performance measures have such a wide range of applications and a large impact on organizational behavior, performance measurement selection is a vital function of organizational leaders (Spitzer, 2007). However, in performance measure selection, pitfalls abound. Although serving as vital signs, routine measures (monitoring metrics) do not engender high performance (Spitzer, 2007)—they simply reflect the overall health of the organization. Too many measures (particularly, if not focusing) send mixed signals as to priorities (Spitzer, 2007). Too many challenging measures may be overwhelming and contribute to loss of self-efficacy and dysfunctional behavior (Locke and Latham, 2002). Measures that are not been strenuously tested for validity and for impact may alienate key stakeholders. As a result, new measures should be introduced as "emergent" and thoroughly tested before being tied to performance (Spitzer, 2007). Consequently, leaders should only select performance measures that drive strategic objectives or track key (process) performance indicators (KPI).

As an example, consider the potential impact of a "length of stay" performance measure that seeks to motivate improved efficiency and better coordination of care processes. If tied to incentives without a balancing measure of readmission rates or patient mortality, the length of stay measure may drive premature discharge with a concomitant decline in patient outcomes and safety.

Not only does healthcare performance measurement contain the pitfalls common to performance measurement in general, but it also involves additional challenges. Healthcare is inherently complex involving thousands of illnesses with outcomes that depend not only on delivery systems but also on interactions of diseases (co-morbidities), prior medical history, patient genetic variability, and patient compliance. Adding to this complexity is a multiplicity of perspectives (providers, patients, payers) and fragmentation of care delivery (inpatient, outpatient, home care, specialization) that lead to performance measures defined by safety, disease-specific processes (timeliness as well as adherence to evidence-based standards of care), patient needs (staying healthy, getting better, living with illness or disability, coping with end of life), delivery system effectiveness and efficiency, and the incorporation of infrastructural elements (electronic health record [EHR], systematic approach to care coordination, and transitions in care). These complexities make assigning performance accountability for healthcare performance measures particularly difficult.

Recognizing this difficulty in measuring healthcare quality and therefore in creating healthcare performance measures, Donabedian (1980, 1988) developed a framework for healthcare measures that differentiates structural, process, and outcomes measures (Table 9.1). As a rationale for his model, Donabedian (1980) suggested that organizational structure influences processes and processes in turn determine outcomes. "Structure" refers to those attributes of the healthcare setting such as space and layout, equipment, human resources, and supporting infrastructure (e.g., electronic medical record system) that are organizationally foundational. "Processes" are the activities that healthcare workers engage in to deliver care. "Outcomes" are the consequences to the patient that can be attributed to the patient's encounter with the healthcare system. Outcomes are characterized as being "distal" (e.g., impact on life expectancy, quality of life, progression of a chronic disease) or "proximal" (sometimes referred to as "intermediate").

Diabetes outcomes measures are illustrative. Diabetes distal outcomes measures include dialysis, leg amputation, and blindness. Diabetes proximal measures include hemoglobin A1C (glycosylated hemoglobin; the extent of hemoglobin glycosylation is a function of mean blood glucose concentration). Process measures would include the frequency of measuring hemoglobin A1C. A structural measure might include the presence of a clinical reminder system that alerts clinicians of the need to measure a hemoglobin A1C level during a clinic visit.

Proximal outcomes measures differ from process measures in that: (1) they are highly correlated with distal outcomes—a patient with hemoglobin A1C levels over 9% has a very high likelihood of developing renal failure requiring dialysis, peripheral neuropathy leading to lower limb amputation, and retinopathy leading to blindness; (2) they depend on a number of processes.

The Donabedian model, although useful for stratifying healthcare performance measures, fails to address a major contributor to poor patient outcomes—fragmentation of care. Healthcare's complexity by necessity leads to specialization. Treatment by multiple providers and systems leads to "handoffs" that create discontinuities in care that contributes to breakdowns in process and outcomes. The

TABLE 9.1 Donabedian Framework Strengths and Limitations

	Strengths	Limitations
Structure	Expedient	Difficult to independently measure (requires auditing)
	Efficient—one measure may cover many processes	Not actionable in short term (often requires substantial redesign and capital investment)
	Often highly predictive of outcomes	
Process	Reflects care received	Sample size constraints—particularly for diseases with low prevalence
	Some are intrinsically valued by patients (e.g., timeliness of access)	Prone to confounding by patient compliance and co-morbidities
	Directly actionable	Subject to manipulation and other forms of dysfunctional improvement behavior
	Attributable to individuals and their actions	Variable linkage to outcomes—a single process measure may not be predictive of overall disease control
	More likely to be accepted by providers particularly if evidence based	May lead to system suboptimization and
	Supportive of a learning organization—improvements can be tracked and shared	May not reflect patient needs (technical quality vs. quality from patient perspective)
	Usually does not require risk adjustment	
Outcomes	Face validity—patients and healthcare providers would agree measure reflects current state	Sample size constraints
	Motivates meaningful improvement	Lag—distal outcomes may not be apparent for years
	Promotes whole-system perspective	Difficulty in establishing proximal outcomes measures
	Stimulates innovation and investment	Difficulty in overtly linking to specific process improvements
		Expense and difficulty of data collection
		Complexity—often requires risk adjustment

Sources: Adapted from IOM Committee on Redesigning Health Insurance Performance Measures, Payment and Performance Improvement Programs & Board on Health Care Services, *Performance Improvement Accelerating Improvement*, National Academies Press, Washington, DC, 2006; Goddard, M. et al., *J. R. Soc. Med.*, 95, 508, 2002.

resulting fragmentation of care delivery and responsibility leads to a natural tendency for individuals in healthcare systems to focus only on performance within their immediate work unit. It also contributes a confounding dimension to healthcare performance measures.

Performance measures directed at individual work units carry substantial risk of compartmentalization and suboptimization (Spitzer, 2007). Consider the following example. A healthcare system has a sophisticated EHR that includes a clinical alerts system that brings unexpected clinical findings to the attention of clinicians. The alerts system is triggered by data elements and has proven effectiveness. The referral department of a medical center within the system sets itself a goal of having patients seen by outside specialists and the reports of that visit in the medical record within 30 days. The referral department develops a strategy for achieving this goal by having the referring specialist fax their reports to the medical center. The faxed reports are scanned into the EHR as images, thereby bypassing the EHR's clinical alerts system, thereby putting patients at risk of providers overlooking critical information. The department while optimizing its system has undermined the overall goal of safety.

The vertical and horizontal integration of performance measures ensures alignment of performance measures in healthcare's fragmented care delivery model but it also adds complexity to healthcare performance measurement. Vertical integration connects departments to organizational strategies; horizontal integration connects the activities of departments to each other (Spitzer, 2007). Organizational strategies are generally abstract (e.g., patient-centered care, effective care, equitable care). Vertical integration translates abstract strategies into performance measures that impact individual work units (Spitzer, 2007). The horizontal integration of performance measures reduces compartmentalization and mitigates suboptimization. Without horizontal integration, performance measures may reinforce departmental "silos" (Spitzer, 2007).

With its interest in transforming healthcare safety, the U.S. Institutes of Medicine (IOM) launched the Redesigning Health Insurance Performance Measures, Payment, and Performance Improvement Project ("IOM PM Redesign") in 2004. Among other goals, the IOM PM Redesign project team focused on developing a framework for selecting of a national set of healthcare performance measures. Building on the work of Donabedian (1980), the IOM PM Redesign team (IOM Committee on Redesigning Health Insurance Performance Measures, Payment and Performance Improvement Programs & Board on Healthcare Services, 2006, p. 99) established the following criteria for healthcare performance measures: scientifically sound; feasible (balance cost of obtaining against impact); important (related to the IOM goals of safety, effectiveness, patient-centeredness, timeliness, efficiency, and equity (IOM Committee on Quality of Healthcare in America, 2000)); aligned with existing recommendations and usage; and comprehensive (not only tracks disease, but also provides information on the delivery system including underuse, overuse, misuse). They advocated the performance measure design principles summarized in Table 9.2.

Healthcare Performance Measurement Systems

Although there is developing interest in a single, unified, independent healthcare performance measurement system (IOM Committee on Redesigning Health Insurance Performance Measures, Payment and Performance Improvement Programs & Board on Health Care Services, 2006), healthcare performance measurement in the United States remains fragmented. A large number of agencies have developed measurement sets that reflect their priorities and interests. Among the more commonly adopted systems are

- HEDIS—Developed by the National Committee on Quality Assurance (NCQA) as the Health Plan Employer Data and Information Data Set, the HEDIS data set focuses primarily on outpatient process measures including prevention, disease management, access, and utilization. The National Quality Forum and the Department of Veterans Affairs use expanded HEDIS data sets (NCQA, 2009).

TABLE 9.2 Healthcare Performance Measure Design Principles

Design Principle	Summary
Comprehensive	Measure all aspects of care: Safety, effectiveness, patient-centeredness, timeliness, efficiency, equity, coherent, robust
Accurate and credible	Supported by high-quality, peer-reviewed, published research; statistically sound; transparent; open and available
Longitudinal	Characterize health and healthcare within delivery systems, across delivery systems, and over time
Support multiple uses	For example, accountability, quality improvement, population health
Intrinsic to care	Data regarding process and outcome should be captured as byproducts of the care process and not require manual collection or extraction. The intrinsic data should facilitate near real-time performance monitoring and feedback and efficient data collection
Express the patient's voice	Healthcare performance measures should include data on patients' perceptions of process and outcomes
Provide multiple perspectives	Demonstrate success for individuals, populations, and systems
Shared accountability	Measures should promote individual and team accountability
Learning system	Measures should advance organizational learning; measures should evolve continuously in response to organizational learning
Independent	Data should be collected and analyzed in such a way that it cannot be manipulated by stakeholders in the outcome
Sustainable	The performance measure system should add value so that funding is assured

Source: Adapted from IOM Committee on Redesigning Health Insurance Performance Measures, Payment and Performance Improvement Programs & Board on Health Care Services, *Redesigning Health Insurance Performance Measures, Payment, and Performance Improvement Project*, National Academies Press, Washington, DC, 2006, pp. 166–169.

- OASIS—Developed by the Centers for Medicare and Medicaid Services (CMS) as the Outcome and Assessment Information Set, OASIS measures adult home care services (OASIS, 2009).
- MDS—Developed by the CMS as the Minimum Data Set (MDS), the MDS 2.0 includes 34 indicators of long-term (nursing home) care quality (CMS, 2009).
- ORYX™—Developed by the Joint Commission, the ORYX measures stipulate a set of performance measures for organizations involved in the entire long-term care process, nursing homes, home care agencies, durable medical equipment suppliers (Joint Commission, 2009b).
- NPSG—Developed by the Joint Commission as the National Patient Safety Goals, the NPSG establishes performance measures and goals for all aspects of patient care directed at reducing morbidity and mortality surrounding high vulnerability care processes identified through the Joint Commission's "sentinel event" root cause analysis reporting system as well as through an ongoing systematic review of the medical literature (Joint Commission, 2009a).
- NQF—The National Quality Foundation, a nonprofit organization representing a wide-range of healthcare stakeholders, endorses 537 healthcare performance measure data sets that encompass a wide range of domains of healthcare (National Quality Foundation, 2009b).
- AHRQ—The Agency for Healthcare Research and Quality maintains the National Quality Measure Clearinghouse™, the Consumer Assessment of Healthcare Providers and Systems (CAHPS), and "AHRQuality Indicators" inpatient care measurement sets (Agency for Healthcare Research and Quality, 2009).

Performance Assessment in the Veterans Health Administration

The Veterans Health Administration (VHA) of the Department of Veterans Affairs (VA), serving 5.34 million veterans in a network of 139 medical centers and more than 880 clinics delivers arguably some of the best and most cost-effective healthcare in the United States (Jha et al., 2003; Asch and McGlynn, 2004; Kerr et al., 2004; Selim et al., 2006; Oliver, 2007). That was not always the case. Starting in 1995, the VHA underwent a remarkable transformation. The key elements of that transformation were: implementation of capitated funding, the development and universal adoption of an EHR, and the implementation of a comprehensive set of performance measures (Jha et al., 2003; Oliver, 2007).

OQP and EPRP

VHA began measuring performance measures in 1996 as part of its multidimensional program to improve quality. Initial measures focused on evidence-based clinic performance measures. Named the "external peer review program" (EPRP), the program initially targeted clinical data from randomly selected charts. While not sufficient to ensure statistical validity on a monthly basis for individual medical centers, the EPRP had statistical validity to measure national performance monthly and medical center performance over the cumulative average for the entire year. In 1997, the VHA Undersecretary for Health established the National Clinical Practice Guideline Council to oversee the adoption, development, and implementation of practice guidelines throughout the VHA. The council, among other functions, identifies and prioritizes clinical areas in need of guidelines and performance measures. Customer satisfaction, access, and administrative (business measures) were added later.

In 2009, the VHA tracked 120 performance measures (81 clinical, 29 access, 7 functional status, and 3 patient satisfaction) and 193 "supporting indicators" (177 clinical, 11 access, and 5 functional). VHA supporting indicators differ from performance measures only in the weight attributed during annual reviews of senior leaders at medical centers, regional networks, and national leaders.

IPEC

With its success in using clinical guidelines and performance measures to transform outpatient care, the VHA launched the Inpatient Evaluation Center (IPEC) in 2005. Initially focusing on critical care, IPEC provides risk-adjusted performance measure data on acute care mortality rates, length of stay, and compliance with evidence-based practice. By focusing on inpatient care performance through the IPEC performance measurement system, the VHA has observed significant and substantial reductions in avoidable inpatient mortality, reductions in length of stay, and increased compliance with evidence-based medicine (Render and Almenoff, 2009).

Healthcare Performance Measure Barrier

As healthcare systems such as the VHA, agencies such as CMS and AHRQ, and organizations such as the IOM, JC, and NQF develop systems for assessing healthcare performance, significant challenges persist.

Establishing Performance Measures

Clinical guidelines drive many healthcare performance measures. However, the process of developing clinical guidelines is neither well standardized nor well controlled (Sniderman and Furberg, 2009), thereby contributing to physician and other clinician skepticism of clinical guideline-derived performance measures. Clinical guidelines in theory are evidence based and not opinion based. However, in many instances, the medical evidence is incomplete or the strength of the evidence is not adequately evaluated by committees and groups establishing clinical guidelines (Sniderman and Furberg, 2009). As a result, committees and groups establishing clinical guidelines often resort to expert consensus and other less scientifically rigorous methods of establishing clinical guidelines.

Not only is the process of developing performance measures suboptimal but also substantive gaps exist in the structure of current measurement systems (IOM Committee on Redesigning Health Insurance Performance Measures, Payment and Performance Improvement Programs & Board on Health Care Services, 2006). The IOM "Crossing the Chasm" (IOM Committee on Quality of Health Care in America, 2001) domains of patient-centered care, equity of care, and efficiency of care are underrepresented; most measures are "points in time" rather than representations of patient health over time; most profile care providers rather than patients (the success of a provider in achieving measurement goals across many measures rather than the success of the provider in achieving multiple measurement goals for individual patients); measures are directed at holding individual providers rather than teams or systems accountable for goals; the effectiveness and efficiency of transitions in care (movement of patients from one care setting to another) is not regularly measured in spite of a literature indicating the risk of transitions in care (IOM Committee on Redesigning Health Insurance Performance Measures, Payment and Performance Improvement Programs & Board on Health Care Services, 2006).

Obtaining Performance Measure Data

Collecting performance data for analysis is an endemic problem in healthcare enterprises. Clinical data is difficult to obtain. In many healthcare systems, not all clinical data is captured electronically. Even when it is, as it is in the VHA, much of it is in the form of unformatted text and, therefore, difficult to extract. Clinical systems are not intended as business process monitoring systems. Much process data is not captured in the EHR, creating substantive gaps in the ability of healthcare organizations to track KPI.

Performance Measure Proliferation

The proliferation of clinical guidelines, and their associated performance measures, is a growing problem. The VHA in 2009 had 259 performance measures tied to clinical guidelines. The National Guideline Clearinghouse maintained by the AHRQ currently lists 2458 clinical guidelines (Agency for Healthcare Research and Quality, 2009). The IOM in its recommendations for a National Quality Coordination Board recommends a "starter set" of 138 performance measures in addition to surveys of services and consumer satisfaction (IOM Committee on Redesigning Health Insurance Performance Measures, Payment and Performance Improvement Programs & Board on Health Care Services, 2006). Not only does tracking a large number of measures impose a substantial overhead on organizations, but it creates problems of focus (Latham, 2004).

Effectiveness of Individual Measures

In time, as individuals and organizations attain performance measures goals, the effectiveness of the measures attenuates as there is too little dispersion between high and low performing sites limiting meaningful comparison and assessment of quality improvement direction. For example, many VHA medical centers scored better than 90% on at least 50% of the 313 VHA's 2009 performance goals and monitors (Francis, 2009). With little dispersion in performance, small, often statistically, insignificant changes in performance can lead to radical changes in rankings, thereby contributing to staff dissatisfaction with the performance measurement system. It also creates a sense of complacency ("we are good"), which undermines the development of a continuous improvement organization.

Performance Measure Aggregation

Aggregation of healthcare performance measures to create "composite scores," "balanced-scorecards," and "dashboards" is an area of active interest and research. Although extensively used in other industries, healthcare does not systematically employ performance measure aggregation.

While proposed as a tool to motivate excellence (Nolan and Berwick, 2006), healthcare systems and performance measurement setting agencies and groups have been slow to adopt the aggregation of individual performance measures into composite scores. For example, the NQF only recently approved criteria for evaluating composite measures (National Quality Foundation, 2009a). In addition to the barriers to developing individual measures, developing composite measure entails additional socio-technical barriers. There is no universally accepted method for aggregating healthcare performance measure into composite scores. Common methods for aggregation of healthcare measures into composite scores include: (1) "all-or-none" (all indicators for a patient must be met for care to be considered a success); (2) "70% standard" (similar to all-or-none but with a more lenient—70%—threshold); (3) "overall percentage" (number of successful indicators for all patients over total number of opportunities); (4) "indicator average" (percentage of time indicators met are averaged across all indicators); and (5) "patient average" (the percentage of time-triggered indicators met for each patient are averaged across all patients) (Reeves et al., 2007). In a comparison of these five methods for aggregating quality measures, Reeves et al. (2007) found that different methods for calculating composite scores led to substantially different conclusions as to performance. They found the differences in conclusions rested not only on differences in the method of aggregation but also on patient populations within the composite measurement cohort.

An additional confounding factor in performance measurement aggregation, is the lack of consensus on how to weigh distal and catastrophic outcomes (e.g., a patient's death), proximal outcomes, process, and structural measures. The degree to which these factors are weighted, how performance measure range of variability, and tracking survival instead of mortality can drastically alter scores and rankings (O'Brien et al., 2007).

According to Kaplan and Norton (1996), while the primary purpose of composite scores is to motivate, the primary purposes of balanced scorecards are to communicate strategic goals objectively and illuminate gaps between strategic goals and current performance. Balanced scorecards are a systemized effort to create horizontal and vertical integration of performance measures and align them with organizational strategic goals. In the balanced scorecard, KPI are grouped into four perspectives: financial, customer, internal process, and innovation and learning. KPI are selected based on their capacity to provide insight as to operational alignment with organizational strategies (Kaplan and Norton, 1992). "Strategy maps" facilitate the identification of balanced scorecard KPI (Kaplan and Norton, 2008). While some healthcare systems have adopted balanced scorecards (Shutt, 2003), most have not (Kocakülâh and Austill, 2007). In addition to the barriers that inhibit performance measurement in healthcare in general, barriers unique to the adoption of balanced scorecards in healthcare include linking the balanced scorecard to positive and negative rewards (Chang, 2007) and challenges with information overload, synthesis of information and judgment bias (Chan, 2009).

Data dashboards enable the aggregation of balanced scorecard KPI that are meaningful from multiple perspectives (Kaplan and Norton, 2008). As such, they serve to motivate performance as well as communicating strategic plans and illuminating performance gaps. Notwithstanding their effectiveness, healthcare organizations have not widely adopted dashboards—perhaps because the aggregation of performance measures is an emerging field.

The Future

Recent developments in medical and business informatics have potential for addressing many of the barriers to healthcare performance measurement. Natural language process (NLP) and "business intelligence" in particular have enormous potential for addressing performance measure data acquisition, performance measure proliferation, the effectiveness of individual measures, and performance measure aggregation.

Natural Language Processing

In the VHA's EHR, as within most EHRs, information about a patient's health status is stored in either structured (e.g., vital sign data, diagnoses, lab results, etc.) or in unstructured (e.g., provider notes, surgical summaries, admit and discharge summaries, etc.) fields. A great deal of essential information about a patient's health that would be useful in performance measures is contained in the unstructured fields. For instance, a patient's vital sign data might tell us that her heart rate was rapid and oxygen saturation was low, but the nursing assessment note would contain additional information such as labored breathing, skin color, and level of consciousness.

Historically, access to this unstructured medical record data meant laborious and expensive chart reviews to extract essential performance measurement information. The VHA EPRP program is one such example. Furthermore, since most chart reviews are focused on a single health indicator, other essential information is passed over as it does not fit the search criteria.

Being able to effectively, efficiently, and consistently mine information from these unstructured notes is the goal of NLP. What NLP promises is the ability to search through unstructured data for relevant terms and the conditional elements around those terms that help define their context and turn these results into useful information. This is not just a simple process of searching for matching strings and extracting them. Since grammar in unstructured text is often ambiguous with multiple variations in interpretation, NLP uses various techniques to weigh the most appropriate interpretation based on semantics and context. Factors such as whether a term is negative or not (negation), in what sequence events occurred (temporality), the sense of a term (simile and morphology), and many others are weighted and that weight is then a value that can be analyzed.

The information gained from NLP can then be used with existing structured data to enhance performance measurement. For example, a patient would self-report that they abstain from tobacco use, which would be stored in a structured health factor field in the EHR. However, a nurse's noted observation that the patient had a pack of cigarettes in his shirt pocket and smelled of tobacco smoke would indicate that he is actually a smoker. This same set of information would be useful in determining the effectiveness of a smoking cessation program, if the patient was given information about the program but subsequent notes indicated that he still smelled of smoke and that he was carrying a pack of cigarettes.

Using NLP to gather information from text stored in the medical record will facilitate data extraction so it can be interpreted, collated, measured, and utilized to improve patient care processes. Academic institutions, private sector healthcare systems, and the VHA are testing current NLP systems so as to understand their effectiveness and to develop algorithms better suited to healthcare. The VHA's Consortium for Health Informatics Research (CHIR) mission is to conduct basic and applied research to advance the effective use of unstructured health record data by VHA clinicians, investigators, and clinician-investigators. The CHIR's work will enable the VHA to extract the vast amount of performance data currently locked within medical record notes.

Operational Business Intelligence

As the healthcare marketplace moves toward widespread adoption of EHR through mandates and market pressures, an opportunity has arisen to improve the accuracy, immediacy, and effectiveness of performance measurement practices through online analytical processing (OLAP) systems and operational business intelligence (OBI) analytics. The goal of OBI is to provide near real-time information to clinicians and care delivery managers regarding the performance of healthcare systems.

As with long standing paper practices, current EHR programs are "transactional" in nature, i.e., they are designed to make individual transactions operate quickly and smoothly. A user can check the status of an individual patient, record events of the current encounter, and store test results for future use. However, this speed and ease of use on the front end does not necessarily present an ideal platform for performance measurement.

OLAP systems take the data gathered by transactional systems and transform it into data that can be rearranged and analyzed so as to generate information. OLAP systems are not designed to speed up a single transaction but, rather, to allow for the grouping of many transactions into views of the processes of the business. With advances in technology providing cheaper access to more storage space and processing power, either locally or in the computer network "cloud," OLAP systems can now be an integral part of any EHR.

OBI analytics is a relatively new term placed upon a very logical but often overlooked practice of applying business rules to data to produce intelligence and, ultimately, knowledge. OBI analytics enables the automation of balanced scorecards, data aggregations, and composite scores, thereby not only addressing the complexity of healthcare performance measurement but also aligning the measures and organizations with strategic plans. Applying OBI to the information produced by OLAP systems creates actionable intelligence that not only communicates performance but enables prediction over time.

Implementing OBI codifies business rules across an organization's information so as to establish the "truth" that the organization as a whole uses to guide its decisions. This "truth" is based on the organization's strategic goals and incorporates the performance criteria that the organization uses as a benchmark. A clear benefit of this codification is that each level of the organization sees the same "truth" because it is realized using the same set of rules. Therefore, if the Chief of Staff is seeing an improvement or degradation in a performance measure, the staff members whose actions impact that measurement can see their piece of that "truth" and how their actions impact the measure. By linking all contributors to outcomes, vertical and horizontal integration is achieved.

KPI are the "canary" metrics that connect processes to outcomes. These are process metrics that indicate the health of the subsystems that contribute to outcomes—much as canaries did in coal mines. As gaps in performance are identified, KPI linked to outcomes through OBI not only track progress but also provide feedback on improvement effectiveness.

One of the significant drawbacks to current performance metric systems is that the reporting of the metric is delayed by weeks and even months, depending on the reporting system, making it very difficult to understand the effect of implemented process changes. OLAP and OBI can alleviate this problem. As patient encounters occur, the OLAP system gathers the data together and analyzes it based on the OBI rules. Depending on how OLAP is implemented, the latency of the data being available for analysis can be almost immediate. This is the case for many manufacturing systems in current use, and is the goal of a project being rolled out in the VHA known as the Corporate Data Warehouse (CDW). Using mirrored server systems, transactions that occur in the production clinical environment are gathered by the structured query language (SQL) OLAP system within seconds. Rapid access to OLAP data and feedback through OBI greatly shortens the cycle time for performance improvement.

OBI enables the integration of data from multiple sources. For instance, comparative data from a national database can be accessed and integrated to report how the local facility's performance compares to like facilities elsewhere. This integration is part of an overall knowledge management platform strategy that applies the same business rules to the information no matter where that information originates from, so a more complete picture of performance can be achieved.

Knowledge management brings together all the sources necessary to complete a picture of the strategic plan and provides a consistent, yet versatile, interface for users to interact with the result.

Summary

Performance measures "motivate, illuminate, communicate" (Metzenbaum, 2006). Developing performance measurement systems in healthcare is a daunting task not only because of the intrinsic complexity of medical care but also because of the resultant complexity in healthcare delivery systems. Healthcare systems such as the VHA have demonstrated that overcoming the barriers to performance measurement yields transformational results. Emerging innovations in medical and business informatics such as NLP and OBI hold promise for overcoming barriers to developing effective healthcare performance assessment systems that meet IOM PM Redesign project team's criteria.

References

Agency for Healthcare Research and Quality. 2009. *Quality & Patient Safety*. http://www.ahrq.gov/qual/, (accessed October 18, 2009).

Asch, S. M. and E. A. McGlynn. 2004. Comparison of quality of care for patients in the Veterans Health Administration and patients in a national sample. *Annals of Internal Medicine* 141:938–945.

Bandura, A. 2004. Cultivate self-efficacy for personal and organizational effectiveness. In *The Blackwell Handbook of Principles of Organizational Behavior*, ed. E. Locke, pp. 120–136. Malden, MA: Blackwell Publishing.

Bandura, A. and D. Cervone. 1983. Self-evaluative and self-efficacy mechanisms governing the motivational effects of goal systems. *Journal of Personality and Social Psychology* 45(5):1017–1028.

Behn, R. D. 2003. Why measure performance? Different purposes require different measures. *Public Administration Review* 63(5):586–606.

Chan, Y.-C. L. 2009. An analytic hierarchy framework for evaluating balanced scorecards of healthcare Organizations. *Canadian Journal of Administrative Sciences* 23(2):85–104.

Chang, L.-C. 2007. The NHS performance assessment framework as a balanced scorecard approach: Limitations and implications. *International Journal of Public Sector Management* 20(2):101–117.

CMS. MDS overview. 2009. http://www.cms.hhs.gov/MDSPubQIandResRep/ (accessed October 18, 2009).

Donabedian, A. 1980. Methods for deriving criteria for assessing the quality of medical care. *Medical Care Review* 37(7):653–698.

Donabedian, A. 1988. The quality of care. How can it be assessed? *Journal of the American Medical Association* 260(12):1743–1748.

Dorner, D. 1991. The investigation of action regulation in uncertain and complex situations. In *Distributed Decision Making: Cognitive models for Cooperative Work*, eds. J. Rasmussen and B. Brehmer, pp. 349–354. Chichester, England: Wiley.

Francis, J. 2009. Personal communication. September 14.

Frese, M. and D. Zapf. 1994. Action as the core of work psychology: A German approach. In *Handbook of Industrial and Organizational Psychology* (2nd edn.), eds. H. C. Triandis and M. D. Dunnette, pp. 271–340. Palo Alto, CA: Consulting Psychologists Press.

Goddard, M., H. T. Davies, D. Dawson, R. Mannion, and F. McInnes. 2002. Clinical performance measurement: Part 1—Getting the best out of it. *Journal of the Royal Society of Medicine* 95:508–510.

Greenburg, J. 2004. Promote procedural justice to enhance acceptance of work outcomes. In *The Blackwell Handbook of Principles of Organizational Behavior*, ed. E. A. Locke, pp. 181–195. Malden, MA: Blackwell Publishing.

Hayward, R. A. and D. M. Kent. 2008. 6 EZ steps to improving your performance: (or How to make P4P pay 4U!). *Journal of the American Medical Association* 300(3):255–256.

IOM Committee on Quality of Health Care in America. 2000. *To Err is Human*. Washington, DC, National Academies Press.

IOM Committee on Quality of Health Care in America. 2001. *Crossing the Chasm: A New Healthcare System for the 21st Century*. Washington, DC: National Academies Press.

IOM Committee on Redesigning Health Insurance Performance Measures, Payment and Performance Improvement Programs & Board on Health Care Services. 2006. *Performance Measurement Accelerating Improvement*. Washington, DC: National Academies Press.

Jha, A. K., J. B. Perlin, K. W. Kizer, and R. A. Dudley. 2003. Effect of the transformation of the veterans affairs health care in the quality of care. *The New England Journal of Medicine* 348:2218–2227.

Joint Commission. 2009a. *National Patient Safety Goals*. http://www.jointcommission.org/patientsafety/nationalpatientsafetygoals/ (accessed October 18, 2009).

Joint Commission. 2009b. *ORYX™*. http://www.jointcommission.org/AccreditationPrograms/HomeCare/ORYX/ (accessed October 18, 2009).

Kaplan, R. S. and D. P. Norton. 1992. The balanced scorecard—Measures that drive performance. *Harvard Business Review*, January–February, 71–79.

Kaplan, R. S. and D. P. Norton. 1996. *Balanced Scorecard: Translating Strategy into Action*. Cambridge, MA: Harvard Business School Press.

Kaplan, R. S. and D. P. Norton. 2008. *The Execution Premium: Linking Strategy to Operations for Competitive Advantage*. Cambridge, MA: Harvard Business School Publishing Corporation.

Kerr, E., R. Gerzoff, and S. Krein. 2004. A comparison of diabetes care quality in the veterans healthcare system and commercial managed care. *Annals of Internal Medicine* 141:272–281.

Klein, H., H. Wesson, M. Hollenbeck, and B. Alge. 1999. Goal commitment and the goal-setting process: Conceptual clarification and empirical synthesis. *Journal of Applied Psychology* 84:885–896.

Kocakülâh, M. C. and A. D. Austill. 2007. Balanced scorecard application in the health care industry: A case study. *Journal of Health Care Finance* 34(1):72–99.

Latham, G. 2004. Motivate employee performance through goal-setting. In *The Blackwell Handbook of Principles of Organizational Behavior*, ed. E. Locke, pp. 107–119. Malden, MA: Blackwell Publishing.

Latham, G. P. and G. H. Seijts. 1999. The effects of proximal and distant goals on performance of a moderately complex task. *Journal of Organizational Behavior* 20:421–429.

Locke, E. A. and G. P. Latham. 2002. Building a practically useful theory of goal setting and task motivation: A 35 year odyssey. *American Psychologist* 57(9):705–717.

Metzenbaum, S. H. 2006. Performance accountability: The five building blocks and six essential practices. IBM Center for the Business of Government, Washington, DC. http://www.businessofgovernment.org (accessed August 1, 2009).

National Quality Foundation. 2009a. *NQF Approves Criteria for Evaluating Composite Measures*. http://www.qualitydigest.com/inside/health-care-news/nqf-approves-criteria-evaluating-composite-measures.htm (accessed October 18, 2009).

National Quality Foundation. 2009b. *NQF-endorsed*® Standards. http://www.qualityforum.org/Measures_List.aspx (accessed October 18, 2009).

NCQA. 2009. What is HEDIS? http://www.ncqa.org/tabid/187/Default.aspx (accessed October 18, 2009).

Nolan, T. and D. M. Berwick. 2006. All-or-none measurement raises the bar on performance. *The New England Journal of Medicine* 295(10):1168–1170.

OASIS. 2009. *OASIS Background*. http://www.cms.hhs.gov/OASIS/02_Background.asp#TopOfPage (accessed October 18, 2009).

O'Brien, S. M., E. R. DeLong, R. S. Dokholyan, F. H. Edwards, and E. D. Peterson. 2007. Exploring the behavior of hospital composite performance measures: An example from coronary artery bypass surgery. *Circulation* 116:2969–2975.

Oliver, A. 2007. The Veterans Health Administration: An American success story? *Milbank Quarterly* 85(1):5–35.

Reeves, D., S. M. Campbell, J. Adams, P. G. Shekelle, E. Kantopantelis, and M. O. Roland. 2007. Combining multiple indicators of clinical quality: An evaluation of different analytic approaches. *Medical Care* 45(6):489–496.

Render, M. L. and P. Almenoff. 2009. The Veterans Health Affairs experience in measuring and reporting inpatient mortality. In mortality measurement. *Agency for Healthcare Research and Quality*. http://www.ahrq.gov/qual/mortality/VAMort.htm (accessed October 31, 2009).

Selim, A. J., L. E. Kazis, and W. Rogers. 2006. Risk adjusted mortality as an indicator of outcomes comparison of the Medicare Advantage Program with the Veterans' Health Administration. *Medical Care* 44:359–365.

Shutt, J. A. 2003. Balancing the health scorecard. *Managed Care* September:42–46.

Sniderman, A. D. and C. D. Furberg. 2009. Why guideline-making requires reform. *Journal of the American Medical Association* 301(4):429–431.

Spitzer, D. R. 2007. *Transforming Performance Measurement: Rethinking the Way We Measure and Drive Organizational Success*. New York: AMACOM.

Tauer, J. M. and J. M. Harackiewicz. 1999. Winning isn't everything: Competition, achievement orientation, and intrinsic motivation. *Journal of Experimental Social Psychology* 39:209–238.

10

Managing Physician Panels in Primary Care

Hari Balasubramanian
University of Massachusetts at Amherst

Brian T. Denton
North Carolina State University

Qi Ming Lin
EInk Corporation

Introduction 10-1
Background and Literature 10-2
Patient Classifications 10-3
Managing Physician Panels 10-5
Emerging Trends in Primary Care 10-8
Team Care • Patient-Centered Medical Home
Summary and Conclusions 10-9
References 10-10

Introduction

Primary care providers (PCPs) are typically the first point of contact between patients and health systems. From a patient's perspective, PCPs provide the majority of care they receive during their lifetime and are responsible for a variety of health services including preventive medicine, patient education, routine physical exams, and the coordination of complex episodes in which patients are referred to medical specialties for secondary and tertiary care. The benefits of a strong primary care system are well documented in the clinical literature. Shi et al. (2005) show that increased access to primary care (1) improves access to health services for relatively deprived population groups; (2) has a strong positive relationship with prevention and early management of health problems; and (3) leads to increased familiarity with patients and, consequently, to less wasteful expenditures due to inappropriate specialist care.

Despite the reported benefits of primary care, a recent study by the American College of Physicians (2006) reports that primary care in the United States "is at grave risk of collapse due to a dysfunctional financing and delivery system." They also emphasize the growing demand for primary care (by 2015, "an estimated 150 million Americans will have at least one chronic condition"), and the steady decline in the supply of primary care physicians over the last decade. This looming crisis in primary care is also at the heart of the policy debate in U.S. healthcare as the nation attempts to reform the healthcare system and provide the roughly 45 million uninsured patients with coverage. As the case of Massachusetts has shown, universal coverage will further strain primary care, as newly insured patients request access to doctors. Several prominent media outlets such as *The New York Times* and *The National Public Radio* recently reported on the severe shortage in primary care physicians in Massachusetts (Brown 2008, Sack 2008). The shortage has been attributed to the state's goal of achieving universal coverage.

Timely access to care and patient–physician continuity have been adversely affected due to these broader trends. The Institute of Medicine has reported "timeliness" as one of the six key "aims for improvement" in its major report on quality of healthcare (Edington, 2001). In one study, nearly 33% of patients cited "inability to get an appointment soon as a significant obstacle to care" (Strunk and Cunningham 2002). More recently, Rust et al. (2008) reported that the inability to get a timely appointment with a primary care physician increases the likelihood of patients visiting the ER. This hinders the appropriate management of chronic diseases that could have been effectively treated in a primary care setting. It is also important that patients see their own physician in order to maintain continuity of care. Indeed, continuity of care is considered one of the hallmarks of primary care. Gill and Mainous (1999) point to several studies which show that patients who regularly see their own providers are (1) more satisfied with their care; (2) more likely to take medications correctly; (3) more likely to have problems correctly identified by their physician; and (4) less likely to be hospitalized. Gill et al. (2000) show a link between lack of continuity and increased emergency department use. Thus, timely access and continuity of care not only have a positive effect on a patient's health, they are also instrumental in reducing healthcare costs.

In this chapter, we look at a case study concerning the Primary Care Internal Medicine (PCIM) practice at the Mayo Clinic in Rochester, Minnesota. Our focus is on improving timely access and continuity of care. The rest of the chapter is organized as follows. We first provide background on the operational aspects of primary care practices and review the relevant literature. We then discuss methods of classifying patients with regard to their appointment request patterns. Next, we investigate how these classifications play a role in the design of a physician's *panel*, where a panel is the set of patients a physician is responsible for. We discuss how timely access and continuity of care can be improved simultaneously by optimizing a physician's panel. Finally, we discuss some of the emerging trends in primary care and their operational implications.

Background and Literature

Primary care practices include family physicians, general internists, and pediatricians. In the United States, more than 66% of all practices are group practices (Hing et al. 2004). As stated earlier, each physician has a *panel*, which is the set of patients he/she is responsible for. Fostering the relationship between a physician and his patients, in other words, improving patient–physician continuity, is one of the foundations of primary care. Patient appointments are typically classifiable into two types: (1) urgent or acute appointments and (2) nonurgent appointments or appointments generally meant for annual exams and to monitor chronic conditions. Physician appointments are generally for 20-minute slots and reimbursement to physicians in primary care (for most practices in the United States) is based largely on the number of 20-minute visits. A physician working full time typically sees about 24 patients a day.

The traditional model of appointment scheduling involved scheduling urgent requests as soon as possible—typically on the same day—while postponing nonurgent visits. However, in recent years, a new paradigm called "advanced access" or "open access" has been adopted by practices nationwide (Murray and Berwick 2003, Murray et al. 2003). Under advanced access, all patients who call are given appointments on the same day: physicians are encouraged to "do today's work today." Thus, the booking of appointments well into the future, which happens frequently for nonurgent appointments, is avoided to a certain extent.

The adoption of open access, which promises patients same-day appointments, has prompted a series of questions. What should physician panel sizes be to allow open access? What if patients prefer to have appointments at some future time rather than see a doctor the same day? These questions have necessitated the use of queuing and stochastic optimization approaches that provide guidelines to practices. For instance, Green et al. (2007) investigate the link between panel sizes and the probability of "overflow" or extra work for a physician under advanced access. They propose a simple probability model that estimates the number of extra appointments that a physician could be expected to see per day as a function of her panel size. The principal message of their work is that for advanced access to work, supply needs to be sufficiently higher than demand to offset the effect of variability. Green and Savin (2008) use a queuing model to determine the effect of no-shows on a physician's panel size. They develop analytical queuing expressions that allow the estimation of physician backlog as a function of panel size and no-show rates. In their model, no-show rates increase as the backlog increases; this results in the paradoxical situation where physicians have low utilization even though backlogs are high. This is because patients, because they have had to wait for long, do not show up.

Gupta et al. (2006) conduct an empirical study of clinics in the Minneapolis metropolitan area that adopted open access. They provide statistics on call volumes, backlogs, number of visits with own physician (which measures continuity), and discuss options for increasing capacity at the level of the physician and clinic. Kopach et al. (2007) use discrete event simulation to study the effects of clinical characteristics in an open access scheduling environment on various performance measures such as continuity and overbooking. One of their primary conclusions is that continuity is care is affected adversely as the fraction of patients on open access increases. The authors mention provider groups (or physicians and support staff) working in teams as a solution to the problem. Gupta and Wang (2008) explicitly model many of the key elements of a primary care clinic. They consider scheduling the workday of a clinic in the presence of (1) multiple physicians, (2) two types of appointments: same-day as well as nonurgent appointments, and (3) patient preferences for a specific slot in a day and also a preference for physicians. The objective is to maximize the clinic's revenue. They use a Markov decision process (MDP) model to obtain booking policies that provide limits on when to accept or deny requests for appointments from patients.

In this chapter, we investigate the effect of panel size and composition on timely access and continuity of care in a primary care group practice. While the effect of the size of a physician's panel has been studied before, there has been no discussion on the type of patients in a physician's panel and its effect on access measures. For instance, females in the age group 55–60 are likely to request twice the number of appointments when compared to males in the group 25–30 (Murray et al. 2007). We first illustrate the differences in appointment request patterns between different categories of patients using examples. We then discuss how the information about patient categories and their appointment request rates are relevant to the design of a primary care physician's panel. Our examples are from the PCIM practice at the Mayo Clinic in Rochester, Minnesota. The PCIM practice is located in downtown Rochester. In all there are 40 physicians in the practice with a total of 20,230 empanelled patients. The majority of the patients are middle-aged or elderly, but the practice also includes young patients between 18 and 40 (pediatric patients are seen in a different practice).

Patient Classifications

Many factors such as age, health status, geographic location, and patterns of historical appointments (appointment types, urgent vs. nonurgent requests, etc.) can be used to define a classification of patient types. The examples we present include two different types of categorizations: the first, a simple categorization based on age and gender, and the second a categorization obtained using classification and regression trees (CART). The purpose of such classifications is to reflect the reality that patient request rates from the different categories may vary significantly.

The first classification uses 28 categories based on age and gender starting with separate groups for males and females aged 18–23 and with the rest of the categories being in 5 year increments. The last two groups are patients aged over 83.

Consider, for example, the empirical distribution of the fraction of total patients in a given category requesting appointments in a week. In Figures 10.1 and 10.2, we contrast the histograms of two different categories: males in the 48–53 age group and females in 73–78 age group. The histograms are based on the weekly visits for the years 2004–2006.

The data can be interpreted as follows. There are in total 708 patients from category 48–53 M empanelled within the PCIM practice. Figure 10.1 shows that an average of 4.8% of these patients will request appointments in a given week. On some weeks as many as 8% of these patients will request appointments.

In contrast, 986 patients from category 73–78 F are enrolled in PCIM (278 more patients than in 48–53 M). Furthermore, from Figure 10.2, on average 8.4% of these patients request appointments in

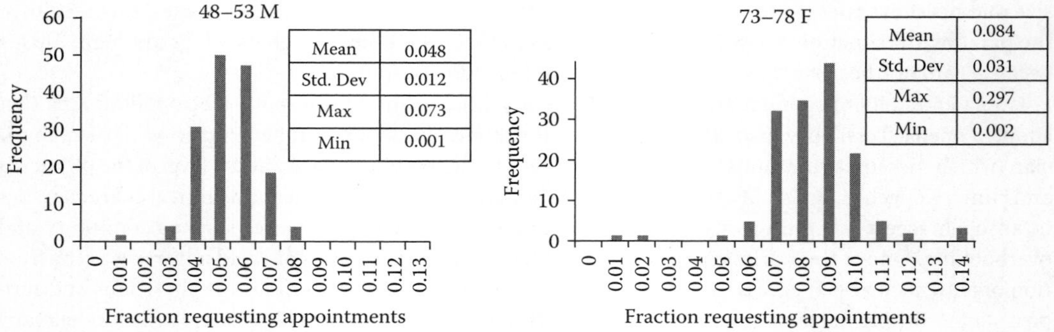

FIGURE 10.1 Comparison of two age and gender categories with regard to fraction total patients requesting appointments per week.

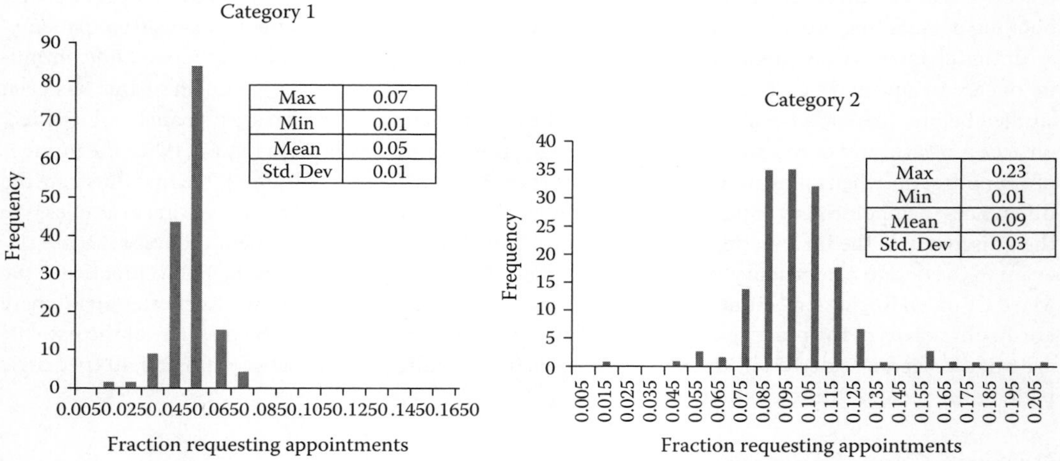

FIGURE 10.2 Comparison of categories 1 and 2 with regard to fraction total patients requesting appointments per week.

a week (as compared to 4.8 for 7 M). Thus, not only is the category size larger but a greater fraction of 73–78 F patients request appointments.

While age and gender serve as a simple proxy for appointment request behavior, specific chronic conditions or diseases may also be useful indicators. Further analysis of the same PCIM patients using CART analysis revealed that in addition to age and gender, coronary artery disease (CAD), hypertension, and depression were significant indicators of high appointment request rates. As an example, Figure 10.2 shows the distribution of the fraction of total patients requesting appointments from two different categories, which we refer to below as categories 1 and 2. Category 1 is comprised of female patients less than 53 years old (2865 total), with none of the aforementioned three conditions. Category 2 is comprised of patients, both male and female, aged above 69 (789 total) and who have CAD. The distributions are clearly different. The mean of the second is double the mean of the first; the second also has a higher variance compared to the first.

Identifying different categories of patients is thus important for understanding patterns in patient demand. Different patients may have different needs—for example, younger patients may not value continuity as much as older patients, and patients with chronic conditions need regular follow-up appointments. The classification of patients helps a practice effectively segment its patients and plan its care delivery models.

Furthermore, classification helps in the design of a physician's panel, which we discuss in the next section. This has an important policy implication. Currently, physicians are reimbursed based on the number of visits. But there are "pay for performance" initiatives (Bohmer and Lee 2009) underway that reimburse not only based on visits but also based on the preventive measures promoted in the population and quantifiable improvement in health outcomes. Any such payment scheme would have to adjust for the type of patients in a physician's panel and mix of diseases.

Managing Physician Panels

Each primary care physician has a panel, which is the set of patients she is responsible for. The demand for appointments a physician has from day to day is a function of the size of the panel. A physician working full time typically has 1500–2000 patients in her panel. But how many patients can one physician accommodate? This has become an important question in primary care (Murray and Berwick 2003). However, based on our observations of differing appointment request patterns among patient categories, it appears that size alone may not be sufficient.

Consider the example of a primary care physician working at the PCIM practice at the Mayo Clinic in Rochester, Minnesota. This physician has 1200 patients in her panel. Using a classification which uses age and gender, CAD, hypertension, and depression as indicators (obtained using CART), we can determine how many patients are from each category. Then, using historical information on the distribution of visit rates from each category (as illustrated in Figure 10.2), it is possible, using a simple simulation, to obtain the distribution of the number of appointments that the physician can expect in a week. For example, the histogram of weekly appointments for this particular physician is shown in Figure 10.3. The histogram is based on 50,000 observations obtained from the simulation.

Can this physician take more patients, assuming the mix of patients remains the same? Table 10.1 shows summary statistics on the number of expected appointment requests in a week for different panel sizes, for the same physician. We also provide the proportion of the estimated distribution that is less than 120. The rationale for choosing this as a reference point is as follows. If the physician works an 8-hour day, then she will have 24 appointments since slots in primary care in the United States are 20 minutes long (even if appointments end up being longer or shorter, as often happens, this is the length of time the physician is billed for). In a week, therefore, she will have approximately 120 slots. Note that this is a conservative estimate since it assumes that the physician is available to see patients all days a week; it also assumes that the physician will accommodate administrative activities, dictations, telephone follow-ups and lunch in time other than the allotted 8 hours to see patients.

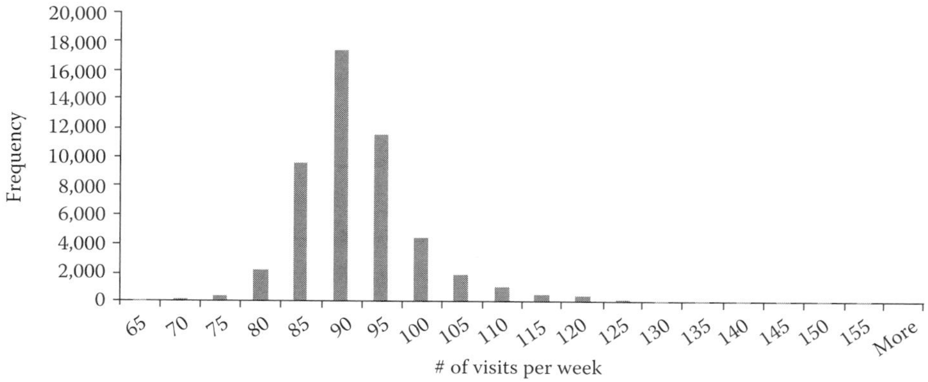

FIGURE 10.3 Empirical distribution of weekly appointments for a typical PCIM physician.

TABLE 10.1 Statistics on Expected Number of Weekly Visits for a PCIM Physician under the Different Panel Sizes

Panel Size	Mean	Standard Deviation	Maximum	Minimum	Less Than 120 (%)
1200	89.71	7.68	153.72	60.32	99.40
1400	104.67	8.96	179.34	70.37	94.18
1600	119.67	10.56	204.96	78.53	59.57
1800	134.57	11.52	230.58	90.48	5.35
2000	149.55	12.80	256.20	100.53	0.36

Table 10.1 shows the proportion of requests is less than 120 for each of the panel size. If this statistic is small, then this means that a significant proportion of the estimated distribution of the total weekly appointments is greater than 120, which in turn implies the physician will either have to put in an unreasonable amount of overtime, or her patients will have to wait, see other physicians, or visit an emergency room. All these are inefficient, high-cost alternatives. Similar statistics can be provided for other limits on the total number of available weekly physician appointments.

Table 10.1 also shows that the average number of appointments increases linearly as the panel size increases. But the proportion of the distribution below 120 decreases nonlinearly. At 1600 patients, the mean is 120 appointments per week, but only 60% of the distribution is below 120. Clinics thus should be careful about planning physician panel sizes with just averages. Recall that 120 is an estimate on the high side; for smaller total available weekly slots, panel sizes larger than 1500 will be untenable. This analysis shows that while nationwide panels tend to be between 1500 and 2000, the mix of disease conditions and the corresponding demand at PCIM imply that a panel size beyond 1500 will not result in an acceptable level of service.

The above discussion pertains to capacity planning at the level of one physician. Most practices, however, are group practices, consisting of more than one physician. Providing timely access and continuity can be viewed as an *optimization* problem, as shown in Figure 10.4. The question is: How many patients from each category should be assigned to each physician's panel? The x_{ij} variables in the figure represent the number of patients assigned from patient category i to physician panel j. In other words, the x_{ij} variables determine the design of physician panels. The demand for any physician j in any week t, denoted in the figure by d_{jt} is clearly a function of how the x_{ij} variables are chosen. Physicians with significant backlogs typically have panels that have a large number of chronically ill patients. Because these patients are unable to obtain timely appointments, they tend to see other physicians. What if the panels were to

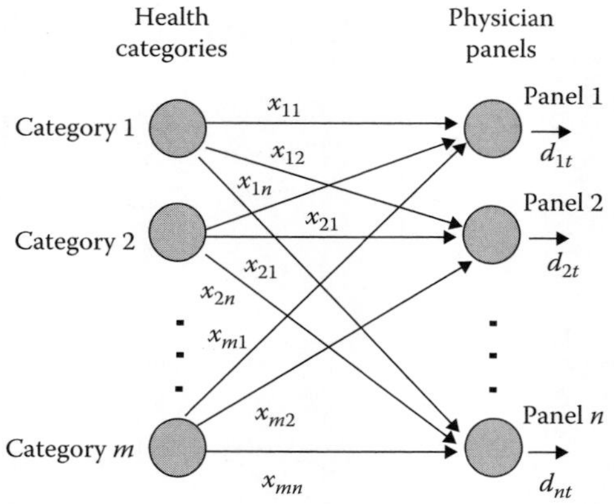

FIGURE 10.4 Panel design framed as an optimization problem.

be redesigned—that is if the excess demand were to be redistributed to other physicians who have some capacity?

Balasubramanian et al. (2007) considered the panel design question using a simulation-optimization framework. They propose a panel design genetic algorithm (PDGA) to generate optimal designs and test it using data from the Mayo Clinic PCIM group practice. For health categories, a simple age and gender classification is used. Each panel design in the PDGA population is evaluated over 52 weeks to calculate waiting time in weeks and average number of redirections to physicians that are not the patient's own. These redirections are viewed as losses in continuity, since an unfamiliar physician will now have to understand the medical history of the patient. This may result in additional follow-up appointments with the patient's own physician, or diagnosis and medication errors.

The simulation works as follows: physician calendars start empty (no appointments) in the first period and move from period to period. In each period, patients request appointments from their PCPs. Patient requests in each period are satisfied on a first-come-first-served basis: requests originating in earlier periods are filled first. Ties between requests arising in the same period to a given physician panel are broken arbitrarily. If the capacity for a particular panel is exhausted, patients have one of two options: to see another provider within the same period or to wait for a future period to see their PCP. We assume that a fixed proportion of patients (40%) are willing to see other providers in the same period. These requests are filled by physicians who have available capacity. For each panel design, we truncate the first 10 weeks of data to remove the initial transient and use 50 replications to obtain our estimates.

The results of the genetic algorithm are compared to the existing panel configuration in the practice, as shown in Table 10.2 and Figure 10.5. Average wait time is improved by more than 30%, while average number of weekly redirections to other physicians is reduced by more than 50%. Figure 10.5 shows graphically the differences in wait times involved in the two solutions. The x-axis indicates the number of weeks. The y-axis indicates the average number of patients who waited i weeks or more, where i is the corresponding value on the x-axis. The PDGA solution performs significantly better but the differences taper off as the number of weeks increases.

Thus, panel redesign shows promise. However, there are several unaddressed issues. Patient and physician preferences about panel choices and compositions have not been considered. We assume that the population of patients remains static during the simulation, that is, no patients leave the system (due to move or death), or no new patients enter the system. Finally, while the current design can be

TABLE 10.2 Comparison of GA Design with Current Practice

	Wait Time	Redirections
	Current Design	
Mean	6.82	531.10
Standard deviation	0.21	26.43
Upper 95% CI	6.87	538.43
Lower 95% CI	6.76	523.78
	PDGA Solution	
Mean	4.50	230.13
Standard deviation	0.18	26.77
Upper 95% CI	4.55	237.55
Lower 95% CI	4.44	222.71

Source: Balasubramanian, H. et al., Improving primary care access using simulation optimization, in *Proceedings of the 2007 Winter Simulation Conference*, Washington, DC, pp. 1494–1500. © 2007 IEEE with permission.

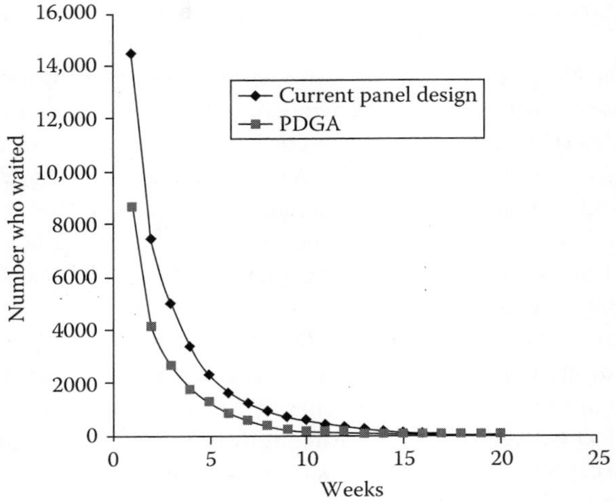

FIGURE 10.5 Comparison of number of weeks waited for the two designs. (From Balasubramanian, H. et al., Improving primary care access using simulation optimization, in *Proceedings of the 2007 Winter Simulation Conference*, Washington, DC, pp. 1494–1500. © 2007 IEEE with permission.)

significantly improved upon, changing panel allocations is difficult in practice. Altering the panel configuration can only be done in the long term, and the practice can use the rate of new patients entering and existing patients leaving to adjust panels so that they are closer to the PDGA solution. Patient and physicians preferences can also be considered in the process. Models that consider such transitions and preferences will be focus of our future research. Additional results and implications for primary care practices can be found in Balasubramanian et al. (2010).

Emerging Trends in Primary Care

Team Care

Primary care physicians are reimbursed less than most other specialties, which discourages medical students from careers in primary care. This is one of main reasons for the current nationwide shortage in primary care (Bodenheimer and Grumbach 2007). As a result, many practices are using support staff such as mid-level physician assistants (PAs) and nurse practitioners (NPs), to fill the void. Indeed, in recent years, there have been increasing calls in the primary care community for practices to adopt the concept of *team care*. The Institute of Medicine in its report *Crossing the Quality Chasm: New Health System for the Twenty-First Century* envisions primary care teams playing a central role (Edington, 2001). Grumbach and Bodenheimer (2004) report several examples of clinics that have adopted team care.

Team care relies heavily on the effective use of support staff. Support staff includes clinical assistants (CAs), receptionists, patient appointment coordinators (PACs), and licensed practical nurses (LPNs). The structure and flows within the framework of a primary team are shown in Figure 10.6. While a patient's PCP will still be her main point of contact, and will coordinate her care, she may be seen by other clinicians in the team. This pooling of the team's capacity allows it to better absorb fluctuations in demand and also direct requests based on the acuity of the case. Future work on patient appointment scheduling in primary care has to consider this team aspect rather than focusing primarily on physicians.

Patient-Centered Medical Home

In recent years, prominent physician organizations have been calling for a fundamental transformation in how primary care is practiced. Specifically, they have been advocating for a patient-centered

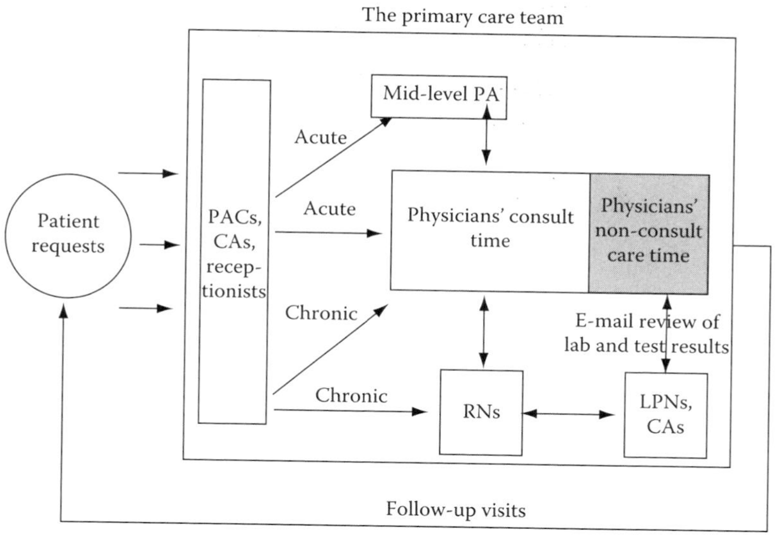

FIGURE 10.6 The team care model in primary care.

medical home (PCMH) which they define as "an approach to primary care… that facilitates partnerships between individual patients, and their personal physicians, and when appropriate, the patient's family" (AAFP/AAP/ACP/AOA 2007). The medical home attempts to counter the increasing fragmentation and lack of coordination that is prevalent in the U.S. healthcare system, by making primary care practices the central point of care. Each patient will have a personal physician, but the physician will also coordinate and will stay informed of the patient's care across other parts of the system: subspecialty care, hospitals, home health agencies, and nursing homes. The medical home model of care will use information technology and electronic medical records to achieve this coordination.

As discussed earlier, physician reimbursement in most practices is currently based on the number of visits. In a medical home, "face-to-face" visits will be complemented by visits with other members of the care team such as nurses and PAs; some exchanges may happen over e-mail and phone. The reimbursement of physicians will thus have to account for "non-visit" care time. This leads to a number of operational questions, since a "capacity" of a clinic now assumes a flexible form rather than being centered solely on physician visits. Furthermore, medical home reimbursement will also "recognize case-mix differences in the patient population being treated within the practice" (AAFP/AAP/ACP/AOA 2007). Such a payment scheme adjusts for the type of disease burdens prevalent in the population. Our discussion regarding patient classifications thus becomes important.

Summary and Conclusions

In summary, we have illustrated approaches for patient appointment scheduling in primary care using a case study involving the PCIM practice at the Mayo Clinic in Rochester, Minnesota. Salient features of our approach include (1) the recognition of the differences in appointments request patterns between patient groups, (2) the use of patient classifications for the effective design of an individual physician's panel, and (3) the discussion of a simulation-optimization framework to redesign panels in a group practice. We have also briefly discussed some of the emerging trends in primary care, specifically team care and the PCMH. Our future work will focus in developing models that evaluate the operational implications of these trends.

References

AAFP/AAP/ACP/AOA (American Academy of Family Physicians, American Academy of Pediatrics, American College of Physicians, and American Osteopathic Association). March 2007. Joint principles of the patient-centered medical home. http://www.acponline.org/advocacy/where_we_stand/medical_home/approve_jp.pdf

American College of Physicians. 2006. The impending collapse of primary care and its implications for the state of the nation's healthcare. Technical report, Philadelphia, PA.

Balasubramanian, H., R. Banerjee, B. Denton, N. Shah, J. Naessens, and J. Stahl. 2010. Improving clinical access and continuity through physician panel redesign. *Journal of General Internal Medicine*, 25(10):1109–1115.

Balasubramanian, H., R. Banerjee, M. Gregg, and B. Denton. 2007. Improving primary care access using simulation optimization. In *Proceedings of the Winter Simulation Conference*, Washington, DC, pp. 1494–1500.

Bodenheimer, T. and K. Grumbach. 2007. *Improving Primary Care: Strategies and Tools for a Better Practice.* New York: McGraw Hill Lange.

Bohmer, R. and T. Lee. 2009. The shifting mission of healthcare delivery organizations. *The New England Journal of Medicine* 361(6):551–553.

Brown, K. 2008. All things considered. Massachusetts health care reform reveals doctor shortage. National Public Radio. http://www.npr.org/templates/story/story.php?storyid=97620520 (November 30, 2008).

Edington, M. ed. 2001. *Crossing the Quality Chasm: A New Health System for the 21st Century.* The Institute of Medicine Report. Technical report, National Academy Press, Washington, DC.

Gill, J. M. and A. Mainous. 1999. The role of provider continuity in preventing hospitalizations. *Archives of Family Medicine* 7:352–357.

Gill, J. M., A. Mainous, and M. Nsereko. 2000. The effect of continuity of care on emergency department use. *Archives of Family Medicine* 9:333–338.

Green, L. V. and S. Savin. 2008. Reducing delays for medical appointments: A queueing approach. *Operations Research* 56(6):1526–1538.

Green, L. V., S. Savin, and M. Murray. 2007. Providing timely access to care: What is the right patient panel size? *The Joint Commission Journal on Quality and Patient Safety* 33:211–218.

Grumbach, K. and T. Bodenheimer. 2004. Can health care teams improve primary care practice? *Journal of the American Medical Association* 291(10):1246–1251.

Gupta, D., S. Potthoff, D. Blowers, and J. Corlett. 2006. Performance metrics for advanced access. *Journal of Healthcare Management* 51(4):246–259.

Gupta, D. and L. Wang. 2008. Revenue management for a primary-care clinic in the presence of patient choice. *Operations Research* 56(3):576–592.

Hing, E., D. K. Cherry, and D. A. Woodwell. 2004. *National Ambulatory Medical Care Survey: 2002 Summary. Advance Data from Vital and Health Statistics; No. 346.* Hyattsville, MD: National Center for Health Statistics.

Kopach, R., P. DeLaurentis, M. Lawley, K. Muthuraman, L. Ozsen, R. Rardin, H. Wan, P. Intrevado, X. Qu, and D. Willis. 2007. Effects of clinical characteristics on successful open access scheduling. *Health Care Management Science* 10:111–124.

Murray, M. and D. M. Berwick. 2003. Advanced access: Reducing waiting and delays in primary care. *Journal of the American Medical Association* 289(8):1035–1040.

Murray, M., T. Bodenheimer, D. Rittenhouse, and K. Grumbach. 2003. Improving timely access to primary care: Case studies of the advanced access model. *Journal of the American Medical Association* 289(3):1042–1046.

Murray, M., M. Davies, and B. Boushon 2007. Panel size: How many doctors can one patient manage? *Family Practice Management*. Downloaded from: http://www.aafp.org/fpm/2007/0400/p44.html

Rust, G., J. Ye, P. Baltrus, E. Daniels, B. Adesunloye, and G. E. Fryer. 2008. Practical barriers to timely primary care access. *Archives of Internal Medicine* 268(15):1705–1710.

Sack, K. 2008. In Massachusetts, universal coverage strains care. *New York Times*, April 5, 2008.

Shi, L., B. Starfield, and J. Macinko. 2005. Contribution of primary care to health systems and health. *The Milbank Quarterly* 83(3):457–502.

Strunk, B. C. and P. J. Cunningham. 2002. *Treading Water: Americans' Access to Needed Medical Care, 1997–2001*. Washington, DC: Center for Studying Health System Change, http://www.hschange.com/ (accessed May 19, 2010).

11

Lean in Healthcare

Philip C. Jones
University of Iowa

Barrett W. Thomas
University of Iowa

Introduction 11-1
Lean Overview 11-2
Historical Perspective 11-4
Does Lean Work in Healthcare? 11-5
Analysis and Discussion 11-8
Causes of Operational Problems • Problems with Implementation
Conclusion 11-12
References 11-12

Introduction

In the United States, spending on healthcare has risen from around 5.2% of gross domestic product (GDP) in 1960 to 13.6% of GDP in 2000 and is currently 16% of GDP in 2007, the most recent year for which data is available (Organisation for Economic Co-operation and Development 2009). The causes for this rapid escalation are varied and complex, and a discussion of them is beyond the scope of this chapter. Nevertheless, concern over rapidly escalating healthcare costs plays a central role in the ongoing debate over healthcare in this country, and regardless of political orientation, virtually everyone agrees that providing high-quality healthcare while simultaneously reining in costs is the desired goal. Many proposed solutions (whether they would actually work or not!) have proven impossible to implement because they require a political consensus that so far has proven elusive. Whether the current healthcare debate will change that is still unknown, and even if political consensus for change is arrived at, whether the resulting changes will actually prove effective is something that will be known for sure only after the fact.

This chapter discusses an approach to improving quality and reducing costs that requires neither all-at-once massive changes to the infrastructure of the healthcare system nor political intervention. The approach is called "Lean." Lean was originally developed and deployed in the manufacturing sector and has begun to be applied in the healthcare sector. Through the use of carefully selected examples, we shall endeavor to point out common features of Lean applications as well as common pitfalls encountered.

This chapter focuses on three key questions. First, can Lean strategies be successfully translated from manufacturing to the healthcare sector? And what does it take to do so? Second, even if Lean can be successfully translated to the healthcare sector, will doing so really be effective at meeting the goal of providing quality healthcare while simultaneously controlling costs? Other strategies, most notably Six Sigma, have their proponents, so a third question is do Six Sigma and Lean complement each other or are they mutually exclusive?

To answer these questions, we would ideally conduct a series of carefully designed and controlled experiments to answer these hypotheses, and we freely admit that we have not done so. The resources we have available preclude our doing so, and indeed, it is probably not feasible to conduct such experimental tests in any event. Rather, we shall rely upon case studies and anecdotal data to illustrate our points and draw our conclusions. While anecdotal data is not ideal, if one anecdote after another all point in the same direction, they do become pretty strong evidence after a certain point. We believe we have reached that point with respect to implementations of Lean in healthcare and can indeed draw reasonably firm conclusions.

The rest of this chapter is organized as follows. The next section provides an overview of Lean principles and tools. The "Historical perspective" section provides a historical perspective by contrasting Lean with the earlier principles of scientific management. The "Does Lean work in healthcare" section establishes that Lean works in healthcare through a review of the literature in Lean healthcare with particular emphasis on those articles reporting implementations. In the "Analysis and discussion" section, we present our analysis of the common features and pitfalls of Lean implementations. The "Conclusion" section contains concluding remarks.

Lean Overview

Lean is a philosophy and a set of tools for driving systematic continuous process improvement within an organization. At its core, the Lean philosophy advocates increasing customer value through the elimination of waste or *muda*, where waste is anything that customer does not value. Lean has its roots in the Toyota Production System, which had its start at Toyota in the late 1940s. Taiichi Ohno (1912–1990) is often credited with being the main developer of the famous Toyota Production System. General overviews of Lean can be found in Womack and Jones (2003) with healthcare-specific introductions given by Spear and Bowen (1999) and Graban (2009).

According to Liker (2004), the Toyota Production System is based on the following 14 principles:

1. Base your management decisions on a long-term philosophy, even at the expense of short-term financial goals.
2. Create a continuous process flow to bring problems to the surface.
3. Use "pull" systems to avoid overproduction.
4. Level out the workload. (Work like the tortoise, not the hare.)
5. Build a culture of stopping to fix problems, to get quality right the first time.
6. Standardized tasks and processes are the foundation for continuous improvement and employee empowerment.
7. Use visual control so no problems are hidden.
8. Use only reliable, thoroughly tested technology that serves your people and processes.
9. Grow leaders who thoroughly understand the work, live the philosophy, and teach it to others.
10. Develop exceptional people and teams who follow your company's philosophy.
11. Respect your extended network of partners and suppliers by challenging them and helping them improve.
12. Go and see for yourself to thoroughly understand the situation.
13. Make decisions slowly by consensus, thoroughly considering all options; implement decisions rapidly.
14. Become a learning organization through relentless reflection and continuous improvement.

These 14 principles are implemented through a set of well-known Lean tools that we shall describe briefly. These tools include

- 7 wastes (current thinking updates this to 8 wastes in many organizations)
- Takt time analysis
- 5S (current thinking updates this to 6S in many organizations)
- 5 Whys
- Value stream mapping (VSM)
- Kaizen events

We recognize that other Lean tools exist, but for the sake of brevity, we have chosen to discuss only those that are most commonly applied. We apologize in advance to those whose favorite Lean tool has been excluded.

The 8 wastes are defined as those activities that take time, energy, and effort, yet do nothing to produce customer value. They are usually identified as follows:

1. Overproduction
2. Waiting
3. Unnecessary transport or conveyance
4. Overprocessing (or incorrect processing)
5. Excess inventory
6. Motion (of workers)
7. Defects
8. Unused employee creativity

Eliminating these kinds of waste (particularly the first 7) helps address the second principle of creating a continuous process flow. These wastes occur in virtually all settings from manufacturing to administrative to healthcare delivery. Manos et al. (2006) spell out precisely how each of these wastes occurs in a healthcare delivery setting.

Takt time analysis targets the fourth principle leveling the workload and rooted in the classical industrial engineering technique of line balancing. The key difference is that Takt time analysis takes as its starting point the need to produce at a rate equal to the rate of customer demand—something that is overlooked or at least hidden in classical line balancing.

The 6S tool consists of steps that help improve the work environment by establishing productive and safe work places. 6S can be regarded as a necessary conditioning step to implementing Lean principles. 6S targets principles 6 and 7 and consists of the following:

1. Sort (separate out unneeded items)
2. Straighten (a place for everything and everything in its place)
3. Shine (clean the workplace up)
4. Standardize (create standard rules, standard work, and standard procedures)
5. Sustain (maintain the improvements you have made)
6. Safety

The 5 Whys is a tool for helping to find and eliminate the root cause of a problem. The 5 Whys addresses principles 13 and 14. The tool is implemented by successively asking "why" until a root cause is uncovered. While exceedingly simple, the 5 Whys helps a practitioner maintain the discipline to look past the superficial causes of a problem to find the more important root cause.

VSM is a tool popularized by Rother and Shook (2003). To understand VSM, first recall the classical industrial engineering tool of process flow mapping in which the physical flow of a product or product family is represented graphically with rectangles denoting process steps, triangles denoting inventory, and arrows representing flows. The innovation of the value stream map is the recognition that the process flow map, while containing information necessary to understand, analyze, and improve a process, does not contain sufficient information to do so. By adding to the process flow map relevant information about the process (cycle times, setup times, batch sizes, number of operators, etc.) as well as information flows, one obtains a value stream map that does contain sufficient information to truly understand and analyze the process. Rother and Shook note that value stream mapping can be done either at the process level, the individual plant level, the corporate level (across plants), or across companies in the supply chain. VSM has been found to be useful not only in manufacturing companies, but in a variety of service organizations including healthcare.

A kaizen event is a structured problem-solving event that targets a specific process for improvement over a two to five day period. Kaizen events directly address principles 13 and 14 as well as, at least indirectly, potentially every other principle. Kaizen events, sometimes called Rapid or Continuous Process Improvement events typically use several of the other Lean tools. The kaizen gathers operators, managers, and owners of a process in one place to develop a value stream map (ideally by observing the existing process in operation) of the existing process, identify waste, determine the underlying causes of waste, develop potential solutions as well as a map of the process' future state (future state value stream map), and implement the selected improvements. A key to the success of the kaizen is that it can help obtain buy-in from all parties related to the process. Kaizen events have been successfully applied in numerous healthcare settings.

In recent years, Lean has become integrated with another process improvement paradigm known as Six Sigma. Six Sigma was developed by Motorola in the 1980s and subsequently popularized by General Electric. To understand Six Sigma, note that the traditional quality paradigm defined a process as capable if the process's natural spread, defined as the process mean plus or minus three standard deviations (three-sigma), lies within the tolerances specified by design. This translates to a process yield of 99.73% if the process output is normally distributed. Motorola, however, noted the output of its processes could shift by as much as 1.5 standard deviations from the original process mean. If the process met only the three-sigma capability requirement of the traditional quality paradigm, a shift of 1.5 standard deviations would imply a drop in the process yield to 93.3%. While this might not seem like an insuperable problem, consider the fact that if multiple parts, say five, all have to be acceptable for an assembly to work (or multiple (five) tasks all have to be done correctly for a medical test to be accurate) then a 93.3% yield for each task would imply a 70.7% overall yield.

Accordingly, Motorola recognized that it was important to have individual processes operating at a Six Sigma quality level, meaning that if the process output is centered on the center of the design specification, then the process will produce approximately two parts per billion that are outside of design tolerances. Further, if the process mean shifts by 1.5 standard deviations, the output will still produce only 3.4 parts per million outside the design tolerances.

The heart of Six Sigma programs is a set of statistical tools that target variance reduction. Some of these tools, design of experiments, for example, are fairly complex and mathematically intense in comparison to the Lean tools mentioned above. Thus, while it is possible to engage the entire workforce with Lean through the aggressive implementation of kaizen events, many of the Six Sigma tools require a degree of statistical sophistication that may not be within every person's range of interest, training, or mathematical ability. As a result, many organizations employing Six Sigma are more heavily reliant on teams of technical experts, whether brought in from outside the organization or developed in-house through Six Sigma green belt and black belt certification programs.

Historical Perspective

To provide some perspective on the application of Lean in healthcare, it is useful to contrast the viewpoints of Frederick Taylor and Taiichi Ohno. Frederick Taylor (1856–1915) is the founder of "scientific management," which forms the basis of the classical industrial engineering techniques that have been used in healthcare settings since the early 1940s. Smalley (1982) provides an excellent historical summary of how classical industrial engineering techniques have been applied within hospitals.

Taylorism was based on the following four fundamental principles (Taylor 1911):

1. Replace rule-of-thumb work methods with methods based on a scientific study of the tasks.
2. Scientifically select, train, and develop each employee rather than passively leaving them to train themselves.
3. Provide "detailed instruction and supervision of each worker in the performance of that worker's discrete task."
4. Divide work nearly equally between managers and workers, so that the managers apply scientific management principles to planning the work and the workers actually perform the tasks.

The flavor of Taylorism can perhaps best be illustrated by the following two quotations from Taylor (Montgomery 1989):

- "With the triumph of scientific management, unions would have nothing left to do, and they would have been cleansed of their most evil feature: the restriction of output."
- "I can say, without the slightest hesitation," Taylor told a congressional committee, "that the science of handling pig iron is so great that the man who is... physically able to handle pig-iron and is sufficiently phlegmatic and stupid to choose this for his occupation is rarely able to comprehend the science of handling pig-iron."

Taylor believed passionately in pursuing efficiencies, and, according to Montgomery (1989),

> Taylor thought that by analyzing work, the 'One Best Way' to do it would be found. He is most remembered for developing the time and motion study. He would break a job into its component parts and measure each to the hundredth of a minute. One of his most famous studies involved shovels. He noticed that workers used the same shovel for all materials. He determined that the most effective load was 21½ lb, and found or designed shovels that for each material would scoop up that amount.

It is also apparent that Taylor's attitudes toward the people who actually do the work would have, insofar as managers adopt them, profound implications.

There are at least three notable distinctions between Lean thinking and Taylor's scientific management. First, while both systems advocate standard work, Taylor's system emphasizes management's determining the "one best way" that is thereupon to be enshrined in the work standard. In Lean thinking, however, standard work is viewed as a starting point upon which to base continuous improvement. For example, Taiichi Ohno once noted, "I told everyone that they weren't earning their pay if they left the standardized work unchanged for a whole month" (Ohno 2001). The very concept of "one best way" is antithetical to the continuous improvement ethic of Lean thinking.

Second, Taylor focused heavily on maximizing efficiency as defined by minimizing the per unit cost. This approach views any worker's idleness as waste, and hence large inventories (of parts in a factory or patients in a waiting room) are to be encouraged so as to accommodate any time variations. In contrast, Lean thinking focuses on producing customer value. From this perspective, the large inventories produced by scientific management cannot be tolerated because they increase lead times for the customer (or patient) and hence detract from customer value. To further illustrate these conceptual differences, imagine that Taylor and Ohno both saw a nurse or medical technician waiting with a patient for a procedure, for example, an x-ray. Both Taylor and Ohno would see waste. To Taylor, the waste would be that the nurse was idle while to Ohno the waste would be that the patient is waiting (Dickson 2008).

Third, Taylor viewed the worker as a cost to be minimized. The worker had nothing to contribute other than his brute labor and indeed, other than his greater manual dexterity, seemingly had nothing to recommend him over a beast of burden. In Lean thinking, however, the worker is viewed as a resource with intimate knowledge of the process whose talents and expertise must be developed and tapped if the organization is to reach its highest potential.

Does Lean Work in Healthcare?

Despite the fact that applications of Lean in healthcare are relatively new, for the most part having begun only within the current decade, there is already a voluminous literature. Most of the papers provide case histories of specific applications with some trying to discern general principles. In what follows, we shall not try to give a complete and encyclopedic coverage of every Lean healthcare application that has ever been performed, but rather we shall provide a sample that gives what we trust is a good flavor of current work in the field. What emerges is that Lean and Six Sigma have been implemented in almost every organizational unit in healthcare across numerous countries making use of the same Lean thinking and tools that have proved so valuable in manufacturing and other service industries. It is worth noting that many of the papers identify that a stumbling block to implementing either methodology appears to be the sense of many healthcare professionals that the healthcare industry is fundamentally different from the manufacturing industry. Hence, they argue, tools developed for manufacturing cannot be successfully applied in our workplace. We believe that the papers discussed here provide, in toto, a convincing counter to this argument.

Correa et al. (2005) discuss the application of radio frequency identification (RFID) technology to help implement Lean in Spanish hospitals. In particular, they provide a categorization of the 7 wastes in healthcare and give examples of each waste. Subsequently, they discuss applications in natal wards, surgery, and document control. Endsley et al. (2006) discuss improving a family practice through the application of Lean tools and provide specific examples or case studies. They emphasize the need to collect information from patients on what they really value (as opposed to what healthcare professionals think they value) and the use of value stream mapping.

Jimmerson et al. (2005) discuss the application of Lean at Intermountain Healthcare in Salt Lake City, Utah. They provide examples of improvements in the cardiology lab, the pharmacy, rehabilitation services, billing, and facility services. They also discuss the use of value stream mapping and provide a detailed case study of the application of Lean to an anatomical pathology lab to reduce the turnaround time of samples from 5 to 2 days. They also make the interesting observation that "...at the root of every operational problem we've studied is a poorly specified activity, a vague unreliable connection, or a complex pathway."

Tragardh and Lindberg (2004) discuss the application of Lean in the Swedish healthcare system. Okolo et al. (2009) discuss the application of Lean tools in the Landstuhl Regional Medical Center in Germany. They claim that improvements due to application of Lean and Six Sigma tools have made it possible for wounded soldiers to return home for further treatment within 3–5 days as opposed to the 30 days it took during the Vietnam War.

Jones and Mitchell (2006) provide an overview of Lean in Great Britain's National Health Service (NHS). They provide specific case studies at a number of different hospitals within the NHS and present some general observations that are extremely interesting. In one case study, for example, Jones and Mitchell report on how staff walking time within the pathology department of a major hospital was cut by 80% and in addition, the turnaround time on samples was cut from 24–30 to 2–3 hours. In another example, they report on how the postoperative mortality rate of patients with fractured hips was cut by 50%. In general, they note that in the processes they studied, there tended to be approximately nine times more non-value-added activity than value-added activity, so improving value-added components in isolation tended not to be an effective strategy. Additionally, they noted the following:

- Lean must by locally led, not imposed from outside.
- Lack of standard work was a frequent and serious problem.
- Disconnects at the gaps between functional silos caused problems.
- Inappropriate metrics encouraged counterproductive behavior.
- Complex processes with many handoffs caused problems.

In one hospital, for example, they noted that the discharge process could involve over 250 steps and handoffs for a single patient.

King et al. (2006) provide a case study of applying Lean in an Australian hospital to improve the flow time of patients through the emergency department. Manos et al. (2006) discuss the applications of Lean to emergency rooms, storage rooms, and staff break rooms. Panchak (2003) discusses rising healthcare costs and presents examples of Lean healthcare applications at Intermountain Healthcare in Salt Lake City, Utah, at Virginia Mason Medical Center in Seattle, Washington, and at Wellmark Blue Cross Blue Shield in Des Moines, Iowa. Kim et al. (2006) present a series of applications of Lean in healthcare settings at Virginia Mason Medical Center in Seattle, Washington, at Park Nicollet Health Services in Minneapolis, Minnesota, and at the University of Michigan Hospital in Ann Arbor, Michigan.

The literature on applications of Six Sigma technology to healthcare is, if anything, even more voluminous than that on Lean applications. Ettinger (2001) discusses the application of Six Sigma methodologies at Virtua Health, a four-hospital system in New Jersey. Christianson et al. (2005) discuss the efforts of Fairview Health Services in Minneapolis to deploy Six Sigma methods. They note the need to find "better ways to engage physicians." Van Den Heuvel et al. (2005) discuss the efforts of a Dutch hospital to implement Six Sigma.

Chassin (1998) explores underlying causes of quality problems in the healthcare system and discusses some of the obstacles to improvement. Chassin notes that the one healthcare specialty that has reduced defects to rates approximating Six Sigma is that of surgical anesthesia. In the 1970s, he observes, there were 25–50 deaths per million due to anesthesia. Since then, anesthesia deaths have been reduced to a rate of 5 deaths per million cases. Chassin presents data to show that other areas of the healthcare system, however, do not fare so well. Chassin also categorizes causes of quality problems into three distinct areas: overuse causes, underuse causes, and misuse causes. He argues that the reasons behind overuse causes include

- Fee for service
- Enthusiasm (e.g., how much fun it is to perform a coronary angioplasty)
- Self-referral
- Malpractice lawsuits

The reasons behind underuse may include lack of insurance, and the fact that there may be either too little information available in some cases or so much information in other cases that physicians cannot keep up to date. He also notes that comparatively little work has been done to discover the reasons behind misuse, but goes on to argue that physicians' resistance to clinical practice guidelines (standard work!) may play a role as do problems with coordination. To explain the coordination issue, Chassin argues

> Consider a woman with early-stage breast cancer, a condition with a five-year survival of greater than 90 percent if high-quality care is provided. At present, in most instances, the woman first receives at one location the mammogram that identifies the suspicious lesion. She is then referred to a surgeon, who performs a lumpectomy at another location; she goes on to visit a radiation oncologist, who performs radiation therapy at still another site; and she finally sees a medical oncologist, who administers multidrug chemotherapy at yet another, separate location. Her care throughout is followed by a primary care physician from a separate office. Nor can she be confident that crucial information will flow reliably from one stage of the process to the next about exactly what was done, what was found, and what was planned.

Chassin also observes that survival rates for surgical patients are much higher when the surgery is performed at a hospital performing high volumes of the surgery in question than when the surgery is performed at a hospital that performs the procedure infrequently.

Guinane and Davis (2004) build the case for Six Sigma quality by noting that a healthcare system operating at a three-sigma level would (in the United States) result in 20,000 incorrect prescriptions per year, 15,000 dropped newborn babies per year, and 12 babies being given to the wrong parents per day. They go on to present a case study from applying Six Sigma techniques to reduce groin injuries from catheterization in a cardiac lab. Lloyd and Holsenback (2006) note that medical errors may impose an annual cost on the U.S. economy in excess of $26 billion. They also present two applications of Six Sigma, one in radiology and one in the process of medication administration.

Bodenheimer (1999) discusses quality problems in healthcare using the three categories of overuse, underuse, and misuse. He states that, depending upon the type, as many as 8%–86% of operations may be unnecessary. Furthermore, in some cases, unnecessary operations have caused death. He also argues that underuse is prevalent in the care of patients with chronic disease and gives the example of diabetics who do not have regular glycohemoglobin measurements and retinal scans. Giving the example that fatal adverse drug reactions in hospitalized patients caused an estimated 106,000 deaths in 1994, he also claims that misuse is a pervasive problem.

Analysis and Discussion

This section presents our analysis of two important questions. First, what are the causes of operational problems we have observed in healthcare settings? Second, what are the impediments to applying Lean principles in healthcare organizations?

Causes of Operational Problems

Jimmerson et al. (2005) claim that one of the following three causes is at the root of every healthcare-related operational problem they have studied:

1. A poorly specified activity
2. A vague unreliable connection
3. A complex pathway

We agree that these three factors are root causes of many operational problems, but in our experience, there are at least three others:

1. Incorrectly identifying what creates customer value
2. Lack of communication
3. Overutilization

The question of utilization deserves additional explanation. Well-known results in queueing (also called waiting lines) show that, as utilization increases, the time that someone or something waits for service increases. Further, not only does the waiting time increase, but it does so in a highly nonlinear fashion (for a detailed discussion of the topic, see Cachon and Terweisch [2009]). In many manufacturing firms, this fact is implicitly recognized in "rules of thumb" that send managers seeking more capacity as utilization moves above 80%.

Our experience indicates that the phenomenon is much less recognized in service industries in general, including healthcare. Thus, particularly when dealing with expensive talent (engineering design personnel, nurses, physicians, etc.), concerns with efficiency ("It's expensive so I must keep it fully utilized!") may lead managers to try to operate systems at high utilizations. What may be missed is that doing so often precludes effective operations with reasonable lead times.

To illustrate and explain these factors, we will present two mini case studies from organizations with which we have worked. Note that the purpose of presenting these two case studies is not to provide yet two more examples of successful applications of Lean. The literature review already completed provides all the examples necessary to convince even a skeptic that Lean can indeed be deployed to good effect in healthcare settings. Rather, our intent here is to present examples to illustrate the three points we make above.

The first mini case study is that of the Infusion Suite at The University of Iowa Hospitals and Clinics (UIHC), and the second mini case study is that of processing doctors' orders at another organization.

The Infusion Suite

The University of Iowa Hospitals and Clinics (UIHC) founded their Infusion Suite in 1993. As its name implies, the purpose of the unit is to serve patients who need infusions of drugs and fluids. While the unit is best known for providing chemotherapy treatments for cancer, it also provides blood and iron transfusions as well as intravenous (IV) medications for the outpatient treatment of such conditions as allergies and rheumatitis.

> Over the last 5 years, as cancer treatments became less surgical and more chemical, the volume of patients in the Infusion Suite had steadily grown. Patient load at the Infusion suite was low when the clinic first opened at 8:00 a.m. and started peaking at around 10:00 a.m. when patients finished their appointments at clinics (e.g., the oncology clinic) elsewhere in the hospital and were sent to the Infusion Suite for an infusion. Patients at the Infusion Suite were assigned a particular nurse on their first visit who always supervised their infusions on subsequent visits. Although the typical processing time for an infusion was in the neighborhood of 2 hours, the average length of stay (flow time) was around 4 hours, so about half of the patient's time was spent simply waiting.
>
> After the patient checked in, he would be routed to the first available chair in the Infusion Suite. When the assigned nurse got to the patient, he would get together the pharmacy order and take it over to the pharmacy where the infusion would be prepared. It is worth noting that it is not uncommon for the infusion itself to cost over $40,000. Once mixed, the infusion has an extremely short shelf life, so preparing the infusion in advance of the patient's arrival was cost prohibitive. After the infusion was ready, the nurse would start the infusion. Nurses were walking over 6 miles per day, much of that walking being between the Infusion Suite and the pharmacy to check whether pharmacy orders were ready.

In this original process, patients were assigned to nurses who they would then see every time they came to the Infusion Suite. The reason behind this assignment was that everyone was sure the patients found it comforting to see a familiar face each time. The effect of this assignment, however, was to create multiple independent queues, one for each nurse. Thus, it was quite common to see one nurse completely overloaded while at the same time one or more other nurses might experience a lull in patient arrivals. This led to both over- and underutilization of nurses. Curiously enough, when data was collected through patient surveys, they found that the patients valued faster service much more than they valued seeing the same nurse. So the entire rationale for not using a pooled queue had been based on an incorrect identification of what created customer value.

The Infusion Suite also had an overly complex flow for the nurses. Because patients were assigned to chairs randomly in order of their vacancy, nurses would frequently be supervising multiple infusions at multiple locations throughout the Infusion Suite. Dividing Infusion Suite chairs into "pods" with each nurse being assigned to one pod obviated this.

Lack of communication also caused many problems. Since there was no direct way to communicate between the pharmacy and the Infusion Suite, nurses were kept busy running back and forth to see if infusions were ready. Additionally, the Infusion Suite saw many patients who did not come from the clinics, but instead had an appointment to come from their home sometime that day. Those patients typically arrived between 10 and 11 a.m., just when the flood of patients was starting to come in from the clinics. Nobody had ever told them that the Infusion Suite was much less busy either early in the morning or late in the afternoon. When this information was communicated to them, they began to come in during the two slack periods, thereby evening out the workload.

Doctors' Orders

> Our second example comes from an in-patient unit at a Midwest hospital. Each morning doctors would gather their charts and do the rounds of their patients. During rounds, the doctors would handwrite their orders and submit them to the charge nurse when they had finished rounds. In a typical day, the nurse would need to process over 300 orders for

the unit. To process the orders, the nurse would need to decipher each of the handwritten orders, which would sometimes require clarification from a doctor. In doing this, the nurse also had to contend with a constant stream of interruptions, which on average occurred at a rate of about 1 per minute. The result was that the average order required just over 7.5 hours to be processed with a range of 1 minute to over 13 hours.

While patient care was never impaired, it is clear that the process was not as effective as it should be. The key issue facing the nurse is that her utilization was nearing 100%. She not only needed to complete the orders but had numerous other responsibilities in the unit. The order lead times were then exacerbated by the fact that the charts were processed in batches during the morning rounds.

While an ideal solution to the problems facing the unit would have been electronic order entry by the doctors, the hospital simply was not in a position to make such a system a reality. Yet, the application of Lean thinking leads to dramatic improvements at a minimal cost. The key was the recognition that the charge nurse's utilization needed to be lowered by removing all unnecessary activity from her job. The process for fulfilling orders was actually left intact, but the other activities were simplified. For one, the nurse's work area was 6S-ed, with the most frequently used items labeled and placed within reach. To eliminate searching, commonly printed forms were given icons on the computer desktop. When possible, forms were consolidated. Perhaps the most important change was creating a system whereby doctors worked a single chart at a time, the equivalent of one-piece flow so often desired in manufacturing settings. The result was that the charge nurse could begin filling orders while the doctors were still on rounds. With the doctors still in the unit while the nurse worked the orders, any clarifications could be made in a timely and face-to-face manner thus facilitating better communication. With these changes, the charge nurse saw a dramatic drop in utilization, thus reducing the time required to fill orders.

Problems with Implementation

We have already noted in the literature review that one frequently cited roadblock to implementation is the concern that Lean, while it may work in manufacturing, simply cannot be applied to healthcare because healthcare is so different from manufacturing. Our view is that this claim is simply no longer credible. Manufacturers in the United States at one time made similar claims. Lean thinking might work for the Japanese, it was argued, but our culture is so different that it cannot possibly work here. That stuff might work well in the automotive industry with its assembly lines and high-volume production, it was claimed, but our industry is so different that it cannot possibly work here. Now, of course, Lean thinking is widely accepted in the U.S. manufacturing industry. We argue that the case studies presented and the literature reviewed in the "Does Lean work in healthcare?" section make similar hash of such claims for the healthcare industry.

That said, there are some significant impediments to implementation that organizations should be aware of before starting down the path to implementing Lean. In our view, the most significant problems include the following:

- Resistance to change
- Narrow focus on tools
- Impatience
- Lack of humility
- Lack of initial and ongoing senior management involvement
- Sustainment is hard

Let us consider these one at a time.

All organizations experience resistance to any changes that are made. As Lean and Six Sigma are by definition about changing the way that people work, many Lean and Six Sigma efforts are met with resistance. In our experience talking with healthcare organizations, this resistance is often viewed as insurmountable. This gloomy view arises because one of the most important and most constrained resources in the hospital is also mostly autonomous in the management structure and thus immune to incentives typically available in other organizations. The resource is doctors. Consequently, in most hospitals that we have observed, successful process improvement efforts have been started with a focus on non-physician-centered processes. The result is that the organization can demonstrate success without interrupting physician care. One of the improvements that often emerges (as in the Infusion Suite example presented earlier) is that patient care improves. Ultimately, this improvement in patient care helps overcome even the most ardent resisters.

Many times, we have seen Lean implementations start with training on and application of various Lean tools discussed in "Lean overview" section. Although this is not necessarily a bad thing, it can become one if that is where the Lean implementation stops. The reason why is that typically at this stage, an organization will have gotten fairly far along the way toward developing 5S (or 6S) and will have started doing kaizen events with a performance metric being the number of kaizen events performed. This in turn leads to the "Kamikaze kaizen" syndrome in which everything gets 5S-ed and kaizened with virtually no thought being given to how it all hooks together. In organizations that focus narrowly on tools, it is common to see pockets of excellence that somehow never produce any impact on ultimate customer value or on the bottom line. It is also common to see tools being misapplied. In one organization, for example, it went so far as to insist that if one had a banana on one's desk, the banana had to be "shadow-boarded." Although this sort of misapplication is easy to spot, others are more difficult. An example is the insistence on using the Takt Time tool in situations where it simply does not apply. Many transactional processes, for example, involve only a single processor, so there is no issue of dividing the work among multiple workstations as in an assembly line. What senior management needs to understand is that part of their job is to go one level above the tools and make certain the organization develops processes for implementing Lean that tie Lean process improvements back to definable organizational strategies or customer value creation.

After starting up Lean implementations, people are understandably anxious to see results. At first, everyone is happy with such metrics as reducing lead-time or reducing inventories. Yet eventually, people want to see how this is impacting the bottom line. As long as the improvements have merely created isolated islands of excellence, there will typically be little to no improvement in either the bottom line or in producing additional customer value. This is where senior management, once they have made certain they have the proper processes in place for organizing their Lean implementation and directing it toward strategic goals, need to have the vision to so see that the improvements they are looking for require fixing their entire value chain. In organizations we have witnessed, 2–3 years is a minimum timeframe for this to occur.

Humility has been defined as the recognition and acknowledgement of the truth. This is where many organizations fall down. Management, adopting a Taylorist philosophy, may believe or act as if they believe that workers have nothing to contribute toward the solution of problems. Organizations may come to believe they are much better than they are. We have encountered several now defunct organizations that insisted, "We've leaned out our entire organization" and truly believed they were world class. All this, mere months before they came tumbling down. Time and again, we have seen that problems arise when one part of the organization hands off to another, and fixing these kinds of relational coordination problems requires not only good communication, but also requires that one part of the organization understands and appreciates what the next does.

Senior management involvement is important from the start. We do mean involvement and not merely buy-in. In every successful Lean implementation with which we are familiar, senior managers from the CEO on down have gotten involved right at the beginning by taking training classes along with workers and working alongside them on kaizen events. By doing so, they lead by example and send a powerful message throughout their organization. In addition to becoming involved in such highly visible demonstrations of hands-on leadership, senior management has simply got to set the stage for success by developing the higher-level processes for implementing Lean as described earlier. Additionally, they need to make sure that incentives and bonuses complement rather than retard what they are trying to accomplish.

Sustainment is hard. It requires management to instill the processes and discipline so that process improvement is the culture of the organization. In our experience, however, the methods that sustain Lean in healthcare have direct analogies in manufacturing. Consider the case of Mercy Hospital in Cedar Rapids, Iowa (Krusie 2009). Mercy has had great success developing a Lean organization and credits Lean with playing an important role in helping the hospital recover from the devastating flooding of the summer of 2008. As they mature as a Lean organization, Mercy has begun to focus on spreading and sustaining their efforts. To do so, they have worked hard to get employees, particularly management, across the organization involved in kaizen activities. They have built a training organization and developed channels for communicating their Lean journey. Mercy has even implemented departmental performance boards. These boards make it possible for anyone passing through the department to see the department's progress in meeting their goals. All of these practices implemented at Mercy are exactly the same as those that we commonly find in manufacturing and other service organizations.

While we have confidence in Mercy's continued success, in our experience, it is not uncommon to see an organization make really tremendous strides toward implementing Lean and seeing really significant improvements in customer value and the bottom line. Then, after a few years of success, the organization tells itself it doesn't need this elaborate system for implementing and tracking Lean. "We don't really need to have a direct report to the CEO be responsible for the organization's Lean efforts," we hear. "It's all so inbred into our culture now that it's self-sustaining," is said. Well, the second law of thermodynamics tells us that nothing is self-sustaining. Organizations share this property of physical systems: without continuing inputs of energy, the Lean system will eventually flame out. That is exactly what we have seen happen.

Conclusion

In the introduction, we posed three questions:

1. Can Lean strategies be successfully translated to the healthcare sector? And what does it take to do so?
2. Even if Lean can be successfully translated to the healthcare sector, will doing so really be effective at meeting the goal of providing quality healthcare while simultaneously controlling costs?
3. Do Six Sigma and Lean complement each other or are they mutually exclusive?

We believe the evidence presented in this chapter provides pretty conclusive answers to these questions. Numerous examples and case studies from the healthcare sector give warrant to the claim that Lean strategies can work in healthcare. To do this requires that the organization avoid the five mistakes discussed in "Problems with Implementation" section. Finally, Lean and Six Sigma are complementary in that Lean focuses on reducing waste while Six Sigma focuses on reducing variance. Together, Lean and Six Sigma provide a powerful set of principles and methods for process improvement that can lead simultaneously to increased customer value and lower costs.

References

Bodenheimer, T. (1999, February), The movement for improved quality in health care, *New England Journal of Medicine*, 340(6), 488–492.

Cachon, G. and Terwiesch, C. (2009), *Matching Supply with Demand*, 2nd edn., New York: McGraw-Hill.

Chassin, M. (1998), Is health care ready for Six Sigma quality?, *The Milbank Quarterly*, 76(4), 565–590.

Christianson, J., Warrick, L., Howard, R., and Vollum, J. (2005), Deploying Six-Sigma in a health care system as a work in progress, *Joint Commission Journal on Quality and Patient Safety*, 31(11), 603–607.

Correa, F., Gil, M., and Redin, L. (2005), Benefits of connecting RFID and Lean principles in healthcare, Working paper 05-44, business economics series 10, Universidad Carlos de Madrid, Department of Business Administration, Madrid, Spain.

Dickson, E. (2008), Applying Lean manufacturing principles in healthcare. Presented to the *Seminar in Lean Practices*, Tippie College of Business, University of Iowa, August 4–8, Iowa City, IA.

Endsley, S., Magill, M. K., and Godfrey, M. M. (2006), Creating a Lean practice, Family Practice Web site, www.aafp.org/fpm

Ettinger, W. (2001), Six Sigma: Adapting GE's lesson to health care, *Trustee*, 54(8), 10–16.

Graban, M. (2009), *Lean Hospitals*, New York: Productivity Press.

Guinane, C. and Davis, N. (2004), The science of Six Sigma in hospitals, *The American Heart Hospital Journal*, 2, 42–48.

Jimmerson, C., Weber, D., and Sobek, D. K. (2005, May), Reducing waste and errors: Piloting Lean principles at Intermountain Healthcare, *Joint Commission Journal on Quality Patient Safety*, 31(5), 249–257.

Jones, D. and Mitchell, A. (2006), Lean thinking for the NHS, http://www.leanuk.org/downloads/health/lean_thinking_for_the_nhs_leaflet.pdf

Kim, C., Spahlinger, D., Kin, J., and Billi, J. (2006), Lean health care: What can hospitals learn from a world-class automaker?, *Journal of Hospital Medicine*, 1(3), 191–199.

King, B.-T., Ben-Tovim, D. I., and Bassham, J. (2006, August), Redesigning emergency department patient flows: Application of Lean thinking to healthcare, *Emergency Medicine Australasia*, 18(4), 391–397.

Krusie, K. (2009), Lean: 'Perfecting the mercy touch.' Presented to the *Seminar in Lean Practices*, Tippie College of Business, University of Iowa, July 27–21, Cedar Rapids, IA.

Liker, J. (2004), *The Toyota Way: 14 Management Principles from the World's Greatest Manufacturer*, New York: McGraw-Hill.

Lloyd, D. and Holsenback, J. (2006), The use of Six Sigma in health care operations: Application and opportunity, *Academy of Health Care Management Journal*, 2, 41–49.

Manos, A., Sattier, M., and Alukal, G. (2006, July), Make healthcare Lean, *Quality Progress*, 39(7), 24–30.

Montgomery, D. (1989), *The Fall of the House of Labor: The Workplace, the State, and American Labor Activism, 1865–1925* (Paperback edition), Cambridge, U.K.: Cambridge University Press.

Ohno, T. (2009), Interview with Koichi Shimokawa and Takahiro Fujimoto. In *The Birth of Lean*, K. Shimokawa and T. Fujimoto, eds. B. Miller and J. Shook, trans., Cambridge, MA: Lean Enterprise Institute, 2009.

Okolo, S., Peeler, C., Rooney, A. J., Yun, J., and Korycinski, D. (2009), Deployed warrior medical management center: A Lean Six-Sigma approach. In *Proceedings of the 2008 IEEE Systems and Information Engineering Design Symposium*, Charlottesville, VA.

Organisation for Economic Co-operation and Development (2009), *OECD Health Data 2009*, Paris, France, published online June 2009.

Panchak, P. (2003), Lean health care? It works!, *Industry Week*, 252(11), 34–40.

Rother, M. and Shook, J. (2003), *Learning to See: Value-Stream Mapping to Create Value and Eliminate Muda*, Cambridge, MA: The Lean Enterprise Institute.

Smalley, H. E. (1982), *Hospital Industrial Engineering: A Guide to the Improvement of Hospital Management Systems*, Prentice-Hall International Series in Industrial and Systems Engineering, Upper Saddle River, NJ: Prentice-Hall.

Spear, S. and Bowen, H. K. (1999), Decoding the DNA of the Toyota Production System, *Harvard Business Review*, September, pp. 96–106.

Taylor, W. T. (1911), *The Principles of Scientific Management*, Sioux Falls, SD: NuVision Publications, LLC, 2007.

Tragardh, B. and Lindberg, K. (2004), Curing a meager health care system by Lean methods—translating 'chains of care' in the Swedish health care sector, *International Journal of Health Planning and Management*, 19, 383–398.

Van Den Heuvel, J., Does, R., and Bisgaard, S. (2005, February), Dutch hospital implements Six-Sigma, *ASQ Six Sigma Forum Magazine*, 4(2), 11–14.

Womack, J. P. and Jones, D. T. (2003), *Lean Thinking: Banish Waste and Create Wealth in Your Corporation*, 2nd edn., New York: Free Press.

12

Patient Safety and Proactive Risk Assessment

Pascale Carayon
University of Wisconsin–Madison

Hélène Faye
Institut de Radioprotection et de Sûreté Nucléaire

Ann Schoofs Hundt
University of Wisconsin–Madison

Ben-Tzion Karsh
University of Wisconsin–Madison

Tosha B. Wetterneck
University of Wisconsin–Madison

Patient Safety and the Need for Proactive Risk Assessment **12**-1
Proactive Risk Assessment **12**-2
Diversity of Proactive Risk Assessment • Proactive Risk Assessment: A Path to Organizational Learning and Sensemaking • Process Analysis in Proactive Risk Assessment • Examples of Proactive Risk Assessment
Practical Considerations of Proactive Risk Assessment **12**-5
Advice for Conducting a Proactive Risk Assessment • Selecting a Proactive Risk Assessment Technique
Case Studies **12**-6
Conclusion **12**-13
References **12**-13

Patient Safety and the Need for Proactive Risk Assessment

Traditionally, patient safety has been approached from one of three paradigms: focus on (1) reducing healthcare professional (HCP) errors, (2) reducing patient injuries, and (3) improving the use of evidence-based medicine. The first paradigm proposed that, to achieve patient safety, errors committed by HCPs must be prevented, eliminated, or reduced. This paradigm is exemplified by the Institute of Medicine (IOM) report that proposed focusing on error reduction through the design of safer systems (Institute of Medicine 2000). A follow-up report by the IOM continued supporting the error prevention paradigm by explaining, "a new delivery system must be built to achieve substantial improvements in patient safety—a system that is capable of preventing errors from occurring in the first place, while at the same time incorporating lessons learned from any errors that do occur" (Institute of Medicine 2004). In an article presenting the second paradigm, Layde et al. (2002) argued that because error and harm are not always linked, patient safety efforts should focus on reducing patient injuries. Errors that do not lead to harm, often called near misses or near hits, may occur when luck is involved, when the error is not clinically significant enough to cause harm, or when the error is caught before harm can be done. The authors argue that since some errors do not result in patient harm, not all errors are worth trying to eliminate. Instead, they propose that individuals in healthcare delivery systems analyze patient harm, determine what factors, including errors, contribute to harm, and then redesign the system of care to eliminate all factors that contribute to harm, including factors that cause errors. The third paradigm proposed by Brennan et al. (2005) focuses on implementing evidence-based practices for quality patient care—if clinicians follow evidence-based practices, then the patients will receive more appropriate, and, therefore, higher quality care. Higher quality care, they argue, will also be safer care. They point out that safety science can contribute to a better understanding of how to design for both safe and effective care. Underlying all three paradigms is the belief that, to achieve safety, changes are needed in the design of the system where patients receive care. The first two, however, are reactive because they require waiting for errors or injuries to occur.

The goal of safety engineering, i.e., to prevent harm to people and property (Karsh et al. 2006, Leveson 1995, Smith et al. 2001, 2003), can be achieved in many different ways. Safety engineers agree on the following hierarchy of good practices (Diberardinis 1998, Hagan et al. 2001a,b, Smith et al. 2001, 2003). First, whenever possible, safety should be built into the design of products, processes, and systems. Second, in the case of an existing system, hazards in the system need to be proactively identified before errors or harm occur; once identified, the hazards can be eliminated, reduced to levels that do not cause harm, or blocked from causing harm. Third, when errors or harm happen, their causes need to be identified and then eliminated. All three approaches are considered necessary, but the first two are proactive as errors and harm have not yet occurred. Healthcare has only recently come to understand the important role of proactive methods (Karsh et al. 2006).

Recently, several authors have proposed proactive methods for addressing patient safety (Battles and Lilford 2003, Carayon et al. 2006, Karsh et al. 2006) that are consistent with the safety engineering ideas of focusing on hazards. A hazard is anything that increases the probability of errors or of patient/employee injury and is analogous to "risk factor" in healthcare or epidemiology. Because hazards occur in the real work environment, they typically interact with each other and can, therefore, lead to other hazards (Battles and Lilford 2003). For example, the computer display of an electronic health record may be difficult to read because of poor contrast between the text and background in the display. The readability of the display could be even worse in situations where room lighting creates glare, further reducing the ability of the physician to read the record. These interactions among the physician, screen, lighting, and text are hazards in that they are potentially detrimental to different types of performance needed to be executed by the physician, i.e., visual perception and decision-making. These in turn may impact patient safety and quality output goals.

The proactive methods focusing on hazards discussed by Battles, Carayon, and Karsh (Battles and Lilford 2003, Carayon et al. 2006, Karsh et al. 2006) are referred to as proactive risk assessment (*note*: in the literature "proactive" is often used interchangeably with "prospective," and "assessment" is often used interchangeably with "analysis"). Battles et al. (2006) framed the pool of methods that make up proactive risk assessment as focusing on: the single event using root cause analysis (RCA) (Gosbee and Anderson 2003); the process level using failure mode and effects analysis, or FMEA (in healthcare also known as healthcare FMEA or HFMEA); and at the system level, using probabilistic risk assessment. In the rest of the chapter, we describe various proactive risk assessment methods and their applications to healthcare and patient safety. We also review the challenges in conducting proactive risk assessment in healthcare.

Proactive Risk Assessment

Diversity of Proactive Risk Assessment

Various risk assessment tools and methods have been developed to identify potential or actual sources of hazards, errors, and accidents in systems and processes. Leveson (1995) describes 12 models and techniques for identifying hazards, including FMEA, fault tree analysis (FTA), and event tree analysis. Unfortunately, very little scientific evaluation of these methods has been conducted (Lehto and Salvendy 1991, Leveson 1995). Lyons (2009) reviewed 35 techniques for error prediction and safety assessment. All of the methods must start with observations and process analysis (Battles and Lilford 2003, Karsh and Alper 2005) and are then followed with prioritization and control strategies and identification of solutions. Several experts have described the advantages and disadvantages of different risk assessment methods, and recommend the use of multiple complementary methods (Israelski and Muto 2007, Leveson 1995, Senders 2004). Risk assessment methods can be retrospective (e.g., analyzing a sentinel event, RCA) or prospective (e.g., analyzing a process and identifying its potential or known failure modes, FMEA), and use either a bottom-up (e.g., FMEA) or top-down (FTA) method.

The methods differ on the continuum of qualitative to quantitative and subjective to objective. They all start qualitatively with observations and process maps; even FTA and probabilistic risk assessment use graphical depictions of components and subsystems, which are qualitative. FMEA adds a quantitative element by assigning scores for severity, probability and detectability, and computing a risk priority score. Probabilistic risk assessment is also quantitative and relies on probabilities. However, in complex sociotechnical systems where humans are involved and given our very limited knowledge on probabilistic contributions of human decisions, behavior, and error and organizational structure and culture, the probabilities will be uncertain and, therefore, highly subjective. Mathematical and statistical methods are currently being developed to deal more robustly with expert judgment uncertainty (Ayyub 2001, Bier 2004, Florin 1999, Kraan and Bedford 2005, Monti and Carenini 2000, Mosleh et al. 1988, Washington and Oh 2006), but there is still much debate and uncertainty about best practices. Marx and Slonim (2003) make the case that probabilistic risk assessment can overcome limitations of FMEA, and that FMEA does not allow for prioritization upon quantitative risk; however, that is a point of debate. FMEA does create risk prioritization using the risk priority number (RPN). While RPN is not a probability per se, experts in probabilistic risk assessment point out that the probabilities used are most often estimates and, therefore, also relative rankings at best, especially when they are based on expert judgments and uncertainty estimates.

Proactive Risk Assessment: A Path to Organizational Learning and Sensemaking

Proactive risk assessment methods can have systemic impact on healthcare organizations, such as improved organizational learning and sensemaking. Battles et al. (2006) have identified seven attributes of "patient safety sensemaking": (1) conversation about a particular issue or event, (2) issue or event that is unexpected, novel, or ambiguous, (3) conversation aimed at reducing ambiguity, (4) involvement of key stakeholders with their own knowledge about the issue or event, (5) using conversation to create new, more understandable knowledge, (6) creation of shared mental models about the issue or event, and (7) development of solutions that can be implemented. These seven attributes are directly related to the use of risk assessment methods and can have beneficial impacts on organizational learning and sensemaking. Organizational learning in healthcare poses unique challenges including the development of shared mental models (Hundt 2007). For the organizational learning to occur, healthcare workers need to understand that they must function as a system of complicated, interdependent parts. The use of risk assessment methods can contribute to organizational learning by helping healthcare providers make sense of their environment and analyze risks of processes and work systems (Battles et al. 2006).

Our own experience of the use of FMEA performed before the implementation of Smart IV pump technology shows the importance of creating a climate of trust and learning, where members of the multidisciplinary FMEA team can share information about risks and develop a better understanding of the process (Hundt et al. 2006, Wetterneck et al. 2004, 2006). The performance of this FMEA very much contributed in establishing a climate, where problems following the implementation of Smart IV pump technology were more likely to be detected, reported, and analyzed (Carayon et al. 2005a, Schroeder et al. 2006). The use of risk assessment methods to analyze and improve systems and processes can, therefore, contribute to the development of high reliability organizing (HRO) characteristics (Weick and Sutcliffe 2001), such as reluctance to simplify interpretations because the FMEA or proactive risk assessment team is attempting to create a more complete, systematic view of the process or system.

Process Analysis in Proactive Risk Assessment

The effectiveness of proactive risk assessment is highly dependent on the characterization of the process under study. In the discipline of human factors and ergonomics, it has long been recognized that the actual work done can be substantially different from the "prescribed" work as defined in job descriptions and procedures (Guerin et al. 2006, Leplat 1989). The discrepancy between the "prescribed" work and the "real" work may be due, for instance, to the need to adapt to local circumstances or context, worker preferences, worker creativity and initiative, and misunderstanding of the work system by the "prescribers" (e.g., people who write policies and procedures). Therefore, whenever conducting a proactive risk assessment, it is critical to gather information about the "real" process in its actual context.

Examples of Proactive Risk Assessment

Cook et al. (2007) conducted a probabilistic risk assessment of the thoracic organ transplantation process with a specific focus on the likelihood of ABO-incompatible organ transplant. The objective of this analysis was to characterize the reliability of the transplantation system during three periods of time: before the March 2003 Jessica Santillan event,* between March 2003 and October 2004, and after October 2004. Using direct observations, interviews, and review of documents, the researchers developed an event tree for organ transplant and three fault trees that produced estimates of the likelihood of an ABO-incompatible transplant during the three periods of time: 0.001384%, 0.000308%, and 0.0000222%, respectively. Changes that were put in place after the March 2003 event included a redesign of the "open" offer process with additional cross checks for ABO compatibility. Matching donor organs to recipients can be done either via a computerized matched list or via an "open" process in which a transplant center proposes recipients to the donor-side coordinators. The results of the probabilistic risk assessment show that the rate of unintentional ABO-incompatible organ transplants was extremely low. The quantitative modeling allowed the evaluation of changes implemented post-March'2003 event, which further reduced the risk of ABO-incompatible transplant. This type of probabilistic risk assessment can be useful to evaluate the risk of rare failures in complex systems that are well-characterized with multiple layers of defense, especially when the failures can have catastrophic consequences (Wreathall and Nemeth 2003).

Karnon et al. (2007) used a quantitative modeling method to evaluate rates of preventable adverse drug events (ADEs) and to identify interventions with the greatest potential for reducing preventable ADEs. Errors were assumed to occur at three stages of the medication use process: prescribing, dispensing, and administration; errors could be detected at the dispensing and administration stages. Only a limited number of error types were considered for the model. Based on existing literature and experts input, several model parameters were estimated: medication error rates, detection rates, probability that undetected errors cause patient harm, and effectiveness of interventions. Three specific interventions were examined: computerized provider order entry (CPOE) technology, pharmacists on hospital units, and bar coding medication administration technology. The quantitative model produced estimates of preventable ADEs for a 400-bed hospital with about 162,000 prescription orders per year. The median number of preventable ADEs per year was around 450 with a range of about 200–700 preventable ADEs per year. This dropped to 300 preventable ADEs per year with CPOE and pharmacists on hospital units. The impact of bar coding medication administration technology was smaller—the median rate of preventable ADEs per year dropped to 400 with a range between 325 and 450 preventable ADEs per year.

Apkon et al. (2004) conducted an FMEA of the process of continuous drug infusion delivery: (1) selecting the drug, (2) selecting a dose, (3) selecting an infusion rate, (4) calculating and ordering the infusion, (5) preparing the infusion, and (6) programming the infusion pump and delivering the infusion. The study was conducted in a pediatric intensive care unit; the objectives were to redesign the process of delivering continuous drug infusion to improve patient safety, efficiency in staff workflow, hemodynamic

* Jessica Santillan is the 17-year old girl who received heart and lungs that were not of her blood type at Duke University Hospital. Jessica Santillan did not survive a second transplant performed.

stability during infusions changes, and efficient use of resources. The researchers also compared the redesigned process to the original process. After the identification of failure modes in each of the six process steps, a multidisciplinary team determined the risk of injury of a failure, the frequency with which failures occur, and the likelihood that a failure would go undetected before an injury results. The multiplication of these three scores led to the calculation of an RPN associated with each failure mode; this led to the identification of the most likely contributors to medically serious failures. Based on the results of the FMEA, the following three main consequences of failure were identified: delivering the wrong drug, delivering the right dose but using too dilute a formulation and resulting in an excessive infusion rate, and delivering the wrong dose of the drug. The RPNs associated with these three consequences were considerably reduced after numerous changes were suggested for improving the process design.

Bonnabry et al. (2008) conducted a failure modes, effects, and criticality analysis (FMECA) to compare the risk of drug prescribing before and after implementation of a computerized patient record, including a CPOE system. The objective was to compare the risks to patient safety in the manual and computerized systems, and to identify any major residual risks in the computerized system that should be the target of additional action. The drug prescribing process included four main steps: (1) therapy selection and prescription modalities, (2) formal prescription, (3) order management by nurses, and (4) treatment follow-up and adaptation. For each failure of each process step, a criticality index was calculated by multiplying the likelihood of occurrence of the failure mode, the severity of the potential effect for the patient, and the chance of detecting the failure before it affected patient safety. Results showed an overall decrease of the criticality by nearly 25% after the implementation of CPOE. The major safety improvements were observed for errors due to ambiguous, incomplete, or illegible orders, wrong dose determination or adaptation, and drug interactions not considered, while the larger increases of criticality were related to vital signs not considered during treatment adaptation and prescription to a wrong patient. The FMECA also identified failure modes for which the risk was considered to be unacceptable, thus, allowing the concentration of efforts on those most critical failure modes.

Practical Considerations of Proactive Risk Assessment

Advice for Conducting a Proactive Risk Assessment

Previous work has identified practical considerations that should be taken into account when preparing for a proactive risk assessment (American Society for Healthcare Risk Management 2002, Spath 2004a,b, Wetterneck et al. 2004, 2009). First and foremost, among the considerations is the need to identify a topic that is both well defined and of limited scope. Initiating a proactive risk assessment with an imprecise objective challenges participants, especially those who may have no prior experience serving on this type of team, and can lengthen and make the team's effort more complicated.

Likewise, a team leader with proven expertise guiding a team from initiation to completion will help render the team to be more successful and team members to be more satisfied with the proactive risk assessment and the outcome of their efforts. Team membership should also include a facilitator or team member with experience in and knowledge of the proactive risk assessment technique that is being utilized. This person must understand and be able to manage group dynamics and ensure open communication with the group. It is highly desirable for the team leader and facilitator to meet between team meetings to discuss progress and strategize how to overcome challenges they may encounter.

Another key participant is a content expert. This person should be actively involved in the process that the risk assessment is addressing. Team members should likewise have a stake in the process under review and recognize the benefit of their participation on the team, both for themselves as well as the department or unit they represent. The team leader and facilitator must ensure that all members are engaged in the team's efforts.

As the proactive risk assessment progresses, it is important for the team to identify other organizations that have addressed a similar issue and either have published about their experience or simply have information to share. Conducting a review of the literature and contacting people from organizations similar to one's own can prove fruitful. Findings and advice can be obtained and shared with the team. When feasible, tests or simulations of the process should be "run" and participants (ultimate end users or individuals who will operate in/work on the process being reviewed) should attempt to "stretch" the process in order to identify potential or actual breakdowns. Similarly, pilot testing a proposed technology being addressed by a proactive risk assessment is valuable (Wetterneck et al. 2006). In a similar fashion, team members can visit another organization or work unit where the process under review is currently operating so that they can observe how the organization addressed challenges or problems the process posed.

A number of constraints must also be taken into account to ensure that the proactive risk assessment method is feasible and its objectives can be met. Time and resource constraints are paramount when considering the expectations and timeline for the team. The amount of time the team is given and team members have available to accomplish the objective will have a significant impact on the amount of work required prior to the team first convening and throughout the proactive risk assessment. Busy healthcare providers and other workers have a limited amount of time to dedicate to such an activity. Thus, more might need to be accomplished outside the formal meeting time. The organization may have a limited number of trained facilitators and individuals with human factors engineering expertise. This may affect the team's level of "sophistication" when selecting various tools or methods to use for mapping processes and/or analyzing data.

On the whole, conducting a proactive risk assessment requires organizational commitment, planning, and expertise to ensure a smooth process and successful outcome. This can be accomplished by selecting a knowledgeable leader, facilitator, and team members and supporting the team with sufficient direction, feedback, and resources to accomplish the task given to them.

Selecting a Proactive Risk Assessment Technique

A major challenge for healthcare organizations is to choose the right proactive risk assessment technique. Lyons (2009) proposed a framework for selecting error prediction techniques, which can be expanded in selecting a proactive risk analysis technique (Figure 12.1). The selection of the technique depends on two major issues: (1) resources and constraints and (2) requirements for what is expected from the technique. A healthcare organization needs to evaluate resources required for applying the technique, such as experts in safety and human factors and ergonomics, and stakeholders or process experts. Time is another major resource that needs to be considered as this has been identified as a major problem with some of the techniques such as FMEA (Wetterneck et al. 2004). Information necessary to use the various techniques can be categorized as information on the physical, cognitive, and psychosocial contributions of the people involved in the process, and information on the rest of the work system, i.e., tools and technologies, and environmental and organizational conditions (Carayon and Smith 2000, Smith and Carayon-Sainfort 1989, Smith and Carayon 2000). Another element regarding resources and constraints that needs to be considered is the need for equipment and software. Some techniques may require collection of data on the process using video or audio taping equipment. Other techniques may require special software for analysis or simulation of complex data (e.g., probabilistic risk assessment). In addition to clearly identifying the resources and constraints about the use of a proactive risk assessment, an organization needs to specify the objectives of the assessment. For instance, if the assessment was used to identify the error recovery opportunities in a process, techniques such as FMEA may be useful.

Case Studies

Table 12.1 summarizes three different case studies of proactive risk assessment that the authors have been involved in. The case studies represent a variety of patient safety issues such as safety of intravenous (IV) medication administration, breakdowns of order-related information in the context of patient transfers from OR to ICU, and ICU nurses' contribution to quality of medication management. FMEA

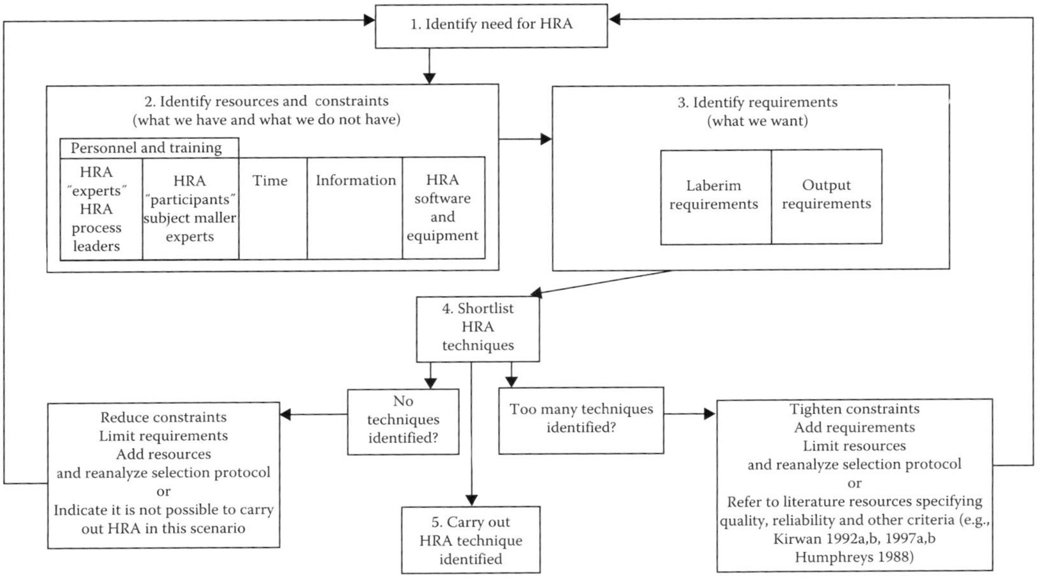

FIGURE 12.1 Process for selecting a proactive risk assessment (or human reliability assessment (HRA)) technique. (Reprinted from Lyons, M., *Appl. Ergonom.*, 40(3), 379, 2009. © 2009; with permission from Elsevier.)

and hybrid FMEA techniques were used in the case studies; the hybrid FMEAs relied on modified and simplified scoring systems. Two of the case studies involved significant preparation (3 months in the case study of CPOE implementation in ICUs and 80 hours of observation and 24 hours of interview in the case study of nurses' contribution to medication management) and only 4 to 5 hours of meeting, whereas the first case study involved 46 hours of meetings spread over 4½ months. Each case study is briefly described in the rest of the section.

Case Study 1: Use of HFMEA to Evaluate the Current IV Medication Administration Process and a Proposed New Process with a Smart IV Pump

An IV pump committee was formed at a 450-bed academic medical center in the Midwestern United States to consider the purchase of a new IV pump with built-in dose error reduction technology after reviewing multiple cases of IV administration errors. The committee developed pump criteria based on safety standards and user needs and selected the Smart IV pump (Cardinal Health) for purchase. The IV pump committee and senior management decided to commit resources to perform an FMEA on the current IV medication administration process

TABLE 12.1 Summary of Case Studies of Proactive Risk Assessment

	Design and Implementation of Smart IV Pump	Implementation of CPOE in ICUs	ICU Nurses' Contributions to Medication Management
Objective	To identify the: (1) risks associated with implementation of the Smart IV pump and (2) solutions to decrease the risk through technology and process redesign	To identify potential breakdowns in order-related information transfer for patients transferred directly to the ICU from the operating room	To identify ICU nurses' contributions to quality of medication management
Process studied	Medication use process, focusing on the current IV medication administration and the expected process after new IV pump implementation	Information transfer of ICU patients postop when transferred directly (back) to the ICU	Nursing medication management process
Organizational context	Hospital and outpatient departments and procedure areas using IV pumps at an academic medical center	Adult and pediatric ICUs in a large regional medical center	Cardiovascular ICU in one hospital
Preparation for proactive risk assessment	Observation of nurses in work environment Review of internal and external data on IV medication administration errors Review of literature on IV pump evaluation Online technology listserv MAUDE database Pilot study of IV pumps	Worked with Director of IT to identify topic and plan for proactive risk assessment based on findings and recommendations of an "FMEA evaluation" conducted as part of previous research project Reviewed process maps constructed by IT staff Three months of planning	Observation of nurses in their work environment Interviews of nurses about decision-making Interviews of nurses about their perceptions of medication management
		Methodology	
Overall Methodology	FMEA	Hybrid FMEA	Hybrid FMEA
Participants (number, disciplines, …)	22 persons from various departments (anesthesia, internal medicine, nursing, biomedical engineering, industrial engineering, central supply, pharmacy, quality improvement) Facilitated by a human factors trained pharmacist, team leader-anesthesiologist	Multidisciplinary team of IT (7), nursing (3), MDs (5), unit clerk (1) Facilitated by a human factors engineer	Seven ICU nurses Facilitated by a human factors engineer
Meetings (number, duration, …)	46 hours of meetings over 4½ months (1–2-hour meetings every week to every other week)	One 5-hour meeting with multidisciplinary team Follow-up meeting with IT team (day after the 5-hour meeting)	Two 2-hour meetings 2 months apart
Focus of proactive risk assessment (failure modes, contributing factors, recovery processes, …)	Failure modes Short- and long-term solutions Contributing factors	Failure modes identified by full group Prioritization and identification of solutions in the design and implementation of CPOE with IT team during a meeting following day	Identification of failure modes Recovery processes Contributing factors

TABLE 12.1 (continued) Summary of Case Studies of Proactive Risk Assessment

	Design and Implementation of Smart IV Pump	Implementation of CPOE in ICUs	ICU Nurses' Contributions to Medication Management
Role of researchers	Two research team members (both participants, one with healthcare background, the other with human factors engineering background)	Two research teams members	Four research team members (1 facilitator, 1 content and process backup, 2 content experts)
Scoring approach	Severity to patient Current process: minor–moderate–major–catastrophic New process: low–moderate–high Probability Both current and new processes: remote, uncommon, occasional, frequent	Efficiency and regulatory compliance: yes–no Quality of care: high–medium–low Patient safety: high–medium–low Medical–legal: high–medium–low	Likelihood: low–moderate–high Impact on patient: low–moderate–high Impact on nurse: low–moderate–high
Evaluation of the proactive risk assessment	Participant survey and structured interview	Four-item questionnaire, subgroup feedback following morning, and review of issues list	Four-item questionnaire administered at the end of the second meeting

using the current IV pump and the proposed process using the Smart IV pump to help minimize the risk of IV medication administration using the new Smart IV pump.

A multidisciplinary committee was assembled, including 22 persons from various departments: anesthesia, internal medicine, nursing, biomedical engineering, industrial engineering, central supply, pharmacy, and quality improvement. The team was facilitated by a human factors trained pharmacist and the team leader was an anesthesiologist end user of IV pumps. The organization had performed one previous FMEA and had used the HFMEA process and, therefore, this process was chosen for the current team and the team received 1–2 hours of FMEA and HFMEA training.

Multiple data sources were used as inputs in the HFMEA process. These included direct observation of nurses administering medications on the nursing units (Carayon et al. 2004, 2005b), review of internal and external reports of IV medication administration errors, and other available literature evaluating IV pumps, nurses' comments about using the new pump from a 2 week pilot study of the Smart IV pump on a cardiovascular medicine unit, replies to a request for information from users of the new Smart IV pump from an academic medical center based technology listserv, and the FDA's MAUDE database, which collects complaints about medical device functioning. These data were combined with the knowledge of team members to develop a process map of the entire medication use process and failure modes for the IV medication administration process. The team evaluated the entire medication use process to understand other parts of the medication use process that would need to be redesigned (i.e., IV medication labeling, ordering of IV pumps, cleaning of IV pumps) and referred these to other hospital committees. The team then focused on identifying failure modes for the IV medication administration process with the current pump and with the new pump. Several team members were trained on the use of the new IV pump and the pump was available at the team meetings; this helped team members to discover new potential failure modes with the technology hardware and software interfaces. The risk priority scores were determined using the HFMEA severity and probability scales for the current pump. A 3-point severity scoring system was used for the new pump as the process was proposed so no actual data existed on which to base the scoring. About 200 failure modes were generated on 38 process steps and about half were selected to proceed to cause generation and solution building. The solutions were categorized into five categories based on the work system (Carayon and Smith 2000, Smith and Carayon-Saintfort 1989): (1) policy and procedure, (2) training or education, (3) environment, (4) people, and (5) technology hardware and software. Technology solutions were further categorized into short- and long-term solutions as a way to present the information back to the organization and to prioritize next steps and the resources needed for those steps. The organization was very receptive to the FMEA team's recommendations and implemented majority of them. A dedicated Smart IV pump nurse was hired to assist with the implementation and to meet with end users after implementation to provide further training and to troubleshoot problems with the pump. A subset of the FMEA team continued to meet after Smart IV pump implementation and reviewed the data collected by the Smart IV pump nurse to understand which failure modes were occurring and any new failure modes that were identified, which had not been anticipated by the team.

Case Study 2: Development and use of a Hybrid Proactive Risk Assessment Prior to Implementation of CPOE/EHR in ICUs

In conjunction with a research project evaluating the implementation of a CPOE/EHR system in ICUs (http://cqpi.engr.wisc.edu/cpoe_home), a large Eastern regional medical center recognized the value of conducting a proactive risk assessment on the forthcoming system. Hospital leadership responsible for the CPOE design and implementation determined that a conventional (H)FMEA would not fit within the time constraints of the IT staff designing the interface and clinical staff caring for patients—all of whom needed to be involved in the proactive risk assessment. Instead, a hybrid proactive risk assessment method was designed and based on the research team's previous experience, as well as the constraints of the regional medical center. This method required considerable preparatory work, one intense 5-hour meeting of all stakeholders, and follow-up by management subsequent to the meeting. Evaluation of the process took various forms.

The two researchers working with the IT manager established ground rules that guided the planning portion of the process. These ground rules resulted from team member (interview) evaluations of two previously conducted FMEAs (Wetterneck et al. 2009). Over a 3 month period, various processes were identified as potential candidates for the proactive risk assessment. The planning process was challenging due to the requirements that the scope of the proactive risk assessment be clearly defined, limited, relevant to the ICUs, and have completed pre- and post-implementation workflows. The order-related information transfer for patients transferred directly to the ICU from the OR was identified as the process for further study. Once stakeholders for this process and team members were nominated, the logistical issues of scheduling, identifying a sufficiently large meeting room, ordering supplies, and selecting a menu were handled by a well-qualified administrative assistant.

The chief medical information officer began the meeting by briefly explaining the process to be followed during the ensuing 5 hours, conveying to the participants the support of hospital leadership, and introducing the IT and research participants. The two researchers served as facilitators and scribes throughout the meeting. One IT staff reviewed the current and proposed workflows that corresponded to the process being analyzed. Aside from directing the focus of the proactive risk assessment for the group, the posted workflow helped reduce any deviations in discussion from the process being reviewed by the team, throughout the 5-hour session. The final introductory activity included a demonstration of the portion of the CPOE system, in its present (unfinished) form, that coincided with the process under scrutiny. All of the introductory activities took approximately 30 minutes.

Discussion and brainstorming of issues ensued. Any issue within the bounds of the proactive risk assessment was recorded on flip chart paper adhered to the walls on the two sides of the room. Duplicate issues were recorded since the facilitators knew that they would be combined at a later step in the process. Whenever an issue was identified that was deemed to be outside the bounds of the proactive risk assessment, the facilitators (two researchers) were able to refer to the workflow and suggest an issue be assigned to the "parking lot"—a list of issues warranting concern at another time but outside the scope of the current proactive risk assessment. After approximately 2½ hours of brainstorming, redundancies were being identified and the team agreed that the list was exhaustive. At this point, there was a 30-minute dinner break. Team members were told that they were excused if they were no longer interested in participating or needed to be elsewhere. Interestingly, no one left the room at that point.

Upon reconvening, the team members grouped like-issues and then began the prioritization process. Priorities were identified according to the extent to which they posed medicolegal, quality, regulatory, safety, or efficiency issues. This grouping and prioritizing took approximately 2 hours. At this point, the facilitators and IT staff told team members that the issues would be referred to the design group, which would then be responsible for dealing with the issues. Overwhelmingly, positive feedback centered around the multidisciplinary nature of the participants and their ability to work together to identify, prioritize, and forward to CPOE designers the issues most critical to them, collectively.

Case Study 3: Proactive Risk Assessment of the Nursing Medication Management Process

Much emphasis has been placed on nursing work and quality, in particular with the goal expressed by the interdisciplinary nursing quality research initiative of the Robert Wood Johnson Foundation to investigate "nursing care processes, the nursing workforce and environment, and the impact of innovation on the quality of patient care" (http://www.inqri.org/).

In this context, a research project was conducted to describe nurses' contributions to the quality of medication management. The goal of the project was to examine various aspects of the nursing medication management process: (1) failure modes that can occur at each step of the process, (2) recovery processes that nurses use to cope with failure modes, and (3) the work-system factors that contribute to the occurrence of failure modes. The major difference between what was done for this study and typical proactive risk assessments is the significant time spent in data collection and analysis before the actual proactive risk assessment took place. About 80 hours of observation of nurses in their work environment, 12 hours of semi-structured interviews on nurses' decision-making in medication management, and 12 hours of interviews about nurses' perceptions of medication management were conducted. The analysis of these data allowed us to specify and clarify the nursing medication management process and its numerous steps.

The study was conducted in a 15-bed cardiovascular ICU (CVICU) of a tertiary referral hospital. We recruited seven volunteering nurses of the CVICU nursing council to participate in the proactive risk assessment, which consisted of two 2-hour focus groups. For the focus groups, members of the research team were assigned specific roles: one facilitator, one content backup, and two content experts who had performed observations and interviews. In the first focus group, nurses were asked to review the failure modes of each step of the medication management process. Nurses were also asked to evaluate the likelihood of failure modes, their impact on patient, and their impact on nurses: each dimension was assigned a score (low, moderate, or high). Finally, nurses listed the different processes used to recover from the failure modes. Two months later, in the second focus group, nurses were asked to list the work-system factors that contribute to the failure modes in the medication management process. At the end of the second focus group, nurses were asked to fill out a questionnaire about the usefulness of the proactive risk assessment methodology, the willingness to participate in a proactive risk assessment again, and the knowledge they gained about nurses' contribution to the quality of medication management.

The most critical failure modes in terms of likelihood, impact on patient, and impact on nurse were as follows: (1) an IV pump is malfunctioning, (2) no line is available to administer an IV medication, (3) the patient's status contraindicates a medication, (4) critical equipment is not working, and (5) the nurse lacks knowledge on medications. Nurses identified a total of 334 contributing factors, such as "the equipment is damaged," "the wrong medication dose is sent to the unit," or "no training has been provided to nurses for material that is not part of their equipment." They also identified 190 recovery processes related to the failure modes. Examples of recovery processes include: "The nurse borrows equipment," "the nurse calls pharmacy," or "the nurse asks questions about a software to a superuser." This information can then be used for developing recommendations for redesigning the medication management process in order to support the recovery processes developed by nurses and reduce barriers to safe, high-quality medication management.

TABLE 12.2 Additional Resources on Proactive Risk Assessment

Resources on Proactive Risk Assessment	References
IHI	http://www.ihi.org/ihi
Joint Commission	http://www.jointcommission.org/
VA National Center for Patient Safety	http://www.va.gov/NCPS/SafetyTopics.html#HFMEA

Conclusion

This chapter presented information about the use and implementation of proactive risk assessment methods in healthcare. Significant attention has been on how various human factors and systems engineering methods can be used to improve patient safety (Carayon 2007). This chapter provides examples of proactive risk assessment applications in healthcare. A number of challenges remain in the effective and efficient application of proactive risk assessment in healthcare, such as reliability of the methods (Shebl et al. 2009) and quantitative versus qualitative approaches (Leveson 1995, Marx and Slonim 2003). Continued effort is necessary to develop proactive risk assessment methods that consider the complexity of healthcare work systems and processes. Various resources on proactive risk assessment are available (see Table 12.2).

References

American Society for Healthcare Risk Management. 2002. Strategies and tips of maximizing failure mode and effects analysis in your organization. http://www.ashrm.org/ashrm/education/development/monographs

Apkon, M., J. Leonard, L. Probst, L. DeLizio, and R. Vitale. 2004. Design of a safer approach to intravenous drug infusions: Failure mode effects analysis. *Quality & Safety in Health Care 13*(4):265–271.

Ayyub, B. M. 2001. *Elicitation of Expert Opinions for Uncertainty and Risk*. Boca Raton, FL: CRC Press.

Battles, J. B., N. M. Dixon, R. J. Borotkanics, B. Rabin-Fastmen, and H. S. Kaplan. 2006. Sensemaking of patient safety risks and hazards. *Health Services Research 41*(4):1555–1575.

Battles, J. B. and R. J. Lilford. 2003. Organizing patient safety research to identify risks and hazards. *Quality & Safety in Health Care 12*:112–117.

Bier, V. 2004. Implications of the research on expert overconfidence and dependence. *Reliability Engineering & System Safety 85*(1–3):321–329.

Bonnabry, P., C. Despont-Gros, D. Grauser, P. Casez, M. Despond, and D. Pugin. 2008. A risk analysis method to evaluate the impact of a computerized provider order entry system on patient safety. *Journal of the American Medical Informatics Association 15*(4):453–460.

Brennan, T. A., A. Gawande, E. Thomas, and D. Studdert. 2005. Accidental deaths, saved lives, and improved quality. *New England Journal of Medicine 353*(13):1405–1409.

Carayon, P. 2007. *Handbook of Human Factors in Health Care and Patient Safety*. Mahwah, NJ: Lawrence Erlbaum Associates.

Carayon, P., A. S. Hundt, B. Karsh, A. P. Gurses, C. J. Alvarado, and M. Smith. 2006. Work system design for patient safety: The SEIPS model. *Quality and Safety in Healthcare 15*(Suppl. I):50–58.

Carayon, P. and M. J. Smith. 2000. Work organization and ergonomics. *Applied Ergonomics 31*:649–662.

Carayon, P., T. B. Wetterneck, A. S. Hundt, M. Enloe, T. Love, and S. Rough. 2005a. Continuous technology implementation in health care: The case of advanced IV infusion pump technology. In *Proceedings of the 11th International Conference on Human-Computer Interaction*, ed. G. Salvendy. Las Vegas, NA: Lawrence Erlbaum Associates.

Carayon, P., T. B. Wetterneck, A. S. Hundt, M. Ozkaynak, P. Ram, J. DeSilvey et al. 2004. Assessing nurse interaction with medication administration technologies: The development of observation methodologies. In *Work With Computing Systems*, eds., H. M. Khalid, M. G. Helander, and A. W. Yeo, pp. 319–324. Kuala Lumpur, Malaysia: Damai Sciences.

Carayon, P., T. B. Wetterneck, A. S. Hundt, M. Ozkaynac, P. Ram, J. DeSilvey. 2005b. Observing nurse interaction with infusion pump technologies. In *Advances in Patient Safety: From Research to Implementation*, eds. K. Henriksen, J. B. Battles, E. Marks, and D. I. Lewin, vol. 2, pp. 349–364. Rockville, MD: Agency for Healthcare Research and Quality.

Cook, R. I., J. Wreathall, A. Smith, D. C. Cronin, O. Rivero, and R. C. Harland. 2007. Probabilistic risk assessment of accidental ABO-incompatible thoracic organ transplantation before and after 2003. *Transplantation 84*(12):1602–1609.

Diberardinis, L. J. 1998. *Handbook of Occupational Safety and Health*. New York: Wiley-Interscience.

Florin, D. 1999. Scientific uncertainty and the role of expert advice: The case of health checks for coronary heart disease prevention by general practitioners in the UK. *Social Science & Medicine 49*(9):1269–1283.

Gosbee, J. and T. Anderson. 2003. Human factors engineering design demonstrations can enlighten your RCA team. *Quality and Safety in Health Care 12*(2):119–121.

Guerin, F., A. Laville, F. Daniellou, J. Duraffourg, and A. Kerguelen. 2006. *Understanding and Transforming Work—The Practice of Ergonomics*. Lyon, France: ANACT.

Hagan, P., G. R. Krieger, and J. F. Montgomery. 2001a. *Accident Prevention Manual: Engineering & Technology*. Chicago, IL: National Safety Council.

Hagan, P., J. F. Montgomery, and J. T. O'Reilly. 2001b. *Accident Prevention Manual for Business & Industry: Administration & Programs*. Chicago, IL: National Safety Council.

Hundt, A. S. 2007. Organizational learning in healthcare. In *Handbook of Human Factors and Ergonomics in Health Care and Patient Safety*, ed. P. Carayon, pp. 127–138. Mahwah, NJ: Lawrence Erlbaum Associates.

Hundt, A. S., P. Carayon, and T. B. Wetterneck. 2006. HRO characteristics as demonstrated through implementation of a smart IV pump. In *Proceedings of the IEA2006 Congress*, eds. R. N. Pikaar, E. A. P. Koningsveld, and P. J. M. Settels Maastricht. Amsterdam, the Netherlands: Elsevier.

Institute of Medicine (ed.). 2000. *To Err is Human: Building a Safer Health System*. Washington, DC: National Academy Press.

Institute of Medicine. 2004. *Patient Safety: Achieving a New Standard for Care*. Washington, DC: National Academies Press.

Israelski, E. W. and W. H. Muto. 2007. Human factors risk management in medical products. In *Handbook of Human Factors and Ergonomics in Health Care and Patient Safety*, ed. P. Carayon, pp. 615–647. Mahwah, NJ: Lawrence Erlbaum Associates.

Karnon, J., A. McIntosh, J. Dean, P. Bath, A. Hutchinson, and J. Oakley. 2007. A prospective hazard and improvement analytic approach to predicting the effectiveness of medication error interventions. *Safety Science 45*(4):523–539.

Karsh, B. and S. J. Alper. 2005. Work system analysis: The key to understanding health care systems. In *Advances in Patient Safety: From Research to Implementation*, ed. Agency for Healthcare Research and Quality, vol. 2, pp. 337–348. Rockville, MD: Agency for Healthcare Research and Quality.

Karsh, B., S. J. Alper, R. J. Holden, and K. L. Or. 2006. A human factors engineering paradigm for patient safety—Designing to support the performance of the health care professional. *Quality and Safety in Healthcare 15*(Suppl I):59–65.

Kraan, B. and T. Bedford. 2005. Probabilistic inversion of expert judgments in the quantification of model uncertainty. *Management Science 51*(6):995–1006.

Layde, P. M., L. M. Cortes, S. P. Teret, K. J. Brasel, E. M. Kuhn, and J. A. Mercy. 2002. Patient safety efforts should focus on medical injuries. *JAMA 287*(15):1993–1997.

Lehto, M. and G. Salvendy. 1991. Models of accident causation and their application: Review and reappraisal. *Journal of Engineering and Technology Management 8*:173–205.

Leplat, J. 1989. Error analysis, instrument and object of task analysis. *Ergonomics 32*(7):813–822.

Leveson, N. G. 1995. *Safeware*. Boston, MA: Addison-Wesley.

Lyons, M. 2009. Towards a framework to select techniques for error prediction: Supporting novice users in the healthcare sector. *Applied Ergonomics 40*(3):379–395.

Marx, D. A. and A. D. Slonim. 2003. Assessing patient safety risk before the injury occurs: An introduction to sociotechnical probabilistic risk modelling in health care. *Quality & Safety in Health Care 12*(Suppl. 2):33–38.

Monti, S. and G. Carenini. 2000. Dealing with the expert inconsistency in probability elicitation. *IEEE Transactions on Knowledge and Data Engineering 12*(4):499–508.

Mosleh, A., V. M. Bier, and G. Apostolakis. 1988. A critique of current practice for the use of expert opinions in probabilistic risk assessment. *Reliability Engineering & System Safety 20*(1):63–85.

Schroeder, M. E., R. L. Wolman, T. B. Wetterneck, and P. Carayon. 2006. Tubing misload allows free flow event with smart intravenous infusion pump. *Anesthesiology 105*(2):434–435.

Senders, J. W. 2004. FMEA and RCA: The mantras of modern risk management. *Quality & Safety in Health Care 13*:249–250.

Shebl, N. A., B. D. Franklin, and N. Barber. 2009. Is failure mode and effect analysis reliable? *Journal of Patient Safety 5*(2):1–9.

Smith, M. J. and P. Carayon. 2000. Balance theory of job design. In *International Encyclopedia of Ergonomics and Human Factors*, ed. W. Karwowski, pp. 1181–1184. London, U.K.: Taylor & Francis.

Smith, M. J. and P. Carayon-Sainfort. 1989. A balance theory of job design for stress reduction. *International Journal of Industrial Ergonomics 4*(1):67–79.

Smith, M. J., P. Carayon, and B. Karsh. 2001. Design for occupational health and safety. In *Handbook of Industrial Engineering: Technology and Operations Management*, ed. G. Salvendy, 3rd edn., pp. 1156–1191. New York: John Wiley & Sons.

Smith, M. J., B. Karsh, P. Carayon, and F. T. Conway. 2003. Controlling occupational safety and health hazards. In *Handbook of Occupational Health Psychology*, eds. J. C. Quick and L. E. Tetrick, pp. 35–68. Washington, DC: American Psychological Association.

Spath, P. 2004a. Worst practices used in conducting FMEA projects. Part 1 of a 2-part series. *Hospital Peer Review 29*(8):114–116.

Spath, P. 2004b. Worst practices used in conducting FMEA projects. Part 2 of a 2-part series. *Hospital Peer Review 29*(9):129–131.

Washington, S. and J. Oh. 2006. Bayesian methodology incorporating expert judgment for ranking countermeasure effectiveness under uncertainty: Example applied to at grade railroad crossings in Korea. *Accident Analysis and Prevention 38*(2):234–247.

Weick, K. E. and K. M. Sutcliffe. 2001. *Managing the Unexpected: Assuring High Performance in an Age of Complexity*. San Francisco, CA: Jossey-Bass.

Wetterneck, T. B., A. S. Hundt, and P. Carayon. 2009. FMEA team performance in health care: A qualitative analysis of team member perceptions. *Journal of Patient Safety 5*(2):102–108.

Wetterneck, T. B., K. A. Skibinski, T. L. Roberts, S. M. Kleppin, M. Schroeder, and M. Enloe. 2006. Using failure mode and effects analysis to plan implementation of smart intravenous pump technology. *American Journal of Health-System Pharmacy 63*:1528–1538.

Wetterneck, T. B., K. Skibinski, M. Schroeder, T. L. Roberts, and P. Carayon. 2004. Challenges with the performance of failure mode and effects analysis in healthcare organizations: An IV medication administration HFMEATM. In *Annual Conference of the Human Factors and Ergonomics Society*, ed. The Human Factors and Ergonomics Society. New Orleans, LA: The Human Factors and Ergonomics Society.

Wreathall, J. and C. Nemeth. 2003. Assessing risk: The role of probabilistic risk assessment (PRA) in patient safety improvement. *Quality & Safety in Health Care 13*:206–212.

13

Toward More Effective Implementation of Evidence-Based Practice: Relational and Contextual Considerations

Priscilla A. Arling
Butler University

Rebekah L. Fox
Texas State University

Bradley N. Doebbeling
Indiana University School of Medicine

Evidence-Based Practice 13-1
Evidence-Based Practice and Implementation Science
Social Capital Theory 13-3
Social Capital in the PARiHS Framework • Social Network Analysis • Communities of Practice
Conclusions 13-11
References 13-11

Evidence-Based Practice

The United States defines the cutting edge in most areas of medical science and technology, particularly in clinical training, research, and practice (Reid et al., 2005; Zerhouni, 2006). However, the lack of true systems for the delivery of healthcare in this country limit the achievements made possible by these advances (Reid et al., 2005). Today's healthcare organizations face challenges of unprecedented breadth and intensity. The current system includes major gaps between evidence and practice, suboptimal quality, inequitable patterns of utilization, poor safety, and unsustainable cost increases. Only a fraction of new scientific discoveries enter day-to-day clinical practice after delays of 17 or more years (Westfall et al., 2007). In contrast, many new drugs, technologies, and devices are quickly adopted into medical practice, often before careful evaluation of safety and cost-effectiveness are conducted.

Evidence-Based Practice and Implementation Science

Gaps in Healthcare Quality, Effectiveness, and Outcomes

Large studies of healthcare delivery demonstrate that only about half (55%) of U.S. citizens receive necessary care; fewer than half of physician practices use recommended processes of care (McGlynn et al., 2003). For example, despite many years of evidence demonstrating the importance of hypertension treatment, only 70% of Americans with hypertension are diagnosed, only 60% are treated, and only

30% are controlled (Hajjar and Kotchen, 2003). This reflects a failure of the system to routinely provide effective, evidence-based delivery of care to the right patients at the right time.

Relatively few resources have been devoted to improving the operations, productivity, and subsequent quality of the U.S. healthcare system (Reid et al., 2005). It is estimated that approximately one-third (30%–40%) of healthcare expenditures, or $600 billion, is spent annually on costs associated with "overuse, underuse, misuse, duplication, system failures, unnecessary repetition, and poor communication and inefficiency" (Reid et al., 2005, pp. 3–4).

Healthcare costs continue to consume a greater proportion of the economy, leaving the public, insurers, industry, and government straining under an increasing financial burden. Unnecessary or inappropriate services are provided far too often because there is little coordination across sites or among providers. Care management, cross-disciplinary care, and preventive care are often not covered or poorly reimbursed. New technologies, drugs, and devices are often adopted quickly with limited or no comparison of their effectiveness versus existing diagnostic approaches or therapies. High administrative costs in health insurance and healthcare delivery contribute to inefficiencies and cost increases (Gauthier and Serber, 2005). To rectify these problems new innovations in healthcare must be implemented.

Innovation Implementation and Uptake

Successful implementation of an innovation locally, like a clinical practice guideline, can lead to improved operational efficiency and patient outcomes. Local implementation projects are often undertaken to overcome a specific clinical or quality problem and are designed to address specific local barriers and facilitators. This approach, however, leads to capturing limited knowledge about effective implementation strategies, since evaluations are often incomplete, post hoc, and not published. Moreover, local efforts in implementation of evidence-based practice (EBP) often do not (1) adequately characterize the intervention and context, (2) determine whether a significant improvement has occurred, (3) account for secular trends, or (4) identify generalizable findings that may apply to other settings. Additionally, assessment of quality improvement efforts may be gathered in a nonrepresentative environment (low ecological validity). Therefore, findings (i.e., implementation strategies) may not be transferable to other environments, depending upon the local barriers, facilitators, and context. As the scope of the problems in the healthcare systems becomes increasingly profound, there is a need not only for local incremental changes, but for system-wide, transformational change.

Complexity of Change in Healthcare Systems

A healthcare system is comprised of multiple levels, including the patient, provider or care team, organization, and the political and economic environment (Ferlie and Shortell, 2001). Each of these levels is nested, representing the interconnections among the levels and the complex nature of healthcare systems. Thus, a system "consists of interacting, interrelated, or interdependent elements that form a complex whole" (Ryan, 2005, p. 5). Elements include, but are not limited to, clinics, units, microsystems, and people. This set of interacting elements behaves differently from the elements acting alone would (Ryan, 2005). In considering healthcare change, it is important to consider a multiple level model of the healthcare system (Reid et al., 2005), in order to focus the implementation effort and ensure the evaluation is appropriately targeted.

To compound this complexity, the system is fragmented by clinical setting (acute care, outpatient, long-term, and palliative care), units, time, and provider subtype which often do not communicate with each other effectively. Thus, the interconnectedness among patients, providers, organizations, and the environment is often not recognized within a healthcare system (Reid et al., 2005). Without recognizing these interconnections, solutions for a sustained system change cannot be considered. Similarly, localized changes may result in unanticipated effects at different levels of the system or in different contexts. A comprehensive review of the multiple levels of factors influencing successful implementation is given by Greenhalgh et al. (2004).

Thus any research that seeks to improve the uptake of EBP innovations must account for multiple elements in the healthcare system, their interrelationships, and the contexts in which the elements are embedded. In addition, in order to support system-wide, transformational change, as opposed to local change, implementation innovations and related research must be based on strong theoretical and scientific foundations. Multiple authors have noted that research in the area of EBP implementation has often lacked the rigorous scientific approach that is the hallmark of EBP research itself. Implementation studies frequently lack a theoretical base that would predict success and would help in applying the findings to different contexts. Even so, it is unlikely that one theoretical approach or model could inform all aspects of implementation (Kitson et al., 2008).

PARiHS Framework for Implementation

One framework for conceptualizing implementation that allows for the leveraging of multiple theoretical positions and models is the PARiHS framework. The PARiHS framework (Kitson et al., 1998, 2008) suggests that successful implementation is the function of interplay between three core elements: evidence, context, and facilitation. *Evidence* combines four related areas: research evidence, clinical experience, patient preferences, and routine data. *Context* is the environment or setting in which the evidence is implemented and also includes culture, leadership, and evaluation. We note the importance of additional contextual subelements including individual roles, team roles, community, history, economics, society, and politics. *Facilitation* describes the action required to help people change their attitudes, behaviors, and practice, given the evidence and context.

Given the PARiHS framework, the challenge remains to find a theoretical perspective that can explain a range of phenomena and inform an understanding of how the elements of the framework interact (Kitson et al., 2008). In this chapter we suggest that one theory, *social capital theory,* is well suited to this purpose. We discuss two specific areas of study within the social capital theory that hold promise for informing EBP implementation and healthcare system transformation: *social network analysis* (SNA) and *communities of practice* (CoPs). We begin by describing the social capital theory.

Social Capital Theory

In any implementation, one of the most important resources to be considered is the relational resource called social capital. Social capital is a resource found in interpersonal relationships, which facilitates and guide actions of people who are connected through those relationships (Coleman, 1988). According to Coleman (1988) social capital occurs in three general forms. *Obligations, expectations, and trustworthiness* are the first form, and are essential to effective healthcare delivery. In some social structures, such as a hospital unit, when Nurse Jones does something for Nurse Smith, she trusts that Nurse Smith will reciprocate in the future. This sets up an expectation in Nurse Jones and an obligation in Nurse Smith. However, for this relationship to be successful and valuable to both parties, trust must exist. Effective quality care requires trust and the fulfillment of obligations. *Information channels* are the second form of social capital. In the fast-paced, information-dependent environment of healthcare, speed, accuracy, and information relationships between providers is critical to good quality care. *Norms and sanctions* are the final form of social capital. In healthcare an individual's profession can establish norms of behavior that are difficult to change (Dopson and Fitzgerald, 2006) and new guidelines for practice are more likely to be adopted if they reflect current norms. Informal norms also emerge from social relationships within the healthcare context. As an example of informal norms in healthcare, Coleman et al. (1957) found that adoption of the use of tetracycline was heavily influenced by which physicians contacted each other for advice on patient care.

Social Capital in the PARiHS Framework

In this section we consider a few examples of social capital's effect on evidence, context, and facilitation.

Evidence

The source of evidence often dictates what type of social capital is created and an individual's subsequent reaction. Depending upon the source an individual may or may not feel an obligation or expectation to act upon the evidence. Evidence derived from patients can and should influence practice, but little is known about the role that patients play in evidence-based healthcare (Rycroft-Malone et al., 2004). Trust in the source is also a key influence. For instance, while randomized controlled trials (RCTs) are often considered the gold standard of evidence in comparing two treatments, trust in that evidence can be further enhanced if the evidence is published in a reputable peer-reviewed journal (Dopson et al., 2002). In terms of information channels, the same evidence is not equally available to all parties. Roles, along with professional standards, can also establish norms for individuals, against which new evidence is judged (Eccles and Grimshaw, 2004; Greenhalgh et al., 2004). Finally, organizations, roles, and professions can determine the rewards and sanctions that may be enforced to either encourage or discourage implementation of the evidence.

Context

Kitson et al. (1998) suggest that implementation success is more likely in organizations where roles are clearly defined and leadership is strong. Strong leaders set expectations for individuals and clear roles aid in individuals understanding their obligations in terms of EBP implementation. Transformational leaders create social capital through the development of trust and the opening of communication channels in organizations. Leaders also help define norms in organizations and can enforce sanctions, both formal and informal.

Another contextual factor that can be found at the individual, team, and organizational levels is culture. In any context there are likely to be multiple cultures and subcultures, each with their own values, assumptions, and beliefs impacting implementation (McCormack et al., 2002). Culture is shaped by the conversations we have each day. Culture shapes the diffusion of innovation by establishing norms that foster or impede the diffusion (Nutley and Davies, 2000). Culture can also determine the channels through which information flows as well as who is trusted by the individual, team, or organization.

The context at the interorganizational, community, and governmental levels are also factors that which influence the effectiveness of implementation and system transformation. Historical relationships between organizations (Dopson et al., 2002) as well as community involvement and support (Fixsen et al., 2005) affect the social capital of implementation by influencing the flow of information, a sense of obligation, norms of cooperation, and trust. Economic and political positions and policies influence reimbursement, incentives, and regulations surrounding an implementation, which are part of the obligations, expectations, norms, and sanctions that can influence EBP implementations.

Facilitation

Given a specific context and the available evidence, facilitators are individuals who work with team members and stakeholders to enhance the implementation process. Some facilitators may also be opinion leaders; however, the emphasis in facilitation is on actively helping others to achieve certain goals and promoting action, and consciously using group and interpersonal skills to effect change (Kitson et al., 1998). The social capital of a given facilitator is expected to play an important role in his or her effectiveness. Implementation success is likely to depend, at least in part, on the extent to which a facilitator can influence a sense of obligation, promote expectations of and instill norms of innovation use among others. The ability to garner this social capital will be influenced by trust in the facilitator. Finally, the information channels available to and used by the facilitator are important to both dissemination and acceptance of the innovation.

Under the umbrella of social capital there are two areas of study that in particular have the potential to aid in the study of EBP implementation: SNA and CoPs. We focus on these two areas because there

TABLE 13.1 Application of SNA and CoP Constructs to Elements Influencing EBP Implementation

PARiHS Element	Application of SNA Constructs	Application of CoP Constructs
Evidence: Multiple forms of evidence influence practice	*Network types and ties*: What actors are involved in the exchange of forms of evidence, how often they exchange that information, with whom; what is the strength of those ties *Network patterns*: Characteristics such as a network's density may influence spread, adoption, nonadoption of evidence *Network boundaries*: Describe who is in/out of team, unit, or profession and thus who exerts influence on social capital	CoPs function as "living" repositories of evidence. CoPs use and produce evidence in a variety of forms. Because of the emphasis on situated learning, evidence used within a CoP often takes the form of personal experience and narrative CoPs can contribute to the overall quality of evidence for a given subject because evidence, in the form of input, is constantly being tested
Context: The setting at multiple levels influences practice: individual, team, unit, organizational, societal, political	*Network types and ties*: Who has contact with certain roles, leaders, evaluators *Network patterns*: Characteristics of network can identify level of influence of contextual components by social structure (e.g., physicians, nurses, staff) *Network boundaries*: Networks can be described by roles, analyze contacts intra- and extra-role; what are the bounds of various types of networks: leaders, feedback, community, or political	CoPs are based on situated learning models therefore the context is necessarily highlighted CoPs rescue tacit knowledge that is often hard to communicate. Diverse membership allows better consideration of contextual factors
Facilitation: Facilitators act upon given evidence and context to affect implementation	*Network types and ties*: Who has contact with facilitator *Network patterns*: How does facilitator's position and others' positions in networks influence outcomes; patterns can evaluate facilitator's perceived power, level of influence *Network boundaries*: What are the bounds of the facilitator's reach; how does reach vary by type of network contact	Facilitation and leadership are split in order to reduce fatigue and allow better focus for both roles Facilitators "breed" facilitators within CoPs Diverse, voluntary membership enables facilitation to be more effective by appealing to multiple forms of source credibility

are well-established models in each area. These models have been successfully applied in a variety of settings, yet are rarely considered in implementing healthcare system change. Table 13.1 describes how constructs in SNA and CoPs could be applied to the elements of the PARiHS framework. We begin by discussing SNA.

Social Network Analysis

SNA is a subfield of study within the broader area of structural sociology that uses graph theory and algebraic notation to define and formalize sociological constructs (Wellman, 1988). Its focus is on the relationship between social entities and the structure of social relations that determine the content of those relationships (Wasserman and Faust, 1994). To ground our discussion of SNA in a healthcare setting, we give the example of network data collected from individuals participating in a healthcare collaborative to reduce the spread of methicillin-resistant *Staphylococcus aureus* (MRSA) in hospital inpatient settings. The project participants who attended the project kick off meeting were asked, "With whom have you previously worked?" Figure 13.1 is a graphical representation of the work relationships between the organizations represented by the individuals. For the purpose of this chapter, each organization's name was changed to a pseudonym. The organizations in the project, or actors, are represented as nodes in a network. In Figure 13.1, each type of node is represented by a different color and

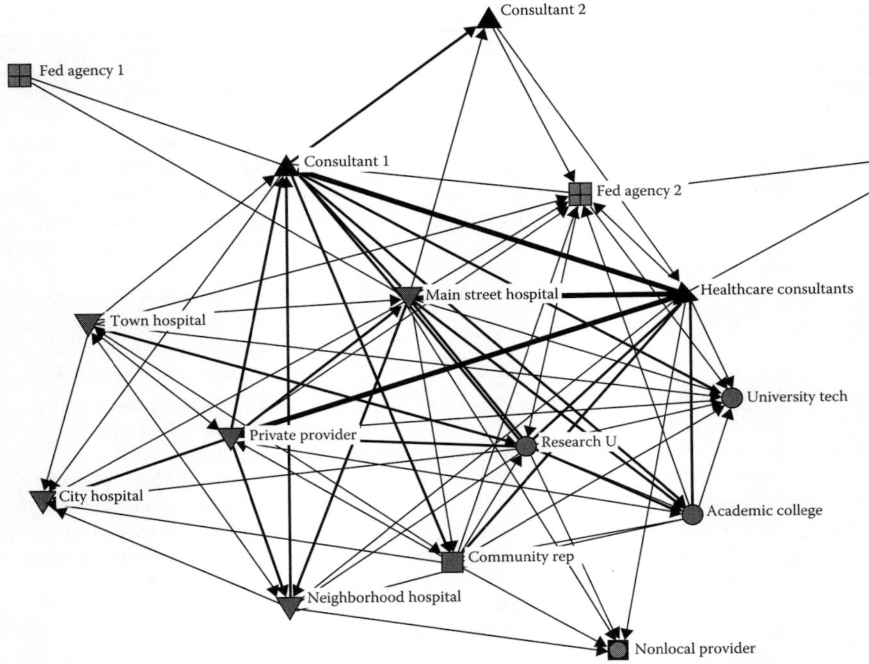

FIGURE 13.1 Sample SNA graph—MRSA project.

shape symbol. For example, "Main Street Hospital" is a local provider and is shown in the diagram as an inverted triangle; "Research U" is a university represented by a circle. Actors can also be individuals, teams, departments, or communities. Actors in a network are connected via their relationships, known as ties. Ties are typically categorized by type such as friendship, advice, and workflow. The ties in Figure 13.1 represent prior working relationships between individuals in organizations. Multiple types of ties between actors are often studied at one time. Each set of ties being studied is considered to be a separate *network* relation, that is, a separate social structure. Each network can exhibit different patterns and have different implications for the actors involved. The determination of who is considered to be in a network and who is outside of the network specifies the *boundary* of each network. The boundary for the network shown was determined by who was participating in the MRSA project. Finally, ties can be valued or given a *strength*. In the MRSA network example, the strength of the tie is the number of contacts who have worked with each other across each relationship. In Figure 13.1, the strength of the relationship is shown by the thickness of the tie line. Heavier lines indicate more contacts. The heavy line between the "private provider" and "healthcare consultants" means there are more individuals involved in that relationship than in the thin line between the "private provider" and "town hospital."

Much of the explanatory power of SNA comes from the ability to describe social relations both qualitatively and quantitatively and to display relations visually. Conceptualizing social structures as networks offers the opportunity to quantitatively analyze patterns in the networks. As an example of how SNA can be used to analyze social relations, we examine a network concept that has been used frequently in healthcare studies, the concept of *density*.

The *density* of a network is the number of actual ties that exist between actors as compared to the number of ties that potentially could exist in the network. West et al. (1999) asked 50 clinical directors of medicine and 50 directors of nursing the question, "With whom do you discuss professional matters?" The nurses' professional networks were less dense than those of the clinical directors. The authors suggest that the lower density in the nurses' networks corresponds to access to a wider range of opinion from others than the opinions available to clinical directors of medicine. In other contexts and studies however, higher density in a network may be desirable. Aydin et al. (1998) found that increased communication network density in a network of nurse practitioners and physicians was associated with higher use of an electronic medical records system.

In the next sections we outline how the analytical concepts discussed above can guide EBP implementation research and practice. Column 2 in Table 13.1 provides an overview on how common SNA constructs could be used to examine factors related to EBP implementation. We first consider a few ways in which SNA constructs could be applied to the MRSA prevention project discussed above, in terms of evidence.

Evidence and Network Analysis

Networks and their ties can be defined by who exchanges evidence with whom. The information obtained depends on the question asked when the analyst collects the network data. In the MRSA project, the network question could ask, "With whom have you exchanged information regarding how to reduce the spread of MRSA?" From this question, a network of ties could be constructed showing how evidence currently flows between individuals in the project. Respondents could also be asked how often they contact each other to exchange MRSA related information: every day, once a week or once a month. This would allow the researcher to assign a strength value to the tie.

We can also analyze each organization's subset of contacts and calculate the density of each subnetwork. Based on the matrix of contact information in Figure 13.1, Health Consultant's subset of the network has the highest density, meaning that many individuals in that subnetwork are in contact with each other. Prior work suggests that dense networks are beneficial for the quick diffusion of existing information within a network, while less dense networks are more likely to bring new information into a network (Burt, 1992). This suggests that less dense networks may be advantageous during the early stages of evidence diffusion, when the evidence needs to be introduced into new networks for it to spread. However, more dense networks later in the evidence's life cycle may promote quicker diffusion in networks where some knowledge of the evidence already exists.

The assessment of patterns in a network relies heavily on the network boundaries chosen. In the MRSA network the analysis is limited to project participants who attended the kick off meeting. Ideally, multiple networks with different types of boundaries should be studied. For example, for evidence dispersion, studying team, unit, professional, and organizational networks would be informative and could show how social capital flows at various levels of analysis.

Context and Network Analysis

Context can be incorporated into network analyses either by specifying the context in the network question or analyzing various contexts after data collection. In the network question, respondents may be asked, "Whom do you look toward for leadership regarding (the implementation or innovation)?" This question might be used to assess the effectiveness of formal leadership or reflect the existence of informal leadership. Additional questions can be used to value the ties in networks. For example, respondents may be asked about their level of trust in each of the members of the network or the timeliness of information they receive from each network contact. Based on prior research, we would expect that an implementation would be positively influenced by high levels of trust and timely information flow. Context may also be derived after data collection by determining the team role, organizational title, position in the organizational hierarchy, or profession of each network respondent.

Network patterns and boundaries can also inform our understanding of the influence of contextual factors. Individuals who are central in a network are frequently chosen as leaders and have the power to get things done in the group. Network patterns can predict the degree to which norms will be shared across network boundaries and the level of cooperation that is likely to occur across groups. In EBP implementations, the boundaries could be formed by roles, professions, organizations, communities, economic, or political contexts. Network patterns would also be useful in assessing the impact and effectiveness of contacts who are evaluators or feedback assessors, identifying the flow of information to and from those contacts.

Facilitation and Network Analysis

The impact of a facilitator in an EBP implementation can be easily assessed by including him or her as a node in each type of network analyzed. The more central the facilitator is in the network, the higher will be his or her influence. Density of the facilitator's network will also indicate whether the network is more apt to spread existing knowledge or introduce new knowledge. We would also expect that facilitators would act as boundary spanners across different network subgroups, and positively impact the EBP implementation in that way. Figure 13.1 shows that in the MRSA project there are many organizations represented in the network and that each organization has at least two ties with another organization in the network. This combination of density and boundary spanning would be expected to facilitate the spread of new information throughout the network.

The examples of network analysis provided above are just a few of the many types of analyses that could inform EBP implementation. The SNA text by Wasserman and Faust (1994) contains not only excellent descriptions on how to analyze network patterns, but can also lead readers to key authors and findings related to various network patterns.

In the next section we discuss another area of study that holds promise for informing EBP implementation, CoPs. We begin by providing an overview of key ideas in the area. We then suggest how those ideas could be applied to the PARiHS framework.

Communities of Practice

A CoP, in general, can be thought of as a group of individuals who share a body of knowledge and work together to solve a common problem. Scholars from a wide range of disciplines including sociology, business, management, and communication, to name but a few, have argued that CoPs demand scholarly attention for their ability to increase effectiveness and reduce organizational costs (Iverson and McFee, 2002; Wenger et al., 2002; Lehaney et al., 2004). In addition, CoPs have gained considerable attention because they serve as forums for practitioners and other interested parties who share a concern for what they do, and wish to improve effectiveness through regular interaction, and because they offer the possibility to save lives (e.g., in high-risk industries such as nursing, firefighting, and the military). A recent research synthesis project in *Implementation Science* revealed that 1421 articles were written about CoPs between 1991 and 2005, 13 of which were primary studies in the health sector (Li et al., 2009).

Because research on CoPs has been carried out in different disciplines, and because there is a lack of consistency in the interpretation of the CoP concept, different definitions have emerged. Jean Lave and EtienneWenger, who are noted as the founders of CoPs explain that CoPs were coined to refer to the "community that acts as a living curriculum for the apprentice" (Wenger, 2006). Wenger et al. (2002) define CoPs as "groups of people who share a concern, a set of problems, or a passion about a topic, and who deepen their knowledge and expertise in this area by interacting on an ongoing basis" (Wenger et al., 2002, p. 4). In 1998, Wenger defined CoPs by three interrelated dimensions: mutual engagement (interaction between individuals that leads to shared meaning about a specific problem or issue), joint enterprise (the process of engagement), and shared repertoire (nomenclature and common resources that enable the community share understanding). Wenger et al. (2002), shifted the focus away from an apprenticeship model, with a focus on the individual's growth, to articulating how CoPs could be tools for organizational change. With this shift, they rearticulated the three elements of CoPs as domain, community, and practice.

Domain refers to the set of issues that bring individuals together. These domains may be based on the profession (cardiologists, teachers, nurses, etc.) or because members face similar problems in different contexts (handling paperwork, workplace motivation, etc.). Whatever creates this common ground is considered the "raison d'etre" (2002, p. 32). This raison d'etre usually represents a topic in which CoP members are passionately interested. Wenger and Snyder (2000) explain that "A community can be made up of tens or even hundreds of people, but typically it has a core of participants whose passion for the topic energizes the community and who provide intellectual and social leadership" (p. 141).

Community refers to the actual people who care about the specific domain. These individuals create the "social fabric of learning" that is based on mutual respect and trust (Wenger et al., 2002, p. 28). The community element also addresses the nature of leadership and membership within CoPs. Generally, leadership is distributed within CoPs creating an "ecology of leadership" (p. 36). Membership in CoPs is dependent on the idea of reciprocation. This is not necessarily give-and-take, but a "pool of goodwill—of social capital—that allows people to contribute to the community while trusting that at some point, in some form, they too will benefit" (p. 37). Individuals trust that membership will be beneficial, but this trust also factors into creating a learning atmosphere. In fact, the learning model represented in CoPs is one of situated learning, in which individuals acquire knowledge within the context that it would be used. Wenger (1996) explains, "Assuming that learning is fundamentally social is not denying that it involves neurological processes, but it is placing these processes in the social context in which we experience them as meaningful? Learning is fundamentally social because we are social beings" (p. 22).

Of the three fundamental elements of a CoP, domain, community, and practice, practice is concerned with shared practices that increase effectiveness (at whatever task) including the "set of frameworks, ideas, tools, information, styles, language, stories, and documents that community members share" (Wenger et al., 2002, p. 29). Iverson and McPhee (2002) identify practice as a "shared repertoire," or the set of resources created by and available to CoPs (p. 261). More specifically, these resources "include a variety of knowledge types: cases and stories, theories, rules, frameworks, models, principles, tools, experts, articles, lessons learned, best practices, and heuristics" (Wenger et al., 2002, p. 38).

These three intertwined fundamental elements—domain, community, and practice help to conceptualize CoPs in general, but CoPs can differ structurally in many ways based on size, location, duration, and types of interaction. Although CoPs are considered fertile sites for learning, they do have weaknesses. CoPs are considered fragile because they can be easily overmanaged thus decreasing their creative capabilities. Lehaney et al. (2004, p. 46) explain that CoPs are "easy to destroy and difficult to construct." The following sections explore the relationship between EBP and communities of practice.

Evidence and Communities of Practice

There are at least two different ways to think about evidence as it applies to CoPs. CoPs both use and produce a variety of evidence. One of the defining features of a CoP is that they serve as repositories of evidence and experiential knowledge. Within the MRSA collaborative, informatics scholars worked directly with nurses and infection control practitioners (ICPs) to develop a consistent and reliable way to collect and analyze MRSA swabs. This information, subsequently, has been shared, updated, and shaped by other members of the community. Information or evidence that is used by a CoP as input can be shaped and tested by the community, who regularly interact and add to the general body of knowledge concerning a particular topic. CoPs that have a diverse, voluntary membership have the opportunity to integrate and test evidence from multiple disciplines. Additionally, information "stored" in CoPs is given context via mentoring. "Newcomers in particular can benefit from having access to the archived material in addition to the experience of and mentoring from experts" (Li et al., 2009, p. 3). Members of the MRSA CoP socialized new members, shared lessons learned, and introduced new individuals to procedures for accomplishing work within the group (e.g., how to access shared computer databases, and how to get in touch with other members). Additionally, knowledge that is shared within CoPs is supported by diverse evidence, often in the form of narrative and personal testimony. The MRSA CoP relied on a shared repertoire of evidence within the community. Individuals would share personal experiential stories to back up suggestions or persuade the group to move in a certain direction. For instance, one very impressive and organized group of nurses researched and decided on a particular brand of personal protective equipment (PPE) for their needs. They shared their story with the community, who could then influence their own hospital's policy based on the experience of the other nurses.

Context and Communities of Practice

Because CoPs emphasize situated learning, context is necessarily in the foreground. Both tacit and explicit knowledge are used and generated, but a CoP is particularly useful for rescuing tacit knowledge. According to Wenger et al. (2002) tacit knowledge refers to the knowledge that individuals have but cannot necessarily communicate easily. For example, explicit knowledge could encompass the on-the-job training that individuals receive when entering an organization or community. Tacit knowledge would represent the unspoken, but important knowledge that does not get formally relayed, such as a deeper understanding of the complex, interdependent system as a whole. CoPs are heralded as providing a context in which tacit knowledge is rescued. For example, within the MRSA CoP, members shared information about the data collection approval processes and whether or not Internal Review Board (IRB) review was needed. The processes were different for the hospitals, the university, and the funding institution. Knowing how these different approval boards functioned, the time needed to get approval, and what the various boards looked for in good proposals, was very important in planning and implementing the proposals for the project. This tacit information was applied within the community setting.

The communal resources used to share explicit and tacit knowledge create "a sort of mini-culture that binds the community together" (Wenger et al., 2002, p. 39). Because this mini-culture is made up of people with diverse backgrounds, members brought with them their own approach to problem solving, which increased the quantity and quality of possible solutions. For instance, one member of the community was trying to figure out ways to determine the number of individuals who acquire MRSA during their time on a specific unit, if no discharge swabbing was performed. Systems engineers and informaticians were able to develop an electronic proxy measure for infection incidence that has proven to be both valid and useful. Additionally, a diverse membership in the CoP increases the ability of a community to produce a solution to a problem that better applies EBP because the solution was created by a variety of individuals who represent a variety of contexts. They also teach each other to become sensitive to contextual and relational issues that they face in their own particular context.

Facilitation and Communities of Practice

Wenger et al. (2002) defined the roles of leaders/champions and facilitators. The leaders/champions function as boundary spanners to raise awareness of the group, recruit new members, provide resources, etc. The facilitator is responsible for day-to-day activities of the group, which is increasingly done online. CoPs help with facilitation because they delineate between day-to-day functioning and longer term leadership. For example, in the MRSA CoP, a group of centralized individuals, who were in contact with a Technical Expert Panel, set long-term goals and functioned as boundary spanners by working with the media, setting standards for recruiting new members, and securing and providing resources in the form of information, finances, and permissions. Project managers, ICPs and other hospital leadership, as well as researchers were responsible for the facilitation of day-to-day activities including conference calls and site visits. CoPs do not have a single unified type of facilitation, and because they are more like "standing committees" they do not end after the facilitation of one particular implementation or campaign. They often provide a model for ongoing facilitation and cautiously warn against facilitator fatigue. Because CoPs are based on situated learning models, facilitators are meant to "breed" new facilitators. The process of knowledge production within CoPs increases the likelihood of broad ownership of ideas, prompting all members to become facilitators. Two of the methods used to increase efficiency on the individual ICU and CCU units were Lean (often associated with the Toyota Production System) and Positive Deviance, both of which are organizational transformation methods. Both processes emphasize the need for leadership to come from "the front lines" if it is to be truly effective and sustainable.

Conclusions

Large studies of healthcare delivery demonstrate that there are major gaps between evidence and practice. Relatively few resources have been devoted to improving the operations, productivity, quality, and cost-effectiveness of the U.S. healthcare system. Successful implementation of an innovation locally, like a clinical practice guideline, can lead to improved operational efficiency and patient outcomes. However, implementation and uptake of EBPs remain suboptimal and greater efforts should be made to study and publish learnings from such efforts.

A healthcare system is composed of multiple levels, including the patient, provider or care team, organization, and the political and economic environment. Research that seeks to reduce the gap between evidence and practice must account for these multiple elements as well as their interconnectedness. Implementation research must also be based on a strong theoretical and scientific foundation. Kitson et al. (2008) suggest in the PARiHS framework that successful implementations are the function of interplay between three core elements: evidence, context, and facilitation.

Social capital provides a theoretical perspective that can inform an understanding of how the elements of the PARiHS framework interact. Under the umbrella of social capital there are two areas of study that in particular have the potential to aid in the study of EBP implementation: SNA and CoPs. SNA is a potentially useful tool to study implementation by focusing on the relationship between social entities and the structure of social relations that determine the content of those relationships. A CoP, in general, can be thought of as a group of individuals who share a body of knowledge and work together to solve a common problem. One of the defining features of a CoP is that they serve as repositories of evidence and experiential knowledge. Because CoPs emphasize situated learning, context is necessarily in the foreground. Thus CoPs can aid in understanding both the interconnectedness and contextual basis of implementation elements.

Both SNA and CoPs hold great promise as theoretical foundations that can inform efforts to improve the uptake of EBP implementation innovations. Greater application of these methods in implementing system change and research, evaluating and identifying effective approaches, are needed.

References

Aydin, C. E., J. G. Anderson, P. N. Rosen, V. J. Felitti, and H. C. Weng. 1998. Computers in the consulting room: A case study of clinician and patient perspectives. *Health Care Management Science* 1: 61–74.

Burt, R. 1992. *Structural Holes: The Social Structure of Competition*. Cambridge, MA: Harvard University Press.

Coleman, J. 1988. Social capital in the creation of human capital. *American Journal of Sociology* 94: 95–120.

Coleman, J. S., E. Katz, and H. Menzel. 1957. The diffusion of an innovation among physicians. *Sociometry* 20(4): 253–270.

Dopson, S. and L. Fitzgerald. 2006. The role of the middle manager in the implementation of evidence-based health care. *Journal of Nursing Management* 14: 43–51.

Dopson, S., L. Fitzgerald, E. Ferlie, J. Gabbay, and L. Locock. 2002. No magic targets! Changing clinical practice to become more evidence based. *Health Care Management Review* 27(3): 35–47.

Eccles, M. and J. M. Grimshaw. 2004. Selecting, presenting and delivering clinical guidelines: Are there any "Magic Bullets"? *Medical Journal of Australia* 180: S52–S54.

Ferlie E. and S. Shortell. 2001. Improving the quality of health care in the United Kingdom and the United States: A framework for change. *Milbank Quarterly* 79(2): 281–315.

Fixsen, D. L., S. F. Naoom, K. A. Blase, R. M. Friedman, and F. Wallace. 2005. *Implementation Research: A Synthesis of the Literature*. Tampa, FL: University of South Florida, Louis de la Parte Florida Mental Health Institute, The National Implementation Research Network.

Gauthier, A. and M. Serber. 2005. A need to transform the U.S. health care system: Improving access, quality, and efficiency. *The Commonwealth Fund* 3: 21.

Greenhalgh, T., G. Robert, F. MacFarlane, P. Bate, and O. Kyriakidou. 2004. Diffusion of innovations in service organizations: Systematic review and recommendations. *Milbank Quarterly* 82(4): 581–629.

Hajjar I. and T. A. Kotchen. 2003. Trends in prevalence, awareness, treatment, and control of hypertension in the United States, 1988–2000. *Journal of the American Medical Association* 290(2): 199–206.

Iverson, J. O. and R. D. McPhee. 2002. Knowledge management in communities of practice: Being true to the communicative character of knowledge. *Management Communication Quarterly* 16: 259–266.

Kitson, A., G. Harvey, and B. McCormack. 1998. Enabling the implementation of evidence based practice: A conceptual framework. *Quality in Health Care* 7: 149–158.

Kitson, A. L., J. Rycroft-Malone, G. Harvey, B. McCormack, K. Seers, and A. Titchen. 2008. Evaluating the successful implementation of evidence into practice using the PARiHS framework: Theoretical and practical challenges. *Implementation Science* 3:1.

Lehaney, B., S. Clarke, E. Coakes, and G. Jack. 2004. *Beyond Knowledge Management*. Hershey, PA: Idea Group Publishing.

Li, L. C., J. M. Grimshaw, C. Nielsen, M. Judd, P. C. Coyte, and I. D. Graham. 2009. Evolution of Wenger's concept of community of practice. *Implementation Science* 4: 11.

McCormack, B., A. Kitson, G. Harvey, J. Rycroft-Malone, A. Titchen, and K. Seers. 2002. Getting evidence into practice: The meaning of 'Context'. *Journal of Advanced Nursing* 38(1): 94–104.

McGlynn, E. A., S. M. Asch, and J. Adams. 2003. The quality of health care delivered to adults in the United States. *New England Journal of Medicine* 348(26): 2635–2645.

Nutley, S. and H. Davies. 2000. Making a reality of evidence-based practice: Some lessons from the diffusion of innovations. *Public Money and Management* 20(4): 35–42.

Reid, P. P., D. Compton, J. H. Grossman, and G. Fanjiang. 2005. Committee on engineering and the health care system. In *Building a Better Delivery System: A New Engineering/Health Care Partnership*. Washington, DC: National Academies Press.

Ryan, J. 2005. Building a better delivery system: A new engineering/health care partnership. In *Building a Better Delivery System: A New Engineering/Health Care*, eds. P. P. Reid, D. Compton, J. H. Grossman, G. Fanjiang, and the Committee on Engineering and the Health Care System, pp. 141–142. Washington, DC: National Academies Press.

Rycroft-Malone, J., K. Seers, A. Titchen, G. Harvey, A. Kitson, and B. McCormack. 2004. What counts as evidence in evidence-based practice? *Journal of Advanced Nursing* 47(1): 81–90.

Wasserman, S. and K. Faust. 1994. *Social Network Analysis: Methods and Applications*. New York: Cambridge University Press.

Wellman, B. 1988. Structural analysis: Some basic principles. In *Social Structures: A Network Approach*, eds. B. Wellman and S. B. Berkowitz. Cambridge, U.K.: Cambridge University Press.

Wenger, E. C. 1996. Communities of practice: The social fabric of the learning organization. *HealthCare Forum Journal* 39(4): 20–26.

Wenger, E. 2006. Where does the concept come from? http://www.ewenger.com/theory/ (accessed December 12, 2006).

Wenger, E., R. McDermott, and W. M. Snyder. 2002. *Cultivating Communities of Practice*. Boston, MA: Harvard Business School Press.

Wenger, E. C. and W. M. Snyder. 2000. Communities of practice: The organizational frontier. *Harvard Business Review* January–February: 139–145.

West, E., D. N. Barron, J. Dowsett, and J. N. Newton. 1999. Hierarchies and cliques in the social networks of health care professionals: Implications for the design of dissemination strategies. *Social Science & Medicine* 48(5): 633–646.

Westfall, J. M., J. Mold, and L. Fagnan. 2007. Practice-based research—"Blue Highways" on the NIH roadmap. *Journal of the American Medical Association* 297(4): 403–406.

Zerhouni, E. A. 2006. Clinical research at a crossroads: The NIH roadmap. *Journal of Investigative Medicine* 54(4): 171–173.

III

System Engineering: Technologies and Methodologies

14 **Computer Simulation in Healthcare** *Sean Carr and Stephen D. Roberts* **14**-1
Introduction • Creating Simulation Models • Simulation Technology • Simulation Modeling Approaches • Experimentation and Optimization • Conclusions • References

15 **An Introduction to Optimization Models and Applications in Healthcare Delivery Systems** *Wenhua Cao and Gino J. Lim* **15**-1
Introduction • Mathematical Models • Solution Techniques • Conclusion • References

16 **Queueing Theory and Modeling** *Linda V. Green* **16**-1
Introduction • Basic Queueing Principles and Models • Analyses of Fixed Capacity: How Many Hospital Beds? • Analyses of Flexible Capacity: Determining Staffing Levels to Meet Time-Varying Demands • References

17 **Markov Decision Processes and Its Applications in Healthcare** *Jonathan Patrick and Mehmet A. Begen* **17**-1
Introduction • MDP Theory • Literature Survey • Conclusion • References

18 **Statistical Analysis and Modeling** *Min Zhang and Mark E. Cowen* **18**-1
Introduction • Hierarchical Model and Bayesian Inference • Conclusion • Acknowledgment • References

19 **Analyzing Decisions Using Datasets with Multiple Attributes: A Machine Learning Approach** *Janusz Wojtusiak and Farrokh Alemi* **19**-1
Introduction • Analyzing Decisions • Building Models for Analyzing Decisions • Generating Alternatives • Application of Decision Analysis to the Evaluation of Medication Outcomes • Conclusion • References

20 The Shaping of Inventory Systems in Health Services *Jan de Vries and Karen Spens* **20**-1
Introduction • Inventory Management Systems: Overview and Background • A Framework for Diagnosing Inventory Management Systems • Discussion and Conclusion • References

21 Facility Planning and Design *Richard L. Miller* **21**-1
Introduction • Strategic and Master Facility Planning Process

22 Work Design, Task Analysis, and Value Stream Mapping *Cindy Jimmerson* **22**-1
Introduction • Deeply Understanding How the Work Currently Happens • Task Analysis • Future State Plan • References

23 Scheduling and Sequencing *Edmund K. Burke, Timothy Curtois, Tomas Eric Nordlander, and Atle Riise* **23**-1
Introduction • Nurse Rostering • Surgery Scheduling • Summary • References

24 Data Mining *Niels Peek* **24**-1
Introduction • Challenges of the Field • Data Exploration • Descriptive Data Mining • Predictive Data Mining • Software • References

25 Applications to HIV Prevention Strategies *Paul G. Farnham and Arielle Lasry* **25**-1
Economic Evaluation Techniques • The Human Immunodeficiency Virus Epidemic • Strategies to Prevent the Spread of HIV • Summary/Conclusions • References

26 Causal Risk Analysis: Revisiting the Vioxx Study *Farrokh Alemi and Manaf Zargoush* **26**-1
Introduction • History of Probabilistic and Causal Analysis • What Is a Cause? • Modeling Multiple Causes: Causal Diagrams • Modeling Multiple Causes: Probability Networks • Modeling Multiple Causes: Simultaneous Equations • Causal versus Noncausal Analysis • References

14

Computer Simulation in Healthcare

Introduction 14-1
Why Simulation in Healthcare? • Where Is Simulation Used in Health Systems?
Creating Simulation Models 14-4
Importance of Validation • Role of Data
Simulation Technology 14-7
Simulation Modeling Approaches 14-7
Monte Carlo Simulation • Discrete-Event Simulation • Object-Oriented Simulation • Systems Dynamics Modeling • Agent-Based Modeling
Experimentation and Optimization 14-12
Conclusions 14-13
References 14-13

Sean Carr
North Carolina State University

Stephen D. Roberts
North Carolina State University

Introduction

Computer simulation is a method that allows experiments on a system through a computer-based model of the system. By experimenting with a model of the system, we avoid all the complications of experimenting with the real system. New equipment is not purchased, people's jobs are not changed, facilities are not renovated, and patterns of practice are not altered. Instead these changes are made to a computer model and the experiments are "simulated." So simulation is a method to "mimic" or "imitate" the real system. It requires no stretch of the imagination to conjure up a simulation that only mimics a real system but makes no attempt to statistically replicate it. That is often referred to as a computer simulation game. In a completely different context, the phrase "healthcare simulation" is used to describe activities in healthcare training often using mannequins, especially as it relates to patient safety and medical procedures. Here, however, computer simulation attempts to reflect a real system, so that the statistical and numerical results of the "experimentation" can legitimately imply consequences to the real system.

Computer simulation is broadly used in healthcare, especially in healthcare delivery. Comprehensive reviews of healthcare simulations are found in England and Roberts (1978), Klein et al. (1993), Fone et al. (2003), and Jacobson et al. (2006). Lowery (1996) and Standridge (1999) discuss the use of simulation in healthcare and present approaches to challenging healthcare issues that are still relevant. A more recent similar discussion is offered by Brailsford (2007). In this chapter, we review a number of ways in which simulation has impacted healthcare operations, healthcare delivery decisions, and health policy. In all of the cases, the basic approach requires that a computer model of the system be built and then subjected to experimentation. The intent here is to present simulation as a technique for the analysis of health systems. We will not attempt to provide a comprehensive compendium of contributions but instead try to illustrate the use of simulation.

Why Simulation in Healthcare?

Of all the quantitative tools that can be used in healthcare, simulation is likely the most popular (as it would be in most industries). There are many reasons for its popularity, particularly in healthcare. In healthcare delivery, the systems of care are characterized as "people serving people." In other words, the "customers" are people and the "servers" are people. In other settings, the customers are things and the servers are machines. The fact that people are the central actors means that the systems have complex behaviors and elements interacting in a wide variety of ways.

Consider the arrivals to a doctor's office. People are supposed to arrive according to a scheduled appointment but they also sometimes "walk in." Appointments may be broken or missed. Some people arrive early, while some arrive late. This arrival process is very difficult to describe by a strict stochastic process due to the various random components affecting the arrivals. Although one case does not make a generality, we will nevertheless assert that *healthcare delivery systems have many random components and that these components interact in complex ways.* Simulation is a tool that invites random variables and is able to combine them in complicated models.

As a second example, consider the problem of determining the staff of nurses needed in the emergency department. Of course many random variables are present and they combine in complex ways, but even if a model of this complexity can be constructed, we still need to know how it can be analyzed. Would we staff the emergency department to minimize patient waiting, to maximize the use of nurses, to minimize the costs, or to maximize the quality of care? And there are probably many other considerations. Hence we must work with many objectives, some of which are in conflict, so: *healthcare systems evaluation requires that attention be given to many objectives.* Simulation does not require the statement of a single objective or some mathematical combination of objectives. Instead, any modeled performance measure can be produced, leaving the determination of how to resolve conflicting objectives to the decision-makers. Nevertheless, the decision-makers will learn from the simulation the operational consequences of a decision or a change in the process of care.

As another example of why simulation is especially useful in healthcare, consider the planning for a new outpatient surgery center associated with a hospital. There are not only many random variables, but also many *unknown* variables which may impact the sizing of this facility. Sometimes these facilities are planned due to advocacy by surgical staff or the need to expand market share by the hospital. A simulation model can be used in advance of any actual facility proposal to explore factors that influence the design of the facility, especially those related to staff and space. When these factors are examined in the context of a simulation model, the debate regarding the advisability of the outpatient surgery center is better informed. For instance, how does the size and staffing affect the capacity of the center to process the expected surgery workload? Is there sufficient waiting space? Is there sufficient recovery capacity? How will the surgeries be scheduled? These questions may not be totally answered by the simulation, but the simulation can clarify the role of various variables.

As noted earlier, *people serve people* in healthcare. The fundamental elements of a healthcare simulation are generally people—patients, nurses, doctors, laboratory technicians, aides, therapists, etc. People are far less predictable than machines and parts. People vary their routine and procedures. People take different amounts of time to perform the same task. When people are the "target" of study, their behavior must become an important element in the simulation. Thus healthcare processes are often difficult to simply specify, and performance measures for the delivery processes are complex. For instance, in a busy outpatient clinic, a nurse may be preferred when gathering height and weight information, but there may be times when the nurse is unavailable and someone else, perhaps the clinic associate, may perform this function. This inability to describe activities and processes simply makes the healthcare environment particularly difficult to model. As a consequence, purely mathematical and statistical models are rarely applicable, and simulation models become the only hope of being able to synthesize the healthcare system.

Finally, it is often observed that the process of constructing a simulation model may be as important as the results from the execution of the simulation. To build a simulation model requires that the system being modeled be fully understood. A simulation model makes patient flow explicit, identifies the skills required of the staff, documents the number of staff available, catalogues the size and use of facilities, etc. In other words, without running a single model, the construction of the model makes for meaningful discussion of how a system works and how changes might improve it. This process permits the stakeholders to participate and build a consensus from the discussions. In healthcare, these accomplishments are not only important but crucial.

Where Is Simulation Used in Health Systems?

Simulation has had widespread use in health systems. Most of the reported uses tend to focus on the improvement of operational issues in healthcare institutions, particularly in hospital systems (Carter and Blake, 2005). Early simulation studies (Hancock et al., 1978; Hancock and Walter, 1984), as well as more recent work (Bagust et al., 1999; Groothuis et al., 2001) addressed the problems of leveling hospital inpatient facilities through admission schedules and the presence of the variability in arrival patterns and treatment requirements. The problem of patient scheduling has been even more extensively examined in the outpatient context, where the appointment rules such as the number of appointment slots, the number of appointments per slot, the number of appointments per session, and so forth are of particular concern (Bailey, 1952; Fetter and Thompson, 1965; Williams et al., 1967; Rising et al., 1973; Smith et al., 1979; Guo et al., 2004).

In essence, the simulation studies of hospital operations focus on capacity and the management of capacity (Smith-Daniels et al., 1988). Scheduling and admissions offer one way to better utilize capacity. Complex systems and nonstationary arrival and service processes make simulation a fitting tool for such an analysis. Appropriate sizing is also a way to deal with capacity. There are many examples of using simulation to assist in the sizing of facilities (Butler et al., 1992a,b; Sepulveda et al., 1999; Akkerman and Knip, 2004) and in hospital design (Gibson, 2007). Another approach to the capacity problem is through staffing and staff scheduling, such as nurse staffing (Sundaramoorthi et al., 2006).

Surgery capacity (Protil et al., 2008) and operating room schedules (Dexter et al., 1999, 2000; Ballard and Kuhl, 2006; Denton et al., 2006; Arnaout and Kulbashian, 2008) provide an important area of investigation since surgery is such an important component of hospital care. In Nova Scotia, Canada, discrete-event simulation was used to plan the necessary amount of surgery bed capacity to achieve shorter wait lists (VanBerkel and Blake, 2007). Effective surgery scheduling is a rather difficult task, especially when subject to high no-show rates and high variability in procedure length and complexity. Simulations have shown the value in certain scheduling rules such as a variation of traditional block scheduling (Fitzpatrick et al., 1993).

Outpatient clinics and ambulatory care are also fertile areas for capacity analysis (Isken et al., 1999; Jun et al., 1999; Morrison and Bird, 2003; Miller et al., 2008). To reduce the complexity in the study of outpatient clinics, it is convenient to separate the scheduling of patients from the capacity constraints (Glenn and Roberts, 1973; Kropp and Carlson, 1977). Like other healthcare operations, scheduling of patients and scheduling of staff (Takakuwa and Wijewickrama, 2008) are popular areas of investigation as is the appointment scheduling in clinics (Wijewickrama and Takakuwa, 2006; Wijewickrama and Takakuwa, 2008). Ho and Lau (1992) used manual simulations to study the costs of several outpatient scheduling rules from the perspectives of both patient and provider and concluded that ultimately the relative costs of idle time affect the choice for the optimal policy.

Probably no single area of the hospital has been studied more thoroughly with simulation than the emergency department (Miller et al., 2004; Sinreich and Marmor, 2004, 2005; Hay et al., 2006; Hoot et al., 2008, 2009; Fletcher and Worthington, 2009). Reducing waiting times (Takakuwa and Shiozaki, 2004; Hung et al. 2007) and reducing length of stay (McGuire, 1997) are common themes, as are fast-track processes (Garcia et al., 1995; Mahapatra et al., 2003; Davies, 2007). Scheduling emergency staff, such as physicians (Rossetti et al., 1999; Carter and Lapierre, 2001) and nurses (Draeger, 1992) and other staff (Evans et al., 1996), improving patient flow (Kirtland et al., 1995), redesigning of facilities

(Wiinamaki and Dronzek, 2003), and integrating with inpatient facilities (Kolb et al., 2007) are among the many changes considered. Other topics include costing (Ruohonen et al., 2006), forecasting of demand (Hoot et al., 2008), lean improvement (Khurma et al., 2008), buffer design (Kolb et al., 2008), team triage (Ruohonen et al., 2006), triage using physicians (Medeiros et al., 2008), and financial impact (Ferrin et al., 2007).

Other areas of simulation applications in hospitals include pharmacy (Vila-Parrish et al., 2008; Yurtkuran and Emel, 2008), outpatient surgery (Huschka et al., 2008), physical exam facility (Song et al., 2008), imaging center (Ramis et al., 2008), hospital interconnections (Gunal and Pidd, 2007), use of medical records (Takakuwa and Katagiri, 2007), and computed tomography (CT) facilities (Bosire et al., 2007).

Many simulation studies go well beyond the wall of a hospital or health institution. These include disease control policies (Brandeau, 2008), spread of influenza (Ekici et al., 2008; Rao and Chernyakhovsky, 2008), enrollment in clinical trials (McGarvey et al., 2007), tuberculosis epidemics (Hughes et al., 2006; Mellor et al., 2007), primary care provision (Balasubramanian et al., 2007), end-stage renal failure resource requirements (Davies, 2006), hospital evacuation (Taaffe et al., 2006), and bioterrorism (Patvivatsiri, 2006). A novel application of simulation is to extend the use of probabilistic sensitivity analysis in medical decision analysis to probabilistic analysis with simulation (Briggs, 2005; Tafazzoli et al., 2009).

Creating Simulation Models

Creating a useful simulation model, whether the model is created in a healthcare setting or elsewhere, employs the same basic steps: (1) the system definition, (2) the development of the conceptual model, (3) the creation of the simulation program, (4) the creation of numerical results, and (5) the final recommendations. From this description, the implication is that the creation of a successful simulation project is a sequential series of steps. However, in fact, these are iterative, and often later stages require revisiting earlier stages and revision of the development. Of these steps, Steps (1) and (2) largely determine the success of the simulation because they define the specific issues to be studied and how these issues will be investigated. It is especially difficult to specify the scope of a simulation study in healthcare since there are so many interacting elements. For example, simulating the scheduling of a surgery suite will require that the model confine itself to a limited set of issues. Otherwise, a comprehensive model will not only include the surgery, but also the limits that the post-anesthesia recovery unit (PACU) capacity has and that the hospital bed capacity has on surgery schedule, which in turn depends on the staffing in these units. This kind of attempt at a "system model" will make it impossible to obtain useful insights within a reasonable amount of time. Also such a model will be almost impossible to parameterize and to validate.

An elaboration of the larger process of creating a simulation model is given in Figure 14.1, which has been adapted from Law and Kelton (2000). In Figure 14.1, several practical aspects of simulation modeling and analysis are highlighted, none more important than the issue of validation, which is discussed in further detail in the following section.

Importance of Validation

For a simulation model to be useful and ultimately used (especially in healthcare), the model must be valid. This means that the model must appear to capture the key behavior of the real system (conceptual validation) and it must be credible to the stakeholders. In healthcare, stakeholders are many and varied, since "management" does not imply the same sense of control that might be expected in another industry. In healthcare, the results of a simulation must be "sold" to several parties. For example, it is common that any serious change to how patients are processed will need to be accepted by the medical staff, the nursing staff, and hospital administration, each of whom brings a different orientation and set of values. Hence it is very important that the "stakeholders" be active participants in all phases of

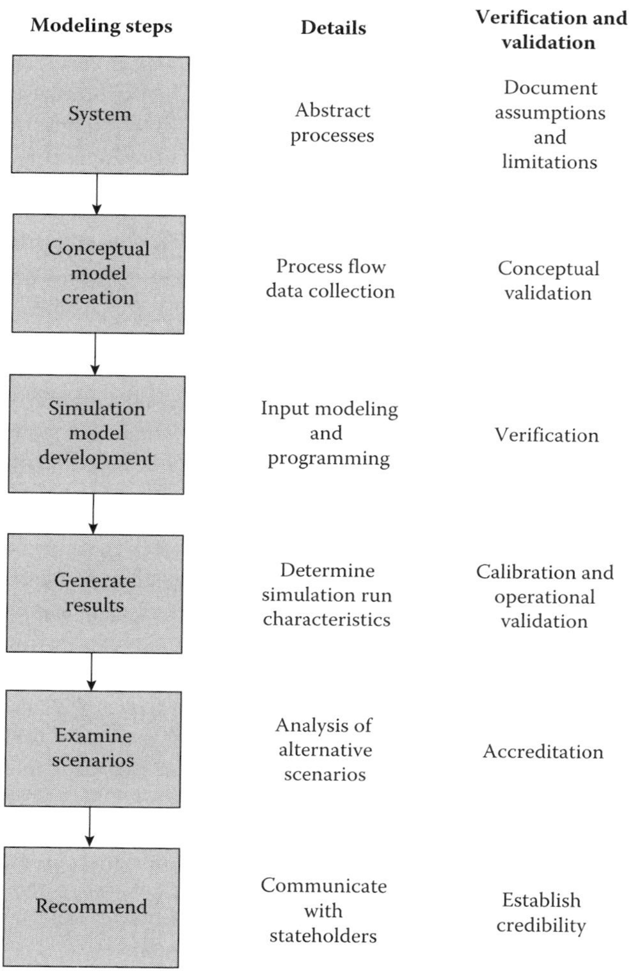

FIGURE 14.1 Creating and using a simulation model.

the simulation project (Eldabi et al., 2002), especially in the early phase of creating a conceptual model from the system description. Also it is rare that the simulation modeler is a healthcare provider, so it is mandatory that the modeler work in a team with "domain experts" to construct models that are relevant and useful.

Simulation models need to be designed for a specific purpose or to answer specific questions, otherwise the model creation process never concludes. In simulation, this is referred to as the "level of detail," and the level of detail will be constrained by the specific purpose of the simulation model. Furthermore, the validation process will be contained by this level of detail. In healthcare, it is critical to involve the subject-matter experts (SMEs), namely, the stakeholders, as early as possible in the statement of the specific questions. Otherwise, a model built with only input from nurses (for example) may not be acceptable to other critical stakeholders, and the results will be either rejected or ignored.

For the validation process to be complete, it needs to produce numbers that are consistent with what would be expected from the actual system. It is difficult to believe the results from a proposed change to the system that has not shown to represent the present systems correctly. Anything that can be done to show the model produces believable numbers will benefit the final recommendations.

Role of Data

Perhaps the greatest limitation to more widespread use of simulation in healthcare is the lack of data. While many manufacturing industries are now discovering the importance of performance data, healthcare information systems are preoccupied with medical records and administrative records needed for reimbursement. Performance data are viewed as an unnecessary burden and so the availability of data often limits model development and use. Certainly, the lack of data is inhibiting, but it need not be.

Data play two important roles in simulation modeling. First, as mentioned earlier, data are needed in the validation process. Second, data are needed to determine model input, that is, the parameters of the model. Data used for validation should not be the same data used for determining simulation input. For example, flow data, queuing data, and utilization can best be used in the validation process, whereas data on the processing times, interarrival times, branching and decisions, and other elements of a simulation can be best employed in determining appropriate simulation input. In the past, data used for parameter estimation in healthcare simulation have come from public databases such as the SEER (http://www.seer.cancer.gov/) and CDC WONDER (http://wonder.cdc.gov/) databases for cancer and mortality data, respectively, as well as from private vendors of healthcare data, such as hospital associations and Medicare databases (http://www.cms.hhs.gov/). And, as always, time studies or work sampling can be performed within one's own unit to determine the distribution of arrival and service times of various healthcare processes.

Inputs to a simulation are usually formed from standard univariate continuous and discrete probability distributions. The selection of a statistical distribution to represent the input to a simulation of a healthcare process usually involves a procedure of first identifying appropriate alternative candidate distributions. These candidate input models are chosen based on how the general properties of the distribution conform to what is known about the input being represented. Parameters for the candidate models are estimated, preferably from data collected from direct observation of the healthcare process. Finally a decision is made for the final input model based on how well the candidate models perform relative to what is known about the actual distribution. This entire procedure is referred to in simulation as "input modeling" because we are identifying a statistical model of the data we have collected.

In the construction of simulation models for healthcare operations, there are two basic kinds of input models that are most often employed—models of arrival processes and models of service processes. Input modeling choices are often based on many factors, including data availability, purpose of input, and structure of the input problem.

In the case of service processes, a histogram of the service time data is helpful in making input model choices. Figure 14.2 shows a histogram with a standard statistical distribution imposed upon it.

In Figure 14.2, the height of each bar represents the number of observed data points whose value lies within the range of the bar's upper and lower limits. This display is rather "typical" of the service times expected in healthcare operations. Notice that this distribution has a right tail longer than the left tail

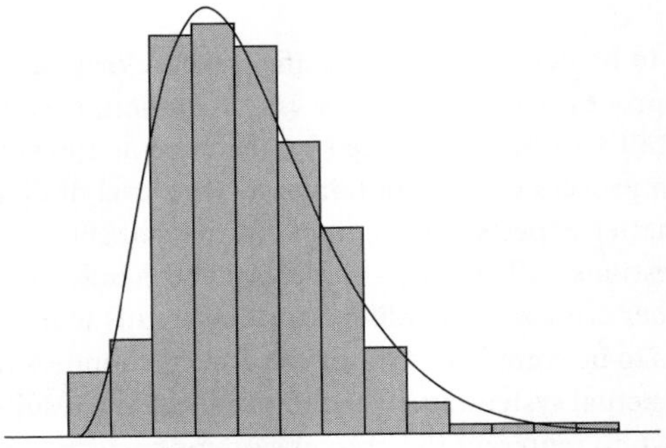

FIGURE 14.2 Histogram of a service time distribution.

and that the mode is less than the mean. The distribution is bounded on the left, unbounded on the right, and is continuous (as opposed to discrete).

As a result, our bias in healthcare operations is to consider standard continuous statistical distributions that match these characteristics such as lognormal, Erlang, gamma, and beta distributions as best representing service times or times in a state. The beta has the advantage of also being bounded on the right, which can prevent the small chance of unrealistically large values. Note that our list does not include the normal, which is symmetric and unbounded in either direction. We also tend to rule out the triangular, which is often recommended, simply because it produces "thick" tails and the data can be better approximated by a beta. An argument for the triangular distribution is that it can be parameterized with a minimum, mode, and maximum; however, if one is willing to make the so-called PERT assumptions about how to compute the variance, then the same three parameters can be used to estimate the beta, sometimes called the BetaPERT.

With regard to the arrival processes, the choices are generally more limited. In many healthcare operations, the arrivals tend to be random and a Poisson arrival process may be appropriate. In such an arrival process, the interarrival times are described by an exponential distribution. The mean of the Poisson is the average arrival rate while the mean of the exponential is the average interarrival time. In a healthcare setting, like an outpatient clinic or the emergency room, the arrival rate may change with time (maybe mornings being busier than afternoons). A Poisson arrival process whose rate changes over time is called a nonhomogeneous Poisson arrival process (NHPP). To describe an NHPP, the user must specify how the arrival rate changes with time. Rate changes are usually estimated over certain periods of time such as the number of arrival per hour during the hours of the day.

There are numerous commercial software packages that can assist in identifying standard statistical distributions. Some simulation software products imbed input modeling packages, such as Arena's *Input Analyzer*. Other software products focus only on input modeling, such as BestFit (http://www.palisade.com/bestfit/), ExpertFit (http://www.averill-law.com/ExpertFit-distribution-fitting-software.htm), EasyFit (http://www.mathwave.com/products/easyfit.html), and Stat::Fit (http://www.geerms.com/).

Simulation Technology

To understand the use of simulation, especially in healthcare, it is necessary to understand some of the fundamental components of simulation technology. Simulation technology is usually embedded within the simulation package or simulation language you are using. In recent years, some commercial simulation software is being oriented to healthcare operations (e.g., MedModel, http://www.promodel.com/products/medmodel/) and Flexsim Healthcare (http://www.flexsim.com/products/healthcare/). Several other vendors are poised to enter this market. For the most part, the healthcare simulation products are adaptations of more general simulation systems that have had their components redesigned or modified to reflect healthcare elements like exam rooms, nurses, medical records, laboratory specimens, radiology films, and so forth.

Each simulation product has its own unique set of concepts and features; however, there are some general characteristics that can be used to classify and describe them. Previously, we have pointed out that some simulation products contain their own input modeling capability, which makes specifying the random components of a simulation in a particular simulation language convenient. Other general features that are particular to a simulation package include the simulation modeling approach, the means of verification and debugging, the output analysis capability, the experimental design options, and the opportunity for optimization.

Simulation Modeling Approaches

The simulation modeling approach refers to the underlying structure of the simulation technology being offered. Some simulation products provide several alternatives. It is convenient to use the following categories of approaches, although it may be argued that these are not inclusive: Monte Carlo, discrete-event, object-oriented, systems dynamics, and agent-based.

Monte Carlo Simulation

A *Monte Carlo simulation* package permits simulations of random variables typically (but certainly not exclusively) within a spreadsheet context. Because in these models, there is no implicit passage of time, they are referred to as static. Examples of Monte Carlo simulations include @Risk (http://www.palisade.com/) and Crystal Ball (http://www.oracle.com/appserver/business-intelligence/crystalball/index.html). Often, all that is required of a Monte Carlo simulation is a definition of the random behavior of variables and any ways that the behavior of one variable affects the behavior of another or output of the system. Then, by generating random variates over the course of many replications, a range of possible output for one system is determined, providing much more information than one single output statistic or average performance metric. Single-period inventory problems, such as the number of transporters required in the hospital on a certain day, the number of surgical suites to be built in a new facility, or the number of spaces in the parking lot, might be modeled with a Monte Carlo simulation. Goitein (1990) used a Monte Carlo simulation to study the trade-off of patient waiting time and physician idle time in outpatient service appointment schedules. A growing use of Monte Carlo simulation is in probabilistic sensitivity analysis of medical decisions (Critchfield and Willard, 1986; Halpern et al., 2000; Briggs et al., 2002). In science, Monte Carlo simulations are used to compute analytically intractable integrals, the now of a new hypothesis test, or stochastic behavior of thermal transfer.

Discrete-Event Simulation

A *discrete-event simulation* forms the basis of many simulation languages and packages and is the most well-developed general simulation modeling approach, although it comes in different forms. It is the dominant approach to simulation of healthcare systems. The applicability of discrete-event simulation to health systems has been recognized for some time (Davies and Davies, 1995). A recent simulation software survey is found in http://www.lionhrtpub.com/orms/surveys/Simulation/Simulation.html which appeared in the October 2009 issue of *OR/MS Today*. Almost all commercial simulation languages are based on the discrete-event simulation technology.

At their lowest level, discrete-event simulations execute time-ordered events, which are points in time where a system changes state. To illustrate, Figure 14.3 is an event graph for a single server model (e.g., patients arriving for registration at an outpatient clinic).

This graph presents the event scheduling rules for the model. In this case, S refers to server availability, Q refers to the number in the queue, t_a is the (random) interarrival time, and t_s is the (random) service time. Here, the rather obvious events are the arrival of the customers and the end of service.

Discrete-event simulation is being more widely used in medical decision-making analysis, even though it has been used for some time, as for example in end-stage renal disease (Roberts et al., 1980). Cooper et al. (2006) note that discrete-event simulation approach to coronary heart disease interventions is preferable when the system is complex and there are resource concerns.

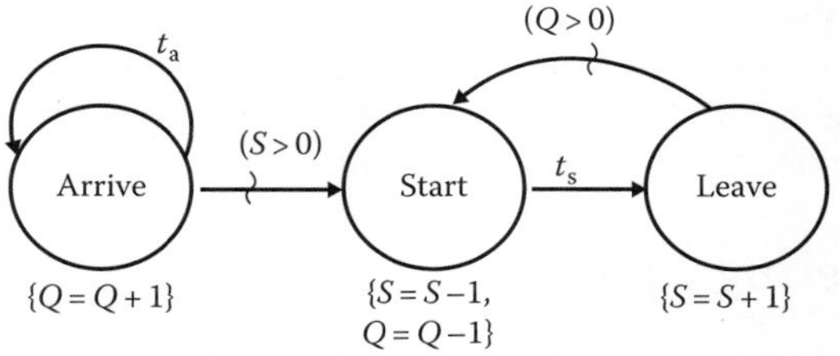

FIGURE 14.3 Event graph for single server model.

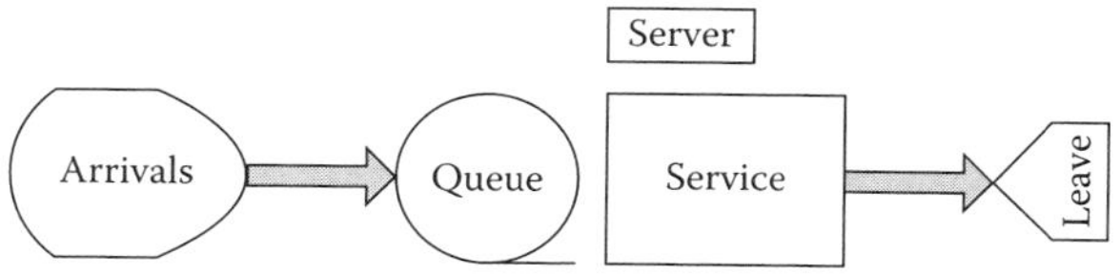

FIGURE 14.4 Process interaction model.

The most popular form of the discrete-event simulation approach is the *process-interaction* framework of discrete-event simulation. Numerous commercial packages implement a version of this, and it is the way most people model healthcare systems. In *process-interaction* simulations, the events are implied and instead of modeling the scheduling of events, the modeler characterizes the processes being modeled (Davies and Davies, 1994). There are many process characterizations, and different simulation products offer their own particular ones. For instance, Figure 14.4 presents one possible representation, in which the arrival of entities (likely representing patients, nurses, doctors, transporters, etc.) is followed as they flow through the system.

The *process-interaction* approach is very compatible with a tool used in business process improvement projects called *process mapping*. In process mapping, the goal is to follow a person or object through a sequence of events while distinguishing and detailing interactions of that object with the environment. At certain points in time, there are processes such as waiting, there are decisions to be made which affect the future course of the object, and there are actions being performed either by or to the object which affect the characteristics of the object and overall length of time the object stays in the system. Often process mapping is used to measure the amount of time spent by the object in both productive and nonproductive periods of waiting as well as the potential total resource usage consumed by an entity. It is easy to see how this tool may be beneficial in exposing some of the inefficiencies in any system, whether a manufacturing facility or a hospital or a clinic. Using this model, simulations employing the *process-interaction* approach can be very useful in identifying healthcare system inefficiencies and testing changes to the ways people or objects move throughout the system.

In process-interaction-based simulation programs, each process or decision is typically defined by a symbol or shape (these shapes and symbols are commonly shared in multiple programs and are often analogous to those used in process mapping). The processes entities encounter and the resources they require throughout their existence from arrival to departure are typically built in sequential fashion by connecting the associated symbols of each process by a directed link within a user-interface and virtual work environment. Within each symbol (often accessed by double-clicking the symbol), process parameters can be further specified. For example, the arrival process may include the interarrival times of entities, the time to begin arrivals, the time to end the arrivals, the number of items per arrival, and so forth, all of which may be random. An action process describes the length of the process and the amount and type of resources needed to carry out the process.

In a *process-interaction* approach, the actual occurrence of events and their sequencing is implicit, letting the modeler concentrate on the way the active members in their simulation interact. Many simulation languages have one basic class of active entities who have a lifetime in the simulation and a set of passive entities called resources that tend to be permanent members of the simulation model. Very often, the *process-interaction* is the interaction among entities of different types. Virtually all the simulation models of healthcare operations (hospital, outpatient clinics, and emergency departments) employ the *process-interaction* approach, although there are important exceptions.

Object-Oriented Simulation

The notion of a single entity type, in part, motivates the development of *object-oriented simulation* (*OOS*) languages. In an OOS, objects interact with each other over time. However, the design and implementation of the objects can be very challenging. Objects are instances of classes, and the class concept is at the

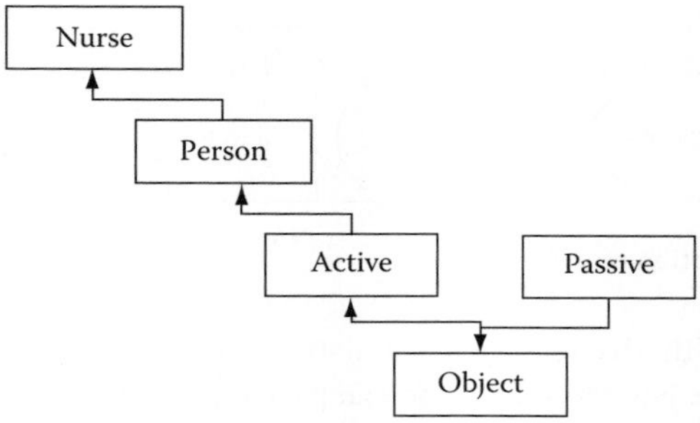

FIGURE 14.5 Example of class structure in OOS.

heart of OOS. A class is composed of properties and methods. The properties provide objects with their unique characteristics, while the methods give the objects their unique behavior. Objects communicate with each other through message passing. For example, an arriving patient object announces its arrival to a particular process object which in turn summands a provider. A class may be constructed from other classes through a process called composition or it may be derived from a parent class through inheritance. Using an OOS requires extra skill from the user because the user now must determine which objects are needed in the simulation and how they will communicate. A simple example of an OOS class structure is shown in Figure 14.5.

This class structure shows the inheritance tree beginning with a base object class from which "active" and "passive" classes may be derived. Next, a person class is derived from the active class, and eventually a nurse class is derived. Because the design of objects adds so much to the burden of modeling, the use of OOS directly in healthcare has been limited. However, this modeling approach has been used to model the behavior and experiences of people affected with colorectal cancer (Roberts et al., 2007). However, OOS is widely used to implement other simulation technologies.

Systems Dynamics Modeling

Another simulation technology is often referred to as *systems dynamics*, although it is a form of continuous simulation. Here the simulation of variables may continuously change with time. In its general form, systems dynamics has a set of state variables that are linked dynamically within a set of differential equations. However, for most applications and those in healthcare, the models consist of "levels" and "rates" where the levels are simply state variables and the rates are first-order differentials (Sterman, 2000). By confining ourselves to this simple form, a wide range of dynamic system problems can be modeled. Figure 14.6 presents a simple causal loop diagram for systems dynamics model.

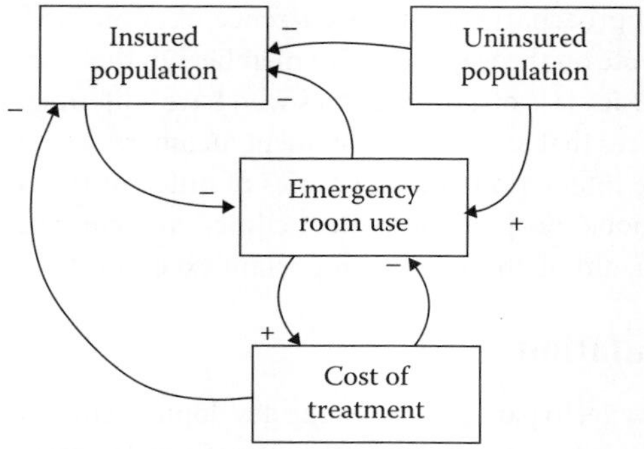

FIGURE 14.6 Causal loop diagram.

In this case, the number of emergency room visits might be modeled as being influenced by the insurance of the population and the cost of being treated at an emergency room. Notice there are positive (+) and negative (–) causal relationships among the variables. For instance, the more visits to an emergency room by the population, the higher the cost. The higher the cost, the higher the insurance, which reduces the number of insured people, and the number of uninsured people increases the use of the emergency room because it is the main source of primary care for them.

Some examples of the use of systems dynamics applied to healthcare include emergency departments (Lane et al., 2000; Lattimer et al., 2004), community care (Lane, 1994), Chlamydia screening (Evenden et al., 2005), and interventions in appointment making (Giachetti, 2008). An introduction to systems dynamics in healthcare is given by Brailsford (2008).

A method related to systems dynamics modeling, compartmental modeling has been used to model communicable disease spread of such diseases as measles, pertussis, rabies, smallpox, as well as several sexually transmitted diseases. This type of modeling segments a general population into different groups of people by common characteristics such as disease state or demographics. The traditional "SIR" compartmental model assumes all people are either "susceptible" (S), "infected" (I), or "recovered" (R). The levels in each subgroup change over time according to defined differential equations. The most basic assumption in this type of modeling is that everyone in the same compartment is identical, and therefore, the average amount of time each person spends in a compartment can be extrapolated to determine the number of people that will enter and leave the compartment. Other simplifying assumptions are that the number of contacts between people in different compartments is proportional to the product of each compartment's percentage of the entire population and that the probability that a contact results in a successful transmission of disease is constant. Many extensions to these types of models have been made over the past years since compartmental models were first studied in 1926 by Kermack and McCormick and mathematical epidemiology was advanced by Bailey in the 1950s. These models can be used to simulate disease spread through a population and "what-if" scenarios can be tested by changing both the demographic and epidemiological parameters as well as introducing healthcare interventions.

Agent-Based Modeling

The last simulation modeling approach that may be used in healthcare is referred to as *agent-based modeling* (*ABM*). ABM (Macal and North, 2006) extends the idea of objects to "agents" whose attributes have a strong association with human behavior, although there is no universal agreement on their definition. This tendency to treat agents as people means that agents need to have intelligent, autonomous characteristics and the capability to make independent decisions. While agents may be independent, they are situated in an environment of other agents, and thus there are rules that govern both the individual decision-making as well as interacting with other agents. Generally, ABM tends to be applied to societal problems which reflect social behavior such as swarming, flocking, following, etc. Some elements of ABM also include systems dynamics (Sterman, 2000; Rahmandad, 2008). Some examples of ABM in healthcare include models of emergency rooms (Stainsby et al., 2009) and epidemics (Burke et al., 2006; Bobashev et al., 2007; Dibble et al., 2007; Hupert et al., 2008; Carpenter and Sattenspiel, 2009). The ABM applications in epidemics reflect not only the recent public health concerns in emergency preparedness, but also in societal action and human behavior.

ABM is computation intensive, as it models each entity individually and captures all defined interactions between different entities. However, with the constant improvement of computational capacity and speed comes the ability to model more and more large-scale and complex systems. Some of the disadvantages or difficulties of ABM lie in model validation. Although the rules and parameters of ABM are based in reality, the output of these models is by nature hypothetical and therefore not easily comparable to real systems.

There are many health examples of several simulation techniques being used together. For instance, Brailsford et al. (2007) combine discrete-event simulation with an ABM to model screening policies for diabetic retinopathy and Bobashev et al. (2007) combine ABM and systems dynamics for modeling epidemics more efficiently, while Roberts and Simoni (2007) use ABM with discrete-event for another epidemiology simulation.

Experimentation and Optimization

A primary reason for simulation is the opportunity to conduct experiments with the simulation model. Experiments can be specified as individual alterations of the present system. Usually these relate to changes in the patient flow, such as a fast-track option in an emergency department. Often there are resource changes like the addition of beds, nurses, laboratories, and so forth. Some simulation languages (environments) make it easy to make systematic changes, like adding and subtracting the number of nurses in the PACU. The rather widespread integration of Visual Basic for Applications (VBA) within the simulation environment allows for pre-run, real-time, and post-run modification of simulation parameters and behavior.

Critical to the development of experimentation is how the simulation will be executed. There are generally two forms of simulations: terminating or transient simulations and steady-state simulations. The terminating simulations have a predefined starting and stopping state. They are most applicable when the simulation has a natural time horizon. Simulation of an individual's medical history is a clear terminating simulation. So would be any operation that was basically an 8- or 16-hour operation, such as a surgery suite or outpatient clinic. Terminating simulations are "replicated," with each replication providing an independent execution of the model with different random numbers being used to sample for the random processes. Therefore, the results of replicated simulation are suitable for standard statistical analysis, and most simulation languages facilitate this kind of analysis. Typically, a terminating simulation is replicated a sufficient number of times that the confidence intervals on the performance measure meet some minimum prespecified width.

Steady-state simulations are designed to be independent of how they are started or stopped. In other words, the results are what we expect to occur after the simulation has run a very long time. Although steady-state simulations appear to be simpler, they are, in fact, problematic. Two statistical issues plague this type of simulation. If the desired result is long-term behavior, we cannot ignore the potential presence of short-term behavior that tends to differ significantly from steady state and is an automatic product of the simulation's startup conditions. No simulation can be executed without startup conditions and so one must determine how to eliminate this startup or warm-up effect. Possible remedies include starting the simulation with resources busy and entities already in the system, or removing the statistics collected during this warm-up period. Second, very few observations of performance measures within a simulation are neither independent nor identically distributed, and thus standard statistics are not immediately appropriate. Considerable simulation research has been devoted to these issues and is beyond the scope of this chapter. However, the interested reader is referred to the standard simulation textbooks (Banks, 1998; Law and Kelton, 2000; Banks et al., 2010).

Generally, in a healthcare simulation, a terminating simulation is used. If the terminating simulation is modeling a nonterminating system, then some appropriate starting and stopping condition is specified (like start on Monday and end the following Monday). A level of precision for the confidence intervals of the chosen performance measures determines the number of replications. Each experiment or alternative is subject to the same experimental design relative to the number of replications and the starting/stopping conditions.

Choosing among the alternatives is done either through a ranking and selection method or through some other statistical analysis of the output. Because ranking and selection require a specified number of alternatives, some simulation packages include an *optimization* feature. This feature will allow the modeler to specify some objective that is a function of the simulation performance measures. Then the modeler is offered the opportunity to put constraints or restrictions on the alternative scenarios to be examined. In this way, a complete optimization problem is specified and the optimization method is allowed to execute. Most optimization methods do not truly optimize, but instead try to find improved scenarios. Usually, a heuristic procedure is used to test the response of the optimization to simulation scenarios being run and to try to find better scenarios based on the accumulated experience.

Simulation optimization is also a topic of considerable active research and the interested reader is referred to the Winter Simulation Conference (http://wintersim.org/). An archive of papers from this conference is found in the web space of the INFORMS Simulation Society (http://www.informs-sim.org/). Many papers from this conference have been cited in this chapter, and it should be noted that special sections of the Winter Simulation Conference have been devoted to healthcare systems. In fact, anyone interested in doing healthcare simulation is referred to this archive.

Conclusions

Computer simulation offers a diverse, powerful, and flexible set of tools for the analysis and improvement of healthcare systems. Models that were too large to be practical a decade ago are now within the computational capability of desktop computers. Problems that were thought to be too complex are now describable in many simulation languages and simulation environments. As simulation has found routine use in many industries, it can also be expected to be used routinely in healthcare, especially as the need to delivery efficient and cost-effective healthcare continues to demand attention. The greatest limitation of simulation is in the insight and capability of the modeler, not the technology. In healthcare, the modeler must work as a member of a team and address the needs and interests of the various stakeholders. To that end, new educational programs will be needed to train and educate people who understand both modeling and healthcare.

References

Akkerman, R. and M. Knip (2004). Reallocation of beds to reduce waiting time for cardiac surgery. *Health Care Management Science* 7(2): 119–126.

Arnaout, J.-P. M. and S. Kulbashian (2008). Maximizing the utilization of operating rooms with stochastic times using simulation. In *Proceedings of the 40th Conference on Winter Simulation*, Miami, FL, Winter Simulation Conference, pp. 1617–1623.

Bagust, A., M. Place et al. (1999). Dynamics of bed use in accommodating emergency admissions: Stochastic simulation model. *BMJ* 319(7203): 155–158.

Bailey, N. T. J. (1952). A study of queues and appointment systems in hospital out-patient departments, with special reference to waiting-times. *Journal of the Royal Statistical Society. Series B (Methodological)* 14(2): 185–199.

Balasubramanian, H., R. Banerjee et al. (2007). Improving primary care access using simulation optimization. In *Proceedings of the 39th Conference on Winter Simulation: 40 years! The Best Is Yet to Come*, Washington, DC, IEEE Press, pp. 1494–1500.

Ballard, S. M. and M. E. Kuhl (2006). The use of simulation to determine maximum capacity in the surgical suite operating room. In *Proceedings of the 38th Conference on Winter Simulation*, Monterey, CA, Winter Simulation Conference, pp. 433–438.

Banks, J. (1998). *Handbook of Simulation: Principles, Methodology, Advances, Applications, and Practice*. New York, Wiley.

Banks, J., I. John, S. Carson et al. (2010). *Discrete-Event System Simulation*, 5th edn. New York, Prentice-Hall.

Bobashev, G. V., D. M. Goedecke et al. (2007). A hybrid epidemic model: Combining the advantages of agent-based and equation-based approaches. In *Proceedings of the 39th Conference on Winter Simulation: 40 years! The Best Is Yet to Come*, Washington, DC, IEEE Press, pp. 1532–1537.

Bosire, J., S. Wang et al. (2007). Comparing simulation alternatives based on quality expectations. In *Proceedings of the 39th Conference on Winter Simulation: 40 years! The Best Is Yet to Come*, Washington, DC, IEEE Press, pp. 1579–1585.

Brailsford, S. C. (2007). Tutorial: Advances and challenges in healthcare simulation modeling. In *Proceedings of the 39th Conference on Winter Simulation: 40 years! The Best Is Yet to Come*, Washington, DC, IEEE Press, pp. 1436–1448.

Brailsford, S. C. (2008). System dynamics: What's in it for healthcare simulation modelers. In *Proceedings of the 40th Conference on Winter Simulation*, Miami, FL, Winter Simulation Conference, pp. 1478–1483.

Brailsford, S., W. Gutjahr et al. (2007). Combined discrete-event simulation and ant colony optimisation approach for selecting optimal screening policies for diabetic retinopathy. *Computational Management Science* 4(1): 59–83.

Brandeau, M. L. (2008). Infectious disease control policy: A role for simulation. In *Proceedings of the 40th Conference on Winter Simulation*, Miami, FL, Winter Simulation Conference, pp. 1578–1582.

Briggs, A. (2005). Probabilistic analysis of cost-effectiveness models: Statistical representation of parameter uncertainty. *Value Health* 8(1): 1–2.

Briggs, A. H., R. Goeree et al. (2002). Probabilistic analysis of cost-effectiveness models: Choosing between treatment strategies for gastroesophageal reflux disease. *Medical Decision Making* 22(4): 290–308.

Burke, D. S., J. M. Epstein et al. (2006). Individual-based computational modeling of smallpox epidemic control strategies. *Academic Emergency Medicine* 13(11): 1142–1149.

Butler, T. W., K. R. Karwan et al. (1992a). An integrative model-based approach to hospital layout. *IIE Transactions* 24(2): 144–152.

Butler, T. W., K. R. Karwan et al. (1992b). Multi-level strategic evaluation of hospital plans and decisions. *The Journal of the Operational Research Society* 43(7): 665–675.

Carpenter, C. and L. Sattenspiel (2009). The design and use of an agent-based model to simulate the 1918 influenza epidemic at Norway House, Manitoba. *American Journal of Human Biology* 21(3): 290–300.

Carter, M. and J. Blake (2005). Using simulation in an acute-care hospital: Easier said than done. In *Operations Research and Health Care*, pp. 191–215. New York, Springer.

Carter, M. W. and S. D. Lapierre (2001). Scheduling emergency room physicians. *Health Care Management Science* 4(4): 347–360.

Cooper, K., S. Brailsford et al. (2006). A review of health care models for coronary heart disease interventions. *Health Care Management Science* 9(4): 311.

Critchfield, G. C. and K. E. Willard (1986). Probabilistic analysis of decision trees using Monte Carlo simulation. *Medical Decision Making* 6(2): 85–92.

Davies, R. (2006). Use of simulation to determine resource requirements for end-stage renal failure. In *Proceedings of the 38th Conference on Winter Simulation*, Monterey, CA, Winter Simulation Conference, pp. 473–477.

Davies, R. (2007). "See and Treat" or "See" and "Treat" in an emergency department. *Proceedings of the 39th Conference on Winter Simulation: 40 years! The Best Is Yet to Come*, Washington, DC, IEEE Press, pp. 1519–1522.

Davies, R. and H. T. O. Davies (1994). Modelling patient flows and resource provision in health systems. *Omega* 22(2): 123–131

Davies, H. T. O. and R. Davies (1995). Simulating health systems: Modelling problems and software solutions. *European Journal of Operational Research* 87(1): 35–44.

Denton, B. T., A. S. Rahman et al. (2006). Simulation of a multiple operating room surgical suite. In *Proceedings of the 38th Conference on Winter Simulation*, Monterey, CA, Winter Simulation Conference, pp. 414–424.

Dexter, F., A. Macario et al. (1999). An operating room scheduling strategy to maximize the use of operating room block time: Computer simulation of patient scheduling and survey of patients' preferences for surgical waiting time. *Anesthesia & Analgesia* 89(1): 7–20.

Dexter, F., A. Macario et al. (2000). Scheduling surgical cases into overflow block time- computer simulation of the effects of scheduling strategies on operating room labor costs. *Anesthesia & Analgesia* 90(4): 980–988.

Dibble, C., S. Wendel et al. (2007). Simulating pandemic influenza risks of US cities. In *Proceedings of the 39th Conference on Winter Simulation: 40 years! The Best Is Yet to Come*, Washington, DC, IEEE Press, pp. 1548–1550.

Draeger, M. A. (1992). An emergency department simulation model used to evaluate alternative nurse staffing and patient population scenarios. In *Proceedings of the 24th Conference on Winter Simulation*, Arlington, VA, ACM, pp. 1057–1064.

Ekici, A., P. Keskinocak et al. (2008). Pandemic influenza response. In *Proceedings of the 40th Conference on Winter Simulation*, Miami, FL, Winter Simulation Conference, pp. 1592–1600.

Eldabi, T., I. Zahir et al. (2002). A proposed approach for modelling health-care systems for understanding. *Journal of Management in Medicine* 16(2): 170–187.

England, W. and S. D. Roberts (1978). Applications of computer simulation in health care. In *Proceedings of the 10th Conference on Winter Simulation*, Vol. 2, Miami Beach, FL, IEEE Computer Society Press, pp. 665–677.

Evans, G. W., T. B. Gor et al. (1996). A simulation model for evaluating personnel schedules in a hospital emergency department. In *Proceedings of the 28th Conference on Winter Simulation*, Coronado, CA, IEEE Computer Society, pp. 1205–1209.

Evenden, D., P. R. Harper et al. (2005). Improving the cost-effectiveness of Chlamydia screening with targeted screening strategies. *Journal of the Operational Research Society* 57(12): 1400–1412.

Ferrin, D. M., M. J. Miller et al. (2007). Maximizing hospital financial impact and emergency department throughput with simulation. In *Proceedings of the 39th Conference on Winter Simulation: 40 years! The Best Is Yet to Come*, Washington, DC, IEEE Press, pp. 1566–1573.

Fetter, R. B. and J. D. Thompson (1965). The simulation of hospital systems. *Operations Research* 13(5): 689–711.

Fitzpatrick, K. E., J. R. Baker, and D. S. Dave (1993). An application of computer simulation to improve scheduling of hospital operating room facilities in the United States. *International Journal of Computer Applications in Technology* 6: 215–224.

Fletcher, A. and D. Worthington (2009). What is a 'generic' hospital model?—A comparison of 'generic' and 'specific' hospital models of emergency patient flows. *Health Care Management Science* 12(4): 374–391.

Fone, D., S. Hollinghurst, M. Temple et al. (2003). Systematic review of the use and value of simulation modelling in population health and health care delivery. *Journal of Public Health* 25(4): 325–335.

Garcia, M., M. A. Centeno et al. (1995). Reducing time in an emergency room via a fast-track. In *Proceedings of the 27th Conference on Winter Simulation*, Arlington, VA, IEEE Computer Society, pp. 1048–1053.

Giachetti, R. E. (2008). A simulation study of interventions to reduce appointment lead-time and patient no-show rate. In *Proceedings of the 40th Conference on Winter Simulation*, Miami, FL, Winter Simulation Conference, pp. 1463–1468.

Gibson, I. W. (2007). An approach to hospital planning and design using discrete event simulation. In *Proceedings of the 39th Conference on Winter Simulation: 40 years! The Best Is Yet to Come*, Washington, DC, IEEE Press, pp. 1501–1509.

Glenn, J. K. and S. D. Roberts (1973). The relationship between resource and utilization factors in an outpatient care system. *AIIE Transactions* 5(1): 24–32.

Goitein, M. (1990). Waiting patiently. *The New England Journal of Medicine* 323(9): 604–608.

Groothuis, S., G. G. van Merode et al. (2001). Simulation as decision tool for capacity planning. *Computer Methods and Programs in Biomedicine* 66(2–3): 139–151.

Gunal, M. M. and M. Pidd (2007). Interconnected DES models of emergency, outpatient, and inpatient departments of a hospital. In *Proceedings of the 39th Conference on Winter Simulation: 40 years! The Best Is Yet to Come*, Washington, DC, IEEE Press, pp. 1461–1466.

Guo, M., M. Wagner et al. (2004). Outpatient clinic scheduling: A simulation approach. In *Proceedings of the 36th Conference on Winter Simulation*, Washington, DC, Winter Simulation Conference, pp. 1981–1987.

Halpern, E. F., M. C. Weinstein et al. (2000). Representing both first- and second-order uncertainties by Monte Carlo simulation for groups of patients. *Medical Decision Making* 20(3): 314–322.

Hancock, W. M., J. B. Martin et al. (1978). Simulation-based occupancy recommendations for adult medical/surgical units using admissions scheduling systems. *Inquiry* 15(1): 25–32.

Hancock, W. and P. Walter (1984). The use of admissions simulation to stabilize ancillary workloads. *Simulation* 43(2): 88–94.

Hay, A. M., E. C. Valentin et al. (2006). Modeling emergency care in hospitals: A paradox—The patient should not drive the process. In *Proceedings of the 38th Conference on Winter Simulation*, Monterey, CA, Winter Simulation Conference, pp. 439–445.

Ho, C. J. and H. S. Lau (1992). Minimizing total cost in scheduling outpatient appointments. *Management Science* 38(12): 1750–1764.

Hoot, N. R., L. J. LeBlanc et al. (2008). Forecasting emergency department crowding: A discrete event simulation. *Annals of Emergency Medicine* 52(2): 116–125.

Hoot, N. R., L. J. Leblanc et al. (2009). Forecasting emergency department crowding: A prospective, real-time evaluation. *Journal of the American Medical Informatics Association* 16(3): 338–345.

Hughes, G. R., C. S. M. Currie et al. (2006). Modeling tuberculosis in areas of high HIV prevalence. In *Proceedings of the 38th Conference on Winter Simulation*. Monterey, CA, Winter Simulation Conference, pp. 459–465.

Hung, G. R., S. R. Whitehouse et al. (2007). Computer modeling of patient flow in a pediatric emergency department using discrete event simulation. *Pediatric Emergency Care* 23(1): 5–10, 10.1097/PEC.1090b1013e31802c31611e.

Hupert, N., W. Xiong et al. (2008). The virtue of virtuality: The promise of agent-based epidemic modeling. *Translational Research* 151(6): 273–274.

Huschka, T. R., B. J. Narr et al. (2008). Using simulation in the implementation of an outpatient procedure center. In *Proceedings of the 40th Conference on Winter Simulation*, Miami, FL, Winter Simulation Conference, pp. 1547–1552.

Isken, M. W., T. J. Ward et al. (1999). Simulating outpatient obstetrical clinics. In *Proceedings of the 31st Conference on Winter Simulation: Simulation—A Bridge to the Future*, Vol. 2, Phoenix, AZ, ACM, pp. 1557–1563.

Jacobson, S. H., S. N. Hall et al. (2006). Discrete-event simulation of health care systems. In *Patient Flow: Reducing Delay in Healthcare Delivery*, pp. 211–252. New York, Springer.

Jun, J. B., S. H. Jacobson et al. (1999). Application of discrete-event simulation in health care clinics: A survey. *The Journal of the Operational Research Society* 50(2): 109–123.

Khurma, N., G. M. Bacioiu et al. (2008). Simulation-based verification of lean improvement for emergency room process. In *Proceedings of the 40th Conference on Winter Simulation*, Miami, FL, Winter Simulation Conference, pp. 1490–1499.

Kirtland, A., J. Lockwood et al. (1995). Simulating an emergency department "is as much fun as…" In *Proceedings of the 27th Conference on Winter Simulation*, Arlington, VA, IEEE Computer Society, pp. 1039–1042.

Klein, R. W., R. S. Dittus et al. (1993). Simulation modeling and health-care decision making. *Medical Decision Making* 13(4): 347–354.

Kolb, E. M. W., T. Lee et al. (2007). Effect of coupling between emergency department and inpatient unit on the overcrowding in emergency department. In *Proceedings of the 39th Conference on Winter Simulation: 40 years! The Best Is Yet to Come*, Washington, DC, IEEE Press, pp. 1586–1593.

Kolb, E. M. W., S. Schoening et al. (2008). Reducing emergency department overcrowding: Five patient buffer concepts in comparison. In *Proceedings of the 40th Conference on Winter Simulation*, Miami, FL, Winter Simulation Conference, pp. 1516–1525.

Kropp, D. and R. Carlson (1977). Recursive modeling of ambulatory health care settings. *Journal of Medical Systems* 1(2): 123–135.

Lane, D. C. (1994). System dynamics practice: A comment on 'A case study in community care using systems thinking.' *The Journal of the Operational Research Society* 45(3): 361–363.

Lane, D. C., C. Monefeldt et al. (2000). Looking in the wrong place for healthcare improvements: A system dynamics study of an accident and emergency department. *The Journal of the Operational Research Society* 51(5): 518–531.

Lattimer, V., S. Brailsford et al. (2004). Reviewing emergency care systems I: Insights from system dynamics modelling. *Emergency Medicine Journal* 21(6): 685–691.

Law, A. M. and D. W. Kelton (2000). *Simulation Modeling and Analysis*, 3rd edn. Boston, MA, McGraw-Hill Higher Education.

Lowery, J. C. (1996). Introduction to simulation in health care. In *Proceedings of the 28th Conference on Winter Simulation*, Coronado, CA, IEEE Computer Society, pp. 78–84.

Macal, C. M. and M. J. North (2006). Tutorial on agent-based modeling and simulation part 2: How to model with agents. In *Proceedings of the 38th Conference on Winter Simulation*, Monterey, CA, Winter Simulation Conference, pp. 73–83.

Mahapatra, S., C. P. Koelling et al. (2003). Emergency departments II: Pairing emergency severity index5-level triage data with computer aided system design to improve emergency department access and throughput. In *Proceedings of the 35th Conference on Winter Simulation: Driving Innovation*, New Orleans, LA, Winter Simulation Conference, pp. 1917–1925.

McGarvey, B. M., N. J. Dynes et al. (2007). A discrete event model of clinical trial enrollment at Eli Lilly and company. In *Proceedings of the 39th Conference on Winter Simulation: 40 years! The Best Is Yet to Come*, Washington, DC, IEEE Press, pp. 1467–1474.

McGuire, F. (1997). Using simulation to reduce length of stay in emergency departments. *Journal of the Society for Health Systems* 5(3): 81–90.

Medeiros, D. J., E. Swenson et al. (2008). Improving patient flow in a hospital emergency department. In *Proceedings of the 40th Conference on Winter Simulation*, Miami, FL, Winter Simulation Conference, pp. 1526–1531.

Mellor, G. R., C. S. M. Currie et al. (2007). Targeted strategies for tuberculosis in areas of high HIV prevalence: A simulation study. In *Proceedings of the 39th Conference on Winter Simulation: 40 years! The Best Is Yet to Come*, Washington, DC, IEEE Press, pp. 1487–1493.

Miller, M. J., D. M. Ferrin et al. (2004). Fixing the emergency department: A transformational journey with EDSIM. In *Proceedings of the 36th Conference on Winter Simulation*, Washington, DC, Winter Simulation Conference, pp. 1988–1993.

Miller, M. J., D. M. Ferrin et al. (2008). Allocating outpatient clinic services using simulation and linear programming. In *Proceedings of the 40th Conference on Winter Simulation*, Miami, FL, Winter Simulation Conference, pp. 1637–1644.

Morrison, B. P. and B. C. Bird (2003). A methodology for modeling front office and patient care processes in ambulatory health care. In *Proceedings of the 35th Conference on Winter Simulation: Driving Innovation*, New Orleans, LA, Winter Simulation Conference, pp. 1882–1886.

Patvivatsiri, L. (2006). A simulation model for bioterrorism preparedness in an emergency room. In *Proceedings of the 38th Conference on Winter Simulation*, Monterey, CA, Winter Simulation Conference, pp. 501–508.

Protil, R. M., J. R. Stroparo et al. (2008). Applying computer simulation to increase the surgical center occupation rate at a university hospital in Curitiba—Brazil. In *Proceedings of the 40th Conference on Winter Simulation*, Miami, FL, Winter Simulation Conference, pp. 1609–1616.

Rahmandad, H. S. J. (2008). Heterogeneity and network structure in the dynamics of diffusion: Comparing agent-based and differential equation models. *Management Science* 54(5): 998–1014.

Ramis, F. J., F. Baesler et al. (2008). A simulator to improve waiting times at a medical imaging center. In *Proceedings of the 40th Conference on Winter Simulation*, Miami, FL, Winter Simulation Conference, pp. 1572–1577.

Rao, D. M. and A. Chernyakhovsky (2008). Parallel simulation of the global epidemiology of Avian influenza. In *Proceedings of the 40th Conference on Winter Simulation*, Miami, FL, Winter Simulation Conference, pp. 1583–1591.

Rising, E. J., R. Baron et al. (1973). A systems analysis of a university-health-service outpatient clinic. *Operations Research* 21(5): 1030–1047.

Roberts, S. D., D. R. Maxwell et al. (1980). Cost-effective care of end-stage renal disease: A billion dollar question. *Annals of Internal Medicine* 92(2 Pt 1): 243–248.

Roberts, D. J. and D. A. Simoni (2007). A teragrid-enabled distributed discrete event agent-based epidemiological simulation. In *Proceedings of the 39th Conference on Winter Simulation: 40 years! The Best Is Yet to Come*, Washington, DC, IEEE Press, pp. 1551–1554.

Roberts, S., L. Wang et al. (2007). Development of a simulation model of colorectal cancer. *ACM Transactions on Modeling and Computer Simulation* 18(1): 1–30.

Rossetti, M. D., G. F. Trzcinski et al. (1999). Emergency department simulation and determination of optimal attending physician staffing schedules. In *Proceedings of the 31st Conference on Winter Simulation: Simulation—A Bridge to the Future*, Vol. 2, Phoenix, AZ, ACM, pp. 1532–1540.

Ruohonen, T., P. Neittaanm et al. (2006). Simulation model for improving the operation of the emergency department of special health care. In *Proceedings of the 38th Conference on Winter Simulation*, Monterey, CA, Winter Simulation Conference, pp. 453–458.

Sepulveda, J., W. Thompson et al. (1999). The use of simulation for process improvement in a cancer treatment center. In *Proceedings of the 31st Conference on Winter Simulation: Simulation—A Bridge to the Future*, Vol. 2, Phoenix, AZ, ACM, pp. 1541–1548.

Sinreich, D. and Y. N. Marmor (2004). A simple and intuitive simulation tool for analyzing emergency department operations. In *Proceedings of the 36th Conference on Winter Simulation*, Washington, DC, Winter Simulation Conference, pp. 1994–2002.

Sinreich, D. and Y. N. Marmor (2005). Emergency department operations: The basis for developing a simulation tool. *IIE Transactions* 37(3): 233–245.

Smith, S. R., B. J. Schroer et al. (1979). Scheduling of patients and resources for ambulatory health care. In *Proceedings of the 11th Conference on Winter Simulation*, Vol. 2, San Diego, CA, IEEE Press, pp. 553–561.

Smith-Daniels, V. L., S. B. Schweikhart et al. (1988). Capacity management in health care services: Review and future research directions. *Decision Sciences* 19(4): 889–919.

Song, W. T., A. E. Bair et al. (2008). A simulation study on the impact of physician starting time in a physical examination service. In *Proceedings of the 40th Conference on Winter Simulation*, Miami, FL, Winter Simulation Conference, pp. 1553–1562.

Standridge, C. R. (1999). A tutorial on simulation in health care: Applications issues. In *Proceedings of the 31st Conference on Winter Simulation: Simulation—A Bridge to the Future*, Vol. 1, Phoenix, AZ, ACM, pp. 49–55.

Stainsby, H., M. Taboada, E. Luque (2009). Towards an agent-based simulation of hospital emergency departments. In *IEEE International Conference on Services Computing*, Bangalore, India, pp. 536–539.

Sterman, J. (2000). *Business Dynamics: Systems Thinking and Modeling for a Complex World*, Boston, MA, Irwin/McGraw-Hill.

Sundaramoorthi, D., V. C. P. Chen et al. (2006). A data-integrated nurse activity simulation model. In *Proceedings of the 38th Conference on Winter Simulation*, Monterey, CA, Winter Simulation Conference, pp. 960–966.

Taaffe, K., M. Johnson et al. (2006). Improving hospital evacuation planning using simulation. In *Proceedings of the 38th Conference on Winter Simulation*, Monterey, CA, Winter Simulation Conference, pp. 509–515.

Tafazzoli, A., S. Roberts et al. (2009). Probabilistic cost-effectiveness comparison of screening strategies for colorectal cancer. *ACM Transactions on Modeling and Computer Simulation* 19(2): 1–29.

Takakuwa, S. and D. Katagiri (2007). Modeling of patient flows in a large-scale outpatient hospital ward by making use of electronic medical records. In *Proceedings of the 39th Conference on Winter Simulation: 40 years! The Best Is Yet to Come*, Washington, DC, IEEE Press, pp. 1523–1531.

Takakuwa, S. and H. Shiozaki (2004). Functional analysis for operating emergency department of a general hospital. In *Proceedings of the 36th Conference on Winter Simulation*, Washington, DC, Winter Simulation Conference, pp. 2003–2011.

Takakuwa, S. and A. Wijewickrama (2008). Optimizing staffing schedule in light of patient satisfaction for the whole outpatient hospital ward. In *Proceedings of the 40th Conference on Winter Simulation*, Miami, FL, Winter Simulation Conference, pp. 1500–1508.

VanBerkel, P. and J. Blake (2007). A comprehensive simulation for wait time reduction and capacity planning applied in general surgery. *Health Care Management Science* 10(4): 373–385.

Vila-Parrish, A. R., J. S. Ivy et al. (2008). A simulation-based approach for inventory modeling of perishable pharmaceuticals. In *Proceedings of the 40th Conference on Winter Simulation*, Miami, FL, Winter Simulation Conference, pp. 1532–1538.

Wiinamaki, A. and R. Dronzek (2003). Using simulation in the architectural concept phase of an emergency department design. In *Proceedings of the 2003 Winter Simulation Conference*, New Orleans, LA, pp. 1912–1916.

Wijewickrama, A. K. A. and S. Takakuwa (2006). Simulation analysis of an outpatient department of internal medicine in a university hospital. In *Proceedings of the 38th Conference on Winter Simulation*, Monterey, CA, Winter Simulation Conference, pp. 425–432.

Wijewickrama, A. and S. Takakuwa (2008). Outpatient appointment scheduling in a multi facility system. In *Proceedings of the 40th Conference on Winter Simulation*, Miami, FL, Winter Simulation Conference, pp. 1563–1571.

Williams, W. J., R. P. Covert et al. (1967). Simulation modeling of a teaching hospital outpatient clinic. *Hospitals* 41(21): 71–75 passim.

Yurtkuran, A. and E. Emel (2008). Simulation based decision-making for hospital pharmacy management. In *Proceedings of the 40th Conference on Winter Simulation*, Miami, FL, Winter Simulation Conference, pp. 1539–1546.

15

An Introduction to Optimization Models and Applications in Healthcare Delivery Systems

Wenhua Cao
University of Houston

Gino J. Lim
University of Houston

Introduction 15-1
Optimization • Applications
Mathematical Models 15-3
Linear Programming Models • Mixed Integer Programming Models • Nonlinear Programming Models • Stochastic Programming Models • Multi-Objective Optimization
Solution Techniques 15-11
Traditional Solution Algorithms • Meta-Heuristic Approaches
Conclusion 15-16
References 15-16

Introduction

Optimization

The term optimization has been well rooted as a field for finding optimal or best possible solutions to complex systems by applying mathematical modeling and computational techniques. The concept of optimization is generally applied to analyzing complex decision problems in which the decision maker aims to achieve single or multiple objectives by determining the values of many decision variables. As a quantitative tool, a specific optimization model is developed to quantitatively represent the problem of interest. Of course, it is not realistic to incorporate all the relationships of a real-world problem into an optimization model. But sophisticated optimization techniques indeed provide a powerful platform to let practitioners approach various decision problems at a great level of breadth, depth, and simplicity.

The implementation of optimization can be divided into three main sequential components: first modeling the problem, then solving the model, and last post-optimization analysis. Frankly, in an optimization model, the decision problem in a complex system is translated as selecting the values of a set of variables such that the objective, representing system performance or quality, is optimized (e.g., minimizing the deviation between supply and demand of nursing shifts, or maximizing nurse working satisfaction in the nurse scheduling problem) and necessary system constraints (e.g., limited number of nurses for nurse scheduling problems) are satisfied. In the form of constrained optimization, a general formulation is

$$\begin{array}{ll} \text{maximize or minimize} & \text{Objective Function} \\ \text{subject to} & \text{Constraints.} \end{array} \tag{15.1}$$

Optimization can be categorized into many subfields according to the different properties of the model. Major ones include linear programming (LP), where objective and constraint functions are all linear; mixed integer programming (MIP), where some of the variables in a linear program are restricted to take integer values; nonlinear programming, where functions do not have to be linear; stochastic programming (SP), where parameters or functions are defined on random variables; and multi-objective programming, where multiple objectives exist in a model and are often conflicting with one another. Other promising areas include robust programming, dynamic programming, convex programming, and semi-definite programming. One problem can be formulated into alternative models of all kinds according to designated purposes. Thanks to the continuous effort of researchers, various algorithms have been developed to systematically solve different optimization models. Also, the modern advancement of computation capabilities empowers practitioners to control sophisticated optimization techniques in a fast and flexible manner.

Applications

The application of optimization techniques was first practiced in the military logistic operations during World War II. After that, many industries—telecommunications, transportation, computer science, engineering, manufacturing, economics, government, biology, healthcare delivery systems—began to utilize optimization techniques to improve their systems to achieve better quality and efficiency. The extensive applications have proven that optimization acts as an indispensable technique for the advancement of various industries. It is superior to other systems in providing rich, systematic, and flexible tools for practitioners to analyze and solve complex decision problems.

The healthcare delivery systems have triggered many emerging optimization problems along with the continuous development of healthcare policies, operations, and equipments. Various rewarding areas include medical facility locations and capacity planning, patient scheduling, medical human resource scheduling, disease prediction, treatment delivery planning, and so on. Unlike optimization problems that arise in other industries, those from healthcare have certain significant characteristics (Pierskalla and Brailler, 1994). For instance, the outcome of a clinical decision-making problem directly affects the health and life quality of patients, sometimes even leads to death. Sometimes, the decision of allocating a medical facility greatly influences the rights of citizens and administrative policies. And often, several decision makers such as physicians, nurses, and administrators participate in the decision-making process. Therefore, inherent dynamics and rigorous requirements add exceptional challenges to optimize healthcare decision problems.

Optimization is such a rich discipline that this chapter cannot possibly provide a broad and thorough discussion on the entire field. Therefore, we intend to present fundamental and well-developed techniques with examples specifically in healthcare delivery systems. The readers of this chapter are expected to have no familiarity with mathematical optimization. The rest of the chapter is organized as follows. The section on mathematical models introduces major mathematical models and illustrates how optimization problems are formulated with examples. Selected benchmark solution methods to various optimization problems are discussed in the section on solution techniques. Optimization methods that are applied to different healthcare delivery problems are listed in the conclusion, where we discuss the importance of optimization techniques in facilitating healthcare delivery systems and the promising outlook of this study and application.

Mathematical Models

Mathematical modeling is crucial in the process of optimization practice. There is often a trade-off in modeling. On one hand, a good optimization model should grasp the essential aspects of a problem in order to naturally and precisely interpret the problem into the mathematical form. On the other hand, an optimization model may become intractable if the model is too complex (Luenberger and Ye, 2008). The balance of the trade-off is necessary to yield a meaningful solution for optimization practice. The selection of models is dependent on the practitioner's experience and specific purpose. Following are some major model formulations that are well studied and adopted.

Linear Programming Models

LP is without question the most popular philosophy in the optimization field because of its simplicity and solvability, as well as its richness in mathematical theories. LP can be used to formulate a wide class of real-world problems. Also, many problems that are virtually nonlinear or of unknown relationships are modeled into alternative LPs, when other models are too complex to present as problems, or too difficult to solve. Thus, LP provides the basis for all other formulations.

A standard LP model, or linear program, includes a set of decision variables, one objective function, and certain constraints (Chvatal, 1983; Murty, 1983; Taha, 2007). The decision variables are the unknown values that the decision maker aims to determine by solving the optimization model. The objective function for maximization or minimization is a linear function of defined decision variables. Constraints are a set of equalities or inequalities that are also linear functions of the decision variables either equal or no greater than or no less than a scalar value. With basic operations, every LP can be formulated in a standard form (Vanderbei, 2008):

$$
\begin{aligned}
\text{maximize} \quad & c_1x_1 + c_2x_2 + \cdots + c_nx_n \\
\text{subject to} \quad & a_{11}x_1 + a_{12}x_2 + \cdots + a_{1n}x_n \le b_1 \\
& a_{21}x_1 + a_{22}x_2 + \cdots + a_{2n}x_n \le b_2 \\
& \vdots \\
& a_{m1}x_1 + a_{m2}x_2 + \cdots + a_{mn}x_n \le b_m \\
& x_1, x_2, \ldots, x_n \ge 0
\end{aligned}
\tag{15.2}
$$

There are n decision variables and m constraints in the LP 15.2. A set of specific values for the decision variables is a solution to the LP. If there exists a solution $x = (x_1, x_2, \ldots, x_n)^T$ that satisfies all the constraints, x is a feasible solution. If the objective function reaches its maximum value (minimum value when LP is a minimization problem) at a feasible solution $x^* = (x_1^*, x_2^*, \ldots, x_n^*)^T$, x^* is an optimal solution. Every LP can be set in one of the following three scenarios:

- *Unbounded.* No finite maximum or minimum value of the objective function exists for the LP. Thus, there does not exist any optimal solution.
- *Infeasible.* No feasible solution exists for the LP.
- *Feasible.* LP is neither unbounded nor infeasible, and has optimal solution(s). The objective function has unique maximum or minimum values, but the optimal solution may not be unique.

Alternatively, an LP is often represented in matrix notation as follows:

$$\begin{aligned} \text{maximize} \quad & c^T x \\ \text{subject to} \quad & Ax \le b \\ & x \ge 0 \end{aligned} \tag{15.3}$$

where

$$x = \begin{bmatrix} x_1 \\ x_2 \\ \vdots \\ x_n \end{bmatrix}, \quad c = \begin{bmatrix} c_1 \\ c_2 \\ \vdots \\ c_n \end{bmatrix}, \quad b = \begin{bmatrix} b_1 \\ b_2 \\ \vdots \\ x_m \end{bmatrix}, \quad A = \begin{bmatrix} a_{11} & a_{12} & \cdots & a_{1n} \\ a_{21} & a_{22} & \cdots & a_{2n} \\ \vdots & \vdots & \vdots & \vdots \\ a_{m1} & a_{m2} & \cdots & a_{mn} \end{bmatrix}$$

One important theory in LP that we need to include is duality. Every LP problem that we refer to as a primal problem has an associated dual problem. In the standard form, problem 15.4 is the dual problem of primal problem 15.3, where $y = (y_1, y_2, \ldots, y_m)^T$:

$$\begin{aligned} \text{minimize} \quad & b^T y \\ \text{subject to} \quad & A^T y \ge c \\ & y \ge 0 \end{aligned} \tag{15.4}$$

It is observed that every feasible solution of the primal problem provides a bound for the optimal objective function value of the dual problem, and vice versa. Two associated theorems are

- *Weak duality theorem.* If $\bar{x} = (\bar{x}_1, \bar{x}_2, \ldots, \bar{x}_n)^T$ is a feasible solution to the primal LP 15.3, and $\bar{y} = (\bar{y}_1, \bar{y}_2, \ldots, \bar{y}_m)^T$ is a feasible solution to the dual LP 15.4, then $c^T\bar{x} \le b^T\bar{y}$.
- *Strong duality theorem.* If $x^* = (x_1^*, x_2^*, \ldots, x_n^*)^T$ is the optimal solution to the primal LP 15.3, and $y^* = (y_1^*, y_2^*, \ldots, y_n^*)^T$ is the optimal solution to the dual LP 15.4, then $c^Tx^* = b^Ty^*$.

The duality is not only theoretically important, but also useful when analyzing and solving certain LP problems. One can check the gap between the primal and dual objective function values to estimate the optimal objective function value of the problem, or to track the progress of the optimization process. Moreover, some primal problems are hard to solve, but their dual problems are easy to solve.

Example 1: IMRT Fluence Map Optimization

Intensity modulated radiation therapy (IMRT) is one of the most advanced cancer treatments in recent years, which uses external radiation beams to irradiate tumors. IMRT can deliver significant radiation dose to precisely conform to the three-dimensional shape of the tumor while sparing the surrounding critical organs and normal tissues. The treatment planning of this technology brings a series of challenging optimization problems for researchers.

Since each of the IMRT beams can be divided into hundreds of sub-beamlets, and the intensity, named fluence, of every beamlet can be modulated independently, one problem called fluence map optimization (FMO) aims to determine optimal beamlet fluence values for every beam used in cancer treatment. With a set of predefined radiation beams, FMO aims to find the optimal intensity profile of each beam. Let (x, y, z) denote a point in the 3D treatment volume including tumor target (T), critical organs (S), and normal tissues (N), i.e., $(x, y, z) \in T \cup S \cup N$. And $(\bar{a}, k)$ denotes the beamlet k of the treatment beam $\bar{a}$, where $\bar{a} \in \bar{a}$, $k = 1, 2, \ldots, t$. Assuming that the dose contribution from beamlet $(\bar{a}, k)$ to point (x, y, z) is available by using separate simulation techniques and is denoted as $d_{(x, y, z, \bar{a}, k)}$, the FMO problem can be formulated as an LP with decision variables as fluence values $w_{\bar{a},k}$:

$$\begin{aligned} \text{minimize} \quad & f(D_{(x,y,z)}) \\ \text{subject to} \quad & D_{(x,y,z)} \geq \sum_{\bar{a} \in \bar{A}} \sum_{k=1}^{t} w_{\bar{a},k} \cdot d_{(x,y,z,\bar{a},k)} \\ & w_{\bar{a},k} \geq 0 \ \forall \bar{a} \in \bar{A}, \ k = 1,2,\ldots,t \end{aligned} \tag{15.5}$$

The objective function for the LP 15.5 can be constructed in various forms according to specific requirements. One example for a minimization LP is an organ-based penalty function that sums the total deviation between the delivered dose and prescribed dose at all points. For illustration, see 15.6, where $f(D_T)$, $f(D_S)$, and $f(D_N)$ are all linear functions of the decision variable $w_{\bar{a},k}$, and λ_T, λ_S, and λ_N are weighting factors. The details of the functions can be found in Lim et al. (2008):

$$f(D_{(x,y,z)}) = \lambda_T f(D_T) + \lambda_S f(D_S) + \lambda_N f(D_N) \tag{15.6}$$

The constraints for the LP 15.5 often include dose distribution constraints to restrict the solution to meet certain requirements. For example, constraints (15.7 and 15.8) limit doses on points within the tumor target to no more than the upper bound T_U, and no less than the lower bound T_L. Similar constraints can be assigned to points in critical organs and normal tissues. More complex constraints for dose–volume requirements are also important to allow better control of dose distribution (Langer and Leong, 1987; Morrill et al., 1991a; Spirou and Chui, 1998):

$$D_T \leq T_U \tag{15.7}$$

$$D_T \geq T_L \tag{15.8}$$

The FMO problem has been extensively studied (Bahr et al., 1968; Rosen et al., 1990; Morrill et al., 1991b; Hamacher and Kfer, 2002; Holder, 2004; Lee et al., 2006). We encourage readers to review articles in which both formulation variants and solution methods are thoroughly discussed.

Mixed Integer Programming Models

The MIP model is defined as LP 15.2 or 15.3 that constrains some or all of x_j to take integer values, i.e., generally $x_j \in Z^+$. Since many real-world decision problems are associated with positive integer valued decision variables and therefore can be formulated as MIP, this branch of optimization has been studied with special interest as it is of practical importance. There are some special cases of MIP that are specifically studied. One is integer programming (IP), sometimes integer linear programming (ILP), which requires all decision variables in an LP to be integers. Other cases are binary (0–1) integer programming (BIP) and binary mixed integer programming (BMIP) when IPs or MIPs have binary (or 0–1) variables that are used to represent common yes/no decisions. A MIP model can be unbounded, infeasible or feasible with optimal solutions, definitions in "Linear programming models" section.

Smith and Taskin (2008) provided a good tutorial of MIP techniques with some examples of applications in medicine and biology. We illustrate the modeling of MIP through a treatment planning problem for brachytherapy, which is another type of radiotherapy.

Example 2: Brachytherapy Treatment Planning

Recent advances in medical devices introduced an internal radiation therapy, named brachytherapy. In brachytherapy, radioactive substances are placed within or close to the tumor region. The aim in brachytherapy treatment planning (BTP) is primarily to determine the location for implantation of radioactive sources. The goal of a brachytherapy plan consists of delivering enough radiation dose to the target tumor mass and sparing surrounding critical organs and normal tissues.

First, modeling the BTP problem requires the dose calculation scheme. Meyer et al. (2003) described an approximation function for dose rate. Let us define the dose rate at a distance l from a single source as $D(l)$, referring Meyer et al. (2003) for calculations. Then, if j indexes the 3D grid of prespecified possible locations of radioactive sources, and an arbitrary point i, the total dose at point i from all source locations is given by

$$D_i = \sum_j y_j D(l_{ij}) \tag{15.9}$$

$$y_j \in \{0,1\} \tag{15.10}$$

where

y_j, the decision variable, is a binary vector indicating the selection or non-selection of location j
l_{ij} is the Euclidean distance from point X_i to point X_j, i.e., $l_{ij} = \|X_i - X_j\|$

The constraints and objective of the BTP optimization model are homogeneously constructed as the IMRT model in Example 1, and so are all radiotherapy optimization models. One can control the dose of radiation on the suspected tumor region (planning target volume (PTV)) by hard constraints:

$$D_i \le T_U \tag{15.11}$$

$$D_i \ge T_L \tag{15.12}$$

or soft constraints

$$D_i - R_U^T \le T_U \tag{15.13}$$

$$D_i + R_L^T \ge T_L \tag{15.14}$$

The specified maximum number of locations for seeds can be controlled by this constraint:

$$\sum_j y_j \le \text{maximum number of locations} \tag{15.15}$$

The objective functions may vary based on the treatment planner's preferences. Lee et al. (2000, 2003) described two kinds of objective functions. One maximizes the total number of points that satisfy specified dose distribution requirements, and the other minimizes the total dose deviation on PTV. See 15.16 for the example of the latter objective function, where $\lambda_{overdose}$ and $\lambda_{underdose}$ are weighting factors:

$$\text{minimize} \quad \sum_i \left(\lambda_{overdose} D_i^{overdose} + \lambda_{underdose} D_i^{underdose} \right) \tag{15.16}$$

Thus, the MIP or BIP model for BTP can be constructed. In addition to the location problem, another optimization problem in BTP is to decide an appropriate amount of time (dwell time) for those sources to stay in the patient's body (Alterovitz et al., 2006). In the dwell-time optimization model, the dose calculation is defined as

$$D_i = \sum_j t_j D(l_{ij}) \tag{15.17}$$

$$t_j \geq 0 \tag{15.18}$$

where t_j is the dwell time. The constraints including 15.9 through 15.12 and objective functions for optimizing locations of radioactive sources can all be used to optimize dwell time. Note that decision variable t_j is not restricted to be an integer, and the resulting model is an LP instead of an MIP.

The MIP modeling techniques have been widely used for most of radiotherapy planning problems as can be found in the literature (Hamacher and Lenzen, 2000; Bednarz et al., 2002; Ferris et al., 2002; Ehrgott et al., 2004; Preciado-Walters et al., 2004; Engel, 2005; Lim et al., 2007, 2008). Since MIP models are more flexible than LP models in formulating real-world decision problems, MIP has been extensively used to deal with practical optimization problems in healthcare delivery systems. Examples include medical resource or hospital location problems (Stummer et al., 2004; Jia et al., 2007; Griffin et al., 2008), medical staffing scheduling problems (Burke et al., 2004; Oddoye et al., 2007; Belien and Demeulemeester, 2008), patient scheduling problems (Denton et al., 2007; Combi et al., 2009), disease prediction problems (Ryu et al., 2007), medical data classification problems (Lee, 2007), and so on.

Nonlinear Programming Models

The nonlinear programming (NLP) model is formulated when the objective function or some of the equalities or inequalities of constraints in the problem 15.1 are nonlinear. For the formal definition, in a mathematical formulation to the problem, we have

$$\begin{aligned} &\text{minimize} \quad f(x) \\ &\text{subject to} \quad x \in X \end{aligned} \tag{15.19}$$

where $f: R^n \rightarrow R$ is a continuous function of n variables, and X is equal to or is a subset of R^n, i.e., $X \subseteq R^n$ (Bertsekas, 1999). If f is linear and X is polyhedral, it is an LP problem; otherwise, it is an NLP problem.

NLP is an important branch in optimization with solid mathematical foundations (Mangasarian, 1994; Ruszczynski, 2006; Luenberger and Ye, 2008), addressing theories like unconstrained and constrained optimization, convex and non-convex optimization, local and global optimal, convergence, and so on. Beyond theoretical significance, NLP problems are generally complex to solve and analyze in practical circumstances. A very simple NLP example in two dimensions can be

$$\begin{aligned} \text{minimize} \quad & x_1^2 + x_2^2 \\ \text{subject to} \quad & x_1 + x_2 \leq 1 \\ & x_1, x_2 \geq 0 \end{aligned} \tag{15.20}$$

where the objective function is quadratic and the constraints are linear.

Example 3: Radiotherapy Treatment Planning

The ultimate goal of all radiotherapy techniques is to deliver a significant amount of dose to the tumor region in order to kill the cancer while avoiding radiation to any other areas. In Examples 1 and 2, the objective functions of LP and MIP formulations interpret the goal in a relatively simple manner and hence have computational strength. However, the biological objectives for radiotherapy treatment planning (RTP) often require nonlinear functions in the optimization model. It can be understood that many biological and physical laws and theories are stated in a nonlinear form. The biologically oriented NLP models have been studied by many researchers (Legras et al., 1982, 1986; Ferris et al., 2003a; Olafsson et al., 2005; Lim et al., 2007).

With the similar constraints and consistent notations in previous examples, the nonlinear objective function for general RTP can be modeled as follows:

$$f(D_\Omega) \leq \|D_\Omega - \theta\|_p \tag{15.21}$$

where $\Omega = T \cup S \cup N$, and $p = 1, 2, \ldots$. Note that θ is the desired radiation dose level for an organ of interest. These problems can be cast as a quadratic programming (QP) problem ($p = 2$), minimizing the Euclidean distance between the dose delivered to each voxel and the prescribed dose (Redpath et al., 1976; Starkschall, 1984; Shepard et al., 1999; Chen et al., 2002).

For example, given θ_T, θ_S, and θ_N are the prescribed dose levels for the tumor target, critical organs, and normal tissues, respectively, a weighted sum of squares objective function is

$$f(D_\Omega) = \lambda_T (D_T - \theta_T)^2 + \lambda_s (D_s - \theta_s)^2 + \lambda_N (D_N - \theta_N)^2 \tag{15.22}$$

Furthermore, the Euclidean norm objective function in a QP can be replaced with a polyhedral one, for which standard reformulations (Lim et al., 2004, 2007) result in LP problems. These models tend to find optimal solutions more quickly than the corresponding QP formulations.

A successful application of NLP can be found in gamma knife radiosurgery for brain cancer (Ferris et al., 2003b; Shepard et al., 2003). The original problems was formulated as mixed integer nonlinear programming (MINLP). The authors propose a novel approach that utilizes NLP reformulation for finding the solution of the MINLP model.

Stochastic Programming Models

SP is an optimization technique that seeks to find an optimal solution to decision-making problems that contain uncertainty. The uncertainty can be understood as uncertain data, or random variables, involved in the objective function or constraints in an optimization model. Ideally, specific joint probability distributions to uncertain parameters are required for SP. But more practical alternatives of probability functions can be several defined outcomes or scenarios of uncertainty. Fuzzy optimization

(Sakawa, 2002) is an option when one does not even have any information about uncertainty. Birge and Louveaux (1997) present the most straightforward method. The idea is to have a solution at the first stage and then optimize the expected outcomes of the solution at the second stage. Based on problem 15.3, a general formulation of the two-stage recourse model can be

$$\begin{aligned} \text{minimize} \quad & c^T x + E\left[\hat{f}(x,\xi)\right] \\ \text{subject to} \quad & Ax \le b \\ & x \ge 0 \end{aligned} \tag{15.23}$$

As $E[\cdot]$ represents expected value, and ξ is a random vector, the function $E[\hat{f}(x, \xi)]$ is called the recourse function. The recourse function incorporates the realization of ξ, resulting from the decision in stage one, to form the minimization or maximization problem toward the final decision.

The recourse model 15.23 can be simply extended to multistage models in the same fashion. The concept of "wait and see" describes the modeling process appropriately. For illustration, a decision is made firstly, then we wait and see the consequence of the previous decision, and re-optimize the problem with inclusion of realized random values. We repeat the procedure until all decisions have been made. Although the SP faces problems closest to real-life scenarios due to the inclusion of the uncertainty nature, the solution difficulty of the SP model is typically significant. For solution algorithms, one may refer to the literature (Birge and Louveaux, 1997; Ruszczynski and Shapiro, 2003).

Example 4: Adaptive Treatment Planning

Adaptive treatment planning (ATP), in contrast to static ones, modifies the treatment plan throughout the treatment delivery horizon based on periodical or continuous feedback. We discuss ATP within the scope of radiation therapy. In general, a radiation treatment plan is implemented during a specific period of time, say 30 days as a session. A small portion of the total prescribed dose, or fraction, is delivered to the patient once daily. Since a range of uncertainties may take place during the long process, such as equipment error, patient setup or positioning variation, organ movement, and so on, these uncertainties can result in a high deviation between dosage actually delivered at the end and optimized dosage based on the original treatment plan. Therefore, ATP is used to counter uncertainties as and when necessary. If the modification of the treatment plan is introduced after delivering a fraction and before the next one, it is called off-line ATP. An online APT adjusts the treatment plan while delivering the fractionated dose.

SP offers a significantly useful method to approach the ATP problem by considering those unavoidable uncertainties that the deterministic modeling techniques are unable to deal with. Thanks to the advance of equipment developments, it has been possible to measure the radiation delivering progress and system errors in real time. Thus, the feedback of associated uncertainties in each fraction can be collected before planning the treatment for the next faction. Complete optimization frameworks for ATP based on SP techniques with solution methods are provided in many recent studies (Lof et al., 1998; Yan et al., 2000; Unkelbach and Oelfke, 2004; Sir et al., 2008; Thongphiew et al., 2008).

The applications of SP are important in many other problems in healthcare delivery systems. Since the demand for heath care is typically uncertain, varying dramatically from regular scenarios to unpredictable emergencies, the medical supply facility location problem, therefore, can be modeled by SP to find a more robust solution (Beraldi et al., 2004; Jia et al., 2007). Studies by Martel and Ouellet (1994) and Punnakitikashem et al. (2008) formulated the nurse assignment problem for hospitals into stochastic optimization models. Colvin and Maravelias (2008) applied SP in optimizing the clinical trial for new drug development by incorporating the uncertainty of body's responses to drugs. From an economic perspective, Gilleskie (1998) developed a stochastic model of a decision-making problem to determine whether to visit a doctor or miss his/her work when experiencing illness. This research can help better understand the behavior of healthcare consumption, and thus the cost of healthcare at a system level.

Multi-Objective Optimization

Multi-objective optimization (MOO), or called multi-criteria optimization, is used to find solutions to problems with multiple objectives that are often conflicting with each other, for instance, minimizing cost while maximizing service, or minimizing risk while maximizing revenue. Such decision problems can be found in many real-world scenarios including the healthcare delivery system. In one example—the nurse scheduling problem—important objectives include maximizing the service level, minimizing the cost, and maximizing the nurse preferences of shifts, and so on. Another example, in the radiation therapy treatment planning optimization, one aims to minimize the deviation between the delivered radiation dose and the prescribed dose on target volumes while minimizing dose on critical and normal tissues at the same time.

A general MOO problem can be represented as follows:

$$\begin{aligned} \text{minimize} \quad & F(x) = \left[f_1(x), f_2(x), \ldots, f_n(x) \right] \\ \text{subject to} \quad & Ax \leq b \\ & x \geq 0 \end{aligned} \tag{15.24}$$

The model 15.24 contains n objective functions: $f_1(x)$, $f_2(x)$, …, $f_n(x)$, where $f_i(x)$, i = 1, 2, …, n can be either linear or nonlinear. The model becomes multi-objective linear programming (MOLP) when all objective functions and constraints are linear. MOLP is the simplest form of MOO models and relatively easy to solve, which have specifically developed algorithms (Ehrgott, 2005). Unlike the single-objective optimization, there is generally no single global optimal solution to a MOO model. Therefore, the MOO solution is often approached by the concept of Pareto optimality, which determines a set of points that satisfy a predefined optimum while identifying optimal points of the MOO model. Other concepts such as efficient frontier and dominant/nondominant are also important to understand characteristics of the MOO model. Details can be found in Deb (2001) and Marler and Arora (2004).

The solution strategies for MOO models have been actively studied. Systematic algorithms exist for MOLP problems to find the efficient frontier but it is still difficult to solve large problems. In order to guarantee a feasible solution with certain quality, more practically useful methodologies are often used to solve real-life MOO problems. Goal programming treats multiple objectives as a set of goals, normally ordered by priority. With required target values to all goals, the deviations between actual values and target values are optimized. Preemptive optimization is a method in which each objective of MOO is optimized separately one at a time. A bound is obtained each time and then a resulting bound is added to the model, until all objectives are optimized. A weighted-sum single-objective method combines multiple objectives into one single-objective function by simply adding each weighted objective up, assuming all individual objectives are either minimization or maximization problems.

Example 5: Nurse Scheduling

Nurse scheduling is a complex personnel scheduling problem that is still largely performed manually in hospitals worldwide. The problem of nurse scheduling sets the task of allocating every nurse to her or his work shifts on a daily basis for a defined period of time under certain requirements. Two major reasons makes the problem particularly difficult. First, nurses have different skill levels and specialties, and the demand for different nurses varies in days and shifts. The scenario leads to an especially large number of decision variables when modeling the problem. Second, addressing job satisfaction is extra important in nurse scheduling, since a satisfied and active workforce is vital to provide quality services. But nurse preferences are often conflicting with the demand of workloads and patterns.

Nurse scheduling is a typical MOO problem. Various objectives include (1) maximizing the service level, e.g., supplying sufficient number of nurses to meet demands and providing nurses with appropriate skill levels and specialties to patients, (2) minimizing operational costs, e.g., avoiding idle or unnecessary personnel time, and reducing hiring and firing costs, (3) maximizing nurse preferences, e.g., nurse requests on willingness to work on particular shifts or days, (4) minimizing unfavorable work patterns, e.g., avoiding isolated working days or isolated day/night shifts for all nurses. The decision variables in a nurse scheduling model often contains integer valued variable for number of nurses, shifts, or work days, also sometimes binary variables meaning selection or non-selection of certain types of nurses or shifts.

Since the formulation of the nurse scheduling problem is not essentially special to our previous examples, and it requires a relatively lengthy explanation of various variables and specific requirements, we do not provide a specific model here. Readers can find more examples in Burke et al. (2001), Azaiez and Al Sharif (2005), Bard and Purnomo (2005), Topaloglu, (2006), and Oddoye et al. (2007). Also, Burke et al. (2004) provided an up-to-date survey of literature in nurse scheduling problems.

Example 6: Medical Resource Planning and Management

Besides the example of the nurse scheduling problem, most decision-making problems in medical resource planning and management are multi-objective, such as hospital location and capacity planning and medical resource scheduling. They are especially exposed in recent researches. Some common objectives include reducing total operational costs, improving quality of service, increasing resource utilization, decreasing patient waiting times, and so on.

Hutzschenreuter et al. (2009) discussed the MOO of hospital resource management with respect to dynamic patient arrival and treatment process. Li et al. (2009a,b) studied the bed allocation problem using MOO models. Cardoen et al. (2009) offered a literature review on operating room planning and scheduling. Stummer et al. (2004) introduced an MOO approach to determine medical resource location and capacity in a region; and the research of Paul and Batta (2008) sought to allocate hospitals and capacities to maximize their access and effectiveness in disaster scenarios. A few more specific problems can also be formulated in the multi-objective scheme, medical waste collection optimization (Shih and Lin, 2003), and mobile medical facility routing optimization (Doerner et al., 2007).

There is a rich body of literature in one important group of problems, i.e., the multi-objective patient (inpatient or outpatient) scheduling problems. Some examples can be found in Vermeulen et al. (2007, 2008) and Combi et al. (2009). Another significant application of MOO is associated with radiotherapy planning, which involves complex medical and biological objectives (Halabi et al., 2006).

Solution Techniques

The chapter has briefly demonstrated modeling variants that can mathematically formulate a problem. While the solution techniques impose no less significance of problem formulation in the optimization field, some important ones are discussed in this section.

Traditional Solution Algorithms

We start this section with some benchmarking and fundamental optimization solution algorithms, which can not only solve problems efficiently, but also provide the bedrock for many other useful variant methods.

Simplex Method

The simplex method was first introduced by George Dantzig in 1947. It is an iteration-based algorithm for generating solutions of LP problems. To demonstrate its methodology, consider a simple LP with two decision variables (x_1, x_2):

$$\begin{aligned} &\text{minimize} \quad f(x_1,x_2) \\ &\text{subject to} \quad g_i(x_1,x_2) \geq 0, \quad i=1,2,\ldots \\ &\qquad\qquad x_1,x_2 \geq 0 \end{aligned} \tag{15.25}$$

The graphical representation of the LP 15.25 is shown in Figure 15.1. The shaded area is the feasible region in which solutions of (x_1, x_2) are satisfied by all constraints of the LP. The simplex method starts from a feasible vertex (point 1 in Figure 15.1), and then moves from one vertex to another until it is proven that either

1. An optimal solution was found (point 4 in Figure 15.1)
2. The problem is unbounded

In the general situation, when there are n decision variables and a set of equalities and inequalities as constraints in an LP problem, the feasible region can be formed as a polytope. The simplex method proceeds, in the same fashion, from one vertex to another through edges of the polytope, until optimum vertex is reached. The detailed operations of the simplex algorithm process can be found in most LP books or tutorials (Murty, 1983; Taha, 2007; Vanderbei, 2008). Other algorithms including primal simplex, dual simplex, network simplex, and interior point (barrier) are also important for certain LP problems.

Branch and Bound

The Branch and Bound algorithm, which originated in 1960, can be used to solve a large range of optimization problems, especially when the decision variables are discreet. It can be an efficient methodology to seek optimal or good solutions for very complex problems. The algorithm contains two main

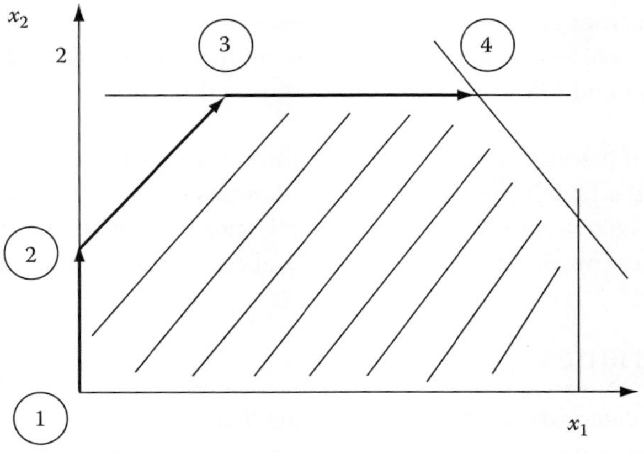

FIGURE 15.1 Illustration of the simplex method in a two-dimension case.

procedures: branching and bounding, like its name. Based on an idea of divide and conquer, the problem is first divided into many subproblems that are easier to solve or have sound efficient solution methods; then the original problem is solved based on information gained from those easy problems. Figure 15.2 illustrates how a branching tree is constructed. Each node stands for a problem. Splitting a node is called branching. Solving the problem at each node (P_1, P_2,..., etc.) will provide a bound (upper or lower) to the original problem (P_0). The branch and bound proceed until no possible node exists.

Let us consider a simple IP problem 15.26. We perform an LP-based branch and bound process to find the optimal solution of the problem:

$$\begin{aligned} \text{maximize} \quad & 17x_1 + 12x_2 \\ \text{subject to} \quad & 10x_1 + 7x_2 \le 40 \\ & x_1 + x_2 \le 5 \\ & x_1, x_2 \in Z^+ \end{aligned} \tag{15.26}$$

Step 0: Initialization. An LP relaxation problem (P_0) is formed by replacing the integral constraint x_1, $x_2 \in Z^+$ by $x_1, x_2 \ge 0$. The optimal LP solution $(x_1, x_2) = (5/3, 10/3)$ provides an upper bound to the original IP problem, i.e., $\bar{z} = 68.33$ (see Figure 15.3a).

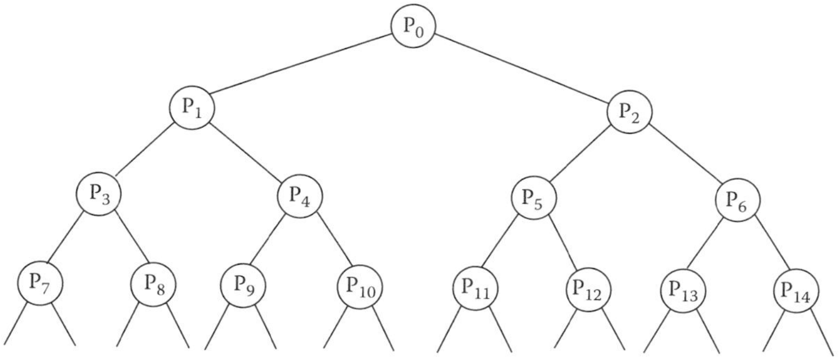

FIGURE 15.2 Problem branching tree.

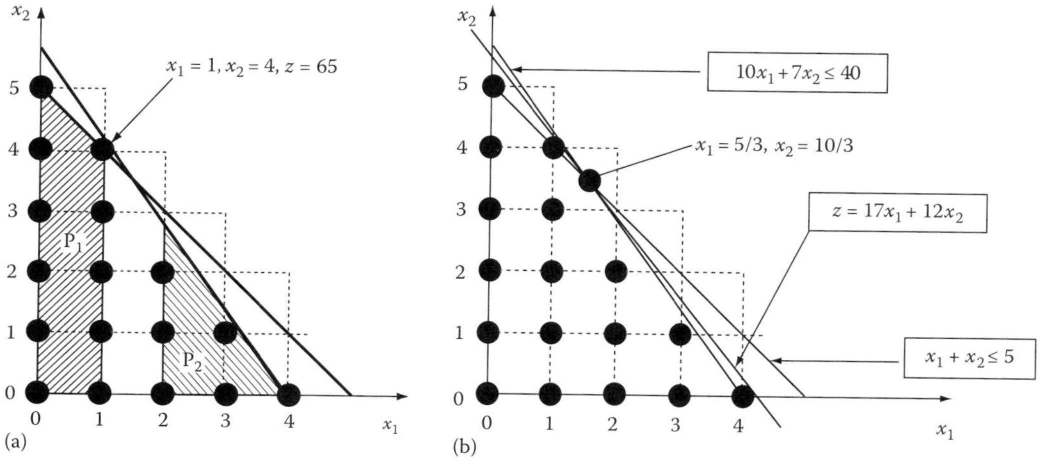

FIGURE 15.3 Branch and bound process illustration: (a) original problem and (b) problem after first branch.

Step 1: Branching. Break the problem (P_0) into two subproblems (P_1 and P_2) by adding one of the constraints ($x_1 \le 1$, $x_2 \ge 2$) to P_0. From optimal solutions of $P_1$and P_2, there is one integer solution, $(x_1^*, x_2^*) = (1,4)$ and $z^* = 65$, which is a solution to the original IP solution (see Figure 15.3b).

Step 2: Bounding. Check the current two subproblems (P_1 and P_2) and update the best upper bound of IP, thus $\bar{z} = 68.29$ with $(x_1, x_2) = (2, 2.86)$ (optimal solution of P_2).

Step 3: Fathoming. Or say, pruning a node in the search tree (Figure 15.2). There are three scenarios to fathom:

- Infeasibility, if the subproblem is infeasible.
- Bound, if the optimal objective value of the subproblem is higher than the current upper bound.
- Optimality, if the optimal solution of the subproblem is an integer. Thus, P_1 is pruned, and no further steps are needed.

Stopping criteria. Stop if no unfathomed subproblem exists, and the incumbent integer solution is optimal to the original IP. Otherwise, return to Step 1. In the example, P_2 returns to the next iteration of branch and bound.

The IP example briefly illustrates how the branch and bound algorithm finds the optimal integer solution by solving LPs. However, it is much more flexible for solving MIP problems (Meyer et al., 2003; Smith and Taskin, 2008). Note that the branching strategy is often vital for the efficiency and effectiveness of the algorithm. Pitfalls lead to exhaustive enumeration. A successful branching decision relies on the good understanding of problem characteristics.

Some variant algorithms such as branch and cut, branch and price, and cutting plane are very useful in solving certain problems. Those algorithms together with branch and bound offer a base for various heuristics. Details are available in literature (Nemhauser and Wolsey, 1988; Floudas, 1995; Barnhart et al., 1998; Wolsey, 1998; Linderoth and Savelsbergh, 1999; Hillier and Lieberman, 2002).

Meta-Heuristic Approaches

When there is no satisfactory algorithm to a specific problem, or it is too difficult to implement such an algorithm, meta-heuristic approaches, or heuristics themselves, are considered as alternatives of solution methods to find a best possible solution within a certain level of effort. Various meta-heuristics often incorporate concepts or experiences from other disciplines, such as biology, physics, mathematics, mechanics, etc. Three well-known methods are local search, simulated annealing (SA), and genetic algorithm (GA).

Local Search

The concept of the local search heuristic is straightforward. It starts from a feasible solution, then searches for another solution from the current solution, in a domain defined in a certain way that improves the incumbent objective function value. The search continues iteratively until no improvement is possible. Note that local search heuristics are meant to converge to a local optimal solution. General steps of local search can be described as follows (supposing a minimization problem and its associated objective function f):

Step 0: Input starting feasible solution S_0, set $S^* = S_0$ and $i = 0$.

Step 1: Construct the neighborhood $N(S_i)$.

Step 2: Search for an improved solution S' in the neighborhood, if $f(S') < f(S^*)$, and $S' \in N(S_i)$, set $S^* = S'$, $i = i + 1$.

Step 3: If all elements in $N(S_i)$ have been tested so that $f(S^*)$ cannot be improved, stop search with S^* as a local optimal solution. Otherwise, return to *Step 1*.

For two practical examples, the local search algorithm was applied to solve the IMRT beam-angle optimization problem (Aleman et al., 2008) and the chemotherapy scheduling problem (Agur et al., 2006).

Simulated Annealing

The SA approach aims to find a global optimal solution to optimization problems, especially combinatorial and discrete ones. The concept, namely, is adopted from the mechanical process. This process initially involves melting a metal or glass at a high temperature and then slowly cooling the substance until it reaches a low-energy stable state with desirable physical properties.

The algorithm of SA initially takes a near-random search to explore as much of the feasible region as possible, and then gradually improves the objective function value. This algorithm can find the global optimal solution if enough time is given for the search. Unlike the local search, SA updates not only the improving solution (with probability 1), but also the non-improving solution (with certain probability between 0 and 1) (Kirkpatrick et al., 1983; Van Laarhoven and Aarts, 1989).

The process of this heuristic can be illustrated as

Step 0: Input starting feasible solution S, set the starting temperature T, the loop length M, and the cooling percentage p.

Step 1: Set $i = 0$.

Step 2: Construct the neighborhood $N(S)$.

Step 3: Select a neighbor $S' \in N(S_i)$, if $f(S') < f(S)$, set $S = S'$; if $f(S') > f(S)$, set $S = S'$ with probability $e[f(S)-f(S')]/T$; set $i = i + 1$.

Step 4: If $i < M$, return to *Step 2*; otherwise set $T = pT$.

Step 5: If $T > 0$, return to *Step 1*; otherwise stop with the best solution found.

Note that the values of several parameters (T, M, or p) are important for the efficiency and solution quality of specific SA algorithms. A range of medical decision problems have been solved by different SA heuristics (Webb, 1989, 1991, 1992; Morrill et al., 1991b; Shu et al., 1998).

Genetic Algorithm

The GA is a known global search heuristic that proceeds from a population (set of solutions) that evolves from one generation (iteration) to the next. For a brief illustration, five procedures are generally conducted in one iteration (Wolsey, 1998):

- *Evaluation*. The fitness of each individual (a solution) in the population is evaluated. The fitness function can be the objective function of the associated optimization model or a specific one.
- *Parent selection*. Parents (solutions) in pairs are selected normally based on their fitness.
- *Crossover*. Each pair of parents produces one or two offspring (new solutions).
- *Mutation*. Some of the offspring are randomly modified.
- *Population selection*. The original population is replaced (partially or entirely) by the offspring with better fitness.

For example, consider the seed location problem in Example 2. A solution of the problem is a binary vector y, with 0 indicating the selected locations and 1 indicating the nonselected locations. The fitness of the solution y can be the objective function 15.16. Assume that we are selecting 4 out of 10 candidate locations. In one iterations, we have two solutions as parents: $y_1 = (0, 0, 1, 0, 1, 0, 0, 1, 1, 0)$ and $y_2 = (0, 1, 0, 1, 0, 0, 0, 1, 1, 0)$. One logical strategy to perform the crossover procedure can be keeping all sharing pattern of 0 and 1, and creating new patterns based on the difference. Thus, there can be four new solutions, offspring, by crossover: i.e., $y_1^c = (0, 1, 1, 0, 0, 0, 0, 1, 1, 0)$, $y_2^c = (0, 0, 1, 1, 0, 0, 0, 1, 1, 0)$, $y_3^c = (0, 0, 0, 1, 1, 0, 0, 1, 1, 0)$, and $y_4^c = (0, 1, 0, 0, 1, 0, 0, 1, 1, 0)$. The mutation procedure for offspring can be defined as a random permutation of the binary decision vector.

Applications of GA for solving radiotherapy optimization problems can be found in Cotrutz and Xing (2003), Lahanas, (1999), Li et al. (2004), and Yu et al. (1997).

Conclusion

It is estimated that the United States spends 15.3% of its GDP on healthcare systems, only second to East Timor-Leste among all the countries worldwide (World Health Organization, 2009). The health share of GDP is still projected to continue increasing in the future. The applications of optimization can help not only reduce healthcare cost but also improve healthcare quality. Optimization techniques have been proved to facilitate complex decision making in the healthcare delivery systems at different levels ranging from strategic planning and systems operations to treatment deliveries (Pierskalla and Brailer, 1994). We have provided an overview of important optimization techniques and their applications in solving decision problems in healthcare delivery systems as an illustration. Main examples included are radiotherapy treatment planning problems. We believe that the research and application of optimization will continue as a significant tool to improve access, efficiency, and effectiveness of our healthcare systems.

References

Agur, Z., R. Hassin, and S. Levy. 2006. Optimizing chemotherapy scheduling using local search heuristics. *Operations Research*, 54(5):829–846.

Aleman, D.M., A. Kumar, R.K. Ahuja, H.E. Romeijn, and J.F. Dempsey. 2008. Neighborhood search approaches to beam orientation optimization in intensity modulated radiation therapy treatment planning. *Journal of Global Optimization*, 42:587–607.

Alterovitz, R., E. Lessard, J. Pouliot, I.J. Hsu, J. O'Brien, and K. Goldberg. 2006. Optimization of HDR brachytherapy dose distributions using linear programming with penalty costs. *Medical Physics*, 33(11):4012–4019.

Azaiez, M.N. and S.S. Al Sharif. 2005. A 0–1 goal programming model for nurse scheduling. *Computers and Operations Research*, 32:491–507.

Bahr, G.K., J.G. Kereiakes, H. Horwitz, R. Finney, J. Galvin, and K. Goode. 1968. The method of linear programming applied to radiation treatment planning. *Radiology*, 91:686–693.

Bard, J.F. and H.W. Purnomo. 2005. Preference scheduling for nurses using column generation. *European Journal of Operational Research*, 164:510–534.

Barnhart, C., E.L. Johnson, G.L. Nemhauser, M.W.P. Savelsbergh, and P.H. Vance. 1998. Branch-and-price: Column generation for solving integer programs. *Operations Research*, 46:316–329.

Bednarz, G., D. Michalski, C. Houser, M.S. Huq, Y. Xiao, P.R. Anne, and J.M. Galvin. 2002. The use of mixed-integer programming for inverse treatment planning with pre-defined field segments. *Physics in Medicine and Biology*, 47(13):2235–2245.

Belien, J. and E. Demeulemeester. 2008. A branch-and-price approach for integrating nurse and surgery scheduling. *European Journal of Operational Research*, 189:652–668.

Beraldi, P., M.E. Bruni, and D. Conforti. 2004. Designing robust emergency medical service via stochastic programming. *European Journal of Operational Research*, 158(1):183–193.

Bertsekas, D.P. 1999. *Nonlinear Programming*, 2nd edn. Athena Scientific, Belmont, MA.

Birge, J.R. and F. Louveaux. 1997. *Introduction to Stochastic Programming*. Springer, New York.

Burke, E.K., P. De Causmaecker, G.V. Berghe, and H.V. Landeghem. 2004. The state of the art of nurse rostering. *Journal of Scheduling*, 7(6):441–499.

Burke, E.K., P.I. Cowling, P. De Causmaecker, and G.V. Berghe. 2001. A memetic approach to the nurse rostering problem. *Applied Intelligence*, 15:199–214.

Cardoen, B., E. Demeulemeester, and J. Belien. 2010. Operating room planning and scheduling: A literature review. *European Journal of Operational Research*, 201(3):921–932.

Chen, Y., D. Michalski, C. Houser, and J.M. Galvin. 2002. A deterministic iterative least-squares algorithm for beam weight optimization in conformal radiotherapy. *Physics in Medicine and Biology*, 47:1647–1658.

Chvatal, V. 1983. *Linear Programming*. W. H. Freeman and Company, New York.

Colvin, M. and C.T. Maravelias. 2008. A stochastic programming approach for clinical trial planning in new drug development. *Computers and Chemical Engineering*, 32(11):2626–2642.

Combi, C., Y. Shahar, and A. Abu-Hanna. 2009. Genetic algorithm based scheduling of radiotherapy treatments for cancer patients. In: V. Barichard, M. Ehrgott, X. Gandibleux, and V. T'Kindt, eds., *Artificial Intelligence in Medicine*, Vol. 5651, pp. 101–105. Springer, Berlin, Germany.

Cotrutz, C. and L. Xing. 2003. Segment-based dose optimization using a genetic algorithm. *Physics in Medicine and Biology*, 48:2987–2998.

Deb, K. 2001. *Multi-Objective Optimization using Evolutionary Algorithms*. Wiley, Hoboken, NJ.

Denton, B., J. Viapiano, and A. Vogl. 2007. Optimization of surgery sequencing and scheduling decisions under uncertainty. *Health Care Management Science*, 10(1):13–24.

Doerner, K., A. Focke, and W.J. Gutjahr. 2007. Multicriteria tour planning for mobile healthcare facilities in a developing country. *European Journal of Operational Research*, 179(3):1078–1096.

Ehrgott, M. 2005. *Multicriteria Optimization*, 2nd edn. Springer, Berlin, Germany.

Ehrgott, M., D. Baatar, H.W. Hamacher, and G.J. Woeginer. 2004. Decomposition of integer matrices and multileaf collimator sequencing. Technical report, Fachbereich Mathematik Technische Universitat, Kaiserslautern, Germany.

Engel, K. 2005. A new algorithm for optimal multileaf collimator field segmentation. *Discrete Applied Mathematics*, 152:35–51.

Ferris, M.C., J. Lim, and D. Shepard. 2003a. An optimization approach for the radiosurgery treatment planning. *SIAM Journal on Optimization*, 13(3):921–937.

Ferris, M.C., J. Lim, and D. Shepard. 2003b. Radiosurgery optimization via nonlinear programming. *Annals of Operations Research*, 119:247–260.

Ferris, M.C., R.R. Meyer, and W.D. D'Souza. 2002. Radiation treatment planning: Mixed integer programming formulations and approaches. Optimization Technical Report 02–08, University of Wisconsin, Madison, WI.

Floudas, C.A. 1995. *Nonlinear and Mixed-Integer Optimization: Fundamentals and Applications*. Oxford University Press, New York.

Gilleskie, D.B. 1998. A dynamic stochastic model of medical care use and work absence. *Econometrica*, 66(1):1–45.

Griffin, P.M., C.R. Scherrer, and J.L. Swann. 2008. Optimization of community health center locations and service offerings with statistical need estimation. *IIE Transactions*, 40(9):880–892.

Halabi, T., D. Craft, and T. Bortfeld. 2006. Dose–volume objectives in multi-criteria optimization. *Physics in Medicine and Biology*, 51:3809–3818.

Hamacher, H.W. and K.H. Kfer. 2002. Inverse radiation therapy planning: A multiple objective optimization approach. *Discrete Applied Mathematics*, 118:145–161.

Hamacher, H.W. and F. Lenzen. 2000. *The Use of Computers in Radiation Therapy*. Springer-Verlag, Berlin, Germany.

Hillier, F.S. and G.J. Lieberman. 2002. *Introduction to Operations Research*, 7th edn. McGraw-Hill Science/Engineering/Math, New York.

Holder, A. 2004. Radiotherapy treatment design and linear programming. In: M. Brandeau, F. Sainfort, and W. Pierskalla, eds., *Operations Research and Health Care: A Handbook of Methods and Applications*, Chap. 29. Kluwer Academic Publishers, Norwell, MA.

Hutzschenreuter, A.K., P.A.N. Bosman, and Han La Poutre. 2009. Evolutionary multiobjective optimization for dynamic hospital resource management. In: M. Ehrgott, C.M. Fonseca, X. Gandibleux, J. Hao, and M. Sevaux, eds., *Evolutionary Multi-Criterion Optimization*, vol. 5467, pp. 320–334. Springer, Berlin, Germany.

Jia, H., F. Ordonez, and M.M. Dessouky. 2007. Solution approaches for facility location of medical supplies for large-scale emergencies. *Computers and Industrial Engineering*, 52(2):257–276.

Kirkpatrick, S., C.D. Gellatt, and M.P. Vecci. 1983. Optimization by simulated annealing. *Science*, 220:671–680.

Lahanas, M., D. Baltas, and N. Zamboglou. 1999. Anatomy-based three-dimensional dose optimization in brachytherapy using multiobjective genetic algorithms. *Medical Physics*, 26(9):1904–1918.

Langer, M. and J. Leong. 1987. Optimization of beam weights under dose-volume restriction. *International Journal of Radiation Oncology Biology Physics*, 13:1255–1260.

Lee, E.K. 2007. Large-scale optimization-based classification models in medicine and biology. *Annals of Biomedical Engineering*, 35(6):1095–1109.

Lee, E.K., T. Fox, and I. Crocker. 2000. Optimization of radiosurgery treatment planning via mixed integer programming. *Medical Physics*, 27(5):995–1004.

Lee, E.K., T. Fox, and I. Crocker. 2003. Integer programming applied to intensity-modulated radiation treatment planning optimization. *Annals of Operations Research*, 119:165–181.

Lee, E.K., T. Fox, and I. Crocker. 2006. Simultaneous beam geometry and intensity map optimization in intensity-modulated radiation therapy. *International Journal of Radiation Oncology, Biology and Physics*, 64(1):301–320.

Legras, J., B. Legras, and J.P. Lambert. 1982. Software for linear and non-linear optimization in external radiotherapy. *Computer Programs in Biomedicine*, 15(3):233–242.

Legras, J., B. Legras, J.P. Lambert, and P. Aletti. 1986. The use of a microcomputer for non-linear optimisation of doses in external radiotherapy. *Physics in Medicine and Biology*, 31(12):1353–1359.

Li, X., P. Beullens, D. Jones, and M. Tamiz. 2009a. An integrated queuing and multi-objective bed allocation model with application to a hospital in China. *The Journal of the Operational Research Society*, 60(3):330–338.

Li, X., P. Beullens, D. Jones, and M. Tamiz. 2009b. Optimal bed allocation in hospitals. In: V. Barichard, M. Ehrgott, X. Gandibleux, and V. T'Kindt, eds., *Multiobjective Programming and Goal Programming*, Vol. 618, pp. 253–265. Springer, Berlin, Germany.

Li, Y., J. Yao, and D. Yao. 2004. Automatic beam angle selection in IMRT planning using genetic algorithm. *Physics in Medicine and Biology*, 49:1915–1932.

Lim, G.J., J. Choi, and R. Mohan. 2008. Iterative solution methods for beam angle and fluence map optimization in intensity modulated radiation therapy planning. *OR Spectrum*, 30(2):289–309.

Lim, J., M.C. Ferris, and D.M. Shepard. 2004. Optimization tools for radiation treatment planning in MATLAB®. In: M.L. Brandeau, F. Saintfort, and W.P. Pierskalla, eds., *Operations Research And Health Care: A Handbook of Methods and Applications*, pp. 775–806. Kluwer Academic Publishers, Boston, MA.

Lim, G.J., M.C. Ferris, S.J. Wright, D.M. Shepard, and M.A. Earl. 2007. An optimization framework for conformal radiation treatment planning. *INFORMS Journal on Computing*, 19(3):366–380.

Linderoth, J. and M.W.P. Savelsbergh. 1999. Search strategies for mixed integer programming. *INFORMS Journal on Computing*, 11:173–187.

Lof, J., B.K. Lind, and A. Brahme. 1998. An adaptive control algorithm for optimization of intensity modulated radiotherapy considering uncertainties in beam profiles, patient set-up and internal organ motion. *Physics in Medicine and Biology*, 43:1605–1628.

Luenberger, D.G. and Y. Ye. 2008. *Linear and Nonlinear Programming*, 3rd edn. Springer, New York.

Mangasarian, O.L. 1994. *Nonlinear Programming*. SIAM, New York.

Marler, R.T. and J.S. Arora. 2004. Survey of multi-objective optimization methods for engineering. *Structural and Multidisciplinary Optimization*, 26(6):369–395.

Martel, A. and J. Ouellet. 1994. Stochastic allocation of a resource among partially interchangeable activities. *European Journal of Operational Research*, 74(3):528–539.

Meyer, R.R., W.D. D'Souza, M.C. Ferris, and B.R. Thomadsen. 2003. MIP models and BB strategies in brachytherapy treatment optimization. *Journal of Global Optimization*, 25(1):23–42.

Morrill, S.M., R.G. Lane, G. Jacobson, and I.I. Rosen. 1991b. Treatment planning optimization using constrained simulated annealing. *Physics in Medicine and Biology*, 36(10):1341–1361.

Morrill, S., R. Lane, J. Wong, and I.I. Rosen. 1991a. Dose–volume considerations with linear programming. *Medical Physics*, 6(18):1201–1210.

Murty, K.G. 1983. *Linear Programming*. John Wiley & Sons, New York.

Nemhauser, G.L. and L.A. Wolsey. 1988. *Integer and Combinatorial Optimization*. Wiley, New York.

Oddoye, J.P., M.A. Yaghoobi, M. Tamiz, D.F. Jones, and P. Schmidt. 2007. A multi-objective model to determine efficient resource levels in a medical assessment unit. *Journal of the Operational Research Society*, 58:1563–1573.

Olafsson, A., R. Jeraj, and S.J. Wright. 2005. Optimization of intensity-modulated radiation therapy with biological objectives. *Physics in Medicine and Biology*, 50:5357–5379.

Paul, J.A. and R. Batta. 2008. Models for hospital location and capacity allocation for an area prone to natural disasters. *International Journal of Operational Research*, 3(5):473–496.

Pierskalla, W.P. and D.B. Brailer. 1994. Applications of operations research in health care delivery. In: S.M. Pollock, M.H. Rothkopf, and A. Barnett, eds., *Handbooks in Operations Research and Management Science*, vol. 6, Chap. 13. Elsevier Science, Amsterdam, the Netherlands.

Preciado-Walters, F., R. Rardin, M. Langer, and V. Thai. 2004. A coupled column generation, mixed-integer approach to optimal planning of intensity modulated radiation therapy for cancer. *Mathematical Programming*, 101:319–338.

Punnakitikashem, P., J.M. Rosenberger, and D.B. Behan. 2008. Stochastic programming for nurse assignment. *Computational Optimization and Applications*, 40(3):321–349.

Redpath, A.T., B.L. Vickery, and D.H. Wright. 1976. A new technique for radiotherapy planning using quadratic programming. *Physics in Medicine and Biology*, 21:781–791.

Rosen, I.I., R. Lane, S. Morrill, and J. Belli. 1990. Treatment plan optimization using linear programming. *Medical Physics*, 18(2):141–152.

Ruszczynski, A. 2006. *Nonlinear Optimization*. Princeton University Press, Princeton, NJ.

Ruszczynski, A. and A. Shapiro. 2003. Stochastic programming. In: *Handbooks in Operations Research and Management Science*, vol. 10. Elsevier, Amsterdam, the Netherlands.

Ryu, Y.U., R. Chandrasekaran, and V.S. Jacob. 2007. Breast cancer prediction using the isotonic separation technique. *European Journal of Operational Research*, 181:842–854.

Sakawa, M. 2002. *Genetic Algorithms and Fuzzy Multiobjective Optimization*. Springer, Norwell, MA.

Shepard, D.M., L. Chin, S. DiBiase, S. Naqvi, J. Lim, and M.C. Ferris. 2003. Clinical implementation of an automated planning system for gamma knife radiosurgery. *International Journal of Radiation Oncology*, 56(5):1488–1494.

Shepard, D.M., M.C. Ferris, G. Olivera, and T.R. Mackie. 1999. Optimizing the delivery of radiation to cancer patients. *SIAM Review*, 41:721–744.

Shih, L. and Y. Lin. 2003. Multicriteria optimization for infectious medical waste collection system planning. *Practice Periodical of Hazardous, Toxic, and Radioactive Waste Management*, 7(2):78–85.

Shu, H.Z., Y.L. Yan, X.D. Bao, Y. Fu, and L.M. Luo. 1998. Treatment planning optimization by quasi-Newton and simulated annealing methods for gamma unit treatment system. *Physics in Medicine and Biology*, 43:2795–2805.

Sir, M.Y., M.A. Epelman, and S.M. Pollock. 2008. Stochastic programming for off-line adaptive radiotherapy. Submitted for publication. Available online at http://www-personal.umich.edu/~mepelman/research/StochProg.pdf (accessed July 13, 2009).

Smith, J.C. and Z.C. Taskin. 2008. A tutorial guide to mixed-integer programming models and solution techniques. In: G.J. Lim and E.K. Lee, eds., *Optimization in Medicine and Biology*, chapter Appendix A, pp. 521–547. Auerbach Publications, Taylor & Francis Group, Boca Raton, FL.

Spirou, S.V. and C.S. Chui. 1998. A gradient inverse planning algorithm with dose-volume constraints. *Medical Physics*, 25(3):321–333.

Starkschall, G. 1984. A constrained least-squares optimization method for external beam radiation therapy treatment planning. *Medical Physics*, 11:659–665.

Stummer, C., K. Doerner, A. Focke, and K. Heidenberger. 2004. Determining location and size of medical departments in a hospital network: A multiobjective decision support approach. *Health Care Management Science*, 7(1):63–71.

Taha, H.A. 2007. *Operations Research: An Introduction*, 8th edn. Prentice Hall, Upper Saddle River, NJ.

Thongphiew, D., V. Chankong, F. Yin, and Q.J. Wu. 2008. An online adaptive radiation therapy system for intensity modulated radiation therapy: An application of multi-objective optimization. *International Journal of Radiation Oncology Biology Physics*, 4(3):453–475.

Topaloglu, S. 2006. A multi-objective programming model for scheduling emergency medicine residents. *Computers and Industrial Engineering*, 51:375–388.

Unkelbach, J. and U. Oelfke. 2004. Inclusion of organ movements in IMRT treatment planning via inverse planning based on probability distributions. *Physics in Medicine and Biology*, 49:4005–4029.

Van Laarhoven, P.J.M. and E.H.L. Aarts. 1989. *Simulated Annealing: Theory and Applications*. Kluwer Academic Publishers, Boston, MA.

Vanderbei, R.J. 2008. *Linear Programming: Foundations and Extensions*, 3rd edn. Springer, New York.

Vermeulen, I., S. Bohte, K. Somefun, and H.L. Poutre. 2007. Multi-agent Pareto appointment exchanging in hospital patient scheduling. *Service Oriented Computing and Applications*, 1(3):1863–2386.

Vermeulen, I., S. Bohte, S. Elkhuizen, P. Bakker, and H.L. Poutre. 2008. Decentralized online scheduling of combination-appointments in hospitals. In: *Proceedings of the International Conference on Automated Planning and Scheduling* (ICAPS-2008), Sydney, Australia.

Webb, S. 1989. Optimization of conformal radiotherapy dose distributions by simulated annealing. *Physics in Medicine and Biology*, 34:1349–1369.

Webb, S. 1991. Optimization by simulated annealing of three-dimensional, conformal treatment planning for radiation fields defined by a multileaf collimator. *Physics in Medicine and Biology*, 36(9):1201–1226.

Webb, S. 1992. Optimization by simulated annealing of three-dimensional, conformal treatment planning for radiation fields defined by a multileaf collimator: II. Inclusion of the two-dimensional modulation of the X-ray intensity. *Physics in Medicine and Biology*, 37(8):1689–1704.

Wolsey, L.A. 1998. *Integer Programming*. John Wiley & Sons, New York.

Yan, D., D. Lockman, D. Brabbins, L. Tyburski, and A. Martinez. 2000. An off-line strategy for constructing a patient-specific planning target volume in adaptive treatment process for prostate cancer. *International Journal of Radiation Oncology Biology Physics*, 48:289–302.

Yu, Y., M.C. Schell, J. Dai, and J.B. Zhang. 1997. Decision theoretic steering and genetic algorithm optimization: Application to stereotactic radiosurgery planning. *Medical Physics*, 24:1742–1750.

World Health Organization. 2009. World health statistics 2009. Available online at http://www.who.int/whosis/whostat/EN_WHS09_Full.pdf (accessed August 14, 2009).

16

Queueing Theory and Modeling*

Introduction 16-1
Why Are Queue Models Helpful in Healthcare? • Queueing Fundamentals
Basic Queueing Principles and Models 16-3
Delays, Utilization, and System Size • Some Simple But Useful Queueing Models
Analyses of Fixed Capacity: How Many Hospital Beds? 16-8
Applying the *M/M/s* Model • The Problem with Using Target Occupancy Levels • Choosing a Delay Standard • Planning for Predictable Changes in Demand • Using Queueing Models to Quantify the Benefits of Flexibility
Analyses of Flexible Capacity: Determining Staffing Levels to Meet Time-Varying Demands 16-14
Data Collection and Model Choices • Constructing the Queueing Models • Choosing a Delay Standard and Applying the Queueing Results • Using Queueing Models to Improve Healthcare Delivery: Opportunities and Challenges
References 16-17

Linda V. Green
Columbia University

Introduction

Why Are Queueing Models Helpful in Healthcare?

Healthcare is riddled with delays. Almost all of us have waited for days or weeks to get an appointment with a physician or schedule a procedure, and upon arrival we wait some more until being seen. In hospitals, it is not unusual to find patients waiting for beds in hallways, and delays for surgery or diagnostic tests are common.

Delays are the result of a disparity between demand for a service and the capacity available to meet that demand. Usually, this mismatch is temporary and due to natural variability in the timing of demands and in the duration of time needed to provide service. A simple example would be a healthcare clinic where patients walk in without appointments in an unpredictable fashion and require anything from a flu shot to the setting of a broken limb. This variability and the interaction between the arrival and service processes make the dynamics of service systems very complex. Consequently, it is impossible to predict levels of congestion or to determine how much capacity is needed to achieve some desired level of performance without the help of a queueing model.

Queueing theory was developed by A.K. Erlang in 1904 to help determine the capacity requirements of the Danish telephone system (Brockmeyer et al. 1948). It has since been applied to a large range of service

* From Green, L.V., Queuing analysis in healthcare, in Randolph, W.H. (ed.), *Patient Flow: Reducing Delay in Healthcare Delivery—Handbook of Healthcare Delivery Systems*, Springer Science+Business Media, LLC, Berlin, Germany, 2006, pp. 281–307. With kind permission from Springer Science+Business Media, LLC.

industries including banks, airlines, and telephone call centers (Stern and Hersh 1980, Holloran and Byrne 1986, Brewton 1989, Brigandi et al. 1994, Brusco et al. 1995) as well as emergency systems such as police patrol, fire, and ambulances (Larson 1972, Kolesar et al. 1975, Chelst and Barlach 1981, Green and Kolesar 1984, Taylor and Huxley 1989). It has also been applied in various healthcare settings as we discuss later in this chapter. Queueing models can be very useful in identifying appropriate levels of staff, equipment, and beds as well as in making decisions about resource allocation and the design of new services.

Unlike simulation methodologies, queueing models require very little data and result in relatively simple formulae for predicting various performance measures such as mean delay or probability of waiting more than a given amount of time before being served. This means that they are easier and cheaper to develop and use. In addition, since they are extremely fast to run, they provide a simple way to perform "what-if" analyses, identify trade-offs and find attractive solutions rather than just estimating performance for a given scenario.

Timely access has been identified as one of the key elements of healthcare quality (Institute of Medicine, Committee on Quality of Healthcare in America 2001) and consequently, decreasing delays has become a focus in many healthcare institutions. Given the financial constraints that exist in many of these organizations, queueing analysis can be an extremely valuable tool in utilizing resources in the most cost-effective way to reduce delays. The primary goal of this chapter is to provide a basic understanding of queueing theory and some of the specific queueing models that can be helpful in designing and managing healthcare delivery systems. For more detail on specific models that are commonly used, a textbook on queueing theory such as Hall (1990) is recommended.

Before discussing past and potential uses of queueing models in healthcare, it is important to first understand some queueing theory fundamentals.

Queueing Fundamentals

A basic queueing system is a service system where "customers" arrive to a bank of "servers" and require some service from one of them. It is important to understand that a "customer" is whatever entity that is waiting for service and does not have to be a person. For example, in a "back-office" situation such as the reading of radiologic images, the "customers" might be the images waiting to be read. Similarly, a "server" is the person or thing that provides the service. So, when analyzing delays for patients in the emergency department (ED) awaiting admission to the hospital, the relevant servers would be inpatient beds.

If all servers are busy upon a customer's arrival, they must join a queue. Though queues are often physical lines of people or things, they can also be invisible as with telephone calls waiting on hold. The rule that determines the order in which queued customers are served is called the queue *discipline*. The most common discipline is the familiar first-come, first-served (FCFS) rule, but other disciplines are often used to increase efficiency or reduce the delay for more time-sensitive customers. For example, in an ED, the triage system is an example of a *priority* queue discipline. Priority disciplines may be preemptive or non-preemptive, depending upon whether a service in progress can be interrupted when a customer with a higher priority arrives. In most queueing models, the assumption is made that there is no limit on the number of customers that can be waiting for service, that is, there is an *infinite waiting room*. This may be a good assumption when customers do not physically join a queue, as in a telephone call center, or when the physical space where customers wait is large compared to the number of customers who are usually waiting for service. Even if there is no capacity limit on waiting room, in some cases, new arrivals who see a long queue may "balk" and not join the queue. This might happen in a walk-in clinic. A similar behavior that is incorporated in some queueing systems is "reneging" or "abandonment," which occurs when customers grow inpatient and leave the queue before being served. An example of this behavior is found in some EDs where the patients who renege are often referred to as "left without being seen."

Finally, queues may be organized in various ways. In most cases, we will consider a *single line* that feeds into all servers. But sometimes each server has his/her own queue as may be the case for a primary care office in which patients have their own physician. This design is usually referred to as queues in *parallel*. In other situations, we may want to consider a *network* design in which customers receive service from different types of servers in a sequential manner. For example, a surgical inpatient requires an operating room (OR), then a bed in the recovery unit, followed by a bed in a surgical intensive care unit (ICU), and/or other part of the hospital. However, it might still make sense to analyze one specific single queue in these situations to determine the capacity requirements of a single type of resource, particularly if there is reason to believe that the resource is a bottleneck.

A queueing model is a mathematical description of a queueing system which makes some specific assumptions about the probabilistic nature of the arrival and service processes, the number and type of servers, and the queue discipline and organization. There are countless possible variations, but some queueing models are more widely used and we focus on these in this chapter. For these models, as well as many others, there are formulae available that enable the fast calculation of various performance measures that can be used to help design a new service system or improve an existing one.

Basic Queueing Principles and Models

Most of queueing theory deals with system performance in *steady state*. That is, most queueing models assume that the system has been operating with the same arrival rate, average service time, and other characteristics for a sufficiently long time that the probabilistic behavior of performance measures such as queue length and customer delay is independent of when the system is observed. Clearly, there are many service systems, including healthcare systems, for which there are time-of-day, day-of-week, or seasonality affects. In this section, we assume that we are looking at systems in steady state and in subsequent sections, we discuss how to deal with systems that have some time-varying characteristics.

Delays, Utilization, and System Size

In queueing theory, utilization, defined as the average number of busy servers divided by the total number of servers times 100, is an important measure. From a managerial perspective, utilization is often seen as a measure of productivity and therefore it is considered desirable for it to be high. For example, in hospital bed planning, utilization is called occupancy level and historically, an average hospital occupancy level of 85% has been used as the minimum level for the states to make a determination under Certificate of Need (CON) regulations that more beds might be needed (see Brecher and Speizio 1995). Since the actual average occupancy level for nonprofit hospitals has recently been under 70%, there has been a widely held perception in the healthcare community that there are too many hospital beds. Largely because of this perception, the number of hospital beds has decreased almost 25% in the last 20 years.

But determining bed capacity based on occupancy levels can result in very long waiting times for beds (Green 2003). In all queueing systems, the higher the average utilization level, the longer the wait times. However, it is important to note that this relationship is nonlinear. This is illustrated in Figure 16.1, which shows the fundamental relationship between delays and utilization for a queueing system. There are three critical observations we can make from this figure. First, as average utilization (e.g., occupancy level) increases, average delays increase at an increasing rate. Second, there is an "elbow" in the curve after which the average delay increases more dramatically in response to even small increases in utilization. Finally, the average delay approaches infinity as utilization approaches 1. (It is important to note that this is assuming that there is no constraint on how long the queue can get and that customers continue to join and remain in the queue.)

The exact location of the elbow in the curve depends upon two critical characteristics of the system: variability and size. Variability generally exists in both the time between arrivals and the duration of service times and is usually measured by the ratio of the standard deviation to the mean, called the coefficient of variation (CV). The higher the degree of variability in the system, the more to the left the elbow will be so that delays will be worse for the same utilization level. System size is defined as the ratio

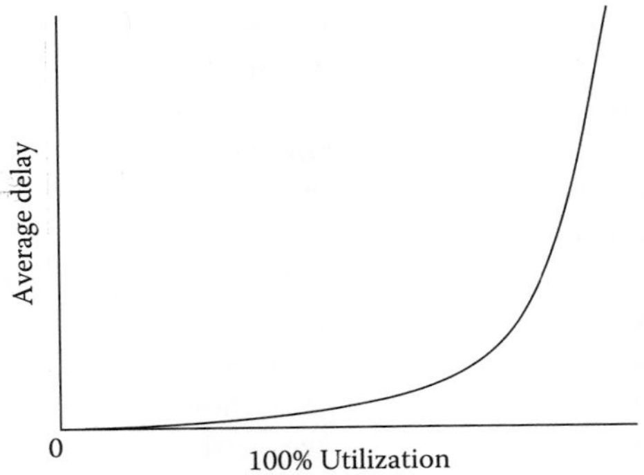

FIGURE 16.1 Trade-off between average delay and utilization in a queueing system. (From Green, L.V., Queuing analysis in healthcare, in Randolph, W.H. (ed.), *Patient Flow: Reducing Delay in Healthcare Delivery—Handbook of Healthcare Delivery Systems*, Springer Science+Business Media, LLC, Berlin, Germany, 2006, pp. 281–307. With kind permission from Springer Science+Business Media, LLC.)

of the average demand over the average service time, which is a determinant of the number of servers needed. The larger the system, the closer the elbow will be to 100%, so that delays will be shorter for the same utilization level.

These basic queueing principles have several important implications for planning or evaluating capacity in a service system. First, the average total capacity, defined as the number of servers times the rate at which each server can serve customers, must be strictly greater than the average demand. In other words, unless average utilization is strictly *less than* 100%, the system will be "unstable" and the queue will continue to grow. Though this fact may appear counterintuitive on the surface, it has been well known by operations professionals for decades. So if an emergency room has 10 patients arriving per hour on average and each healthcare provider (physician or physician assistant) can treat 2 patients per hour on average, a minimum of 6 providers is needed. (Of course, in many contexts, if arrivals see a long queue, they may not join it or they may renege after waiting a long time. If so, it may be possible to have stability even if the average demand exceeds the average capacity.) Second, the smaller the system, the longer the delays will be for a given utilization level. In other words, queueing systems have economies of scale so that, for example, larger hospitals can operate at higher utilization levels than smaller ones yet maintain similar levels of congestion and delays. Finally, the greater the variability in the service time (e.g., length-of-stay), the longer the delays at any given utilization level. So a clinic or physician office that specializes in, for example, vision testing or mammography will experience shorter patient waits than a university-based clinic of the same size and with the same provider utilization that treats a broad variety of illnesses and injuries. These properties will be more specifically illustrated when we discuss applications of queueing models.

Some Simple But Useful Queueing Models

Poisson Process

In specifying a queueing model, we must make assumptions about the probabilistic nature of the arrival and service processes. The most common assumption to make about arrivals is that they follow a *Poisson* process. The name comes from the fact that the number of arrivals in any given time period has a Poisson distribution. So if $N(t)$ is the number of arrivals during a time period of duration t then $N(t)$ has a Poisson distribution

$$\text{Probability}\{N(t)=n\}=\frac{e^{-\lambda t}(\lambda t)^n}{n!}$$

where λ is called the *rate* and is the expected number of arrivals per unit time. For example, if $\lambda = 10$ customers per hour, then the expected number of arrivals in any 60-minute interval is 10 and the expected number to arrive in a 15-minute interval is 2.5. Notice that these are averages so that λ need not have an integer value. Another way to characterize the Poisson process is that the time between consecutive arrivals, called the interarrival time, has an *exponential* distribution. So if *IA* is the interarrival time of a Poisson process with rate λ,

$$\text{Probability}\ \{IA \le t\} = 1 - e^{-\lambda t}$$

and $1/\lambda$ is the average time between arrivals.

An important property of the exponential distribution is that it is "memoryless." This means that the time of the next arrival is independent of when the last arrival occurred. This property also leads to the fact that if the arrival process is Poisson, the number of arrivals in any given time interval is independent of the number in any other nonoverlapping time interval. Conversely, it can be shown analytically that if customers arrive independently from one another, the arrival process is a Poisson process. For this reason, the Poisson process is considered the most "random" arrival process.

In determining whether the Poisson process is a reasonable model for arrivals in a specific service system, it is useful to consider its three defining properties:

1. Customers arrive one at a time.
2. The probability that a customer arrives at any time is independent of when other customers arrived.
3. The probability that a customer arrives at a given time is independent of the time.

In most contexts, customers generally do arrive one at a time. Though there may be events, such as a major accident, that trigger multiple simultaneous arrivals, this is likely to be an exceptional circumstance which will not significantly affect the effectiveness of this modeling assumption. Intuitively, the second property is also often a reasonable assumption. For example, in an emergency room, where the population of potential patients is very large, it is unlikely that someone arriving with a broken arm has anything to do with someone else's injury or illness, or that the fact that the number of patients who arrived between 9 a.m. and 10 a.m. was four provides any information about the number of patients that are likely to arrive between 10 a.m. and 11 a.m. Again, there may be occasional exceptions, such as a flu outbreak, which violate this assumption, but in the aggregate, it is likely to be reasonable. However, the third property may be more suspect. More typically, the average arrival rate varies over the day so that, for example, it is more likely for an arrival to occur in the morning than in the middle of the night. Certain days of the week may be busier than others as well. However, we may be able to use the standard Poisson process as a good model for a shorter interval of time over which the arrival rate is fairly constant. We discuss this in more detail in a subsequent section.

So the assumption of a Poisson process will generally be a good one when the three properties above are a reasonable description of the service system in question. However, it is possible to perform more rigorous tests to determine if it is a good fit. The simplest tests are based on the relationship of the standard deviation to the mean of the two distributions involved in the Poisson process. Since the variance (square of the standard deviation) of the Poisson distribution is equal to its mean, we can examine the number of arrivals in each fixed interval of time (e.g., 30 minutes) and determine whether the ratio of the mean to the variance is close to 1. Alternatively, since the exponential distribution is characterized by its standard deviation being equal to its mean, we can look at the interarrival times and compute the ratio of the standard deviation to the mean to see if it is close to 1. Hall (1990) describes goodness of fit tests in greater detail.

Many real arrival and demand processes have been empirically shown to be very well approximated by a Poisson process. Among these are demands for emergency services such as police, fire, and ambulance, arrivals to banks and other retail establishments, and arrivals of telephone calls to customer service call centers. Because of its prevalence and its assumption of independent arrivals, the Poisson process is the most commonly used arrival process in modeling service systems. It is also a convenient assumption to make in terms of data collection since it is characterized by a single parameter—its rate λ. In healthcare, the Poisson process has been verified to be a good representation of unscheduled arrivals to various parts of the hospital including ICUs, obstetrics units, and EDs (Young 1965, Kim et al. 1999, Green et al. 2005).

M/M/s Model

The most commonly used queueing model is the *M/M/s* or *Erlang delay* model. This model assumes a single queue with unlimited waiting room that feeds into *s* identical servers. Customers arrive according to a Poisson process with a constant rate, and the service duration (e.g., LOS or provider time associated with a patient) has an exponential distribution. (These two assumptions are often called Markovian, hence the use of the two "M's" in the notation used for the model.)

One advantage of using the *M/M/s* model is that it requires only three parameters, and so it can be used to obtain performance estimates with very little data. Given an average arrival rate, λ, an average service duration, $1/\mu$, and the number of servers, *s*, easy-to-compute formulae are available to obtain performance measures such as the probability that an arrival will experience a positive delay, p_D, or the average delay, W_q:

$$p_D = 1 - \sum_{n=0}^{s-1} p_n \tag{16.1}$$

$$W_q = \frac{p_D}{\left[(1-\rho)s\mu\right]} \tag{16.2}$$

for

$$\rho = \frac{\lambda}{s\mu} \tag{16.3}$$

and

$$p_n = \begin{cases} \dfrac{\lambda^n}{n!\mu^n} p_0 & (1 \le n \le s) \\ \dfrac{\lambda^n}{s^{n-s}s!\mu^n} p_0 & (n \ge s) \end{cases} \tag{16.4}$$

where

$$p_0 = \left[\sum_{n=0}^{s-1} \frac{(\rho s)^n}{n!} + \frac{\rho^s s^{s+1}}{s!(s-\rho s)}\right]^{-1} \quad \rho < 1 \tag{16.5}$$

Note that ρ is the average utilization for this queueing system and the equation is only valid when the utilization is strictly less than 1. Also note that average delay increases as utilization approaches 1. These quantitative observations support the discussion of utilization and delays in the previous section.

Many other measures of performance can be calculated as well and many of the formulae for both the *M/M/s* and other common queueing models are available in software packages or are easily programmable on spreadsheets. One common performance constraint is often referred to as the *service level*—a requirement that x% of customers start service within y time units. For example, many customer call centers have a target service level that 85% of calls be answered within 20 seconds. The delay is always measured from the time of the demand for service (e.g., patient registered in the ED) to the time at which service begins (e.g., a provider is available to treat that patient). It is important to note that the model's delay predictions pertain only to waiting times due to the unavailability of the server.

Some Useful Extensions of the M/M/s Model

There are several variations on the basic *M/M/s* queueing model. One such important variation for many healthcare organizations is the *M/M/s* with priorities (Cobham 1954). While the fundamental model assumes that customers are indistinguishable and are served FCFS, the priority model assumes that customers have differing time sensitivities and are allocated to two or more service classes $i = 1,2,\ldots N$, and that customers are served in priority order with 1 being the highest priority and N the lowest. Within any given class, customers are served FCFS. But when there is a queue and a server becomes available, a customer belonging to class $i > 1$ will be served only if there are no waiting customers of class 1, …, $i - 1$. A priority queueing model would be appropriate if a facility is interested in identifying the capacity needed to assure a targeted service level for the highest priority customers. For example, in an ED, while many arriving patients would not incur any particular harm if they had to wait more than an hour to be seen by a physician, some fraction, who are emergent or urgent, need a physician's care sooner to prevent serious clinical consequences. In this case, a priority queueing model could be used to answer a question like, "How many physicians are needed to assure that 90% of emergent and urgent patients will be seen by a physician within 45 minutes?"

There are two types of priority queueing disciplines: preemptive and non-preemptive. In the preemptive model, if a higher priority customer arrives when all servers are busy and a lower priority customer is being served, the lower priority customer's service will be interrupted (preempted) so that the higher priority customer can begin service immediately. The preempted customer must then wait for another server to become free to resume service. In the non-preemptive model, new arrivals cannot preempt customers already in service. While priority queueing models are usually either purely preemptive or non-preemptive, it is possible to model a service system that has both preemptive and non-preemptive customer classes. This might be appropriate for a hospital ED where the normal triage system which classifies patients as emergent, urgent, or nonurgent is generally assumed to be non-preemptive, but a preemptive discipline is used for certain urgent patients whose conditions are extremely time-sensitive, such as stroke victims. In addition to the usual input parameters for the *M/M/s* model, priority models also require data on the fraction of customers in each of the priority classes.

Another common variant of the *M/M/s* model assumes a finite capacity $K \geq s$ and is notated as *M/M/s/K*. In this model, if a customer arrives when there are K customers already in the system (being served and waiting), the customer cannot join the queue and must leave. A common application of this would be a telephone trunk line feeding into a call center. Such a system has a finite number of spaces for calls being served or on hold and when a new call comes in and all the spaces are already filled, the new arrival hears a busy signal and hangs up. A similar phenomenon might occur in a walk-in health clinic, which has a waiting room with a fixed number of seats. Though some patients may choose to wait even if there is no seat available upon arrival, many patients may leave and try to return at a less busy time. Customers who are "blocked" from joining the queue are called "lost" and may show up again or never return. In these types of systems, queueing analysis might be used to help determine how large the waiting or holding area should be so that the number of customers who are blocked is kept to an acceptably low level.

A specific special case of these finite capacity models is the one where $K = s$ so that there is no waiting room for those who arrive when all servers are busy. These are called pure "loss" models and they are often used to analyze service systems in which it is considered either impractical or very undesirable to have any customers wait to begin service. For example, Shmueli et al. (2003) used a loss model to analyze the impact of various admissions policies to hospital intensive care units.

M/G/1 and *G/G/s* Models

An important characteristic of the exponential distribution used in the *M/M/s* is that the standard distribution equals the mean and so the CV of the service time equals 1. If the actual CV of service is a bit less than or greater than 1, the *M/M/s* will still give good estimates of delay. However, if the CV is substantially different than 1, the *M/M/s* may significantly underestimate or overestimate actual delays. (Recall that if variability is lower, the model will overestimate delays while the converse is true if variability is greater.) In this case, if the arrival process is Poisson, and there is only one server, the average delay can still be calculated for any service distribution through use of the following formula for what is known as the *M/G/1* system:

$$W_q = \left[\frac{\lambda\rho}{1-\rho}\right]\left[\frac{1+CV^2(S)}{2}\right] \tag{16.6}$$

where $CV^2(S)$ is the square of the coefficient of variation of the service time. Clearly, this formula requires knowledge of the standard deviation of the service time in addition to the mean in order to compute $CV^2(S)$. This formula also illustrates the impact of variability on delays. Notice that, as mentioned previously, as the coefficient of variation of the service time increases, so does the average delay.

Though there are no exact formula for non-Markovian multi-server queues, there are some good, simple approximations. One such approximation (Allen 1978) is given by

$$W_q = W_{q,M/M/s}\frac{\left[CV^2(A)+CV^2(S)\right]}{2} \tag{16.7}$$

where

$CV^2(A)$ is the square of the coefficient of variation of the arrival time
$W_{q,M/M/s}$ is the expected delay for an *M/M/s* system (Equation 16.2)

So this formula requires the standard deviation of the interarrival time as well and again demonstrates that more variability results in longer delays.

Analyses of Fixed Capacity: How Many Hospital Beds?

Many resources in healthcare facilities have a fixed capacity over a long period of time. These are usually "things" rather than people: beds, operating rooms, imaging machines, etc. Queueing models are not always appropriate for analyzing such resources. In particular, if the patients for a resource are scheduled into fixed time slots, there is little or no likelihood of congestion unless patients routinely come late or the time slots are not large enough to accommodate most patients. An example of this would be a magnetic resonance imaging (MRI) facility, which is only used by scheduled outpatients.

However, the difficulty of managing many healthcare facilities is that the demand for resources is unscheduled and hence random, yet timely care is important. This is the case for many parts of a hospital that deal primarily with nonelective admissions. In these cases, queueing models can be very helpful in identifying long-term capacity needs.

Applying the *M/M/s* Model

To illustrate the use of a queueing model for evaluating capacity, consider an obstetrics unit. Since it is generally operated independently of other services, its capacity needs, for example, number of postpartum beds can be determined without regard to other parts of the hospital. It is also one for which the use of a standard *M/M/s* queueing model is quite good. Most obstetrics patients are unscheduled and the assumption of Poisson arrivals has been shown to be a good one in studies of unscheduled hospital admissions (Young 1965). In addition, the *CV* of length of stay is typically very close to 1.0 (Green and Nguyen 2001) satisfying the service time assumption of the *M/M/s* model.

A queueing model may be used either descriptively or prescriptively. As an example of the descriptive case, we can take the current operating characteristics of a given obstetrics unit, that is, arrival rate, average LOS, and number of beds, and use these in Equation 16.1 to determine the probability that an arriving patient will not find a bed available. Let us assume that the Big City Hospital's obstetrics unit has an average arrival rate of $\lambda = 14.8$ patients per day, an average LOS of $1/\mu = 2.9$ days, and $s = 56$ beds. Then, the *M/M/s* formula for probability of delay (1) produces an estimate of approximately 4%. To use the *M/M/s* prescriptively to find the minimum number of beds needed to attain a target probability of delay, we can enter Equation 16.1 in a spreadsheet and produce a table of results for a broad range of bed capacities to find the one that best meets the desired target. Table 16.1 is a partial table of results for our example obstetrics unit.

TABLE 16.1 Probability of Delay and Utilization for Obstetrics Unit

No. of Beds	Pr(Delay)	Utilization
45	.666	.953
46	.541	.933
47	.435	.913
48	.346	.894
49	.272	.875
50	.212	.858
51	.163	.841
52	.124	.825
53	.093	.809
54	.069	.794
55	.051	.780
56	.037	.766
57	.026	.753
58	.018	.740
59	.013	.727
60	.009	.715
61	.006	.703
62	.004	.692
63	.003	.681
64	.002	.670
65	.001	.660

Though there is no standard delay target, Schneider (1981) suggested that given their emergent status, the probability of delay for an obstetrics bed should not exceed 1%. Applying this criterion, Table 16.1 indicates that this unit has at least 60 beds. Table 16.1 also shows the utilization level for each choice of servers and that at 60 beds, this level is 71.5%. This is what hospitals call the average occupancy level and it is well below the 85% level that many hospitals and healthcare policy officials consider the minimum target level. It is also below the maximum level of 75% recommended by the American College of Obstetrics and Gynecology (ACOG) to assure timely access to a bed (Freeman and Poland 1997). So does this example show that as long as an obstetrics unit operates below this ACOG occupancy level of 75%, the fraction of patients who will be delayed in getting a bed will be very low?

The Problem with Using Target Occupancy Levels

Hospital capacity decisions traditionally have been made, both at the government and institutional levels, based on target occupancy levels—the average percentage of occupied beds. Historically, the most commonly used occupancy target has been 85%. Estimates of the number of "excess" beds in the United States, as well as in individual states and communities, usually have been based on this "optimal" occupancy figure (Brecher and Speizio 1995, p. 55). In addition, low occupancy levels are often viewed as indicative of operational inefficiency and potential financial problems. So hospital administrators generally view higher occupancy levels as desirable. However, as we saw previously in this chapter, higher occupancy levels result in longer delays and so basing capacity on target occupancy levels can lead to undesirable levels of access for patients.

In Green (2003), the basic *M/M/s* model was used to demonstrate the implications of using target occupancy levels to determine capacity in both obstetrics and ICU units in New York State. Figure 16.1

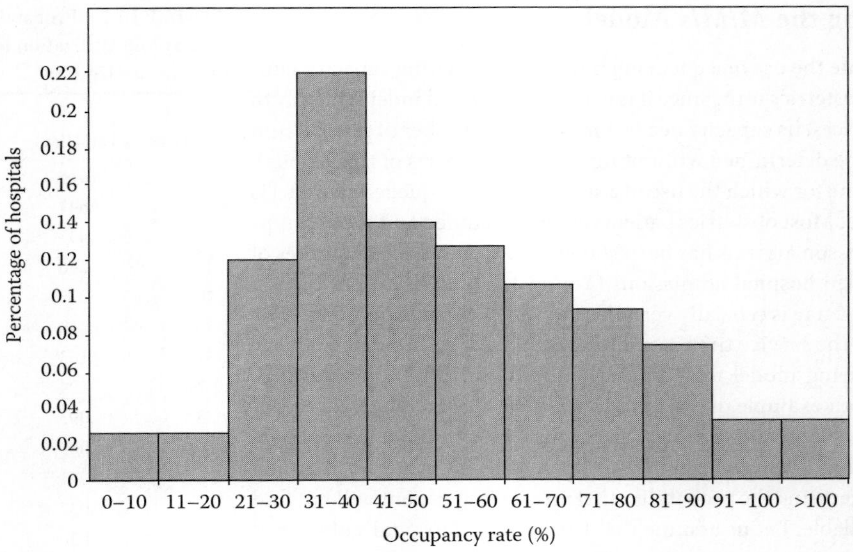

FIGURE 16.2 Average occupancy rates of New York maternity units. (From Green, L.V., Queuing analysis in healthcare, in Randolph, W.H. (ed.), *Patient Flow: Reducing Delay in Healthcare Delivery—Handbook of Healthcare Delivery Systems*, Springer Science+Business Media, LLC, Berlin, Germany, 2006, pp. 281–307. With kind permission from Springer Science+Business Media, LLC.)

from that paper (shown here as Figure 16.2) shows the distribution of average occupancy rates for 148 obstetrics units in New York State for 1997. These data, representing nearly all obstetrics units in New York, were obtained from Institutional Cost Reports (ICRs), and unlike most other published data, reflect staffed beds rather than certified beds. The graph shows that many maternity units had low average occupancy levels and the overall average occupancy level for the study hospitals was only 60%, which, based on the ACOG standard, would imply significant excess capacity. Applying this 75% standard to the 1997 data, 117 of the 148 New York state hospitals had "excess" beds, while 27 had insufficient beds.

However, if one considers a bed delay target as a more appropriate measure of capacity needs, the conclusions can be quite different. Now the number of beds in each unit becomes a major factor since, for a given occupancy level, delays increase as unit size decreases. While obstetrics units usually are not the smallest units in a hospital, there are many small hospitals, particularly in rural areas, and the units in these facilities may contain only 5–10 beds. Of the New York state hospitals considered here, more than 50% had maternity units with 25 or fewer beds.

In the *M*/*M*/*s* model, probability of delay is a function of only two parameters: s and ρ, which in our context are the number of beds and occupancy level, respectively. Each of the three curves shown in Figure 16.3 represents a specific probability of delay as a function of these two variables, as generated by Equation 16.1. Thus, using the unit size and occupancy level reported on the ICR report for a given maternity unit, we can determine from this figure if the probability of delay meets or exceeds any one of these targets. For example, if a maternity unit has 15 beds and an occupancy level of 45%, it would fall below all three curves and hence have a probability of delay less than .01 or 1%, meeting all three targets.

Doing this for every hospital in the database, 30 hospitals had insufficient capacity based on even the most slack delay target of 10%. (It is interesting to note that two of the hospitals that would be considered overutilized under the 75% occupancy standard had sufficient capacity under this delay standard.) Tightening the probability of delay target to 5% yields 48 obstetrics units that do not meet this standard. And adopting a maximum probability of delay of 1% as was suggested in the only publication identified

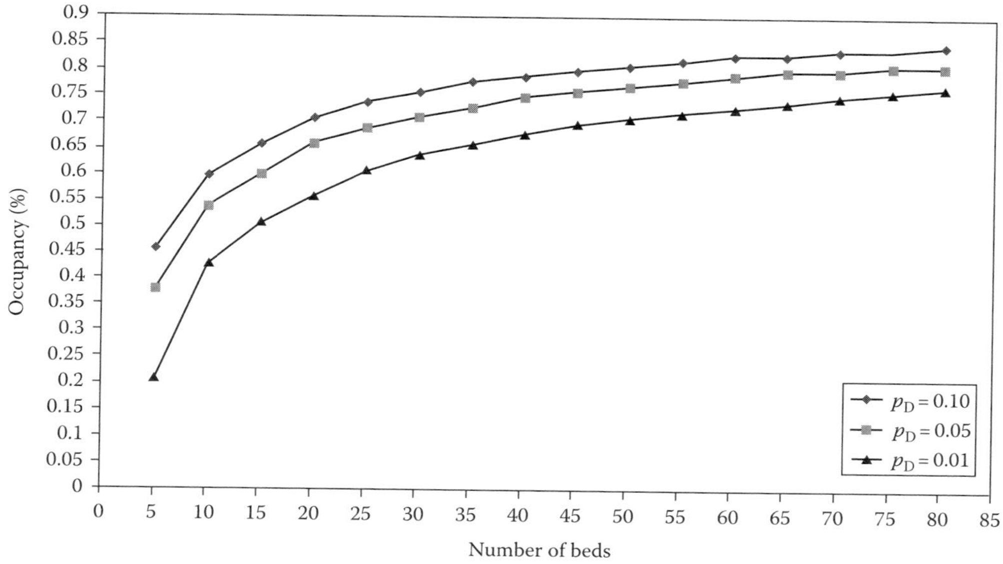

FIGURE 16.3 Probability of delay (p_D) by occupancy level and unit size. (From Green, L.V., Queuing analysis in healthcare, in Randolph, W.H. (ed.), *Patient Flow: Reducing Delay in Healthcare Delivery—Handbook of Healthcare Delivery Systems*, Springer Science+Business Media, LLC, Berlin, Germany, 2006, pp. 281–307. With kind permission from Springer Science+Business Media, LLC.)

as containing a delay standard for obstetrics beds (Schneider 1981) results in 59 or 40%, of all New York state maternity units with insufficient capacity.

How many hospitals in New York State had maternity units large enough to achieve the ACOG-suggested 75% occupancy level and also meet a specified probability of delay standard? Using Figure 16.3, we see that for a 10% target, an obstetrics unit would need to have at least 28 beds, a size that exists in only 40% of the state hospitals. For a 5% standard, the minimum number of beds needed is 41, a size achieved in only 14% of the hospitals; for a 1% standard, at least 67 beds are needed, leaving only three of the 148 or 2% of the hospitals of sufficient size.

Choosing a Delay Standard

As the previous analysis illustrates, the number of required beds can change substantially depending upon what level of delay is considered tolerable. There is no single right choice and in choosing a delay standard, several factors are relevant.

First, what is the expected delay of those patients who experience a delay? This performance measure can be easily calculated once both the probability of delay (Equation 16.1) and the average or mean delay (Equation 16.2) are known. Specifically,

$$\text{Expected delay of delayed customers} = \frac{W_q}{p_D} \qquad (16.8)$$

So returning to our obstetrics example above, Table 16.1 shows that the average delay is 0.008 days (note that since the input was expressed in days, so is the output) which multiplying by 24 gives us 0.19 hours. So dividing this by the probability of delay of .04 results in an expected delay for delayed patients of about 4.75 hours. This may indicate that the probability of delay standard should be lower. This, of course, should be considered in light of what this level of congestion means for the particular hospital.

What are the possible consequences of congestion? In the obstetrics case, while patients in some hospitals remain in the same bed through labor, delivery, recovery, and postpartum, in most maternity units, there are separate areas for some or all of these stages of birth. Therefore, a delay for an obstetrics bed often means that a postpartum patient will remain in a recovery bed longer than necessary. This, of course, may cause a backup in the labor and delivery areas so that newly arriving patients may have to wait on gurneys in hallways or in the emergency room. Some hospitals have overflow beds in a nearby unit that is opened (staffed) when all regular beds are full. (This is likely the case for the five hospitals that reported average occupancy levels exceeding 100%.) While these effects of congestion likely pose no medical threat for most patients who experience normal births, there could be adverse clinical consequences in cases in which there are complications. In particular, whether patients are placed in hallways or overflow units, the nursing staff is likely to be severely strained, thereby limiting the quantity and quality of personal attention. Even if a hospital is able to obtain additional staffing, it is usually by using agency nurses who are more expensive and not as familiar with the physical or operating environment, thereby jeopardizing quality of patient care. In addition, telemetry devices such as fetal monitors that are usually in labor and delivery rooms may be unavailable in other locations, thus compromising the ability to monitor vital signs of both mother and baby. Finally, it is worth noting that such results of congestion may negatively affect patients' perceptions of service quality.

Of course, all major capacity decisions need to be made in light of financial constraints, competing demands, and predictions concerning future demands for the service.

Planning for Predictable Changes in Demand

When making capacity decisions about resources that will be used over several years, it is clearly necessary to consider how conditions may change over that period of time. So in determining the choice of arrival rate or average LOS for a queueing analysis of a hospital unit, it would be important to engage in analyses and discussion to gauge how these parameters may change and then run the model to determine the sensitivity of capacity levels to these changes.

However, what may not be so obvious is the need to consider the changes in the arrival rate that are likely to occur on a regular basis due to predictable day-of-week or time-of-year patterns. For example, obstetrics units often experience a significant degree of seasonality in admissions. An analysis performed on data from a 56-bed maternity unit at Beth Israel Deaconess Hospital in Boston (Green and Nguyen 2001) revealed that the average occupancy levels varied from a low of about 68% in January to about 88% in July. As indicated by Figure 16.4, the *M*/*M*/*s* model estimate of the probability of delay of getting a bed for an obstetrics patient giving birth in January is likely to be negligible with this capacity. However, in July, the same model estimates this delay to be about 25%. And if, as is likely, there are several days when actual arrivals exceed this latter monthly average by say 10%, this delay probability would shoot up to over 65%. The result of such substantial delays can vary from backups into the labor rooms and patients on stretchers in the hallways to the early discharge of patients. Clearly, hospitals need to plan for this type of predictable demand increase by keeping extra bed capacity that can be used during peak times, or by using "swing" beds that can be shared by clinical units that have countercyclical demand patterns.

Most hospital units experience different arrival rates for different days of the week. For example, in one surgical intensive care unit, the average admissions per day over a 6 month period varied from a low of 1.44 for Sundays to a high of 4.40 for Fridays. Using the average arrival rate over the week of 3.34 in a queueing model would indicate that given the 12 bed capacity of this unit, the probability of delay for a bed was about 39%, indicating serious congestion. However, this is very misleading because delays will be significantly greater in the middle of the week and quite small earlier in the week due to the large differences in the admissions rates (Green and Nguyen 2001). This illustrates a situation in which a steady-state queueing model is inappropriate for estimating the magnitude and timing of delays and for which a simulation model will be far more accurate.

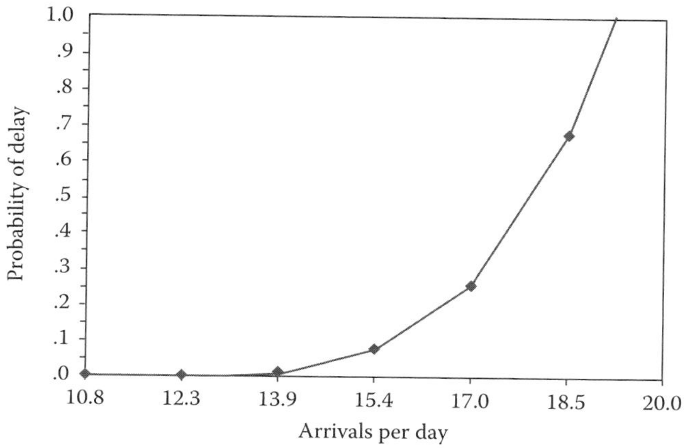

FIGURE 16.4 Probability of delay as a function of arrivals per day for a 56-bed obstetrics unit. (From Green, L.V., Queuing analysis in healthcare, in Randolph, W.H. (ed.), *Patient Flow: Reducing Delay in Healthcare Delivery—Handbook of Healthcare Delivery Systems*, Springer Science+Business Media, LLC, Berlin, Germany, 2006, pp. 281–307. With kind permission from Springer Science+Business Media, LLC.)

Using Queueing Models to Quantify the Benefits of Flexibility

Healthcare facilities often have to make a choice as to the extent to which resources should be dedicated to specific patient types. For example, should there be an imaging facility just for the use of inpatients, or for emergency patients? Should there be a "fast-track" unit in the emergency room to deal with simpler, nonurgent cases. How many distinct clinical service units should be used for hospital inpatients? In many of these situations, a queueing analysis can be useful in evaluating the potential trade-offs between more flexible and more specialized facilities.

For example, seriously ill patients arriving at a hospital ED often experience serious delays in being admitted due to highly variable patient demands and insufficient inpatient bed capacity. Yet, hospitals are often reluctant or unable to add capacity because of cost pressures, regulatory constraints, or a shortage of appropriate personnel. This makes it extremely important to use existing capacity most efficiently. Increasing bed flexibility can be a key strategy in alleviating congestion. For example, hospitals vary in the degree to which they segregate patients by diagnostic type. While all hospitals have separate units for pediatrics, obstetrics, and psychiatric patients, some also have distinct units for clinical services such as cardiology, neurology, oncology, urology, neurosurgery, etc. Other hospitals may make no such distinctions and simply designate all of these as medical/surgical beds. What are the implications of these differing bed assignment policies on delays for beds?

As mentioned in the "Delays, utilization, and system size" section, service systems have economies of scale and so in general, the less specialized the beds, the larger the pool of beds that can be used for any type of patient, and therefore the fewer beds should be needed to achieve a given standard of delay. In other words, if one hospital has 100 general medical/surgical beds, and another has the same 100 beds, but allocated into 10 distinct clinical services, each of which can only be used for patients falling into the appropriate category, the second hospital will likely have considerably longer delays for beds (which usually show up as longer stays in the ED) and lower average occupancy levels than the first. This is pretty clear once you consider that by creating separate categories of beds, there is the possibility of patients waiting for beds even when beds are available if they are the "wrong" kind. This also happens when beds are distinguished by capability, for example, telemetry beds.

Clearly, there are many instances in which there are compelling clinical and/or managerial reasons for maintaining particular patient types in specialized units. From a medical perspective, there may be benefits derived from having patients clustered by diagnostic categories in dedicated units managed and staffed by specialized nurses. These include shorter LOS, fewer adverse events and fewer readmits. Yet, many hospital managers believe that nurses can be successfully cross-trained and that increasing bed flexibility is ultimately in the best interests of patients by increasing speedy access to beds and minimizing the number of bed transfers. By incorporating waiting times, percentage of "off-placements" and the effects on LOS, queueing models can be used to better evaluate the benefits of greater versus less specialization of beds or any other resource. This would be done by simply modeling the general-use unit as a single multi-server queueing system fed and comparing the results to those from modeling each distinct service as an independent queue. In the latter case, the overall patient delay can be obtained from an arrival rate weighted average of the individual queue delays (Green and Nguyen 2001).

Analyses of Flexible Capacity: Determining Staffing Levels to Meet Time-Varying Demands

As mentioned previously, healthcare facilities generally experience very different levels of demand over the day, over the week, and even over the year. Many facilities adjust their staffing—for example, physicians, nurses, technicians, housekeeping staff—in order to respond to the demands in a timely fashion at minimal cost. This is often done without the help of a quantitative model and can lead to an inefficient and ineffective allocation of resources. Here we use the example of determining physician staffing levels in an ED to illustrate how queueing models can be used to improve performance in these types of situations.

Data Collection and Model Choices

In order to use a queueing model to determine how to adjust staffing to meet time-varying demands, it is first necessary to collect fairly detailed data on the volume of demand that must be handled by that staff by time of day and day of week. In collecting demand data, the goal is twofold. First, and most obviously, the data will be used to parameterize the queueing model. However, before that can be done, it must first be determined how many staffing models are needed. That is, will staffing be identical for all days of the week or vary from day to day? For example, in a study conducted in the ED of a midsize urban hospital in New York City (Green et al. 2005), the overall volume varied from a low of 63 patients per day on Saturdays to a high of 72 per day on Monday. This degree of variation indicated that the then-current policy of identical staffing levels for all days of the week was likely suboptimal. However, it was deemed impractical to have a different provider schedule every day and so it was decided to use queueing analyses to develop two schedules: weekday and weekend. This required aggregating ED arrival data into these two groups. For each, demand data was then collected for each hour of the day using the hospital's admissions database to understand the degree of variation over the day (see Figure 16.5). This level of detail also allows for the use of queueing analysis to determine the impact of different shift starting times on delays and/or staffing levels.

A queueing model also requires an average provider service time per patient, which must include the times of all activities related to a patient. In the ED, these activities include direct patient care, review of x-rays and lab tests, phone calls, charting, and speaking with other providers or consults. In many, if not most, hospitals, these data are not routinely collected. At the time of the study, provider service times were not recorded and had to be estimated from direct observation and historical productivity data.

Constructing the Queueing Models

Since the *M*/*M*/*s* model assumes that the arrival rate does not change over the day, actual service systems that have time-varying demands typically use this model as part of a *SIPP* (stationary independent period-by-period) approach to determine how to vary staffing to meet changing demand. The *SIPP* approach begins by dividing the workday into staffing periods, for example, 1, 2, 3, or 8 hours. Then a series of *M*/*M*/*s* models are constructed, one for each staffing period. Each of these period-specific

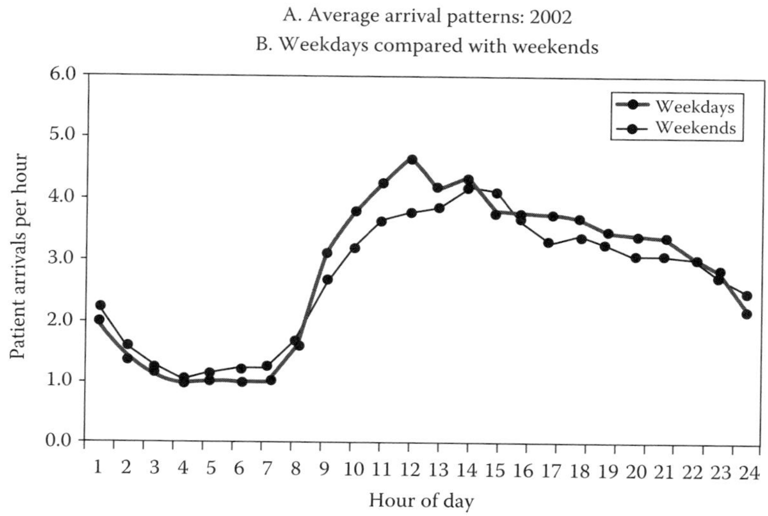

FIGURE 16.5 Average arrival rate by hour of the day. (From Green, L.V., Queuing analysis in healthcare, in Randolph, W.H. (ed.), *Patient Flow: Reducing Delay in Healthcare Delivery—Handbook of Healthcare Delivery Systems*, Springer Science+Business Media, LLC, Berlin, Germany, 2006, pp. 281–307. With kind permission from Springer Science+Business Media, LLC.)

models is independently solved for the minimum number of servers needed to meet the service target in that period. The service target might be a desired maximum mean delay or probability of delay standard. However, recent research has shown that the *SIPP* approach is often unreliable, particularly when average service times are 30 minutes or more, and that a simple modification, called *Lag SIPP*, is often more effective in identifying staffing levels that achieve the desired performance standard (Green et al. 2001). This is because in many service systems with time-varying arrival rates, the time of peak congestion significantly lags the time of the peak in the arrival rate (Green et al. 1991). While the standard *SIPP* approach ignores this phenomenon, the *Lag SIPP* method incorporates an estimation of this lag and thus does a better job of identifying staffing levels to limit delays. For the *M*/*M*/*s* model, the lag can be well approximated by an average service time.

Choosing a Delay Standard and Applying the Queueing Results

In our ED physician staffing study, the *Lag SIPP* approach was applied by first advancing the arrival rate curve by our estimate of the average physician time per patient, 30 minutes. We then constructed a series of *M*/*M*/*s* models for each 2-hour staffing interval, using the average arrival rate for each based on the time-advanced curve and the average 30-minute service time. The delay standard we choose was that no more than 20% of patients wait more than 1 hour before being seen by a provider. The use of 1 hour is consistent with the time standards associated with emergent and urgent patient groups used in the National Hospital Ambulatory Medical Care Survey (McCaig and Burt 2004). The 20% criterion reflects the approximate percentage of nonurgent arrivals at the study institution.

The modeling results gave the number of ED physicians needed in each of the 2-hour staffing intervals to meet the delay standard. In total, 58 physician hours were needed on weekdays to achieve the desired service standard, which represented an increase of 3 hours over the existing staffing level of 55 hours. Model runs for the weekend indicated that the target performance standard could be achieved with a total of 53 provider-hours. In both these cases, the queueing analyses suggested that some physician hours should be switched from the middle of the night to much earlier in the day. A more subtle change suggested by the model was that the increase in staffing level to handle the morning surge in demand needed to occur earlier than in the original schedule. Though resource limitations and physician availability prevented the staffing suggested by the queueing analyses from being implemented exactly, the insights gained from these analyses were used to develop new provider schedules. More specifically, as a result of the analyses, one physician was moved from the overnight shift to an afternoon shift, 4 hours were moved from the weekends and added to the Monday and Tuesday afternoon shifts (since these were the two busiest days of the week) and a shift that previously started at noon was moved to 10 a.m. These changes led to shorter average delays and a reduced fraction of patient that left before being seen by a physician.

Using Queueing Models to Improve Healthcare Delivery: Opportunities and Challenges

As this chapter has illustrated, service systems are very complex due to both predictable and unpredictable sources of variability in both the demands for service and the time it takes to serve those demands. In healthcare facilities, decisions on how and when to allocate staff, equipment, beds, and other resources in order to minimize delays experienced by patients are often even more difficult than in other service industries due to cost constraints on the one hand and the potentially serious adverse consequences of delays on the other hand. Therefore, it is imperative that these decisions should be as informed as possible and rely upon the best methodologies available to gain insights into the impact of various alternatives.

Queueing theory is a very powerful and very practical tool because queueing models require relatively little data and are simple and fast to use. Because of this simplicity and speed, they can be used to quickly evaluate and compare various alternatives for providing service. Beyond the most basic issue of determining how much capacity is needed to achieve a specified service standard, queueing models can also be useful in gaining insights on the appropriate degree of specialization or flexibility to use in organizing resources, or on the impact of various priority schemes for determining service order among patients.

On the other hand, though queueing models do not require much data, the type of operational data needed as input to a queueing model is often unavailable in healthcare settings. Specifically, though demand or arrival data are often recorded, service times are usually not documented. So a queueing analysis might require a data collection effort to estimate, for example, the time that a care provider spends with a patient. However, as information technology systems become more prevalent in healthcare, this type of data will be increasingly available.

In developing the data inputs for a model, it is also very important to make sure that all of the data needed for the model is collected and/or estimated. On the demand side, this means including all demands for care, including the ones that may not have been met in the past because of inadequate capacity. For example, in a hospital ED, some patients who are forced to wait a long time before seeing a physician leave the ED before being seen. If these are not captured in the data collection system that is being used to measure demands, the model will underestimate the capacity needed to meet the desired performance standard. On the service side, it is important to include all of the time spent by the servers that is directly associated with caring for the patient. For a physician, this may include reviewing medical history and test results in addition to direct examination of the patient.

In addition to data, a queueing analysis of a particular healthcare system requires the identification of one or more delay measures that are most important to service excellence for that facility. These measures should reflect both patient perspectives as well as clinical realities. For example, though hospital ED arrivals with nonurgent problems may not require care within an hour or so from a clinical perspective, clearly very long waits to see a physician will result in high levels of dissatisfaction, and perhaps even departure, which could ultimately lead to lost revenue. Trying to decide on what might be a reasonable delay standard in a specific healthcare facility is not trivial due to a lack of knowledge of both patient expectations as well as the impact of delays on clinical outcomes for most health problems.

In summary, healthcare managers are increasingly aware of the need to use their resources as efficiently as possible in order to continue to assure that their institutions survive and prosper. This is particularly true in light of the growing threat of sudden and severe demand surges due to outbreaks of epidemics such as SARS and avian or swine flu, or terrorist incidents. As this chapter has attempted to demonstrate, effective capacity management is critical to this objective as well as to improving patients' ability to receive the most appropriate care in a timely fashion. Yet, effective capacity management must deal with complexities such as trade-offs between bed flexibility and quality of care, demands from competing sources and types of patients, time-varying demands, and the often differing perspectives of administrators, physicians, nurses, and patients. All of these are chronic and pervasive challenges affecting the ability of hospital managers to control the cost and improve the quality of healthcare delivery. To meet these challenges, managers must be informed by operational and performance data and use these data in models to gain insights that cannot be obtained from experience and intuition alone. Queueing analysis is one of the most practical and effective tools for understanding and aiding decision-making in managing critical resources and should become as widely used in the healthcare community as it is in the other major service sectors.

References

Allen, A.O. 1978. *Probability, Statistics and Queueing Theory, with Computer Science Applications*. Academic Press, New York.

Brecher, C. and S. Speizio. 1995. *Privatization and Public Hospitals*. Twentieth Century Fund Press, New York.

Brewton, J.P. 1989. Teller staffing models, *Financial Manager's Statement*, July–August: 22–24.

Brigandi, A.J., D.R. Dargon, M.J. Sheehan, and T. Spencer III. 1994. AT&T's call processing simulator (CAPS) operational design for inbound call centers, *Interfaces*, 24: 6–28.

Brockmeyer, E., H.L. Halstrom, and A. Jensen. (eds.) 1948. The life and works of A.K. Erlang, *Transactions of the Danish Academy of Technical Science 2*. Copenhagen Telephone Company, Copenhagen, Denmark.

Brusco, M.J., L.W. Jacobs, R.J. Bongiorno, D.V. Lyons, and B. Tang. 1995. Improving personnel scheduling at airline stations, *Operations Research*, 43: 741–751.

Chelst, K. and Z. Barlach. 1981. Multiple unit dispatches in emergency services, *Management Science*, 27: 1390–1409.

Cobham, A. 1954. Priority assignment in waiting line problems, *Operations Research*, 2: 70–76.

Freeman, R.K. and R.L. Poland. 1997. *Guidelines for Perinatal Care*, 4th edn. American College of Obstetricians and Gynecologists, Washington, DC.

Green, L.V. 2003. How many hospital beds? *Inquiry*, 39: 400–412.

Green, L.V. 2006. Queuing analysis in healthcare, in Randolph, W.H. (ed.), *Patient Flow: Reducing Delay in Healthcare Delivery—Handbook of Healthcare Delivery Systems*. Springer Science+Business Media, LLC, Berlin, Germany, pp. 281–307.

Green, L.V., J. Giulio, R. Green, and J. Soares. 2006. Using queueing theory to increase the effectiveness of physician staffing in the emergency department, *Academic Emergency Medicine*, 13: 61–68.

Green, L.V. and P.J. Kolesar. 1984. The feasibility of one-officer patrol in New York City, *Management Science*, 20: 964–981.

Green, L.V., P.J. Kolesar, and A. Svoronos. 1991. Some effects of nonstationarity on multi-server Markovian queueing systems, *Operations Research*, 39: 502–511.

Green, L.V., P.J. Kolesar, A. Svoronos. 2001. Improving the SIPP approach for staffing service systems that have cyclic demands, *Operations Research*, 49: 549–564.

Green, L.V. and V. Nguyen. 2001. Strategies for cutting hospital beds: The impact on patient service, *Health Services Research*, 36: 421–442.

Hall, R.W. 1990. *Queueing Methods for Service and Manufacturing*. Prentice Hall, Upper Saddle River, NJ.

Holloran, T.J. and J.E. Byrne. 1986. United Airlines station manpower planning system, *Interfaces*, 16: 39–50.

Institute of Medicine, Committee on Quality of Health Care in America. 2001. *Crossing the Quality Chasm: A New Health System for the 21st Century*. National Academy Press, Washington, DC.

Kim, S., I. Horowitz, K.K. Young, and T.A. Buckley. 1999. Analysis of capacity management of the intensive care unit in a hospital, *European Journal of Operational Research*, 115: 36–46.

Kolesar, P.J., K. Rider, T. Crabill, and W. Walker. 1975. A queueing linear programming approach to scheduling police cars, *Operations Research*, 23: 1045–1062.

Larson, R.C. 1972. *Urban Police Patrol Analysis*. MIT Press, Cambridge, MA.

McCaig, L.F. and C.W. Burt. 2004. National hospital ambulatory medical care survey: 2002 emergency department summary, *Advance Data from Vital and Health Statistics*, 340: 1–35.

Schneider, D. 1981. A methodology for the analysis of comparability of services and financial impact of closure of obstetrics services, *Medical Care*, 19: 395–409.

Shmueli, A., C.L. Sprung, and E.H. Kaplan. 2003. Optimizing admissions to an intensive care unit, *Health Care Management Science*, 6: 131–136.

Stern, H.I. and M. Hersh. 1980. Scheduling aircraft cleaning crews, *Transportation Science*, 14: 277–291.

Taylor, P.E. and S.J. Huxley. 1989. A break from tradition for the San Francisco police: Patrol officer scheduling using an optimization-based decision support system, *Interfaces*, 19: 4–24.

Young, J.P. 1965. Stabilization of inpatient bed occupancy through control of admissions, *Journal of the American Hospital Association*, 39: 41–48.

17

Markov Decision Processes and Its Applications in Healthcare

Jonathan Patrick
University of Ottawa

Mehmet A. Begen
University of Western Ontario

Introduction 17-1
MDP Theory 17-2
Decision Epochs • States and State Spaces • Actions and Action Sets • Transition Probabilities • Reward or Cost Functions • Solving a Finite Horizon MDP • Solving Infinite Horizon Models • Continuous Time Models • Limitations of Markov Decision Processes
Literature Survey 17-8
Operational Healthcare Applications • Clinical Healthcare Applications
Two MDP Applications 17-10
Healthcare Management: Multi-Priority Patient Scheduling • Clinical Decision Making: Liver Transplantation Decision Models
Conclusion 17-16
References 17-16

Introduction

John Kitto once said that "The human mind is much given to the thrilling exercise of leaping across chasms as if they were not there." He no doubt did not mean it as a compliment and yet, in some instances, the courage necessary to do so is a prerequisite to any action whatsoever. It would seem prudent however to do as much as possible to determine how big a chasm it is that we are seeking to jump and to attempt by all means possible to reduce that chasm to a more reasonable size!

In healthcare, as in most human endeavors, we are inevitably forced to make decisions with less than complete information and thus in one sense, we are necessarily "jumping over chasms [of ignorance] as if they were not there." As an example, consider the surgical department of a hospital. Each time a surgery is booked, a certain amount of operating room (OR) time and a certain number of beds days are consumed. The problem is that, prior to the surgery, the amount of OR time is not known with any certainty and, prior to the patient's discharge from the hospital, the number of bed days consumed is not known with any certainty. Thus, we have to make the booking decision prior to knowing with certainty the resource consumption implicit in that decision! Moreover, the decision as to what type and when to book surgeries today has an inevitable impact on what decisions one can make tomorrow and what costs/profits might be incurred in the future. In fact, booking decisions made today may cause unwanted cancellations months from now. Such a problem is a classic example of a stochastic, sequential decision problem.

Sequential decision problems (SDPs), as the name implies, are problems in which a series of decisions are made in sequence and where each subsequent decision is impacted by the preceding set of decisions. Stochastic sequential decision problems are simply SDPs where at least some outcomes are known only probabilistically. Such problems abound in healthcare from management decisions such as scheduling and capacity planning to treatment decisions such as when to initiate, or how long to continue, a certain treatment. Unfortunately, these decision problems are often negotiated with limited empirical understanding of what the future consequences might be. To continue with the metaphor, those involved in healthcare decision making are often to forced to leap with limited knowledge of the width of the chasm they are being forced to jump!

Markov decision processes (MDPs) are a set of mathematical models that seek to provide optimal solutions to precisely such sequential decision problems. If the SDP is stochastic, an MDP model cannot remove the uncertainty but it can help the decision maker to make the best possible decisions in light of what knowledge is available. MDP models cover a wide range of potential applications divided broadly into finite and infinite horizon models (based on whether we are dealing with a finite or infinite number of decisions) as well as discrete and continuous time models (based on whether decisions are made at regular, discrete intervals or are triggered by a random occurrence). In the rest of this chapter, we first set out the basic theory of MDPs before moving into a brief discussion of a variety of applications of MDP to healthcare with a special focus on two in particular—one in healthcare management and another in clinical decision making.

MDP Theory

Decision Epochs

All MDP models have five basic components. First, the decision maker must determine how often a decision is made and whether those decisions are made at fixed intervals (a discrete model) or varying intervals (a continuous model). The time at which a decision is made is called the decision epoch. For instance, a hospital might check the inventory of a certain medical device each night and determine whether to order any additional items. In that case, we would have a discrete MDP where decisions are taken once a day. A typical inventory management problem is usually defined as an infinite horizon MDP unless the item being stocked is being phased out (i.e., a medical device where a new version is going to hit the market in the near future). Conversely, treatment decisions are often made in continuous time, in response to a patient's condition. Such a SDP would have to be modeled as a continuous-time, finite horizon model.

States and State Spaces

Second, the decision maker must determine what relevant information needs to be tracked in order to make an informed decision. Thus, in the inventory example, it is clear that the relevant information is the current inventory in stock. Should the price of the device vary that might also be a necessary piece of information to track. The current values of the relevant information at decision epoch t is called the state (usually represented by s_t) and forms the basis upon which decisions are made. The state space, S, is the set of all possible states of the system. Note that the state need only contain the relevant information that changes from decision epoch to decision epoch. All other relevant information can simply be used as input into the model.

Actions and Action Sets

Third, it is necessary to determine what actions are available to the decision maker in each potential state of the system. Thus, in our example, the decision maker must determine how much, if any, new items to order. Most likely there is a limit on how much inventory can be stored and thus the set of available actions depends on the state (as inventory on hand plus order quantity cannot exceed the holding capacity). The action at decision epoch t is most often represented by a_t, and the set of all possible actions in state s_t by the term, $A_t(s_t)$.

Transition Probabilities

Fourth, a MDP would be a poor model for a SDP, if it did not consider the evolution of the system. The transition probabilities determine the probability with which each possible state is visited at the next decision epoch based on the current state and action. To return once again to the inventory model, the transition probabilities depend on the probability of new demand and the action taken. The next state is determined by

$$s_{t+1} = s_t + a_t - D_t$$

where D_t is a random variable representing new demand. Notice that in this formulation we are assuming back orders are allowed as new demand may be bigger than current and new inventory thus allowing the new state to be negative. Thus, the transition probability matrix has the form

$$p(s_{t+1} \mid s_t, a_t) = \begin{cases} p(d) & \text{if } s_{t+1} = s_t + a_t - d \\ 0 & \text{otherwise} \end{cases}$$

where $p(d)$ is the probability of there being d new demand requests. We will assume that the probability of reaching a given new state is dependent only on the current state and the current action and not on the history of past states and actions. This is accomplished by simply including in the state definition any relevant information from the past history.

Reward or Cost Functions

Finally, taking a given action in a given state may result in a reward (or cost). These are what distinguish a good action from a poor one. For instance, there will be a cost for ordering more inventory and for holding inventory that is balanced against the cost of stocking out. In this case, the reward will depend both on the action (how much to order) and the state (how much inventory is on hand). Thus, the reward function might be written as

$$r(s_t, a_t, s_{t+1}) = f\left([s_t + a_t - s_{t+1}]^+\right) - O(a_t) - h(s_t)$$

where $O(\ )$ is the ordering cost, $h(\ )$ is the holding costs (if s_t is positive), or the stock-out costs (if s_t is negative) and $f(\ )$ represents revenue from procedures performed. Notice that in this formulation we are assuming that new inventory arrives before any demand is realized. Of course, the state of the system at the next decision epoch is not known in advance (since demand is random) and therefore, the decision maker must decide based on the expected reward which is written as

$$r(s_t, a_t) = \sum_d p(s_{t+1} \mid s_t, a_t) r(s_t, a_t, s_{t+1})$$

Solving a Finite Horizon MDP

The above five components formally define an MDP model. The next step is to determine the optimal decision policy. We begin with the easier finite horizon case. We define a *decision rule*, d_t, as a function that dictates what decision to take for each possible state at decision epoch t. Decision rules may depend on the entire history up to that decision epoch or they may depend only on the current state of the system. If they depend only on the current state they are called *Markovian*. Decision rules may also be *deterministic* if they dictate only one given action for each state or they may be *probabilistic* if they give a probability distribution over the set of possible actions that is used to randomly determine the appropriate action. A *policy*, $\pi = (d_1, d_2,\ldots, d_N)$, is a set of decision rules (one for every decision epoch) that dictates what action to take for any given state and any given decision epoch. A policy is Markovian if the decision rule for each decision epoch is Markovian and deterministic if each decision rule is deterministic. Since it is possible, under mild assumptions, to show that there always exists an optimal policy that is Markovian and deterministic (given the objectives we discuss below), we restrict discussion to this subset of all possible policies.

The natural goal is to find the policy, π^*, that gives the greatest total reward over the length of the horizon. Formally, we define the total reward of a policy π over a finite horizon of length N and starting at state s as

$$v_N^{\pi}(s) = E_s^{\pi}\left\{\sum_{t=1}^{N-1} r_t(X_t, Y_t) + r_N(X_N)\right\}$$

where

X_t is a sequence of random variables representing the progression of the state
Y_t is a sequence of random variables representing the actions taken at each decision epoch based on policy π

The term $r_N(X_N)$ represents the salvage value of being in state X_N at the end of the planning horizon. v_N^{π} is called the *value function* of the policy π. Ideally, we would like to find a policy π^* such that

$$v_N^{\pi^*}(s) \geq v_N^{\pi}(s)$$

for all starting states s and for all alternative policies π. This would seem to be a fairly daunting task, especially if the planning horizon is long. The genius of MDP theory was to realize that such a problem could be solved one decision epoch at a time rather than trying to solve the whole decision problem at once. The process is called backward induction as it starts in the last period in which there is a decision, period $N - 1$, and moves back to period 1. We define $u_t^{\pi}(s)$ as the total reward achieved from period t onward:

$$u_t^{\pi}(s) = E_s^{\pi}\left\{\sum_{n=t}^{N-1} r_t(X_t, Y_t) + r_N(X_N)\right\}$$

If we define $u_t^{*}(s)$ as the maximum reward achievable if in state s at decision epoch t, then we can recursively determine $u_t^{*}(s)$ for each state s by solving

$$u_t^{*}(s) = \max_{a\in A(s)}\left\{r_t(s,a) + \sum_{j\in S} p_t(j \mid s,a)u_{t+1}^{*}(j)\right\} \tag{17.1}$$

These are called *Bellman's optimality equations* after Richard Bellman, one of the founding figures in MDP theory. When faced with a SDP (i.e., playing chess), one knows that it is important to take into account not only present rewards but also where an action might lead (i.e., future states). This is precisely what Bellman's equations do as they find the action for each state that maximizes the combination of the present reward *and* the expected future rewards assuming one acts optimally for all future decision epochs.

As with any induction method, one needs a starting point but for a finite horizon model that is easy as there is no decision to be made in the final epoch and thus $u_N^*(s) = r_N(s)$ for all s. We can therefore proceed to find $u_{N-1}^*(s),\ldots,u_1^*(s)$ for all s recursively using Equation 17.1. The optimal decision at any given epoch and for any given state is an action a such that

$$a \in \arg\max_{a \in A(s)} \left\{ r_t(s,a) + \sum_{j \in S} p_t(j \mid s,a) u_{t+1}^*(j) \right\}$$

Formally, we can set out the backward induction algorithm in the following steps:

1. Set $t = N$ and $u_N^*(s) = r_N(s)\ \forall s \in S$.
2. Let $t = t - 1$ and compute for each s in the state space:

$$u_t^*(s) = \max_{a \in A(s)} \left\{ r_t(s,a) + \sum_{j \in S} p_t(j \mid s,a) u_{t+1}^*(j) \right\}.$$

3. For each s in the state space, find an action a in $A(s)$, such that

$$a \in \arg\max_{a \in A(s)} \left\{ r_t(s,a) + \sum_{j \in S} p_t(j \mid s,a) u_{t+1}^*(j) \right\}.$$

4. If $t = 1$ then stop else return to step 2.

The function $u_1^*(s)$ is the maximum expected reward over the entire planning horizon given that the system starts in state s. The optimal policy is constructed from the actions a found in step 3 and can be presented to the manager as either a look-up table that gives the optimal action for each state and every decision epoch or, if possible, as a function that accomplishes the same.

Let us return to the inventory management problem and assume that the terminal rewards are zero (or at least less than the ordering costs) and that the ordering function includes both a fixed cost and a variable cost. In this case, if we use backward induction to find the optimal policy, it returns a well-known (s_t, S_t) policy. An (s_t, S_t) policy orders as soon as the inventory drops below the value s_t and always orders enough so that the post-decision (pre-demand) inventory is S_t. The subscript t implies that the actual values may differ for each decision epoch. As the end of the horizon approaches, the policy shifts so that fewer items are ordered so that the final inventory can be as close to zero as possible.

Solving Infinite Horizon Models

What allows backward induction to work in the finite horizon setting is that we can easily determine the starting point $u_N^*(s)$. However, a significant number of SDPs in healthcare do not fit the finite horizon model as the decision process is ongoing. Obviously, as N goes to infinity we lose the starting point for the backward induction algorithm.

One might also suppose that writing down an optimal solution to the infinite horizon problem is unachievable as there are now an infinite number of decision epochs and thus the look-up table would have infinite dimensions. Fortunately, for a great many problems the optimal solution turns out to be independent of the decision epoch. This makes intuitive sense as there is really no difference, in the infinite horizon setting, between the decision problems at decision epoch t and at decision epoch $t + 1$, provided that the transition probabilities and rewards are independent of t. This is born out in the finite inventory management model discussed earlier in that the policy has the same trigger value, s, for ordering and the same order up to value S provided the end of the planning horizon is sufficiently far away. Policies that do not change from decision epoch to decision epoch are said to be *stationary*.

To even begin to talk about solving an infinite horizon MDP, we need to first redefine our objective. The natural extension of the finite horizon model would be to attempt to find a policy π that maximizes

$$v^{\pi}(s) = E_s^{\pi}\left\{\sum_{t=1}^{\infty} r_t(X_t, Y_t)\right\}$$

However, this objective is problematic on three accounts.

1. It may not even exist.
2. If it does exist, there may be no policy that achieves the maximum.
3. It may be infinite for a number of different policies that are not all equally good policies. (For instance, it would be infinite both for a policy that yields a reward of \$1 every decision epoch and one that yields \$100 every decision epoch.)

Two solutions have been proposed. First, we can assume that upfront rewards are generally preferred to deferred rewards. This is most easily incorporated into the model by discounting future rewards by a number $\lambda \in (0, 1)$. Thus, we would seek to find a policy π that maximizes

$$v_{\lambda}^{\pi}(s) = E_s^{\pi}\left\{\sum_{t=1}^{\infty} \lambda^{t-1} r_t(X_t, Y_t)\right\}$$

for each s in S. Even though this remains an infinite sum, it has the advantage of being guaranteed to converge to a finite number provided that all rewards are bounded.

If we make the following four assumptions

1. All rewards and transition probabilities are independent of t.
2. All rewards are bounded.
3. Future rewards are discounted.
4. The state space is finite or countable.

then we can be assured that there exists an optimal stationary, Markovian, deterministic policy. A number of methods have been developed for determining the optimal policy for an infinite horizon MDP but the three basic methods are called value iteration, policy iteration, and a linear programming version of Bellman's equations. The reader is referred to some classic textbooks (e.g., Puterman 1994) on MDP for the details.

If it does not make sense to discount future rewards then the alternative objective is to find a policy π that maximizes the *average* reward. Formally, this can be written as

$$g^{\pi}(s) = \lim_{N\to\infty} \frac{1}{N} v_{N+1}^{\pi}(s) = \lim_{N\to\infty} \frac{1}{N} \sum_{n=1}^{N} P_{\pi}^{n-1} r_{d_n}.$$

In general, there is no guarantee that the average reward as defined above will exist. However, for stationary policies it is guaranteed to exist. Our ability to actually determine the optimal policy for the average reward objective depends on the form of the Markov chain induced by the deterministic, stationary policies available in the decision model (Puterman 1994).

Continuous Time Models

So far we have assumed that decisions are taken at regular intervals. However, there are plenty of decisions within healthcare that are triggered by random events such as the arrival or departure of a patient or a change in the patient's condition. In such cases, decisions are often taken every time the state of the system changes. This brings us into the realm of continuous-time Markov decision processes.

In discrete MDPs, the rewards depend only on the current state and action as well as possibly the next state. In a continuous time model, this is no longer sufficient as costs may also depend on how long the system stays in the present state until the next state transition. Thus, we consider two rewards—a lump sum reward for taking action a when in state s and a reward rate that is paid out for every time unit spent in state s given action a was taken at the last decision epoch. For instance, in an outpatient clinic, there may be a waiting cost dependent on the size of the queue that would be incorporated into the *rate cost* and a fixed cost for changing the number of nurses or doctors on duty.

Surprisingly, in most cases, a continuous time model can be reduced to one that has the same form as in the discrete discounted reward case and thus, all the methodologies developed for discrete time can be equally well applied here. Again, we refer the reader to some classic textbooks (Bellman 1957, Puterman 1994, Bertsekas 2001, Feinberg and Schwartz 2002) for further details.

Limitations of Markov Decision Processes

The major challenge facing MDP theory has been termed the "curse of dimensionality." In many applications, the size of the state space is simply too large to allow even modern computing capabilities to solve the MDP model directly. For instance, consider a scheduling problem where clients are scheduled up to 30 days in advance and where there are three priority classes. To make an informed decision, the state space must include the current capacity available on each of the 30 days as well as the current number of clients waiting in each priority class. Even if there is only room for 10 appointments in a day and the maximum number in the queue is 10 per priority class, one still gets a state space that contains 10^{33} different values.

In recent decades, a field of research called approximate dynamic programming (ADP) has developed in an attempt to solve larger MDP models. The fundamental idea is to assume that the value function has a given functional form that can be characterized by a reasonable number of parameters. Thus, rather than seeking to present a look-up table that outlines the optimal action for every state, the ADP methodology seeks to find the optimal parameter values that characterize the assumed form of the value function in order to get the best approximation possible.

It remains somewhat of an open question as to how to determine the appropriate value function characterization though often the nature of the application gives some distinct clues. A simple approximation that is linear in the state variables often suffices. Once that form has been chosen, there are two main methods for determining the optimal parameter values. The first is to simulate the evolution of the system in order to fine-tune the parameters (Sutton and Barto 1998, Bertsekas 2001, Powell 2007). The second is to use the approximate value function characterization in the linear programming (LP) version of Bellman's optimality equations and to solve for the optimal parameter values using the LP (Adelman 2005, de Faris and Van Roy 2003). Using this methodology, much larger MDP models have been "solved" with simulations used to show the benefits of the derived policies. However, there remain a number of unsolved questions in ADP theory that make this an interesting field of research.

Literature Survey

As discussed in the previous section, MDPs, also sometimes referred to as (stochastic) dynamic programming, is a strong analytical tool to analyze decision-making problems under uncertainty. MDP has proven useful in many applications of operations research, computer science, finance, engineering, and other disciplines. In this section, we focus on healthcare operations research applications of MDP.

Healthcare problems often involve uncertainty and sequential decision making. They involve uncertainty due to the many sources of randomness such as patient arrivals, resource availability, treatment durations, reactions of patients to drugs/treatments, disease progress, size of a tumor and vaccine supply to name but a few. Examples for such stochastic SDPs are the acceptance/rejection of an organ for a transplant, a choice between starting and waiting (for another month/until the next test) for a (drug or radiation) treatment, the acceptance or rejection of a patient for an appointment (e.g., surgery, CT scan), a selection of a treatment option from a set of alternatives and the number of elective patients to be booked for a surgery in the presence of emergency surgeries. One common theme in these examples is that the decision maker is interested in a collection of decisions, not particularly in a single day/time decision. Usually, this collection of decisions is called a decision policy such as a booking policy for elective surgeries and a treatment policy on when to start a drug therapy.

Uncertainty, (sequential) decision making and the need for a decision policy are all clues that should immediately recommend MDP as a solution method. In the healthcare literature, MDPs have become increasingly popular. This may be due to the fact that healthcare challenges—increasing costs, lack of resources to achieve reasonable service levels, increasing need for complicated clinical decision making—are continuously growing in almost every country in the world. The application areas of healthcare research involving MDP are diverse. They range from operational studies, e.g., Patrick et al. (2008) and Green et al. (2006) to revenue management applications such as Gupta and Wang (2008) to purely clinical decisions such as determining therapy start times and deciding when/if to accept an organ offer for a transplant (Alagoz et al. 2004, Sandikci et al. 2008, Shechter et al. 2008). In the following sections, we briefly describe a few of the MDP applications in the healthcare field broadly categorized into operational and clinical.

Operational Healthcare Applications

Probably, one of the first researchers to formulate a hospital admission scheduling problem as a MDP is Kolesar (1970). The author defined the system state as the number of beds occupied (at a certain time, e.g., daily) and the decision (or the action) to be number of admissions. The model includes discharges as well as scheduled and unscheduled arrivals to the system. He introduces a few possible optimization problems using the linear programming formulation but neither solves nor analyzes them due to the sheer size of any practical instance of these problems.

Gerchak et al. (1996) develop a stochastic dynamic programming model to determine the number of elective surgeries booked for a day in the presence of both elective and emergency surgery demand. Ideally, elective surgeries would be done immediately (i.e., as soon as their demand is realized) but accepting too many elective patients may cause overtime as well as leave insufficient capacity for emergency patients. The authors use the number of outstanding (unbooked) surgeries as their state variable and they determine how many elective surgeries to accept each day. They investigate the properties of their model, characterize the optimal policy (which is not a strict booking limit type), and perform numerical examples.

Another operational healthcare MDP example comes from Green et al. (2006) in which authors study the problem of admitting outpatients and inpatients in the presence of emergency patients to a diagnostic facility such as a MRI. One has to schedule outpatients in advance without knowing the demand from inpatients and emergency patients that may arise later. The problem is complicated by outpatient no-shows and cancellations. Emergency patients usually have the highest priority bumping any previously booked appointment. In the case of inpatients and outpatients, a decision has to be made to determine which one to scan next (if they are both waiting before an exam slot). Selecting an outpatient for the scan increases the wait time and hence hospital stay of an inpatient, whereas selecting an inpatient for the scan makes the outpatient wait, decreases the service quality, and affects the business. In this article, the authors develop dynamic priority rules to determine a control policy for inpatients and outpatients before an exam slot. Their model is a single period finite-horizon MDP where the system state is the number of nonscheduled inpatients and scheduled outpatients. They also develop a heuristic for the control policy and test it with numerical studies under a range of parameters. Even though they do not develop an optimal policy for outpatient booking, they provide a heuristic that works reasonably well in a variety of scenarios.

Patient choice in booking a primary-care clinic appointment is considered in Gupta and Wang (2008). Besides the random arrivals of patients, the authors consider the different preferences of patients such as choice of physician and time of day for their appointments. They divide the patients into two groups: regular and same-day patients. Regular patients have preferences for a physician as well as a certain time of day whereas same-day patients will accept any available appointment for that day but may still have a physician preference. The authors formulate this capacity management problem as a MDP in order to determine which appointment requests to accept with the objective of maximizing revenue (their objective also includes a cost function to penalize the clinic if it cannot meet the request of a patient). Under a mild condition on the patient choice probabilities and in the case of a single physician clinic the optimal policy is a threshold-type policy. In the case of multiple physicians, they provide a partial structure to the optimal policy and propose heuristics.

Another paper that takes into account patient choice in healthcare is Su and Zenios (2004). The authors investigate the effect of patient choice on a kidney transplant system which has a high rate of kidney refusals. (Patients who are on the kidney transplant wait list may decline an organ offer if they expect to receive better future offers.) They specifically study the effect of the queuing discipline on organ allocation efficiency (i.e., less organ wastage and less waiting times). The authors use a queuing model (an M/M/1 queue) with two independent arrival streams (patients and organs). Organs differ in their quality whereas patients are homogeneous and the states are dialysis, post-transplant, or death. Patients may decline a kidney offer, in which case they remain on dialysis, or accept it. Transplant takes place once there is a matching kidney available and the patient chooses to proceed. A patient may leave the queue either post-transplant or due to death. Each patient maximizes his/her own total expected discounted QALYs (quality adjusted life years) by solving an optimal stopping problem: when to accept an organ offer. The authors assume complete information and employ dynamic programming and game-theoretical approaches to characterize the equilibrium under various scenarios. They find that under the FCFS (first-come, first-serve) rule, patients become more selective resulting in unnecessary organ wastage since new arrivals to the queue do not affect the existing patients. On the other hand, under the LCFS (last-come, first-served) rule, the system achieves socially optimal organ allocation but with serious equity concerns. The authors also provide a numerical example using data from the U.S. transplantation system to show a 25% potential increase in the supply of kidneys with a better control of patient choice.

Two interesting applications of dynamic programming that somehow lie on the boundary of operational and clinical healthcare decisions are Wu et al. (2005) and Alterovitz et al. (2005). The first paper studies the influenza vaccine selection problem (to evaluate the prospective benefit of history-based vaccination) whereas the second one develops an optimal motion plan for the steering of an image-guided medical needle.

Clinical Healthcare Applications

Schaefer et al. (2004) provides a good survey of MDP applications in clinical decision making prior to 2004. The authors summarize the applications of MDP under the following titles: epidemic control, drug infusion, kidney transplantation, spherocytosis treatment, treatment of ischemic heart disease, breast cancer screening and treatment, and liver transplantation. Since 2004, there have been more examples of MDP applied to medical/clinical decision making, especially to patient decision-making models (patients usually make their decisions with their physicians). MDPs are well suited to these problems since a patient (with his/her physician) should make a decision, which not only has immediate effects but also influences the future outcomes and decisions. For example, Alagoz et al. (2004, 2007a,b) and Sandikci et al. (2008) develop MDP models to solve the liver acceptance problem, (Shechter et al. 2008) determines when to start HIV drug therapy, and (Kurt et al. 2008) use MDPs to determine lipid ratios to initiate the statin treatment for patients with type 2 diabetes.

An interesting MDP study comes from Shechter et al. (2008). The authors provide a framework to answer the question of "When to initiate HIV therapy?" Patients may choose to delay the therapy due to the side effects and toxicities related to the drugs as well as the potential of the virus to develop resistance to the therapy and thus severely limit the number of treatment options that remain available to the patient. However, the therapy cannot be delayed forever since there is a possibility of irrecoverable damage to the patient's immune system, the development of other AIDS-related problems and death. The authors develop a MDP model to find the optimal timing for the start of a therapy to maximize the expected lifetime (or quality-adjusted lifetime) of a patient. They think of the problem as an optimal stopping problem where the trade-off for a patient (and/or the patient's physician) is that the patient may choose to wait one more time period (e.g., 1 month) or start the HIV therapy and accept the expected remaining life associated with the patient's current health state (when initiating therapy). The authors provide structural properties to their optimal solution and solve with clinical data. Their results support the early treatment of HIV, which contradicts some of the recent trends toward later treatment.

Similar to Shechter et al. (2008), Kurt et al. (2008) investigates the initiation of statin treatment for patients with type 2 diabetes in order to maximize the patient's quality-adjusted lifetime before coronary heart disease (CHD) or stroke. Type 2 diabetes may have serious complications such as CHD and stroke. CHD and stroke are responsible for the majority of the diabetic deaths in the United States. Type 2 diabetes can multiply the patient's risks for CHD and stroke by fivefold. Therefore, in type 2 diabetes treatment decisions, CHD and stroke considerations play a crucial role. Statin-based cholesterol management has been clinically proven to decrease the risks of CHD and stroke (of type 2 diabetes patients). However, this statin treatment has significant side effects of its own such as pain in muscles and problems in the liver. Some other observed side effects are headaches, fever, fatigue, and memory loss. It is recommended that once a patient starts statin treatment she/he should stay with the treatment for the rest of her/his life. Therefore, initiating the statin treatment too soon may cause unnecessary and serious side effects while initiating treatment too late may be deadly. The authors formulate the problem as a MDP to balance the trade-off between adverse side effects and the benefits of statins. They derive structural properties (sufficient conditions for control limit treatment policies) to their model and perform computational experiments (with clinical data from the Mayo Clinic). They report results on two hypothetical patients, one male and one female. The numerical tests show that the optimal policy is of a control-limit type, and although the male patient's optimal treatment policy is more aggressive than the female's treatment policy, his quality-adjusted survival prior to his first terminal event is less than that of the female patient. We now go into detail on two specific applications: one management and one clinical.

Two MDP Applications

Healthcare Management: Multi-Priority Patient Scheduling

This application is based on research done by one of the authors, Jonathan Patrick, along with Martin Puterman and Maurice Queyranne. The research was published in *Operations Research* in December 2008 (Patrick et al. 2008). A less technical version was published in *Health Policy* in 2008 (Patrick and Puterman 2008). This research developed from an applied project (involving both authors) with a local hospital in Vancouver. The project was primarily concerned with capacity planning and patient flow through a CT department. The team provided the hospital with a detailed analysis of current

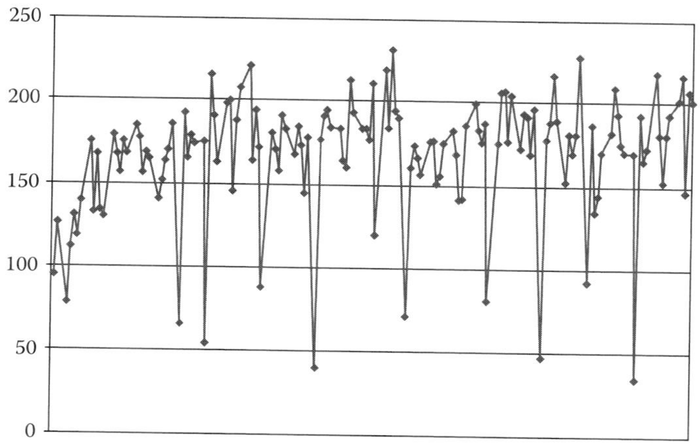

FIGURE 17.1 Variability in daily inpatient demand for CT scans.

wait times, demand, supply, and utilization. We provided a scenario analysis tool that compared the cost-effectiveness of various potential methods for increasing throughput with the recommendation that an additional CT tech be hired in order to cover breaks. What became apparent through the analysis was that the current scheduling system lacked consistency. Wait times even within the same priority class varied tremendously suggesting that insufficient planning resulted in varying levels of congestion. The variability in demand, as shown in Figure 17.1, demonstrates the significant potential of a more intelligent scheduling policy to improve efficiency. The research described in this section in more generality was designed to provide such a scheduling policy.

Problem

A common challenge facing healthcare managers is the allocation of a single resource to competing patient classes. For instance, consider a CT scanning department. Patient requisitions for a scan arrive daily and are classified by a radiologist according to urgency. A typical hospital will have a number of patient priority classes each one with a unique wait time target. The booking manager must therefore decide where in the booking horizon (how long in advance the radiology department books scans) to book the current waiting demand.

Such scheduling problems are classic SDPs as the booking decisions made today clearly impact on what booking decisions can be made tomorrow. In addition, there are at least two potential sources of uncertainty: the length of each scan and the rate of new demand. Clearly, in the multi-priority setting, a FCFS policy may not perform well as it will undoubtedly mean that some patients receive their scan very quickly while other clients may end up waiting beyond their wait time target. The challenge is to determine how much of a delay to give to lower priority demand in order to insure that there is always sufficient capacity for higher priority demand.

Model

To develop this into an MDP model, we provide some general notation. We assume that there are I priority classes and that the booking horizon is N days long. Decisions are assumed to be made once a day—once all demand for that day has arrived and been prioritized. Thus we are dealing with a discrete time, infinite horizon MDP. For ease of illustration, we assume that service times are deterministic and of equal length. (The model can be modified to remove these simplifications.)

To make a rational decision, the booking manager must know both the current state of the booking slate (i.e., how many clients are already booked into each day) as well as the current waiting demand in each priority class. Thus, we will define the state as $\vec{s} = (\vec{x}, \vec{y})$, where $\vec{x} = (x_1, \ldots, x_N)$ represents the number of clients already booked into each day and $\vec{y} = (y_1,\ldots, y_I)$ represents the number of waiting clients in each priority class.

The action consists of how many of each priority class to book into each day. We represent this by the vector $\vec{a} = (a_{11},\ldots, a_{IN})$, where a_{in} represents the number of priority i clients to book for a scan in n days. We assume that there is a fixed regular hour capacity (i.e., C clients can be booked into each day) and that there is a limited amount of overtime available. Thus, we will give the booking manager the ability to relieve any stress on the system by performing some scans through overtime. We let $\vec{z} = (z_1,\ldots, z_I)$ represent demand serviced through overtime. Actions are clearly constrained to not exceed capacity constraints (both regular and overtime) and not to exceed waiting demand (though it can be less than waiting demand representing the possibility of delaying the booking decision).

What makes this an infinite horizon MDP is that even though there is a finite number of days in advance that one can book, each day the booking slate rolls over with day N becoming day $N - 1$, day $N - 1$ becoming day $N - 2$ and so on. Day N therefore always starts off empty. We can represent the transition of the state by

$$(\vec{x};\vec{y}) \rightarrow \left(x_2 + \sum_{i=1}^{I} a_{i2},\ldots,x_N + \sum_{i=1}^{I} a_{iN},0; y_1 - \sum_{n=1}^{N} a_{1n} + y_1',\ldots,y_I - \sum_{n=1}^{N} a_{IN} + y_I' \right)$$

where y_i' represents new priority i demand. Thus, the only stochastic element in the transition is the new demand.

The last piece in defining this as an MDP is to determine the rewards/costs. Since we are seeking to determine an optimal schedule for meeting the wait time targets, there clearly needs to be a cost associated with booking a client beyond the wait time target. In addition, there is a cost associated with servicing clients with overtime and a cost associated with delaying the booking decision of a client. We represent the costs to the system as

$$c(\vec{s},\vec{a}) = \sum_{n=1}^{N}\sum_{i=1}^{I} b(i,n)[n - T(i)]^{+} a_{in} + \sum_{i=1}^{I} h(i)z_i + \sum_{i=1}^{I} f(i)\left(y_i - \sum_{n=1}^{N} a_{in} \right)$$

where

$T(i)$ is the wait time target for priority class i.

$b(i, n)$, $h(i)$, and $f(i)$ are the costs associated with booking, overtime, and delaying the booking decision, respectively.

Note that we are assuming a straight linear cost to overtime (each additional overtime client costs the same amount) and that there is zero cost associated with booking a client into any day up to the wait time target.

The challenge with attempting to solve this MDP is that it runs into the curse of dimensionality as the size of the state space is much too large for traditional MDP algorithms to solve. We thus are forced to resort to ADP that simplifies the problem by assuming that the value function in the MDP has a specific form. A common and usually quite successful approximation is to assume that the value function is linear in the state. That is

$$v(\vec{s}) = V_0 + \sum_{n=1}^{N} V_n x_n + \sum_{i=1}^{I} W_i y_i$$

The parameter V_n can be interpreted as the marginal cost of having an additional booking on day n and W_i as the marginal cost of having an additional priority i client waiting to be booked. We can then use the methods from ADP theory to solve for the optimal parameter values V_0, V_n, W_i in order to get the optimal linear value function approximation. This can be inserted into the optimality equation and used to determine the appropriate action for a given state.

Results

The policy that results from solving this MDP using ADP has an easily implementable form. For each priority class, it gives a booking window in which clients of that priority can be booked. The upper bound on that window is always the wait time target while the lower bound depends on a number of factors including demand rates for higher priority classes. Clients from each priority class are booked into the appropriate window starting from the closest day to the furthest away for the highest priority class but starting from the furthest day and moving forward to the closest for all other priority classes. This gives the booking manager the greatest flexibility in terms of insuring capacity that is available for the highest priority class while still meeting the targets of the lower priority classes. The solution to the model also gives a threshold priority class such that if a patient is from a priority class that is classified as more urgent than the threshold priority class and there is no scanning slot available in the appropriate booking window, then that client is serviced through overtime. (Should there not be sufficient overtime to service all eligible clients then the lower priority clients booking decision is delayed to tomorrow.) All other clients simply have their booking decision delayed should there be no capacity available in the appropriate booking window. Figure 17.2 gives a picture of the booking policy for a hospital with five priority classes. Day 0 represents overtime so that only the first three classes are ever served through overtime if required. All classes are potentially booked into day 1 as any capacity not used is lost by tomorrow. Otherwise, each class has a booking window, with the upper bound on the window being the wait time target for that class.

As a bonus, the researchers were also able to give a lower bound on the amount of overtime capacity required (for a given regular hour capacity) in order for this policy to remain the optimal policy based on the affine approximation of the value function. Failure to meet this lower bound meant that the wait time targets could not be met. The research also provides an upper bound on regular hour capacity above which the optimal policy switched to a FCFS policy simply because there was sufficient capacity for there to be no need to do anything more fancy. Thus, the MDP model turns out to provide both scheduling and capacity planning.

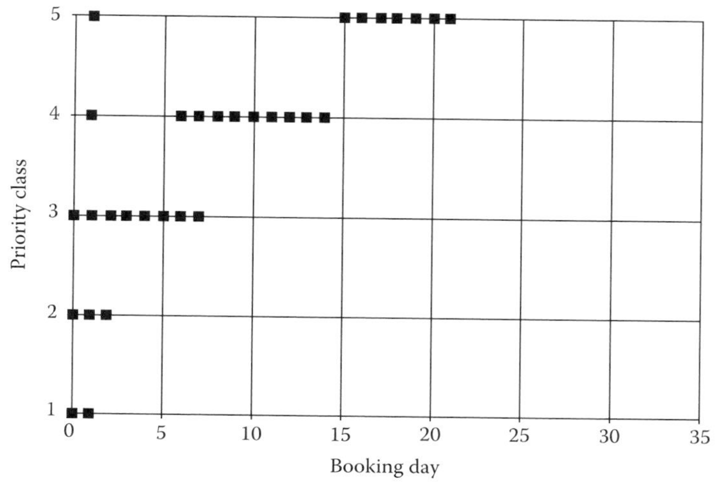

FIGURE 17.2 Booking windows for the multi-priority patient scheduling.

Challenges and Future Research

These type of scheduling and management challenges abound in healthcare. Surgical scheduling, for instance, would be another instance but in that case one clearly cannot rely on a deterministic service time and would also have to expand to include multiple surgical types as well as priority classes. Radiation treatment scheduling provides another twist on the problem. In this case, clients are booked not simply into one appointment but into a series of daily appointments that are not necessarily all of the same length. Clearly, the curse of dimensionality is a huge issue in these types of problems and thus the improvement of ADP theory becomes crucial to providing the healthcare community with better and more efficient scheduling policies.

Clinical Decision Making: Liver Transplantation Decision Models

Alagoz et al. (2004) developed a model to determine when to perform a living-donor liver transplantation to maximize the expected remaining life of a patient who has end-stage liver disease. Transplantation is the only viable therapy for these patients. Cadaveric liver supply is not sufficient to satisfy the increasing demand of livers for transplantation and hence living donors are becoming more important (and increasing) sources for patients with end-stage liver diseases. Liver has an exceptional ability to regenerate allowing a living donor to have his/her entire lobe implanted into a patient. The donor's liver reaches its previous size in a matter of weeks.

In this study, it is assumed that the patient does not receive any cadaveric offers, the donor (most likely a relative of the patient) is known, and the quality of the organ is constant during the horizon of the model. Moreover, it is also assumed that the transplantation carries no risks for the donor. The patient has to decide when to have the transplantation (if ever) given that there is always a liver (of known quality) available. An immediate transplant may not be the best option given the patient's health condition and the quality of the organ. As an example, if the patient is presently in good health and the organ quality is poor, it makes more sense to wait. On the other hand, if the patient's condition deteriorates and the quality of the organ is good then it may be better to do the operation immediately.

The authors developed an MDP model to solve this control problem. The model has states representing patient health, actions (transplant or wait), rewards (expected life expectancy based on a given action and state), and transition probabilities, which determine the state of the system in the next decision epoch. The objective is to choose the action that maximizes the life expectancy of the patient given the donor organ quality. By using this analysis, it is also possible to generate control policies to answer questions such as: (1) Given the quality of the organ, what is the threshold for a patient's health below which it is optimal to transplant? or (2) What is the minimum organ quality that will result in immediate transplantation for a specified health state of the patient?

The authors derive some structural properties of optimal policies for the model and provide numerical results based on real patient data. They compare different patients' and disease groups' optimal control policies. In their numerical tests, the optimal policy is of a control-limit type. In some cases, when the quality of liver is low, it is optimal for the patient to avoid transplantation entirely.

In a following paper (Alagoz et al. 2007a), the same authors consider the decision problem faced by patients who are on the cadaveric liver waiting list: should a liver offer be accepted or refused? There is a list of patients waiting for liver transplantation. The available organ is offered to a suitable patient in the waiting list but the transplant surgeon/patient can decline the organ offer without any penalty. It is mentioned in the paper that 45% of liver offers are declined by the first transplant surgeon/patient to whom they are offered. For a patient whose health is not very critical (and hence who can wait longer for transplantation), it may be better to wait for future offers if the quality of the current organ offer is low. Even for a more critical patient, if the future prospect for higher quality organs is very high, then it may still be better for the patient to wait. Given a particular patient with a current health state and organ offer, should she accept or reject the organ for transplantation? The answer to this question depends on the current patient heath, disease progression, quality of the current liver offer, and prospect for future organ offers.

Patients who are at the top of the waiting list are expected to be sicker but will also have more organ offers. All these factors as well as the uncertainty of future organ availability and quality make the cadaveric-donor case more complicated than the living-donor problem.

The authors formulate a MDP model where the state is given by the patient's health and the quality of the offered liver. They implicitly take into account the waiting list by allowing the liver arrival probabilities to depend on the patient's health (the sicker patient is more likely at the top of the list and hence will receive more offers). The decisions are either to accept the offer or to wait (for one more period). If the patient accepts the offer than she moves to the absorbing state of transplant and receives a reward based on the expected QALYs post-transplant. If the patient chooses to wait, then she receives an intermediate reward and the system moves to a new state based on the transition probabilities (which depend on the patient's health and the offered liver). As in the previous paper, the authors provide structural and computational results of their study. The model presented in Alagoz et al. (2004) is a special case of the model given in Alagoz et al. (2007a).

The authors combine the living donor and cadaveric donor problem into one in Alagoz et al. (2007b) to answer the following questions for a patient with end-stage liver disease with an available living donor: should the patient wait or have a liver transplantation now? If the patient goes for transplantation then should she use a cadaveric liver or the liver of the living donor? As in the previous papers, they formulate the problem as a MDP (in fact they extend the state space of Alagoz et al. (2007a) to include the living donor liver option), characterize the optimal policy, and perform computational experiments. They find conditions so that their optimal policies are of a "at-most-three-region" (AM3R) type. We can visualize this AM3R type of policy with a chart where one of the axis is patient health level and the other one is cadaveric organ quality, and the area of this chart is divided into three with line segments, and each separated area represents the conditions when it is optimal to choose precisely one of the three possible actions: wait, transplant with living donor, and transplant with cadaveric donor. A patient may use this chart to decide his/her optimal decisions given his/her health status and the cadaveric liver quality. The authors also include in their analysis a disutility factor if a living donor is used (this is due to the fact that most living donors are somehow related to the patient who receives the liver). This paper can be viewed as a generalization of Alagoz et al. (2004, 2007a).

In the studies of Alagoz et al. (2007a,b), one of the assumptions is that patients do not know their position in the waiting list. In reality, a patient may infer her position in the waiting list based on the number of organ offers in a time interval (the higher the number of organ offers, the more likely she is at the top of the list). The closer to the top of the waiting list the more selective the patient gets in accepting a liver. Sandikci et al. (2008) extends the Alagoz et al. (2007a) MDP model by including a patient's rank in the waiting list to estimate the price of privacy in the liver transplantation process. The authors define the price of privacy as the number of expected life days lost due to the lack of complete waiting list information. They estimate, with their clinical-based numerical studies, that the price of privacy is on the order of 5% of the optimal value—i.e., if patients knew the complete waiting list information they would improve their expected life expectancy by 5% on average. For example, patients who are close to the top of the list receive more frequent organ offers and hence may choose to be selective and wait for a higher quality organ if they knew their rank on the list. On the other hand, patients who are not at the top are not receiving that many organ offers and therefore may decide to accept an organ with a lower quality that otherwise they would have rejected.

The authors assume that patients optimize their own decisions without considering how other patients act. In reality, a patient's actions may be influenced by what other patients do. This calls for a game-theoretical approach and in our opinion would be a nice extension to the current literature.

Conclusion

MDP is a powerful and eminently suitable modeling approach to handle uncertainty in sequential decisions. As has been demonstrated above, such SDPs abound in healthcare. While the research described in this chapter has demonstrated significant success, there remain a number of challenges to the continued application of MDPs to healthcare.

One major challenge is the frequent scarcity of good data. Healthcare data systems are most often centered around clinical needs while failing to capture the necessary information to adequately answer managerial questions. It is often challenging to collect sufficient data to adequately determine the transition probability matrices or to get reasonable estimates for the reward functions. This problem is hardly unique to MDPs but plagues any attempt to apply quantitative methods within healthcare.

A second major challenge concerns the size of the SDPs that are often of interest in healthcare. Quite often the size of the state space makes traditional algorithms for solving MDPs intractable. Thus, the tools of ADP will, we believe, become crucial to the advancement of MDP applications in healthcare.

Most often in healthcare management in particular, decisions are based on a combination of experience and trial and error. These decisions are often based on insufficient evidence and are therefore often reactive in that they are responding to crises that have already appeared rather than proactively avoiding crisis. While expert opinion can often be quite good, it is rarely optimal and on occasion disastrously wrong. MDPs allow for greater advance planning as it is not necessary to guess at the impact of particular decisions regarding scheduling and capacity planning, for instance. It is one of the many tools that operations research can offer to the healthcare community in order to improve evidence-based decision making.

References

Adelman, D. 2005. Dynamic bid-prices in revenue management. *Operations Research* 55: 647–661.

Alagoz, O., L. M. Mailart, A. J. Schaefer, and M. S. Roberts. 2004. The optimal timing of living-donor liver transplantation. *Management Science* 50(10): 1420–1430.

Alagoz, O., L. M. Mailart, J. Schaefer, and M. S. Roberts. 2007a. Determining the acceptance of cadaveric livers using an implicit model of the waiting list. *Operations Research* 55(1): 24–36.

Alagoz, O., L. M. Mailart, A. J. Schaefer, and M. S. Roberts. 2007b. Choosing among living-donor and cadaveric livers. *Management Science* 53(11): 1702–1715.

Alterovitz, R., M. Branicky, and K. Goldberg. 2005. Constant-curvature motion planning under uncertainty with applications in image-guided medical needle steering. *Proceedings of the IEEE/RSJ International Conference on Intelligent Robots and Systems (IROS)* 1: 120–125.

Bellman, R. E. 1957. *Dynamic Programming*. Princeton, NJ: Princeton University Press.

Bertsekas, D. P. 2001. *Dynamic Programming and Stochastic Control*. Belmont, MA: Athena Scientific.

de Faris, D. and B. Van Roy. 2003. The linear programming approach to approximate dynamic programming. *Operations Research* 51: 850–865.

Feinberg, E. and A. Schwartz. 2002. *Handbook of Markov Decision Processes*. Boston, MA: Kluwer.

Gerchak, Y., D. Gupta, and M. Henig. 1996. Reservation planning for elective surgery under uncertain demand for emergency surgery. *Management Science* 42(3): 321–334.

Green, L., S. Savin, and B. Wang. 2006. Managing patient service in a diagnostic medical facility. *Operations Research* 54(1): 11–25.

Gupta, D. and L. Wang. 2008. Revenue management for a primary-care clinic in the presence of patient choice. *Operations Research* 56(3): 576–592.

Kolesar, P. 1970. A Markovian model for hospital admission scheduling. *Management Science* 16(6): 384–396.

Kurt, M., B. Denton, A. J. Schaefer, N. Shah, and S. Smith. 2008. At what lipid ratios should a patient with type 2 diabetes initiate statins? Working paper, available from http://www.ie.pitt.edu/~schaefer/ (accessed October 2009).

Patrick, J. and M. L. Puterman. 2008. Reducing wait times through operations research: Optimizing the use of surge capacity. *Healthcare Policy/Politiques de Sante* 3(3): 75–88.

Patrick, J., M. L. Puterman, and M. Queyranne. 2008. Dynamic multipriority patient scheduling for a diagnostic resource. *Operations Research* 56(6): 1507–1525.

Powell. W. B. 2007. *Approximate Dynamic Programming: Solving the Curses of Dimensionality*. Hoboken, NJ: John Wiley & Sons.

Puterman, M. 1994. *Markov Decision Processes*. New York: John Wiley & Sons.

Sandikci, B., L. M. Maillart, A. J. Schaefer, O. Alagoz, and M. S. Roberts. 2008. Estimating the patient's price of privacy in liver transplantation. *Operations Research* 56(6): 1393–1410.

Schaefer, A. J., M. D. Bailey, S. M. Shechter, and M. S. Roberts. 2004. Modeling medical treatment using Markov decision processes, in *Handbook of Operations Research/Management Science Applications in Health Care*, eds. M. Brandeau, F. Sainfort, and W. Pierskalla, pp. 597–616. Dordrecht, the Netherlands: Kluwer Academic Publishers.

Shechter, S. M., M. D. Bailey, A. J. Schaefer, and M. S. Roberts. 2008. The optimal time to initiate HIV therapy under ordered health states. *Operations Research* 56(1): 20–33.

Su, X. and S. Zenios. 2004. Patient choice in kidney allocation: The role of the queueing discipline. *MSOM* 6(4): 280–301.

Sutton, R. S. and A. G. Barto. 1998. *Reinforcement Learning: An Introduction*. Cambridge, MA: MIT Press.

Wu, J. T., L. M. Wein, and A. S. Perelson. 2005. Optimization of influenza vaccine selection. *Operations Research* 53(3): 456–476.

18

Statistical Analysis and Modeling

Min Zhang
Purdue University

Mark E. Cowen
St. Joseph Mercy Health System

Introduction 18-1
Background • Classical Statistical Approaches to Provider Profiling
Hierarchical Model and Bayesian Inference 18-5
Two-Part Hierarchical Model • Bayesian Inference • Summary Measure
Conclusion 18-13
Acknowledgment 18-13
References 18-14

Introduction

Background

Statistical analyses are becoming increasingly utilized within the healthcare industry whether the institution is considered academic or not, and whether the results of the analyses are published in the peer-reviewed literature or used solely for internal purposes. The structure of the analyses can vary depending on the type of question or vantage point of the requestor. For this chapter, we assume a health system, payor, or managed care-related organization is the decision maker and audience for the findings of a particular analysis, but similar efforts could be done to help individual patients or a group of clinicians in their decision making. We will describe issues and examples of analyses within two broad categories defined according to focus: those where the patient population and their outcomes are of primary interest, and those pertaining to comparisons of provider performance, commonly referenced as profiles or report cards. We will review some common statistical tests utilized within the healthcare industry, and conclude with a more detailed example of provider profiling to illustrate some of the concepts. This chapter cannot substitute for formal coursework in statistics and epidemiology, but should provide a context for applying previous lessons or motivation to pursue additional learning.

Before proceeding further, we note the choice of which statistical approach to take, or whether or not to perform a statistical test in the first place, depends on the question being asked and how the results may be applied for decision making in other settings or circumstances in the future. This is the concept of statistical inference. Not all quantitative questions in healthcare require statistical testing, nor will p values establish the veracity of the interpretation or application of the findings. For an example of a common question that does not require a test of statistical significance, consider a hospital wishing to know whether or not it achieved its financial target in the past fiscal year. The answer does not depend on whether $10,000 on either side of the target represents a statistically significant difference from the target or not. A similar example from outside the healthcare field is the relevance of a p value to the final outcome of an election if the challenger won by one or by 100,000 votes. In either of these scenarios, the answer can be known definitively at the end of the fiscal period or when the last ballot has been counted and statistical testing is not necessary. The opposite extreme of performing an unnecessary statistical test is over-relying on or over-interpreting the results. For example, consider the situation in which Hospital C has a lower mortality rate than Hospital D, and suppose the difference can be considered statistically significant. A low *p* value by itself in this circumstance is not sufficient to support a conclusion that patients were safer in Hospital C. Other information such as how severity of illness was addressed in the analysis is needed. Flaws in the design of analyses, even if performed strictly for internal purposes, should be addressed or acknowledged when interpreting the findings. In contrast, statistical testing is appropriate and may be helpful when attempting to answer the following types of questions: What can we expect of our financial performance next year in light of previous years' performance? Do the results of the preelection poll suggest one candidate would win if the election were held today? Is the difference in length of stay from last year due to chance or a more systematic influence? To what extent is the mortality rate explained by factors outside of our control, for example, the severity of the patients' illness on arrival? Does physician A's performance from last year suggest he will perform better than physician B next year?

The first category of analyses we are considering concerns a population of patients and their outcomes, and distinguishing the impact of an individual hospital or physician is unimportant. These studies can be multi-institutional as in the case of clinical trials, cohort and survival analyses, and will not be discussed further here. Similar analyses can also be conducted within an organization regarding its performance, and concern the understanding, and improvement of healthcare outcomes over time, be they financial or clinical. Here, techniques and approaches from clinical epidemiology can be useful. For an example, consider a hospital wishing to understand and improve the incidence of postsurgical infections. The risk or likelihood of a patient developing an infection might be expected to depend on the baseline level of health, the nature of the surgical procedure, and timing and types of antibiotics given. The outcome might also reflect the quality of the surgical and nursing care processes experienced. If the literature provides only a partial explanation for the underlying causes of infections, then a hospital might wish to conduct its own study, identifying additional, potential factors that could promote or prevent infections, and test the strength of the association using univariate and or multivariate statistical techniques. On the other hand, if all relevant factors were known and identified in the published literature on infections, then a hospital might simply track the proportion of its patients receiving the evidence-based processes of care. Hypothesis testing in this case might be performed to see if this year's performance, compared to last year's, represents a change over that expected by chance alone.

Some organizations prefer assessing improvement with a statistical process control approach using a graphical time series of data points rather than formal hypothesis testing. This approach is suitable if the main goal is to achieve a particular level of performance by continually refining and tracking the overall effect of a quality improvement project, rather than to elucidate the precise effect of the individual components of the intervention. We will touch upon this approach only briefly here. Two common and related statistical process control techniques are run and control charts (http://www.ihi.org/IHI/Topics/Improvement/ImprovementMethods; Wheeler and Chambers, 1992). Originally developed for the manufacturing industry, these charts are graphs of data over time, such as the proportion of patients prescribed a given preventive medication each month, the percent of operating room cases that start on time, the average hospital stay for patients each month, the total accounts receivable by month, or the number of falls on a nursing unit per month. Such time series of data points naturally follow a pattern, with data points usually falling near or on either side of a line indicating the average. The challenge is in understanding if the pattern merely represents chance fluctuations or demonstrates a more deliberate or predictable process. Evidence of variability, or a certain amount of change or deviation from what could be considered the average, occurs all the time within and without the healthcare industry (Blumenthal, 1994). The likelihood that the pattern of data points over time represents chance events, that is, the expected level of day-to-day variation, versus a true shift or trend in performance is determined by how many of the points fall on one side of the average line or the other, and how far a data point is from the average line (distance expressed in terms of "sigma" units or standard deviations) (Wheeler and Chambers, 1992). The underlying concept is similar to the card game of poker in which the value of a particular set of cards, such as being all spades or being in sequence of ascending order, is in indirect proportion to the probability of its occurrence.

The second general category of statistical analyses common in the healthcare industry concerns provider (generally physicians or hospitals) profiling or report cards. These can be generated for both intra and interinstitution purposes. An example of a hospital's internal profiling activities is the Joint Commission standard MS.08.01.03 requires the medical staff to assess the competence of its members, an initiative referenced as "ongoing physician performance evaluation" (Joint Commission, 2009). Examples of external comparisons of hospital performance include the publically reported performance measures for processes and outcomes of care for patients with acute myocardial infarction, heart failure, and pneumonia (see http://www.hospitalcompare.hhs.gov, accessed August 31, 2009), and various proprietary, comparative reports aimed to influence consumer choice. For any profiling activity, some type of decision rule is needed to distinguish good performance from bad, adequate from subpar. The decision rule can be a threshold, a line of demarcation that separates acceptable from unacceptable performance, as could be used for hospital mortality rates (Austin, 2002). Or, providers can be evaluated according to their comparative ranking relative to other providers on the outcome measure of interest (Austin, 2002). Importantly, the assessment of the same provider's performance can be different depending on which profiling approach used (Austin, 2002; Iezzoni, 2003). This suggests caution is needed when making decisions based on a single profiling report. The findings are more likely to be trustworthy if similar results are found in a series of reports, and if the underlying methodology is sound.

Because it is unlikely that all hospitals or physicians care for identical patient populations with the same severity and complexity level, risk adjustment techniques are often used to elucidate true performance differences. Usually the risk-adjusted outcome takes the form of an "O:E" ratio of the observed (i.e., the actual, unadjusted, "raw" or "crude") quantity of interest to that which would be expected (projected, derived, or attributed) based on the illness burden. For example, if a hospital's unadjusted mortality rate was 6.0% whereas that expected based on the case mix was 3.0%, then the O:E ratio would be 2, indicating the particular hospital had twice the mortality of that anticipated by the type and severity of illness of its patients. Conversely, if the hospital's actual mortality rate was 2.0%, then its ratio of 0.67 would indicate fewer outcomes than expected.

The risk adjustment process has two major components. The first is the choice of variables (covariates or comorbidities) that are taken into account when performing the risk or severity adjustment, such as, the age of the patient and the presence or absence of certain chronic diseases. The second aspect is the choice of statistical model or approach to use, which will be addressed in more detail later. Both components can impact the inference drawn from a risk-adjusted outcome. The interpretations of the O:E ratios (or similar summaries) often imply that all of the excess or reduced mortality in relation to that expected is attributable to the hospital or physician being profiled. However, the extent and adequacy of the risk adjustment may also impact the results. So, perhaps, a more practical question than whether the results have been risk adjusted or not, is the question of to what extent or how well the risk adjustment has been done. The answer can be complex but includes evaluating the appropriateness of the statistical approach used, measuring the extent to which the variability in the provider outcomes can be accounted for by the risk factors considered, and comparing results within strata of risk levels (Iezzoni, 2003). The underlying methodologies for provider profiles are increasing in sophistication, so some level of understanding of these approaches is needed by academic and nonacademic healthcare systems in order to understand and respond appropriately to the findings. A good reference for learning more about the practice and implications of risk adjustment is provided (Iezzoni, 2003).

For either population studies or profiling activities, the starting point for statistical testing is determined by the numerical property of the outcome of interest. Common outcomes in healthcare generally take the form of a binary variable or a continuous outcome. Binary variables take the value of yes or no, present or absent, pertaining to each unit of analysis (such as a patient), and can be summed for a group to yield a proportion or percent, such as the mortality, complication, or readmission rate. Common statistical tests for comparing binary outcomes include the chi-square test for testing the association between a single explanatory variable (such as time period) and a binary outcome (dead versus alive), and multivariable logistic regression to account for the effect of a number of potential influences on the outcome of interest such as age and coexisting illnesses. Common examples of continuous outcomes are hospital length of stay and cost per case. The common statistical tests for continuous outcomes will be described shortly. Although the outcomes mentioned above are straightforward, the choice and format of other healthcare outcomes may not be defined clearly by the requestor initially. Dialog is often needed with the analyst to refine and clarify the endpoint used to answer the clinical, managerial, or policy question. In addition to binary or continuous outcomes, another type of outcome is the time to an event, such as the time to relapse or the time to response to treatment, often labeled as survival analyses. These analyses are common in the peer-reviewed literature, particularly for clinical trials, but they are less commonly performed for routine, non-published reports within the industry.

Healthcare-related analyses pose a few particular challenges to the statistician. A number of statistical tests are based on assumptions that may not be applicable to the types of questions or analyses mentioned. Failure to account for or address exceptions to these assumptions can lead to erroneous conclusions. For example, a symmetrical, bell-shaped, or normal (also referenced sometimes as Gaussian) distribution is often assumed for continuous outcomes. In this circumstance, the most common occurrence (or highest point in the bell-shaped curve) is at or near the center or average value for the population of interest. If the outcome of interest is distributed in such a fashion, a common statistical test, the *t*-test, can be used to compare outcomes between two groups (e.g., between two time periods or between genders). If there is more than one explanatory variable to consider, then ordinary least squares regression may be used. However, healthcare costs or hospital stays do not generally follow the familiar bell-shaped form. Instead, the distribution of costs is lopsided or skewed to one end or the other because a proportionately small number of patients or procedures generate a disproportionate amount of the expenses or hospital stays. For this circumstance, the statistician either needs to use a test that does not assume the outcome follows a normal distribution (e.g., a nonparametric test such as the Wilcoxon sign rank test), or needs to transform the outcome (often done by taking the logarithm of costs or hospital stays, etc.) so that the resulting pattern more closely resembles the normal distribution. Use of an inappropriate test could impact the conclusion regarding the effectiveness of a program or the performance of a particular provider. Another assumption often violated in healthcare analyses is that the outcome for each unit of analysis (e.g., cost per patient) is independent of, unrelated, or not influenced by the outcomes of other units (e.g., costs incurred by other patients) in the study population. In fact, for many analyses, particularly those related to provider profiling, patients do share some common influences on their outcomes, for example, being cared for by the same physician, a situation often described as clustering. Performing a statistical analysis that incorrectly ignores clustering of cases also could lead to erroneous conclusions.

Classical Statistical Approaches to Provider Profiling

Ordinary Least Squares Regression

Ordinary least squares regression has been one of the most popular approaches in profiling physician performance (Salem-Schatz et al., 1994; Chang and McCracken, 1996; Fowles et al., 1996) because it can include variables representing the age and severity of illness of the patients. However, its use requires the assumption that the outcome variable (e.g., costs) is normally distributed, and that clustering (i.e., patients are nested within their primary care physicians) is not present. When used for physician profiling, an indicator variable for each physician can be included in the ordinary least squares model (Feinglass et al., 1991; Bryce et al., 2000), representing a *fixed effects regression.*

However, there are several issues for this fixed-effects approach. In addition to the confounded within- and between-physician effects, this model fails to account for the correlation structure of the data and is unable to incorporate any physician-specific characteristics that are often collected in real data (Normand et al., 1997; Hofer et al., 1999; Normand, 2008).

Random Effects Approach

As a further improvement, Cowen and Strawderman (2002) employed the mixed-effects model where the physician (i.e., cluster) effects are treated as random effects, that is, the physician effects are regarded as a random sample of the effects of all physicians in the entire population (i.e., the universe of physician's past, present, future, even those not represented in the particular dataset). The relative contribution to pharmacy costs attributable to a physician's practice style is represented by an intercept for each physician in the equation, with the intercept representing the "average" physician assigned a value of zero. These random effects can be further decomposed into effects attributable to specific physician characteristics and to random error. Correspondingly, the intraclass correlation coefficient was used to measure the extent of the variability between physicians relative to the overall variability in total pharmacy costs among the patients (Cowen and Strawderman, 2002). Results from the two population showed that the range of intraclass correlation coefficients was rather low (Cowen and Strawderman, 2002), suggesting differences in physician prescribing habits played a minor role in the differences in pharmacy expenditures for the patients. Other studies also presented the low range of intraclass correlation coefficient in similar settings (Sixma et al., 1998; Hofer et al., 1999; Beaulieu et al., 2001). Cowen and Strawderman (2002) detailed the comparisons of the ordinary least squares regression, fixed-effects model, and random-effects approach.

Hierarchical Model and Bayesian Inference

As shown in the data presented by Cowen and Strawderman (2002), the pharmacy expenditure data for a managed care population usually have a large percentage of patients with zero pharmacy costs and a small number with very high expenses, in addition to the clustered nature of the data. Such properties prevent us from using the classical linear (i.e., ordinary least square) regression models. Ignoring the fact that a sizeable number of patients have zero expenses may throw away information about physician's performance and bias the corresponding estimation. It is preferable to employ a different and more appropriate model that takes into account the zero inflated data, for example, a two-part hierarchical model consisting of two levels. The first or patient level has two parts, the first part models the initial decision by a physician to prescribe drugs or not for the patient, the second part of the model examines the intensity of the prescribing (given a prescription has been written) due to multiple or expensive medications. The second or physician level of this model incorporates physician characteristics such as gender that may influence prescribing patterns (Zhang, 2003; Zhang et al., 2006).

Two-Part Hierarchical Model

Suppose that the pharmacy cost data are available from a total of M physicians, let Z_{ij} be the observed cost of patient j within physician i, and X_{ij} be the patient characteristics such as age and the presence or absence of diabetes or heart disease, where $i = 1, \ldots, M$ and $j = 1, \ldots, n_i$. Further, let W_i represent the vector of physician specific characteristics. To account for the zero-inflated nature of the cost data, we assume that

$$Z_{ij} = I\left(Y_{ij}^{(1)} > 0\right) \times \exp\left(Y_{ij}^{(2)}\right),$$

where $Y_{ij}^{(1)}$ and $Y_{ij}^{(2)}$ represent the two latent variables that are not observed. In essence, $Y_{ij}^{(1)}$ represents the tendency to write (or not write) a prescription for the condition, and $Y_{ij}^{(2)}$ represents the expense of the prescriptions written. As a function of $Y_{ij}^{(1)}$ and $Y_{ij}^{(2)}$, Z_{ij} is zero if $Y_{ij}^{(1)} \le 0$ and equals to $\exp(Y_{ij}^{(2)})$ if $Y_{ij}^{(1)} > 0$.

The first level is to model the cost at the patient level (using the two components above), where we adjust the patient characteristics as well as the random effects from individual physicians. More specifically, we have

$$\begin{cases} Y_{ij}^{(1)} = \beta_0^{(1)} + \gamma_i^{(1)} + \beta^{(1)} X_{ij}^{(1)} + \varepsilon_{ij}^{(1)} \\ Y_{ij}^{(2)} = \beta_0^{(2)} + \gamma_i^{(2)} + \beta^{(2)} X_{ij}^{(2)} + \varepsilon_{ij}^{(2)}, \end{cases}$$

where $\gamma_i^{(1)}$ and $\gamma_i^{(2)}$ represent how far the performance of the ith physician deviates from that of an average physician, represented by the values of $\beta_0^{(1)}$ and $\beta_0^{(2)}$ in each part, respectively, $\beta^{(1)}$ and $\beta^{(2)}$ are the parameters (i.e., the cost weights) corresponding to the patient characteristics $X_{ij}^{(1)}$ and $X_{ij}^{(2)}$ that may differ in the two parts. For the two error terms in both parts, we further assume

$$\begin{pmatrix} \varepsilon_{ij}^{(1)} \\ \varepsilon_{ij}^{(2)} \end{pmatrix} \sim N\left(\begin{pmatrix} 0 \\ 0 \end{pmatrix}, \begin{pmatrix} 1 & 0 \\ 0 & \sigma_e^2 \end{pmatrix} \right).$$

Note that the variance of $\varepsilon_{ij}^{(1)}$ is set to be 1 for identifiability, and the variance of $\varepsilon_{ij}^{(2)}$ is σ_e^2.

In the second level of the hierarchical model, the physicians' effects are partitioned into systematic effects and random effects, where the former is modeled via physicians' characteristics and the latter is modeled by putting a distribution on the random error term

$$\begin{pmatrix} \gamma_i^{(1)} \\ \gamma_i^{(2)} \end{pmatrix} \sim N\left(\begin{pmatrix} \alpha^{(1)} W_i^{(1)} \\ \alpha^{(2)} W_i^{(2)} \end{pmatrix}, V \right).$$

Here $W_i^{(1)}$ and $W_i^{(2)}$ are the characteristics of physician i (e.g., physician age, physician gender) and they are allowed to be different. V is a positive definite matrix and its non-diagonal elements may not be zero if $\gamma_i^{(1)}$ and $\gamma_i^{(2)}$ are not independent.

Bayesian Inference

There are two major approaches for statistical inference, one is the frequentist approach (examples include the chi-square and t-tests mentioned previously) and the other is called Bayesian approach (Bolstad, 2007; Koch, 2007). Due to the recent advances in computing, Bayesian approach is emerging as an effective alternative to frequentist methods for data analysis in a variety of fields (Carlin and Louis, 2000). As shown in Normand et al. (1997), Bayesian approach has certain advantages in physician profiling. For example, we can obtain both the point estimate of the parameters (i.e., $\beta^{(1)}$ and $\beta^{(2)}$ in the model) and the uncertainty associated with the point estimate for each parameter in the model. Such uncertainty is important to account for when assessing performance. In addition, any prior information can be formally incorporated into the statistical model. Therefore, we employed Bayesian inference for the two-part hierarchical model defined above.

Unlike the frequentist approach, Bayesian analyses incorporate prior knowledge or beliefs regarding a hypothesis along with the information contained in the dataset being analyzed. Essentially, this means that the estimate of a particular parameter (such as the impact of patient age or physician performance) obtained from the posterior distribution of the Bayesian inference, reflects the updated information of the prior beliefs (i.e., what this parameter's value is likely to be) using the information extracted from the actual dataset (i.e., the observed data). With Bayesian inference, both the observed data and parameters of interest (e.g., $\beta^{(1)}$ and $\beta^{(2)}$ in the example above representing the relative cost weights of patient age or other risk factors) are considered random variables drawn from their corresponding distributions. To understand this in a general sense, conceptualize a graph of values where the possible values are on the horizontal axis and the proportion of the population having those values is on the vertical axis. This represents the distribution of the parameters of interest. Therefore, we need a statistical model to model the observed data, and specify the prior distributions (i.e., the starting points based on previous studies or assumptions) regarding the parameters of interest. Then, the estimation of parameters can be obtained from the posterior distribution.

For example, let $z = (z_1, \ldots, z_n)$ be the observed data and θ be the parameters of interest to be estimated. Further, let $P(z|\theta)$ represent the likelihood of observing the dataset z given θ were the true parameters, and $\pi(\theta|\eta)$ be the prior belief regarding the distributions for the parameters θ. Then, the posterior distribution $p(\theta|z)$ for the parameters θ, can be obtained using Bayes' theorem

$$p(\theta|z) = \frac{p(\theta,z)}{p(z)} = \frac{\int p(z,\theta,\eta)d\eta}{\iint p(z,\theta,\eta)d\eta d\theta} = \frac{\int p(z|\theta)\times\pi(\theta|\eta)\times g(\eta)d\eta}{\iint p(z|\theta)\times\pi(\theta|\eta)\times g(\eta)d\eta d\theta}.$$

In essence, the equation says the posterior probability distributions are proportional to the product of the prior distributions and the likelihood function. Therefore, to estimate the parameters through their posterior distributions as shown above, one needs to specify the prior distributions (i.e., the probability distribution representing the prior belief of the parameter) for the parameter θ and hyperparameters η using the functional form of $\pi(\theta|\eta)$ and $g(\eta)$. Then, the integrations involved in both numerator and denominator can be performed using a computer-based sampling method.

To avoid inappropriately influencing the posterior results $p(\theta|z)$ due to the choices of distribution functions and the corresponding parameter values for the prior distributions, "non-informative priors" are employed in the following analyses. More specifically, a normal distribution with a mean of zero and variance of one million, $N(0, 10^6)$ is specified for all the β parameters (including $\beta_0^{(1)}, \beta^{(1)}, \beta_0^{(2)}, \beta^{(2)}$), inverse Wishart (diag(10,10),2) is chosen for the variance–covariance matrix V, and the prior for σ_e^2 is its conjugate prior, inverse Gamma, with both shape and scale parameters as 10^{-3}. Statistical inferences are performed using Markov chain Monte Carlo method. The package BUGs (Bayesian inference Using Gibbs Sampling) written by Spiegelhalteret al. (2000) was employed for implementation. For each parameter, we can get the following outputs from BUGs: the density of the posterior distribution, the summary statistics (e.g., mean, median, standard deviation) of the posterior distribution, as well as information to evaluate the convergence of the Markov chain such as time series plots and autocorrelation plots. In addition, the convergence was evaluated using CODA (Best et al., 1996) using the samples drawn from the Markov chain.

Summary Measure

On the basis of the two-part hierarchical model, we proposed a summary measure, namely physician-explained variation (*PEV*) to evaluate and quantify the physician's contribution to variations of the total pharmacy cost.

Let $\theta_i = (\gamma_i^{(1)}, \gamma_i^{(2)})^T$ and $T = \sum_{i=1}^{M}\sum_{j=1}^{n_i} Z_{ij}$ be the total observed cost, where Z_{ij} is assumed to follow the two-part hierarchical model previously described. Then, we propose to construct

$$\text{PEV} = \frac{\text{Var}(E[T\,|\,\theta_1,\ldots,\theta_M])}{\text{Var}(T)}$$

as a measure of the contribution of all physicians to the variation in the total cost T. Given the fact that the physicians are assumed to be independent and that, for $j \neq k$, Z_{ij} and Z_{ik} are independent conditional on θ_i, we have

$$\text{PEV} = \frac{\sum_{i=1}^{M} \text{Var}\left(\sum_{j=1}^{n_i} E\left[Z_{ij}|\theta_i\right]\right)}{\sum_{i=1}^{M} \text{Var}\left(\sum_{j=1}^{n_i} E\left[Z_{ij}|\theta_i\right]\right) + \sum_{i=1}^{M}\sum_{j=1}^{n_i} E\left[\text{Var}\left(Z_{ij}|\theta_i\right)\right]}.$$

Note that all expectations and variances are conditional on the model parameters.

The numerator of *PEV* is the variance of the conditional expectation of the total cost given the vector of physician random effects, and thus is intended to capture the "between physician" component of the variation, and correspondingly, the denominator is the variance of the total cost (consisting of the variability between physicians and among patients within the physicians' practices). The proposed *PEV* measure appears to be useful in an asymptotic sense provided that $M \to \infty$ and n_i with $i = 1, \ldots, M$ remain bounded. This assumption is reasonable in a managed care context since a physician serving patients in an health maintenance organization (HMO) will eventually limit the enrollment. However, *PEV* as proposed may represent a less reasonable measure in other situations. For example, when the panel size within a cohort varies significantly, the estimation of the *PEV* might be dominated by those physicians with large number of patients. To avoid this issue, it is worth to consider alternatives. A potentially interesting class of measures is provided by the following averaged *PEV* (*APEV*):

$$\text{APEV} = \frac{1}{M}\sum_{i=1}^{M} w_i \sum_{j=1}^{n_i} \frac{\text{Var}\left(E\left[Z_{ij}|\theta_i\right]\right)}{\text{Var}(Z_{ij})}$$

where $w_1, \ldots, w_M$ are the non-negative weights for each physician. Note that *APEV* reduces to the intraclass correlation coefficient in the mixed model (Cowen and Strawderman, 2002) if $w_i = 1/n_i$ is chosen. In the case that a summary measure independent of both i and j is preferred, one can take some kind of average as defined in the *APEV*. Besides $w_i = 1/n_i$, other choices for the weight can be taken in different situations. Our analyses here are performed on the basis of $w_i = 1/n_i$.

In terms of the significance of the results, if *PEV* is high, it might be worthwhile for healthcare managers to emphasize interventions focused on the physician in order to reduce the pharmacy expenditures. On the other hand, if *PEV* is low, other potential patient-level factors such as the type and severity of the diseases or conditions may play an important role, so investigating and attenuating those potential factors when possible might be helpful.

Case Study

DATA

The case study is set in a physician hospital organization in the late 1990s that contracted with a local HMO to provide all necessary healthcare services on a fixed budget. This arrangement meant the organization would incur the financial risk (or gain) relative to budget for an approximately 100,000 member population. Pharmacy costs represented a sizeable and increasing portion of the total expenditures and therefore, an important area of financial risk. This motivated analyses to understand the underlying causes of the pharmacy expenditures and to inform the design of interventions to control them. Because the medications paid for by the health plan required the authorization of a physician, a goal of the project was to create a performance-based incentive program for physicians that would encourage cost-effective prescribing. The incentive in this instance represents a consequence or application of the profiling exercise. The illness burden of the patients was taken into account. Diseases or conditions likely to require medical therapy were identified and grouped into clinically relevant categories to serve as risk-adjustment covariates. The unit of analysis in the dataset was a managed care patient, the outcome of interest was the pharmacy expenditures for the year for that patient, and the potential explanatory variables were patient age, gender, the presence or absence of the disease categories of interests, the assigned primary care physician, and the corresponding physician's age, gender, and time from graduation from medical school.

STATISTICAL INFERENCE

To fit the Bayesian two-part hierarchical model, WinBUGs (version 1.3) was employed with the non-informative prior distributions described previously. The initial values of intercepts and coefficients of all covariates were set to zero. The initial value of σ_e^2 is 10^3 and an identity matrix is used as initial value for the variance–covariance matrix *V*. Results showed that the inferences were robust to other choices of initial values. On the basis of the convergence diagnostics, we found that it is sufficient to discard the first 10,000 samples of the chain (burn-in period), and saved the following 10,000 samples for inference.

RESULTS

For all parameters in both parts of the model, Table 18.1 shows the posterior mean and its standard deviation, as well as the 95% credible interval.

Although the ultimate goal of the project was to derive an incentive program for physicians based on their prescribing habits, the parameter values for the risk-adjusting covariates (Table 18.1) also provide important information to the organization. As expected, all nine covariates describing the patients' disease types have positive effect on the pharmacy cost because medications are often used to treat these conditions (it would be highly unusual that the presence of any of diseases would make a patient less likely to receive a prescription). In addition, the older patients are more prone to be sick and thus incur more expenditures than younger ones. Surprisingly, the patients of female physicians have higher pharmacy costs than those of male physicians. A possible explanation would be that female physicians tend to care for a higher proportion of female patients who are more likely to generate higher pharmacy costs than male patients. However, the interaction between patient gender and physician gender is not significant if we include it in the model. Therefore, it would be worthwhile for healthcare managers for this organization to further investigate the possible reasons for higher expenditures associated with female physicians.

There does not seem to be much differences among the parameter values for the different types of diseases in part I of the model, the tendency of these to be treated with medications (as opposed to being managed by some other modality). A healthcare organization could use the part I results to examine the appropriateness of medication use within these categories or identify areas where prescriptions might not be needed. In contrast to part I, however, we observed a wide range in the values of the parameter coefficients in part II, reflecting the quantity and expense of prescriptions written for these conditions. This indicates that the pharmacy expenditures attributed to some diseases, such as affective disorders, a neuropsychiatric diagnosis, epilepsy, or HIV condition, and

TABLE 18.1 Results for the Two-Part Hierarchical Model Estimation

Variable	Parameter	Mean (SD)	95% CI
Infection	$\beta_1^{(1)}$	0.78 (0.01)	(0.76, 0.81)
Diabetes	$\beta_2^{(1)}$	0.49 (0.03)	(0.43, 0.56)
Affective disorders	$\beta_3^{(1)}$	0.58 (0.04)	(0.49, 0.67)
A neuropsychiatric diagnosis, epilepsy, or HIV condition	$\beta_4^{(1)}$	0.47 (0.07)	(0.33, 0.61)
Anxiety	$\beta_5^{(1)}$	0.50 (0.03)	(0.43, 0.56)
Hypertension and/or hyperlipdemia	$\beta_6^{(1)}$	0.48 (0.02)	(0.44, 0.52)
Coronary artery disease or heart failure	$\beta_7^{(1)}$	0.22 (0.05)	(0.13, 0.31)
Asthma, COPD, or allergic rhinitis	$\beta_8^{(1)}$	0.59 (0.03)	(0.54, 0.65)
Collagen vascular disease	$\beta_9^{(1)}$	0.55 (0.09)	(0.38, 0.73)
Age (patient)	$\beta_{10}^{(1)}$	0.01 (0.00)	(0.01, 0.01)
Gender (physician)	$\alpha_1^{(1)}$	−0.15 (0.03)	(−0.21, −0.09)
Infection	$\beta_1^{(2)}$	0.37 (0.02)	(0.34, 0.40)
Diabetes	$\beta_2^{(2)}$	0.98 (0.03)	(0.92, 1.04)
Affective disorders	$\beta_3^{(2)}$	1.20 (0.04)	(1.12, 1.27)
A neuropsychiatric diagnosis, epilepsy, or HIV condition	$\beta_4^{(2)}$	1.25 (0.06)	(1.12, 1.38)
Anxiety	$\beta_5^{(2)}$	0.76 (0.03)	(0.70, 0.82)
Hypertension and/or hyperlipdemia	$\beta_6^{(2)}$	0.67 (0.02)	(0.63, 0.70)
Coronary artery disease or heart failure	$\beta_7^{(2)}$	0.62 (0.04)	(0.54, 0.69)
Asthma, COPD, or allergic rhinitis	$\beta_8^{(2)}$	0.79 (0.03)	(0.74, 0.84)
Collagen vascular disease	$\beta_9^{(2)}$	1.33 (0.07)	(1.19, 1.47)
Age (patient)	$\beta_{10}^{(2)}$	0.04 (0.00)	(0.04, 0.04)
Gender (physician)	$\alpha_1^{(2)}$	−0.18 (0.04)	(−0.26, −0.11)
$\mathrm{Var}\left(\gamma_i^{(1)}\right)$	V_{11}	0.02 (0.00)	(0.01, 0.02)
$\mathrm{Var}\left(\gamma_i^{(2)}\right)$	V_{22}	0.03 (0.01)	(0.02, 0.04)
$\mathrm{Corr}\left(\gamma_i^{(1)}, \gamma_i^{(2)}\right)$	ρ	0.76 (0.07)	(0.60, 0.87)
Random error	σ_e^2	2.34 (0.02)	(2.31, 2.37)

Source: Reprinted from Zhang, M. et al., *J. Am. Stat. Assoc.*, 101, 934. With permission.

Notes: The superscript $^{(1)}$ represents the first part of the model, the tendency that the condition(s) of a patient requires a prescription. The superscript $^{(2)}$ represents the second part of the model, the expense of the prescriptions written for the conditions of interest.

collagen vascular disease are much higher than for other diseases, such as infection and heart-related conditions. A healthcare organization might recommend cost-effective medication regimens for some of the more expensive conditions, or examine the areas closely for redundancy or overlap in the types of prescriptions written. The results also indicate a high degree of correlation between the two random terms, indicating physicians who are likely to write a prescription for a particular condition are also likely to prescribe more intensely for that condition (either due to issuing more prescriptions, more refills, or prescribing relatively more expensive medications than average).

Understanding the sources that contribute to the observed variation and representing their contributions quantitatively is one of the major issues in healthcare, and the results can be used to serve as the basis to further improve the strategy. For the two-part hierarchical model, we defined

TABLE 18.2 Estimation of PEV and APEV

Parameter	Integration Method	Mean	SD	Median
PEV	Simpson	0.396	0.033	0.396
	Gauss–Hermite	0.417	0.032	0.416
APEV ($W_i = 1/n_i$)	Simpson	0.011	0.001	0.011
	Gauss–Hermite	0.011	0.001	0.011

PEV and *APEV* to estimate the percentage of variability in the total cost that can be explained by the physician effect. As there is no closed form for the calculation for either *PEV* or *APEV*, two numerical methods were employed for approximation, that is, Gauss–Hermite integration and Simpson's rule. We used 10 points for Gauss–Hermite integration and 21 points for Simpson's rule. The results are shown in Table 18.2.

Note that *APEV* is much smaller than *PEV*, and the estimates using two methods are quite close. The distributions of *PEV* and *APEV* are shown in Figure 18.1. The *APEV* is similar to the ICC in Cowen and Strawderman (2002), and indicates that variability in prescribing habits among the physicians in this organization is fairly small relative to the widely varying level of pharmacy expenditures at the patient level. Physicians appear to be prescribing in a similar fashion and intensity. An implication of this finding is that the healthcare organization needs more than an incentive program aimed at individual physician prescribing to manage its growing expenses.

Each physician' performance index can be calculated using the samples drawn from the parameter chains, and correspondingly, ranking these physicians on the basis of performance indices provides a rank chain for each physician as discussed in Zhang et al. (2006). The mean

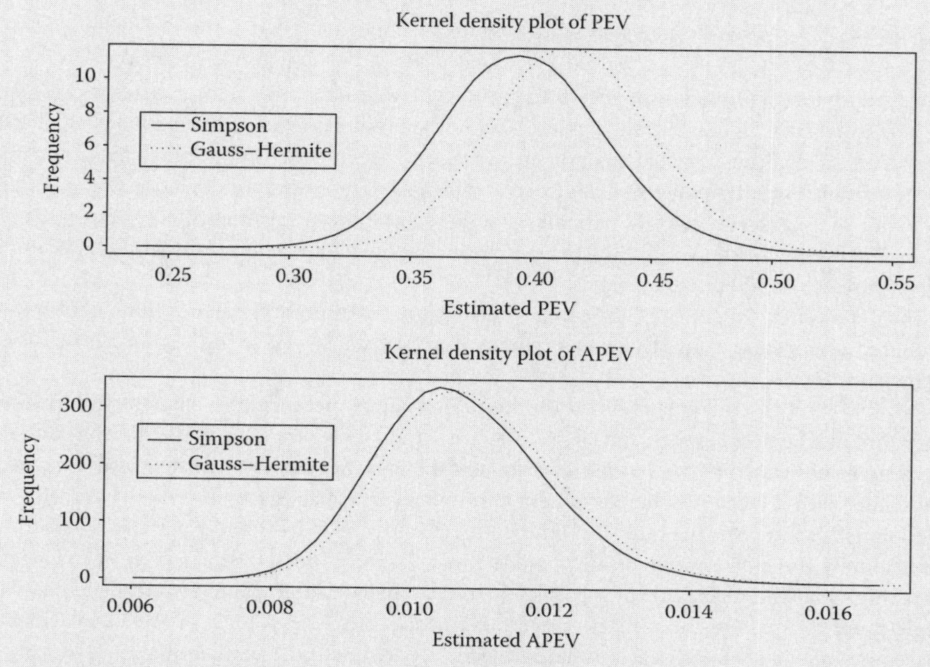

FIGURE 18.1 Posterior distribution of PEV and APEV.

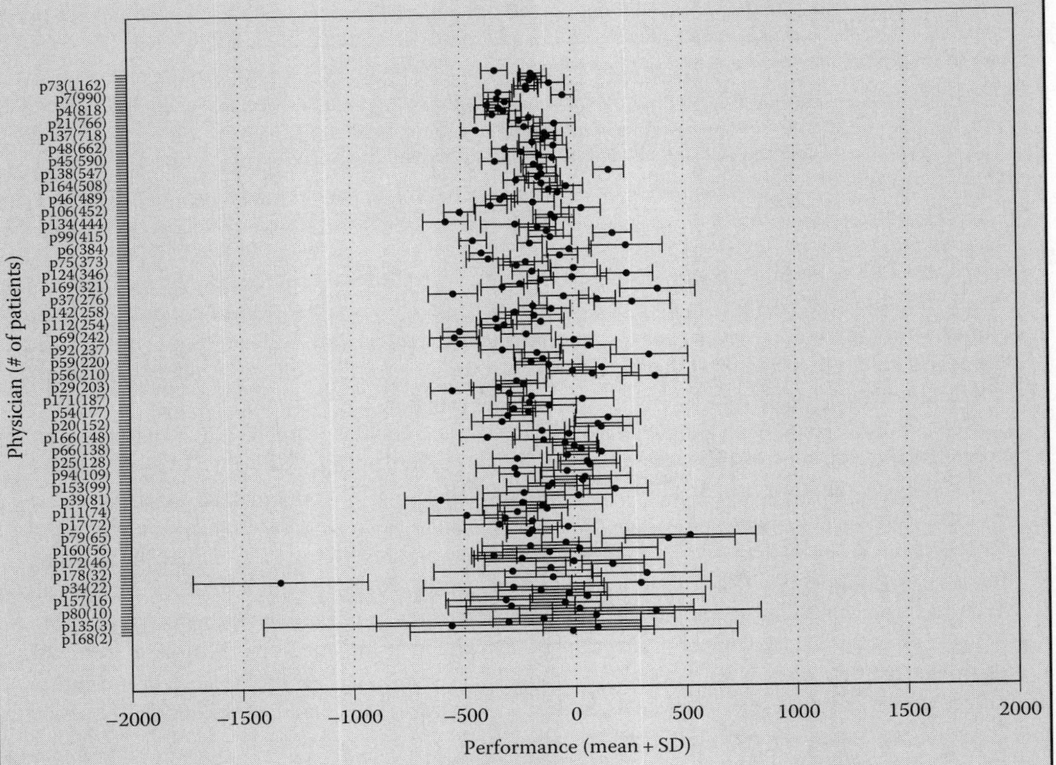

FIGURE 18.2 Performance plot for all physicians.

performance for all physicians is shown in Figure 18.2 where for *y*-axis, the physicians are sorted by their panel size. Figure 18.2 shows that most of the physicians' risk-adjusted, per-patient costs are within $500 of the expected cost for the average physician, and that the extremes are usually physicians with smaller panel size and correspondingly, large standard deviations. For example, physician 34, who serves only 22 patients, generated $1330 less per patient than the average physician. As a result of the wide standard deviation, one needs to be careful when evaluating the physicians with smaller panel sizes.

The *x*-axis shows the mean (indicated by dot) ± the corresponding standard deviation of the estimated performance, and the *y*-axis represents the physician ID with the number of patients in the parenthesis.

We also rank the physicians based on the performance measure (i.e., smaller rank indicates better financial performance), and the results are shown in Figure 18.3. Note that the rank does not seem to be related to the sample size, though the variance of the estimated rank is small for physicians with a large number of patients and vice versa. Especially for physicians with very small panel size, such as the ranks for physicians 135 and 168 (with 3 and 2 patients, respectively) cover almost the entire range of all possible ranks (1–180), indicating the level of uncertainty regarding what the true rank of a particular physician is. Making inference on the basis of a single point estimate of the rank is dangerous in this case. As Bayesian inference provides the uncertainty associated with each estimated rank, we will be more confident about the rank for physicians with large panel size. Furthermore, we can increase the number of samples in Gibbs sampling in order to estimate the rank with a desirable accuracy.

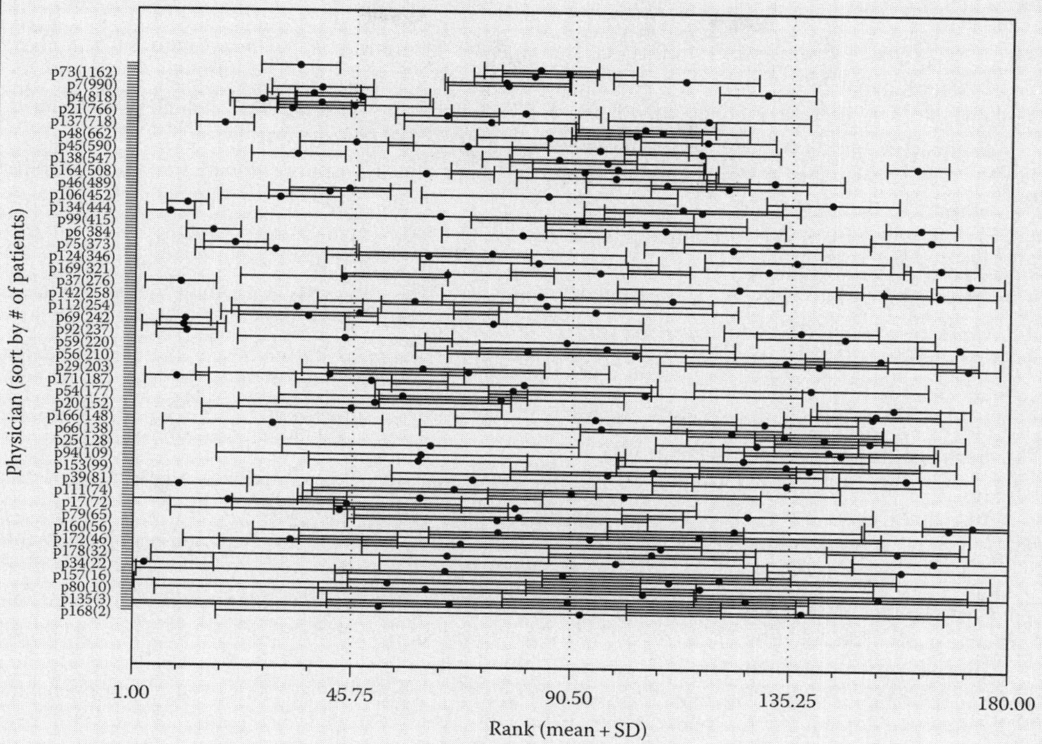

FIGURE 18.3 Rank plot for all physicians.

The x-axis shows the mean (indicated by dot) ± the corresponding standard deviation of the estimated rank, and the y-axis represents the physician ID with the number of patients in the parenthesis.

Conclusion

Healthcare organizations have the dual challenge of improving the quality and effectiveness of the care delivered in the face of staggering costs. The management decisions within this high-stakes environment will become increasingly dependent on appropriate and valid inferences from data. Useful statistical approaches can range from fairly simple hypothesis testing and the charting of performance measures over time to sophisticated multilevel regression models that account for the non-normal distribution of outcomes in addition to clustering. For an example of the latter as a step in the profiling process, we presented a two-part hierarchical model to fit the clustered, highly skewed, and zero-inflated pharmacy expenditure data of a managed care organization. The fully Bayesian inference was employed to obtain the posterior distributions of the model parameters, the summaries derived from them, and rankings of physicians. The summary measures, *PEV* and *APEV*, are defined to quantify the physician contribution to the total cost variability. Attention to the appropriate statistical assumptions and modeling increases the likelihood that the results and inferences are valid and can be trusted.

Acknowledgment

Part of the work is Min Zhang's thesis under supervision of Drs. Robert Strawderman and Martin Wells from Cornell University.

References

Austin, P.C. 2002. A comparison of Bayesian methods for profiling hospital performance. *Med. Decis. Making* 22:163–172.

Beaulieu, M.-D., R. Blais, A. Jacques, R.N. Battista, R. Lebeau, and J. Brophy. 2001. Are patients suffering from stable angina receiving optimal medical treatment? *QJM* 94:301–308.

Best, N., M.K. Cowles, and K. Vines. 1996. Convergence diagnosis and output software for Gibbs sampling output. Version 0.40.

Blumenthal, D. 1994. The variation phenomenon in 1994. *N. Engl. J. Med.* 331:1017–1018.

Bolstad, W.M. 2007. *Introduction to Bayesian Statistics*, 2nd edn. Wiley-Interscience, Hoboken, NJ.

Bryce, C.L., J.B. Engberg, and D.R. Wholey. 2000. Comparing the agreement among alternative models in evaluating HMO efficiency. *Health Serv. Res.* 35:509–528.

Carlin, B.P. and T.A. Louis. 2000. *Bayes and Empirical Bayes Methods for Data Analysis*, 2nd edn. Chapman and Hall/CRC, Boca Raton, FL.

Chang, W. and S.B. McCracken. 1996. Applying case mix adjustment in profiling primary care physician performance. *J. Health Care Finance* 22:1–9.

Cowen, M.E. and R.L. Strawderman. 2002. Quantifying the physician contribution to managed care pharmacy expenses: A random effects approach. *Med. Care* 40:650–661.

Fowles, J.B., J.P. Weiner, D. Knutson, E. Fowler, A.M. Tucker, and M. Ireland. 1996. Taking health status into account when setting capitation rates. *JAMA* 276:1316–1321.

Hofer, T.P., R.A. Hayward, S. Greenfield, E.H. Wagner, S.H. Kaplan, and W.G. Manning. 1999. The unreliability of individual physician "report cards" for assessing the costs and quality of care of a chronic disease. *JAMA* 281:2098–2105.

Iezzoni, L.I. 2003. *Risk Adjustment for Measuring Health Care Outcomes*, 3rd edn. Health Administration Press, Chicago, IL.

Joint Commission Resources Accreditation Manual Plus, http://amp.jcrinc.com (accessed September 21, 2009).

Koch, K.R. 2007. *Introduction to Bayesian Statistics*, 2nd edn. Springer, Berlin, Germany.

Normand, S.L. 2008. Some old and some new statistical tools for outcomes research. *Circulation* 118:872–884.

Normand, S.L., M.E. Glickman, and C.A. Gatsonis. 1997. Statistical methods for profiling providers of medical care: Issues and applications. *J. Am. Stat. Assoc.* 92:803–814.

Salem-Schatz, S., G. Moore, M. Rucker, and S.D. Pearson. 1994. The case for case-mix adjustment in practice profiling. *JAMA* 272:871–874.

Sixma, H.J., P.M. Spreeuwenberg, and M.A. van der Pasch. 1998. Patient satisfaction with the general practitioner: A two-level analysis. *Med. Care* 36:212–229.

Spiegelhalter, D., A. Thomas, and N. Best. 2000. *WinBUGs Version 1.4.3 User Manual.*

Wheeler, D.J. and D.S. Chambers. 1992. *Understanding Statistical Process Control*, 2nd edn. SPC Press, Knoxville, TN.

Zhang, M. 2003. Profiling pharmacy expenditures in managed health care: A two-part hierarchical model and Bayesian inference. PhD Dissertations, Cornell University, Ithaca, NY.

Zhang, M., R.L. Strawderman, M.E. Cowen, and M.T. Wells. 2006. Bayesian inference for a two-part hierarchical model: An application to profiling providers in managed health care. *J. Am. Stat. Assoc.* 101:934–945.

19

Analyzing Decisions Using Datasets with Multiple Attributes: A Machine Learning Approach

Introduction 19-1
Analyzing Decisions 19-2
Building Models for Analyzing Decisions 19-4
Attributional Rule-Based Models
Generating Alternatives 19-7
Application of Decision Analysis to the Evaluation of Medication Outcomes 19-8
Conclusion 19-9
References 19-10

Janusz Wojtusiak
George Mason University

Farrokh Alemi
Georgetown University

Introduction

Let us start with some definitions. A decision maker is a person who makes a decision. A decision is the process of choosing among different alternatives. Decision analysis is a process of formulating and analyzing alternatives according to a set of criteria. There are many advantages of the decision analysis process:

- *Describes possible alternatives*. An important advantage of decision analysis is that it describes many alternatives that might be missed by decisions makers because they are too closely involved in the problem or because the problem is too complex.
- *Documents the decision*. Decision analysis describes and documents how the decision was made: What were the alternatives considered? What were the data collected? What were the decision makers' preferences? What was the recommended course of action?
- *Shows the logic of the decision-making process*. Decision analysis breaks complex multidimensional problems into smaller components that can be aggregated to represent the problem using mathematical and analytical rules. It clearly indicates why one alternative is preferred to another and reduces misinterpretation.
- *Quantifies uncertainty and preferences*. Decision analysis uses mathematical or computational models to deal with uncertain events and decision makers' preferences. It is able to assign specific numbers to different events and preferences, thus making the process clear and repeatable.

Traditionally, decision analysis literature is concerned with analysis, but decision analysis could be misleading if it analyzes wrong alternatives. The first and foremost important role of an analyst is to focus the problem on the correct set of alternatives. The correct set of alternatives is not always clear. One way to help the decision maker articulate different alternatives is to describe the cause and effect in the data. Once the causal structure is understood, then alternatives can be generated to address each of the causes. Machine learning can help decision makers understand the causal structure within their environment. This chapter describes how attributional rules can be used to understand a problem environment and generate a new set of alternatives. The key in decision analysis is to articulate the alternatives, and the key to generating alternatives is to understand the cause and effects.

Decision analysis can be used both to support human decision makers and to help computers make automated and autonomous decisions. Automated methods for analyzing decisions are particularly useful when available data is very large or described using many attributes. In such situations, humans are not able to deal with the complexity of the problem and only specialized computer systems can be used. Traditional human-centered or "manual" methods of analyzing decisions are very widely described in the literature, while less attention is paid to automated methods able to deal with large amounts of data.

This chapter discusses methods for analyzing decisions for problems in which alternatives are described using many attributes. This corresponds to the situation in which the modeled world is complex, and many parameters contribute to outcomes of alternatives among which the decision is to be made.

Methods described in this chapter are illustrated by an example about post-release monitoring of medications. In this example, the Food and Drug Administration (FDA) is faced with the problem of withdrawing a medication from the market because it causes excess mortality. Specifically, we discuss the use of decision analysis in the context of the withdrawal of Vioxx from the market because it was believed that it led to cardiac events (Bresalier et al. 2005). Vioxx was the brand name for Rofecoxib, a nonsteroidal anti-inflammatory drug that was available in the market between 1999 and 2004, and was prescribed to over 84 million people (Knox 2004). The manufacturer withdrew the medication abruptly after it was linked to excess cardiac events.

Analyzing Decisions

Decision analysis is a multistep iterative process involving analysis of available data, interviewing experts, building models for predicting outcomes for different alternatives, and using these models to arrive at the final decision. The following steps describe a typical decision analysis process. Each step is briefly illustrated using the problem of benchmarking hospitals.

1. *Define goal.* Before starting the analysis process, it is important to clearly specify the goal of the decision. In particular, why is there a need to decide? A related question is, who is deciding? Answers to these questions are not always clear. In many organizations, it is difficult to locate the actual person or group of people who are responsible for making the decision. Extensive literature is available on how to specify goals of the analysis and how to deal with groups of decision makers.

   Healthcare administrators, policy makers, private and government organizations, and pharmaceutical companies are often interested in answering questions, such as: Which of the given medications of therapies work the best for a specific group of patients? Is a specific medication safe? What are the adverse events related to the use of specific medication? Should that medication be removed from the market or be available to patients? Decision analysis methods provide a systematic way of answering such questions.
2. *Define alternatives.* Once the goal of the analysis is specified, alternatives need to be defined to specify possible options, among which the decision maker needs to make a selection. In some cases, there may be only two alternatives (a binary decision), for example, (a) to remove medication from the market or (b) to keep that medication available to customers. In other cases,

there are several considered alternatives: (a) to permanently remove medication from the market, (b) to temporarily remove medication from the market and request further studies, (c) to keep medication on the market but issue a warning, (d) to create strict guidelines for the use of that medication, or (e) to keep the medication on the market as is. A good decision analysis generates alternatives that might have not been considered at the start of the analysis. For example, the analysis of data might indicate a subset of patients for whom Vioxx is effective—in which case the medication may not be withdrawn uniformly from the market.

3. *Define perspective of the analysis*. Analysis can be performed from different perspectives. Important questions that an analyst needs to answer concern (a) what is to be measured in the analysis? (b) what are the outcomes to be used? or more generally, (c) what is the perspective of the analysis?

   One can imagine a hypothetical decision regarding change in an insurance plan. If the decision is modeled from the point of view of an insurance company, an analyst would concentrate on outcomes such as profit to the company, number of new customers attracted, or customers potentially lost, etc. The same analysis performed from the perspective of a patient would consider the patient's quality of care, satisfaction, cost of care (i.e., co-payment, premiums), etc. Results of the analyses may be very different and potentially in favor of different alternatives.

   In the simplest case, one measure of outcomes is used in single-criterion decision analysis. When more than one measure of outcome is used, then the analysis is called *multi-criteria decision analysis* (MCDA), which is widely studied in the literature (Lootsma 1999).

   In the medication effects analysis example, analysis can be done from the perspective of the FDA, consumer organizations, pharmaceutical companies, etc. Depending on the perspective of the analysis, different preferences are used.

4. *Select data sources*. Selecting the perspective of analysis as described in the previous step allows the analyst to start searching for relevant data. Different sources of data can be considered: patient information available in electronic medical records (EMR), data collected during clinical trials available in the original form or as a summary from web services, such as ClinicalTrials.gov, results of studies published in peer-reviewed journals, results of surveys, and others.

   In some cases, there may be no relevant data available for the analysis. There may be several reasons for this, such as no relevant data was ever collected, the data is not accessible by the analyst, the data may be made accessible but not soon enough (i.e., using the data requires multiple levels of review including IRB approval), and no experts with relevant knowledge are accessible. In such a case, an analyst must revise the perspective of the analysis and find a way of analyzing the problem using what data is available. In the case of complete lack of relevant data, the analysis cannot be performed.

   The decision to withdraw Vioxx was based on multiple sources of data including retrospective data from electronic health records and prospective data from new clinical studies.

5. *Build models for alternatives*. With available data sources and a clear problem definition, an analyst can start building models for all alternative choices. This is usually a complicated process that involves analyzing available data and interviewing experts to acquire their domain knowledge.

   Models for all alternatives are assembled into a decision tree, as illustrated in Figure 19.1. On the left side of the tree, the root node represents the decision to be made. Branches coming from the root represent possible alternatives. Each of the alternatives is described using its own model built from data and background knowledge. Note that models for different alternatives do not need to be decision trees themselves. Different types of models can be used, such as sets of rules, Bayesian networks, logistic regression, support vector machines, or neural networks.

   A method for building rule-based models from data and background knowledge is described in detail in "Building models for analyzing decisions" section. The process of acquiring models for experts is well studied and described in the literature. Knowledge of many experts can be combined to form one coherent model (Merrick 2008).

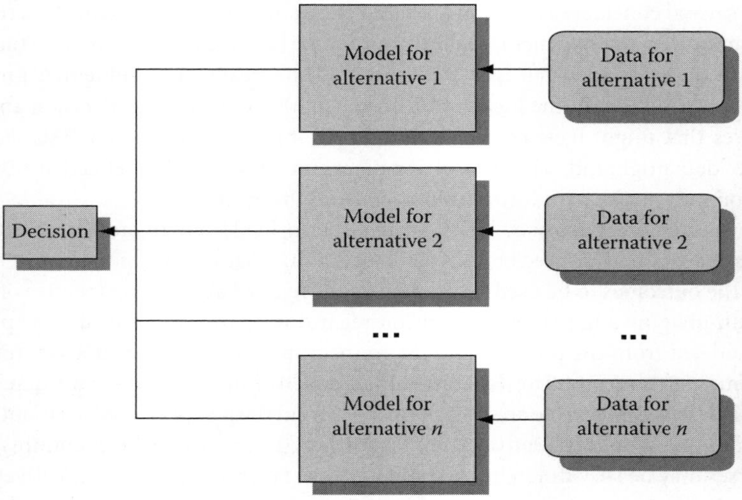

FIGURE 19.1 A decision followed by models for n different alternatives and their models.

6. *Use models to make predictions/evaluate alternatives*. Each alternative is represented by its model. These models can be applied to evaluate results of each alternative in an unknown situation of interest. This application may be simple when models directly correspond to the situation of interest, or may involve repetitive application of these models with the need to aggregate results at the end. The latter is illustrated by the problem of evaluating medications, in which repetitive application of models to different patients' data is performed ("Application of decision analysis to the evaluation of medication outcomes" section). Aggregation of individual results at the end may be done through simple counts or more advanced statistics.
7. *Perform sensitivity analysis of the obtained results*. Results of the analysis may be biased by data, experts' judgments, or imprecision of making measurement. Sensitivity analysis is the process in which created models are perturbed in order to check how large changes are needed in order to change decision. For example, minor changes to a medication effect model may reverse the result of the analysis. This means that either the model needs to be changed or that there is no true difference in the value of the compared alternatives. In the medication effect example, the latter would mean that the medication has no effect on cardiac events.

   Additionally, statistical analysis of obtained results can be performed. The statistical significance of obtained results can be calculated, and tests can be performed on previously unseen datasets.
8. *Make a recommendation*. Results of the final analysis are to be presented to decision makers in the form of a recommendation. In this paper, we assume that the decision analysis goal is to support decision making, not replace the decision maker. The recommendation should clearly state the purpose of the analysis, the assumption made, the sources of data, and the results of evaluating different alternatives. For example, the result of analysis may state that the use of a specific drug increases the chance of cardiac events.

Building Models for Analyzing Decisions

All steps described in the previous section are critical to a successful decision analysis process. However, this chapter's focus is on using machine learning to build models that are used to analyze alternative choices, which may consequently lead to discovery of new alternatives. Because building models is tidily coupled with selecting and preprocessing data, the two will also be briefly described. Other steps of decision analysis briefly discussed in the previous section, such as the definition of the goal and the perspective of the analysis, are fairly standard and widely covered in the literature (Skinner 2005, Alemi and Gustafson 2006, Rakus-Andersson et al. 2009). They are also part of typical courses on healthcare decision analysis. Materials for one course offered at the George Mason University is available at http://hap.gmu.edu/730.

We now describe in more detail the task of generating alternatives. The key to formulating new alternatives is in understanding causes of the events of interest. In the Vioxx example, the event of interest was excess mortality from cardiac events. It was important to understand if Vioxx was causing the excess mortality or if Aspirin (another medication) had a protective effect. Once the cause and effect are understood then alternatives can be generated. For example, we might come up with the alternative that patients in the last phases of rheumatoid arthritis might be helped with Vioxx even though some might have an increased risk of cardiac events. To understand cause and effect, we need to analyze existing data and find "if-then" rules that describe the data accurately. When these rules describe cause and effect, we refer to them as attributional rules.

Usually, the analyst has access to multiple sources of data, some with overlapping and contradictory information. It is often not easy to understand the causes of events. Some data point to one cause and other data point to alternative causes. For example, excess mortality associated with Vioxx might be due to the fact that this medication was prescribed to the frail elderly with severe arthritis pain. Vioxx could be the cause of cardiac events or the cardiac event could have occurred anyway. A patient's cardiac event may be due to the use of medication, or other existing conditions. It is not always clear what the cause of the patient's safety problems is. Before a decision can be made regarding how to improve a hospital's operation, patient safety problems should be attributed to specific causes. By analyzing data and background knowledge, machine learning methods are able to select relevant attributes, corresponding to causes and effects, and to use them in building models for decision alternatives. A risk analysis-based approach to discovering casual relationships is described by Alemi in Chapter 26.

Attributional Rule-Based Models

Decision support systems, expert systems, and management systems are often based on knowledge represented in the form of rules. This chapter describes automated methods for deriving rules from data and background knowledge. Medical and healthcare expert systems, dating a few decades back, are well known for their use of rules. One of the most well-known examples is the first medical expert system, MYCIN (Buchanan and Shortliffe 1984), built in the 1970s. Most current medical decision support systems are also based on different forms of rules, such as those defined in the Arden syntax, which is part of HL7.

This section describes a special form of *if ... then ... except* rules called attributional rules (Michalski 2004). Such rules, given by Equation 19.1, can be automatically induced from data and background knowledge. They are also more expressive than rules created by most automated rule-induction programs.

$$CONSEQUENT \Longleftarrow PREMISE \mid\_ \; EXCEPTION : ANNOTATION \tag{19.1}$$

$$[L \; rel \; R : A] \tag{19.2}$$

CONSEQUENT and *PREMISE* are conjunctions of attributional conditions; *EXCEPTION* is either a conjunction of attributional conditions or an explicit list of examples that are exceptions to the rule, and *ANNOTATION* lists additional information about the rule (e.g., its coverage, quality, complexity). Attributional conditions are in form 19.2, where L is an attribute, an internal conjunction or disjunction of attributes, a compound attribute, or a counting attribute; *rel* is one of $=$, $:$, $>$, $<$, $\leq$, $\geq$, or $\neq$, R is an attribute value, an internal disjunction or conjunction of attribute values, or an attribute, and A is an optional annotation that lists information about the condition. The symbols <== and |_ indicate implication and exception, respectively. In English, Equation 19.1 says that the *CONSEQUENT* is true (or likely to be true) if the *PREMISE* is true, except for when the *EXCEPTION* is true. The rule does not say anything about the status of *CONSEQUENT* when the *PREMISE* is not satisfied.

Over the past four decades, AQ programs pioneered several new directions in machine learning (Michalski 1983). AQ21, the newest program in the family, implements many of the features developed over the years (Wojtusiak et al. 2006). The system is still being extended with new features tailored toward healthcare data analysis. Other well-known programs from the AQ family are AQ7 (Michalski and Larson 1975), AQ11 (Michalski and Larson 1983), AQ15c (Wnek et al. 1996), AQ17 (Bloedorn et al. 1993), and AQ19 (Michalski and Kaufman, 2001). Wojtusiak et al. (2006) described basic algorithms used by AQ21.

The following describe basic guidelines for preparing data for learning rules by AQ21. Although some details may differ, similar guidelines apply for most other rule-induction programs, and programs that create other forms of knowledge (decision trees, Bayesian networks, etc.):

1. *Define representation space by selecting input and output attributes, their types, and domains.* Output attributes, known in statistics as dependent variables, represent classes or values being predicted or modeled. For example, when discovering characteristics of patients with cardiac events after taking medication, an output attribute may represent two possible outcomes: cardiac event and no cardiac event. Input attributes, known in statistics as independent variables, represent characteristics based on which prediction or classification is made. In the medication effects example these would be different patients' characteristics relevant to the problem, such as primary and secondary diagnoses, length of stay, other medications, and so on.

   Based on Michalski and Wojtusiak (2007), there are seven basic types of attributes. Their semantics affect model induction processes, thus type selection should be done carefully. These types are *nominal attributes* whose domains are unordered finite sets of elements, *structured attributes* whose domains are partially ordered finite sets of elements representing hierarchies, *ordinal attributes* whose domains are fully ordered finite sets of elements, *interval attributes* whose domains include numbers with defined addition and subtraction operations, *ratio attributes* defined as interval attributes but with multiplication and division, *absolute attributes* representing integer numbers without any defined operations, and *set-valued attributes* whose domains represent sets of items. Additionally, all numeric attributes can be discretized into a (usually small) number of ranges. A correct specification of attribute types is very important as it provides problem knowledge about the structure of the problem domain, which allows the learning algorithm to select a right set of induction operators.

   Only relevant attributes should be present in the data. Based on expert knowledge, attributes that are clearly not relevant to the process should be removed from the data in order not to introduce additional complexity and noise. For example, when analyzing effects of medications, patients' social security numbers, emergency contact information, and street addresses are clearly irrelevant. In many databases such irrelevant attributes are, however, mixed with relevant ones. After removing attributes based on experts' knowledge, the next step is to apply statistical methods for attribute selection. In their books, Liu and Motoda (1998, 2007) presented details of many computational methods for selecting attributes.

   Attributes available in the data may not be directly relevant to the decision problem, but their combination is. For example, if a dataset consists of three waiting times at three different locations in a hospital, each one of them may not directly influence a negative outcome, but the sum of the three times (say, total waiting time) might. Thus, one needs to define additional attributes not present in the original data. This can be done either manually, based on expertise, or automatically using constructive induction methods (Bloedorn and Michalski 1998). Created attributes can then be inserted into the data and used in rule induction.
2. *Select representative examples.* When the available dataset is very large, there is often no need to use all of it. In fact, when dealing with extremely large databases, it may not be possible to apply a

machine learning algorithm on the entire dataset. For this reason, statisticians and data miners, developed efficient methods for selecting a representative subset of data. This process, known in statistics as *sampling* and *instance selection* in data mining (Liu and Motoda 2001), is well documented and many methods are available. After selecting a representative subset of data, the learning algorithm can be run more efficiently and can provide good results.

3. *Resolve missing values.* It is not uncommon that many values in the database are not available. According to Michalski and Wojtusiak (2005), there are three possible reasons for values not being present. These values are referred to as meta-values. First, the most common, reason is that a value exists, but it is not known because it was not entered into the database (i.e., a patient did not provide some information, or a nurse did not record some value). This type of meta-value is called *unknown*, and is often denoted in data as "?." It is usually handled by most machine learning and statistical software by replacing "?" by an average, a mean, or some other estimation of the actual value (imputation of values). The second type of meta-values is used when the true value does not exist, as logically impossible. For example, a patient's prostate specific allergen (PSA) test results are not present for female patients in a database, but may be present for males. This type of meta-value is called *not-applicable* and is denoted as "N/A" in the data. Despite the obvious difference from the unknown meta-value, most analytical software do not distinguish between the two, and incorrectly apply imputation methods for not-applicable values. Finally, the third meta-value represents expert knowledge. Some values in the database may be deliberately removed as not relevant to the considered problem. Such values are called *irrelevant*, and are denoted as "*." AQ learning uses meta-values as a form of background knowledge and treats them accordingly to the values' semantics.
4. *Apply a machine learning method.* After data preprocessing briefly described in points 1–3, one can finally apply a rule induction method to build models for each decision. There are many available programs for learning rules from data, including the earlier mentioned programs from the AQ family, CN2 (Clark and Niblett 1989), slipper (Cohen and Singer 1999), LERS (Grzymala-Busse 2005), and others. The Weka system created by Witten and Frank (2005) implements several rule learning methods along with other machine learning algorithms under one coherent graphical interface.

   Based on the selected output attribute(s), an analyst needs to define classes for which models will be learned. For example, a class may represent patients for whom cardiac events are present, and another class may represent those for whom no cardiac events are present. Often, classes are defined by domains of an output attribute. In the above example, an output attribute is nominal with two values, "present" and "not present." Different learning programs require data in slightly different formats. In most cases, these are variants of flat databases, given as comma-separated text files.
5. *Review and test learned rules.* Results of learning need to be verified. This can be done by manually inspecting learned rules, testing them on a previously unseen dataset, or by combination of the two. The most commonly used process of validating decision rules identified from the data is based on setting aside some of the data to test the accuracy of the learned rules. For example, when validating rules for predicting deaths associated with the use of Vioxx, a randomly selected sample of patients' data can be put aside and used for testing.

After the process of learning rules is completed, they can be immediately used for classification of examples, or presented to decision makers.

Generating Alternatives

Once the causal structure of the data is understood, meaning that we have a complete set of attributional rules, then the analyst needs to work with the decision maker to check if new alternatives emerged from the data.

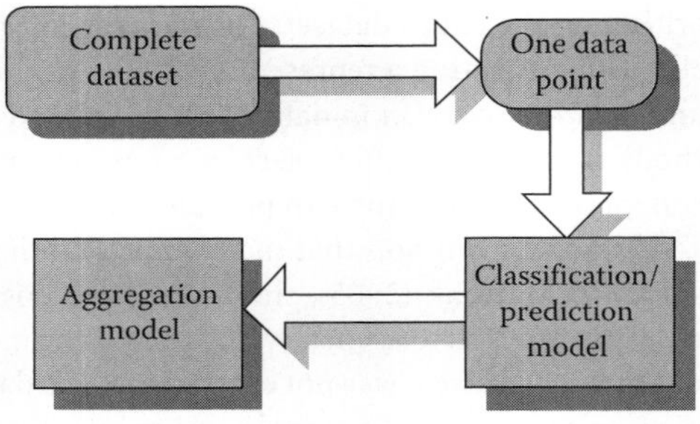

FIGURE 19.2 Applying classification or prediction models to individual data points to arrive at a total model score.

The simplest possible case is when rules correspond directly to the decision being modeled. Then, all that needs to be done is to insert specific data for the given situation and calculate values associated with different alternatives of the decision. For example, one can imagine a situation in which models were learned to predict if a medication should be (a) removed from the market, (b) temporarily suspended until more studies are completed, or (c) left on the market. From a dataset containing characteristics of medications and information about the success and the failure for all three approaches in previous cases, three models for the three alternatives can be derived. Given the characteristics of a specific medication and the results of its trials, the models are able to answer if that medication should be removed from the market. Additional numerical scores associated with matching data against rule-based models can be calculated to provide the strength of the decision (i.e., its support).

A more complicated situation is when the learned rules do not directly correspond to the decision but, rather, values for the alternatives need to be calculated by applying them to the collected datasets. Such a situation appears when rules are built for parts of the problem, and need to be aggregated. For example, when evaluating a medication, one may discover rules for predicting if a given patient is likely to have complications after using that medication. To evaluate that medication, a global answer for all possible patients is needed. Figure 19.2 presents the flow of data when models are applied. From a complete dataset, an individual data point is selected. This data point is then classified using created models. Finally, an aggregation model is used to store results of classification. This is repeated for all data points in the dataset.

To aggregate classification results for multiple data points, several methods can be used. The simplest way is to count how many data points were classified to the class of interest.

An important aspect of the more complicated case is that it can lead to the identification of alternatives that were not previously considered. An analyst may discover that there are subsets of data for which the outcomes are opposite. This may lead to the creation of additional alternatives for the modeled decision, namely, starting to do it differently for different cases—create individualized models.

The next section describes how to apply methods described in “Building models for analyzing decisions” and “Generating alternatives” sections to the evaluation of medication outcomes, exemplified by Vioxx and its effect on cardiac events.

Application of Decision Analysis to the Evaluation of Medication Outcomes

This section illustrates the application of machine learning—based decision analysis to the prediction of medication outcomes. Specifically, it shows how to apply the methodology to the problem of predicting if the use of a medication causes adverse events. This work is inspired by the recent case of Rofecoxib (known under brand names Vioxx and Ceoxx) that is believed to increase the risk of excess cardiac events. This application area is closely related to Chapter 26 in which Alemi presents a casual risk analysis used to discover the root causes of cardiac events related to Vioxx.

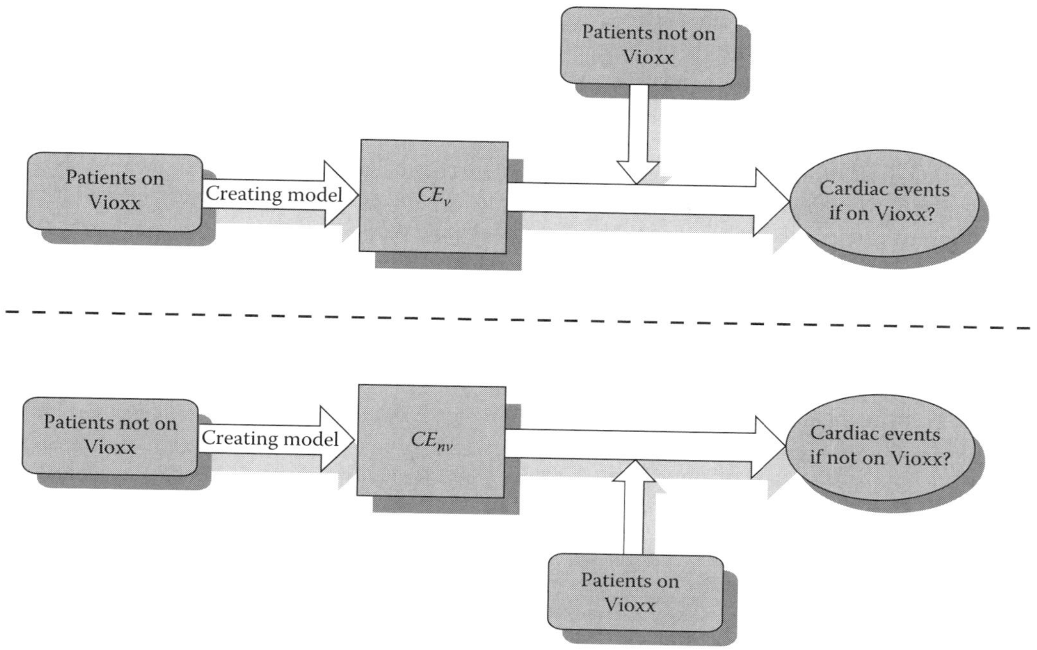

FIGURE 19.3 Building and applying models for Vioxx as a cause of cardiac events.

Following the methodology outlined in "Building models for analyzing decisions" and "Generating alternatives" sections, we will show how to construct rule-based models for assessing if Vioxx is the cause of cardiac events in patients. To do so, the analyst needs to answer the question: Would a patient have a heart attack if he didn't take the medication? In order to do so, two models need to be constructed. The first model, CE_V, is built to describe the characteristics of patients who had cardiac events and had taken Vioxx. The second model, CE_{nV}, is built to describe characteristics of patients who had cardiac events and had not taken Vioxx. Next, these models are cross-applied to the data of patients who had and had not taken Vioxx. The model CE_{nV} is applied to patients who had taken Vioxx and did have cardiac events. This application allows one to assess if these patients would have had cardiac events if they had not taken Vioxx. Then, the model CE_V is applied to patients who had not taken Vioxx and did not have cardiac events. This application allows one to assess if these patients would have cardiac events if they had taken Vioxx. The application can be performed as described in "Generating alternatives." It results in numbers of patients who would have a heart attack if on Vioxx and those who would not have a heart attack if not on Vioxx. This process is illustrated in Figure 19.3.

The application of models as illustrated above can lead to the identification of subpopulations of patients for whom the use of Vioxx is not dangerous. If such a population is well-defined and its properties are easy to measure (i.e., it is easy to assess if Vioxx will be dangerous for a given patient), then an additional alternative can be added to the decision being modeled to allow for partial use of the medication.

The application of machine learning to analyze decisions automatically suggested new possible alternatives to be considered in the analysis. The presented method can be applied to analyze other medications and treatments, and their adverse events.

Conclusion

Computers can be used to analyze and support decision making for problems that involve many attributes and large datasets. Because of their complexity and size, such problems cannot be addressed by traditional decision analysis methods. This chapter presented a rule-based approach to construct models for different alternatives, and the use of these models to calculate values for different alternatives. Based on these values, a decision maker can make an informed choice based on evidence and supported by data. Moreover, rule-based models of data may automatically suggest new alternatives, which were not considered in the original decision.

By creating decision models, the presented methodology is able to answer if some factor causes an adverse event. To do so, models are constructed to check if the adverse event would be present with a lack of presumed cause. This problem has been exemplified by showing how to analyze if Vioxx causes cardiac events. Data for performing this type of analysis is typically collected and available from clinical trials.

References

Alemi, F. and D. H. Gustafson. 2006. *Decision Analysis for Healthcare Managers*. Chicago, IL: Health Administration Press.

Bloedorn, E. and R. S. Michalski. 1998. Data-driven constructive induction. *IEEE Intelligent Systems, Special issue on Feature Transformation and Subset Selection* 13: 30–37.

Bloedorn, E., J. Wnek, R. S. Michalski, and K. Kaufman. 1993. AQ17 a multistrategy learning system the method and users guide. Reports of the Machine Learning and Inference Laboratory, MLI 93-12. Fairfax, VA: School of Information Technology and Engineering, George Mason University.

Bresalier, R. S., R. S. Sandler, H. Quan, J. A. Bolognese, B. Oxenius, K. Horgan, C. Lines, R. Riddell, D. Morton, A. Lanas, M. A. Konstam, and J. A. Baron. 2005. For the adenomatous polyp prevention on Vioxx (APPROVe) trial investigators, cardiovascular events associated with Rofecoxib in a colorectal adenoma chemoprevention trial. *The New England Journal of Medicine* 352: 1092–1102.

Buchanan, B. G and E. H. Shortliffe. 1984. *Rule Based Expert Systems: The Mycin Experiments of the Stanford Heuristic Programming Project*. Reading, MA: Addison-Wesley.

Clark, P. and T. Niblett. 1989. The CN2 induction algorithm. *Machine Learning* 3: 261–289.

Cohen, W. W. and Y. Singer. 1999. A simple, fast, and effective rule learner. In *Proceedings of the Sixteenth National Conference on Artificial Intelligence*, Orlando, FL.

Grzymala-Busse, J. W. 2005. *LERS—A Data Mining System in the Data Mining and Knowledge Discovery Handbook*. Heidelberg, Germany: Springer, pp. 1347–1351.

Knox, R. 2004. Merck pulls arthritis drug Vioxx from market. NPR. http://www.npr.org/templates/story/story.php?storyId=4054991 (accessed October 5, 2009).

Liu, H. and H. Motoda. 1998. *Feature Extraction, Construction and Selection: A Data Mining Perspective*. New York: Springer.

Liu, H. and H. Motoda. 2001. *Instance Selection and Construction for Data Mining*. Berlin, Germany: Springer.

Liu, H. and H. Motoda. 2007. *Computational Methods of Feature Selection*. Boca Raton, FL: Chapman & Hall/CRC.

Lootsma, F. 1999. *Multi-Criteria Decision Analysis via Ratio and Difference Judgement*. Dordrecht, the Netherlands: Kluwer Academic Publishers.

Merrick, J. R. W. 2008. Getting the right mix of experts. *Decision Analysis* 5(1): 43–52.

Michalski, R. S. 1983. A theory and methodology of inductive learning. *Artificial Intelligence* 20: 111–161.

Michalski, R. S. 2004. Attributional calculus: A logic and representation language for natural induction. Reports of the Machine Learning and Inference Laboratory, MLI 04-2, George Mason University, Fairfax, VA, April.

Michalski, R. S. and K. Kaufman. 2001. The AQ19 system for machine learning and pattern discovery: A general description and user's guide. Reports of the Machine Learning and Inference Laboratory, MLI 01-2, George Mason University, Fairfax, VA.

Michalski, R. S. and J. Larson. 1975. AQVAL/1 (AQ7) user's guide and program description. Report No. 731, Department of Computer Science, University of Illinois, Urbana, IL, June.

Michalski, R. S. and J. Larson. 1983. Incremental generation of VL1 hypotheses: The underlying methodology and the description of program AQ11. Reports of the Intelligent Systems Group. ISG 83–5. UIUCDCS-F-83-905, Department of Computer Science, University of Illinois, Urbana, IL, January.

Michalski, R. S. and J. Wojtusiak. 2005. Reasoning with meta-values in AQ learning. Reports of the Machine Learning and Inference Laboratory, MLI 05-1. George Mason University, Fairfax, VA, June.

Michalski, R. S. and J. Wojtusiak. 2007. Semantic and syntactic attribute types in AQ learning. Reports of the Machine Learning and Inference Laboratory, MLI 07–1, George Mason University, Fairfax, VA.

Rakus-Andersson, E., R. R. Yager, N. Ichalkaranje, and L. C. Jain. (Eds.). 2009. *Recent Advances in Decision Making*. Berlin/Heidelberg, Germany: Springer-Verlag.

Skinner, D. C. 2005. *Introduction to Decision Analysis: A Practical Guide to Improving Decision Quality*, 2nd edn. Gainesville, FL: Probabilistic Publishing.

Witten I. H. and E. Frank. 2005. *Data Mining: Practical Machine Learning Tools and Techniques*, 2nd edn. San Francisco, CA: Morgan Kaufmann.

Wnek, J., K. Kaufman, E. Bloedorn, and R. S. Michalski. 1996. Inductive learning system AQ15c: The method and user's guide. Reports of the Machine Learning and Inference Laboratory, MLI 96-6. George Mason University, Fairfax, VA, August.

Wojtusiak, J., R. S. Michalski, K. Kaufman, and J. Pietrzykowski. 2006. The AQ21 natural induction program for pattern discovery: Initial version and its novel features. In *Proceedings of The 18th IEEE International Conference on Tools with Artificial Intelligence*, Washington, DC, November 13–15.

20

The Shaping of Inventory Systems in Health Services

Jan de Vries
University of Groningen

Karen Spens
Hanken School of Economics

Introduction **20**-1
Inventory Management Systems: Overview and Background **20**-2
A Framework for Diagnosing Inventory Management Systems **20**-3
Physical Infrastructure • Inventory Planning and Control • Information System • Organizational Embedding
Discussion and Conclusion **20**-10
References **20**-11

Introduction

Without doubt, the healthcare sector has changed significantly during the last decades. A stronger necessity to deliver healthcare services in a more efficient and effective way together with a growing need to improve the quality of care has forced many healthcare organizations to start projects in the area of patient logistics, care pathways, information systems, and quality management (Mahmoud and Rice, 1998; Stock et al., 2007). It will be of no surprise, therefore, that in many countries, the healthcare sector undergoes radical changes on both a political, institutional, and organizational level. Moreover, numerous governmental initiatives are taken to stimulate healthcare organizations to reduce costs and improve the delivery of health services. The Dutch Government, for instance, in 2004 introduced a quality program entitled "Faster better" aiming at making the healthcare sector safer, more efficient, and patient centered. Following this program, more than 24 Dutch hospitals started projects in the area of quality management, patient logistics, and materials management. All projects concentrated on reducing costs and creating a more care-focused organization by means of integrated care pathways, establishing a stronger integration between the planning systems being used, optimizing goods flows for medicines and improving hospital logistics processes. Recent studies on this program indicate that the organizations can benefit significantly from a more systematic approach (de Vries, 2007). At the same time, however, studies also show (Towill and Christopher, 2005; Schneller and Smelter, 2006) that the development and implementation of improvement programs in the healthcare sector is far from simple due to the complex nature of the care delivery process and the strong interconnectedness between the management areas involved.

Inventory management is a well-covered area in literature and during the last four decades, inventory control has been the topic of numerous publications in the area of operational research, business administration, operations management, and logistics (e.g., Blinder and Maccini, 1991; Silver et al., 1998; Razi and Tarn, 2003). Notwithstanding the impressive body of knowledge regarding inventory management in an industrial setting, some gaps and holes exist in our knowledge with respect to inventory management in a healthcare setting (Oliveira and Pinto, 2005). Only few studies have addressed the question of how the design and implementation of inventory management systems in a health service setting takes place (Beier, 1995; Novek, 2000; Nicholson et al., 2004). Additionally, only few frameworks are available with respect to the shaping of hospital supply chains and the underlying mechanisms of this process as well as the way how hospital supply chains should be shaped and designed are still subject to debate and study (Miller and Arnold, 1998). Clearly, the shaping of inventory management systems strongly relates to areas like management accounting, business logistics, planning and control and information management (Bonney, 1994; Chikan, 2001). Moreover, the design of inventory management systems often includes an organizational dimension as well (Zomerdijk and de Vries, 2003). The allocation of authorities and responsibilities concerning the inventory system confronts organizations with important challenges that, in many cases, cannot be solved easily. It will be of no surprise therefore that many projects in the area of inventory management are characterized by a high degree of complexity. The strong necessity to balance various aspects and to make adequate trade-offs between requirements originated in different management areas seem to be almost inherent to the (re)shaping of inventory management systems (Kisperska-Moron, 2003).

Despite the fact that hospitals carry large amounts of a great variety of products, studies suggest that healthcare organizations still pay little attention to the management of inventories (Nicholson et al., 2004). Having some unique characteristics, the shaping of inventory systems in a healthcare setting is far from a clear, straightforward design process and it is for this reason, why in this chapter a framework is presented, which can be of help to healthcare organizations when assessing and (re)designing their inventory management system.

In "Inventory management systems: overview and background," first an overview is presented of important issues related to the design of inventory management systems. Starting from this literature overview, a framework is presented, aiming at being supportive when assessing and reshaping inventory systems. The underlying rationale of the framework is grounded in the necessity for applying an integrated approach when inventory systems need to be (re)designed. In "A framework for diagnosing inventory management systems," the framework is further explained and worked out. In "An illustrative example: The case of a Dutch hospital," an application of the framework is presented.

We view the contribution of this chapter from two perspectives. First, this chapter aims to advocate the role of clear, well-defined design frameworks when assessing and reshaping inventory systems. Second, some tentative conclusions are drawn about the applicability of the framework outlined in this chapter. In doing so, we concentrate on identifying critical factors when applying the framework.

Inventory Management Systems: Overview and Background

Studies suggest that inventory costs in the healthcare sector are substantial and are estimated to be between 10% and 18% of net revenues (Jarett, 1998). Similar to industrial companies, healthcare organizations are for this reason increasingly compelled to reassess their inventory management system in order to reduce costs (Brennan, 1998). Within the area of operations research and operations management, many contributions can be found with respect to inventory control in the industrial sector (Blinder and Maccini, 1991; Rabinovich and Evers, 2002; Lutz et al., 2003). Generally, these contributions concentrate on three important topics. The first topic many studies focus on regards the question of how much of an item needs to be ordered. In order to determine the economic order quantity (EOQ), several costs associated with the ordering process can be taken into account and it is for this reason why in literature a huge amount of models address the trade-off problem between ordering costs and stockholding costs (Plossl, 1985; Silver et al., 1998). Strongly related to the topic of order quantity is the issue of ordering interval. Clearly, the performance of inventory management systems is closely connected to the availability of the stock-keeping products, which in itself is heavily influenced by the ordering policy. Numerous studies have modeled this issue and many models can be found related to the timing of orders (Minner, 2003). Finally, many studies in the area of inventory management have focused on the inventory control system itself. Subjects related to this research area are the usage and applicability of ABC classifications (Reid, 1987; Nagarur et al., 1994), the role and impact of information systems (Rabinovich and Evers, 2002), and the embedding of the inventory control system in the overall planning and control system of the company (Kisperska-Moron, 2003; Zomerdijk and de Vries, 2003).

Without doubt, the three topics mentioned are very valuable and research in this area has improved our understanding of inventory problems significantly. Many contributions in the area of inventory management, however, are based on mathematics, statistics, and sophisticated techniques of modeling, and the underlying assumptions of the models and techniques are often not met in practice. Moreover, several authors have argued that the quantitative methods from the fields of operations management and operations research are insufficient to cope with today's organizational complexity, and that a more qualitative approach is what we need with respect to important inventory management issues (Hayes, 1998; Lovejoy, 1998). Additionally, it is often argued that it is highly important to take the organizational context of inventories into account during the process of (re)shaping inventory systems (Kisperska-Moron, 2003; Zomerdijk and de Vries, 2003). Amongst others, an organizational perspective on inventory management includes issues like the allocation of tasks and responsibilities with respect to the inventory system, decision making and communication processes, as well as the (political) behavior of the parties involved. Despite the growing attention in the field of operations management to organizational issues, existing inventory management frameworks still seem to lack a clear focus regarding the link between the organizational embedding of the inventory system and the technical aspects of the inventory system.

Clearly, a number of problems appear when trying to transfer the existing body of knowledge developed for industrial companies to the management of inventories in hospitals. In a hospital setting, patient caregivers must be sure that particular products and items, like drugs, are always available. However, in many hospitals it is not always clear which party is responsible for the money tied up in inventories. Additionally, in hospitals, decision-making processes regarding inventory systems are heavily influenced by many different stakeholders having different scopes on the inventory setting. Nurses, pharmacists, doctors, financial managers, and care managers often have diverse perceptions and interests with respect to the inventory system and it will be of no surprise that recent studies have indicated a severe impact of this diversity on the shaping and functioning of inventory systems in a healthcare setting (Kuljis et al., 2007). Compared to industrial companies, the process of (re)shaping inventory management systems in a healthcare setting is probably more affected by political and organizational processes (Nicholson et al., 2004). In general, it is well known that various groups of people in organizations may have different perceptions of management systems and studies performed in the field of information systems indicate that the design of these systems can often be explained by the actions and attitudes of the stakeholders involved (Coakes and Elliman, 1999; Boonstra, 2006). This finding is confirmed by the results of an exploratory case study on the shaping of inventory systems in hospitals (de Vries, 2008). A strong focus of the stakeholders on patient-oriented care and cure processes, a federated-type meritocracy character of hospitals, and the multidimensional nature of inventory systems easily leads to a fragmented process of reshaping the inventory system, which is more based on negotiation than on a logistical-oriented design rationale.

In "A framework for diagnosing inventory management systems," a framework is presented, which can be of help during the process of assessing and (re)shaping inventory management systems in hospitals. The main idea behind this framework is that inventory management systems are multidimensional in character, which needs to be reflected in the design as well as in the process of (re)shaping the inventory system.

A Framework for Diagnosing Inventory Management Systems

Inventory management has been subjected to a huge amount of studies during the last decades. Traditionally, many of these studies focus on developing quantitative models and techniques in order to determine optimal order quantities and balancing trade-off questions regarding timing and volume decisions (Blinder and Maccini, 1991). During the last decade, however, some studies have indicated that more attention should be paid to organizational issues regarding inventory control. Clearly, these studies reflect the growing awareness in practice that the performance of inventory management systems is not only influenced by the technical aspects of the inventory system but also by the organizational embedding of the inventory system. Starting from this notion, some authors have argued that a more integrated approach is what we need when developing and shaping inventory management systems (Chikan, 2001).

The approach described in this section aims to be supportive when an inventory management systems needs to be (re)assessed and (re)shaped. Although applicable in both manufacturing and service settings, in this contribution, we will concentrate on inventory systems in a healthcare setting. The starting point for the advocated approach is the process of defining an *inventory management concept.* An inventory management concept can be considered as a blueprint of an inventory system including the physical infrastructure, the planning and control system, the management information infrastructure, as well as the organizational embedding of the inventory system. An inventory management concept in other words encompasses four main decision areas that highly affect the performance of inventory systems. One of the basic assumptions underlying the necessity of defining an inventory management concept is that by taking these four decision areas explicitly into account during the process of diagnosing and (re)shaping inventory systems, a more integrated approach is safeguarded. Additionally, defining an inventory management concept can help healthcare organizations in checking the completeness of the redesign. As already has been stated, in practice, many inventory management projects are characterized by a rather partial and incomplete approach. By taking the definition of an inventory management concept as a starting point for inventory management projects, healthcare organizations are forced to include key decision areas into account during the process of analyzing and (re)shaping the inventory system. Consequently, a more integrated and systemized approach hopefully can be achieved. Figure 20.1 outlines the basic idea behind an inventory management concept (de Vries, 2007). It is noticed here that the approach described below has some similarities with the framework developed by Verstegen (1989). His framework, however, concentrates on defining and implementing a logistical concept and not as much on an inventory management concept.

It will be of no surprise that the internal as well as external performance objectives, which need to be achieved, are taken as a starting point when defining an inventory management concept. In general, internal performance objectives relate to the requirements defined by the healthcare organization itself. Hospitals, for instance, normally have large quantities of many different medicines in stock. In case of emergency, specific medicines need to be available at once. For this reason, safety stocks and reorder levels of medicines and drugs are highly influenced by the "critical character" of the medicines.

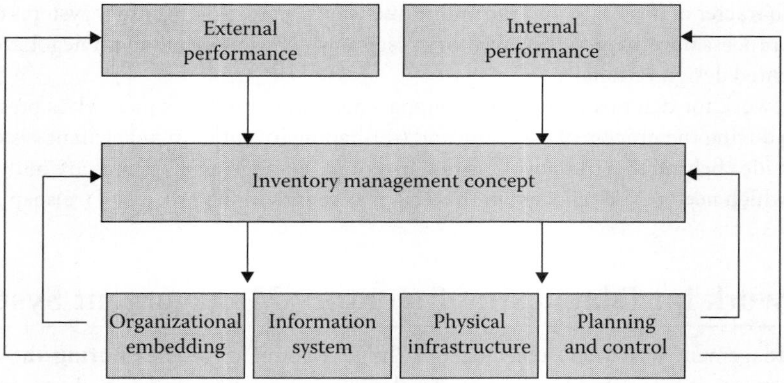

FIGURE 20.1 Overview of an inventory management concept.

In many cases, internal performance objectives are often operationalized in terms of quality, cost- and speed-related goals. However, not only do internal performance objectives play an important role when assessing and (re)shaping inventory systems in a healthcare setting; external performance objectives frequently have a significant influence on the inventory system as well. Government regulations, the influence of insurance companies on stock-keeping products, the necessity to comply with standards set by professional associations, and the requirements set by audit committees for instance, also have an important (external) impact on inventory systems.

Without doubt, linking internal objectives to external objectives is an important second step when defining an inventory management concept. In the case of inventory management systems for drugs, for instance, the process of balancing internal and external performance objectives sets the overall target for open as well as for closed stock items. Open stock items relate to items that are dispensed directly to patients; closed stock items relate to items that are kept in a secure store from where they are distributed to local departments and treatment areas. In practice, the assessment of internal and external performance objectives, addressing the impact of the inventory system to these objectives, and balancing all the different trade-offs probably is the most difficult part of defining an inventory management concept.

Once the overall contribution of the inventory system toward achieving the internal and external performance objectives has been assessed, the achievement of the objectives is further worked out. Starting from an overall blueprint of the inventory system, four main decision areas as well as their interrelationships need to be addressed when defining an inventory management concept:

- The physical infrastructure
- The planning and control system
- The information system
- The organizational embedding

At this stage, the overall blueprint of the inventory system is further operationalized for each of these four decision areas.

Physical Infrastructure

The physical infrastructure encompasses the physical setting of the inventory system and consists of the main goods flows and stock points of the products and items that are subjected to the analysis and (re) shaping process. In hospitals, these goods flows can relate to, for instance, medicines, drugs, medical devices, health aids (e.g., bandage) and surgical supplies. Within hospitals, therefore, many different flows of goods can be distinguished and the overall physical infrastructure of the inventory system is often quite complex. Amongst other issues, decisions on the physical shaping of the infrastructure includes issues as whether or not "stockless schemes" should be applied, the amount of stock points, and the way the emergency sourcing of items is dealt with. The number and location of stock points is closely related to the supply structure of the products. In the case of medicines for instance, hospitals often have an internal pharmacy producing medicines and other pharmaceuticals. At the same time, many pharmaceuticals are directly delivered from a medical wholesaler or pharmaceutical industry to the hospital. The characteristics of the supply chain of pharmaceuticals, therefore, directly influence the number of stock points and the way medicines are distributed to and within the hospital.

Starting from the internal and external performance objectives of the health service organization, an inventory management concept includes clear and well-defined statements about the physical setting of the inventory system. The inventory management concept, in other words, addresses the way how the overall objectives of the healthcare organization ought to be achieved by means of the physical setting of the inventory system. Recent studies on this topic illustrate the complexity of this issue (Pedersen, 2006). The physical infrastructure of drug inventory systems, for instance, is closely connected to the way medicines are dispensed and prepared in the hospital. Many medicines for inpatient use are dispensed and prepared in a centralized pharmacy. However, within hospitals, frequently satellite pharmacies exist in patient care areas. Clearly, this infrastructure has a huge impact on the number of stock points and the drug distribution system. The physical infrastructure of the inventory system, therefore, cannot be considered in isolation but ought to be assessed and defined as an integrated part of the flow of goods and products within the hospital.

Inventory Planning and Control

A second decision-making area that needs to be taken into account when defining an inventory management concept encompasses the planning and control of inventory items. As already mentioned, inventory decisions include both timing and quantity decisions. Clearly, these decisions depend on the demand characteristics of the stock-keeping products, the amount of uncertainty with respect to the inventory system, and the required performance of the inventory system. In hospitals for instance, patient caregivers must be sure that critical medicines and drugs are available all the time. Replenishment levels for these critical items, therefore, are mainly based on the necessity of being available and not as much on inventory costs. Obviously, inventory planning and control cannot be considered in isolation either and closely relate to the overall planning system of the health service organization. A trigger of a drug running out of stock, for instance, normally will induce a signal to produce or procure the drug. The inventory planning system, therefore, needs to be linked to the planning system of the medicine-producing facility of the hospital (Dellaert and Van de Poel, 1996).

Although in literature many sophisticated models are described, in practice, often the EOQ and/or the economic batch quantity (EBQ) approach is used. Despite the fact that these models have been heavily criticized (Schonberger and Knod, 1994), the straightforward approach of these models as well as the simplicity of the underlying planning mechanism justifies the fact that these models still are considered as being best practices in hospitals.

Inventory decisions not only include decisions on how much or when to order but also on how the inventory system ought to be controlled. In hospitals, logistics and operations managers need to cope with many thousands of different stock-keeping products that are supplied by many different suppliers and/or produced internally by many different departments. The control of these stock-keeping products, therefore, is a complex and dynamic task including many different issues like

- What procedures should be used to support the inventory planning system?
- What priorities should be allocated to different stock-keeping products?
- How should inventories be measured and assessed?

Clearly, these issues also should be addressed when defining an inventory management concept in a health service delivery setting.

Information System

In practice, the structuring of the planning and control system is closely related to the information system to be used. Many studies in the area of operations management have revealed that the performance of inventory systems highly depends on the availability of accurate and timely information (Manthou et al., 1996). Moreover, in practice, inventory decision-support systems and management information systems are often integrated by means of a computerized, company-wide system (Lowell and Celler, 1998; Siau et al., 2002). Software in the area of enterprise resource planning, for instance, is built around several modules, amongst them financial, inventory, and production planning modules. Following the development in manufacturing companies, nowadays hospital information systems are also increasingly characterized by an integrated approach, including modules in the area of pharmacy, inventory management, registration of patients, and financial management. Studies in the field of hospital information systems indicate, however, that a lack of integration between different information systems, the usage of several platform technologies, and a lack of information sharing still often is the reason for a lack in the performance of hospital inventory systems (Mahmoud and Rice, 1998). It will be of no surprise therefore that projects in the area of inventory systems often have a strong information-oriented focus, aiming at implementing sophisticated software in order to improve the performance of the inventory system of the health service delivery organization.

Inventory management systems in hospitals require information from several sources. Examples of important data necessary to make inventory-related decisions are time-phased requirements for the products and stock-keeping items, demand for all items, receipts of each stock number, stock on hand, and data on costs associated with the stock-keeping products. When defining an inventory management concept, the information system related to the inventory system should be taken into account explicitly. In doing so, the information dimension cannot be separated from the planning and control dimension and it is for this reason why both areas are considered as crucial for achieving external as well as internal performance objectives.

Organizational Embedding

Recent studies in the area of inventory management indicate that little to no attention is paid to the organizational embedding of inventory systems (de Vries, 2007). Clearly, the organizational setting of inventories often have a significant influence on the performance of inventory systems and for this reason cannot be disregarded when assessing and (re)shaping inventory systems. In their study on inventory systems, Zomerdijk et al. (2003) address four areas of importance with respect to the organizational context of inventory systems. The allocation of tasks, authorities and responsibilities to employees, the way decision-making processes are organized, the communication patterns as well as the behavior of the stakeholders involved in the decision-making processes in practice are key issues affecting the performance of inventory systems. Recent studies on the role stakeholders play during inventory projects reveal that the outcomes of projects in the area of inventory management are frequently influenced by the interests of different stakeholders (de Vries, 2009). Moreover, decisions made during the course of these projects are only partly based on a rational straightforward decision-making process. Various stakeholders often have different perceptions of the inventory projects, which can easily lead to political processes, conflicting interests, negotiation behavior, and opportunistic power play of the stakeholders involved in the project. There are some strong indications that the same accounts for inventory projects in health service delivery settings. Especially in a healthcare setting, the existence of multiple stakeholders having multiple goals regarding the inventory system may easily result in different perceptions and expectations. Unit managers, for instance, often emphasize a fast delivery of medicines and stress the importance of accurate and reliable inventory data. Medical staff employees also have a clear interest in a fast delivery of special medicines and avoidance of the risk of running out of stock. Logistical managers in hospitals, on the other hand, strongly focus on minimizing inventory costs, avoiding obsolete medicines, and optimizing the trade-off between service delivery and efficiency. Next to the physical infrastructure, the planning and control structure and the information system, the organizational setting of inventory systems is a fourth important dimension, which also needs to be addressed explicitly when defining an inventory management concept.

In this section, four dimensions have been introduced, which are considered as being of eminent importance when assessing and (re)shaping inventory systems in general, and inventory systems in a healthcare setting in particular. The underlying rationale of these dimensions is that the performance of inventory systems is influenced by various elements. In addition, inventory systems are clearly a multi-dimensional phenomenon and it is for this reason why it is considered to be important to include these dimensions when defining a blueprint of the inventory system in a healthcare setting. Obviously, the four dimensions should not only be addressed separately but have to be related to each other. Moreover, shaping an inventory system also includes the process of aligning the four dimensions in order to achieve a fit between the items. The information system being used as well as decision-making processes with respect to inventory system for instance, should be in line with the authorities and responsibilities of the employees involved in the inventory system. Management practices in hospitals indicate that a misalignment between the four dimensions mentioned above, is often the reason for a lacking performance of the inventory system and it is therefore important to take the issue of alignment explicitly into account when defining an inventory concept.

In "An illustrative example: The case of a Dutch hospital," an illustration of how the approach outlined above can be applied in practice is provided. In doing so, an inventory project of a medium-sized hospital in the Netherlands is taken as a starting point.

An Illustrative Example: The Case of a Dutch Hospital

During the period February 2006–December 2008, a case study was performed aiming at assessing the strengths and weaknesses of the advocated approach described in the previous sections. Additionally, the study aimed at improving the inventory system in a medium-sized hospital. The empirical research can be characterized as mix of a case study approach and action research. The case study part of the research concentrated on the question to what extent inventory management systems can be improved by applying an integrated and systemized approach including the four decision areas addressed in "A framework for diagnosing inventory management systems." Additionally, the action research part of the study focused on the application and improvement actions undertaken during the inventory project. In doing so, the model outlined in Figure 20.1 was followed.

Clearly, the approach advocated in "A framework for diagnosing inventory management systems" encompasses a diagnostic part as well as a redesign phase. In this section, however, we will concentrate on illustrating how the framework can be used when diagnosing an inventory system.

The hospital where the inventory project has taken place employs about 1500 employees and has 400 beds. The hospital covers about 80 medical specializations and each year around 20,000 patients are admitted to the hospital and more than 180,000 treatments in an outpatients' department take place. The inventory project started in February 2006 and aimed at improving the performance of the inventory system of pharmaceuticals in the hospital. The inventory project consisted of three phases. During the first phase, an analysis was made of the strengths and weakness of the inventory system. An overall assessment of the performance of the inventory system made during the startup of the project revealed that during a 6 month period, stock levels of 43% of the products were below the minimum safety stock level for 20 days on average. Additionally, 16% of the products was facing the risk of running out of stock, resulting in many rush orders to produce medicines and the necessity to take additional measures to prevent from dangerous situations. Additionally, an assessment of the external objectives revealed that the hospital had the ambition to become the main supplier of medicines for other hospitals in the region. The improvement of the overall inventory system of the hospital was therefore considered to be of strategic importance by the board of directors of the hospital. Moreover, the hospital aimed at becoming a good manufacturing practice (GMP) certified production facility of medicines and for this reason, it was decided by the board that the overall inventory system of medicines needed to be assessed thoroughly and improved whenever necessary.

During the second phase of the project, an assessment was made of the four areas described in "A framework for diagnosing inventory management systems." Clearly, different stakeholders had different perceptions of the strengths and weakness of the inventory system. The head of the laboratory, for instance, considered the planning process of making medicines as the main reason for the lacking performance of the inventory system. The managing director of the hospital pharmacy, on the other hand, strongly believed that this planning process was appropriate, but judged the hospital information system as being the main reason for the products running out of stock. It is interesting to note that different stakeholders assigned different meanings to the reshaping of the inventory system, and during the course of the project, it became clear that the project team consisted of delegated stakeholders having a clear interest in the way medicines were stored and distributed. By applying a systemized approach during this second phase and making a clear distinction between the physical infrastructure of the inventory system, the planning and control of the stock items, the information dimension, and the organizational embedding of the inventory system, discussions between the stakeholders involved could, to a certain extent, be structured and guided.

Starting from the analyses made with respect to the four areas and based on several internal studies, at the end of 2007, it was concluded that four main reasons were considered to be accountable for the lacking performance of the inventory system:

- Generally, it was agreed upon that too many stock points existed at the patient care units.
- The inventory information system used was characterized by a great variety of different platforms and many loosely coupled information systems. In addition, the information system used by the hospital pharmacy and the information system of pharmaceutical suppliers showed a lack of integration resulting in inefficiencies and inadequate management reports.
- Although clear and well-defined decision rules existed, the process of releasing production orders of medicines by the central hospital pharmacy appeared to be somewhat intransparent and was characterized by a rather ad hoc nature of the decisions being made.
- Authorities and responsibilities regarding the production, storage and distribution of medicines showed to be very fragmented and not clearly defined. Moreover, in some cases, a clear misfit existed between the authorities and responsibilities allocated to employees regarding inventory costs and replenishment levels.

By applying the framework, the four dimensions of the inventory system were not only studied and assessed separately but also analyzed in coherence. In doing so, it was concluded that the above-mentioned issues were strongly interconnected to each other and that this interaction could be considered as a dominant factor in explaining the overall performance of the inventory system of medicines. A detailed study of the shortcomings of the inventory system indicated that a strong negative interaction between the dimensions existed. Apparently, shortcomings with respect to one dimension were reinforced by the shortcomings of some of the other dimensions. The fragmented character of the organizational embedding of the inventory system, for instance, induced the usage of a fragmented inventory information system. The severe shortcomings in the information systems being used, in turn, had a strong negative influence on the decision-making processes with respect to the control of stock levels and inventory costs. Additionally, the complexity of the physical infrastructure consisting of many small-scale stock points and a high degree of complexity with respect to the distribution process of medicines in the hospital reinforced this negative interaction.

During the third phase, the project group concentrated on conceiving an inventory management concept. In line with the aim of an inventory management concept, a blueprint was made of the inventory system consisting of a detailed plan on how the overall performance objectives of the inventory systems could be achieved by means of the four decision areas. Additionally, an improvement plan was made encompassing all the actions that should be undertaken in order to improve the overall performance of the inventory system. This blueprint as well as the improvement steps defined in the action plan formed the basis of a redesign process that was finished mid-2008. Starting from the analyses made in the second phase of the project, this redesign process was built on three pillars:

- A redesign of the physical infrastructure including the distribution process as well as the number of stock points of medicines and pharmaceuticals. In doing so, the ambitions of the board of directors with respect to the hospitals' ambition to become a major supplier of medicines for hospital in the region, was taken into account.
- All stakeholders strongly believed that the shortcomings regarding the organizational embedding of the inventory system had a strong negative influence on the other dimensions of the inventory system as well as on the overall performance of the inventory system. For this reason, authorities and responsibilities with respect to stock levels, the distribution of medicines as well as inventory costs were reallocated and streamlined. Additionally, communication and coordination procedures were also reorganized.
- Finally, a start was made with respect to the implementation of software linkages between the hospital information system and the inventory information system.

An internal survey conducted in 2008 showed that despite the fact that some improvement plans had not been implemented yet, all respondents believed that due to the changes made, significant improvements have been established with respect to the reduction of inventory costs, a more efficient way of working, and increasing service delivery performance.

Discussion and Conclusion

Although associated with industrial companies, nowadays a strong focus on inventory management has also become paramount in the healthcare sector. The healthcare sector in general and hospitals in particular are confronted with a growing necessity to reduce costs and it is for this reason that many hospitals have started projects in the area of patient logistics, materials handling, and inventory management. Projects in the area of inventory management in the health sector, however, are complex in nature due to the many different stakeholders involved and the wide variety of perceptions of these stakeholders on inventory issues. Additionally, hospitals often have large amounts of many different products in stock, which makes decisions on inventory management related issues often to a complex subject.

The approach described in this chapter indicates that hospitals can benefit from a more systemized assessment and redesign process with respect to the inventory system. Clearly, an inventory management concept can be a helpful tool for organizations to improve the performance of the inventory system. The framework described is based on the view that inventory systems are a multidimensional phenomenon. The physical infrastructure, the planning and control system, the information architecture as well as the organizational embedding of the inventory system highly influence the overall performance of the inventory system and for this reason should be taken into account when assessing and reshaping the inventory system. As has been illustrated by our case example, not only the dimensions separately but also the interdependence between the dimensions needs to be taken into account explicitly.

The framework outlined in this chapter can be helpful when structuring projects in the area of inventory systems. By addressing specific aspects based on the dimensions of the framework and by making a clear distinction between a descriptive, diagnostic, and redesign phase, different stakeholders are able to identify themselves more profoundly with the overall aim of the inventory project. The application of an inventory management concept in other words, prevents the stakeholders from having a too narrow focus and safeguards a more integrated approach with respect to inventory management issues.

Despite the promising benefits of the advocated approach, some practical lessons can be derived from our illustrative case study. In summary, the following lessons seem to be important when applying the framework:

- In a healthcare setting, decisions made during the process of analyzing and reshaping an inventory system are often heavily influenced by the dynamics and interactions between the stakeholders involved. Defining and applying an inventory management concept, therefore, can easily become the subject of negotiation and conflicts. On the one hand, the application of an inventory management concept can be of help when channeling the power and interest positions of parties involved in the project. On the other hand, defining an inventory management concept can also reinforce potential conflicts by making opposing standpoints and interests more visible. Clearly, project management should be aware of this potential danger.
- Although not explicitly addressed in "An illustrative example: The case of a Dutch hospital," the case study indicates that defining an inventory management concept can easily become a goal in itself. Obviously, an inventory management concept should be an instrument to help stakeholders when assessing and reshaping an inventory system. However, in some cases, the approach described can easily become the subject of discussions keeping the hospital away from implementing improvement actions. Moreover, describing an inventory management concept can easily become the main target of the project group. It will be clear that project managers and the main stakeholders involved in the project should be aware of the aim of an inventory management concept and of the potential risk of the project drifting away from improving the inventory system toward writing a paper document.
- A third important lesson learned from other case studies performed in the field of inventory systems and the application presented in this chapter relates to the heaviness of the approach. Sometimes, the problems that need to be resolved with respect to inventory systems in a healthcare setting are rather straightforward and well defined. In these cases, the framework might be too profound and a more straightforward approach could be more appropriate.

Without doubt, the conclusions mentioned above are only a first step toward a more integrated design methodology regarding inventory systems in a healthcare setting. Although further research is required, we hope that the groundwork presented in this chapter may help hospitals in guiding inventory projects and aid managers in deciding whether to apply the framework presented or to use other approaches.

References

Beier, F.J. 1995. The management of the supply chain for hospital pharmacies: A focus on inventory management practices. *Journal of Business Logistics* 16:153–173.

Blinder, A.S. and L.J. Maccini. 1991. Taking stock: A critical assessment of recent research on inventories. *Journal of Economic Perspectives* 5(1):73–96.

Bonney, M.C. 1994. Trends in inventory management. *International Journal of Production Economics* 25:107–114.

Boonstra, A. 2006. Interpreting an ERP-implementation project from a stakeholder perspective. *International Journal of Project Management* 24:38–52.

Brennan, C.D. 1998. Integrating the healthcare supply chain. *Healthcare Financial Management* 52(1):31–34.

Chikan, A. 2001. Integration of production and logistics—In principle, in practice and in education. *International Journal of Production Economics* 69:129–140.

Coakes, E. and T. Elliman. 1999. The role of stakeholders in managing change. CAIS: Focus issue on legacy information systems and business process change. *Communications of the Association Information Systems* 2(4):2–30.

Dellaert, N. and E. Van de Poel. 1996. Global inventory control in an academic hospital. *International Journal of Production Economics* 46–47:277–284.

Hayes, R.H. 1998. Developing POM faculties for the 21st century. *Production and Operations Management* 7(2):94–98.

Jarett, P.G. 1998. Logistics in the health care industry. *International Journal of Physical Distribution and Logistics Management* 28(9/10):741–742.

Kisperska-Moron, D. 2003. Responsibilities for inventory decisions in polish manufacturing companies. *International Journal of Production Economics* 81–82:129–139.

Kuljis, J., R. Paul, P. Lampros, and K. Stergioulas. 2007. Can health care benefit from modeling and simulation methods as business and manufacturing has? In: *Proceedings of the 2007 Winter Simulation Conference*, S.G. Henderson, B. Biller, M.-H. Hsieh, J. Shortle, J.D. Tew, and R.R. Barton (eds.), Washington, DC: IEEE Press, pp. 1449–1453.

Lovejoy, W.S. 1998. Integrated operations: A proposal for operations management teaching and research. *Production and Operations Management* 7(2):106–124.

Lowell, N.H. and B.G. Celler. 1998. Information technology in primary health care, *International Journal of Medical Informatics* 55(1):9–22.

Lutz, S., H. Loedding, and H. Wiendahl. 2003. Logistics-oriented inventory analysis. *International Journal of Production Economics* 85:217–231.

Mahmoud, E. and G. Rice. 1998. Information systems technology and healthcare quality improvement. *Review of Business* 19(3):8–13.

Manthou, V., P. Notopoulus, and M. Vlachopoulou. 1996. Information systems design requirements for inventory management: A conceptual approach. *International Journal of Production Economics* 45:181–186.

Minner, S. 2003. Multiple-supplier inventory models in supply chain management: A review. *International Journal of Production Economics* 81–82:265–279.

Miller, J.G. and P. Arnold. 1998. POM teaching and research in the 21st century. *Production and Operations Management* 7:99–105.

Nagarur, N.N., Hu, T.-S., and N.K. Baid. 1994. A Computer-based inventory management system for spare parts. *Industrial Management & Data Systems* 94(9):22–28.

Nicholson, L., A.J. Vakharia, and S.S. Erenguc. 2004. Outsourcing inventory management decisions in healthcare: Models and applications. *European Journal of Operational Research* 154:271–290.

Novek, J. 2000. Hospital pharmacy automation: Collective mobility or collective control? *Social Science & Medicine* 51(4):491–503.

Oliveira, F.J. 2005. Enabling long term value added partnership in the healthcare industry, MSc thesis, MIT Center for Transportation and Logistics, Cambridge, MA.

Oliveira, M.D. and C.G. Pinto. 2005. Health care reform in Portugal: An evaluation of the NHS experience. *Health Economics* 14:203–220.

Pedersen, C.A., P.J. Schneider, and D.J. Scheckelhoff. 2006. ASHP national survey of pharmacy practice in hospital settings: Dispensing and administration—2005. *American Journal of Health-System Pharmacy* 63:327–345.

Plossl, G.W. 1985. *Production and Inventory Control: Principles and Techniques*. Englewood Cliffs, NJ: Prentice-Hall.

Rabinovich, E. and Ph.T. Evers. 2002. Enterprise-wide adoption patterns of inventory management practices and information systems. *Transportation Research Part E: Logistics and Transportation Review* 38(6):389–404.

Razi, M.A. and J. Michael Tarn. 2003. An applied model for improving inventory management in ERP systems. *Logistics Information Management* 16(2):114–124.

Reid, R. 1987. The ABC method in hospital inventory management: A practical approach. *Production and Inventory Management Journal* 28(4):67–70.

Schneller, E.S. and L.R. Smeltzer. 2006. *Strategic Management of the Health Care Supply Chain*. San Francisco, CA: Jossey-Bass.

Schonberger, R.J. and E.M. Knod. 1994. *Operations Management: Continuous Improvement*. Homewood, IL: Irwin.

Siau, K., P.B. Southard, and S. Hong. 2002. E-healthcare strategies and implementation. *International Journal Healthcare Technology and Management* 4(1/2):118–131.

Silver, E.A., D.F. Pyke, and R. Peterson. 1998. *Inventory Management and Production Planning and Scheduling*. New York: John Wiley & Sons, Inc.

Stock, G.N., K.L. McFadden, and C.R. Gowen III. 2007. Organizational culture, critical success factors, and the reduction of hospital errors. *International Journal of Production Economics* 106:368–392.

Towill, D. and M. Christopher. 2005. An evolutionary approach to the architecture of effective healthcare delivery systems. *Journal of Health Organisation and Management* 19(2):130–147.

Verstegen, M.F.G.M. 1989. Ontwikkeling van een logistiek concept. *Tijdschrift Voor Inkoop & Logistiek* 7–9:23–29 (in Dutch).

de Vries, J. 2007. Diagnosing inventory management systems: An empirical evaluation of a conceptual approach. *International Journal of Production Economics* 108:63–73.

de Vries, J. 2008. Understanding the shaping of inventory systems in health services: Results of an exploratory case study. In: *Paper presented the 15th International Symposium on Inventories*, August 22–26, 2008, Budapest, Hungary.

de Vries, J. 2009. Assessing inventory projects from a stakeholder perspective: Results of an empirical study. *International Journal of Production Economics* 118:136–145.

Zomerdijk, L.G., J. de Vries. 2003. An organizational perspective on inventory control: Theory and practice. *International Journal of Production Economics* 81–82:173–183.

21

Facility Planning and Design

Richard L. Miller
Earl Swensson Associates, Inc. (ESa)

Introduction 21-1
Strategic and Master Facility Planning Process 21-1
Facility Needs Assessment • Physical Plant Evaluation • Site Evaluation • Master Facility Plan Deliverables • Initiating a New Design and Construction Project • Facility Design Process

Introduction

Plan to create a plan, examine the plan, plan the plan, select the planners, and work the plan. Planning cannot be too involved or too careful when a hospital or healthcare system is considering a capital building project. All stakeholders need to weigh in on the critical decisions before the first ceremonial shovel hits the dirt.

Stakeholders in the planning and design process will vary from institution to institution, dependent upon the type of facility and whether the owner falls into the private or public category or is for-profit or not-for-profit. No matter if the healthcare project in question involves construction of a new facility from the ground up, replacement of an outdated facility, or an expansion and renovation, careful planning is essential to ensure its success.

An organization's leadership is responsible for setting a clear vision and making timely decisions throughout the life of the capital building project. Development of a strategic operational plan and a master facility plan create the framework for making these decisions.

Strategic and Master Facility Planning Process

The master facility plan provides a comprehensive view of the overall program and facility improvement needs of the organization to provide services consistent with its mission and vision.

Before the master facility planning process begins with an architect, it is important for an organization to validate its mission and strategic vision as established by its leadership.

This includes an organizational assessment and a review of the organization's competitive position within the market. Such an analysis leads to the development of key business strategies for the future and long-range operational goals with a prioritized implementation plan, financial and resource allocation strategy, marketing plan, and a schedule for meeting these goals.

The strategic planning phase is often the time in which an organization identifies the need to expand existing programs and initiate new ones, leading to discussions about expanding the capacity of its facilities. A strategic plan is based upon identifying service line needs and the hospital's ability to fill those needs that benefit the community and the hospital's revenue. At this stage, a hospital often develops preliminary ideas regarding the physical plant and creates an early business plan. However, further analysis is required before determining if a facility should be renovated, enlarged, or replaced.

Facility Needs Assessment

A facility needs assessment is an important next step in this process. Feasibility studies include analysis and benchmarking of patient volumes and demographics, market share, physician recruiting goals and strategies, patient and staff satisfaction data, strategic goals, projected growth for existing programs, and plans for new programs. It is also important to evaluate operational planning assumptions such as patient acuity, average length of stay for inpatients, treatment times for clinical areas and to review current available evidence linking specific design elements to improved outcomes.

Analyzing all of this data and understanding the organization's mission, long-range goals, and operational vision ultimately lead to establishing key planning units (number of patient rooms, operating rooms, emergency department treatment rooms, diagnostic imaging rooms, etc.). These are the key space drivers for a facility and they are the primary elements that drive the facility size.

Once the key planning units are established, the space program is developed. This document lists all of the physical space requirements for a facility—the key planning units in addition to all of the support spaces. This tool is used by the architect to determine the gross square footage requirements for the facility.

Physical Plant Evaluation

Evaluating the existing physical plant is another important element in this process.

Evaluation of an existing facility involves due diligence on the part of architects and engineers to conduct a thorough evaluation of zoning restrictions, existing site conditions and utilities, traffic and parking, building infrastructure systems (e.g., mechanical, electrical, plumbing, information technology and low voltage systems), and structural restrictions and functional challenges.

After completing an evaluation of the existing physical plant, the architect and engineer develop options for the organization to consider in order to meet planning goals, which may include renovations, additions, a combination of additions and renovations, or facility replacement. These recommendations may include options for adaptive reuse or demolition of functionally obsolete portions of existing facilities.

Site Evaluation

If the decision is made to replace the facility, site selection and evaluation are critical and should encompass several key factors. Visibility of the site is important for marketability and easy access by patients, families, and visitors. A parcel of land should be chosen that is adequate in size for long-range growth on a new campus. Site grading, the amount of cut or fill work required on the site and access to utilities can impact project costs.

It is also important to evaluate geometry of the land for functional, effective design to support operational programs that will be included in the facility. Efficient operations are influenced by proper building relations. Solar orientation of the building is an important element in the evaluation and has an impact on the ability to provide access to natural light, a factor that evidence-based research has shown to be important in creating a healing environment.

Providing an efficient parking layout with access near entries and convenient wayfinding is essential. Separating distinct zones for public and patient parking versus support and employee parking is another factor in the site evaluation. It is important to consider access for food service, materials management, pharmaceutical deliveries, linen and trash pickup, and other support services. These back-of-house functions are vital to hospital operations and require access near the loading dock; however, the location should be carefully considered and ideally placed away from the main hospital entrance and public view when approaching the facility.

In addition, careful consideration must be given to separate emergency department access for ambulance traffic and emergency walk-in patients. Helipad access with approved FAA flight patterns and easy access to the emergency department cannot be overlooked. Finally, site masterplan opportunities and expansion zones that provide minimal disruption and rework must be evaluated for all buildings being considered for the site, including the hospital, physician office building, freestanding specialty centers (cancer, outpatient surgery center, etc.), ambulance service building, powerhouse, among others.

Master Facility Plan Deliverables

At the end of the master facility planning process, the architect's finished product is comprised of several elements: a description of the master facility plan methodology, demographics data, analysis and findings, summary of existing conditions, proposed drawings that include blocking and stacking diagrams, space program, preliminary budget figures, and a summary of recommendations. This report will include options for growth of the campus over time, and it will often include construction phasing considerations, particularly for larger campuses (see Figure 21.1).

Initiating a New Design and Construction Project

When an organization decides to initiate a new design and construction project, one of the first steps is to define the project's scope, preliminary budget, and schedule. The completed master facility plan is an informative tool in this decision-making process. At this stage a request for qualifications and/or a request for proposals is often sent out to prospective architecture firms for response and a selection process is defined.

Once the selected architect is on board, project goals and guiding principles are established, a project schedule is developed, and the budget parameters are confirmed. User groups are formed to work with the design team during the design process. Involvement of key users such as clinicians (physicians, nurses, pharmacists, therapists, etc.), administrators, department directors, unit managers, safety and infection control representatives, plant operations, and environmental staff is important. Patient input is another critical element and may be obtained through focus groups and feedback from patient advisory council members and patient satisfaction surveys.

Depending on the level of detail that was addressed in prior stages, the architect or a program consultant will lead the programming effort to develop a detailed functional and space allocation program. If the program is well developed, the architect will validate and test the program assumptions during the transition period from programming to facility design. It is important to have consistency in those involved in the process, and the user groups established during the early stages should remain involved throughout the design.

Facility Design Process

The facility design process is made up of four key phases: conceptual design, schematic design, design development, and construction documents. During the conceptual design phase, design ideas are tested against the project goals or guiding principles and the organization's mission, vision, values, and

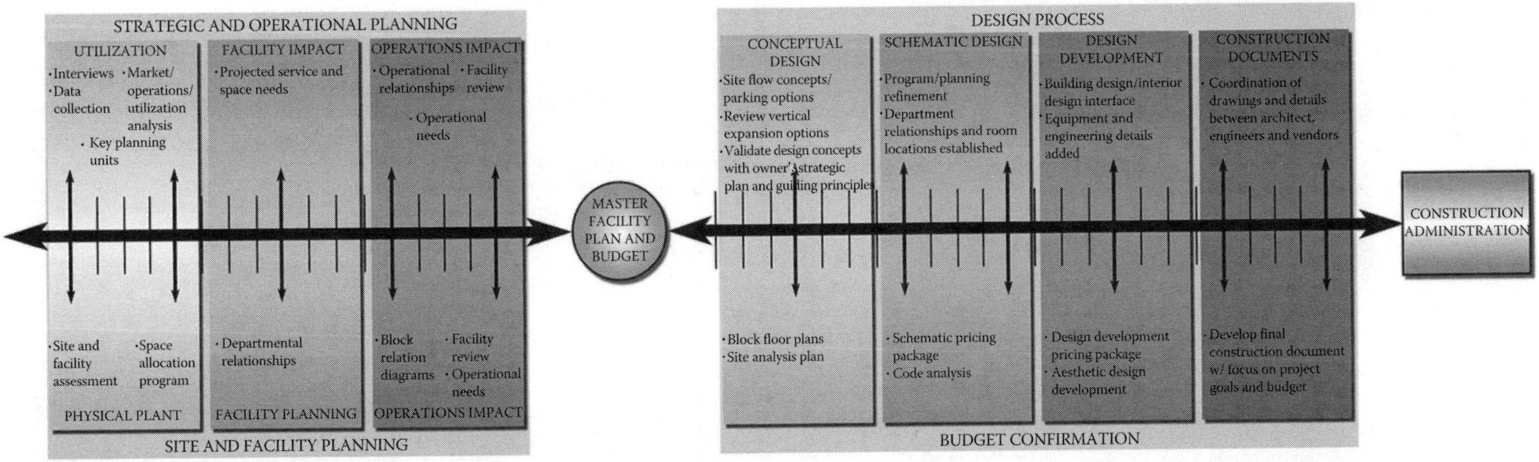

FIGURE 21.1 Integrated strategic planning, facility planning, and design processes. (Courtesy of Earl Swensson Associates, Inc. (ESa), Nashville, TN. With permission.)

strategic plan. Locations of departments and their relationships to other departments are discussed and tested in block diagrams to confirm basic operational flow and identify functional relationships.

In schematic design, the design team develops drawings that illustrate the scale and relationship of a project's components to each other. Work flow and operational efficiencies are key discussion points that drive the design. Relationships of departments to each other, both horizontally and vertically, and room locations are finalized within the plans.

Design development is the phase in which details are determined and added to the drawings. Architectural details include the building's exterior elevations, roof plans, stair and elevator sizes and minimum clearances, and the identification and location of specialty systems (i.e., pneumatic tubes, conveying systems, etc.). Architects and interior designers work together to coordinate interior elements such as casework, doors and windows, materials and finishes, clinical room wall elevations, and key ceiling details and heights. Other elements involve (1) fixed and major equipment models and locations within a space; (2) special structural, mechanical, electrical, and plumbing data; (3) building systems; and (4) material specifications.

In the construction documents phase, the design team completes detailed specifications and drawings which will be used by the contractor to complete construction of the project. This phase requires less user group input and more coordination of architectural, mechanical, electrical, plumbing, and structural details necessary for construction.

Throughout the design process, safety and infection control issues should be considered in the layout of spaces as well as in the selection of materials to be used for construction. Durability and cleanability of materials are important factors that must be taken into account during the design process.

As an architectural firm designing all manners of healthcare projects from coast to coast, we consistently see the value of owners' early involvement of all the key players including the project's manager/owner representative, design team, and construction team. The project's manager/owner representative may be an employee of the hospital or health system or may be a consultant hired by the organization in the role of program manager or project manager. The design team includes not only architects and engineers (civil, structural, mechanical, electrical, and plumbing), but also other professional consultants who bring expertise to the project.

These consultants often include the following: geotechnical codes and Americans with Disabilities Act (ADA) compliance, sustainability, traffic and parking, elevator, medical equipment planner, signage and wayfinding, building skin, acoustics, and lighting. Throughout the planning and design process, all of the design team members work collaboratively to incorporate best practices into the design and coordinate details on the design documents. These details will ultimately be used by the contractor as a "detailed assembly kit" for construction of the facility.

Case Study

To better illustrate facility planning and design concepts in a step-by-step process, the complex expansion and renovation of an existing hospital in a high-growth market in the southeastern United States is a demonstrated example. Williamson Medical Center (WMC) in Franklin, Tennessee, began as a county hospital in 1957. In 1987, the hospital moved to its current site as a four-story facility with a high mix of semiprivate rooms and limited services (see Figure 21.2).

At the turn of the millennium, it became painfully evident that the county and surrounding market had outgrown the existing hospital. It could no longer adequately fulfill its purpose, vision, and values.

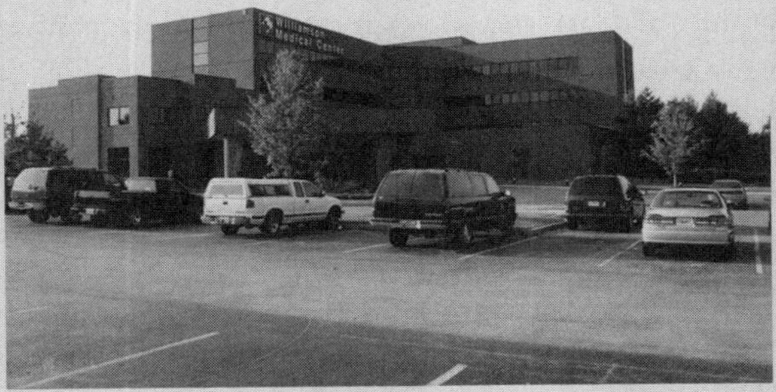

FIGURE 21.2 The county hospital's existing four-story facility needed to expand and add services to accommodate the high-growth area. (Courtesy of Earl Swensson Associates, Inc. (ESa), Nashville, TN. With permission.)

Although the hospital had particularly strong service lines in orthopedics, urology, general surgery, and obstetrics (OB), and its clinical staff enjoyed a good reputation in bedside manner, these assets were not enough to support the county's exploding population in the areas surrounding the historic town of Franklin and nearby Brentwood and Spring Hill. Needs outnumbered capacity and services. The county's population grew from 126,638 in 2000 to an estimated 172,252 in 2008. That number is projected to be near 185,000 by 2013.

While its vision was to strive "to be the preferred provider of healthcare services to the residents of Williamson County, and the acute care center of excellence for the surrounding region," there was concern that some of the county's residents were bypassing the closer facility to drive to Nashville for healthcare services.

Not only had WMC outgrown its emergency department, OB was identified as an opportunity for market share growth. In order to be competitive with Nashville facilities, a few of which were poised to set up satellite facilities in the county, the medical center needed to quickly take steps to enlarge its emergency department, add services, increase inpatient accommodations, and convert all patient rooms to private rooms.

TEAM INITIATES FEASIBILITY PHASE

It was at this juncture that the hospital's board hired our architectural firm ESa to further develop a strategic and master facility plan. All primary stakeholders, including executive administrators, board, and a select group of key physicians, engaged in an all-day planning session to look at the facility's strengths, weaknesses, opportunities, and obstacles. The baseline data of the hospital's volumes, market, and demographics were analyzed.

The medical center, through its board, management staff, and its physicians had the advantage of strong leadership. All were open-minded and receptive to examining different ideas and options for establishing better market positioning for the hospital. Everyone agreed the emergency department needed changes related to size and a more obvious entry to its physical positioning. There was also consensus that expansions and changes were necessary in the key services of OB, outpatient surgery, diagnostic imaging, registration, preadmission testing, lab, pharmacy, physical therapy, and the main lobby/dining/public amenities areas. As previously mentioned, there was a desire for the hospital to have an all-private-room model as well as a need for a connection between the hospital and the medical office building (MOB). Bringing all users and stakeholders to the table was critical to the thorough planning process.

SITE EVALUATION

While a number of physicians, members of the board, and the administrative team felt the existing hospital's limited site would not allow for expansion, we looked at the pros and cons of total relocation versus expansion on site to position the hospital for the next 20–30 years. Three important factors entered into the equation: (1) The existing location's proximity to the nearby interstate with accessibility and visibility as well as its strategic positioning between two growing communities in the county were significant advantages, (2) expansion at the current site would be more cost effective than replacement on another site, and (3) as the existing facility was less than 20 years old, functional issues could be overcome through renovation and expansion. Additionally, by remaining on the site where it had relocated just two decades earlier, the hospital would avoid political fallout within the community.

After careful evaluation, we were able to show them that an expansion-in-place could be accomplished, saving millions of dollars in capital costs to the institution while still meeting their strategic goals. A pros and cons list was compiled, and an assessment was made of the costs already invested in the site (site development, facility and infrastructure costs, powerhouse) as well as usable life of the existing site. From these steps, a campus concept was then developed that could support future growth, including specialty clinics as services expanded. A MOB would be attached at all levels of the hospital for physical and operational integration. One street located on the property would be closed, and a cul-de-sac added on the south end to provide contiguous growth opportunities to the west without street separation (see Figure 21.3).

The site was challenging with grade drops and the fact that it was also bordered by two secondary roads at the east and west boundaries. There was also the issue of additional parking as

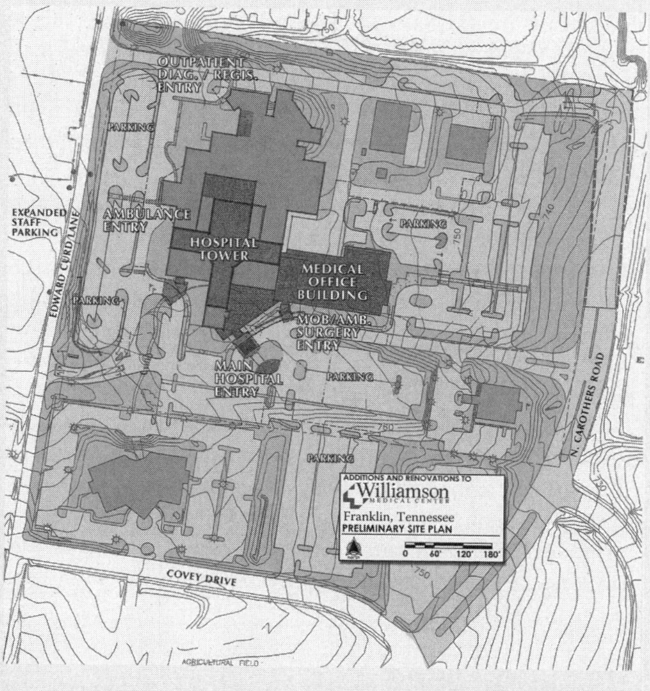

FIGURE 21.3 The medical center's expanded services required additional surface parking, which was extended across Edward Curd Lane (figure left). (Courtesy of Earl Swensson Associates, Inc. (ESa), Nashville, TN. With permission.)

limited land was left for surface parking, and structured parking was cost prohibitive at this phase of planning. Designing the entry at an angle would address both streets, while also providing straight access to outpatient services. Parking would be addressed by surface lots initially and a future parking garage as volumes grew.

MASTER FACILITY PLAN RECOMMENDATIONS

To satisfy immediate priorities, our team recommended to the board's planning committee that two floors be added to the hospital's existing four-story inpatient tower. Secondly, we presented an expansion of the south end of the first floor that would yield the necessary space for the emergency, imaging, and dietary departments. Imaging, in fact, could be expanded in-place via vacated emergency department space.

The emergency department expansion could be accomplished in three phases without ever shutting it down. All three phases would be contiguous with the only new construction for this department being the canopy. A dedicated drive would remain for ambulance traffic with a new drive for public entry.

A north addition would include expanded registration, preadmissions testing, a cath lab addition and an improved link to surgery staging beds. This north-end work would not begin until the emergency department registration was opened and was able to serve as an interim registration area for the hospital. The dietary expansion would also require close coordination among the designers, general contractor and owner with a temporary shutdown of the hospital's food service.

While only one of the two floors would initially be built, with the sixth floor shelled for future use, costs and disruptions would be minimized if both floors were added at the same time. The availability of another floor would allow the hospital to convert all beds to private rooms, decommission semiprivate beds, and stay within its licensed bed count. Ahead of its time, this conversion actually prepared the hospital to be in compliance with the *2006 Guidelines for Design and Construction of Health Care Facilities*, published by the American Institute of Architects. These guidelines set single-bed rooms as the minimum standard for typical nursing units in general hospitals and inpatient primary-care hospitals. (During the course of the project, approval was obtained for an additional 40 beds, which allowed the sixth floor to be built.)

In addition to the offering of private rooms, the inclusion of an ambulatory surgery center, medical office space, and more parking would place the medical center in a more competitive position. The hospital already had a strong outpatient program and performed a significant amount of outpatient surgery. With it currently being located within the hospital, outpatients were required to go through the normal hospital processing minus the ease and convenience of a separate outpatient center. While the option of building a separate, freestanding ambulatory surgery center was weighed, an integrated facility appeared to be the most advantageous solution given the limitations of the site. As an anchor tenant of the MOB, the surgery center, with four operating rooms, would have the benefit of the proximity of the physician tenants and ease of access for staff and surgeons working in both inpatient and outpatient surgery areas.

Additionally, the tower's connection, via a corridor, to the hospital would allow the outsourcing—avoiding duplication—of such support services as central sterile, lab, materials management, pharmacy, and environmental services for both the ambulatory surgery center and the hospital (see Figure 21.4).

PROJECT PHASING PLAN

For the purpose of immediately addressing need and also initiating physician recruitment, the decision was made to fast-track the seven-story tower that would house the MOB, support

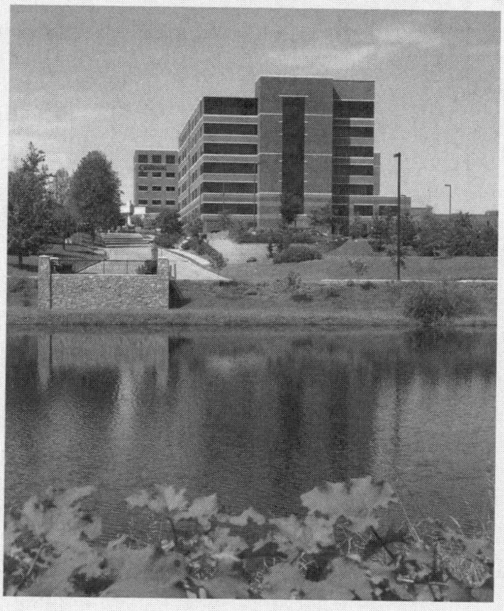

FIGURE 21.4 The new medical office building connects to the hospital, cost effectively avoiding duplication of support services. (Photo courtesy of Chad Alan. With permission.)

services, and the first-floor surgery center. The lab, physical and occupational therapies, medical records, and physicians' lounge would be among the first build-outs on the ground floor of the addition (see Figures 21.5 and 21.6).

Through the recommended purchase of additional property across an adjoining street, the facility was ensured future expansion availability for the existing location through this addition and for the next 20–30 years.

Anticipated population growth in the county mandated that the hospital's expansion and reconfiguration be designed to flexibly grow with the area. The flexibility of the MOB's design could also be translated for other future uses as it was the same construction type as the hospital, would have the same floor-to-floor heights as the bed tower, wide structural column bays, elevators at two ends to allow future conversion, and the north end could expand outwardly, if necessary.

In order to accomplish these goals for the hospital without ceasing operations and with minimal disruption, our team recommended that the construction be done in phases. If the board, however, wanted to proceed with all of the recommendations at once, the construction would be shortened to approximately 16 months. The plan allowed for the early selection of the general contractor, Medical Construction Group, to provide preconstruction services. Parsons-META was program manager.

Including the contractor as part of the team early in the design process provided opportunities not only to evaluate schedule and phasing options, but also to price the project at each stage of design, validating design details against the project budget targets, and fine-tuning the construction schedule and project phasing as decisions were being made. The contractor's role also includes maintaining a clean construction site and addressing infection control measures, particularly when renovating existing areas of a facility or constructing an addition that directly connects to existing space. Maintaining safe means of exiting from the facility during construction

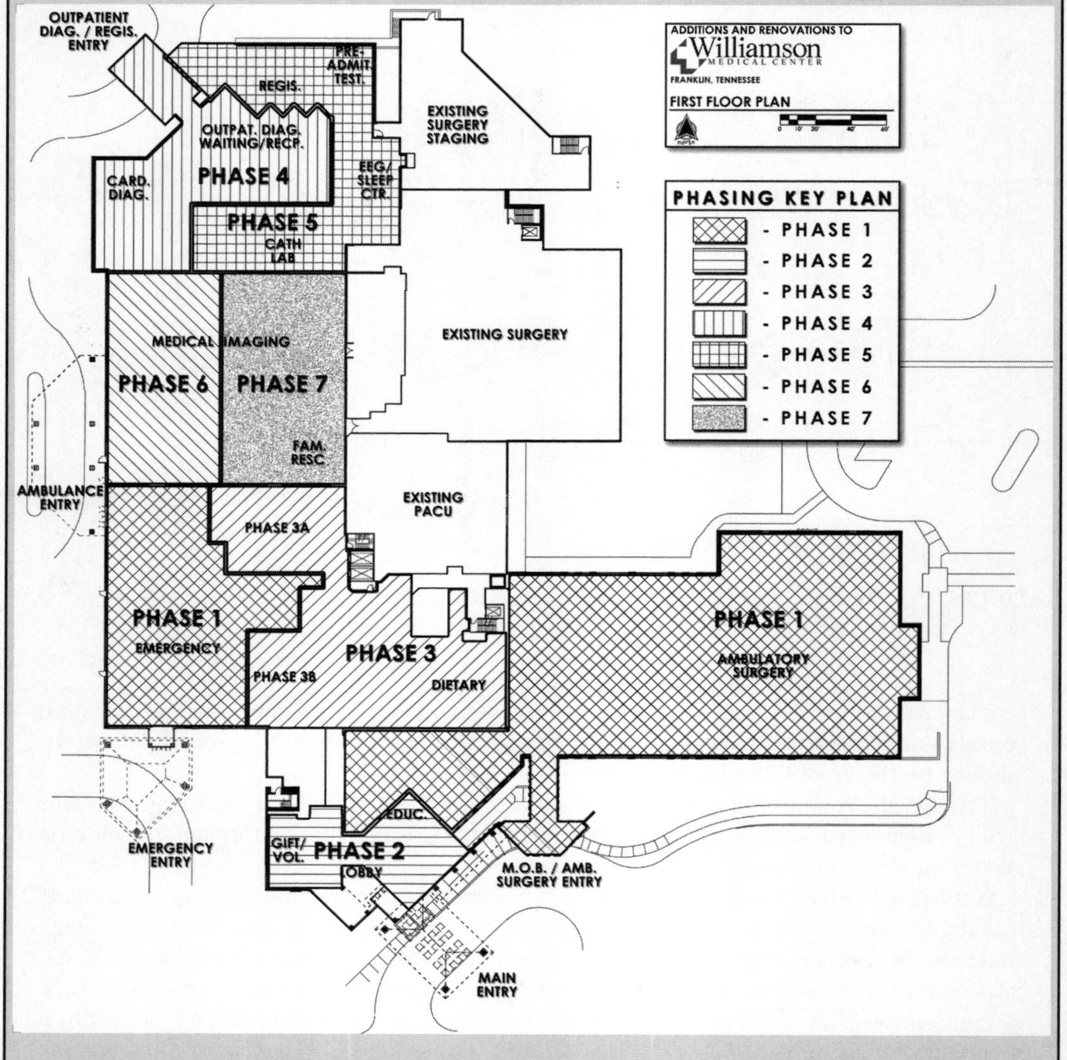

FIGURE 21.5 Accomplishing the expansions and renovations in seven phases allowed the hospital to remain operational without shutting down its services. (Courtesy of Earl Swensson Associates, Inc. (ESa), Nashville, TN. With permission.)

is another key life safety measure that the team must address. These factors illustrate the importance of making the contractor selection early in the process and the value of a collaborative team approach to address the challenges of a complex phased project.

Numerous meetings were held. Efficiencies and proximities of departments were evaluated as were improvements in wayfinding. The hospital's administrative team remained very involved throughout these discussions and decided to proceed with the phased plan approach. The owner took an aggressive approach to temporarily relocate several departments to portable buildings to streamline the process. These displaced departments included admitting, physical therapy/occupational therapy, medical records, administration, physicians' lounge, and public/staff dining services.

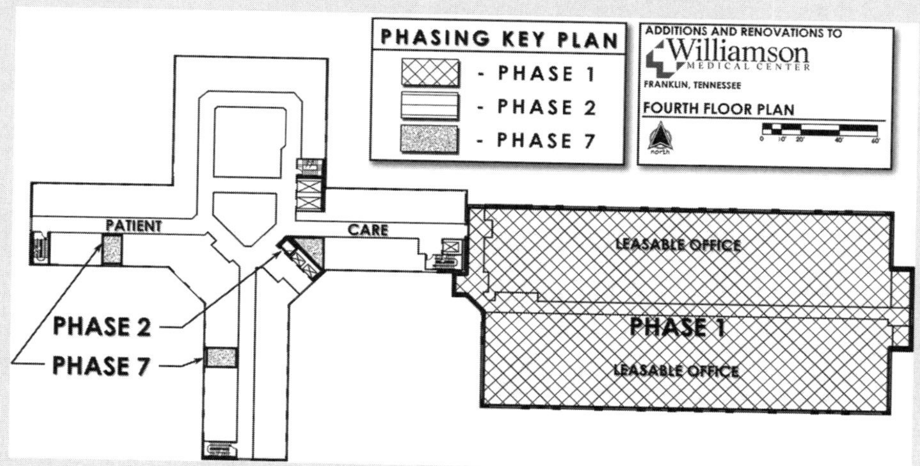

FIGURE 21.6 Accomplishing the expansions and renovations in seven phases allowed the hospital to remain operational without shutting down its services. (Courtesy of Earl Swensson Associates, Inc. (ESa), Nashville, TN. With permission.)

All departments, realizing that the hospital's very survival was at stake, bought into the plan of short-term displacement of spaces in order to be moved, at completion of construction, into the *right* location. The end result was a shorter construction time and less disruption to patient care than would have occurred if the departments had remained in place during the renovation work (see Figure 21.7).

The emergency department moved into vacated spaces rather than into new construction in order to protect land usage and to allow further expansion. The pharmacy and lab moved one time into their new home (see Figure 21.8).

Throughout the complexity of the planning, conscious thought was given to patient service. In the OB unit, for instance, noise, inefficient flow, and security were concerns in the hospital's

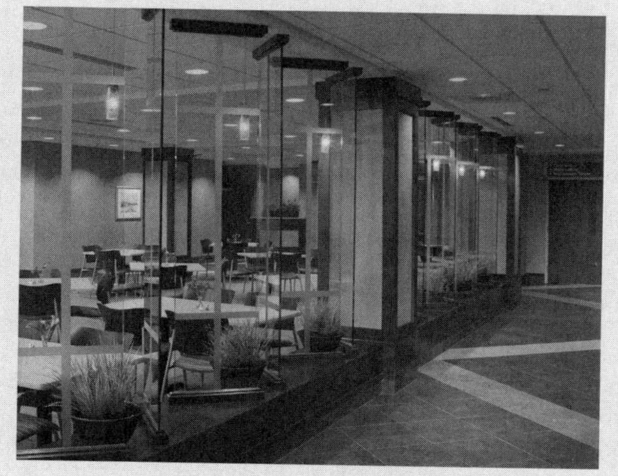

FIGURE 21.7 The new dining on the main public corridor of the first floor is designed to emulate a café setting. (Photo courtesy of Kieran Reynolds. With permission.)

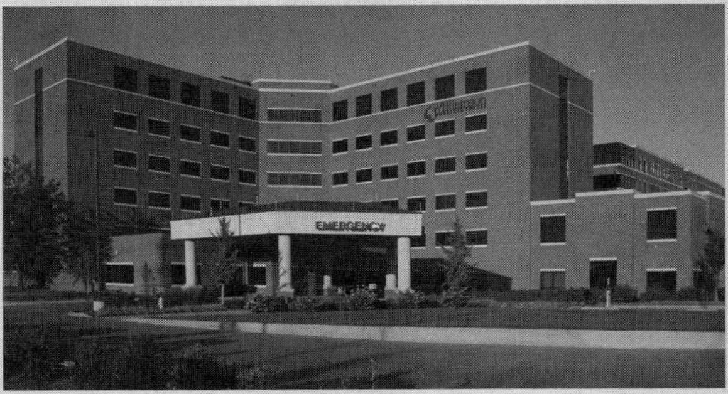

FIGURE 21.8 A new canopy introduces WMC's Emergency Department, which moved into vacated spaces to protect land usage and allow further expansion. (Photo courtesy of Chad Alan. With permission.)

existing layout. For correction of these issues, the unit was temporarily moved. The OB unit was one of the last phases to be completed, and its sequencing was successfully accomplished.

During the schematic design and design development stages, Dennis Miller, the new CEO, arrived. The Certificates of Need (CON) for a level IIb neonatal intensive care unit (NICU) and an additional 40 inpatient beds were added under Miller's administration. The structural platform for both of these additions was already included in the original expansion plan.

The renovation and expansion encompassed three sides of the existing facility on top, and internally. Except surgery, recovery and the existing support services on the ground floor, every department was affected with construction work while the hospital remained in full operation. This was accomplished by close partnering with the contractor in order to provide adequate staging and temporary housing of displaced departments.

The master facility plan has enabled WMC to remain true to its goals of providing care, showing compassion, and serving its community. This plan continues to support growth and future planning initiatives on the medical center campus. Today WMC offers comprehensive inpatient and outpatient services, 24-hour emergency care, preventive health screenings, and wellness activities (see Figure 21.9).

VALUE OF PLANNING

This case study is a good illustration of how a project design and construction team can work with an organization's leadership to be successful when planning, designing, and executing construction of a healthcare capital building project. This project is more complex than some, because of the amount of phasing involved in order to replace-in-place rather than relocate the facility to a new site. This example demonstrates such valuable lessons as

1. The impact of an experienced, dedicated, and supportive board
2. The importance of an administration's engagement in phasing discussions and willingness to make timely decisions in order to keep the process moving
3. The importance of early general contractor selection, which allows participation in pricing at key milestones and early development of phasing plans
4. The value of an owner's willingness to temporarily relocate departments in order to decrease construction time and cause fewer disruptions to patient care
5. The critical nature of effective team communication and coordination
6. The necessity of planning for flexibility and growth to accommodate the market

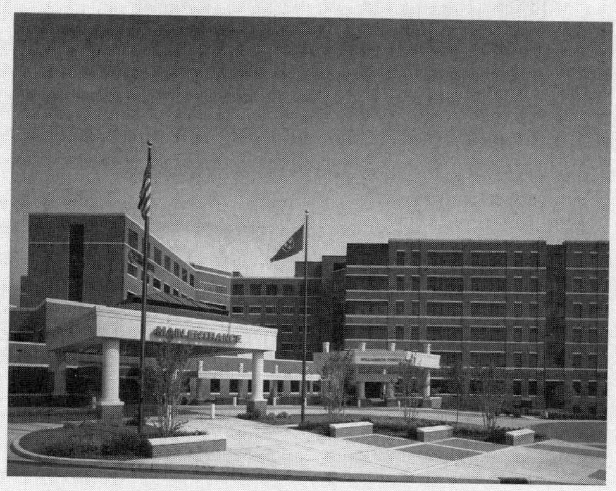

FIGURE 21.9 With its phased expansions and renovations complete, WMC is positioned to serve the community well into the future. (Photo courtesy of Kieran Reynolds. With permission.)

The opportunity to lead a capital building project is significant and does not occur often in the career of a healthcare executive or a board member's tenure. Careful, deliberate planning, which is forward thinking and flexible, is vital for an organization's future success. It begins with a clear strategic vision and dedicated leaders willing to be engaged in the process to collaborate with the design and construction team in achievement of the project's vision.

22

Work Design, Task Analysis, and Value Stream Mapping*

Cindy Jimmerson
Lean Healthcare West

Introduction 22-1
Deeply Understanding How the Work Currently Happens 22-2
High-Level View: Value Stream Mapping • Moving from the Current State to Future State
Task Analysis 22-7
Future State Plan 22-9
References 22-11

Introduction

The way an organization functions is the backbone of its culture. Solid work design permits the more traditional interpretations of culture (mission, values, and organizational philosophy) to grow as the heart and muscle of an organization and refines the definition to "how we work here." Only the most robust of organizations recognize the value of this cultural structure. Without clearly articulated design of work, inconsistency and unreliability in the delivery of services creates unrest, distrust, and unclear expectations of workers and the outcomes of work. In healthcare, lack of specification of work translates to unhappy caregivers, nervous administrators, and potentially unsafe and definitely dissatisfied patients.

The author of this chapter and others† (Sobek and Jimmerson 2003) estimate that the cost of poor work design in healthcare in the United States stands at a staggering 60%, that is, 60% of work performed by caregivers and support services in the current system does not add value to the patient/customer or the business enterprise. Given the crisis states of healthcare access, quality, and funding today, the opportunities for improving healthcare delivery through work redesign are limitless and only recently being considered with a grave eye. Rather than funding more of the same, prospecting a better way to work based on deep understanding of how the work is currently designed offers an affordable way to capture some of the wasted resources that currently exist in our system and improve in every medical organization, *how we work here*.

* In this chapter the author will use the term "worker" to refer to the person who carries out any piece of work. It is critical for understanding the concepts that will be explored in this chapter for the reader to know that "the person who does the work," be it performance of a surgical procedure, meal preparation, or hospital administration, will be recognized as the subject matter expert because he or she does this work every day. Acknowledgment of the worker as the person who knows the work best as a function of their experience in daily work is a critical factor in creating successful work design for improving healthcare delivery.

† NSF Grant #0115352.

In this chapter we will discuss concepts and methods borrowed from the Toyota Motor Company and other organizational greats who have recognized consistent and reliable work as a standard of success. In consideration of the brevity of a single chapter to highlight this work, references to the Toyota Production System (TPS) *for this chapter only* will include accumulated practices of Lean, Six Sigma, and other programs developed from TPS-based concepts. Applications to healthcare with case studies to illustrate the techniques, talent engaged, and outcomes will support arguments regarding the measurable value of improving work design, *using TPS/Lean thinking.* This chapter will focus on deeply understanding how work currently happens through task analysis and value stream mapping, and redesigning work to capture currently wasted potential using the same methods.

Deeply Understanding How the Work Currently Happens

Every activity of work in healthcare, from the CEO's responsibility of hiring a new medical director to the laundry worker's duties of supplying correct volumes of clean linen to a nursing unit, fits somewhere in a scheme of work and has observable steps. When those steps are not standardized, clearly understood, and accepted by the people who are affected and engaged in any one of the linked activities, inconsistency in recurring work is a likelihood. Random work produced without work design creates confusion, discomfort, and tenuous reliability that the task will be completed, let alone completed to a recognized standard and the satisfaction of the patient/customer. Standard work that secures the process and is easy to visualize and communicate insures the exact opposite: reliable and consistent practice that produces satisfying and predictable outcomes, created in a safe environment by confident workers. To get to that desired state of function, the processes of work must be transparent with a mechanism to insure that problems will be identified and mended, and an onward plan for improved service communicated.

Historically, we in healthcare have been eager to fix problems as they present but have not always engaged the people doing the work with a pragmatic method to really understand and ferret out the root causes of urgently occurring issues. This firefighting approach has resulted in less than ideal improvements, usually directed by decisions made away from where the work happens, thus not maximizing the talent of the people who know the work best, that is, those who do the work. Therefore, let us explore a better way to work that will move the work closer to ideal (Lee and Woll 2003).*

Ideal

- Exactly what the patient needs, *defect free*
- One by one, customized to each individual patient
- On demand, exactly as requested
- Immediate response to problems or changes
- No waste
- Safe for patients, staff, and clinicians: physically, emotionally, and professionally

The reader can no doubt bring to mind personal experiences where time was wasted, frustration mounted, and less than satisfactory results were achieved with this approach. Consider the illustration below as the first step in looking at problematic work differently (Figure 22.1).

* Ideal: The concept of Ideal is originally credited to Dr. Russell L. Ackoff.

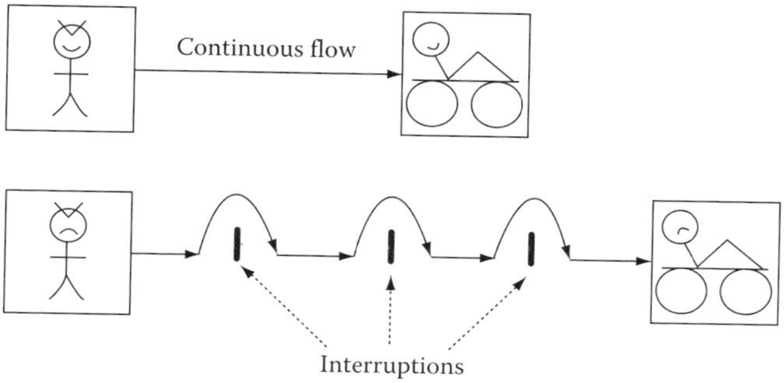

FIGURE 22.1 Observing work in action and recognizing where roadblocks occur that prevent work from happening with continuous flow is the first activity of discovering how to redesign current work.

If the nurse in Figure 22.1 set out to change a dressing for the patient in the leanest of situations he or she would do *exactly* what was ordered, using a checklist to remind/insure that all steps were carried out using the right techniques, materials, and medications (all at hand, clearly marked) with personal protection to prevent infection or injury of the nurse and patient, at the time prescribed. The patient would get exactly what he or she needed (no more, no less), when it was needed, delivered in a safe environment, creating no waste of materials or talent.

Perhaps more familiar to the reader is the scenario illustrated by the lower drawing in Figure 22.1; in a less than ideal situation, the nurse may arrive at the bedside and discover that the information he or she had received is not relevant to the patient's condition (creating a trip or a phone call away from the bedside to clarify the order) and dressing material or medication is missing (requiring another trip to collect necessary gear). If the caregiver is unaware that the patient is unable to turn himself or herself before entering the room, he or she has to leave again to find staff assistance to move the patient.

Each one of these frequently occurring interruptions in work creates wasted time, risk, declining confidence of the patient in the organization's ability to care for him or her and frustration for the worker. While these seemingly small complications in work seem insignificant, they are an unfortunate norm in most healthcare practice and recur hundreds if not thousands of times a day in every organization. This simple illustration could be applied to almost any process of work, assigning a different label to the worker, the customer, and the many work-arounds that are created by ineffective process steps.

Given the option, anyone would choose to do their work with continuous flow; beginning any task of work with clear direction and expectations, all the required information and materials to do the work on hand, moving to safe and satisfactory completion without interruptions. We can likely recall the sense of accomplishment that we have experienced with work that has progressed in such a manner and we can more likely recollect the frustration and anxiety that has marred work littered with interruptions, confusion, rework, and errors. Observing these obstacles in work is the first step in removing them; recognizing how they inhibit effective flow of work is the single primary step in creating work design that eliminates waste and risk.

Direct observation of work in motion stands above all other methods for deeply understanding the steps required to accomplish a task and recognizing work-arounds. We frequently rely on file data or emotional testimony to assume understanding of a work process, but direct observation of work cannot be underestimated as true information on which improvements can be built with confidence.

High-Level View: Value Stream Mapping

One visual method used for understanding the way work happens is the *value stream map* (VSM). As the name suggests, it illustrates the stream of steps that must occur to produce a requested product or service (value) to the requestor. The VSM clarifies the activities and order of the *flow of work*. Multiple occurrences can be evaluated to determine variation in practice. Let us take the image in Figure 22.2 apart to clarify the way it works.

In Figure 22.3, the unhappy patient is represented on the right upper corner (dotted lines), arriving at the Emergency Department for treatment of a laceration.

The steps in making the request for treatment flow from the patient on the right to the left side of the page.

Next, each of the major steps required to complete the request is illustrated on the VSM as a "process box," in which several activities occur to produce each essential step. (Figure 22.4)

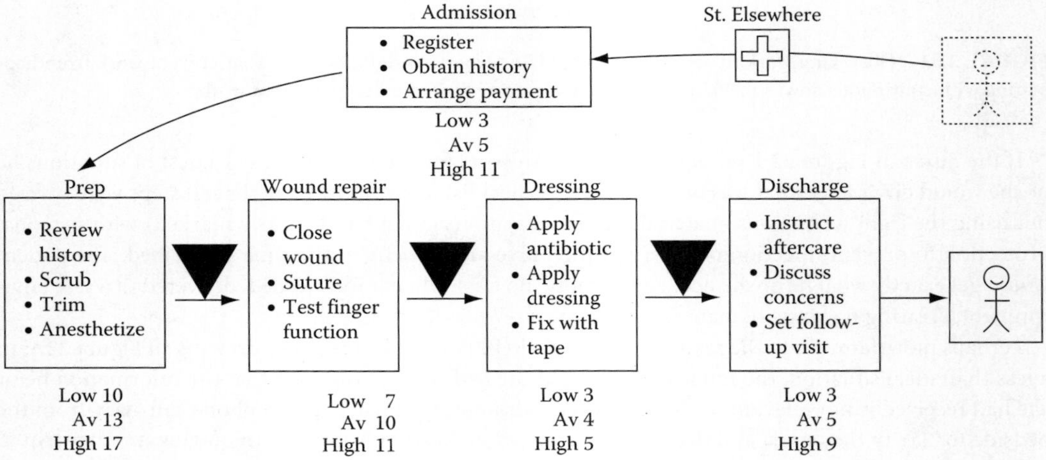

FIGURE 22.2 VSM for an unhappy patient arriving at the emergency department for treatment of a laceration.

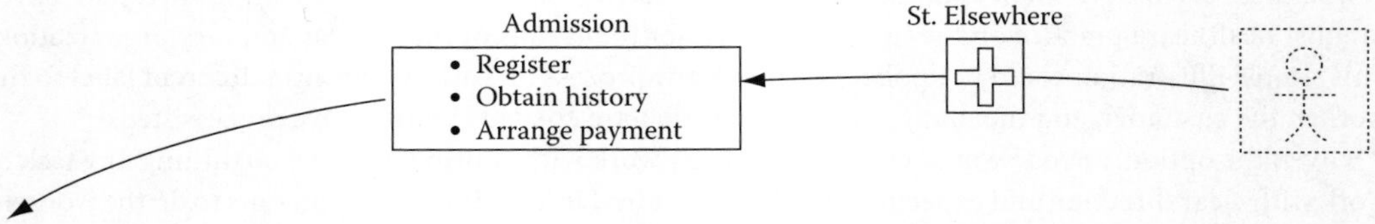

FIGURE 22.3 Understanding the entire process, including all the steps in the *request* for a service or product, beginning with the *requester* (on the right of this illustration), is essential to get the big picture of how the work is initiated.

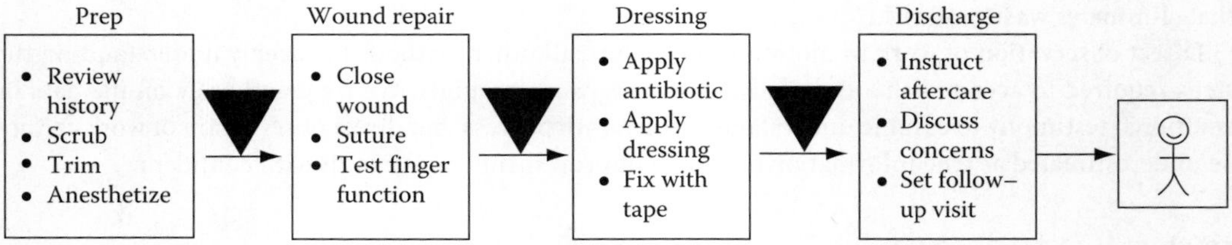

FIGURE 22.4 Once the request and all its steps are clear, it is easier to then map all the steps in *answering* the request. Note that the customer ends up on the right side of the VSM, directly below where he or she initiated the request. *Ideal* for the requester would be the shortest route between when the request was made and when it was satisfied.

The black inverted deltas between the process boxes indicate breaks in the work when nothing is happening to move the process along. These interruptions or delays may be due to a myriad of events such as a handing off of responsibilities that require waiting for another worker or a delay imposed by interrupting a set schedule (e.g., getting an emergency x-ray). See process boxes and the activities that occur within them in Figure 22.4. The arrows indicate the flow of work from left to right; if work in an earlier box is repeated as the process progresses, backward-directing arrows may be drawn to accurately indicate loops in the flow of work.

Analysis of the time spent completing each of those steps creates a *time and motion* study of what is happening that *adds value* to the process and how much of the that time is *not adding value*. The measurement/analysis of several samples of the process gives us additional information about how consistently and reliably the same work occurs. Recognizing where inconsistencies occur on the map points to where we can focus work design improvements. Simple averaging of the samples will provide a snapshot of the best-case scenario (the lowest time a step can be performed to the standard), the worst case, and the average of the samples times. Consider the data on the map (Figure 22.5), shown here again as in Figure 22.2.

As we create VSMs to better understand and evaluate the processes of daily work, the ability to see and measure each of the steps for its true value, *through the eyes of the patient/customer* is the beginning of correcting work design. Objectively evaluating the steps for value highlights what should be left in the revision of the process and what activities can be changed or eliminated. In this recognition is the opportunity to eliminate waste. In the elimination of waste, an increase in capacity is created in addition to a decrease in worker frustration and most importantly, *a quicker, safer delivery of the care a patient requires* (Jimmerson 2009).

VSMs provide elemental information from which specific task analysis and problem solving is directed. In turn, A3 problem solving reveals opportunities to use 5S, standardized work and other Lean methods to maximize flow and improve quality. VSMs compose visual and articulate vectors for policy deployment (*hoshin kanri*), which leads to the structure for improving work design across the healthcare business enterprise. While no one activity of Lean is more essential than another, the vital foundation that value stream mapping information provides is a sound conceptual element in improving the design of work.

VSMs differ from familiar flowcharts because they do not illustrate what *should* happen, based on an organizational policy or a procedure described in a manual; instead they visualize how the work is

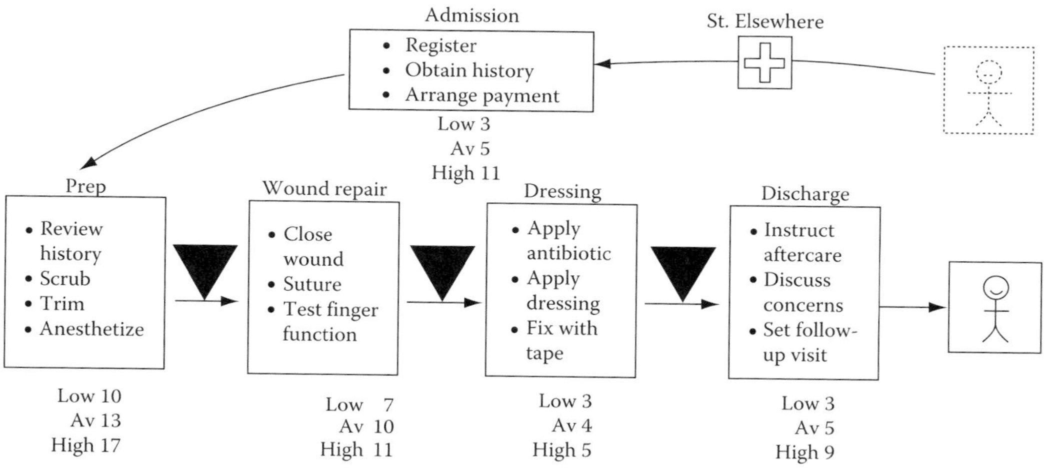

FIGURE 22.5 Seeing the steps and time passing on the map gives the user the information needed to design out redundant or ambiguous work and add essential valuable activities toward the goal of best quality and fewest steps/time.

observed to be *really* happening now. Likewise, they differ from conventional *process maps* commonly used in industrial engineering in that they also point out when *nothing* is happening to move the process along (indicated in the illustrations by the inverted deltas (▼) between the process boxes). This is significant as it immediately recognizes waste disguised as *delay* between work steps, a substantial consumer of worker time in most processes.

VSMs are created from a combination of historical knowledge and direct observation, with observation being the validating step. This keeps the information in the map objective and accurate and is the first step toward straightforward collaboration for process improvement. Mapping the current condition may start at a staff meeting but the work needs to be observed *in action* to validate for accuracy. Validation of revisions of the work is equally important to continually insure that the work is indeed true and to generate momentum and buy-in for the corrections with the people who do the work.

Moving from the Current State to Future State

The first objective with completing a current state map is to document all the steps in the process from request to satisfaction. Because the request occurs "upstream" in the overall process, sometimes recognizing the complexity and simplifying this part of the process positively affects the operations downstream.

Once the steps are completely documented the process can be assessed for opportunities to improve the flow of work. Because the method is visual (done on a whiteboard with a group or on 11″ × 17″ paper) obstacles in flow of work will be apparent. Redundant or ambiguous work will be visible and ideas for improving the flow will be forthcoming. Sometimes moving an activity from one step to another makes a significant improvement with little or no cost, training or addition of resources.

As problems with flow are eliminated, consideration of the data for variation in the samples measured will point to steps that are inconsistent. Simply recording the time spent finishing the activities within the process boxes will reflect the difference between the best-case scenario (lowest time spent completing the step) and longest time required for the same activities in another sample. If the lowest and highest numbers are very close, this will confirm that variation in the performance of that step is low and the need to focus improvement activities on that step are a lower priority; likewise, a great variation in the time required to complete activities will point directly at the most available opportunity to make improvements. Hence, understanding the design of current work leads us to the next step, formulating a better work design by creating a *future state map*.

The future state map is the proposed better design of work that is created after the current state map has been validated and evaluated for failings. In the collective activity of creating this new vision the good ideas of the staff can be mined for improving the work design.

More than one person, perhaps representing more than one department within or even outside the organization, will need to participate in creating maps of both current state and future state that are accurate and whose redesign is supported by all the parties affected by the work in mention. A collaborative advantage of value stream mapping is drawing the first rendition with a pencil (in a meeting, the initial work can be done on a whiteboard for visibility and inclusion of all participants). The pencil-and-paper version assures easy validating with the affected parties not in attendance and archives the details of discoveries from the collaborative work. The on-the-spot changeability of the pencil-drawn document allows for completeness, accuracy, and involvement of the people who will use the changed process in a quick and informal but thorough way.

When choosing the first process to map, consider the following:

- It must be observable; a process that can be followed and the activities of the process seen.
- For the sake of accelerating observations, data collection, and testing changes, it is best if it occurs frequently. Observing a process that only repeats a few times a month may have value,

but is likely not a good place to start. One of the most gratifying features of this work is that it is quick and results can be seen and understood while the work is fresh and problems are relevant.

- The process should involve work that is recognized by the staff and the administrative team as worthy of the resources being dedicated to the improvement efforts. Establishing the importance to the patient/customer, the worker, and the business enterprise is critical in determining its worth.

VSMs can be modified in scope to fit the focus requirements of any group that is interested in improving work processes. For organizational planners and administrators the views may be very high, with greater scope and less detail. For the surgeon in the operating room, the details on the map may be finer and the scope much narrower to address a particular process of very specific work.

Task Analysis

Seeing work as it happens allows us to recognize roadblocks that a worker has to work around and to measure the staggering waste that is created by ineffective processes. Many tools have been developed to prompt and record sources of waste; Figure 22.6 illustrates one simple but useful form for capturing the good information acquired when work is observed, minute by minute, as it occurs.

Note that with the form below, the *activity* that is being observed is recorded with other demographic data and there is an area to sketch or describe the physical layout of the work area. Minute by minute documentation of work (time is noted when the worker changes activities) is made and described in the first two columns. Analysis of that work is done at the completion of the observation by reflection and assignment of an appropriate icon that best indicates the nature of each work/time entry. The recommended observation time is 30–60 minutes but should be adjusted for the circumstances of the work and the intended use of the information.

Figure 22.7, although perhaps difficult to read in content, makes the point of the value of using this kind of tool. It is a personal *worksheet* onto which the observer times, visually diagrams, questions, and recognizes issues (note the "storm cloud" written in the left margin...a safety threat was recognized that needs immediate attention!). In the reflection summary the observer colored in the icons that best related to work/time entries and then added the number of minutes spent in each of the iconic categories. The calculations objectively supported what the worker knew in his or her gut: of the total time of 27 minutes observed, only 10 minutes was spent doing the actual work of the activity and 17 minutes passed walking, clarifying unclear information, making/receiving phone calls, and looking for required supplies and meds that were not on hand. When we start to analyze tasks with this degree of scrutiny it is easy to see the waste (and opportunities!) created when a poor design of work, facility, and information goes unchecked.

Again, any similar tool that supports task analysis at this level will be priceless in revealing wasted time and talent and is a very inspirational place to begin revising work design.

Once the tasks of work have been observed with this attention to detail, engaging the observed workers in the analysis of the activities is both enlightening for all parties and offers a sound and objective foundation of knowledge from which obstacles can be removed and improvements made.

Frequently if we work in a silo-like system we may attempt to fix a problem for our own selves and not be aware of the upstream effects to our work and the effects we may be creating for the steps downstream of us in the process. Current and future state VSMs illustrate the adjacencies of the consecutive steps and how each step can be affected by the neighboring work. The greatest challenge when difficulties are exposed is avoiding "band-aid" fixes to the identified problems. Workers will eagerly jump to fix an apparent problem, inadvertently (and with the best intentions for improvement) creating more work-arounds and adding unintended but real complexity to a process. Removing the root cause and doing

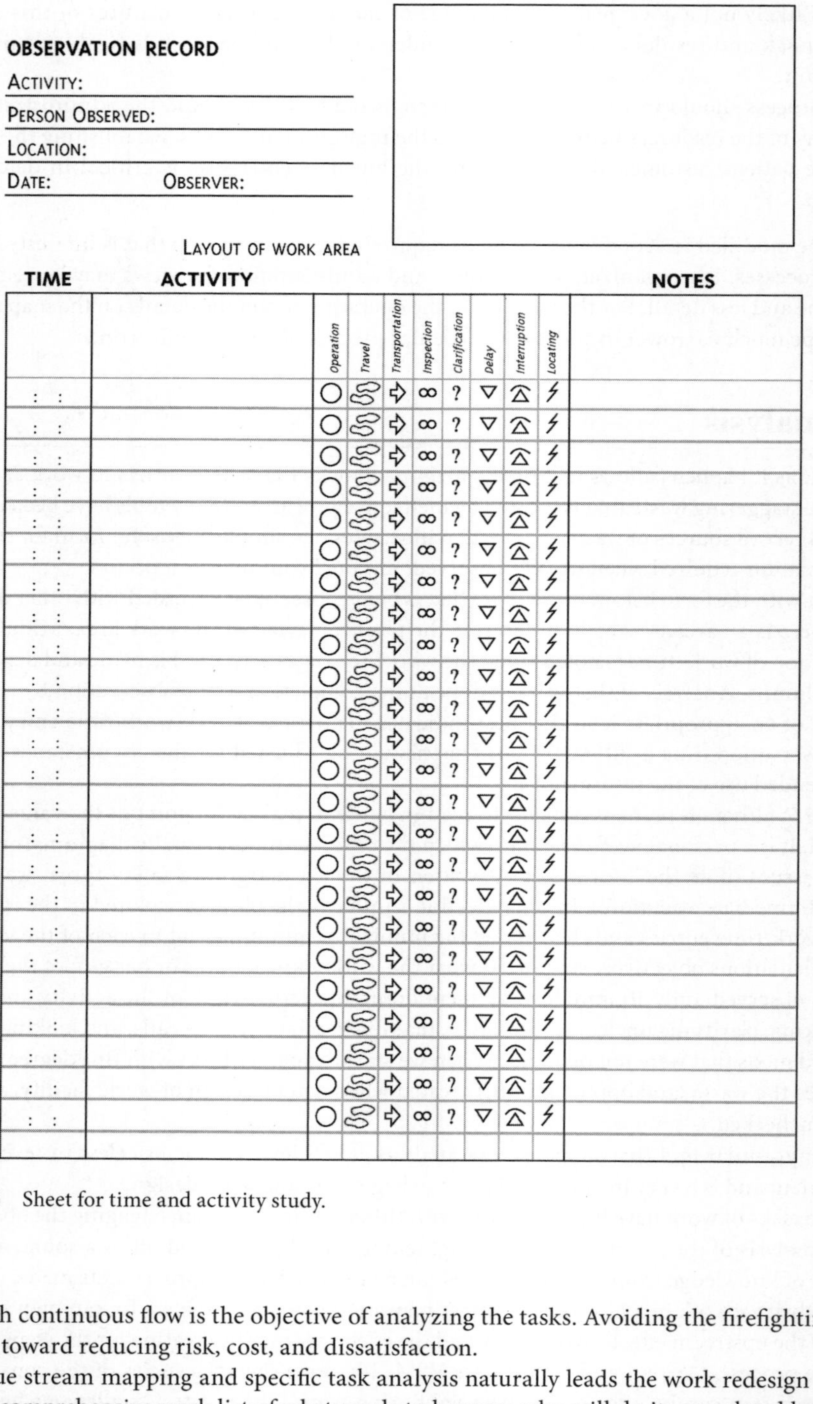

FIGURE 22.6 Sheet for time and activity study.

the work with continuous flow is the objective of analyzing the tasks. Avoiding the firefighting mode is the first step toward reducing risk, cost, and dissatisfaction.

Using value stream mapping and specific task analysis naturally leads the work redesign to a *future state plan*, a comprehensive work list of what needs to happen, who will do it, completed by when and a clear expectation of the results of each improvement task. This plan details what needs to be done to adjust the tasks of work to move from the how the work happens now (diagrammed on the current state map) to the proposed better way to work (the future state map).

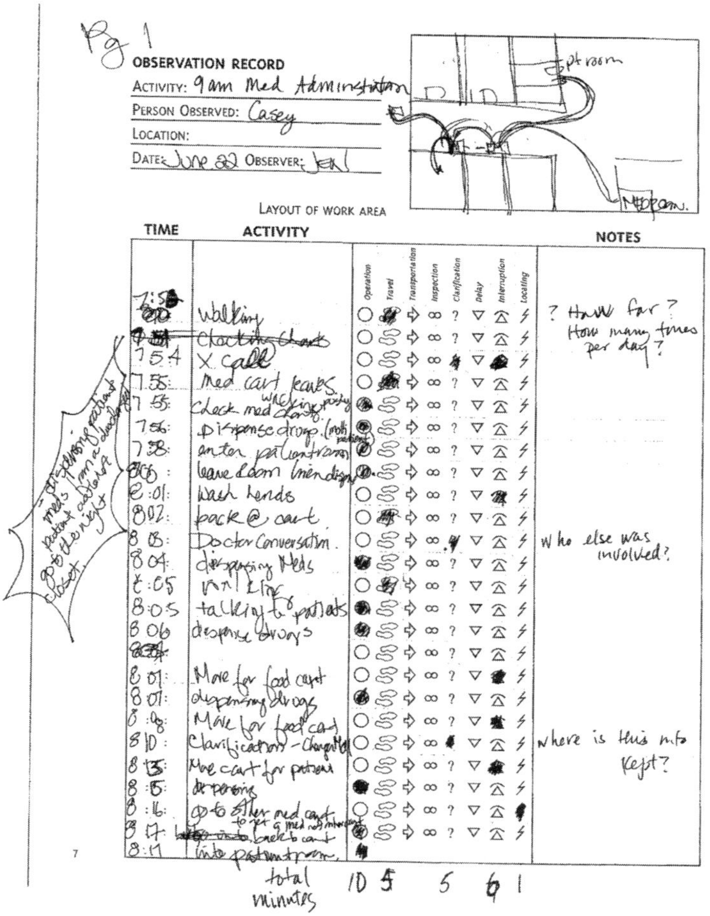

FIGURE 22.7 Example of time and activity study for medicine administration in a hospital.

Future State Plan

The author would be remiss not to mention the progression of the TPS/Lean process as it relates to the design of work. Ideally, each assigned improvement in the future state plan would be addressed with a standard approach to solving the problems identified. The value of having one problem solving method that is accepted by all workers with the confidence that they will have a voice (and a responsibility!) in being part of the improvement process deserves the reader's attention. The thinking that will have been learned and practiced with value stream mapping and task analysis experience can be applied to solving specific problems of work, all of which culminate in better work design (Table 22.1).

TABLE 22.1 Future State Action Plan

What	Who	When	Expected Outcome
1. Standardize room stock	CJ,LR	December 4, 2008	POU supplies
2. Standardize room set-up	JT, LO	November 28, 2008	Improve room turnover
3. Computerize discharge plan	PR,ST, JP	December 15, 2008	Expedite on-time discharge

ISSUE Pt. measurement of glucose delayed in truama ICU

BACKGROUND

Intensive Glucose Testing research depends on regular and timely blood glucose analysis. In the 12 bed-ICU the average number of patients on the Intensive Glucometry protocol = 9
Observed nurses took average of 17 minutes to draw/measure/treat when glucometer not in room

CURRENT CONDITION

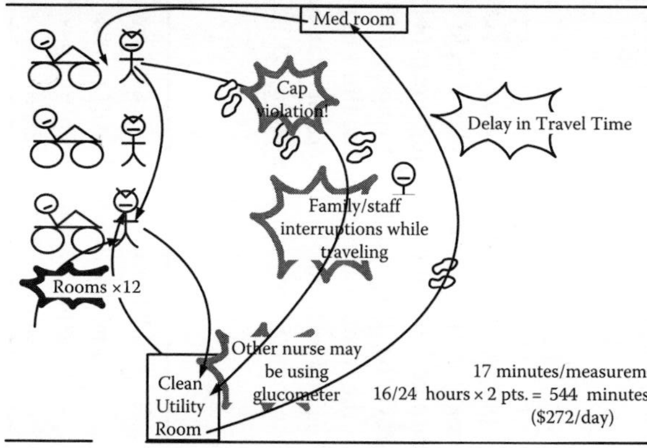

17 minutes/measurement
16/24 hours × 2 pts. = 544 minutes/day (9.1 hours)
($272/day)

PROBLEM ANALYSIS

1. CAP violation
   Why? unlabeled blood is out of the patient room
      Why? glucometer is housed in clean utility room
         Why? must be shared by 12 patient rooms

2. Delay in treatment
   Why? Travel time to use glucometer in clean utility room
      Why? one glucometer is shared and must be centrally stored
         Why? glucometers not at bedside
            Why? not enough glucometers
   Why? Distractions between drawing blood, checking value and treating patient
      Why? often stopped by family/staff when traveling
         Why? glucometer not in room

3. Potential for error
   Why? Blood not labeled when taken from room
      Why? glucometer not in room

TARGET CONDITION Title: Glucometer availability

To	Lorie
By	Kathy
Date	October 12, 2006

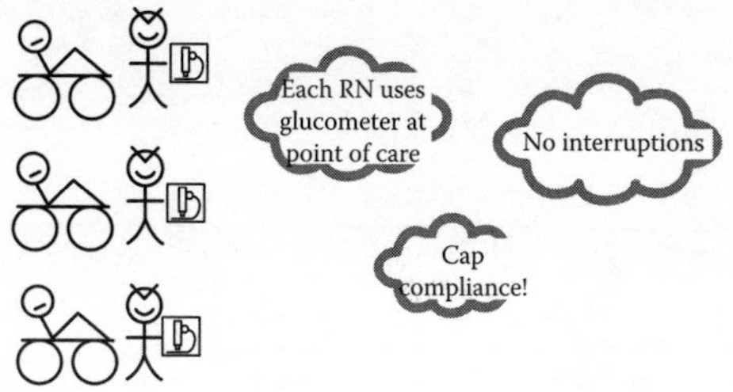

3 minutes = 1 Glucose measurement
16 measurements/24 hours × 2 pts = 96 minutes/day
($48/day)

COUNTERMEASURES

1. Place glucometers at bedside
2. Review glucose protocol and new glucometer use with staff

IMPLEMENTATION PLAN

What	Who	When	Outcome
Get approval for additional glucometer purchase	Lorie	10/13/06	Initiate purchase of 8 glucometers
Get funding	Dr. K	10/20/06	Purchase glucometers
Orient staff to new machines/policy at staff meeting	Kathy	11/1/06	Staff prepared to use new process!

COST/BENEFIT

Cost	$$$
Staff time to travel/share glucometer	$ 99,280/year
Benefit	**$$$**
Staff time ($$) with glucometer in the room	$ 17.520
Consistent measurement and treatment of glycemic variance	Quality

TEST

Measure time it takes to do glucose testing at bedside vs. travel time and sharing one machine in

FOLLOW UP

November 12, 2006
Staff time measuring blood glucose at beside: 3 minutes

FIGURE 22.8 A3 problem solving example.

While the limits of this chapter do not allow for expanded discussion of A3 Problem Solving (Jimmerson 2008) it is highly recommended that the inquisitive reader explore this method for addressing *specific problems* identified with value stream mapping and task analysis. A3 documents act both as a template for completing every step of the problem understanding, root cause analysis, and correction plan but also as a detailed archive of the tasks and individuals involved in constantly advancing the design of work on a specific level. A sample A3 appears in Figure 22.8.

References

Lee, T. and T. Woll. 2003. Reflections on the idealized design planning process. *Center for Quality of Management Journal* 11(2): 4–5.

Jimmerson, C. 2008. *A3 Problem Solving for Healthcare*. Productivity Press. NYC, New York. www.coe.montana.edu/IE/faculty/sobek/A3/index.htm

Jimmerson, C. 2009. *Value Stream Mapping made Easy for Healthcare*. Productivity Press. NYC, New York.

Sobek, D.K. and C. Jimmerson. 2003. Applying the Toyota production system to a hospital pharmacy. In *Proceedings of the 2003 Industrial Engineering Research Conference*, Portland, OR.

23

Scheduling and Sequencing

Edmund K. Burke
University of Nottingham

Timothy Curtois
University of Nottingham

Tomas Eric Nordlander
SINTEF Information and Communication Technology

Atle Riise
SINTEF Information and Communication Technology

Introduction 23-1
Nurse Rostering 23-2
Methodologies
Surgery Scheduling 23-9
Patient Mix Planning • Creating a Master Surgery Schedule • Operational Surgery Scheduling
Summary 23-13
References 23-13

Introduction

Healthcare management includes many different planning tasks. These tasks are often interconnected by the flow of patients through clinical pathways, or the use of resources across such pathways. Many of these planning tasks involve the creation of schedules and sequences. Some of the more common scheduling scenarios include:

- Creating rosters for nurse and physicians
- Scheduling patient appointments
- Scheduling the use of operating theatres
- Scheduling regular treatment (for example, radiotherapy and chemotherapy)

Often the schedules are still created by hand. Producing them manually without the help of a decision support system has two significant disadvantages:

1. The schedules produced are suboptimal and do not utilize precious resources as efficiently as possible. This can have a number of adverse effects such as unnecessary expenditure, inferior quality of patient care, and dissatisfied employees.
2. The scheduling is in itself a time consuming and sometimes a frustrating task, which often falls on employees who could use their time more productively, especially as they are frequently already overloaded. For example, it is usually a responsibility of head nurses to create rosters. Asking nurses to solve these very challenging problems distract them from their primary duty of healthcare. As such, it is not a welcome assignment.

Fortunately, these undesirable situations can be greatly improved. Since the early 1950s, researchers have been analyzing these problems and utilizing theory from fields such as mathematics, computer science, economics, and engineering. There is now a large and growing body of research into technologies for automating and optimizing these scheduling processes. With the ubiquity of powerful personal computers, these systems are increasingly being adopted in many environments and the associated benefits realized.

In this chapter, we will look at two commonly occurring scheduling problems in healthcare environments—nurse rostering and surgery scheduling. In the following sections, we will examine the problems in more depth and present a variety of techniques that have been developed to solve them.

Nurse Rostering

Unlike many other well-studied optimization problems, no standard model or formulation for the nurse-rostering problem exists. This may be because constraints and objectives for each problem instance vary widely, not just between different countries and hospitals but also between different departments and wards within a hospital. This lack of a single version of the nurse-rostering problem has had two effects on the research and development of technologies and methodologies for the nurse-rostering problem: (1) there are very few commonly used benchmark data sets that researchers can use to develop and gauge the success of different approaches (this is unusual for such a widely researched problem); and (2) a large variety of techniques have been developed for the problem, often with each approach tailored to a particular situation.

Although there is no single, standard formulation of the problem, it *is* possible to identify a common general structure, which can be stated as follows:

> For a set of employees (for example, belonging to a single ward) and a given planning period, decide for each employee on which shift (if any) they are assigned each day.

This is of course subject to a large number of constraints and objectives. As mentioned, these constraints and objectives vary significantly between organizations. Also, a constraint for one instance may be an objective in another. For example, in one situation there may be a constraint on the number of hours an employee can work within the planning period, whereas in another, the employee may exceed this limit but the overtime should be minimized.

The constraints and objectives for the nurse-rostering problem can be broadly split into two groups:

1. *Employees' working requirements*: These affect the schedule (work pattern) for each employee. Examples include:
   a. Minimum/maximum number of hours worked
   b. Minimum/maximum number of consecutive days with work
   c. Minimum/maximum number of consecutive days without work
   d. Minimum/maximum number of consecutive weekends with work
   e. Minimum/maximum number of weekends with work
   f. Minimum/maximum number of shifts of a certain type (e.g., a maximum number of night shifts)
   g. Annual leave or requests for certain days or shifts off or on
   h. Rest requirements after a series of night shifts
   i. Subpatterns to avoid (for example an early shift after a late shift)
   j. Requests to work at the same times as other employees (e.g., to enable carpooling or supervision of trainee nurses)
2. *Cover requirements*: These constraints ensure that the correct number of employees are present during each shift for each day. They may also consider skill mixes and may be expressed as minimum, maximum, and/or preferred numbers of employees working.

In the case study that follows in the next section, we provide an integer programming (IP) model of a nurse-rostering problem in which some of these constraints are formalized. In the following sections, we discuss three popular methodologies and approaches that have been successfully applied to the nurse-rostering problem—mathematical programming, constraint programming (CP), and heuristic approaches.

Methodologies

The methods used to solve the problems can be placed in one of two broad categories: exact and heuristic optimization methods. Exact methods (e.g., mathematical programming and CP) have the advantage that they will guarantee to produce optimal solutions. The disadvantage is that, for many real world nurse-rostering problems, the time required to find these solutions is impractically large. As a result, most exact optimization methods applied to real world nurse-rostering problems do one or more of the following:

- Solve a relaxation of the problem.
- Use a number of heuristics.
- Terminate before the optimal solution is found.

Yet, exact optimization techniques are very successful. For example, often it is only necessary to model the problem and then use a highly developed algorithm such as CPLEX's (http://www.ilog.com/products/cplex/) mixed-integer programming (MIP) solver to solve it. On the other hand, designing the model or formulation is not always trivial and can have a critical effect on the success of the algorithms.

Approaches that do not guarantee to produce optimal solutions are broadly categorized as heuristic methods. Heuristic approaches are commonly applied to, and are particularly suited to, nurse-rostering problems for a number of reasons. First, it is actually very difficult to define what would be an optimal solution. The problem formulations are often based on subjective decisions and vague preferences such that an "optimal" solution may not actually be the best or most preferable solution. For example, an employee might say "I would quite like a day off on…" or "I don't really want a night shift on…" These sorts of statements are difficult to translate into exact mathematical expressions. Secondly, users are often impatient and want short waiting times for solutions. As such, they are willing to trade optimal solutions for near optimal solutions in order to reduce computation times. This is particularly the case for nurse rostering that may need new solutions at short notice due to absences and sickness. A criticism of heuristic approaches is that they can be inconsistent between problem instances and may require more programming. On the other hand, complicated objective functions may be easier to handle with higher level programming languages. Another major criticism is, of course, that you cannot, in general, guarantee optimality.

Mathematical Programming

Before solving the nurse-rostering problem using a mathematical programming approach, it is necessary to decide on the formulation of the problem. There are two common formulations. The first one is to model the decision variables as nurse to shift assignments. In other words, the variable takes the value 1 if the nurse is assigned to that shift and 0 if not (here, we refer to a shift as a shift type (e.g., night shift) on a specific day). See "Case Study: Solving a Nurse-Rostering Problem Using a VNS Approach" of this chapter for an example of this formulation. The second formulation is to model the decision variables as nurse to pattern assignments. Here, the patterns are generally predefined. As the number of possible patterns for each nurse is exponentially large, a subset of acceptable patterns is generated for each nurse at the start of the algorithm. This approach indicates that the final solution is not necessarily optimal but in our experience MIP solvers such as CPLEX 10 can solve this formulation of the problem quite quickly (even if the number of patterns for each nurse is >1000). Using the nurse-shift formulation does guarantee optimality but even powerful solvers such as CPLEX and Xpress-MP (http://www.dashoptimization.com/) are often ineffective on real-world sized problems.

An alternative approach is branch and price, in which, in effect, new patterns are generated as required. In this approach, a linear programming (where integrality constraints are relaxed) nurse-pattern formulation is used at each node in a branch and bound tree. The branching is usually performed by progressively assigning shifts in the overall roster. Using the dual costs from the cover constraints, subproblems are then generated and solved to find new reduced cost patterns (columns) to add to the original problem. The column generation subproblem can be modeled as a shortest path problem with resource constraints. Although this is also NP-hard, it can often be solved efficiently by using a dynamic programming approach. Examples of branch and price approaches for nurse rostering are provided by Jaumard et al. (1998), Mason and Smith (1998), and Eveborn and Rönnqvist (2004).

Constraint Programming

The word "programming" in mathematical programming is related to the planning and scheduling problems it was originally used on (i.e., to create a program or schedule for a specific task). In contrast, "programming" in CP relates to programming computer languages, using constraints. The field started in the 1960s (Jebali et al. 2006) and matured for industrial use in the 1990s. The CP combines reasoning and computing techniques over constraints and its main subfield, constraint satisfaction, applies techniques to find solutions to constraint satisfaction problems (CSPs). As in the mathematical models, CSPs are defined in terms of variables, domains (possible values) for these variables, and constraints, which restrict the simultaneous values that the variables can take. A solution to a CSP, is the assignment of a value to every variable in such a way that all constraints are satisfied.

Most search algorithms systematically assign possible values to the variables using simple heuristics to control the order in which variables should be considered (variable order) and the order in which to assign domain values (value order); these heuristics can be either static or dynamically changed during search. In addition, the main CSP search technique interleaves various forms of backtracking search with consistency enforcement, in which infeasible values are removed from the domains of the variables through reasoning about the constraints. Today, there are CP libraries in many programming languages (e.g., C++, Java, Python, Prolog, LISP, etc.) and toolkits (e.g., ILOG (http://www.ilog.com and http://www.sics.se/sictus/)) are available. Examples of CP approaches applied to nurse rostering include those provided by Meisels et al. (1997), Meyer auf'm Hofe (2000), and Weil et al. (1995).

Heuristic Approaches

The largest proportion of approaches in nurse-rostering literature can be categorized as heuristic, local search, or metaheuristic methods. Heuristics may be constructive and build solutions step-by-step or by improving, for example, repairing violations in randomly generated rosters. Local search and metaheuristics use the idea of neighborhood search. In a neighborhood search, new solutions are created by making small changes to existing solutions. For example, by swapping assignments between two nurses or adding or removing assignments to or from a single nurse. These types of swaps and moves are called neighborhood operators. Local search terminates when no improving neighborhood moves/swaps can be found for the best solution found so far (i.e., the solution is locally optimal). Metaheuristics extend local search by providing mechanisms for allowing unimproving changes (small and large) to solutions in order to *escape* from local optima. However, for both metaheuristics and local search, identifying efficient neighborhood operators can often have a significant impact on the performance of the algorithm.

The popular metaheuristic framework tabu search has been applied to nurse rostering a number of times (e.g., Dowsland and Thompson 2000). Another type of metaheuristic, evolutionary algorithms, are also often used for nurse rostering. Like most metaheuristics, there is no strict and universally accepted definition for evolutionary algorithms. However, evolutionary algorithms are sometimes loosely inspired by natural or biological processes and often use one or more of the following:

- Generations (algorithmic iterations)
- Populations (multiple concurrent solutions)
- Crossover (combining features from two solutions to produce new solutions)
- Mutation (random changes to solutions)
- Population management (e.g., elitism, survival of the fittest, diversification strategies)

These features are not exclusive to evolutionary algorithms though and may appear in other metaheuristics in one form or another too. For example, "shuffles" or "kicks" in the metaheuristics variable neighborhood search and iterated local search could be described as mutations. Examples of evolutionary algorithms include genetic algorithms, memetic algorithms (genetic algorithms plus local search), and scatter search. For examples of these approaches applied to nurse rostering, see Burke et al. (2001) and Dias et al. (2003).

Other heuristic approaches that have been used to successfully solve nurse-rostering problems include case based reasoning (Beddoe and Petrovic 2007) and hyperheuristics (Burke et al. 2003).

Case Study: Solving a Nurse-Rostering Problem Using a VNS Approach

We will now discuss a metaheuristic approach, which was used to solve a challenging scheduling problem provided by a software company, who specialize in workforce management solutions. The problem contains a large number of objectives many of which are common in nurse-rostering problems. An IP model of the problem is provided below.

Parameters:

I = Set of nurses available
$I_t|t \in \{1,2,3\}$ = Subset of nurses who work 20, 32, 36 hours per week, respectively, $I = I_1 + I_2 + I_3$
J = Set of indices of the last day of each week within the scheduling period = {7, 14, 21, 28, 35}
K = Set of shift types = {1(*early*), 2(*day*), 3(*late*), 4(*night*)}
K' = Set of undesirable shift type successions = {(2,1), (3,1), (3,2), (1,4), (4,1), (4,2), (4,3)}
d_{jk} = Coverage requirement of shift type k on day j, $j \in \{1,\ldots,7|J|\}$
m_i = Maximum number of working days for nurse i
n_1 = Maximum number of consecutive *night* shifts
n_2 = Maximum number of consecutive working days
c_k = Desirable upper bound of consecutive assignments of shift type k
g_t = Desirable upper bound of weekly working days for the tth subset of nurses
h_t = Desirable lower bound of weekly working days for the tth subset of nurses

Decision variables:

x_{ijk} = 1 if nurse i is assigned shift type k for day j, 0 otherwise.

The constraints are

1. Shift cover requirements.

$$\sum_{i \in I} x_{ijk} = d_{jk}, \quad \forall j \in \{1,...,7|J|\}, k \in K$$

2. A nurse may not start more than one shift each day.

$$\sum_{k \in K} x_{ijk} \leq 1, \quad \forall i \in I, j \in \{1,...,7|J|\}$$

Other requirements are formulated as (weighted w_i) goals. The overall objective function is:

$$\text{Min } \bar{G}(x) = \sum_{i=1}^{15} w_i \bar{g}_i(x),$$

where the goals are:

1. Complete weekends (i.e., Saturday and Sunday are both working days or both off).

$$\bar{g}_1(x) = \sum_{i \in I} \sum_{j \in J} \left| \sum_{k \in K} \left[x_{i(j-1)k} - x_{ijk} \right] \right|$$

2. Minimum of two consecutive nonworking days.

$$\bar{g}_2(x) = \sum_{i \in I} \sum_{j=2}^{7|J|-1} \max \left\{ 0, \sum_{k \in K} \left[-x_{i(j-1)k} + x_{ijk} - x_{i(j+1)k} \right] \right\}$$

3. A minimum number of days off after a series of shifts.

$$\bar{g}_3(x) = \sum_{i \in I} \sum_{j=2}^{7|J|-1} \max \left\{ 0, \sum_{k \in K} \left[x_{i(j-1)k} - x_{ijk} + x_{i(j+1)k} \right] - 1 \right\}$$

4. A maximum number of consecutive shifts of type early and late.

$$\bar{g}_4(x) = \sum_{i \in I} \sum_{r=1}^{7|J|-c_k} \sum_{k \in \{1,3\}} \max \left\{ 0, \sum_{j=r}^{r+c_k} x_{ijk} - c_k \right\}$$

5. A minimum number of consecutive shifts of type early and late.

$$\bar{g}_5(x) = \sum_{i \in I} \sum_{j=2}^{7|J|-1} \sum_{k \in \{1,3\}} \max \left\{ 0, -x_{i(j-1)k} + x_{ijk} - x_{i(j+1)k} \right\}$$

6. A maximum and minimum number of working days per week.

$$\bar{g}_6(x) = \sum_{t=1}^{3} \sum_{i \in I_t} \sum_{w=1}^{|J|} \left[\max\left\{0, \sum_{j=7w-6}^{7w} \sum_{k \in K} x_{ijk} - g_t \right\} + \max\left\{0, h_t - \sum_{j=7w-6}^{7w} \sum_{k \in K} x_{ijk} \right\} \right]$$

7. A maximum of three consecutive working days for part-time nurses.

$$\bar{g}_7(x) = \sum_{i \in I_1} \sum_{r=1}^{7|J|-3} \max\left\{0, \sum_{j=r}^{r+3} \sum_{k \in K} x_{ijk} - 3\right\}$$

8. Avoiding certain shift successions (e.g., an *early* shift after a *day* shift).

$$\bar{g}_8(x) = \sum_{i \in I} \sum_{j=1}^{7|J|-1} \sum_{(k_1,k_2) \in K'} \max\left\{0, x_{ijk_1} + x_{i(j+1)k_2} - 2\right\}$$

9. Maximum number of working days.

$$\bar{g}_9(x) = \sum_{i \in I} \max\left\{0, \sum_{j=1}^{7|J|} \sum_{k \in K} x_{ijk} - m_i\right\}$$

10. Maximum of three working weekends.

$$\bar{g}_{10}(x) = \sum_{i \in I} \max\left\{0, \sum_{j \in J} \sum_{k \in K} \max\left\{x_{i(j-1)k}, x_{ijk}\right\} - 3\right\}$$

11. Maximum of three night shifts.

$$\bar{g}_{11}(x) = \sum_{i \in I} \max\left\{0, \sum_{j=1}^{7|J|} x_{ij4} - 3\right\}$$

12. A minimum of two consecutive night shifts.

$$\bar{g}_{12}(x) = \sum_{i \in I} \sum_{j=2}^{7|J|-1} \max\left\{0, -x_{i(j-1)4} + x_{ij4} - x_{i(j+1)4}\right\}$$

13. A minimum of two days off after a series of consecutive night shifts. This is equivalent to avoiding the pattern: night shift–day off–day on.

$$\bar{g}_{13}(x) = \sum_{i \in I} \sum_{j=2}^{7|J|-1} \max\left\{0, x_{i(j-1)4} - \sum_{k \in K} x_{ijk} + \sum_{k \in K} x_{i(j+1)k} - 1\right\}$$

14. Maximum number of consecutive night shifts.

$$\overline{g}_{14}(x) = \sum_{i \in I} \sum_{r=1}^{7|J|-n_1} \max\left\{0, \sum_{j=r}^{r+n_1} x_{ij4} - n_1\right\}$$

15. Maximum number of consecutive working days.

$$\overline{g}_{15}(x) = \sum_{i \in I} \sum_{r=1}^{7|J|-n_2} \max\left\{0, \sum_{j=r}^{r+n_2} \sum_{k \in K} x_{ijk} - n_2\right\}$$

The data for this instance (and others) are also available at the recently developed rostering benchmark website (http://www.cs.nott.ac.uk/~tec/NRP/).

The algorithm used to solve this problem was a hybrid approach that combined heuristic ordering with variable neighborhood descent. The first step is to create an initial roster which is done using heuristic ordering of shifts to be assigned. As the cover requirements cannot be violated, it is possible to precreate all the shifts that need to be assigned in order to produce a feasible solution. These shifts are, then, heuristically ordered based on an estimate of how difficult they may be to assign. For example, there are many high priority objectives related to night shifts; so a successful heuristic was to assign night shifts first. Similarly, objectives related to weekends conflict with many other objectives; so weekend shifts are given a higher order. Once the shifts are ordered they are assigned one by one using a greedy method, which operates as follows: Before assigning a shift to an employee, all employees are tested as the possible assignee and the employee that causes the least gain in the objective function on receiving this shift is chosen. After this initial roster is created it is improved (according to the objective function) using a variable neighborhood descent.

Variable neighborhood descent gradually improves a solution by testing neighborhood operators and applying the improving changes. The algorithm finishes when all neighborhood operators have been tested on the current best known solution and when a better solution was not found. In other words, the current best is locally optimal for all the neighborhoods being used. For this problem two simple neighborhood operators were used:

- Moving a shift from one employee to another.
- Swapping the employees assigned to a pair of shifts.

Using additional operators may provide further benefit, depending on the instances being solved. After the variable neighborhood descent, the best known solution can be returned or a simple diversification mechanism can be used to continue the search. This mechanism is a solution disruption method in which a small number of employees are selected and all their shifts unassigned. The roster is then repaired by reassigning these shifts over all the employees using the

TABLE 23.1 Hybrid VNS Outline

1. Create initial roster (using heuristic ordering)
2. REPEAT
3. Variable neighbourhood descent
4. Un-assign shifts of a set of nurses
5. Repair roster (using heuristic ordering method)
6. UNTIL max computation time exceeded

heuristic ordering method. After this, the variable neighborhood search is again applied. It was observed that regardless of the instance size, it was most effective to select three or four nurses to unassign the shifts from. When selecting the nurses it was also found useful to introduce bias toward those with the worst individual schedules (i.e., work patterns with the higher objective function values). The overall algorithm is outlined in Table 23.1.

More information on this problem and algorithm can be found in Burke et al. (2008). For further reading on the nurse rostering problem see Burke et al. (2004).

Surgery Scheduling

In many hospitals, the surgery department is a significant cost driver (Cardoen et al. 2008, Macario et al. 1995), partly due to the expensive resources directly involved in surgery. In addition, the operating room (OR) management influences other activities and associated resources in the hospital. For these reasons, surgery planning is crucial for cost efficient treatment and care, both in the surgery department and in other parts of the hospital. Better surgery planning can improve resource efficiency, reduce staff workload, reduce patients' waiting time, reduce the number of surgery cancellations, and improve overall performance in the hospital. Surgery planning is, however, a very complex task. This is because of the many resources that are involved, their involvement in other hospital activities, as well as the high degree of dynamics and uncertainty that is inevitable in most hospitals.

Surgery scheduling is getting increasing attention from researchers. There is already a sizeable literature on topics related to surgery scheduling, both in the operations research community and in the healthcare management community. A number of these publications apply discrete event simulation, and typically evaluate various simple sequencing heuristics for surgery scheduling based on their effect on OR performance and resource utilization (Blake and Carter 1997). In recent years, a number of authors have applied more advanced optimization methods for surgery-scheduling problems. Apart from the references found herein, a good overview of the existing literature is found in the surveys of Blake and Carter (1997), Magerlein and Martin (1978), Przasnyski (1986), and—more recently—Cardoen et al. (2008).

The term surgery planning covers planning tasks at different levels of detail and time scale. Following Blake and Donald (2002), we divide these into three levels; strategic, tactical, and operational surgery planning. Below, we give examples of planning tasks found at each level.

Patient Mix Planning

At the strategic level, we find the problem of determining the best distribution of OR time between the different medical specialties (or surgeons). This is often referred to as patient mix (or case mix) and relates closely to manufacturing product mix decisions (Hughes and Soliman 1985, Robbins and Tuntiwongbiboon 1989), where the objective is to decide the type and quantity of products to maximize profit. In the literature, most hospital–patient mix models are based on patient throughput maximization while in practice many more (often conflicting) objectives are considered, such as satisfying funding restrictions, care demand; OR, bed, and staff capacity; staff skills and interests; etc. (Rifai and Pecenka 1989, Blake and Carter 2002, 2003). Different solution techniques have been applied to the patient-mix problem, including linear programming (Hughes and Soliman 1985, Robbins and Tuntiwongbiboon 1989, Adan and Vissers 2002, Dexter et al. 2002), mixed linear programming (Vissers et al. 2005), and goal programming (Rifai and Pecenka 1989, Blake and Carter 2003).

A solution to the patient-mix problem provides a target quantity for each type of surgery that the hospital desires to handle. This translates into the proportion of the total OR time needed for each patient group (Beliën and Demeulemeester 2007, Blake and Donald 2002). This, in turn, gives the target proportion of total OR time for each medical specialty (or surgeon); let us call this the *target* OR time distribution.

Creating a Master Surgery Schedule

At the tactical planning level, some hospitals create a cyclic timetable that distributes OR time for each medical specialty over days and ORs. Such a timetable is often called a master surgery schedule (MSS). In the MSS, the OR time is divided into blocks, which in turn is allocated to medical specialties (or surgeons).

In Figure 23.1, we show an MSS with three ORs over a period of 1 week. Each OR day is divided into two blocks; morning and afternoon. The blocks are allocated to seven different medical specialties (orthopedic surgery, gynecological surgery, etc.).

Note that the existence of an MSS is not necessary—to use such a preallocation of OR time to specialties is a choice made by the hospital. The admission planner (see the section "Operational surgery scheduling") use the MSS as a template when conducting block scheduling—assigning elective cases to the blocks. The MSS guaranties that each specialty has available OR time on given days, and the need to prebook far in advance to reserve the OR time is less pressing. Block scheduling has been shown to produce higher resource utilization and less cancellations than open scheduling (Pham and Klinkert 2008). However, using an MSS has noted drawbacks. For example, an MSS might require redesign if the size of a medical specialty changes. Also, booking vacations and meetings have to be done around the blocks. If demand fluctuations leave blocks of OR time poorly utilized, it is important that the OR time is released to other specialties. The blocks often have a "block release time" that says how much earlier before the block starting time should the allocated block be released to other specialties (Malhotra 1999).

Developing an MSS involves creating and allocating blocks of OR time to each specialty in such a way that it best satisfies the objectives. The main objective is to minimize the deviation from the target OR time distribution. Others can be to minimize the changes to the existing MSS, minimize OR—or ward—staff cost (overtime), or maximize OR utilization. The MSS is often preferred to be as simple and repetitive as possible, which entails to have as few changes as possible from week to week (Blake et al. 2002). Often, the desired length of the cyclic period is given; when it is not, the length becomes a variable in the optimization problem. The generated MSS must satisfy a set of constraints like, always schedule infectious surgeries at the end of day, respect OR capabilities, etc. Also, when determining practical block sizes, one must take into account the uncertainty of surgical procedure durations, OR cleaning time, etc.

An MSS should be revised whenever changes in patient mix, staff or equipment availability, or demand occur; depending on the particular hospital, these changes might take place once or several times in a year. In reality, the MSS is more static and is sometimes used for years before being updated (case study by Beliën et al. 2005). Often this is not because the existing MSS is optimal, but because it continues to be feasible. Furthermore, the creation and maintenance of an MSS is a combinatorial

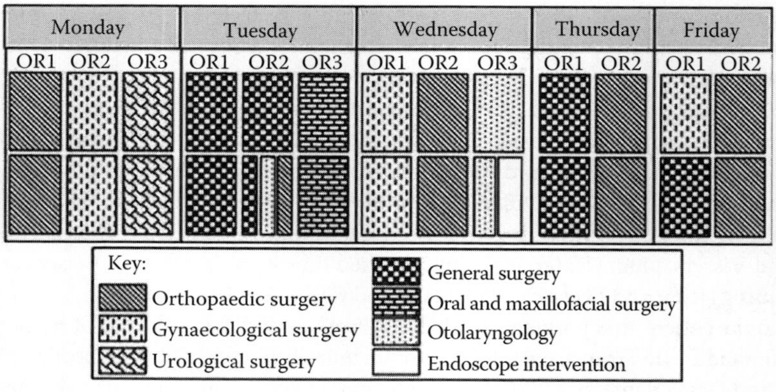

FIGURE 23.1 The MSS of a Norwegian hospital.

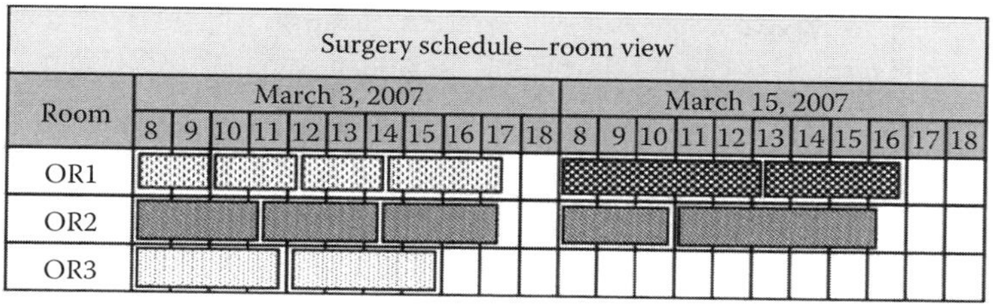

FIGURE 23.2 Snapshot from a simplified surgery schedule, showing the allocation of surgeries to rooms and days.

optimization problem that is difficult to solve manually. Without an optimization based planning, it is difficult to assess how far the existing MSS is from the optimal.

In the literature, different optimization techniques have been used to design MSSs: IP (Blake et al. 2002), mixed linear programming (Vissers et al. 2005, Santibanez et al. 2007), and metaheuristic methods (Beliën and Demeulemeester 2007) among others.

Operational Surgery Scheduling

Operational surgery scheduling includes a variety of planning problems—with different time horizons—that are solved on a daily (or weekly) basis. The resulting surgery schedule contains dates and times of surgery; as well as the allocation of critical resources, such as surgeons, ORs (see Figure 23.2), operation teams, equipment, or postoperative bed capacity.

These problems concern the allocation of dates and times of surgery to a set of given interventions, while reserving capacity for these interventions on a set of critical resources.

The formulation of surgery-scheduling problems varies considerably between hospitals. Variations also occur between planning at different time scales. In the following, we discuss the optimization problems encountered at different planning stages.

Intervention Assignment

The intervention assignment problem—also known as advance scheduling—concerns the assignment of interventions to ORs and days (Ozkarahan 2000, Guinet and Chaabane 2003, Ogulata and Erol 2003, Jebali et al. 2006, Chaabane et al. 2008, Hans et al. 2008). The problem occurs in admission planning, which is the first stage of operational surgery scheduling. Before describing the intervention assignment problem, let us provide some context through a typical example of admission planning from a Norwegian hospital.

After being referred for surgery by a specialist, the patients are registered on a waiting list. Every second or third day, the admission planner goes through these unserved referrals, and assigns a date of surgery to each one. Note that prior to this planning, a surgery schedule already exists from previous admission planning. The admission planner also communicates planned dates with some of the patients before "fixing" the surgery date. However, these surgeries can still be moved between rooms during subsequent planning. The date chosen for a surgery may be anything from a few days to several months into the future, depending on the queue length, the clinic capacity, and the surgery due dates.*

The assignment of dates to surgeries requires the resolution of the intervention assignment problem, which can be described as follows:

- The input information includes
    - A set of unplanned elective surgeries
    - An initial plan, in which the date of some of the surgeries are already fixed
    - A model of the hospital, including information about all critical resources

* Due dates are based on the patient's medical condition.

- The task is, then, to choose a date and a room for each surgery, in a way that optimizes certain objectives, while respecting certain constraints. The most common constraints are related to:
  - OR opening hours
  - Surgeon availability
  - An MSS (see previous section)
  - Time-lag constraints, such as cleaning times, surgery durations, and due dates
  - Precedence constraints, such as requiring infected patients to be treated as the last case in the day

If an MSS is used, this constrains the days and rooms into which the surgeries belonging to a given medical specialty can be assigned. This is often referred to as "block scheduling" (Ozkarahan 2000), as opposed to "open scheduling," where this constraint is absent (Chessare 2004). Common objectives of the intervention assignment problem include patient waiting time, personnel overtime, hospitalization costs, expected number of cancellations, workload leveling, and resource utilization. However, there are many variations, as will be discussed below.

Most versions of the intervention assignment problem are NP-hard. Hans et al. (2008) argue that the intervention assignment problem is a generalization of the so-called general bin packing problem with unequal bins, and thus strongly NP-hard. When planning is done by hand, this complexity is handled by simplifying the problem. This simplification is often done by introducing simple rules of the thumb such as "plan two hip surgeries in R 5 on Thursdays." Of course, what is lost is the flexibility to find (near) optimal solutions based on the real-problem formulation. This is one reason why the introduction of decision support systems can be of great value, provided it employs suitable optimization methods.

Intervention Scheduling

Intervention scheduling—also known as "allocation scheduling"—is the problem of scheduling previously assigned interventions within the respective rooms and days (Ozkarahan 2000, Jebali et al. 2006). This problem is usually considered at later stages of the planning process, such as in weekly planning of the following week's interventions, or daily planning of the following day's interventions. At this stage, more information about critical resources (e.g., individual surgeons or equipment) becomes available. The demand may also have changed, due to the arrival of emergency patients or late cancellations of scheduled surgeries. Intervention scheduling may also assign surgeons to interventions, if this has not been done at some earlier stage. The constraints of the "intervention assignment problem" are normally still respected with the possible exception of block scheduling constraints. In addition, the intervention scheduling has to respect additional constraints, e.g., concerning the availability and skills of individual surgeons and the availability of mobile equipment. Common objectives include overtime; resource utilization; and patient or personnel preferences, such as waiting time in the morning for young children.

Note that the above clean cut separation between intervention assignment and scheduling is not always desirable, or even possible. In some cases, the admission planning will involve objectives that depend on the sequence of surgeries during each day. Examples are the preference of treating children early, or the use of critical bottleneck postoperative resources such as recovery beds or intensive care unit capacity. In addition, if surgeons are chosen during admission planning, surgeon overtime will also depend on the sequencing of interventions. In all such cases, admission planning will involve an optimization problem with both assignment and scheduling aspects.

In the literature, we only find this combination addressed in connection with short-term scheduling, typically with 1 day or 1 week planning horizons (Pham and Klinkert 2008). Jebali et al. (2006) show that the flexibility to reassign interventions during scheduling gives improved solutions at the price of a considerably higher calculation effort.

Variations

We have described the basic versions of operational surgery-scheduling problems. There are, however, many variations and additional aspects to consider, such as:

- Hospital bed availability (Blake and Carter 1997).
- Postoperative resources (Jebali et al. 2006).
- Availability of stationary and mobile equipment, and the necessary sterilization time between uses of such. For example, Jebali et al. (2006) consider stationary equipment that is present in some, but not all, of the ORs in the operation theatre.
- Human resources, including working time regulations, team assignment, and various other preferences.
- Uncertainty, e.g., in surgery recovery durations, resource availability, cancellations, and emergency care disruptions (Marcon et al. 2001, Denton et al. 2007, Hans et al. 2008).
- Different objectives, such as resource utilization, idle time, peak reduction, and load balancing.
- Multiobjective treatment of independent conflicting objective functions.
- Assigning interventions to teams, instead of—or in addition to—rooms (Krempels and Panchenko 2006). This is relevant for hospitals where the surgical teams are the critical resource.

The rich diversity of surgery-scheduling problems dictates that efficient decision support tools for OR management must incorporate optimization methods that are robust across problem variations and sizes. So far, this need for robustness has not received a lot of attention in the optimization literature. Rather, the focus has been on tailored methods for selected surgery-scheduling applications. A large selection of optimization methods have been investigated, including linear programming, MIP, goal programming, column generation, branch-and-price, constructive heuristics, and metaheuristic methods. For a comprehensive review, see Cardoen et al. (2010).

Summary

In this chapter, we have examined two complex and challenging scheduling problems from the healthcare domain. A large and growing body of research exists on how to efficiently manage these complex processes. The scheduling problems found in the healthcare domain are often of high computational complexity. Future application driven research will, therefore, likely have an increased focus on heuristic optimization algorithms, as well as hybrid combinations of various existing methods. A compilation of standard benchmark problems for healthcare scheduling problems is needed for a more quantitative comparison of methods. However, given the many differences found between healthcare institutions, researchers should also evaluate new methods with respect to their robustness across problem variations.

Increasingly, hospitals are exploiting research results along with the latest technologies to facilitate and improve their scheduling decisions. We believe this trend will continue, resulting in more efficient utilization of hospital resources, and thus resulting in better healthcare.

References

Adan I and JMH Vissers. 2002. Patient mix optimisation in hospital admission planning: A case study. *International Journal of Operations and Production Management*. 22(4): 445–461.

Beddoe GR and S Petrovic. 2007. Enhancing case-based reasoning for personnel rostering with selected tabu search concepts. *Journal of the Operational Research Society*. 58(12): 1586–1598.

Beliën J and E Demeulemeester. 2007. Building cyclic master surgery schedules with leveled resulting bed occupancy. *European Journal of Operational Research*. 176(2): 1185–1204.

Beliën J, E Demeulemeester, and B Cardoen. 2005. Building cyclic master surgery schedules with leveled resulting bed occupancy: A case study: SSRN.

Blake JT and MW Carter. 1997. Surgical process scheduling: A structured review. *Journal of the Society for Health System*. 5(3): 17–30.

Blake JT and MW Carter. 2002. A goal programming approach to strategic resource allocation in acute care hospitals. *European Journal of Operational Research*. 140(3): 541–561.

Blake JT and MW Carter. 2003. Physician and hospital funding options in a public system with decreasing resources. *Socio-Economic Planning Sciences*. 37(1): 45–68.

Blake J, F Dexter, and J Donald. 2002. Operating room managers' use of integer programming for assigning block time to surgical groups: A case study. *Anesthesia & Analgesia*. 94(1): 143–148.

Blake JT and J Donald. 2002. Mount Sinai hospital uses integer programming to allocate operating room time. *Interfaces*. 32(2): 63–73.

Burke EK, P Cowling, P De Causmaecker, and G Vanden Berghe. 2001. A memetic approach to the nurse rostering problem. *Applied Intelligence*. 15(3): 199–214.

Burke EK, T Curtois, G Post, R Qu, and B Veltman. 2008. A hybrid heuristic ordering and variable neighbourhood search for the nurse rostering problem. *European Journal of Operational Research*. 188(2): 330–341.

Burke EK, P De Causmaecker, G Vanden Berghe, and H Van Landeghem. 2004. The state of the art of nurse rostering. *Journal of Scheduling*. 7(6): 441–499.

Burke EK, G Kendall, and E Soubeiga. 2003. A tabu-search hyperheuristic for timetabling and rostering. *Journal of Heuristics*. 9(6): 451–470.

Cardoen B, E Demeulemeester, and J Beliën. 2010. Operating room planning and scheduling: A literature review. *European Journal of Operational Research*. 201(3): 921–932.

Chaabane S, N Meskens, A Guinet, and M Laurent. 2008. Comparison of two methods of operating theatre planning: Application in Belgian hospital. *Journal of Systems Science and Systems Engineering*. 17(2): 386–392.

Chessare JB. 2004. Maximizing throughput: Smoothing the elective surgery schedule to improve patient flow. http://urgentmatters.org/346834/318807/318808/318811 (accessed July 30, 2008).

DashOptimization, Xpress-MP. http://www.dashoptimization.com/ (accessed February 18, 2009).

Denton B, J Viapiano, and A Vogl. 2007. Optimization of surgery sequencing and scheduling decisions under uncertainty. *Health Care Management Science*. 10(1): 13–24.

Dexter F, JT Blake, DH Penning, B Sloan, P Chung, and DA Lubarsky. 2002. Use of linear programming to estimate impact of changes in a hospital's operating room time allocation on perioperative variable costs. *Anesthesiology*. 96(3): 718–724.

Dias TM, DF Ferber, CC de Souza, and AV Moura. 2003. Constructing nurse schedules at large hospitals. *International Transactions in Operational Research*. 10(3): 245–265.

Dowsland KA and JM Thompson. 2000. Solving a nurse scheduling problem with knapsacks, networks and tabu search. *Journal of the Operational Research Society*. 51(7): 825–833.

Eveborn P and M Rönnqvist. 2004. Scheduler – A system for staff planning. *Annals of Operations Research*. 128: 21–45.

Guinet A and S Chaabane. 2003. Operating theatre planning. *International Journal of Production Economics Planning and Control of Productive Systems*. 85(1): 69–81.

Hans E, G Wullink, M van Houdenhoven, and G Kazemier. 2008. Robust surgery loading. *European Journal of Operational Research*. 185(3): 1038–1050.

Hughes WL and SY Soliman. 1985. Short-term case mix management with linear programming. *Hospital & health services administration*. 30(1): 52–60.

ILOG, ILOG Solver. ILOG Inc.: Paris, France. http://www.ilog.com/ (accessed Febraury 18, 2009).

ILOG, CPLEX mathematical programming optimizer http://www.ilog.com/products/cplex/ (accessed February 18, 2009).

Jaumard B, F Semet, and T Vovor. 1998. A generalized linear programming model for nurse scheduling. *European Journal of Operational Research*. 107(1): 1–18.

Jebali A, AB Hadj Alouane, and P Ladet. 2006. Operating rooms scheduling. *International Journal of Production Economics Control and Management of Productive Systems*. 99(1–2): 52–62.

Krempels KH and A Panchenko. 2006. An approach for automated surgery scheduling. *The Practice and Theory of Automated Timetabling*. 209–233.

Macario A, TS Vitez, B Dunn, and T McDonald. 1995. Where are the costs in perioperative care?: Analysis of hospital costs and charges for inpatient surgical care. *Anesthesiology*. 83(6): 1138–1144.

Magerlein JM and JB Martin. 1978. Surgical demand scheduling: A review. *Health Services Research*. 13(4): 418–433.

Malhotra V. 1999. Getting the schedule done. *Seminars in Anesthesia, Perioperative Medicine and Pain*. 18(4): 300–305.

Marcon E, S Kharraja, and G Simonnet. 2001. Minimization of the risk of no realization for the planning of the surgical interventions into the operation theatre. *Eighth IEEE International Conference on Emerging Technologies and Factory Automation*. Antibes-Juan les Pins, France, pp. 675–680.

Mason AJ and MC Smith. 1998. A nested column generator for solving rostering problems with integer programming. *International Conference on Optimisation: Techniques and Applications*. Perth, Australia, pp. 827–834.

Meisels A, E Gudes, and G Solotorevsky. 1997. Combining rules and constraints for employee timetabling. *International Journal of Intelligent Systems*. 12(6): 419–439.

Meyer auf'm Hofe H. 2000. Solving rostering tasks as constraint optimization. Selected papers from the *Third International Conference on Practice and Theory of Automated Timetabling*, Springer Lecture Notes in Computer Science, Konstanz, Germany. 2079: 191–212.

Ogulata SN and RZ Erol. 2003. A hierarchical multiple criteria mathematical programming approach for scheduling general surgery operations in large hospitals. *Journal of Medical Systems*. 27(3): 259–270.

Ozkarahan I. 2000. Allocation of surgeries to operating rooms by goal programing. *Journal of Medical Systems*. 24(6): 339–378.

Pham DN and A Klinkert. 2008. Surgical case scheduling as a generalized job shop scheduling problem. *European Journal of Operational Research*. 185(3): 1011–1025.

Personnel scheduling benchmarks. http://www.cs.nott.ac.uk/~tec/NRP/ (accessed March 27, 2009).

Przasnyski ZH. 1986. Operating room scheduling – A literature review. *AORN Journal*. 44(1): 67–76.

Rifai AK and JO Pecenka. 1989. An application of goal programming in healthcare planning. *International Journal of Production Management*. 10(3): 28–37.

Robbins WA and N Tuntiwongbiboon. 1989. Linear programming is a useful tool in case-mix management. *Healthcare Financial Management*. 43(6): 114–116.

Santibanez P, M Begen, and D Atkins. 2007. Surgical block scheduling in a system of hospitals: An application to resource and wait list management in a British Columbia health authority. *Health Care Management Science*. 10(3): 269–282.

SICStus, SICStus Prolog. 2007. Swedish institute of computer science: Kista, Sweden. http://www.sics.se/sicstus/ (accessed Febraury 18, 2009).

Vissers JMH, IJBF Adan, and JA Bekkers. 2005. Patient mix optimization in tactical cardiothoracic surgery planning: A case study. *IMA Journal of Management Mathematics*. 16(3): 281–304.

Weil G, K Heus, P Francois, and M Poujade. 1995. Constraint programming for nurse scheduling. *IEEE Engineering in Medicine and Biology Magazine*. 14(4): 417–422.

24

Data Mining

Niels Peek
University of Amsterdam

Introduction 24-1
Challenges of the Field 24-2
Data Exploration 24-4
Descriptive Data Mining 24-7
Predictive Data Mining 24-10
Software 24-15
References 24-15

Introduction

The widespread application of information technology in our society has led to a revolutionary growth in processes where data is acquired, stored, and retrieved in electronic format. This development covers many areas of human endeavor, and also applies to the healthcare field where clinical and health-related information is increasingly stored in electronic databases. The abundant volumes of electronic data available can be used to discover new medial knowledge and improve the process of care, by uncovering relations and structures in the data that were previously unknown. The discipline concerned with this task has become known as data mining.

Data mining is generally defined as the analysis of (large) observational data sets to find unsuspected relationships and to summarize the data in novel ways that are both understandable and useful to the data owner (Hand et al. 2001, Giudici 2003, Witten and Frank 2005, Han and Kamber 2006). It is a young and interdisciplinary field, drawing from disciplines such as database systems, data warehousing, machine learning, statistics, signal analysis, data visualization, information retrieval, and high-performance computing. And rather than comprising a clear-cut set of methods, the term "data mining" refers to an eclectic approach where choices are led by pragmatic considerations concerning the problem at hand. Data mining has been successfully applied in diverse areas such as marketing, finance, engineering, security, games, and science. It is often applied in the context of knowledge discovery in databases (KDD) (Fayyad et al. 1996a,b), which, loosely defined, is a process with four stages: (i) selecting the relevant data sources to address the knowledge discovery questions at hand, (ii) preprocessing (integrating, cleaning, filtering, and, if necessary, transforming) data from these sources, (iii) applying data mining techniques to extract potentially interesting structures from the data, and (iv) interpreting, validating, and appraising the discovered structures, and presenting them to end users.

In medicine, data mining is usually applied to analyze large observational sets of patient data, with the objective of increasing our knowledge of the patients' disease and the treatment that was given to them or to build a model that can be used to diagnose or prognosticate similar patients. Data mining has expanded the toolset of medical data analysts, which was traditionally dominated by statistical regression methods. Conversely, medical data analysis applications have inspired data mining researchers to develop methods that accurately address the typical problems that are associated with medical data.

And thanks to the recent integration of molecular and clinical data taking place in genomic medicine, the area has gained a fresh impulse and a new set of complex problems it needs to address.

As appears from the above, the goals of data mining extend over two broad categories: description and prediction (Hand et al. 2001, Giudici 2003). Descriptive data mining attempts to discover implicit and previously unknown knowledge. Typical descriptive tasks are discovery of frequent patterns, finding interesting associations and correlations in data, cluster analysis, outlier analysis, and evolution analysis. To arrive at valuable results, it is essential that the structures that are derived from the data can be present in a format that is comprehensible by humans. Predictive data mining seeks to find a model or function that predicts some crucial but (yet) unknown property of a given object, given a set of currently known properties. In applications of predictive data mining in medical diagnosis, for instance, one seeks to predict a patient's disorder based on clinical signs and symptoms, medical history, physical examination, and findings from diagnostic tests. Predictive data mining is related to the supervised machine learning paradigm, and well-known algorithms in this area are decision tree learners, Bayesian classifiers, linear and logistic regression analysis, artificial neural networks, and support vector machines (SVMs). The models that result from predictive data mining may be embedded in information systems and need not, in that case, be comprehensible by end users.

The distinction between descriptive and predictive data mining is not always clear-cut. Interesting patterns that were found with descriptive data mining techniques can sometimes be used for predictive purposes. Conversely, a comprehensible predictive model (e.g., a decision tree) may highlight interesting patterns and thus have descriptive qualities. It may also be useful to alternate between descriptive and predictive activities within a data mining process. In all cases, the results of descriptive and predictive data mining should be valid on new, unseen data in order to be valuable to, and trusted by, end users.

Following Hand et al. (2001), we distinguish two types of structures, models and patterns, that may be derived from data. A model is a high-level, global representation of reality, based on summarizing an entire data set. It describes general rules and therefore allows one to make inferences, that is, to make statements about the population from which the data were drawn or about likely future data values. In contrast, a pattern is a local feature of the data, perhaps holding for only a few records or a few variables. The significance of patterns is found in the fact that they describe departures from general rules: a particular interaction between two diagnostic variables, a subgroup of patients with exceptional outcomes, an episode with remarkable variation, etc. Where models are frequently used for predictive purposes, patterns are often employed in descriptive data mining.

The remaining sections are organized as follows. First, in the next section, we discuss the main challenges for the field of medical data mining. The "Data Exploration" section reviews methods for exploratory data analysis, while the "Descriptive Data Mining" section considers descriptive data mining methods and the section after that discusses methods for predictive data mining. The chapter is concluded with an overview of data mining software.

To illustrate the described techniques we will use a fictitious data set of 10,000 intensive care unit (ICU) patients. The patients in this fictitious example have a mean age of 61.6 years and 3651 (36.9%) are females. Furthermore, 2977 (29.8%) patients were admitted to the ICU for medical reasons, and 7023 (70.2%) after surgery. From all 10,000 patients, 8598 (86.0%) survived.

Challenges of the Field

Since its inception, the field of data mining has faced four major challenges: (i) handling very large data sets; (ii) dealing with observational data that were collected for other purposes than data mining; (iii) analyzing data from multiple sources, including relational and multimedia data; and (iv) representation of domain knowledge. Below we address each of these challenges in more detail, with particular attention to the medical context.

Many traditional data analysis methods, such as those stemming from statistics, assume that the data under scrutiny have a limited size, in terms of both the number of variables involved and the number of data records. For instance, these methods assume that the number of variables in the data set is small enough to be inspected one-by-one by the analyst (e.g., with data visualization techniques) and that the data set fits into working memory of the computer that is used to conduct the analysis. With the rapidly increasing number of data items that is recorded in care processes, this is no longer realistic. Clinical biochemical analysis, a routine diagnostic procedure, can provide concentrations of up to 100 different chemicals in bodily fluids (blood, urine, sputum). Signal datasets from operating theaters and ICU contain monitoring parameters that have been recorded with high sampling frequencies, yielding sets with megabytes of data per patient per day. And modern genome-wide association studies include data on several hundred thousands of single nucleotide polymorphisms in the human DNA. These data volumes imply that traditional data analysis procedures need to be extended, modified, and also supplemented by different kinds of procedures. Modern data sets typically do not fit into the working memory of a PC and can therefore not be handled by most statistical software packages. But even if they could, the analysis would often take days or weeks to complete because many of the traditional algorithms are not computationally efficient enough to deal with such data volumes. A popular data mining solution is to use algorithms that perform computations separately on each of the rows or each of the columns of the data set. Furthermore, in data mining many steps that were traditionally carried out manually by the analyst are automated.

Large volumes of data increase the opportunities for data mining. They allow to discover patterns that are rare but interesting, and to prove effects that are small but nevertheless significant. But size, as the statistician David Hand has put it, is a "two-edged sword" (Hand et al. 2000). One can always find apparent structures in data, but many of these structures will not be "real" in the sense that they represent aspects of the actual process in which the data was collected. Instead, these structures will represent noise, random fluctuations, or misrecordings in the data. Unfortunately, it is not a good idea to test each potentially interesting model or pattern for statistical significance, as the large number of statistical tests will also produce chance findings. To summarize, size is the main opportunity for data mining but also a major computational and statistical challenge.

Data mining is often concerned with data that were collected as secondary to some other activity. Once collected, they clearly represent a resource: it is likely that the mountains of data contain valuable or interesting information, if one can identify and extract it. However, there are serious risks involved with this type of analysis, because of inadequacies in the data (Hand 1998). Individual records may be distorted by missing values, misrecordings, and other anomalies. Routinely collected medical data are notorious for missing values, which will often (but certainly not always) mean that for the variables in question there was nothing unusual noted and therefore nothing recorded. A data field for recording "complications," for instance, may be empty because there were none. But also the data set as a whole may be inadequate because the data collection process was based on convenience or opportunity. It is a well-known phenomenon that emergency cases are often underrepresented in medical databases, simply because there was no time for data registration. This will result in a selection bias (i.e., whether or not a record is included in the database depends on the values the variables take), and conclusions that are drawn from the data should be approached with caution. Finally, data that was collected in nonexperimental settings (such as routine care) will often misrepresent causal relationships due to a phenomenon called "confounding by indication." In routine care, patients with more serious conditions receive more intense treatments but still they may experience worse outcomes than other patients that are less ill. The data then seem to tell us that more intense treatments lead to worse outcomes but this is not a sound conclusion. Also dealing with these problems of secondary analysis is a major challenge for medical data mining.

Another assumption that is typically made by traditional data analysis methods is that the data can be represented in a two-dimensional ("flat") $n \times m$ table, where the rows describe n independent data records (in a medical context typically corresponding to different patients) and the columns contain measured values of m variables for each record. In practice, data will often stem from a variety of different sources and may have a structure that is far more complicated than can be expressed in a flat table. Data from digital signal and imaging techniques typically have a higher dimensional spatiotemporal structure. But also "ordinary" clinical data is often based on sequences of clinical observations at subsequent hours, days, or clinical visits, with the time between and number of subsequent observations varying from patient to patient. Analyzing temporal sequence data is therefore a topic that has received considerable attention in the medical field.

As data mining is concerned with knowledge discovery, a final challenge for the field is proper, accurate, and intuitive representation of domain knowledge. Knowledge representation has, in fact, a dual role in data mining, as it is both needed to encode background knowledge that is available prior to the analysis and to communicate the results of the analysis to domain experts and end users. Exploiting background knowledge can improve the quality of results and speed up the data mining process. For instance, many medical datasets reflect facts such as "only women can become pregnant" and "only men may get prostate cancer." There is no point in bothering the data mining user with these well-established facts. By incorporating them into the analysis as "background knowledge," we can avoid such well-established facts being presented as novelties. Of course, the data mining algorithm in question should allow one to do so, and there must be a convenient format for encoding all the relevant background knowledge. Avoiding the regurgitation of trivialities may not only improve the relevance of the results, but also speed up the knowledge discovery process.

The format that is used by data mining algorithms to represent knowledge is also important for the communication of results with domain expert and end users. As will be explained later in this chapter, there exists much variation in the communicability of data mining results. Some algorithms produce symbolic rules or tree structures that are easy to interpret while others deliver inextricable "black box" models. In knowledge discovery processes, domain experts are often crucial to validate the results that are produced by automated data mining algorithms. In such cases, these "black box" models are certainly not a good choice.

Data Exploration

A first step in most data mining projects is to explore the data set at hand, often without clear ideas of what one is looking for. Exploratory data analysis methods are therefore typically interactive and visual.

Exploratory data analysis usually starts with computing statistical summaries of the variables in the data. Categorical variables, including binary variables, are conveniently summarized by relative frequencies. Numerical variables are often summarized by statistics such as the minimum, maximum, mean, median, and standard deviation (Hand et al. 2001). Table 24.1 lists these summary statistics for 32 variables in the example data set, computed over all 10,000 instances. The table also lists the number of missing values per variable.

A number of conclusions can immediately be drawn from the table. The number of missing values varies widely among the variables, with nine variables apparently being complete and others have tens, hundreds, or even thousands of missing values. A number of missing values were coded differently, with the values −99 and +9999, and were therefore not recognized as missing by the software that was used to summarize the data. And some of the values in the data set are obviously wrong, such as the negative age (−22 years).

Another striking observation is that for some of the numeric (i.e., noncategorical) variables, the mean value is quite different from the median, and the standard deviation is very large. This usually indicates that the values do not follow a Gaussian distribution. Because many data analysis methods assume that variables follow (at least approximately) such a distribution, it is a good idea to investigate this further by visualizing the measured values in the data set. A simple yet powerful tool to do so is the histogram,

TABLE 24.1 Summary Statistics for 32 Variables in the Example Dataset

Variable	Min	Max	Mean	Median	s.d.	NAs
Age (years)	−22	117	61.55	65.00	15.86	0
Female sex	0	1	0.37			0
Length (cm)	−99	208	171.20	172.00	18.69	829
Weight (kg)	0	190	77.01	75.00	15.33	748
Chronic renal failure	0	1	0.03			0
Admission type						311
Medical	0	1	0.28			
Surgical	0	1	0.72			
Emergency	0	1	0.32			2557
Acute renal failure	0	1	0.04			0
Cardiovascular insufficiency	0	1	0.11			0
Respiratory insufficiency	0	1	0.05			0
Sepsis	0	1	0.01			185
Heart rate	−99	300	83.10	85.00	45.64	300
Respiratory rate	−99	60	4.88	11.00	27.06	350
Systolic blood pressure (mm Hg)	−99	300	100.63	105.00	54.26	356
Mean blood press. (min. 24 hours)	−99	170	53.70	60.00	39.68	330
Mean blood press. (max. 24 hours)	0	9999	623.15	100.00	2215.89	339
Body temperature (min. 24 hours)	−99	40.1	24.13	35.80	37.93	341
Body temperature (max. 24 hours)	−99	9999	758.48	37.60	2584.90	367
Prothrombin time	−99	9999	1188.75	15.00	3249.70	1255
paO_2	−99	9999	136.28	85.00	687.25	1744
fiO_2	−99	9999	523.69	40.00	2156.39	1870
Serum creatinine (min. 24 hours)	−99	1395	88.20	80.00	106.39	494
Serum creatinine (max. 24 hours)	4	9999	828.14	92.00	2557.60	630
Hb (min. 24 hours)	−99	10.7	−7.89	5.50	35.37	8501
Hb (max. 24 hours)	−99	11.2	−7.21	6.50	35.99	8505
Platelet count (min. 24 hours)	−99	1100	158.38	150.00	105.40	1082
Serum glucose (min. 24 hours)	−99	96	0.04	7.00	27.67	2087
Serum glucose (max. 24 hours)	0.26	9999	690.41	10.80	2513.63	1921
Use of vasoactive medication	0	1	0.56			0
Mechanical ventilation	0	1	0.66			0
ICU length-of-stay	0	144.2	3.39	0.99	7.33	46
Survival	0	1	0.86			0

Notes: Min, minimum value; max, maximum value; mean, mean value; median, median value; s.d., standard deviation; NAs, number of missing values.

showing the number of values that lie in consecutive intervals. Figure 24.1a shows a histogram of the paO_2 variable, after removal of the (impossible) negative values and all occurrences of the value +9999. The minimum value is now +2, and the maximum value +5512. As can be seen from the histogram, the distribution of values is not Gaussian but highly skewed, with most values lying relatively close to zero. Often such variables can be transformed to a Gaussian distribution by taking the natural logarithm of the measured values. In the case of the paO_2 variable, the transformed distribution is indeed much closer to a Gaussian, with mean, median, and standard deviation of 4.55, 4.47, and 0.54, respectively (Figure 24.1b).

While tools for summarizing and displaying single variables are typically used to clean and transform the data, tools for summarizing and displaying relationships between two or more variables are used to formulate hypotheses about the problem domain that is represented by the data. A simple

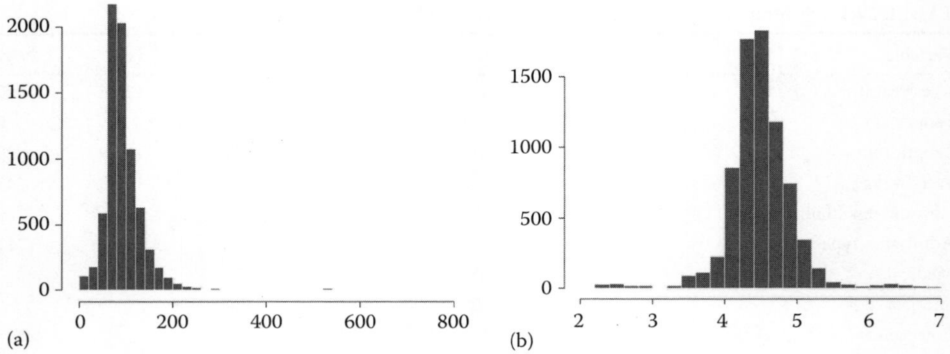

FIGURE 24.1 Histograms of arterial oxygen pressure (paO_2) values in the example data set, before (a) and after (b) applying a logarithmic transformation.

way to investigate pairwise relationships between variables is to compute Pearson's product-moment correlation coefficient (Pearson 1895), defined as

$$r_{xy} = \frac{\sum_{i=1}^{n} (x_i - \bar{x})(y_i - \bar{y})}{(n-1)s_x s_y}$$

where

$\bar{x}$ and $\bar{y}$ are the sample means of the variables X and Y
s_x and s_y are their sample standard deviations

Pearson's correlation coefficient r_{xy} expresses the degree of linear dependence between X and Y. It is 1 in the case of a perfect positive linear dependency between the two variables, −1 in the case of a perfect negative linear dependency, and some value between −1 and 1 in all other cases. The closer r_{xy} is to 0, the weaker the correlation between the variables.

By computing all pairwise correlations in a dataset and selecting the ones that exceed some predefined threshold (e.g., below −0.75 or above +0.75) one can systematically search for pairs of strongly related variables. Unfortunately, such an approach will often yield a lot of information that is trivial for anyone who is knowledgeable in the domain in question. In the ICU data set, for example, the highest correlation (0.95) is found between minimum and maximum serum creatinine measured in the first 24 hours of ICU stay. This is not surprising, as for many patients the serum creatinine will hardly change in such a time span. Similarly, high correlations are found between the arterial oxygen pressures (paO_2) measured at admission and the same variable measured after 24 hours (0.90), and between the minimal systolic blood pressure and minimal mean blood pressure measured during the first 24 hours of ICU stay (0.82).

Pearson's product-moment correlation assumes Gaussian distributions and a linear dependency between the variables X and Y. When these assumptions are wrong, then r_{xy} will be closer to 0, and may erroneously suggest that there exists no association between the two variables. In such cases, it is better to apply a nonparametric statistical test of association, such as the Wilcoxon rank sum test (Lehmann 1975). For categorical variables, one can use Pearson's χ^2 test (1890). A disadvantage of both procedures is that they only provide a test statistic, and not a pure quantification of the strength of association: with large data sets they consider even the weakest associations to be "significant." It is generally a good idea to visually inspect all pairwise associations that stand out in numerical exploration of correlation and association. An example is given in Figure 24.2, which provides a scatterplot of the minimal mean blood pressure in the first 24 hours of ICU stay versus the minimal systolic blood pressure in the same period. These variables have a Pearson's correlation coefficient of 0.79. The scatterplot confirms a strong linear dependency between them.

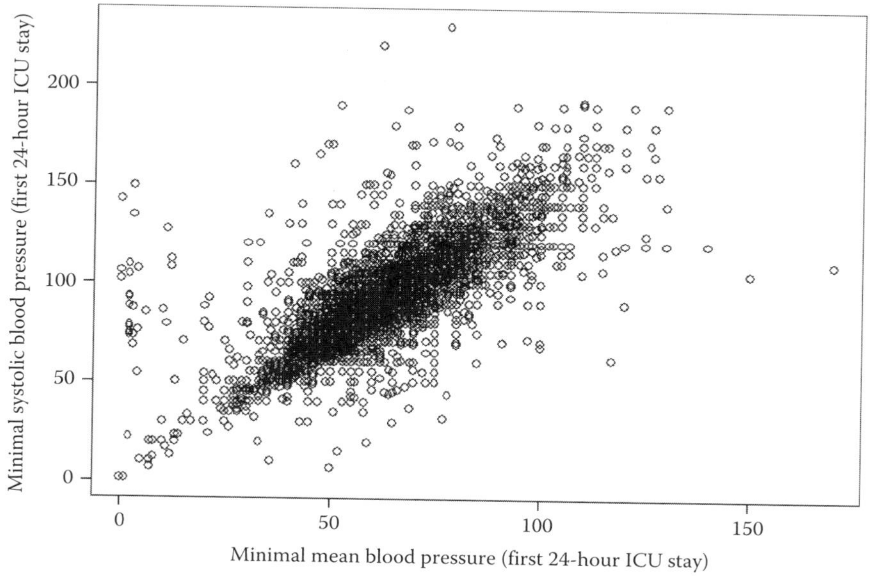

FIGURE 24.2 Scatterplot of minimal mean blood pressure versus minimal systolic blood pressure in the first 24 hours of ICU stay.

Descriptive Data Mining

Descriptive tools for summarizing and visualizing data such as the ones presented in the previous section typically fail to be useful when the number of variables in the data is large. When there are hundreds or thousands of variables, it becomes laborious and time-consuming to inspect their individual distributions manually. Even more problematic is the fact that the number of pairwise correlations (and scatterplots) grows quadratically in the number of variables. Possible solutions for this problem are to project high-dimensional data to lower-dimensional spaces (principal component analysis [PCA]), to identify clouds of similar data points (cluster analysis), and to identify frequently occurring patterns in the data (market basket analysis). These methods are jointly referred to as descriptive data mining methods and discussed in this section.

PCA (Pearson 1901, Jolliffe 2002) is a procedure to transform a large number of correlated, numerical variables into a smaller number of uncorrelated variables called principal components. Each principal component is a linear combination of the original variables, chosen such that it maximizes the sum of squared distances (i.e., variability) between the data points after taking previous principal components into account. So the first principal component accounts for most variability in the data, and each succeeding component accounts for as much of the remaining variability as possible. Mathematically, the first principal component is the eigenvector corresponding to the largest eigenvalue of the covariance matrix **V** of the data, the second principal component is the eigenvector corresponding to the second largest eigenvalue of **V**, and so on.

PCA has the same disadvantages as Pearson's product-moment correlation: it assumes that the variables in the data set are numerical and Gaussian distributed, and that there mainly exist linear dependencies between them. If this is true, and there exist many variables in the data set that are highly correlated, then PCA can achieve an effective dimensionality reduction. When the assumptions are not true, it will be much less effective. PCA is often applied in biomedical research, for example, for analyzing DNA microarray data (Peterson 2003), infrared spectroscopy and mass spectrometry data (Stoyanova and Brown 2001), multi-response questionnaires (Cork et al. 1998, Maclellan-Wright et al. 2007), and medical image data (Eyal and Degani 2009).

A rather different approach to exploring the relationships in high-dimensional data is cluster analysis (Kaufman and Rousseeuw 1990). In contrast to PCA, which assumes that there is a single cloud of data points, cluster analysis tries to identify clouds (clusters) of similar data points. The objective is to find grouping of data points in clusters such that intracluster distances are small and intercluster distances are large. A simple but popular algorithm for cluster analysis is k-means clustering (MacQueen 1967). This algorithm initially chooses k points at random from the data set to locate k centroids, the middle points of the clusters, and assigns each other point to its closest centroid. Then, the centroids are relocated by computing the geometrical mean of the points assigned to each cluster (and they will no longer correspond to actual points in the data set). This process is repeated until the positions of the centroids have stabilized. Because all computations are performed on a point-by-point (i.e., row-by-row) basis, k-means clustering easily scales up to large data sets (with many records).

Table 24.2 shows the results of applying the k-means clustering algorithm to the example data set, with $k=4$. The first cluster consists of patients that were admitted to the ICU for medical reasons. These patients differ in multiple respects from the other patients that were admitted for recovery after a surgical procedure. In particular, the survival rate is relatively low (69.8%) in this group. The three other clusters are more similar to each other. Cluster 2 consists of patients with relatively high serum creatinine values and platelet counts and a lower survival than in the other two surgical clusters. Cluster 4 is distinguished from Cluster 3 by the fact that it is dominated by patients who underwent emergency surgery. The treatment regimen was quite intense for these patients (mechanical ventilation and use of vasoactive medication), but their survival rate was remarkably good.

A disadvantage of k-means clustering is that the value of k must be set in advance, and in general it will not be clear which value is appropriate. Hierarchical clustering algorithms (Ward 1963) alleviate this problem by creating a nested hierarchy of partitional clusterings. The top level clustering in the hierarchy always consists of one large cluster that contains all data points, the bottom level clustering always consists of n singleton clusters each containing one data point, and the clusterings at intermediate levels represent different compromises between unity and diversity. Once the cluster hierarchy is complete, one can decide which level provides the most interesting grouping of data points, thus choosing the number of clusterings k. Furthermore, the cluster hierarchy itself, which is often depicted as a dendrogram, may be a valuable source of knowledge about the domain in question. Hierarchical clusterings can be produced in a top-down (divisive hierarchical clustering) and bottom-up fashion (agglomerative hierarchical clustering), of which the latter is more common. This type of algorithm sets out with n singleton clusters each containing one data point and then recursively merges the two clusters that are closest together until a single large cluster remains. An important difference with k-means clustering

TABLE 24.2 Description of Four Data Clusters Obtained with k-Means Clustering ($k=4$)

Variable	Cluster 1	Cluster 2	Cluster 3	Cluster 4
Admission type	Medical	Surgical	Surgical	Surgical
Emergency	No	No	No	Yes
Mean age	62.6	58.5	59.5	66.7
Heart rate	102.2	89.8	86.1	83.9
Systolic blood pressure	103.8	123.8	113.9	102.6
Serum creatinine (max. 24 hours)	143.2	116.2	95.7	98.6
Platelet count (min. 24 hours)	167.4	193.7	171.4	141.6
Use of vasoactive medication	Yes	No	No	Yes
Mechanical ventilation	Yes	No	Yes	Yes
ICU length-of-stay	5.77	2.37	2.36	2.43
Survival rate	69.8%	90.3%	93.4%	95.4%

is that the notion of distance now applies to clusters instead of individual data points. Furthermore, hierarchical clustering does not easily scale up to large data sets.

Cluster analysis is a very popular technique to derive gene expression profiles from DNA microarray data sets (Eisen et al. 1998), and it is also frequently applied in the field of medical image analysis (Wismüller et al. 2004). In both fields, data sets are typically very large and have little apparent structure. Cluster analysis is then a convenient way to find structure. It should be noted, however, that there exists a serious risk of chance findings because cluster analysis will always produce a result (i.e., a partitional or a hierarchical clustering), regardless whether there exists any structure in the data. Even if the data points are uniformly and randomly distributed over the feature space, clustering algorithms will produce a result that suggests that there exist clouds of related data points. In recent years, researchers are therefore increasingly developing methods to distinguish "genuine" clusters from chance results (e.g., see Tibshirani et al. 2001).

A third popular method to discover structures in high-dimensional data is market basket analysis (Agrawal et al. 1996). This method is very different from PCA and cluster analysis. It employs a symbolic rather than numeric representation, and focuses entirely on local patterns in the data. Market basket analysis was developed in the 1990s for the retail industry, which had started to store electronic logs of supermarket transactions. Each logged transaction consisted of a description of the items that the customer had in his or her basket, a subset of all the available items in the shelves of the supermarket. Retailers were interested in discovering which sets of items were often sold together, to improve their marketing strategies. Market basket analysis therefore seeks to find so-called frequent itemsets in the data. The user must specify in advance the minimum support (relative frequency of occurrence in the data set) that is required to deem an itemset as "frequent." The algorithm starts with finding all frequent 1-itemsets, that is, sets with one item and the required minimum support. From these, it recursively constructs the frequent 2-itemsets, frequent 3-itemsets, and so on. It can easily handle large datasets because the computations are performed on a strict column-by-column basis. The algorithm further takes advantage of the fact that all subsets of a frequent k-itemset must itself be smaller frequent itemsets and is therefore computationally very efficient.

Market basket analysis algorithms cannot handle numeric data, and therefore numeric variables need to be transformed to ordinal categorical variables first, for instance by creating equally spaced range categories. This procedure was applied to the ICU data set, after which frequent itemsets with a minimum support of 65% where enumerated. With this minimum support threshold, there were 21 frequent 1-itemsets, 33 frequent 2-itemsets, 12 frequent 3-itemsets, and no frequent itemsets larger than that.

The second step in market basket analysis is to derive association rules, which are rules of the form

$$\{I_1,\ldots,I_k\} \Rightarrow \{I_{k+1},\ldots,I_m\}$$

describing associations between frequently co-occurring itemsets. The proportion of all records containing items $I_1, \ldots, I_k$ where also items $I_{k+1}, \ldots, I_m$ occur is called the confidence of the rule, and the most frequently applied statistic to rank association rules. Table 24.3 shows the 10 association rules that were derived from the frequent 2- and 3-itemsets with highest confidence values. All rules describe very strong associations (with confidence values above 0.90) and support values around 0.70.

A distinctive asset of association rules is their symbolic format. Association rules are easily communicated to domain experts and can be inspected by them for appraisal. However, a drawback is that the algorithm is unaware of any background knowledge, often resulting in a counter-intuitive placement of items in the rules. For instance, the fourth rule in the table says that patients with relatively low first-day peak potassium values that survived their ICU stay mostly did not have an infection at admission. But of course we will not know whether patients have survived before they have left the ICU. From an application perspective, it does not make sense to predict infection at onset after the ICU treatment has finished; the converse would be more logical. Another drawback, caused by optimization of the confidence metric, is illustrated by the "infection = no" item in the table. Infections are rare in our data set (just 7.6%

TABLE 24.3 The 10 Association Rules with Minimum Support 0.65 and Highest Confidence Values Listed in Decreasing Order of Confidence Value

No.	Rule	Support	Confidence
1	{min_mean_blood_press_24h > 54.5} ➡ {syst_blood_press_adm > 70.5}	0.68	0.97
2	{resp_rate_adm < 30.5, survival = yes} ➡ {infection = no}	0.70	0.95
3	{survival = yes} ➡ {infection = no}	0.86	0.94
4	{max_potas_24h < 5.07, survival = yes}➡ {infection = no}	0.71	0.94
5	{syst_blood_press_adm > 70.5, survival = yes} ➡ {infection = no}	0.74	0.94
6	{resp_rate_adm < 30.5, syst_blood_press_adm > 70.5} ➡ {infection = no}	0.72	0.94
7	{resp_rate_adm < 30.5} ➡ {infection = no}	0.80	0.94
8	{min_temp_24h > 33.85, survival = yes} ➡ {infection = no}	0.73	0.93
9	{min_creat_24h < 118.5, survival = yes} ➡ {infection = no}	0.72	0.93
10	{resp_rate_adm < 30.5, min_temp_24h} > 33.85 ➡ {infection = no}	0.72	0.93

Abbreviations: min_mean_blood_press_24h, minimal mean blood pressure (during first 24 hours of ICU stay); syst_blood_press_adm, systolic blood pressure (at ICU admission); resp_rate_adm, respiratory rate (at ICU admission); max_potas_24h, maximal serum potassium value (during first 24 hours of ICU stay); min_temp_24h, minimal body temperature (during first 24 hours of ICU stay); min_creat_24h, minimal serum creatinine value (during first 24 hours of ICU stay).

of all patients had an infection), and therefore the "infection = no" item is very common in most subsets of the data. As a result, nearly any frequent itemset $\{I_1, \ldots, I_k\}$ can be used to produce an association rule $\{I_1, \ldots, I_k\}$ ➡ {infection = no} with a high confidence value. In our example, 9 out of 10 association rules have this form. Unfortunately, these are not describing interesting associations but merely repeating the fact that infections are uncommon. For this reason, much of the research in this area has focused on measures for quantifying the "interestingness" of association rules (Silberschatz and Tuzhilin 1996, Tan et al. 2002). One alternative measure is lift, which divides confidence by the background frequency of the rule consequent $\{I_{k+1}, \ldots, I_m\}$. If the lift is above 1, the antecedent $\{I_1, \ldots, I_k\}$ at the left-hand side of the rule describes a situation where the consequent is more likely to occur than in general. It is similar to the notion of relative risk that is frequently used in epidemiology.

To illustrate the difference between the two measures of association, we present the results of a second run of the market basket analysis algorithm on the ICU dataset, now requiring a minimum support of 0.40 and maximizing the lift value, in Table 24.4. The rules that were found are quite different and in general more complex than the rules from the first run. Confidence values of the 10 best rules are between 0.79 and 0.88, and the lift values are all close to 1.73.

Market basket analysis has primarily been used for cross-selling applications in the retail industry. In the medical domain, it has been applied for biosurveillance (Brossette et al. 2000), to find clinical patterns of obstructive sleep apnea (Huang et al. 2008), and to find temporal association rules in administrative and clinical data of diabetes patients (Concaro et al. 2009).

Predictive Data Mining

Descriptive data mining methods summarize data to increase understanding of the underlying problem domain. In doing so, there is no specific focus or target. Predictive data mining methods, in contrast, have the specific aim of foretelling the value of one specific variable (called response variable), based on measured values of other variables (called predictors). When the response variable is numerical, the prediction task is called regression, and when the response variable is categorical, it is called classification. Here, we will focus on binary classification, that is, prediction of the value of a binary response variable, while noting that the data mining process applied to regression and classification problems is quite similar. In the medical field, the goal of classification is to use patient-specific

TABLE 24.4 The 10 Association Rules with Minimum Support 0.40 and Highest Lift Values Listed in Decreasing Order of Lift Value

No.	Rule	Support	Confidence	Lift
1	{syst_blood_press_adm > 70.5, min_creat_24h < 118.5, max_gluc_24h < 15.95} ➡ {max_creat_24h < 120.5, 3.55 < min_gluc_24h < 16.85}	0.46	0.88	1.73
2	{max_creat_24h < 120.5, 3.55 < min_gluc_24h < 16.85} ➡ {syst_blood_press_adm > 70.5, min_creat_24h < 118.5, max_gluc_24h < 15.95}	0.51	0.79	1.73
3	{min_creat_24h < 118.5, max_potas_24h < 5.07, max_gluc_24h < 15.95} ➡ {max_creat_24h < 120.5, min_creat_24h < 118.5}	0.47	0.88	1.73
4	{max_creat_24h < 120.5, 3.55 < min_gluc_24h < 16.85} ➡ {min_creat_24h < 118.5, max_potas_24h < 5.07, max_gluc_24h < 15.95}	0.51	0.81	1.73
5	{min_creat_24h < 118.5, max_gluc_24h < 15.95, infection = no} ➡ {max_creat_24h < 120.5, 3.55 < min_gluc_24h < 16.85}	0.46	0.88	1.73
6	{max_creat_24h < 120.5, 3.55 < min_gluc_24h < 16.85} ➡ {min_creat_24h < 118.5, max_gluc_24h < 15.95, infection = no}	0.51	0.80	1.73
7	{min_creat_24h < 118.5, max_gluc_24h < 15.95} ➡ {max_creat_24h < 120.5, max_potas_24h < 5.07, 3.55 < min_gluc_24h < 16.85}	0.50	0.83	1.73
8	{max_creat_24h < 120.5, max_potas_24h < 5.07. 3.55 < min_gluc_24h < 16.85} ➡ {min_creat_24h < 118.5. max_gluc_24h < 15.95}	0.48	0.86	1.73
9	{min_temp_24h > 33.85, min_creat_24h < 118.5, max_gluc_24h < 15.95} ➡ {max_creat_24h < 120.5, 3.55 < min_gluc_24h < 16.85}	0.46	0.88	1.72
10	{max_creat_24h < 120.5, 3.55 < min_gluc_24h < 16.85} ➡ {min_temp_24h > 33.85, min_creat_24h < 118.5, max_gluc_24h < 15.95}	0.51	0.80	1.72

Abbreviations: syst_blood_press_adm, systolic blood pressure (at ICU admission); min_creat_24h, minimal serum creatinine value (during first 24 hours of ICU stay); max_creat_24h, maximal serum creatinine value (during first 24 hours of ICU stay); min_gluc_24h, minimal serum glucose value (during first 24 hours of ICU stay); max_gluc_24h, maximal serum glucose value (during first 24 hours of ICU stay); max_potas_24h, maximal serum potassium value (during first 24 hours of ICU stay); min_temp_24h, minimal body temperature (during first 24 hours of ICU stay).

information to predict the most probable response class and thereby support clinical decision making. Typical applications of binary classification are to distinguish diseased from nondiseased people on the basis of their medical features and test results (diagnosis) (Kononenko 2001, Lavrac et al. 1998), or to predict whether or not patients will survive medical treatment, based on their diagnoses and illness characteristics (prognosis) (Abu-Hanna and Lucas 2001). Predictive data mining methods usually derive a predictive model from the data set, which is a general recipe or formula to predict the value of the response variable for some arbitrary new case. Some methods that derive predictive patterns also exist, each focusing on a specific group of cases, but this is less common. Both predictive models and patterns should be validated on a separate data set (usually called validation set or test set) before deployment.

Researchers in pattern recognition (Duda et al. 2001) and statistics (Hastie et al. 2001) have worked on classification and regression problems since the 1960s, generally approaching these problems from a statistical estimation perspective and using numerical mathematics as the principal toolset. The classical approach to binary classification stemming from these fields is discriminant analysis. Discriminant analysis searches for the boundary that separates the two classes of data points (e.g., diseased and nondiseased patients) by estimating, for each of the two classes separately, the distribution of the predictor variables. For instance, the mean age of survivors in the ICU dataset is 61.0 years, and the mean age of nonsurvivors is 66.6 years, indicating that age is a predictor of ICU survival. Using this variable only, we would predict that patients older than 63.8 ((66.6 + 61.0)/2) years are more likely to die than to survive, and whereas for patients younger than 63.8 years the converse would hold. The threshold value of 63.8 years is called the decision boundary. Of course this model is far too simple for the complex ICU domain and it does not accurately predict survival (it is in fact wrong in 49.8% of all cases). But we can generalize it to two or more predictors, replacing the estimates of the class-conditional means by estimates of class-conditional multivariate Normal (i.e., Gaussian) distributions. With two predictors, this will replace the classification threshold (63.8 years) by a line, and with $m > 2$ predictors the decision boundary becomes an $(m-1)$-dimensional hyperplane in the m-dimensional space that is spanned by the predictor variables. Furthermore, if the variances of the two class-conditional distributions are assumed to be equal, the decision boundary will be a linear hyperplane, and if they are not assumed to be equal it will be quadratic. The latter choice is by definition more expressive and will always achieve, in principle, a separation between the two classes that is equally good or better. But it also requires that more parameters are estimated from the data. If the data set is not large enough to support reliable estimation of these parameters, the former choice (called linear discriminant analysis) will perform better in practice.

With its roots in the theory of multivariate normal distributions, the application of discriminant analysis is limited to classification problems with only numerical predictor variables. A different approach was developed in the field of Bayesian statistics and is called the naive Bayesian classifier (Russek et al. 1983, Kononenko 1993). This method estimates the class-conditional distribution of each predictor individually from the data set, and also estimates the prior (i.e., marginal) distribution of the response variable. To make predictions for new cases, it applies Bayes' theorem to compute the posterior distribution of the response variable. We can do this not only for numerical predictor variables, but also for binary and categorical variables. For instance, $P(\textit{medical} \mid \textit{survival}) = 0.225$ in the ICU dataset. Because the prior probability of survival is 0.860, the posterior probability of survival for patients that are admitted for medical reasons equals

$$P(\text{survival} \mid \text{medical}) = \frac{P(\text{medical} \mid \text{survival}) \cdot P(\text{survival})}{P(\text{medical})} = \frac{0.225 \cdot 0.860}{0.275} = 0.704$$

(Note that this probability is close to the survival rate of Cluster 1 in Table 24.2, as expected.) When there are multiple predictor variables, the same formula is applied repeatedly, implicitly assuming that the class-conditional distributions of predictors are mutually independent. In words, a naive Bayes classifier assumes that the presence (or absence) of a particular feature of a class is unrelated to the presence (or absence) of any other feature. This is a strong assumption and usually an over-simplification of reality, hence the name naive Bayesian classifier. But in spite of this, naive Bayesian classifiers often work surprisingly well. It is also computationally attractive because the model is built on a column-by-column basis. It is therefore still a popular classification method in data mining.

Researchers in the field of machine learning have traditionally focused on symbolic prediction methods, that is, methods that derive predictive models or patterns in a symbolic format. A most popular example are recursive partitioning methods that derive a model that can be expressed as a decision tree (Breiman et al. 1984, Quinlan 1993). In brief, recursive partitioning methods seek to find a division of the data set into subsets where the response variable is constant ("pure"). The division itself is based on predictor variables. This is accomplished by first splitting the data set into two subsets with the relatively purest distribution of response values, and subsequently splitting these subsets into further subsets, and so on, hence the name recursive partitioning. The resulting hierarchy of splits is expressed as a tree

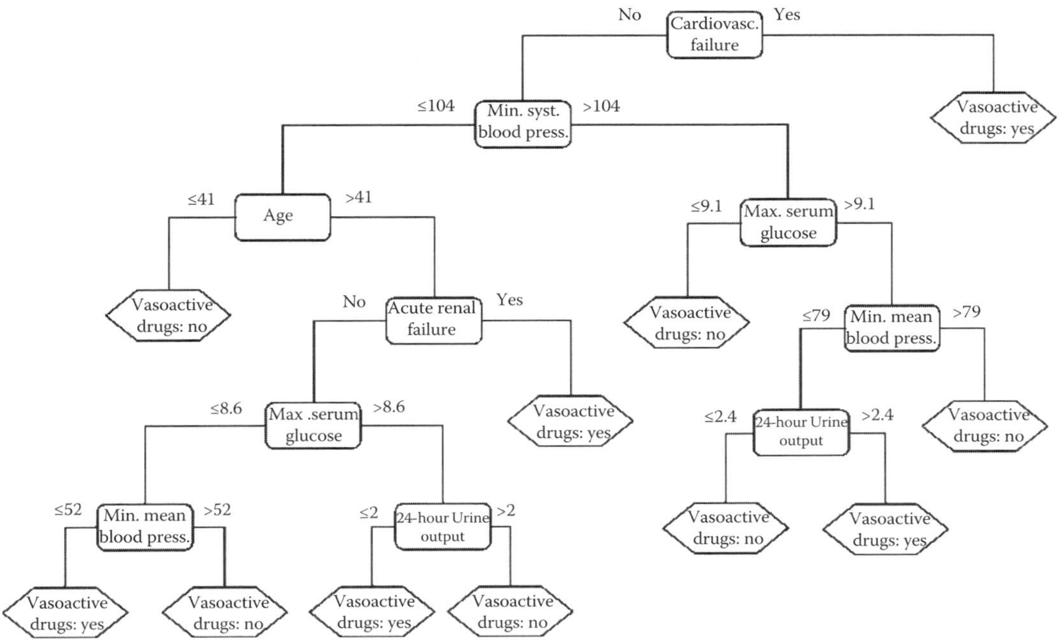

FIGURE 24.3 Decision tree to predict the use of vasoactive medication during the first 24 hours of ICU stay.

and effectively provides a means to foretell the variable of the response variable based on the values of predictor variables.

An example decision tree for the ICU domain is depicted in Figure 24.3. In this tree, the response variable is "use of vasoactive medication during the first 24 hours of ICU stay" (which is true for 55.9% of all patients), so it essentially models the policy of ICU clinicians regarding this type of treatment at the site where the data were collected. The primary predictor is occurrence of cardiovascular failure: patients with cardiovascular failure were very often (1118 out of 1306 cases, or 85.6%) treated with vasoactive medication. For patients without cardiovascular failure, the minimal systolic blood pressure is important: if it was above 104 mm Hg, use of vasoactive medication was uncommon (32.6%), and if it was below 104 mm Hg, it was common (64.6%). In both situations further splits, based on other predictor variables, are used to refine the classification (e.g., patients with a lower minimal systolic blood pressure are further divided by their age, and patients with a higher minimal systolic blood pressure by their maximum serum glucose). Note that the threshold of 104 mm Hg was automatically determined by the decision tree induction algorithm. A common way to quantify the predictive accuracy of a classification model is to compute the error rate, that is, the percentage of misclassified cases on an independent test set. The decision tree of Figure 24.3 has an error rate of 38.3%, which means that it is probably not acceptable for use in clinical practice.

As appears from the example, decision trees are very transparent and can therefore be used for communication with and verification by domain experts. Instead of presenting the entire model, it is also possible to regard each path in the tree as a separate pattern that corresponds to a decision rule, for example,

IF cardiovasc. failure = no AND min. syst. blood press. ≤ 104 AND age ≤ 41 THEN vasoactive drugs = no,

corresponding to the leftmost path in the example tree. From a data mining perspective, decision tree induction algorithms are attractive because they are well able to handle data sets with many records. However, when there are many variables in the data set, decision trees have the tendency to model peculiarities of the data set instead of the underlying relationship between predictors and response variable, a phenomenon called overfitting. The same may happen when the data contain much random variation ("noise"), which is true for many medical data sets.

An interesting type of predictive model that combines symbolic and numerical representation is the Bayesian network (Pearl 1988, Cowell et al. 1999, Lucas et al. 2004). Formally, a Bayesian network is a graphical representation of a multivariate probability distribution on a set of discrete random variables. The network structure codes information about conditional independence relations between the variables, while information about the probability distribution is coded as a set of numeric parameters or functions. Algorithms exist for learning both network structure and parameters from data. Once the model is complete, a Bayesian network allows for computing any marginal or conditional probability regarding the variables involved. By focusing on the prediction of a response variable, we obtain a special specific class of Bayesian networks, called Bayesian network classifiers. The expressiveness of this type of model has led to some impressive achievements for well-known classification problems. Furthermore, the network structure is expressed as a directed acyclic graph and amenable to an intuitively appealing, causal interpretation. Learning Bayesian networks from data is computationally prohibitive, but over the last two decades much effort has been invested in improving the efficiency of learning algorithms.

Three more classification methods are worth mentioning. Logistic regression is a powerful and well-established method from statistics (Hastie et al. 2001). It is an extension of ordinary linear regression to binary classification problems. Similar to the naive Bayesian classifier, the underlying model for probability is multiplicative but uses a more sophisticated method based on a maximum likelihood estimation to determine the coefficients in its probability formula. These coefficients represent strength of association and can be translated to odds ratios. The multilayer perceptron (Cybenko 1989) is a type of artificial neural network (Bishop 1995) which allows to model complex, nonlinear decision boundaries in multivariate feature spaces. The theoretical properties of this model are impressive and multilayer perceptrons outperform other models on most classification problems in terms of predictive accuracy. Moreover, an interesting feature is that the learning algorithm allows processing the data set on a record-by-record basis, thus easily scaling up to large data volumes. However, multilayer perceptrons also suffer from a number of deficiencies (Schwarzer et al. 2000), including a tendency to "overfit" the data, similar to decision trees. SVMs (Cristianini and Shawe-Taylor 2000), finally, are perhaps today's most powerful classification method in terms of predictive accuracy. They are based on statistical learning theory (Vapnik 1998). Central to the method is a procedure that finds a linear decision boundary in an arbitrarily complex, higher-order transformation of the original feature space. As a result, SVMs can induce highly complex, nonlinear decision boundaries in the original space. Both multilayer perceptrons and SVMs are so-called black box models: their form and complexity prohibits interpretation by human domain experts or end users. They can be used for prediction, but not for knowledge discovery.

Table 24.5 lists the error rates of five classification models that were developed on the ICU data set for predicting the use of vasoactive medication. The error rates were computed with 10-fold cross-validation, a computational procedure that avoids the use of a separate test set (Hastie et al. 2001). In this case, the multilayer perceptron outperformed the other classification methods with an error rate of 25.7%.

All classification methods that were mentioned above have been applied extensively to medical prediction problems. Comprehensive overviews of such applications are found in (Lavrac et al. 1998, Abu-Hanna and Lucas 2001, Kononenko 2001, Lucas et al. 2004, Bellazzi and Zupan 2008).

TABLE 24.5 Error Rates of Five Classification Models That Were Developed on the Example Data Set for Predicting the Use of Vasoactive Medication in the First 24 hours of ICU Stay

Model Type	Error Rate %
Decision tree	38.3
Naive Bayes classifier	30.4
Bayesian network	26.9
Logistic regression	27.6
Multilayer perceptron	25.7

Note: The error rates were estimated with 10-fold cross-validation.

Software

A substantial number of commercial and noncommercial data mining software systems exists. Some systems only implement specific algorithms; examples are the See5 (http://www.rulequest.com) and CART (http://www.salford-systems.com) systems for learning decision trees. Others offer an integrated data mining environment that allows the use and comparison of different algorithms, sometimes integrated with database management software. A popular open-source data mining environment is Weka, written in Java and developed at the University of Waikato in New Zealand (http://www.cs.waikato.ac.nz/ml/weka). It implements most of the algorithms discussed in this chapter, and also includes procedures for statistically validating the mining results and a graphical programming module. Similar functionalities are offered by the open-source environment Orange, written in C++ and developed at the University of Ljubljana, Slovenia (http://www.ailab.si/orange). Orange was specifically developed for mining data from the biomedical domain, and has attractive visualization methods and offers both a graphical programming module and a scripting language.

Over the last decade, most commercial fabricants of statistical software products have extended their catalog with data mining software. Examples are SPSS Clementine (http://www.spss.com), SAS Enterprise Miner (http://www.sas.com), and TIBCO Sportfire Miner (http://spotfire.tibco.com/). Many data mining algorithms have also been implemented for the open-source statistical software environment R (cran.r-project.org). An up-to-date list of data mining software is maintained at the KDnuggets website (http://www.kdnuggets.com).

References

Abu-Hanna, A. and P. J. Lucas. 2001. Prognostic models in medicine: AI and statistical approaches. *Methods Inf Med*. 40(1): 1–5.

Agrawal, R., H. Mannila, R. Srikant, H. Toivonen, and A. I. Verkamo. 1996. Fast discovery of association rules. In: Fayyad, U. M. et al. (eds.), *Advances in Knowledge Discovery and Data Mining*, pp. 307–328. Menlo Park, CA: American Association for Artificial Intelligence.

Bellazzi, R. and B. Zupan. 2008. Predictive data mining in clinical medicine: Current issues and guidelines. *Int J Med Inform*. 77(2): 81–97.

Bishop, C. M. 1995. *Neural Networks for Pattern Recognition*. Oxford, UK: Oxford University Press.

Breiman, L., J. H. Friedman, R. A. Olshen, and C. J. Stone. 1984. *Classification and Regression Trees*. Belmont, CA: Wadsworth.

Brossette, S. E., A. P. Sprague, W. T. Jones, and S. A. Moser. 2000. A data mining system for infection control surveillance. *Methods Inf Med*. 39(4–5): 303–310.

Concaro, S., L. Sacchi, C. Cerra, and R. Bellazzi. 2009. Mining administrative and clinical diabetes data with temporal association rules. *Stud Health Technol Inform*. 150: 574–578.

Cork, R. D., W. M. Detmer, and C. P. Friedman. 1998. Development and initial validation of an instrument to measure physicians' use of, knowledge about, and attitudes toward computers. *J Am Med Inform Assoc*. 5(2): 164–176.

Cowell, R. G., A. P. Dawid, S. L. Lauritzen, and D. J. Spiegelhalter. 1999. *Probabilistic Networks and Expert Systems*. New York: Springer.

Cristianini, N. and J. Shawe-Taylor. 2000. *An Introduction to Support Vector Machines and Other Kernel-Based Learning Methods*. Cambridge, U.K.: Cambridge University Press.

Cybenko, G. 1989. Approximation by superpositions of a sigmoidal function. *Math Control Signals Syst*. 2(4): 303–314.

Duda, R. O., P. E. Hart, and D. G. Stork. 2001. *Pattern Classification*, 2nd edn. New York: Wiley.

Eisen, M. B., P. T. Spellman, P. O. Brown, and D. Botstein. 1998. Cluster analysis and display of genome-wide expression patterns. *Proc Natl Acad Sci USA*. 95: 14863–14868.

Eyal, E. and H. Degani. 2009. Model-based and model-free parametric analysis of breast dynamic-contrast-enhanced MRI. *NMR Biomed*. 22(1): 40–53.

Fayyad, U. M., G. Piatetsky-Shapiro, and P. Smyth. 1996a. The KDD process for extracting useful knowledge from volumes of data. *Commun ACM*. 39(11): 27–34.

Fayyad, U. M., G. Piatetsky-Shapiro, P. Smyth, and R. Uthurusamy. 1996b. *Advances in Knowledge Discovery and Data Mining*. Menlo Park, CA: AAAI Press.

Giudici, P. 2003. *Applied Data Mining Statistical Methods for Business and Industry*. London: John Wiley & Sons.

Han, J. and M. Kamber. 2006. *Data Mining: Concepts and Techniques*. San Francisco, CA: Morgan Kaufmann Publishers.

Hand, D. J. 1998. Data mining—Reaching beyond statistics. *Res Offic Statist*. 2: 5–17.

Hand, D. J., G. Blunt, M. G. Kelly, and N. M. Adams. 2000. Data mining for fun and profit. *Statist Sci*. 15(2): 111–131.

Hand, D. J., H. Mannila, and P. Smyth. 2001. *Principles of Data Mining*. Cambridge, MA: MIT Press.

Hastie, T., R. Tibshirani, and J. Friedman. 2001. *The Elements of Statistical Learning*. New York: Springer.

Huang, Q. R., Z. Qin, S. Zhang, and C. M. Chow. 2008. Clinical patterns of obstructive sleep apnea and its comorbid conditions: A data mining approach. *J Clin Sleep Med*. 4(6): 543–550.

Jolliffe, I. T. 2002. *Principal Component Analysis*, 2nd edn. New York: Springer.

Kaufman, L. and P. J. Rousseeuw. 1990. *Finding Groups in Data: An Introduction to Cluster Analysis*. New York: Wiley.

Kononenko, I. 1993. Inductive and Bayesian learning in medical diagnosis. *Appl Artif Intell*. 7: 317–337.

Kononenko, I. 2001. Machine learning for medical diagnosis: History, state of the art and perspective. *Artif Intell Med*. 23: 89–109.

Lavrac, N., I. Kononenko, E. Keravnou, M. Kukar, and B. Zupan. 1998. Intelligent data analysis for medical diagnosis: Using machine learning and temporal abstraction. *AI Commun*. 11: 191–218.

Lehmann, E. L. 1975. *Nonparametrics: Statistical Methods Based on Ranks*. San Francisco, CA: Holden and Day.

Lucas, P. J. F., L. C. Van der Gaag, and A. Abu-Hanna. 2004. Bayesian networks in biomedicine and health care. *Artif Intell Med*. 30: 201–214.

Maclellan-Wright, M. F., D. Anderson, S. Barber, N. Smith, B. Cantin, R. Felix, and K. Raine. 2007. The development of measures of community capacity for community-based funding programs in Canada. *Health Promot Int*. 22(4): 299–306.

MacQueen, J. 1967. Some methods for classification and analysis of multivariate observations. In: *Proceedings of the Fifth Berkeley Symposium on Mathematical Statistics and Probability*, pp. 281–297. Berkeley, CA: University of California Press.

Pearl, J. 1988. *Probabilistic Reasoning in Intelligent Systems: Networks of Plausible Inference*. San Mateo, CA: Morgan Kaufmann.

Pearson, K. 1890. On the criterion that a given system of deviations from the probable in the case of a correlated system of variables is such that it can be reasonably supposed to have arisen from random sampling. *Phil Mag*. 50(5): 157–175.

Pearson, K. 1895. Note on regression and inheritance in the case of two parents. *Proc R Soc Lond*. 58: 240–242.

Pearson, K. 1901. On lines and planes of closest fit to systems of points in space. *Phil Mag*. 2(6): 559–572.

Peterson, L. E. 2003. Partitioning large-sample microarray-based gene expression profiles using principal components analysis. *Comput Methods Programs Biomed*. 70(2): 107–19.

Quinlan, J. R. 1993. *C45: Programs for Machine Learning*. San Mateo, CA: Morgan Kaufmann.

Russek, E., R. A. Kronmal, and L. D. Fisher. 1983. The effect of assuming independence in applying Bayes' theorem to risk estimation and classification in diagnosis. *Comput Biomed Res*. 16: 537–552.

Schwarzer, G., W. Vach, and M. Schumacher. 2000. On the misuses of artificial neural networks for prognostic and diagnostic classification in oncology. *Stat Med*. 19: 541–561.

Silberschatz, A. and A. Tuzhilin. 1996. What makes patterns interesting in knowledge-discovery systems. *IEEE Trans Knowl Data Eng.* 8(6): 970–974.

Stoyanova, R. and T. R. Brown. 2001. NMR spectral quantitation by principal component analysis. *NMR Biomed.* 14(4): 271–277.

Tan, P. M., V. Kumar, and J. Srivastava. 2002. Selecting the right interestingness measure for association patterns. In: *Proceedings of the 8th ACM SIGKDD International Conference on Knowledge Discovery and Data Mining*, pp. 32–41. New York: ACM Publishers.

Tibshirani, R., G. Walther, and T. Hastie. 2001. Estimating the number of clusters in a dataset via the Gap statistic. *J Royal Statist Soc B.* 63: 411–423.

Vapnik, V. N. 1998. *Statistical Learning Theory*. New York: Wiley.

Ward, J. H. 1963. Hierarchical grouping to optimize an objective function. *J Am Statist Assoc.* 58(301): 236–244.

Wismüller, A., O. Lange, D. R. Dersch, G. L. Leinsinger, K. Hahn, B. Pütz, and D. Auer. 2004. Cluster analysis of biomedical image time-series. *Int J Comput Vision.* 46: 103–128.

Witten, I. and E. Frank. 2005. *Data Mining: Practical Machine Learning Tools and Techniques*. San Francisco, CA: Morgan Kaufmann Publishers.

25

Applications to HIV Prevention Strategies

Paul G. Farnham
Centers for Disease Control and Prevention

Arielle Lasry
Centers for Disease Control and Prevention

Economic Evaluation Techniques **25**-1
The Human Immunodeficiency Virus Epidemic **25**-2
Strategies to Prevent the Spread of HIV **25**-3
Summary/Conclusions **25**-10
References **25**-11

Economic evaluation techniques have been used since the late 1960s to evaluate healthcare programs to assist in resource allocation and policy-making decisions (Grosse, 1970). These techniques all focus on comparing some measure of the output, outcomes, or consequences of a program with the costs of the inputs used to provide those outcomes. Policy makers can use the techniques to identify alternatives to a given policy and to focus on the consequences of providing additional resources to one program compared with another (Grosse et al., 2007).

In this chapter, we begin with a description of the use of economic evaluation techniques in healthcare. We then provide an overview of the human immunodeficiency virus/acquired immune deficiency syndrome (HIV/AIDS) epidemic, the policy area for discussion, and we describe the most important HIV prevention interventions. Finally, we discuss two HIV prevention case studies, one focusing on preexposure prophylaxis (PrEP) and the other on a risk-reduction program. We conclude with a comparison of the economic evaluation techniques in the two case studies.

Economic Evaluation Techniques

Three main techniques are used for economic evaluation: (1) cost-effectiveness analysis (CEA); (2) cost–utility analysis (CUA); and (3) cost–benefit analysis (CBA) (Gold et al., 1996; Haddix et al., 2003; Drummond et al., 2005). These techniques differ in how the measurement, valuation, and comparison of costs and consequences are undertaken. In CEA, program outcomes or consequences are measured in the most appropriate natural effects or physical units. For healthcare, the number of cases of disease prevented or the number of life years saved by a medical or prevention intervention are often used as outcome measures. Because no valuation is placed on the outcomes, these measures can be simply counted to determine the effectiveness of the intervention. The use of CEA is most appropriate where there is already general agreement on the type of program outcomes or where the outcomes of the alternatives being considered are the same or very similar. Thus, when comparing two programs for preventing HIV infection, the number of infections prevented may be an appropriate outcome measure.

If a federal agency or a state health department attempts to make comparisons between allocating additional funds for HIV prevention versus lung cancer prevention, then comparing cases prevented of these two different diseases is problematic. One approach would be to measure the cost per life-year saved in each case. However, this approach focuses solely on the extension of life years and does not capture any of the issues relating to the quality of those life years or the values individuals attach to them. Thus, CEA is limited to comparisons within policy areas, when there are similar outcomes of interest in each alternative program, and when outcomes are valued equally.

In the healthcare arena, CUA has been developed as a variant of CEA that focuses on quality of life issues. In CUA, the outcome measure is typically a quality-adjusted life year (QALY) in which the number of life years gained through the intervention has been adjusted for factors relating to the quality of those life years. QALYs are based on utility weights ranging in value from zero (death) to one (perfect health) that are assigned to each year of life gained from the intervention and then summed.

Although CUA helps in making comparisons across alternative healthcare programs, decision makers may have to evaluate more diverse alternatives, such as comparing healthcare programs with education and job training programs, all of which have outcomes that are not directly comparable. CBA may be the most appropriate evaluation technique in these cases because it attempts to put a monetary valuation on the consequences of these different interventions, which reflects the amount of money society is willing to pay for the output of these programs. Dollars thus become the common metric for making comparisons across programmatic areas. Decision makers can assess benefit-cost ratios or net benefits (benefits minus costs) of alternative programs to devise a rank ordering of priorities. However, there are numerous conceptual and empirical problems in developing these willingness-to-pay estimates that often include the problem of placing a value on the lives saved by a given program (Fisher et al., 1989; O'Brien and Gafni, 1996; Mrozek and Taylor, 2002).

Health researchers have traditionally favored the use of CEA and CUA over CBA. However, recent methodological developments incorporate the concept of willingness to pay for a QALY and summarize variation in this willingness to pay with threshold analyses and cost-effectiveness acceptability curves, thus making closer links among CEA, CUA, and CBA (Tolley et al., 1994; Pauly, 1995; Briggs et al., 2006; Willan and Briggs, 2006).

The components of an economic evaluation of a healthcare program or intervention have been well defined in several publications (Gold et al., 1996; Haddix et al., 2003; Drummond et al., 2005). These include the following steps: (1) Define the problem or question to be analyzed. (2) Clearly indicate the alternative strategies being evaluated including the strategy that best represents current practice or the most relevant alternative. (3) Indicate the perspective of the analysis that will influence which costs and outcomes are included. (4) Determine the time frame in which the intervention will be evaluated and the analytic horizon over which the costs and the effects of the intervention will be measured. (5) Indicate what evaluation methods will be used and how costs and outcomes will be determined. (6) Specify the discount rate that will be used to calculate the present value of costs and outcomes that occur in the future. (7) Identify the sources of uncertainty in the model and the sensitivity analyses that will be used to determine the impact of this uncertainty.

Modeling techniques are often used in economic evaluation, given that the goal is to measure the final impact of the program on a given population (Briggs et al., 2006). Models are particularly useful when some of the alternatives being considered have not actually been implemented or when there is great uncertainty about the effectiveness of the intervention. Because data are often collected only on intermediate outcomes, models are used to relate these measures to the final outcomes of interest to decision makers. Modeling in economic evaluation allows an analyst to combine information from a variety of sources and to account for events occurring over time (Barton et al., 2004). Modeling forces a decision maker to explicitly confront alternatives and to examine the logic of what might happen under each alternative.

The Human Immunodeficiency Virus Epidemic

One healthcare area where there has been extensive use of these economic evaluation techniques to analyze alternative disease prevention strategies is the HIV epidemic, given the significant health and monetary impacts of this disease. The Centers for Disease Control and Prevention (CDC) estimates that more than 1.1 million people in the United States are currently living with HIV infection, while approximately 232,700 persons are undiagnosed and unaware of their infection (CDC, 2008a, 2009b). Approximately 56,300 persons were newly infected with HIV in 2006, an increase from previous estimates of 40,000 infections per year (Hall et al., 2008). By the end of 2007, 583,298 persons had died of AIDS, the end-stage of HIV infection (CDC, 2009a), although the mortality rate has decreased substantially since the mid-1990s given the advent of antiretroviral therapy (ART).

HIV disease stage is measured in part by an individual's CD4 cell count, which declines as the disease progresses. Low CD4 counts may make individuals with HIV more susceptible to various opportunistic infections. CD4 count is an important measure of the status of an individual's immune system with a count below 200 cells/μL indicating serious immune damage or AIDS (AIDS InfoNet, 2009a).

Current guidelines call for patients to be treated with ART when their CD4 count falls below 350 cells/μL. Treatment regimens are a function of both the CD4 count and a patient's viral load or the amount of HIV in the blood. The goals of therapy are to reduce the viral load as much as possible for as long as possible, restore or preserve the immune system, improve the patient's quality of life, and reduce the sickness and death caused by HIV (AIDS InfoNet, 2009b). The issue of whether ART should be started at a CD4 count as high as 500 cells/μL is under debate (Granich et al., 2009; Zolopa et al., 2009).

HIV prevalence is defined as the number of existing cases of disease, while incidence is defined as the number of new cases within a time frame. In the United States, the highest prevalence and incidence of HIV are observed among men who have sex with men (MSM) and members of racial minority groups. Of the estimated annual 56,300 new infections in 2006, 45% were among blacks, 53% were among MSM, and 27% were among women. HIV incidence for blacks was seven times that of whites and almost three times that of Hispanic persons (Hall et al., 2008; Buchacz et al., 2009).

From 1996 to 2005, 38.3% of those diagnosed with HIV received a diagnosis of AIDS within the subsequent 12 months indicating a late diagnosis; an additional 6.7% received an AIDS diagnosis from 1 to 3 years after their HIV diagnosis (CDC, 2009b). Individuals who are unaware of their HIV infection are more likely to engage in high-risk sexual behavior that results in further transmission than those who have learned their status and have had the opportunity to modify these behaviors (Marks et al., 2006).

Schackman et al. (2006) have estimated a projected life expectancy of an HIV-infected person of 24.2 years from the time of entering care and a discounted (3%) total lifetime treatment cost per person of $385,000 (2004 $) for adults initiating ART at a CD4 count of 350 cells/μL or less. The undiscounted lifetime cost was $618,900 or an average of $2100 monthly. The monthly cost of HIV care ranged from $2000 for those with a CD4 count greater than 300 cells/μL to $4700 for those with a CD4 count less than 50 cells/μL. Discounted costs estimated from the time of infection were $303,100 with a life expectancy of 32.1 years, given the estimate that infection on average occurs 8.1 years before entry into care. Of the $23.3 billion the U.S. federal government spent on HIV in FY 2008, 50% was for care and treatment, 12% for research, 10% for cash and housing assistance, 4% for prevention, and 25% for the international epidemic (Kaiser Family Foundation, 2009). Funds spent on HIV prevention help to offset money that would have been spent on treatment, illustrating the importance of economic evaluation in this policy area.

Strategies to Prevent the Spread of HIV

Approaches for preventing HIV can be classified under two broad headings. Biomedical approaches include the use of ART to prevent mother-to-child or perinatal transmission; postexposure prophylaxis (PEP) with ART to prevent the development of HIV from both occupational and nonoccupational exposures; PrEP with ART for high-risk uninfected persons; the use of topical microbicides; male circumcision; and vaccine development. Behavioral approaches include all those interventions designed to reduce risky behavior and decrease the likelihood of HIV transmission and infection. These include individual-level, group-level, and community-level risk-reduction programs; interventions to promote the use of condoms and other barrier methods; school and community education programs; the treatment and prevention of drug and alcohol abuse; and needle exchange programs (Schreibman and Friedland, 2003; Fauci, 2007; Global HIV Prevention Working Group, 2008). HIV counseling and testing programs may also lead to behavior change that reduces the risk of infection (Holtgrave and McGuire, 2007; Janssen, 2007).

To illustrate the different approaches to preventing HIV and to outline how economic evaluation methods can be applied, we present a case study of a biomedical intervention, PrEP, and a case study focusing on a behavioral intervention, an adaptation of the popular opinion leader (POL) intervention to reduce HIV risk behaviors among black MSM.

Case Study of Preexposure Prophylaxis

DESCRIPTION OF THE STRATEGY

Chemoprophylaxis is the provision of a medicine or vaccine to individuals before they are exposed to an infectious agent. For example, malaria prophylaxis has been standard practice for travelers to malaria-endemic countries. Antimalaria medications are administered in anticipation of a potential exposure and are thus present in the bloodstream should the traveler become exposed to the disease. Studies of mother-to-child HIV transmission have shown that providing antiretroviral treatment to HIV-infected women during labor and delivery and to their newborns immediately following birth can reduce the risk of transmission by about 50%. Antiretroviral regimens among healthcare workers following needle stick and other accidental exposures to HIV have been associated with an 80% reduction in the risk of infection when treatment is initiated promptly and continued for several weeks (CDC, 2008b). These developments led researchers to explore whether HIV transmission could be decreased further if antiretroviral treatment is delivered before exposure to HIV (Paxton et al., 2007).

HIV PrEP had long been thought not feasible for human beings because there were no drugs that had high potency against HIV, simple dosing schedules, low rates of adverse effects, and a low frequency of drug-induced resistance. However, in 2001, tenofovir, a nucleotide reverse transcriptase inhibitor with these qualities, was approved. The combination treatment of tenofovir and emtricitabine, another nucleoside reverse transcriptase inhibitor, was approved in 2004 (Paxton et al., 2007). Daily oral doses of tenofovir (Viread) or tenofovir plus emtricitabine (Truvada) are being used in clinical trials of HIV PrEP.

The CDC sponsored three ongoing clinical trials of PrEP involving heterosexuals in Botswana, injection drug users in Thailand, and MSM in the United States. The Botswana trial focuses on the safety and efficacy of tenofovir plus emtricitabine and is enrolling 1200 HIV-negative heterosexual men and women ages 18–39. The Thailand study examines the safety and efficacy of tenofovir with an enrollment of 2400 HIV-negative intravenous drug users (IDUs) at 17 drug treatment clinics in Bangkok. The U.S. study has enrolled 400 HIV-negative MSM who reported having anal intercourse in the prior 12 months. Two arms of the trial receive either tenofovir or the placebo immediately, while the other two arms receive the drug or placebo after 9 months of enrollment. The U.S. trial is designed to assess the clinical and behavioral safety of tenofovir among HIV-negative MSM, but is not large enough to evaluate the drug's efficacy in reducing HIV transmission. However, it will provide information for the development of implementation guidelines if drug efficacy is demonstrated in the other trials. All three CDC studies are randomized, double-blind, placebo-controlled trials where participants also receive risk-reduction counseling and other prevention services. The trials will assess the effects of PrEP on HIV risk behaviors, adherence to and acceptability of the regimens, and the resistance characteristics of the virus for those who become infected (CDC, 2008b).

MODELING OUTCOMES AND COSTS

Because the PrEP clinical trials are ongoing, there is a need for economic and disease modeling to estimate the impacts of implementing a PrEP program in the United States and its cost-effectiveness. Desai et al. (2008) developed a compartmental model to simulate the acquisition of HIV, disease progression, and the effects of HIV treatment and care on survival and HIV transmission. Compartmental models are population-based epidemic models where individuals are grouped into various disease and/or treatment states, and the flow of individuals to and from these states can be simulated (Bailey, 1975; Hethcote and Yorke, 1984). These models can be deterministic where event occurrence is not subject to chance, or stochastic where event occurrences are determined by probability distributions (Garnett, 2002).

Desai et al. (2008) adapted their model to simulate a once-daily, self-administered PrEP regimen among high-risk uninfected MSM in New York City. The model was divided into four age groups and four sexual activity classes based on the annual number of new sexual partners. The HIV infection rate, calculated by age and sexual activity class, depended on the annual number of new sex partners, HIV infection status in the chosen partner, and HIV transmission probabilities that were a function of the partner's infection stage and the duration of the partnership. Model parameters, drawn from the literature, were validated by comparing HIV prevalence, incidence, and the number of MSM living with HIV/AIDS generated by the model to HIV/AIDS surveillance data from the CDC and the New York City Department of Health and Mental Hygiene. The outcome measure, the number of HIV infections prevented, was derived by comparing the number of model-generated new infections with and without the PrEP regimen.

Desai et al. (2008) analyzed 36 hypothetical scenarios that varied by the mechanism of protection, efficacy, adherence, and population coverage. They defined adherence as the proportion of all MSM who adhered completely to a daily PrEP regimen. Efficacy, or the reduction in susceptibility to HIV infection upon exposure to an HIV-infected partner, was varied among the scenarios as were assumptions about the effects of partial drug adherence. The model considered either 1,500 or 15,000 individuals that corresponded to coverage rates of 2.5% and 25% of the very high-risk MSM population in New York City. All simulations began in 2008 and projected the epidemic and the impact of PrEP until 2013.

Desai et al. (2008) conducted the economic evaluation of PrEP from the perspective of the U.S. healthcare system. They included the costs for drug administration and monitoring and the treatment cost savings associated with HIV infections prevented as determined by the model. The authors used the 2007 U.S. average wholesale price from the producer of Tenofovir plus emtricitabine of $31 per 500 mg tablet taken daily. They also estimated the costs of medical screening to determine eligibility for potential chemoprophylaxis candidates and the costs of ongoing medical and adherence monitoring, valued at $1300 per person for the first year and $1020 per person per year thereafter. Costs for medical services were based on Medicare reimbursement rates. The researchers assumed that all participants incurred these costs regardless of their actual adherence or involvement with medical monitoring.

The outcome of the analysis was the incremental cost per QALY saved for the infections prevented by the PrEP intervention compared with no intervention. Net costs of the intervention were defined as the program costs of chemoprophylaxis and monitoring less the lifetime treatment costs for those HIV infections prevented by the intervention. These were divided by the number of QALYs saved to determine the incremental cost-effectiveness ratio (ICER) for the intervention.

ESTIMATING HIV TREATMENT COSTS SAVED

For their base-case analysis, Desai et al. (2008) assumed that a lifetime HIV-related treatment cost of $343,130, based on the work of Schackman et al. (2006), was saved for each infection prevented. The lifetime cost of treating a case of HIV is estimated by simulating monthly or quarterly changes in disease stage for large cohorts of HIV-infected patients based on changes in viral load and CD4 counts derived from clinical studies and varying assumptions about the impact of ART on disease progression. Schackman et al. (2006) updated the Cost-effectiveness of Preventing AIDS Complications (CEPAC) model (Freedberg et al., 1998; 2001; Paltiel et al., 2005) with cost and utilization data from HIV Research Network (HIVRN) sites. The HIVRN is a network of 18 primary HIV care clinics and offices that treat more than 14,000 patients. These providers collect longitudinal clinic and health services utilization data on their patients including demographic characteristics, medications prescribed, frequency of outpatient visits, and the number of inpatient admissions.

Schackman et al. (2006) obtained HIVRN data on the number of outpatient visits and hospitalizations. Because data on emergency room visits were not captured by HIVRN, the researchers used the ratio of emergency room to outpatient visits reported in an earlier survey, the HIV Cost and Services Utilization Survey or HCSUS, to estimate this variable (Frankel et al., 1999; Shapiro et al., 1999). Costs included all inpatient visits and medications for patients with an ICD-9 code indicative of HIV infection. The researchers assumed that patients used four sequential ART regimens derived from existing clinical guidelines, and that the optimal selection of individual drugs was based on HIV drug resistance testing. The costs of ART and opportunistic infection medications were calculated using 2004 average wholesale prices adjusted for the average state Medicaid reimbursement rate to retail pharmacies. These costs were applied to the disease state-transition model to project the lifetime medical costs for HIV-infected adults from the time of infection. The researchers assumed that patients received care according to U.S. guidelines for ART and that patients remained in care for the rest of their lives.

ESTIMATING QALYS SAVED

Using the utility weights derived from the meta-analysis of Tengs and Lin (2002), Desai et al. (2008) estimated that 6.95 QALYs were saved for each HIV infection prevented through the chemoprophylaxis regimens. Tengs and Lin (2002) had noted the variation in the published utility weights for various stages of HIV infection. These weights ranged from 0.69 to 0.88 for asymptomatic HIV infection, 0.48 to 0.82 for symptomatic HIV infection, and 0.24 to 0.79 for AIDS. The variation in these weights is likely due to differences in the methods used for eliciting utility weights, variability in the respondents used for elicitation, or variation in the ways researchers defined the lower and upper bounds of utility scales. The three major methods for eliciting preferences are the standard gamble, time trade-off, and rating methods (Patrick and Erickson, 1993; Gold et al., 1996; Haddix et al., 2003; Drummond et al., 2005). The standard gamble method often yields higher utility estimates than the time trade-off method, while the latter results in higher weights than the rating method. People who have experienced the health condition in question generally report higher weights than those who have not experienced the condition. The zero and one end points of the utility scale have also been defined differently in various studies.

Tengs and Lin (2002) undertook a meta-analysis of HIV/AIDS utility estimates, based on 25 published articles reporting 74 utilities elicited from 1956 respondents, to pool the results from multiple studies and obtain a combined estimate. Tengs and Lin estimated the following values using patients as respondents: 0.94 for asymptomatic infection; 0.82 for symptomatic infection; and 0.70 for AIDS. The corresponding values for non-patients were the following: 0.68 for asymptomatic HIV infection; 0.56 for symptomatic infection; and 0.44 for AIDS. Desai et al. (2008) used the patient-based set of weights for their analysis.

Both future costs and QALYs were discounted at a rate of 3% in the analysis to calculate the present value of these variables. Discounting is used because costs and outcomes occurring in the future are weighted differently from those occurring at the present time. Although earlier healthcare evaluation studies used a 5% discount rate, there has been a general consensus since the mid-1990s that a 3% real rate is appropriate (Gold et al., 1996; Haddix et al., 2003).

SENSITIVITY ANALYSIS

Desai et al. (2008) performed sensitivity analyses by analyzing the 36 scenarios described above that varied efficacy, the mechanism of protection, coverage, and adherence. They estimated ICERs and daily chemoprophylaxis threshold prices above which the ICER would exceed $50,000 and $100,000 per QALY saved, willingness-to-pay thresholds that have been commonly used in the literature, for all combinations of program parameters, three estimates of lifetime treatment costs, and low and high limits of the expected number of HIV infections prevented.

RESULTS

The results for the base-case scenario indicated that 1710 new cases of HIV infection, or 8.7% of the 19,510 new cases of HIV predicted in the model from current incidence rates, would be prevented by chemoprophylaxis assuming coverage of 15,000 high-risk MSM, the basic mechanism of protection, an efficacy of 50%, and program adherence of 50% (Desai et al., 2008). Seven hundred cases would be directly prevented by the chemoprophylaxis program, whereas the remaining 1010 are secondary cases that would be prevented indirectly by reducing HIV prevalence in the community. This large number of indirectly prevented cases resulted primarily from a reduction in the prevalence of sexually active individuals in the short primary stage of HIV infection. Under base-case assumptions, the chemoprophylaxis program costs $31,970 per QALY saved. The daily drug price would have to exceed $39 (compared with the base-case value of $31) for the $50,000 per QALY willingness-to-pay threshold to be surpassed.

Sensitivity analysis showed that program coverage levels bear an important influence on the results (Desai et al., 2008). If only 2.5% of high-risk MSM were enrolled, the PrEP regimen did not prevent enough HIV infections to justify the intervention. However, at 25% program coverage, expected reductions in HIV infections ranged from 4% to 23% depending on assumptions about efficacy and the mechanism of protection. Variations in lifetime HIV treatment costs did not have a substantial impact on the cost-effectiveness results.

Key concerns about a PrEP program include the possible increases in participants' risk behavior resulting from the sense of security provided by the program, the development of antiretroviral drug resistance among those for whom PrEP failed to prevent HIV infection, and renal impairment related to long-term use of tenofovir. Desai et al. (2008) found that a 4.1% increase in sexual partners could offset the number of infections prevented by the program. Due to the uncertainty surrounding the issue of drug resistance, the authors decided not to include this factor in their model until more data became available. The authors also assumed that there was no significant renal impairment associated with the drug usage, given medical screening to exclude at-risk patients and the current safety profile of the drugs.

Desai et al. (2008) concluded that a PrEP program for high-risk MSM in the United States could be effective in preventing HIV infections and cost-effective over a broad range of values for the epidemiologic, programmatic, and cost variables. Although the authors noted the uncertainty regarding a number of important variables in their analysis, they argued that the study results should encourage policy makers to discuss potential program implementation.

Case Study of the Popular Opinion Leader Intervention Applied to Black MSM

DESCRIPTION OF THE STRATEGY

Given the importance of MSM for the U.S. HIV epidemic, many behavioral interventions have focused on this group. Several reviews have shown that HIV behavioral interventions are effective in reducing risky sexual behavior and maintaining safer sex practices for adult MSM (Herbst et al., 2005; 2007; Lyles et al., 2007). Person-to-person behavioral interventions vary by several characteristics: the level of delivery (individual, group, or community); the type of personnel delivering the program (volunteers or paid professionals); and the specific content of the intervention (partner negotiation, risk-reduction decision making, or instruction on condom usage). Most of the evaluations of these interventions focus on the following outcomes: unprotected anal intercourse, the consistent use of condoms during anal intercourse, and the number of sex partners, all of which are linked to HIV acquisition (Herbst et al., 2007).

Individual-level and group-level interventions assist clients in changing their HIV-risk behaviors through changes in beliefs, motivation, and self-efficacy, and they provide information about HIV and STDs. In addition, group-level interventions include discussions that promote the support of group members and the influence of peers to help change behavior. Group-level interventions can be delivered by a counselor, facilitator, or peer. Community-level interventions attempt to change individuals' risk behaviors by modifying the attitudes, norms, and values within a defined community. The rationale is that individuals may be better able to change their behaviors if there are peer norms supporting safer sex practices within the community. These interventions have longer implementation periods than individual-level and group-level interventions. The crucial issue for the evaluation of community-level interventions is measuring the diffusion of behavior change (Herbst et al., 2007).

One example of a community-level intervention is the POL model (Kelly et al., 1991; 1992; Kelly, 2004). This intervention, whose goal is to increase safer-sex norms among a well-defined community, uses ethnographic techniques both to identify the community and those individuals within the community who are the most well-liked, popular, and trusted by other members. These individuals are trained as POLs who will initiate HIV risk-reduction messages to friends and acquaintances in everyday conversations. These leaders personally endorse the benefits of safer behavior and make recommendations on how others can implement change. Logos, such as a traffic light symbol worn by the POL, or other devices are used as mechanisms to start conversations. POLs meet in weekly groups to develop their skills and increase their confidence in delivering HIV prevention messages. They then set goals for the number of risk-reduction conversations with others in the target population between the weekly sessions. These outcomes are reviewed and reinforced at subsequent training sessions. Although opinion leaders are paid a modest stipend for attending the weekly sessions, they are not paid for having the conversations. Program designers argued that this type of payment would convert the opinion leaders into paid outreach workers, which would alter the nature of the intervention (Kelly, 2004).

BEHAVIORAL INTERVENTION OUTCOMES

Kelly et al. (1991, 1992) conducted evaluations of the POL model in Biloxi and Hattiesburg, Mississippi and in Monroe, Louisiana. Each of these cities had one or two large gay bars that served as a primary social setting for MSM in those communities. Kelly et al. (1991) randomly selected Biloxi to receive the POL intervention, while the other two cities served as comparison groups. The opinion leaders were trained, and the intervention was implemented as described above. Behavioral surveys of male club patrons were completed at baseline and 3 and 6 months later. The risk characteristics of the populations in the intervention and control cities were initially comparable. The post-intervention surveys indicated that unprotected anal intercourse decreased by about 30% from initial levels, whereas much less change occurred among the men in the control cities. There was an increase in the use of condoms and a decrease in the number of men reporting multiple sexual partners in the previous 2 months only among men in the intervention city.

Using the same cities, Kelly et al. (1992) completed baseline surveys in all three cities. They then implemented the intervention in city 1, repeated the surveys in all cities, introduced the intervention in city 2, and so on, until all cities had received the same intervention. The results of the analysis indicated reductions of 15%–29% from baseline levels in the proportion of men who engaged in any unprotected anal intercourse. Reductions in the number of sexual partners were reported for two of the three cities.

Given the high rates of infection reported among black MSM, Jones et al. (2008) adapted the POL model to focus on this group in three North Carolina cities (Raleigh, Greensboro, and Charlotte) in which the target population could be assessed, recruited, and trained. The researchers conducted four equally spaced cross-section surveys during the 1-year study period. Exposure to the intervention was measured by asking respondents how many times they had seen the project logo. Although there were high levels of risk among participants in this sample, at the final assessment there were significant decreases in the proportion of individuals reporting unprotected anal intercourse, the number of partners for unprotected anal intercourse, and the mean number of partners for and episodes of unprotected sex. There were also significant increases in the percent reporting consistent condom use. Although this study illustrated the adaptation of an existing community intervention to a high-risk group, it was limited by the fact that it did not include a control group for comparison.

MODELING OUTCOMES AND COSTS

Given that the POL model has shown effectiveness in reducing HIV risk behaviors, there is the further question of the impact of these behavior changes on the number of infections prevented and of the cost of the intervention. Pinkerton et al. (1998) analyzed both of these questions in their evaluation of the Kelly et al. (1991) intervention. Because only behavioral outcome data were reported, Pinkerton et al. (1998) used a mathematical modeling technique, the Bernoulli process model, to translate this behavior change data into an estimate of the number of infections prevented by the intervention. In this model, each act of intercourse is treated as an independent event with a small, fixed probability of HIV transmission. The number of infections prevented, including secondary infections among the partners of already-infected intervention participants, is a function of (1) the number of individuals and their partners whose behavior is affected by the intervention; (2) the number of acts of protected and unprotected receptive and insertive anal intercourse and the number of partners for each of these behaviors; (3) HIV prevalence in the community; (4) the per-act transmission probabilities associated with each type of unprotected intercourse; and (5) the effectiveness of condoms in preventing HIV transmission. These models have become standard in the literature examining the impact of behavior changes on HIV infections prevented (Pinkerton and Abramson, 1998; Pinkerton and Holtgrave, 1998).

Pinkerton et al. (1998) used the sexual behavior parameters derived from the surveys in the original study by Kelly et al. (1991) combined with other parameters derived from the literature to estimate model outcomes. They used the number of individuals completing surveys in the original study as a measure of the size of the affected population. The researchers noted that this was a conservative estimate as it assumed that the impact of the intervention was limited to the subpopulation sampled in the bars where the intervention occurred. Intervention costs, measured in 1996 dollars, were collected retrospectively and included staff compensation (four weekly 90–120 minute sessions) ($6700), monetary incentives given to the POLs ($5300), materials and other expenses such as rental fees, catering, and staff travel ($4100), and an estimate for overhead ($1000). The overall cost was about $40 per affected individual. HIV treatment costs and QALYs saved by the intervention were derived using methods similar to those discussed above for the PrEP case study.

RESULTS

Pinkerton et al. (1998) concluded that this intervention prevented 0.262 infections and saved just under three QALYs discounted at 3%. This small impact resulted from the fact that the researchers assumed only a very limited 2-month period of intervention effectiveness. However, the base-case cost per HIV infection averted was approximately $65,000, which was less than the treatment cost per case of HIV, thus making the intervention cost-saving. The intervention remained either cost-effective or cost-saving in all the sensitivity analyses. Pinkerton et al. (1998) found that their results were not very sensitive to the particular model used to estimate the number of infections averted or to other parameters including condom effectiveness. The per-contact probability of transmission and HIV prevalence in the community did have a larger impact on the cost-effectiveness results.

Summary/Conclusions

Economic evaluation techniques can be applied to a wide range of healthcare programs as illustrated by the two case studies in this chapter. Although both case studies focus on HIV prevention, the use of a drug regimen for PrEP contrasts sharply with a behavior change/risk-reduction intervention among MSM as alternative prevention strategies. Because HIV prevention is such a complex process, both of these strategies may be necessary. However, this conclusion raises the economic question of how best to allocate resources among these and other HIV prevention strategies.

The economic evaluation techniques discussed in this chapter can assist decision makers in this process. They are a general set of techniques comparing costs and outcomes that can be applied to a wide range of programs. Both of the case studies developed in this chapter follow the economic evaluation steps described in the "Economic Evaluation Techniques" section. The alternatives for comparison are defined, and the strategies are outlined in detail. In both cases, mathematical modeling is used to estimate the relevant outcomes for the analysis. For PrEP, there are no program outcomes that can be directly observed because the efficacy results of the clinical trials have not been reported yet. For risk-reduction interventions, the data typically collected are intermediate outcomes or changes in specific behaviors related to the acquisition and transmission of HIV. Trials and quasi-experiments of most behavioral interventions are not run long enough or are not of sufficient size to detect significant impacts on HIV incidence. Thus, mathematical modeling is used to estimate how measures of behavior change translate to HIV infections prevented.

Intervention costs are measured similarly in both approaches. The goal is to account for the value of the resources used in implementing the intervention. How costs are measured depends on whether the analysis takes the perspective of society as a whole or that of various payers in the system. Cost measurement also depends on the specific program alternatives being compared.

The estimation of HIV treatment costs and QALYs saved in both approaches is based on standard techniques developed in the literature. Although there are varying models that are used to project disease progression and the costs associated with different disease stages, these models provide estimates that are relatively comparable. Estimates of QALYs saved may vary due to differences in the utility weights applied to the life years gained from an intervention. However, there is a reasonable consensus on the methods used to estimate QALYs.

Economic evaluation of healthcare programs is a multidisciplinary process that builds on the underlying scientific evidence for intervention effectiveness. If an intervention is found to be effective, the next question for decision makers usually relates to the costs associated with achieving program outcomes. The techniques discussed in this chapter illustrate the approaches that can be taken to provide evidence on these questions for HIV prevention interventions and other healthcare programs.

References

AIDS InfoNet. 2009a. CD4 cell tests. Fact Sheet No. 124, March 11. www.aidsinfonet.org

AIDS InfoNet. 2009b. U.S. antiretroviral therapy guidelines. Fact Sheet No. 404, April 28. www.aidsinfonet.org

Bailey, N.T.J. 1975. *The Mathematical Theory of Infectious Diseases and Its Applications*, 2nd ed. U.K.: Charles Griffin and Company.

Barton, P., S. Bryan, and S. Robinson. 2004. Modelling in the economic evaluation of health care: Selecting the appropriate approach. *Journal of Health Services Research & Policy* 9(2): 110–118.

Briggs, A., K. Claxton, and M. Sculpher. 2006. *Decision Modeling for Health Economic Evaluation*. New York: Oxford University Press.

Buchacz, K., M. Rangel, R. Blacher, and J.T. Brooks. 2009. Changes in the clinical epidemiology of HIV infection in the United States: Implications for the clinician. *Current Infectious Disease Reports* 11: 75–83.

CDC. 2008a. HIV prevalence estimates—United States, 2006. *MMWR* 57(39): 1073–1076.

CDC. 2008b. CDC trials of pre-exposure prophylaxis for HIV prevention. Fact Sheet.

CDC. 2009a. *HIV/AIDS surveillance report, 2007*, vol. 19. Atlanta: U.S. Department of Health and Human Services, Centers for Disease Control and Prevention; [inclusive page numbers]. http://www.cdc.gov/hiv/topics/surveillance/resources/reports/

CDC. 2009b. Late HIV testing—34 states, 1996–2005. *MMWR* 58(24): 661–665.

Desai, K., S.L. Sansom, M.L. Ackers et al. 2008. Modeling the impact of HIV chemoprophylaxis strategies among men who have sex with men in the United States: HIV infections prevented and cost-effectiveness. *AIDS* 22: 1829–1839.

Drummond, M.F., M.J. Sculpher, G.W. Torrance, B.J. O'Brien, and G.L. Stoddart. 2005. *Methods for the Economic Evaluation of Health Care Programmes*, 3rd ed. New York: Oxford University Press.

Fauci, A.S. 2007. Pathogenesis of HIV disease: Opportunities for new prevention interventions. *Clinical Infectious Diseases* 45(Suppl 4): S206–S212.

Fisher, A., L.G. Chestnut, and D.M. Violette. 1989. The value of reducing risks of death: A note on new evidence. *Journal of Policy Analysis and Management* 8(1): 88–100.

Frankel, M.R., M.F. Shapiro, N. Duan et al. 1999. National probability samples in studies of low-prevalence diseases. Part II: Designing and implementing the HIV cost and services utilization study sample. *Health Services Research* 34(5 Part I): 969–92.

Freedberg, K.A., E. Losina, M. Weinstein et al. 2001. The cost effectiveness of combination antiretroviral therapy for HIV disease. *The New England Journal of Medicine* 344(11): 824–831.

Freedberg, K.A., J.A. Scharfstein, G.R. Seage III et al. 1998. The cost-effectiveness of preventing AIDS-related opportunistic infections. *JAMA* 279(2): 130–136.

Garnett, G.P. 2002. An introduction to mathematical models in sexually transmitted disease epidemiology. *Sexually Transmitted Infections* 78: 7–12.

Global HIV Prevention Working Group. 2008. Behavior change and HIV prevention: [Re]Considerations for the 21st century. www.globalhivprevention.org

Gold, M.R., J.E. Siegel, L.B. Russell, and M.C. Weinstein. 1996. *Cost-Effectiveness in Health and Medicine*. New York: Oxford University Press.

Granich, R.M., C.F. Gilks, C. Dye et al. 2009. Universal voluntary HIV testing and immediate antiretroviral therapy as a strategy for elimination of HIV transmission: A mathematical model. *The Lancet* 373(9657): 48–57.

Grosse, R.N. 1970. Problems of resource allocation in health. In *Public Expenditure and Policy Analysis*, R.H. Haveman and J. Margolis (eds.), pp. 518–548. Chicago, IL: Markham Publishing Company.

Grosse, S.D., S.M. Teutsch, and A.C. Haddix. 2007. Lessons from cost-effectiveness research for United States public health policy. *Annual Review of Public Health* 28: 365–391.

Haddix, A.C., S.M. Teutsch, and P.S. Corso. 2003. *Prevention Effectiveness: A Guide to Decision Analysis and Economic Evaluation*, 2nd edn. New York: Oxford University Press.

Hall, H.I., R. Song, P. Rhodes et al. 2008. Estimation of HIV incidence in the United States. *JAMA* 300(5): 520–529.

Herbst, J.H., C. Becker, A. Mathew et al. 2007. The effectiveness of individual-, group-, and community-level HIV behavioral risk-reduction interventions for adult men who have sex with men: A systematic review. *American Journal of Preventive Medicine* 32(4S): S38–S67.

Herbst, J.H., R.T. Sherba, N. Crepaz et al. 2005. A meta-analytic review of HIV behavioral interventions for reducing sexual risk behavior of men who have sex with men. *Journal of Acquired Immune Deficiency Syndromes* 39(2): 228–241.

Hethcote, H. and J. Yorke. 1984. Gonorrhea transmission dynamics and control. In *Lecture Notes in Biomathematics*, vol. 56, 111pp. Berlin, Germany: Springer-Verlag.

Holtgrave, D. and J. Maguire. 2007. Impact of counseling in voluntary counseling and testing programs for persons at risk for or living with HIV infection. *Clinical Infectious Diseases* 45: S240–S243.

Janssen, R.S. 2007. Implementing HIV screening. *Clinical Infectious Diseases* 45: S226–S231.

Jones, K.T., P. Gray, Y.O. Whiteside et al. 2008. Evaluation of an HIV prevention intervention adapted for black men who have sex with men. *American Journal of Public Health* 98(6): 1043–1050.

Kaiser Family Foundation. 2009. HIV/AIDS policy fact sheet. The HIV/AIDS Epidemic in the United States. Menlo Park, CA, www.kff.org

Kelly, J.A. 2004. Popular opinion leaders and HIV prevention peer education: Resolving discrepant findings, and implications for the development of effective community programmes. *AIDS Care* 16(2): 139–150.

Kelly, J.A., J.S. St. Lawrence, Y.E. Diaz et al. 1991. HIV risk behavior reduction following intervention with key opinion leaders of population: An experimental analysis. *American Journal of Public Health* 81(2): 168–171.

Kelly, J.A., J.S. St. Lawrence, L.Y. Stevenson et al. 1992. Community AIDS/HIV risk reduction: The effects of endorsements by popular people in three cities. *American Journal of Pub Health* 82(11): 1483–1489.

Lyles, C.M., L.S. Kay, N. Crepaz et al. 2007. Best-evidence interventions: Findings from a systematic review of HIV behavioral interventions for US populations at high risk, 2000–2004. *American Journal of Public Health* 97(1): 133–143.

Marks, G., N. Crepaz, and R.S. Janssen. 2006. Estimating sexual transmission of HIV from persons aware and unaware that they are infected with the virus in the USA. *AIDS* 20: 1447–1450.

Mrozek, J.R. and L.O. Taylor. 2002. What determines the value of life? A meta-analysis. *Journal of Policy Analysis and Management* 21(2): 253–270.

O'Brien, B. and A. Gafni. 1996. When do the 'dollars' make sense? Toward a conceptual framework for contingent valuation studies in health care. *Medical Decision Making* 16: 288–299.

Paltiel, A.D., M.C. Weinstein, A.D. Kimmel et al. 2005. Expanded screening for HIV in the United States—An analysis of cost-effectiveness. *The New England Journal of Medicine* 352(6): 586–595.

Patrick, D.L. and P. Erickson. 1993. *Health Status and Health Policy: Allocating Resources to Health Care*. New York: Oxford University Press.

Pauly, M.V. 1995. Valuing health care benefits in money terms. In *Valuing Health Care: Costs, Benefits, and Effectiveness of Pharmaceuticals and Other Medical Technologies*, F.A. Sloan (ed.), pp. 99–124. New York: Cambridge University Press.

Paxton, L.A., T. Hope, and H.W. Jaffe. 2007. Pre-exposure prophylaxis for HIV infection: What if it works? *Lancet* 370: 89–93.

Pinkerton, S.D. and P.R. Abramson. 1998. The Bernoulli-process model of HIV transmission: Applications and implications. In *Handbook of Economic Evaluation of HIV Prevention Programs*, D.R. Holtgrave (ed.), pp. 13–32. New York: Plenum Press.

Pinkerton, S.D. and D.R. Holtgrave. 1998. A method for evaluating the economic efficiency of HIV behavioral risk reduction interventions. *AIDS and Behavior* 2(3): 189–201.

Pinkerton, S.D., D.R. Holtgrave, W.J. DiFranceisco et al. 1998. Cost-effectiveness of a community-level HIV risk reduction intervention. *American Journal of Public Health* 88(8): 1239–1242.

Schackman, B.R., K.A. Gebo, R.P. Walensky et al. 2006. The lifetime cost of current human immunodeficiency virus care in the United States. *Medical Care* 44(11): 990–997.

Schreibman, T. and G. Friedland. 2003. Human immunodeficiency virus infection prevention: Strategies for clinicians. *Clinical Infectious Diseases* 36: 1171–1176.

Shapiro, M.F., M.L. Berk, S.H. Berry et al. 1999. National probability samples in studies of low-prevalence diseases. Part I: Perspectives and lessons from the HIV cost and services utilization study. *Health Services Research* 34(5 Part I): 951–968.

Tengs, T.O. and T.H. Lin. 2002. A meta-analysis of utility estimates for HIV/AIDS. *Medical Decision Making* 22: 475–481.

Tolley, G., D. Kenkel, and R. Fabian. 1994. *Valuing Health for Policy: An Economic Approach*. Chicago, IL: The University of Chicago Press.

Willan, A.R. and A.H. Briggs. 2006. *Statistical Analysis of Cost-effectiveness Data*. West Sussex, England: John Wiley & Sons, Ltd.

Zolopa, A.R., J. Andersen, L. Komarow et al. 2009. Early antiretroviral therapy reduces AIDS progression/death in individuals with acute opportunistic infections: A multicenter randomized strategy trial. *PLoS ONE* 4(5): e5575.

26

Causal Risk Analysis: Revisiting the Vioxx Study

Farrokh Alemi
Georgetown University

Manaf Zargoush
ESSEC Business School

Introduction 26-1
History of Probabilistic and Causal Analysis 26-2
What Is a Cause? 26-3
Modeling Multiple Causes: Causal Diagrams 26-5
Modeling Multiple Causes: Probability Networks 26-5
Modeling Multiple Causes: Simultaneous Equations 26-7
Causal versus Noncausal Analysis 26-8
References 26-9

Introduction

The purpose of this chapter is to model risks of adverse events using causal probability models. To infer a cause and an effect, an experiment is needed where the cause is introduced and withdrawn and the effect is examined. Most risk analysis is not based on experimental data and uses observational data from naturally occurring variation in occurrences of causes and effects. For example, to infer that an environmental pollutant has led to an adverse event, experimental data are needed. The pollutant must be introduced in randomly chosen subjects or circumstances and the effect monitored. Because putting people at increased risk of adverse events is unethical, experimental data is seldom used in risk analysis. Instead, the analyst relies on observational data. But causal inferences from observational data are suspect. The observed increased risk of adverse events may be due to another variable not studied. It may, for example, show that an individual exposed to a pollutant has increased risk for breast cancer. The patient's breast cancer might have been caused by her smoking habit and not by the external pollutants. In analysis of observational data, it is difficult to control for alternative explanations of the adverse event. In recent years, progress has been made in making causal inferences from observational data. The purpose of this chapter is to review this progress and provide a blueprint of how causal risk analysis should be done.

Risk analysis is risk analysis, meaning that the methods of risk analysis are the same even when applied to many different application areas. In predicting the risk of adverse hospital events (e.g., wrong side surgery), risk of security breaches, risk of privacy violations, health risk of pollutants, risk of excess mortality from medications, and many other non-healthcare applications (e.g., risk of space disaster, risk of flood, risk of nuclear accidents), the methods are the same. All of these applications share a common problem structure. First, there is an adverse event of interest, for example, mortality, cardiac event, operating room fire, terrorist action, or nuclear accident (Figure 26.1).

Second, there are a set of causes often referred to as risk factors (e.g., smoking, slippery floors, new medication). Each of these causes could lead to the adverse event. Third, the impact of the causes (risk factors) may be moderated by various circumstances, which we refer to as moderating factors. Some factors may enhance the impact of the causes and others may prevent it. For example, in environmental risk

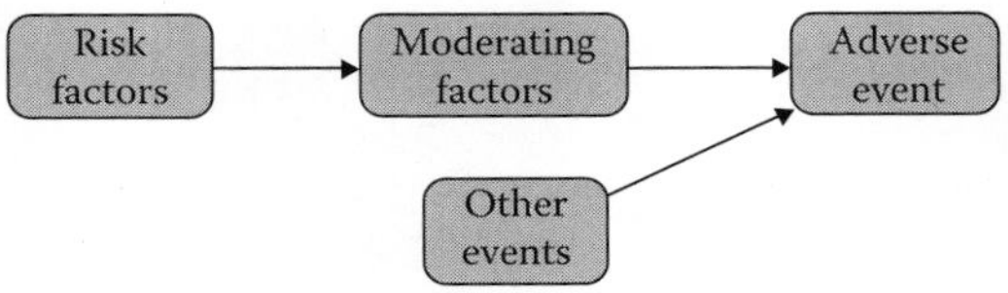

FIGURE 26.1 Common structure of risk analysis problems.

analysis, the moderating factors are the way the pollutant spreads in the environment and is absorbed by the population. Analysts need to model how the dispersion and absorption processes mitigate the impact of the pollutant. In patient safety, patient falls may be caused by slippery floors. Some patients wake up at night and would like to go to bathroom and fall in the process. The impact of slippery floors may be mitigated by lowering the height of the patient beds at nights and thereby enabling patients more control over their movements. For still another example, new medications may cause unanticipated excess mortality. In analysis of impact of medication on excess cardiac events, the impact may be mitigated by the patient's genetic predispositions. While the application of risk analysis varies, the structure of the problem at hand is similar and the methods of analysis are the same.

To illustrate the methods of causal risk analysis, we show how it can be applied to the determination of risk of excess cardiac events caused by the use of Rofecoxib (commonly known as Vioxx). Merck & Co. discovered and marketed Vioxx for treatment of osteoarthritis, acute pain conditions, and dysmenorrhea. The Food and Drug Administration (FDA) approved the use of Vioxx on May 20, 1999. It quickly gained a large market share, particularly among physicians treating patients with arthritis. A series of small studies of the long-term impact of Vioxx raised concerns that it might increase cardiac events. Two large-scale prospective studies were undertaken (Bombardier et al. 2000, Bresalier et al. 2005), one of which was stopped before the end of the study because preliminary analysis indicated that experimental patients were at increased risk of cardiac events. Finally, a very large study of patients in Kaiser Permanente involving 2.3 million person-years of follow up indicated that Vioxx increased the risk of cardiac events (Graham et al. 2005). This is the study that we will use throughout this chapter because it made causal inferences from observational data within electronic health records. On September 30, 2004, Merck voluntarily withdrew Vioxx from the market. Vioxx was the largest drug to be withdrawn from the market. In the year before withdrawal, Merck had sales revenue of $2.5 billion from Vioxx (Reuters 2006). At the time of withdrawal, Merck and Co. also disclosed that their earlier unpublished studies had shown an increased risk of cardiac events, but that findings were not significant. Merck and Co. was criticized for failing to disclose data on adverse events of Vioxx to FDA. Congressional hearing led to interest in development of methods of monitoring impact of medications after FDA approvals, the so-called post-release monitoring. Congress passed a law empowering FDA to create the sentinel database for monitoring impact of medications. Later, the American Recovery Act funded the widespread use of electronic health records, which increased the availability of observational data on impact of medications. Thus, it made it easier to analyze the impact of medications from observational data within electronic health records. We selected the Vioxx case as an example for demonstrating causal risk analysis because it is a model for how risk of medications can be analyzed and because it demonstrates the issues and difficulty associated with causal inferences from observation data.

History of Probabilistic and Causal Analysis

Probabilistic risk analysis started in 1967 in the space industry, where, except for a short period of time, it has been the standard approach for analysis of risks associated with shuttle flights (Colglazier and Weatherwax 1986, Bell and Esch 1989, Planning Research Corporation 1989, Science Applications International Corporation 1989, Pate-Cornell and Fischbeck 1994, Hoffman et al. 1998, Cooke and Jager 1998). In nuclear safety, probabilistic risk analysis has been used to assess reactor safety

(Environmental Protection Agency 1976, Union of Concerned Scientists 1977, Kemeny 1979, Rogovin and Frampton 1980, Kaplan and Garrick 1981). Probabilistic risk analysis has been applied to cyber terrorism (Taylor et al. 2002), earthquake predictions (Chang et al. 2000), floods and coastal designs (Voortman et al. 2002, Kaczmarek 2003, Mai and Zimmermann 2003), environmental pollution (Slob and Pieters 1998, Moore et al. 1999), waste disposal (Garrick and Kaplan 1999, Ewing et al. 2004), and environmental health (Cohen 2003, Sadiq et al. 2003). Applications to healthcare problems have been less common (Marx and Slonim 2003, Wreathall and Nemeth 2004, Alemi 2007). Probabilistic risk analysis has been applied to medication errors in a hospital (Hover and O'Donnel 2007), falls in an assisted living home (Song 2007), and infant mortality (Yang and Kitsantas 2007). In healthcare, many probabilistic risk analysis studies are reported under other headings, for example, as statistical analysis of adverse effects of new medications.

In recent decades, probabilistic analysis has evolved into causal analysis. The early causal analysis focused on path analysis and simultaneous equations (Wright 1921). Judea Pearl used probabilistic networks for causal analysis (Pearl 1986, 1988, Rebane and Pearl 1987). More recent works have highlighted how causal graphs, probability networks, and simultaneous equations are interrelated and can be used interchangeably for causal analysis (Pearl 2000).

The application of causal analysis to risk analysis is rare. Cox reports one of the earliest applications of causal risk analysis to the understanding of the impact of environmental pollutants (Cox 2001).

What Is a Cause?

For more than a millennium, scientists have been clarifying what can legitimately be considered a cause of an event. Aristotle, for example, speaks of classes of causes more than a millennium ago. Furthermore, many psychologists believe that humans think through causal reasoning (Sloman 2005). We say that a spark causes a forest fire, smoking causes lung cancer, or Vioxx leads to excess cardiac events. Despite widespread use of the term, despite a long history of active research in this area, a great deal of confusion remains about what is a cause. When we ask people to list the causes of excess cardiac events, we were surprised by the answers they gave. Much of what they said could not be considered a cause at all. Some listed the goals of the healthcare system—e.g., one person said that she wanted to reduce excess cardiac events in order to improve quality of care. Improving quality of care maybe a reason why we reduce excess cardiac events but it is not a cause of it.

When asked what causes cardiac events, some responded "being male." While it is true that men have more cardiac events, it is hard to imagine the Y-chromosome plays an active role in creating cardiac events. Being male has a probabilistic but not a causal relationship to cardiac events.

So many people make errors in listing causes of cardiac events that it occurred to us that we need to distinguish a cause from other concepts such as goals, reason, and motivation. We need to define a cause so that independent observers can judge if claims of causality are plausible.

At the simplest possible level, we can imagine a world in which there is one cause and one effect (Figure 26.2). The cause and the effect are shown in two separate nodes and an arrow shows the direction of the influence. Given this simple cause and effect diagram, the question is what we need to show that supports our claim that one event causes the other. For example, what evidence is necessary to claim that the medication Vioxx led to excess cardiac events.

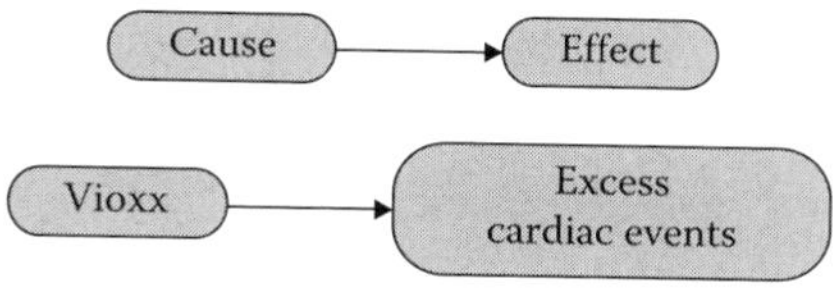

FIGURE 26.2 A simple causal diagram.

First, to clarify what is a cause, we need to be clear about what is an event. Events are physical or mental changes that have a start and an end. In this sense, taking the Vioxx medication is considered an event. This event causes another event called "cardiac event." Causes link events to each other. It is easy to talk of events causing other events because an event marks a change. It is hard to say the same about non-events—e.g., physical objects. Physical objects do not typically cause changes because they seldom change themselves. It is hard to imagine that hospital walls cause cardiac events (even though some hospitals have more cardiac events than others) because these walls do not change and therefore cannot be considered events. The very definition of events and the association between cause and change leads to the obvious statement that causes are temporary events. They are absent at one point in time and present at another point in time. The statement that being male is a cause of cardiac events does not sound reasonable to us because it is always present, even when a man has no cardiac event. On the other hand, the statement that smoking is a cause of cardiac events could be reasonable because a person might change his smoking habit and see the consequence of it in terms of lower cardiac events. A legitimate candidate for causes of cardiac events needs to be a temporary event.

Second, we expect causes and effects to be associated with each other. The relationship between a cause and effect might be measured in terms of a correlation or the conditional probability of observing the effect given the presence of the cause. It is important to point out that the relationship between a cause and an effect is often not deterministic. A cause does not always lead to the same effect. A previous heart attack increases the risk of cardiac events but it is not true that everyone who has a history of heart attacks will have new cardiac events.

Third, causes describe a mechanism where an event leads to another (Susser 1991, Morabia 2005). A series of events can cause each other. The process continues until the effect emerges. The original event can be called the root cause. The cause immediately preceding the effect is called direct cause. The more the mechanism from the cause to the effect is clear, the stronger the claim that one has found a cause and not merely two associated events. We are more likely to believe that Vioxx leads to excess cardiac events if it is clear how the active ingredient in Vioxx creates the heart attack.

Fourth, another point that should be obvious is that causes must precede the effect (in Figure 26.2, the cause node should precede the effect node and the direction of the arrow should be from cause to the effect). One cannot talk of Vioxx causing a cardiac event if the heart attack preceded taking the medication. Nor can one talk of cardiac events causing the taking of Vioxx. Even if aspirin is taken as a preventive measure, still it is the aspirin that is the cause and not the future cardiac events.

Fifth, and perhaps most important, if one claims that an event causes the other, then the counterfactual should also be true. A counterfactual refers to the claim that for individuals that the effect has occurred, the effect would not have happened if the cause was not present. This is perhaps key criterion that separates a causal event from other types of events. For our example, where we claim that Vioxx leads to excess cardiac events we also need to show that for patients who had a heart attack, they would have not had the heart attack if it were not for the Vioxx. Here is a scenario under which a counterfactual does not hold. Suppose that the intervention occurs only among patients who are severely ill. For these patients, removing the cause will not lead to improvements. They are likely to die, anyway. The intervention was a shot in the dark, it could help but it could not make the situation worse. For example, suppose that we give Vioxx to patients who have such severe arthritis pain that they cannot function well. These patients tend to be much older and also at increased risk of cardiac events in any case. If we see excess cardiac events among patients who took Vioxx compared to patients who took an alternative medication, it is now difficult to attribute the excess cardiac events to Vioxx. In fact, in these circumstances, the counterfactual claim is no longer valid. It is not true that if we had not given the medication these patients would not have had the cardiac event. Blaming Vioxx for death of these patients is akin to blaming the fireman for the fire. It blames a treatment of last resort for outcomes that would have occurred anyway. Thus, the verification and testing of counterfactual claims is central to causal risk analysis.

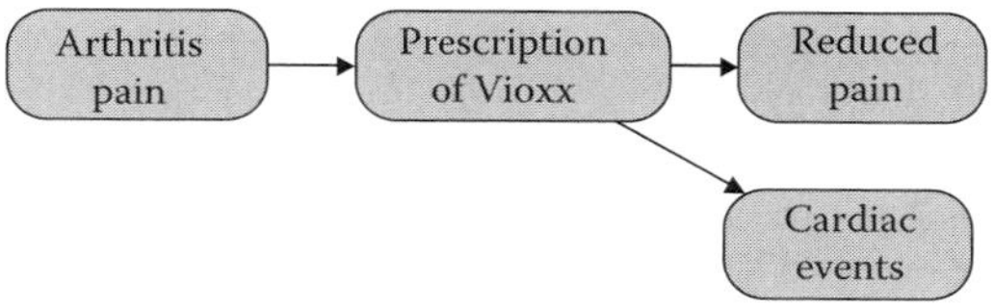

FIGURE 26.3 A causal diagram showing side effects of Vioxx medication.

Modeling Multiple Causes: Causal Diagrams

Most events have multiple causes, and one task of the risk analyst is to sort out which of the many causes is the central reason for the occurrence of the adverse event. At the same time, while one cause is too few, too many causes could make the analysis much more difficult. It is possible to claim that everything has an effect on something else, and in the end—despite several degrees of separation—everything is a cause. This type of thinking is not very helpful. It is important to limit the analysis of causes to events that have a large impact and are under the control of the decision maker. From a practical perspective, a select few causes are likely to explain most of the effect. Being struck by lightning can lead to cardiac events, but the event is so rare as not to be relevant in most causal analysis.

Simple cause–effect relations are known from intuition or can be verified using the five criteria we presented earlier, but more complex situations require modeling to track the many interactions among the causes of various events. There are three ways to do so: causal diagram, probabilistic network, and simultaneous equations.

A causal graph shows events as nodes and the cause and effect relationship as a directed link between the nodes. For example, the graph in Figure 26.3 shows that patient's arthritis pain leads to the prescription of Vioxx, which in turn leads to both reduced pain and the side effect of excess cardiac events.

In a causal diagram, every arrow specifies a cause and effect relationship. Missing arrows also tell a great deal. The absence of an arrow shows the lack of a direct cause and effect. As we will see in a later section, each missing arrow shows an assumption of conditional independence. For example, in Figure 26.2, there is no direct link between arthritis pain and cardiac events. This suggests that, if it were not for the Vioxx, arthritis pain and cardiac events were independent events.

Modeling Multiple Causes: Probability Networks

A probability network goes a step beyond causal diagrams by assigning a specific probability to each direct cause and by using the calculus of probabilities to measure the impact of a change somewhere in the causal diagram on the entire network of nodes. As before, the nodes represent events, arrows indicate causality (now measured in terms of conditional probabilities), and missing arrows encode conditional independencies between the events. A Bayesian probability network is assumed to be a directed and acyclic graph. By "directed," we mean that any two events that are related to each other have a direction of influence on each other. By "acyclic," we mean that it is not possible to start at any node on the graph and return to the same point by going through other nodes in the analysis. In this sense, Bayesian probability networks cannot model causes that feed into themselves. For example, poor care leads to lower market share (see Figure 26.4). Lower market share leads to lower volume of services, which in turn leads to less practice and thus more poor care.

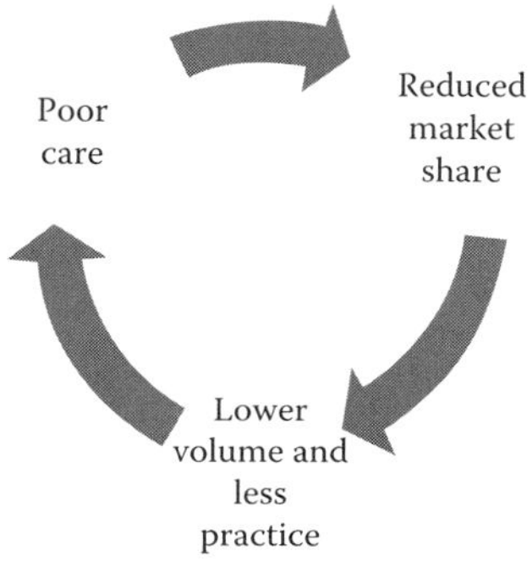

FIGURE 26.4 A possible cyclic causal diagram.

Strictly speaking, probability network are not causal networks unless we restrict the variables listed as causes and consequences.

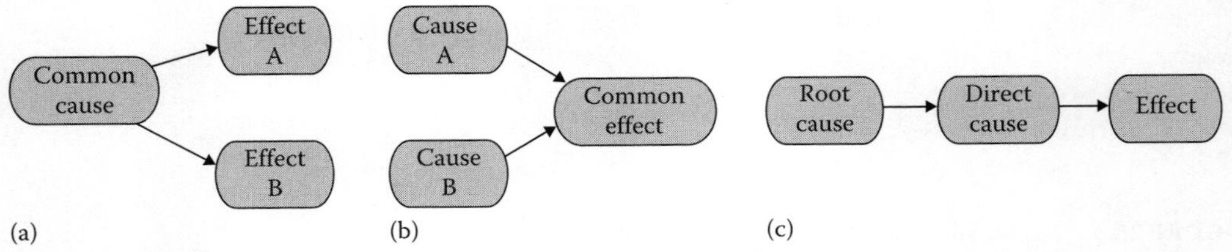

FIGURE 26.5 Possible causal relations among three events. (a) Diverging, (b) converging, and (c) serial.

A key component of probability networks is how multiple causes interact. One way to understand this is to examine three possible ways that three nodes can be represented in a causal relationship. Between any three events, three possible relationships are possible: serial, diverging, or converging structures.

A serial structure (right side of Figure 26.5) identifies the root and the direct cause of the adverse event. Figure 26.3 also contains an example of a serial structure. In this example, the root cause "arthritis pain" is an indirect cause of cardiac events. There is no direct arc from the root cause to the adverse event. This means that the impact of the root cause on the adverse event is indirect, operating through an intermediate cause. That is, the direct cause of cardiac event is the medication Vioxx. If one removes the Vioxx medication, then there is no longer any relationship between arthritis and cardiac events. A serial graph structure can be identified by examining conditional independence. In a serial structure, the root cause (left node) is conditionally independent of the adverse event (right node) given the direct cause (middle node). In Figure 26.3, the serial drawing implies that among patients who received Vioxx, arthritis pain and cardiac events are independent from each other. This assumption can and should be tested in the data to verify that the sequence assumed in the causal model is accurate.

A diverging structure (left side of Figure 26.5) depicts a situation where one cause leads to multiple effects. Whether a common cause is leading to multiple effects can also be detected by examining conditional independence of the effects. As can be expected, effects that have a common cause are correlated and dependent on each other. Furthermore, these effects are conditionally independent of each other given the common cause. Figure 26.3 also shows an example where Vioxx is leading to two effects: the intended reduction of pain and the unintended cardiac event. In this example, reduction of pain and cardiac events are independent from each other among patients who took Vioxx.

Finally, middle of Figure 26.5 shows a diverging causal structure. In these structures, two causes lead to the same effect. In a diverging or common effect, the causes are independent from each other except when conditioned on the effect. Another and perhaps more intuitive way of saying the same thing is that when the effect has been observed and we know that one cause is not present, then probability that the alternative cause is present is increased. Figure 26.6 gives an example where patients are assumed to die through two separate and independent causes: severity of cardiac illnesses and severity of other diseases (e.g., cancer). If we know that the patient has died and we know that there was no cardiac event, then we would think it very likely that the patient has died from the other cause, i.e., from other diseases such as cancer. Likewise, if we know that the patient has cancer and the patient has died, then it is likely that the patient did not die from cardiac events.

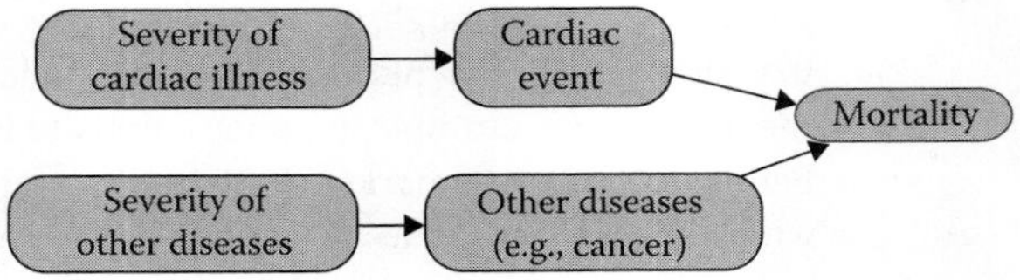

FIGURE 26.6 Two different causes of mortality.

Once a causal probability network has been constructed, it can be used to predict the occurrences of the adverse event. The way causal networks simplify the calculation of probability of an event is through the use of conditional independence among the events. The probability of the adverse events is assumed to be a function of its direct causes and nothing else. In this fashion, the probability of each node can be written as a function of few causes. The probability of the adverse event, S, can be predicted from the presence of various causes. Even if a cause has not yet occurred but has a chance of occurring (unobserved causes), this information can be used in the predictions. The probability of the adverse event given a set of different unobserved (C_U) and observed causes (C_i) can be calculated using the following formula:

$$P(S \mid C_1, C_2, \ldots, C_n) = \sum_{C_U} P(S \mid C_1, C_2, \ldots, C_n) P(C_{U1}) P(C_{U2}) \ldots P(C_{UN})$$

In this fashion, a large complicated causal diagram could be easily distilled into a set of probabilistic relationships, which can then be used to estimate the probability of the adverse event.

Modeling Multiple Causes: Simultaneous Equations

A third approach to causal analysis is to use simultaneous equations. In this approach, the effect is the dependent variable in the equation and the direct causes are the independent variables. For each node, a different equation is written showing the relationship of the events that directly lead to it. For example, we may start with the adverse event and write an equation that predicts the adverse event from its direct causes. Then, an equation is written to predict the direct causes of the adverse event from events that lead to these causes. The process is continued until every node (except nodes without a direct cause) has an associated equation. Simultaneous solutions of these equations allow one to predict how changes in one event affect the frequency of the adverse event.

Figure 26.7 shows a causal diagram for how Vioxx leads to excess cardiac events. Figure 26.7 assumes that patients who have arthritis pain are prescribed Vioxx, in order to reduce their pain. Some patients develop cardiac events. These patients may also have cardiac events because of their underlying unrelated illness (shown as a direct link between patient's severity of cardiac illness and occurrence of cardiac events). In Figure 26.7, cardiac events are assumed to cause mortality. In addition, mortality may be caused by other noncardiac events (e.g., cancer). Given the structure of Figure 26.7, a number of equations can be written.

We start with equations relevant for predicting mortality (note that in all of the following equations the English letters correspond to the letters within Figure 26.7 and all of the Greek letters correspond to constants that can be estimated from the data):

$$M = \alpha + \beta C + \gamma O$$

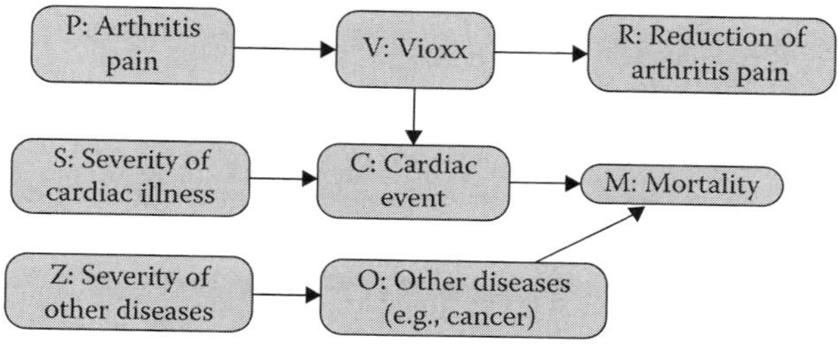

FIGURE 26.7 A model of relationship between Vioxx and cardiac events.

This equation says that mortality is a function of patients with cardiac, C, and other, O, diseases. Next, we write the equations for predicting cardiac events:

$$C = \delta + \varepsilon V + \theta S$$

This equation states that cardiac events are a function of the patient's severity of cardiac illness and the use of Vioxx. This is the core relationship of interest. The equation, in essence, shows what percent of cardiac events can be attributed to the use of Vioxx. Next, we write the equations for frequency of observing other disease:

$$O = \vartheta + \mu Z$$

This equation states what might be obvious, that frequency of other diseases is a function of severity of other illnesses in the patient. Finally, an equation links the use of Vioxx to the level of pain among patients with arthritis:

$$V = \pi + \rho P$$

Simultaneous solution of the above five equations allows one to detect whether Vioxx has led to excess mortality.

Causal versus Noncausal Analysis

Causal risk analysis starts with a hypothesized model of the relationships anticipated in the data. For the study of Vioxx this is Figure 26.7. Within this model, we want to estimate how much of excess mortality can be attributed to the use of Vioxx. The first step is to verify that the causal relationships depicted in the model meet the criteria discussed earlier (i.e., causes must change over time, there should be association between cause and effect, causes must precede effects, and the counterfactual statements should be true). All of these conditions are easily verified except the counterfactual claim. To verify the counterfactual claim, we need to show that patients who had a cardiac event would not have had the event if it were not for the Vioxx. We can predict what might have happened to these patients by examining the severity of their illness. This is simply the situation in Figure 26.6. The predictions of what might have happened is done through the analysis of simultaneous equations described in the previous section (through use of path analysis) or through use of Bayesian probability networks.

What was actually done in the study by Graham and colleagues was different. They classified patients in 10 cardiac risk categories through the use of patients' diagnoses, previous medication use, and unexplained mortality. They then conducted a matched case study where patients within the same cardiac risk category were compared to each other based on whether the patient used Vioxx or alternative medications. The study showed that Vioxx led to increased risk of cardiac events compared to the alternative medication.

The two approaches may lead to different conclusions. One reason for the difference is that the causal analysis takes into account risk not related to cardiac events. It does so because elderly patients (most of the patients who received high-dose Vioxx were elderly) present with multiple illnesses. Ignoring mortality through other causes besides cardiac risks would ignore a major risk factor for mortality among these patients. Information about patients' mortality from other diseases changes the probability that Vioxx caused the cardiac events (in the context of earlier discussion this is a converging structure with two causes of a common effect).

The accuracy of both the causal and the Graham and colleague's approach relies on the ability to predict cardiac events from patient's severity of illness. Unfortunately, Graham and colleagues do not publish the accuracy of their severity index. They do mention that the highest and the lowest severity scores differed by 12-fold. But this does not tell us what percentage of variance in cardiac events are explained by the severity index. In previous studies of myocardial infarction, several commercial severity indices did not correctly predict more than 76% of cases (Alemi et al. 1990). Since in severity-adjusted outcome studies, the adverse outcomes not explained by the patient's severity is attributed to quality of care, this suggests that 24% of cases may have received poor care. This is an unreasonably high percentage that is not supported by medical record reviews. Therefore, the existing severity indices may not have been sufficiently accurate to correctly test for the counterfactual claim.

This issue has been settled through a number of experimental studies. The study by Graham and colleagues was based on observational data, from which it is difficult to make causal inferences. The procedure described here was intended to improve the methods of Graham and colleagues. In particular, we hope that, in the future, investigators will use causal risk analysis to make more informed decisions from observational data.

Like the Vioxx study, risk analysis, in general, can benefit from use of causal models. The analyst and the policymakers make causal interpretation of the risk analysis whether causal assumptions are explicitly discussed in the report. Since these studies are interpreted in causal terms, it is important to use causal methods for risk analysis.

References

Alemi, F. 2007. Probabilistic risk analysis is practical. *Qual. Manag. Health Care* October–December; 16(4):300–310.

Alemi, F., J. Rice, and R. Hankins. 1990. Predicting in-hospital survival of myocardial infarction. A comparative study of various severity measures. *Med. Care* September;28(9):762–775.

Bell, T. E. and K. Esch. 1989. The space shuttle: A case study of subjective engineering. *IEEE Spectr.* June;42–46.

Bombardier, C., L. Laine, A. Reicin, D. Shapiro, R. Burgos-Vargas, B. Davis, R. Day, M. B. Ferraz, C. J. Hawkey, M. C. Hochberg, T. K. Kvien, and T. J. Schnitzer; VIGOR Study Group. 2000. Comparison of upper gastrointestinal toxicity of rofecoxib and naproxen in patients with rheumatoid arthritis. VIGOR Study Group. *N. Engl. J. Med.* November;343(21):1520–1528, 2 page following 1528.

Bresalier, R. S., R. S. Sandler, H. Quan, J. A. Bolognese, M. Stat, K. Horgan, C. Lines, R. Riddell, D. Morton, A. Lanas, M. A. Konstam, and J. A. Baron. 2005. Cardiovascular events associated with rofecoxib in a colorectal adenoma chemoprevention trial. *N. Engl. J. Med.* 352(11):1092–1102.

Chang, S. E., M. Shinozuka, and J. E. Moore. 2000. Probabilistic earthquake scenarios: Extending risk analysis methodologies to spatially distributed systems. *Earthq. Spectr.* 16(3):557–572.

Cohen, B. L. 2003. Probabilistic risk analysis for a high-level radioactive waste repository. *Risk Anal.* October;23(5):909–915.

Colglazier, E. W. and R. K. Weatherwax. 1986. Failure estimates for the space shuttle. In: Abstracts for Society for Risk Analysis Annual Meeting, November 9–12, 1986, Boston MA, p. 80.

Cooke, R. and E. Jager. 1998. A probabilistic model for the failure frequency of underground gas pipelines. *Risk Anal.* August;18(4):511–527.

Cox, L. A. 2001. *Risk Analysis: Foundations, Models and Methods. Series: International Series in Operations Research & Management Science.* Boston, MA: Kluwer.

Environmental Protection Agency. 1976. Reactor safety study oversight hearings before the subcommittee on energy and the environment of the committee on interior and insular affairs. In *House of Representatives, 94th Congress*, 2nd Session, Serial No. 84-61, Washington DC, June 11.

Ewing, R. C., C. S. Palenik, and L. F. Konikow. 2004. Comment on "Probabilistic risk analysis for a high-level radioactive waste repository" by B. L. Cohen in *Risk Analysis*, volume 23, 909–915. *Risk Anal.* December;24(6):1417–1419.

Garrick, B. J. and S. Kaplan. 1999. A decision theory perspective on the disposal of high-level radioactive waste. *Risk Anal.* October;19(5):903–913.

Graham, D. J., D. Campen, R. Hui, M. Spence, C. Cheetham, G. Levy, S. Shoor, and W. A. Ray. 2005. Risk of acute myocardial infarction and sudden cardiac death in patients treated with cyclo-oxygenase 2 selective and non-selective non-steroidal anti-inflammatory drugs: Nested case-control study. *Lancet* February 5–11;365(9458):475–481.

Hoffman, C. R., R. Pugh, and F. M. Safie. 1998. Methods and techniques for risk prediction of space shuttle upgrades. In *AIAA Conference*, April 20–23, 1998, Long Beach, CA.

Hover, C. and L. O'Donnel. 2007. Causes of medication error. *Qual. Manag. Health Care* 16(4): 349–353.

Kaczmarek, Z. 2003. The impact of climate variability on flood risk in Poland. *Risk Anal.* June; 23(3):559–566.

Kaplan, S. and B. Garrick. 1981. On the quantitative definition of risk. *Risk Anal.* 1:11–27.

Kemeny, J. 1979. Report of the President's Commission on the Accident at Three Mile Island, Washington, DC.

Mai, S. and C. Zimmermann. 2003. Risk analysis-tool for integrated coastal planning. In *Proc. of the 6th Int. Conf. on Coastal and Port Engineering*, Colombo, Srilanka.

Marx, D. A. and A. D. Slonim. 2003. Assessing patient safety risk before the injury occurs: An introduction to sociotechnical probabilistic risk modelling in health care. *Qual. Saf. Health Care* December;12(Suppl 2):ii33–ii38.

Moore, D. R. J., B. E. Sample, G. W. Suter, B. R. Parkhurst, and T. R. Scott. 1999. A probablistic risk assessment of the effects of methylmercury and PCBs on mink and Kingfishers along East Fork Poplar Creek, Oak Ridge, Tennessee, USA. *Environ. Toxicol. Chem.* 18(12):2941–2953.

Morabia, A. 2005. Epidemiological causality. *Hist. Philos. Life Sci.* 27(3–4):365–379.

Pate-Cornell, M. E. and P. S. Fischbeck. 1994. Risk management for tiles of the space shuttle. *Interfaces* 24(1):64–86.

Pearl, J. 1986. Fusion, propagation, and structuring in belief networks. *Artif. Intell.* 29(3):241–288.

Pearl, J. 1988. *Probabilistic Reasoning in Intelligent Systems*. San Mateo, CA: Morgan Kaufmann.

Pearl, J. 2000. *Causality: Models of Reasoning and Inference*. Cambridge, U.K.: Cambridge University Press.

Planning Research Corporation. 1989. Independent assessment of shuttle accident scenario probabilities for Galileo mission and comparison with NSTS program assessment.

Rebane, G. and J. Pearl. 1987. The recovery of causal poly-trees from statistical data. In *Proceedings, 3rd Workshop on Uncertainty in AI*, Seattle, WA, pp. 222–228.

Reuters 2006. Merck sees slightly higher 2007 earnings. *New York Times*, p. A1. December 7, 2006. http://www.nytimes.com/2006/12/07/business/07drug.html?ex=1323147600&en=19d27b5814f1c1e8&ei=5088&partner=rssnyt&emc=rss

Rogovin, M. and G. T. Frampton. 1980. Three Mile Island, a Report to the Commissioners and to the Public, Government Printing Office, Washington, DC.

Sadiq, R., T. Husain, B. Veitch, and N. Bose. 2003. Distribution of arsenic and copper in sediment pore water: An ecological risk assessment case study for offshore drilling waste discharges. *Risk Anal.* December;23(6):1309–1321.

Science Applications International Corporation. 1995. *Probabilistic Risk Assessment of the Space Shuttle*. Washington, DC: Center for Aerospace Information.

Slob, W. and M. N. Pieters. 1998. A probabilistic approach for deriving acceptable human intake limits and human health risks from toxicological studies: General framework. *Risk Anal.* December;18(6):787–798.

Sloman, S. 2005. *Causal Models: How People Think about the World and Its Alternatives*. Oxford, U.K.: Oxford University Press.

Song, L. 2007. Tutorial on analysis of causes of falls within an assisted living setting. *Qual. Manag. Health Care* 16(4): 349–353.

Susser, M. 1991. What is a cause and how do we know one? A grammar for pragmatic epidemiology. *Am. J. Epidemiol.* April 1;133(7):635–648.

Taylor, C., A. Krings, and J. Alves-Foss. 2002. Risk analysis and probabilistic survivability assessment (RAPSA): An assessment approach for power substation hardening. In *Proc. ACM Workshop on Scientific Aspects of Cyber Terrorism*, Washington, DC.

Union of Concerned Scientists. 1977. *The Risk of Nuclear Power Reactors: A Review of the NRC Reactor Study*, WASH-1400. Cambridge, MA: Union of Concerned Scientists.

Voortman, H. G., P. van Gelder, and J. K. Vrijlin. 2002. Risk-based design of large-scale flood defense systems. In *28th International Conference on Coastal Engineering*, Cardiff, Wales.

Wreathall, J. and C. Nemeth. 2004. Assessing risk: The role of probabilistic risk assessment (PRA) in patient safety improvement. *Qual. Saf. Health Care* June; 13(3):206–212.

Wright, S. 1921. Correlation and Causation. *J. Agri. Res.* 20(7):557–585. http://www.ssc.wisc.edu/soc/class/soc952/Wright/Wright_Correlation%20and%20Causation.pdf

Yang, L. and Y. Kitsantas. 2007. Monitoring causes of infant mortality. *Qual. Manag. Health Care* 16(4): 349–353.

[illegible]er, M. 1997. [illegible] A grammar of planning [illegible] [illegible].

[illegible], L. [illegible] Kurtz, and [illegible]. [illegible] Methods and procedures [illegible] (KAPSA). [illegible] assessment [illegible] Washington, DC.

United [illegible] Nuclear Regulatory [illegible]. 1975. Reactor Safety Study. WASH-1400. [illegible]

Voortman, H. G., van Gelder, and J. K. Vrijling. 2002. Risk-based design of large-scale flood defence systems. In 28th International Conference on Coastal Engineering, Cardiff, Wales.

Wilhelmi, [illegible] and [illegible]. 2004. [illegible] The role of [illegible] risk assessment [illegible] intervention. [illegible]

Wright, S. 1921. Correlation and Causation. J. Agric. Res. 20: [illegible] Wright [illegible]

Yang, [illegible] and [illegible]. [illegible] [illegible] 159.

IV

Design, Planning, Control, and Management of Healthcare Systems

IV.A Preventive Care

27 **Vaccine Production** *Karen M. Polizzi and Cleo Kontoravdi* **27**-1
Introduction • Overview of Production Systems • Cell Culture–Derived Vaccines • Product Purification • References

28 **Economic Implications of Preventive Care** *George H. Avery, Kara E. Leonard, and Steve P. McKenzie* **28**-1
Introduction • Examples of the Economic Implications of Prevention • Discussion • References

27

Vaccine Production

Introduction 27-1
Market Overview and Applications • Vaccine Evolution • Types of Vaccines
Overview of Production Systems 27-5
Production in Eggs • Production in Plants • Production in Non-Plant Cells
Cell Culture–Derived Vaccines 27-7
Host Systems and Current Applications • Plant Cells • Bacterial Cells • Yeast Cells • Insect Cells • Mammalian Cells • Reverse Genetics
Product Purification 27-13
Overview of Purification Process • Quality Control • Methods for Assessing Product Quality • Planning and Scheduling
References 27-15

Karen M. Polizzi
Imperial College London

Cleo Kontoravdi
Imperial College London

Introduction

Vaccines are biological preparations that improve an organism's immunity to a particular disease. They can be prophylactic, such as influenza vaccines or Cervarix®, which is currently administered to girls aged 12–13 in the United Kingdom to prevent cervical cancer due to infection with the human papilloma virus (HPV). Alternatively, vaccines can be therapeutic, such as BiovaxID™, which is in clinical trials for prolonging disease-free survival in follicular non-Hodgkin's lymphoma. Vaccines contain an agent that acts by stimulating the immune system to recognize this agent as a foreign entity. The immune system is then better prepared to recognize this agent and destroy it if the organism is infected with it in the future.

Market Overview and Applications

The rate of development of vaccines has significantly accelerated, bringing with it improvements in manufacturing techniques that will enable further expansion. In the past 25 years, the rate of development of new vaccines has increased from one every 5 years to approximately one every year (Ulmer et al. 2006). According to a report published in 2007, the global vaccine market is expected to reach $23.8 billion by 2012 (Mitchell 2007). The list of top selling vaccines currently includes many against influenza, for children and adults, and some against MMR and hepatitis (Business Insights 2005). The key manufacturers are Wyeth, Merck & Co., Sanofi-Aventis, Chiron, and GSK. Pediatric vaccines such as for measles, mumps, and rubella (MMR), meningitis, and polio, have so far dominated the market, but adult vaccines are expected to gain an increased market share (Business Insights 2005). Specifically, vaccines for influenza, hepatitis, and sexually transmitted diseases are projected to drive growth in the future.

Influenza vaccines have been available for over 50 years, but have received increased interest since 2000 due to the outbreaks of highly pathogenic strains of avian flu (H5N1) and swine flu (H1N1), which was declared a pandemic by the WHO in June 2009. Because the flu virus is changing its antigenic shape constantly, the composition of the flu vaccine needs to be adapted to these changes regularly. The Global Influenza Surveillance Network of the WHO monitors these changes and makes recommendations for the strains to be included into the vaccine for the coming influenza season.

Cancer vaccines are also predicted to become a major player in the vaccine market, attracting revenues of more than $8 billion by 2012 (Kalorama Information 2007). They offer an attractive option for cancer prevention or the therapy of cancer patients thanks to their ability to deliver treatment of high specificity, low toxicity, and prolonged activity. Some cancers are caused by viruses and can thus be prevented by appropriate vaccines, such as the HPV, which is known to cause cervical cancer. In 2006, Merck received Food and Drug Administration (FDA) approval for the first prophylactic vaccine against the HPV, while other prophylactic and therapeutic HPV vaccines are currently in clinical trials. Ongoing research to identify biomarkers of cancer that will elicit an immune response will aid in the development of vaccines that are able to help the body eliminate cancerous cells (Offringa et al. 2000). Patient-specific (autologous) and generic (allogenic) whole-cell cancer vaccines represent another strategy that has shown success in early clinical trials (Copier et al. 2007). Finally, research in DNA vaccines, an alternative to conventional vaccines, is hoped to provide a breakthrough for diseases such as malaria and HIV, for which no efficacious vaccines currently exist.

Vaccine Evolution

Edward Jenner used the fluid obtained from blisters from those infected with cowpox virus to successfully protect individuals from subsequent infection with smallpox in the 1790s. This is widely considered the first use of vaccination (the name is derived from the Latin for cow, "vacca"), although there is evidence of an ancient Chinese practice of intentionally inflicting smallpox on oneself in order to avoid severe disease, which began as early as 200 BC and was introduced to Europe in the early eighteenth century. The first burst of active research into vaccines as a prophylactic device, however, was not until the end of the nineteenth/beginning of the twentieth centuries with the development of vaccines for cholera, tetanus, and rabies by Louis Pasteur in the 1879–1880s, followed by vaccines for typhoid fever, plague, and a host of other infectious diseases by the end of the first part of the twentieth century. Demonstrable production of viral propagation in chicken eggs was first demonstrated in 1931 and became adopted for the production of vaccines for influenza, measles, mumps, and rubella (Hilleman 2000). Many of these early vaccines were redeveloped or underwent further refinements as time went on in order to improve their safety or efficacy.

The exact composition and purity of early vaccines were often poorly understood. Certainly, in the course of vaccination with material from cowpox blisters, other pathogenic organisms, most notably the causative agent of syphilis, were also transmitted. However, in some sense, the high degree of morbidity and mortality from infectious diseases mitigated the risks of vaccination. On the other hand, in the modern era, at least in developed countries, the majority of those vaccinated in mass campaigns would not encounter the disease over their lifetime. Thus, there is considerable pressure from the public to develop vaccines that are side effect free (Stern and Markel 2005). Unfortunately, even after the advent of modern microbiological techniques, our understanding of the molecular components of whole cell vaccines is still not complete (Spier 1992). However, current regulations on vaccine manufacturing do ensure a high degree of purity, uniformity, and safety in modern vaccines (Buckland 2005). Additionally, the shift toward cell culture production systems, recombinantly produced subunit vaccines, and chemically synthesized agents will lead to further improvements in these areas (Spier 1990).

Types of Vaccines

There are a wide variety of types of vaccines which can be broadly characterized into three groups: (1) whole organism vaccines, including live, attenuated/inactivated strains, and recombinant organisms;

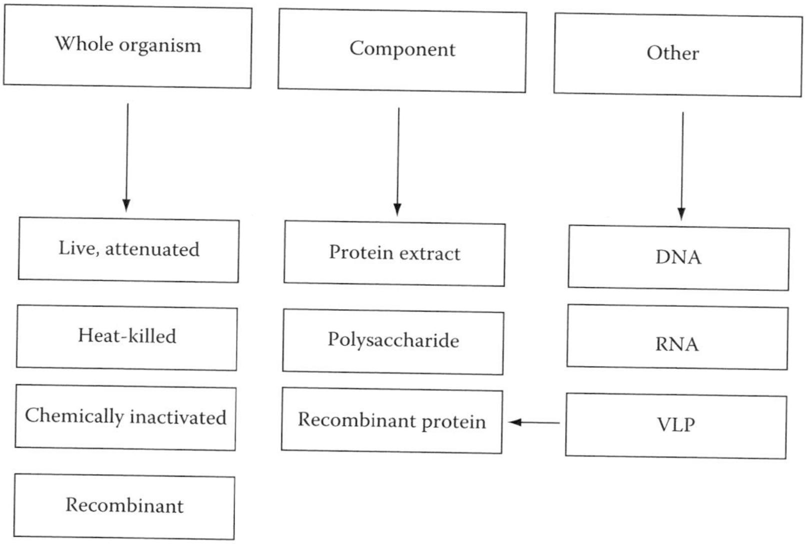

FIGURE 27.1 Types of vaccines.

(2) component vaccines consisting of one or several antigens from the organism being vaccinated against; and (3) other vaccines containing nontraditional components such as DNA, RNA, or nanoparticles (Figure 27.1).

Whole Organism Vaccines

The first successful instances of vaccination were achieved through the use of whole organism vaccines. For example, the active agent in the pustular fluid Edward Jenner used to confer immunity to smallpox was the antigenically similar, but non-infectious, cowpox virus (although Jenner did not realize this, since the germ theory of disease was still nearly a century away). Other well-known whole organism vaccines include the Salk and Sabin polio vaccines and the combined MMR childhood vaccine. Whole organism vaccines efficiently generate immunity because they are very similar to the pathogenic organism itself and contain the same molecular patterns which are recognized by various parts of the immune system. Live, attenuated vaccines have the added benefit that they mimic the invasion of the host in that same manner that the pathogenic strain would (Ulmer et al. 2006). For example, live, attenuated influenza vaccines that are currently licensed in the Russian Federation and the United States appear to be safe and efficacious and may possibly induce a broader and more long-lasting protection than do inactivated vaccines (WHO 2005).

In order to prevent whole organism vaccines from causing the disease that they are designed to prevent, they must be impaired in some way. This can consist of inactivating the virus or bacterium using a chemical agent such as formalin or by the application of heat, or genetically modifying the organism to create an auxotrophy that impairs its ability to replicate in the host (Detmer and Glenting 2006). For example, an oral vaccine consisting of live, attenuated *Vibrio cholerae*, Orochol Berna®, is licensed for vaccination against cholera in several countries, although it is not currently being produced (Hill et al. 2006). The strain of *V. cholerae* used in this vaccine has been modified in two ways. First, the gene for the production of the cholera toxin subunit A, the portion which causes disease symptoms, has been deleted. Second, this strain also has a resistance marker inserted into the hemolysin gene that diminishes its ability to multiply in the intestinal tract, preventing colonization (Levine et al. 1988). These mechanisms ensure that the strain cannot accidentally reactivate to produce the harmful toxin and limiting its ability to spread in the host and among the general population.

More recently, recombinant organisms have been created that produce the antigens of a disease-causing agent in a relatively harmless organism. These recombinant bacterial vaccines often employ organisms that are generally recognized as safe (GRAS), such as strains of lactic acid bacteria expressing the antigen of a disease-causing pathogen. Since lactic acid bacteria are widely used as probiotics, an added advantage to their use in vaccine production is that they can be administered orally and naturally survive the journey through the stomach to the intestinal mucosa. On the other hand, since the bacteria do not invade the intestinal cells, generating high levels of immunity can be problematic and often requires a prohibitively large dose of the organism (Detmer and Glenting 2006). This field is currently under development, but initial animal trials show promise. In one example, *Lactobacillus acidophilus* expressing the *Bacillus anthracis* protective antigen was used to induce immunity to anthrax in mice by targeting dendritic cells in the intestine via a protein fusion. Upon subsequent challenge with the Sterne strain of *B. anthracis*, survival rates in mice given the oral *L. acidophilus* vaccine were comparable to those given a subcutaneous injection of a recombinant anthrax vaccine (75% versus 80%) (Mohamadzadeh et al. 2009).

Component Vaccines

Component vaccines are composed of one or more antigen-stimulating compounds such as proteins, peptides, or polysaccharides which are the part of the pathogen that elicits the immune response. The antigens can either be from the pathogen itself (secreted toxins or extracts of killed organism) or produced recombinantly by another organism. Component vaccines can be produced very efficiently on a large scale using bioreactors, and because they do not contain cells, they often have reduced chance of inducing an allergic reaction. If there are multiple serotypes of an organism, a component vaccine can easily be adjusted to include broad coverage of the different groups. However, there can be difficulties with the production of components in the correct antigenic conformation, particularly with recombinant protein vaccines, and the purification and downstream processing of the component vaccines is sometimes very complex. Also, clearly, in order to produce an effective component vaccine, the antigen that elicits the immune response must be known and relatively well characterized (Ulmer et al. 2006).

Most of the commercially available component vaccines are produced directly from the pathogenic organism. For example, the combined vaccine for diphtheria, tetanus, and pertussis (DPT or DTP), routinely administered during childhood vaccination protocols, usually consists of inactivated toxins harvested from *Corynebacterium diphtheriae* and *Clostridium tetani* grown in bioreactors as well as four purified toxins from *Bordetella pertussis* (Bae et al. 2009). However, an increasing amount of research into the use of cell culture to produce recombinant component vaccines suggests a future shift toward this technology because of its increased safety (no involvement of pathogenic organisms) and efficiency (quickly growing hosts can be chosen and their growth and production optimized). For example, some have capitalized on the benefits of the yeast *Saccharomyces cerevisiae* as a host strain to produce several recombinant antigens including hepatitis antigens and anthrax toxin (Inamura et al. 1986, Dehoux et al. 1986, Hepler et al. 2006). Because yeast is easy to culture, multiplies rapidly, and contains very few endogenous proteins with immunogenic potential, it represents an ideal system for the production of protein subunit vaccines. In the anthrax example, the recombinant antigen that was produced was shown to elicit a protective response in both rabbits and rhesus monkeys, highlighting the promise of such an approach (Hepler et al. 2006).

Other Types of Vaccines

A third class of vaccines encompasses other, less traditional formulations. Of these, spontaneously self-assembling nanoparticles produced from recombinant viral capsid proteins have seen the most applications in the commercial market. These virus-like particles (VLP) often mimic all or part of the naturally occurring virus which opens up applications as a form of purified subunit vaccine. Often the immunogenic response of a VLP is stronger than vaccines made from individual protein subunits because of the spatial presentation of the antigens. Examples include some early Hepatitis B vaccines (Grgacic and

Anderson 2006) and, more recently, the anti-cervical cancer vaccines such as Gardasil®, which form VLPs of mixed antigens from four serotypes of HPV (McLemore 2006). VLPs can also be used as a delivery system for other antigens, including nucleic acids (Grgacic and Anderson 2006).

Vaccines based on purified nucleic acids, DNA and RNA, can be used to elicit an immune response in a process that mimics some types of viral infection. DNA-based vaccines can be introduced into the cell as a plasmid that contains the gene coding for one or more antigens. The host cell then expresses the antigen itself, as it would following viral infection, via transcription of mRNA and translation to protein. The antigen is then displayed for the immune system and cellular immunity is developed. In particular, strong reactions from the cytotoxic T-cell-mediated immunity can be elicited. DNA-based vaccines are very simple to manufacture on a large scale, afford easy downstream processing, are stable during storage, and developing vaccines for different diseases is simply a matter of changing the gene for the antigen. Thus, DNA-based vaccines are a very promising area of future research (Shirmbeck et al. 2001). RNA-based vaccines behave similarly, but deliver mRNA to the cytoplasm of cells where it is translated directly. The amount of antigen produced depends in part on the stability of the mRNA construct, which is often a limiting factor. RNA-based vaccines that are capable of self-replication have also been developed, aimed at prolonging the response (Cannon and Weismann 2002).

Overview of Production Systems

A variety of systems can be used for vaccine production, ranging from chicken eggs to plants and cultures of prokaryotic and eukaryotic cells. A summary of the available production methods and examples of their applications is shown in Table 27.1. This section will review each of these methods, their advantages, and challenges.

Production in Eggs

Traditionally, vaccines, such as for MMR and influenza, are produced in fertilized chicken eggs in a process that lasts approximately 6 months. Fertilization is followed by injection of the virus into the eggs, which accumulates in the fluid surrounding the embryo. The embryo becomes infected so that the virus can multiply. After several days of incubation, the eggs are opened and the virus is harvested. On average, one to two eggs yield one dose of vaccine.

Egg-based production of flu vaccines is well established and cost-effective. However, it presents a number of drawbacks. Specifically, in terms of vaccine supply, there is a lack of year-round availability of high-quality eggs or on-the-spot accessibility in the case of high demand due to a pandemic. The supply of healthy chicken eggs could further be reduced or diminish in the case of a bird flu pandemic. Moreover, the presence of adventitious agents in eggs can jeopardize the quality and safety of the produced vaccine.

A further disadvantage of the egg-based method specifically for the production of influenza vaccines is the low susceptibility of summer eggs to influenza virus infection (Monto et al. 1981), which poses a limit to year-round production. In addition, there is evidence that human influenza viruses isolated and passed on chick embryos may lose one of the antigenic hemagglutinin domains (Schild et al. 1983, Katz et al. 1987, Robertson 1993), which is not observed in the isolation and passage of human influenza viruses on mammalian cells (Katz et al. 1990, Robertson et al. 1990).

Production in Plants

Plant-made vaccines are one of the alternative vaccine production methods that are currently being evaluated. It offers the significant advantage of involving no animal components and thus overcomes the risk of contamination with mammalian pathogens. Two options are currently being investigated: vaccine production from plant cell culture and from whole plants. Both methods involve the transformation

TABLE 27.1 Summary of Vaccine Production Methods and Examples of Application

Production Method	Cell Line/Type	Examples of Application
Chicken eggs	N/A	Influenza, MMR
Whole plant	Tobacco	Hepatitis B surface antigen (Mason et al. 1992)
		Cholera toxin B subunit (Daniell et al. 2001)
Plant cell culture	*Nicotiana tabacum*-1	Hepatitis B surface antigen (Kumar et al. 2007)
		Staphylococcus Enterotoxin B (Hefferon and Fan 2004)
Whole bacterial cells	*Salmonella typhi*	Typhoid vaccine (Berna Biotech; Levine et al. 2007)
	Vibrio cholerae O1	Cholera vaccine (Leyten et al. 2005)
Bacterial cell culture	*Escherichia coli*	*Schistosomiasis japonica* (Solomon et al. 2004)
		Merozoite surface protein 1 for malaria (Epp et al. 2003)
		Cysteine–Cysteine type chemokine receptor 5 for HIV (Wu et al. 2006)
Yeast cell culture	*Pichia pastoris*	P30P2MSP1_{19} for malaria (Brady et al. 2001)
	Saccharomyces cerevisiae	Hepatitis B virus surface antigen (Imamura et al. 1986)
		Hepatitis B virus envelope proteína (Dehoux et al. 1986)
		Bacillus anthracis protective antigen (Hepler et al. 2006)
		Human papilloma virus VLPs (Buckland 2005)
Insect cell culture	*Spodoptera frugiperda*	Influenza H5 (Treanor et al. 2001)
Mammalian cell culture	HEK 293	*Schistosoma japonicum* (Yuan et al. 2007)
		HIV pseudovirion (Devitt et al. 2007)
	MDCK	Influenza H5N1 (Hu et al. 2008)
	MDBK	Bovine parainfluenza 3 (Conceição et al. 2007)
	Vero	Influenza A and B viruses (Govorkova et al. 1996)
		Rabies (Kumar et al. 2005)
	MRC-5	Hepatitis A (Peetermans 1992)
	CHO	Pre S/S hepatitis B virus vaccine (Argentini et al. 2005)
		Receptor-binding domain of SARS coronavirus spike protein (Du et al. 2009)
	Chicken fibroblasts	Rabies (Novartis, www.rabavert.com)
	PER.C6	Influenza virus (Boon 2009)

of the plant or plant cells with the gene(s) encoding an immunogenic protein capable of preventing infection by a pathogenic agent. The vaccines can be made from transient or stable transformation of the plant cells or plant.

A major drawback of whole plant-made vaccines and pharmaceuticals in general is the associated concern about food safety. Specifically, pollen from transgenic plants can cross-contaminate food crops if adequate containment measures are not taken. Such measures, which are essential for obtaining approval from regulatory agencies, would involve geographical isolation, buffer plants, physical containment in glasshouses, isolated harvest, processing and transport of the plants and their products, as well as decontamination of equipment used for the above operations (Rigano and Walmsley 2005). Further suggestions for containment would be to allow for an uncultivated period before production is switched from pharmaceuticals to food crops, and to insert the transgenes into the genome of the chloroplast, which would ensure that the gene would not be present in pollen.

Production in Non-Plant Cells

An alternative way of producing vaccines is based on the culture of bacterial, insect, yeast or mammalian cells. Producing component vaccines by this method is similar to other biotechnological processes used for the supply of recombinant proteins and antibodies. Whole organism viral vaccines can be produced in mammalian cells. The virus is injected into these cells, enabling it to multiply as the cells grow. Once the fermentation process is complete, a series of purification steps follows for the removal of host proteins, DNA material, and other potentially adventitious agents, before the final product formulation is achieved.

An advantage of this method is that the cells can be grown in chemically defined, animal component-free media therefore reducing the risk of impurities such as other viruses, which are present in egg-derived vaccines. This also minimizes the risk of allergic reactions to foreign proteins and simplifies the purification of the product, which reduces to the separation of host proteins and nucleic acid material from the product. Cell cultures offer the possibility of carrying out regular checks for adventitious agents and ensuring that cell stocks and production population are contaminant free. Moreover, the cell-based technology avoids the need to work with potentially pathogenic live viruses, which are necessary when working with eggs, making the production process inherently safer. Finally, cell-based vaccine supply can draw on existing fermentation know-how to rapidly meet demand.

Cell Culture–Derived Vaccines

Host Systems and Current Applications

Various cell types have been reported to be suitable for the production of whole or component vaccines or vaccine candidates. Figure 27.2 depicts their classification into prokaryotic and eukaryotic microorganisms based on their internal structure. Eukaryotes have a membrane-bound compartment, the nucleus, where their DNA is kept, whereas prokaryotes have no distinct compartment for their genetic material. The properties of these cell types and examples of their use for the production of component or whole vaccines will be discussed in this section.

Plant Cells

Plant cells are eukaryotic cells that have certain structural differences from other eukaryotes. For example, they are contained within a cell wall similar to that of bacterial cells, which is mainly composed of cellulose and lignin. Transgenic plants have been used in the form of plant cell cultures, whole plants, and tissue (hairy roots) cultures for the production of proteins such as antibodies, enzymes, and hormones. Examples include the production of avidin (Hood et al. 1997) and b-glucuronidase (Witcher et al. 1998) from whole plants. Whole plant production is believed to be the cheapest alternative; however, plant tissue and plant cell culture are also available as quicker production methods or when containment is essential (Sharp and Doran 2000). Sharp and Doran (1999) have reported one critical issue

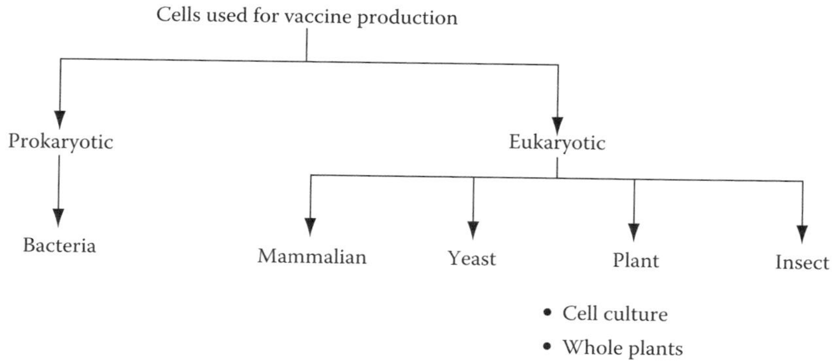

FIGURE 27.2 Classification of cells used for vaccine production.

with plant-based protein production, that of foreign protein degradation. This can reduce the levels of recovered protein and can make its separation from fragments difficult.

Regarding vaccine/vaccine component production from plant cell cultures, *Nicotiana tabacum*-1 cells appear to be the most widely used hosts. Kumar et al. (2007) reported the production of a hepatitis B surface antigen and Hefferon and Fan (2004) described the synthesis of Staphylococcus enterotoxin B both from the culture of *N. tabacum*-1 cells. Concerning whole tobacco plants, these have been used to produce a hepatitis B surface antigen (Mason et al. 1992) and cholera toxin B subunit (Daniell et al. 2001), both candidate vaccine antigens. A significant advantage of this method is that oral administration of such transgenic plant tissues has been shown to induce immune responses (Haq et al. 1995, Arakawa et al. 1998, Richter et al. 2000). It has been suggested that plant cells containing an oral vaccine may, in fact, protect against premature digestion of the antigen (Walmsley and Arntsen 2000). This can simplify vaccine delivery and possibly decrease the cost of immunization.

However, despite these benefits, nuclear transgenes often yield inadequate antigen levels. There are two methods for inducing foreign protein production in plants, via the nuclear genome or the chloroplast genome. Daniell et al. (2001) compared the two methods by evaluating the gene expression of an unmodified B subunit of cholera toxin of *V. cholerae* integrated in chloroplast genomes and that of an unmodified B subunit of enterotoxigenic *Escherichia coli* expressed via the nuclear genome of tobacco plants. They found that the expression levels via chloroplast integration were 410-fold higher than those via the nuclear genome. This therefore shows that large-scale vaccine production via transgenic plants is possible. The same researchers further showed that the foreign proteins were properly expressed and assembled in transgenic chloroplasts, which is an essential prerequisite for their correct in vivo function. Finally, the authors estimated the cost of producing 1 kg of recombinant protein in transgenic plants and found it to be 50 times lower than that of producing the same amount by *E. coli* fermentation as reported in Petridis et al. (1995). Plant cell-based production may therefore be an attractive alternative for vaccine production in the future, which may also offer the potential benefit of oral administration.

Bacterial Cells

Bacterial cells are prokaryotic microorganisms, as shown in Figure 27.2. They belong to a group of unicellular microorganisms, which are enclosed within a tough layer of carbohydrates, the cell wall, which lies around their plasma membrane. Various bacterial cells, such as *E. coli* and *Streptococcus*, are known pathogens responsible for food poisoning, meningitis, and pneumonia. Certain bacterial cell lines, most notably *E. coli*, have been used for many decades for the production of protein drugs such as insulin.

With regards to vaccines, *E. coli* cultures have been reported to be suitable production systems. For example, Solomon et al. (2004) used *E. coli* to produce a *Schistosoma japonicum* surface membrane protein, which was then assessed as a potential vaccine candidate for human schistosomiasis. Epp et al. (2003) used the same host cell system to successfully express the C-terminal 42 kDa portion of a merozoite surface protein 1 of the human malaria parasite *Plasmodium falciparum*, which, after purification, was shown to meet key criteria for clinical use. This protein was put forward as an essential component of a future anti-malaria vaccine. A final example is the production of the *E. coli*-produced recombinant vaccine candidate for HIV infection (Wu et al. 2006). This consists of a T helper epitope coupled to the N-terminus of cysteine–cysteine type chemokine receptor 5 extracellular domains.

An alternative to the expression of vaccines in bacterial cell cultures and subsequent parenteral administration is the use of live bacterial vaccines. Whole bacterial vaccines have been marketed against a multitude of diseases since the beginning of the twentieth century, with vaccines against cholera and the plague based on inactivated bacteria licensed in the United States as early as 1914 and 1911, respectively (Guttormsen and Kasper 2001). Live bacteria can be administered orally or nasally to induce an immune response to themselves or to carry a vaccine component into an organism. This administration method is considered particularly advantageous as it mimics the route of entry of many pathogens and reduces the reliance on the healthcare infrastructure necessary for parenteral administration (Detmer and Glenting 2006), which, although successful with some diseases, is less effective with enteric and respiratory diseases (Rigano and Walmsley 2005).

Both pathogenic and nonpathogenic bacteria, such as food bacteria, can be used; however, the former need to be attenuated to reduce their virulence. The use of bacteria as vehicles of an antigen, a therapeutic protein, or DNA vaccines raises a number of concerns such as the possibility of transfer of undesired genes via the plasmid, spread of antibiotic resistance genes, or formation of anti-DNA antibodies (Detmer and Glenting 2006). Even though the development of bacteria carrying heterologous genes still faces some challenges, live vaccines based on attenuated *S. typhi* and *V. cholera* are currently available.

Yeast Cells

Yeast cell cultures are used to produce subunit vaccines because of their ability to process recombinant proteins in a manner similar to that of the native organism. Yeast cells are eukaryotic microorganisms that belong to the kingdom Fungi. They are employed in the production of recombinant proteins as well as for the production of biofuels. Among the most widely used yeast species are *S. cerevisiae*, also known as Baker's yeast, and *Pichia pastoris*.

With regards to component vaccines, both of these species have been used in experimental studies. Brady et al. (2001) reported the production of $P30P2MSP1_{19}$, a recombinant subunit vaccine derived from merozoite surface protein 1 (MSP1) of the causative agent of malaria, *P. falciparum*, in *P. pastoris* yeast cells. Imamura et al. (1986) reported the production of a surface antigen of the hepatitis B virus and Dehoux et al. (1986) the production of a large envelope protein of the same virus, both in *S. cerevisiae*. There have further been recent studies on the use of heat-killed *S. cerevisiae* cells as vaccines. Specifically, Capilla et al. (2009) have reported evidence that the heat-killed cells induced immunity against *Coccidioides*, a disease endemic in the Americas, in mice. However, the exact mechanism by which immunity is effected remains to be elucidated.

Insect Cells

Insect cells are successfully used for protein production, as they exhibit high specific productivity, have simple cultivation requirements, and have the ability to post-translationally modify the proteins. Commonly used cell lines include SF9, SF21, *Drosophila* Schneider 2 (S2), and High-Five cells, for which there are serum-free media commercially available. Expression systems successfully employed with insect cells include the *Baculovirus* expression system and the InsectSelect stable expression system. The *Drosophila* stable expression system is also used with S2 cells.

An example of the use of insect cells for vaccine production is that of an experimental trivalent influenza virus hemagglutinin (HA; a molecule that sticks out of the surface of the influenza virus) vaccine produced in insect cells using recombinant baculoviruses (Treanor et al. 2007). This was evaluated in a randomized controlled trial, which provided preliminary evidence of protection against influenza infection and disease in adults. This study also concluded that the trial results of this vaccine suggest that in adults, the minor differences in HA glycosylation seen in insect cells compared with mammalian cells do not have a major effect on the actual protection provided by the vaccine.

Recently, the U.S.-based vaccine company Protein Sciences Corporation has been awarded a contract by the U.S. Health department to develop an influenza vaccine against type A(H1N1) flu (swine flu) using their insect cell technology. They report that their vaccine production method is based on infecting caterpillar cells with a baculovirus carrying the gene for HA and propose that this technology is safer than using mammalian cells as there is no possibility for the insect cells to learn how to propagate human viruses. They also suggest that vaccine production from insect cells can be easily and rapidly scaled up because it does not require the same specialized infrastructure or media formulation necessary for mammalian cell cultures (Pollack 2009).

Mammalian Cells

In the case of glycoprotein-based vaccines, suitably modified structures can only be generated by expression in mammalian cells. Their production can be achieved by stable or transient infection/transduction or transfection. Last but not least, the strains grown in cell cultures equal the original clinical isolates, while the growth of epidemic viruses in eggs results in variants that are antigenically distinct from the original viruses. Emerging endemic viruses sometimes do not grow at all in eggs. Virus grown in mammalian cell culture is therefore more representative of the circulating wild type virus than that grown in eggs.

MDCK Cells

The Madin-Darby canine kidney (MDCK) cell line is an adhesive line that has been adapted to grow in synthetic, hormone-supplemented, serum-free media (Taub et al. 1979). It has been used for the production of an inactivated whole-virus H5N1 vaccine (Hu et al. 2008) in a microcarrier culture system. The microcarriers were shown to provide the adhesive cells with adequate support in a 5L system and were being tested in pilot-scale facilities (30 and 150L) to establish this as a viable method for large-scale vaccine production. Recently, it was reported that Novartis obtained approval to manufacture the first influenza vaccine using MDCK cells in 2007 (Boon 2009).

Vero Cells

Vero cells were developed from kidney epithelial cells extracted from an African green monkey in 1962 (Yasumura and Kawakita 1963). Vero cells are susceptible to a broad range of viruses and are widely used to develop vaccines against associated diseases. Studies have shown that Vero cells constitute a suitable system for the isolation and cultivation of influenza A and B viruses (Govorkova et al. 1995, 1996). Continuous Vero cell lines have further been used for the production of the rabies virus PV-11 (Kumar et al. 2005) and for polio virus vaccine production (Litwin 1992). Vero cells are anchorage dependent but can be grown as cell aggregates or in microcarriers in suspension culture and serum-free media (Litwin 1992, Wressnigg et al. 2009).

MDBK Cells

The Madin-Darby bovine kidney (MDBK) line was derived from the renal tissue of an adult steer (*Bos taurus*). They are epithelial-like cells that are used both for vaccine production (Conceição et al. 2007) and for performing antiviral drug studies (Guo et al. 2007). As adherent cells, they can be grown in microcarriers for suspension cultures in spinner flasks or bioreactors, as outlined in Conceição et al. (2007).

HEK-293 Cells

The human embryonic kidney (HEK) 293 cell line was developed from the sheared adenovirus 5 (Ad5) DNA transformation of the human embryonic kidney cell (Graham et al. 1977). HEK293 cells are used for transient transfection (Yuan et al. 2007) and are widely employed in research for vaccine production, adenovirus and adeno-associated viral vectors, and gene therapy. Their extended use in expression experiments stems from their ease of maintenance and high transfection efficiency. HEK293 cells can be grown in adherent mode, but have also been adapted to suspension conditions. The main limitation with the latter is their tendency to aggregate in suspension, which can be overcome with the use of specially designed cell culture media (e.g., ExCell 293® by SAFC Biosciences and FreeStyle 293™ by Invitrogen).

MRC-5 Cells

The human diploid MRC-5 cell line was derived from normal lung tissue of a 14-week-old male fetus (Jacobs et al. 1970). This cell line has been adapted to serum-free conditions and meets the requirements of WHO and National Control Authorities for continuous cell lines suitable for the production of vaccines. It has been reported to be free of extraneous agents, shows normal karyology, and lacks tumorigenicity (Peetermans, 1992). These cells are widely used to study viruses *ex vivo* (e.g., Yamagishi et al. 2008, Falkenhagen et al. 2009) and for vaccine production (e.g., Peetermans 1992, Alirezaie et al. 2008).

CHO Cells

Chinese hamster ovary (CHO) cells (Puck, 1985) are the most widely used cell line for the industrial production of recombinant proteins and monoclonal antibodies. They are the preferred host cell line thanks to their high rate of protein production and their ability to accurately glycosylate these products. CHO cells were originally adherent but have been adapted to grow in suspension and serum-free conditions. More recently, researchers have reported the development of vaccines with CHO cells. For example, Argentini et al. (2005) reported the development and successful testing of a non-adjuvanted vaccine against woodchuck hepatitis virus, while Du et al. (2009) reported the production of a receptor-binding domain of SARS coronavirus spike protein, a candidate subunit SARS vaccine, in CHO-K1 cells.

Avian Fibroblasts

Fibroblast cells of avian origin are regarded as an alternative to egg use for virus isolation and research, which potentially avoids structural changes often seen in egg-based production of influenza vaccine in particular (Lee et al. 2008). Avian cell lines can be of chicken or quail origin and are thought to be the most suitable hosts for the study of avian viruses as they maintain species specificity. Regarding vaccine production, there is currently one licensed product of avian fibroblast cultures, which is a chicken fibroblast–derived vaccine against rabies (RabAvert™, Novartis) produced by Chiron Behring GmbH & Co.

PER.C6 Cells

PER.C6, a human cell line that was originally created for the generation of adenoviral vectors for gene therapy applications, is derived from human embryonic retinoblasts (Fallaux et al. 1998). Developed by Crucell in compliance with Good Laboratory Practice with complete documentation from the beginning (Pau et al. 2001), and licensed by Merck and Sanofi-Aventis, PER.C6 cells have many features that make them ideal for production of purified subunit vaccines as well as a good host for live viral vaccines. Some of the benefits of PER.C6 include a high transfection efficiency, lack of adventitious viruses or retroviruses, high levels of recombinant protein production, and ability to adapt to a wide variety of growth conditions (Jones et al. 2003). The ability of PER.C6 cells to endow proteins with human-like glycosylation patterns could be advantageous in the manufacture of antigen-specific vaccines for tumor cells. In addition, the cells can be grown in serum-free suspension culture to a high density (up to 10^7 cells/mL) without the need for solid support (Pau et al. 2001) and large culture volumes can be easily attained, with 20,000 L scale already achieved (Boon 2009). Currently, PER.C6 cells are being explored for the manufacture of influenza vaccines (Phase II trials, Sanofi-Aventis; Bae et al. 2009).

Mammalian Cell Transfection

There are two options for the transfer of foreign genes into eukaryotic cells: stable or transient transfection. Stable transfection is a methodology that yields cell lines with moderate to high levels of gene expression and is typically used for large-scale production. In this method, the expression vector is inserted into the host cell genome or is maintained as an extrachromosomal element. The former highly depends on the position of the host cell's DNA at which the foreign vector is integrated, while the latter allows the transfection of large pieces of DNA and is independent of position effects. In both cases, a selectable marker on the expression vector needs to be used to ensure that the cells contain the gene of interest.

Transient gene expression (TGE) is a rapid method that is often used to analyze the properties of genes and the expression of recombinant proteins and to produce experimental results or material for analysis in a short time. Under transient transfection, expression of the inserted gene takes place between 12 and 72 hours after DNA transfer, after which there is a rapid deterioration in expression due to cell death or loss of expression plasmid. Early large-scale transient transfections were limited by the relatively short lifespan of the culture. This was overcome, however, by the use of better cell lines, predominantly HEK 293, which lead to the production of large quantities of recombinant proteins. CHO and HEK 293 cells are the major hosts for large-scale TGE as they are readily transfected with low-cost delivery agents such as calcium phosphate (CaPi) and polyethylenimine (PEI).

For regulatory reasons, biologically derived products for therapeutic applications need to be produced in chemically defined, animal component-free conditions. The elimination of additives such as serum reduces the risk of contamination with infectious agents and facilitates the purification of secreted product, which is currently the most costly part of the production process. However, for transient transfections, the absence of serum substantially reduces the efficiency of calcium phosphate-mediated DNA transfer (Jordan et al. 1996), while PEI-mediated transfection is serum-independent (Derouazi et al. 2004, Pham et al. 2005). The extent of product glycosylation has been reported to be comparable under both stable and transient transfection (Muller et al. 2007).

Reverse Genetics

Reverse genetics is a process by which whole viruses can be created from DNA inserted into a host cell. This is analogous to the process of using nucleic acids as a vaccine, but yields the production of an intact virus rather than just display of the viral antigen. The use of reverse genetics to generate influenza vaccines is especially promising as it would allow for tailoring of the viral antigens by changing the sequence of the DNA used in the production process. Thus, changes in response to antigenic variation could be handled more rapidly than with the traditional reassortment process and the possibility of generating novel antigens exists. However, since influenza is a negative (anti)-sense RNA virus, the process is complicated by the need to produce the anti-sense RNA for each of the viral genes, along with the viral proteins necessary to form the intact virus.

Early systems for reverse genetics of negative-sense RNA viruses relied on the use of helper viruses that were cotransfected either with a viral RNA complex that had been synthesized *in vitro* (Palese et al. 1996) or with a plasmid that could be used to generate the viral genes *in vivo* (Neumann et al. 1994). However, these systems were relatively inefficient, as the presence of the helper viruses complicates the process of selecting successful transformants. Later systems replaced the helper viruses with a series of plasmids. Neumann et al. (1999) showed efficient viral production from cells transfected with plasmids for the production of the viral RNA (8) as well as plasmids to produce all of the viral proteins (9). Experiments where only plasmids necessary to produce the viral genes (8) and the viral proteins related to RNA synthesis (4) were transfected into cells did yield viral production, although it was very inefficient (Neumann et al. 1999). In either case, the requirement to transfect 12 or 17 different plasmids into cells made this system somewhat unwieldy experimentally. Thus, there have been significant efforts to streamline the process and reduce the number of plasmids necessary to create intact viruses (Hoffmann et al. 2000, Neumann et al. 2005). The number of necessary plasmids was reduced to eight by using the same plasmid to create the viral RNA and an mRNA transcript, which is used by the host cell to create viral proteins by transcription from two different promoters (Hoffmann et al. 2000). The same system was used to create recombinant viruses that combine the currently circulating viral antigens with the core genes from strains which produce a high viral yield to generate efficient vaccine production without the need to select for successful reassortments (Hoffmann et al. 2002). Finally, recently, the number of plasmids was further reduced by combining multiple genetic elements onto a single plasmid. Some production of intact viruses was achieved by using a single plasmid, but the best system used three plasmids—one to produce all eight viral RNAs and two to produce the necessary viral proteins. Splitting the viral RNAs onto two separate plasmids would allow this system to be adapted for creating viruses without reassortment (Neumann et al. 2005).

Product Purification

Overview of Purification Process

Regardless of the type of vaccine, the first steps in downstream processing are to separate the vaccine from the cell used to produce it and to concentrate it into a small volume before beginning subsequent purification steps. This is usually done by centrifugation and/or filtration (Wolff and Reichl 2008). Additional purification steps depend on the host production system as well as the type of vaccine, but include the traditional unit operations of chromatography, filtration, extraction, and centrifugation. In cases where DNA contamination needs to be reduced, a nuclease digestion step may be applied. A typical flow diagram for vaccine purification can be seen in Figure 27.3.

Purification of Whole-Virus Vaccines

Many whole-virus vaccines including rabies (Kumar et al. 2005) and influenza vaccines from whole eggs and from cell culture (Wolff and Reichl 2008) are traditionally purified using gradient-density centrifugation or zonal ultracentrifugation to isolate the viral pellet. However, size-exclusion chromatography of influenza viruses is a viable alternative to centrifugation because the virus particles tend to aggregate into particles on the order of 100,000 kDa, which is much larger than most host cell biopolymers (except for genomic DNA, which in most studies remains a contaminant) (Wolff and Reichl 2008). Recent work has shown that size-exclusion chromatography to remove small molecules, proteins, and other debris, followed by an anion exchange chromatography step to remove host-cell DNA could be a viable option for purification of virus from cell culture (Kalbfuss et al. 2007). Some studies have applied anion exchange chromatography in the absence of size exclusion treatment, but there appear to be significant behavioral differences between different influenza strains. Therefore, the anion exchange method has to be developed and applied on a case-by-case basis, making it inconvenient for industrial process development (Wolff and Reichl 2008). On the other hand, ion exchange chromatography works well for poliovirus purification. The industrial process to produce inactivated polio vaccine used by GSK employs two ion exchange steps, one anionic and one cationic (van Wezel et al. 1984, Duchêne 2006). Other types of chromatography used in the purification of whole viruses include specific affinity chromatography steps, such as in the case of purification of herpes simplex viral vaccines using heparin-based resin (O'Keeffe et al. 1998).

Split Purification of Egg-Based Viral Vaccines

Inactivated whole viruses from egg-based production are rarely used because of the immunogenic potential of viral lipids. Instead, it is more common to subject them to a process called split purification. In split purification, viruses purified using one of the methods outlined above are subsequently extracted with ether or detergent and the viral proteins are recovered by ultracentrifugation, followed by heat or chemical inactivation (Bae et al. 2009).

Purification of Antigens from Cell Culture

The downstream processing of antigens produced in cell culture for component vaccines is very similar to the purification of proteins for other medical uses, such as antibodies and other therapeutic proteins. If the antigen is associated with the cell (either intracellular or part of the membrane), steps must be taken to extract it, but wherever possible antigens are targeted to be secreted into the culture medium to

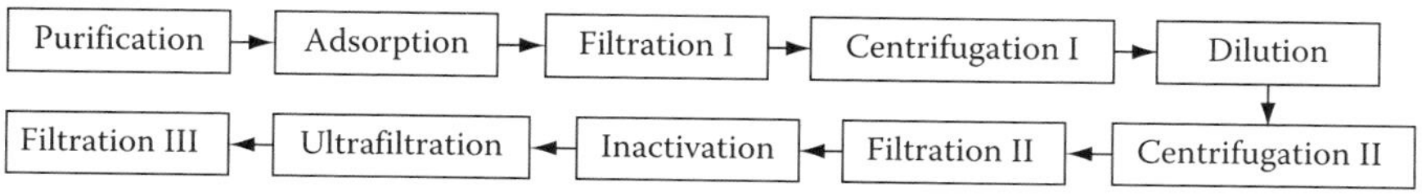

FIGURE 27.3 Typical process flow diagram for downstream processing of vaccines.

ease downstream purification, eliminating the need for this step. However, secreted antigens are usually quite dilute and will need to be concentrated. In addition, any components of the medium that might interfere with further purification will need to be removed, often by diafiltration. Subsequent processing steps usually focus on various types of chromatography including ion exchange, hydrophobic interaction, and affinity varieties.

In a recent paper, chromatographic assays were miniaturized to allow for the high throughput analysis of the final product following fermentation to produce an HPV capsid antigen followed by two purification steps. Because the product in question self-assembles into a VLP, it was necessary to completely purify the protein from the fermentation to understand the impact of changing variables on the final product. Micropipette tips packed with resin on the scale of less than 100 μL served as "mini columns" and robotic liquid handling was used to increase throughput. On the whole, the volumes handled were 1000-fold less than on laboratory scale preparation and throughput was increased 10-fold (Wenger et al. 2007). Such a system could be amenable to routine process monitoring.

Quality Control

Quality control in the vaccine industry, as with the production of any medicinal compound, begins with the sourcing of materials for fermentation through to ensuring low batch-to-batch variability in the final product. Quality control of the final vaccine is complicated by the size of the molecule and the need to be able to ensure adequate potency. In contrast with small molecule pharmaceuticals, it is nearly impossible to fully characterize each vial of vaccine because the size of the molecule is greater by 4–6 orders of magnitude. Thus, to satisfy regulatory requirements, the product is usually defined by the process used to produce it. This means that any changes in production process, including changes of scale, require the manufacturer to show that the product remains unchanged in terms of safety and efficacy and may require them to complete new clinical testing (Buckland 2005).

In order for the final process to be certified, certain criteria must be fulfilled. In most countries, including those in the European Union and the United States, these include minimizing the use of animal-derived components, particularly those of bovine origin, in order to reduce the risk of transmissible spongiform encephalopathies (U.S. Food and Drug Administration 2002, Fuchs 2002). In addition, if any genetic manipulation has taken place (e.g., introduction of a heterologous gene by recombinant technology, deletion of a native gene), the genetic stability of the construct must be assessed throughout the process and over time to ensure that no unintended changes will result. Similarly, since variations in culture conditions will almost certainly result in changes to the yield, purity, or posttranslational modification of the final product, process monitoring procedures at various stages of growth must be utilized to detect any deviations from the norm. Finally, purification procedures must be demonstrated to remove any harmful agents that might be introduced during vaccine production including adventitious viruses, naked DNA, or foreign proteins (Fuchs 2002). Extensive documentation for all aspects of the process is usually required.

One method of scientifically reviewing and monitoring processes is called process analytical technology (PAT). In PAT, the components of a process are systematically varied and the result on the outcome is used to determine which of the possible sources of variation have the largest effect on the product yield, quality, and/or other characteristics. These are then defined as the parameters which are critical for process control and the online monitoring and correction of these processes should ensure the quality of the product. PAT has been widely applied to a variety of processes in the chemical industry (as process analytical chemistry), and to a lesser extent, to the synthesis of pharmaceuticals (Workman et al. 2009). Applying PAT to processes usually requires a deep understanding of the variables that can affect the outcome, so processes where the biology is complex or ill-defined are difficult to handle within a PAT framework. Nonetheless, the early stages of PAT are beginning to be applied to vaccine production using the process to manufacture a whole-cell *B. pertussis* vaccine as an example (Streefland et al. 2007, 2009). In both cases, DNA microarray analysis was used to monitor the cellular metabolism and levels of antigen production in response to changes in conditions. In the first example, preculture conditions were fixed that minimized variability in antigen production by using a chemically defined medium and regular harvest times (Streefland et al. 2007). In the second example, the effect of dissolved oxygen limitation during the fermentation was assessed for its impact on the final product (Streefland et al. 2009). Through other similar step-wise investigations and a final assessment of interactions using statistical design of experiments, PAT can be implemented even for complex biological processes.

Methods for Assessing Product Quality

The final product must be assayed for its sterility, antigenicity, and the level of contaminants such as production host DNA or proteins. Infectivity can be tested either in cell culture by calculating the $TCID_{50}$ or using live animals or embryos with an LC_{50}. Antigenicity usually requires live animals for testing. Live vaccines must also be tested for the level of infectivity and specific vaccines may have other specific properties that need to be tested (e.g., HA activity for influenza vaccines) (Wolff and Reichl 2008). Inactivated vaccines must be proven to be completely inactivated (Duchêne 2006). The level of purity is often assessed using standard assays for nucleic acids and proteins, although some newer methods such as capillary electrophoresis (CE) are gaining use.

CE is an automated electrophoretic technique by which molecules of different size, charge, and shape are separated from each other in a capillary of small width, but long diameter. The use of a capillary affords improved resolution over traditional electrophoretic techniques and also allows the analysis of relatively small sample volumes, ideal for high throughput analyses or routine testing of many samples (Gordon et al. 1988). CE has been widely applied in the analysis of therapeutic proteins and is increasingly applied to the analysis of vaccines, both for initial characterization of the protein and for process monitoring. Virtually any antigen is suitable for analysis using CE, including polysaccharides, proteins, and nucleic acids and the technique allows determination of both the concentration and purity of the vaccine, replacing sodium dodecyl sulfate polyacrylamide gel electrophoresis (SDS-PAGE) gels as a means to determine the mass, quantity, charge, and purity of protein-based vaccines. Because CE is a relatively rapid technique, it can also be employed as a means of monitoring the steps in downstream processing (Nunnally and Yao 2007).

Planning and Scheduling

Batch processing is widely used in the manufacture of vaccines, similarly to the production of most cell culture–derived products. Scheduling is hence an important aspect of manufacturing, particularly in the case of vaccines for which demand is subject to seasonal changes. The advantage of batch scheduling is that the same type or even piece of equipment can be used to process many different products. As analyzed in Tsang et al. (2006), scheduling requires detailed knowledge of demand and delivery requirements as well as information on the sequence, duration, and constraints of equipment use, and is therefore specific to each product and manufacturing site. Previous studies in this field include the proposal of an optimization-based methodology for planning and scheduling of an egg-derived influenza vaccine production facility by Tsang et al. (2006), while a general strategy for modeling and scheduling cell culture–based processes has been presented by Gosling (2003).

References

Alirezaie, B, K Aghaiypour, and A Shafyi. 2008. Genetic characterization of RS-12 (S-12), an Iranian isolate of mumps virus, by sequence analysis and comparative genomics of F, SH, and HN genes. *J. Med. Virol.* 80:702–710.

Arakawa, T, DKX Chong, and WHR Langridge. 1998. Efficacy of a food plant-based oral cholera toxin B subunit vaccine. *Nat. Biotechnol.* 15:248–252.

Argentini, C, R Giuseppetti, E D'Ugoa, V La Sorsa, E Tritarelli, S Orobello, A Canitano, R Glück, and M Rapicetta. 2005. A pre-S/S CHO-derived hepatitis B virus vaccine protects woodchucks from WHV productive infection. *Vaccine* 23:3649–3656.

Bae, KD, JY Choi, YS Jang, SJ Ahn, and BK Hur. 2009. Innovative vaccine production technologies: The evolution and value of vaccine production technologies. *Arch. Pharm. Res.* 32:465–480.

Boon, L. 2009. Companies claim to fame and their scientific challenges in vaccine development. *Immunol. Lett.* 122:122–125.

Brady, CP, RL Shimp, AP Miles, M Whitmore, and AW Stowers. 2001. High-level production and purification of P30P2MSP1_{19}, an important vaccine antigen for malaria, expressed in the methylotropic yeast *Pichia pastoris*. *Prot. Exp. Purif.* 23:468–475.

Buckland, BC. 2005. The process development challenge for a new vaccine. *Nat. Med.* (Suppl.) 11:S16–S19.

Business Insights. 2005. *The Vaccines Market Outlook: Market Analysis of Future Growth and Leading Players by Sector*, Dallas, TX.

Cannon, G and D Weissman. 2002. RNA based vaccines. *DNA Cell Biol.* 21(12):953–961.

Capilla, J, KV Clemonsa, M Liua, HB Levinea, and DA Stevens. 2009. *Saccharomyces cerevisiae* as a vaccine against coccidioidomycosis. *Vaccine* 27:3662–3668.

Conceição, MM, A Tonso, CB Freitas, and CA Pereira. 2007. Viral antigen production in cell cultures on microcarriers Bovine parainfluenza 3 virus and MDBK cells. *Vaccine* 25:7785–7795.

Copier, J, S Ward, and A Dangleish. 2007. Cell based cancer vaccines: Regulatory and commercial development. *Vaccine* (Suppl.) 25S:B35–B46.

Daniell, H, SB Lee, T Panchal, and PO Wiebe. 2001. Expression of the native cholera toxin B subunit gene and assembly as functional oligomers in transgenic tobacco chloroplasts. *J. Mol. Biol.* 311:1001–1009.

Dehoux, P, V Ribes, E Sobczak, and RE Streeck. 1986. Expression of the hepatitis B virus large envelope protein in *Saccharomyces cerevisiae*. *Gene* 48(1):155–163.

Derouazi, M, P Girard, F Van Tilborgh, K Iglesias, N Muller, M Bertschinger, and FM Wurm. 2004. Serum-free large-scale transient transfection of CHO cells. *Biotechnol. Bioeng.* 87:537–545.

Detmer, A and J Glenting. 2006. Live bacterial vaccines—A review and identification of potential hazards. *Microb. Cell Fact.* 5:23.

Devitt, G, M Thomas, AM Klibanov, T Pfeiffer, and V Bosch. 2007. Optimized protocol for the large scale production of HIV pseudovirions by transient transfection of HEK293T cells with linear fully deacylated polyethylenimine. *J. Virol. Methods* 146:298–304.

Du, LY, GY Zhao, L Li, YX He, YS Zhou, BJ Zheng, and SB Jiang. 2009. Antigenicity and immunogenicity of SARS-CoV S protein receptor-binding domain stably expressed in CHO cells. *Biochem. Biophys. Res. Commun.* 384:486–490.

Duchêne, M. 2006. Production, testing, and perspectives of IPV and IPV combination vaccines: GSK's biological view. *Biologicals* 34:164–166.

Epp, C, CW Kauth, and HBR Lutz. 2003. Expression and purification of *Plasmodium falciparum* MSP-1_{42}: A malaria vaccine candidate. *J. Chromatogr. B* 786:61–72.

Falkenhagen, A, J Heinrich, and K Moelling. 2009. Short hairpin-loop-structured oligodeoxynucleotides reduce HSV-1 replication. *Virol. J.* 6:43.

Fallaux, FR, A Bout, I van der Velde, DJM van den Wollenberg, KM Hehir, J Keegan, C Auger et al. 1998. New helper cells and matched early Region-1 deleted adenovirus vectors prevent generation of replication competent adenoviruses. *Hum. Gene Ther.* 9:1909–1917.

Fuchs, F. 2002. Quality control of biotechnology-derived vaccines: Technical and regulatory considerations. *Biochimie* 84:1173–1179.

Genzel, Y, M Fischer, and U Reichl. 2006. Serum-free influenza virus production avoiding washing steps and medium exchange in large-scale microcarrier culture. *Vaccine* 24:3261–3272.

Gordon, MJ, X Huang, SL Pentoney, and RN Zare. 1988. Capillary electrophoresis. *Science* 242:224–228.

Gosling, I. 2003. Process simulation and modelling strategies for the biotechnology industry: Optimizing productivity in multiproduct batch facilities. *Genet. Eng. News,* www.chemsim.com/GENArticleSept03pdfprep.pdf.

Govorkova, EA, NV Kaverin, LV Gubareva, B Meignier, and RG Webster. 1995. Replication of influenza A viruses in a green monkey kidney continuous cell line (Vero). *J. Infect. Dis.* 172:250–253.

Govorkova, EA, G Murti, B Meignier, C De Taisne, and RG Webster. 1996. African green monkey kidney (Vero) cells provide an alternative host cell system for influenza A and B viruses. *J. Virol.* 70:5519–5524.

Graham, JSFL, WC Russell, and R Nairn. 1977. Characteristics of a human cell linetransformed by DNA from human adenovirus type 5. *J. Genet. Virol.* 36:59–74.

Grgacic, EVL and DA Anderson. 2006. Virus like particles: Passport to immune recognition. *Methods* 40:60–65.

Guo, JT, T Zhou, H Guo, and TM Block. 2007. Alpha interferon-induced antiviral response noncytolytically reduces replication defective adenovirus DNA in MDBK cells. *Antivir. Res.* 76:232–240.

Guttormsen, HK and DL Kasper. 2001. Bacterial vaccines, In: *Therapeutic Immunology*, 2nd edn. pp. 401–412. Edited by, TB Strom, KF Austen, SJ Burakoff, and F Rosen. Malden, MA: Blackwell Science.

Haq, TA, HS Mason, JD Clements, and CJ Arntzen. 1995. Oral immunization with a recombinant bacterial antigen produced in transgenic plants. *Science* 268:714–716.

Hefferon, KL and Y Fan. 2004. Expression of a vaccine protein in a plant cell line using a geminivirus-based replicon system. *Vaccine* 23:404–410.

Hepler, RW, R Kelly, TB McNeely, H Fan, MC Losada, HA George, A Woods et al. 2006. A recombinant 63 kDa fragment of anthrax protective antigen produced in the yeast *Saccharomyces cerevisiae* provides protection in rabbit and primate inhalational challenge model of anthrax infection. *Vaccine* 24:1501–1514.

Hill, DR, L Ford, and DG Lalloo. 2006. Oral cholera vaccines: Uses in clinical practice. *Lancet Infect. Dis.* 6:361–373.

Hilleman, MR. 2000. Vaccines in historic evolution and perspective: A narrative of vaccine discoveries. *Vaccine* 18(15):1436–1447.

Hoffmann, E, S Krauss, D Perez, R Webby, and RG Webster. 2002. Eight plasmid system for rapid generation of influenza virus vaccines. *Vaccine* 20:3165–3170.

Hoffmann, E, G Neumann, Y Kawaoka, G Hobom, and RG Webster. 2000. A DNA transfection system for the generation of influenza A virus from eight plasmids. *Proc. Natl. Acad. Sci.* 97:6108–6113.

Hood, EE, DR Witcher, S Maddock, T Meyer, C Baszczynski, M Bailey, P Flynn et al. 1997. Commercial production of avidin from transgenic maize: Characterization of transformant, production, processing, extraction and purification. *Mol. Breed.* 3:291–306.

Hu, AYC, TC Weng, YF Tseng, YS Chen, CH Wu, S Hsiao, AH Chou et al. 2008. Microcarrier-based MDCK cell culture system for the production of influenza H5N1 vaccines. *Vaccine* 26:5736–5740.

Imamura, T, M Araki, A Miyanohara, J Nakao, H Yonemura, N Ohtomo, and K Matsubara. 1986. Expression of hepatitis B virus middle and large surface antigen genes in *Saccharomyces cerevisiae. J. Virol.* 61(11):3543–3549.

Jacobs, JP, CM Jones, and JP Baille. 1970. Characteristics of a human diploid cell designated MRC-5. *Nature* 227:168–170.

Jones, D, N Kroos, R Anema, B van Montfort, A Vooys, S van der Kraats, E van der Helm et al. 2003. High level expression of recombinant IgG in the human cell line PER.C6. *Biotechnol. Prog.* 19:163–168.

Jordan, M, A Schallhorn, and FM Wurm. 1996. Transfecting mammalian cells: Optimization of critical parameters affecting calcium-phosphate precipitate formation. *Nucleic Acids Res.* 24:596–601.

Kalbfuss, B, M Wolff, R Morenweiser, and U Reichl. 2007. Purification of cell-culture derived human influenza A virus by size exclusion chromatography and anion-exchange chromatography. *Biotechnol. Bioeng.* 96:932–944.

Kalorama Information. 2007. *Vaccines: The World Market*, Rockville, MD.

Katz, JM, CW Naeve, and RG Webster. 1987. Host cell mediated variation in H3N2 influenza viruses. *Virology* 156:386–395.

Katz, JM, M Wang, and RG Webster. 1990. Direct sequencing of the HA gene of influenza (H3N2) virus in original clinical samples reveals sequence identity with mammalian cell-grown virus. *J. Virol.* 64:1808–1811.

Kumar, GBS, TR Ganapathi, L Srinivas, CJ Revathi, and VA Bapat. 2007. Hepatitis B surface antigen expression in NT-1 cells of tobacco using different expression cassettes. *Biol. Plantarum* 51(3):467–471.

Kumar, AAP, KR Mani, C Palaniappan, LNR Bhau, and K Swaminathan. 2005. Purification, potency and immunogenicity analysis of Vero cell culture-derived rabies vaccine: A comparative study of single-step column chromatography and zonal centrifuge purification. *Microbes Infect.* 7:1110–1116.

Lee, CW, K Junga, SJ Jadhaoc, and DL Suarez. 2008. Evaluation of chicken-origin (DF-1) and quail-origin (QT-6) fibroblast cell lines for replication of avian influenza viruses. *J. Virol. Meth.* 153: 22–28.

Levine, MM, C Ferreccio, RE Black, R Lagos, O San Martin, and WC Blackwelder. 2007. Ty21a live oral typhoid vaccine and prevention of paratyphoid fever caused by *Salmonella enterica* Serovar Paratyphi B. *Clin. Infect. Dis.* 45:S24–S28.

Levine, MM, JB Kaper, D Herrington, J Ketley, G Losonsky, CO Tacket, B. Tall, and S Cryz. 1988. Safety, immunogenicity, and efficacy of recombinant live oral cholera vaccines CVD103 and CVD103-HgR. *Lancet* 332:467–470.

Leyten, EMS, D Soonawala, C Schultsz, C Herzog, RJ Ligthelm, S Wijnands, and LG Visser. 2005. Analysis of efficacy of CVD 103-HgR live oral cholera vaccine against all-cause travellers' diarrhoea in a randomised, double-blind, placebo-controlled study. *Vaccine* 23:5120–5126.

Litwin, J. 1992. The growth of Vero cells in suspension as cell-aggregates in serum-free media. *Cytotechnology* 10:169–174.

Mason, HS, DMK Lam, and CJ Arntzen. 1992. Expression of hepatitis B surface antigen in transgenic plants. *Proc. Natl. Acad. Sci.* 89:11745–11749.

McLemore, MR. 2006. Gardasil®: Introducing the new human papilloma virus vaccine. *Clin. J. Oncol. Nurs.* 10:559–560.

Mitchell, S. 2007. Global vaccine market to top 23 billion dollars. United Press International, Washington, DC.

Mohamadzadeh, M, T Duong, SJ Sandwick, T Hoover, and TR Klaenhammer. 2009. Dendritic cell targeting of *Bacillus anthracis* protective antigen expressed by *Lactobacillus acidophilus* protects mice from lethal challenge. *Proc. Natl. Acad. Sci.* 106:4331–4336.

Monto, AS, HF Maassab, and ER Bryan. 1981. Relative efficacy of embryonated eggs and cell culture for isolation of contemporary influenza viruses. *J. Clin. Microbiol.* 13:233–235.

Muller, N, M Derouazi, F Van Tilborgh, and S Wulhfard. 2007. Scalable transient gene expression in Chinese hamster ovary cells in instrumented and non-instrumented cultivation systems. *Biotechnol. Lett.* 29:703–711.

Neumann, G, K Fuji, Y Keno, and Y Kawaoka. 2005. An improved reverse genetics system for influenza A virus production and its implications for vaccine production. *Proc. Natl. Acad. Sci.* 102:16825–16829.

Neumann, G, T Watanabe, H Ito, S Watanabe, H Goto, P Gao, M Hughes et al. 1999. Generation of influenza viruses entirely from cloned cDNAs. *Proc. Natl. Acad. Sci.* 96:9345–9350.

Neumann, G, A Zobel, and G Hobom. 1994. RNA polymerase-I mediated expression of influenza viral RNA molecules. *Virology* 202:477–479.

Nunnally, BK and K Yao. 2007. The use of capillary electrophoresis in vaccines. *Anal. Lett.* 40:615–627.

Offringa, R, SH van der Burg, F Ossendorp, REM Toes, and CJM Melief. 2000. Design and evaluation of antigen-specific vaccination strategies against cancer. *Curr. Opin. Immunol.* 12:576–582.

O'Keeffe, RS, MD Johnston, and NKH Slater. 1998. The affinity adsorptive recovery of an infections herpes simplex virus vaccine. *Biotechnol. Bioeng.* 62:537–545.

Palese, P, H Zheng, OG Engelhardt, S Pleschka, and A García-Sastre. 1996. Negative-strand RNA viruses: Genetic engineering and applications. *Proc. Natl. Acad. Sci.* 93:11354–11358.

Pau, MG, C Ophorst, MH Koldijk, G Schouten, M Mehtali, and F Uytdehaag. 2001. The human cell line PER.C6 provides a new manufacturing system for the production of influenza vaccines. *Vaccine* 19:2716–2721

Peetermans, J. 1992. Production, quality control and characterization of an inactivated hepatitis A vaccine. *Vaccine* 10:S99–S101.

Petridis, D, E Sapidou, and J Calandranis. 1995. Computer aided process analysis and economic evaluation for biosynthetic human insulin production: A study case. *Biotechnol. Bioeng.* 48:529–541.

Pham, PL, S Pettet, B Cass, E Carpentier, G St-Laurent, L Bisson, A Kamen, and Y Durocher. 2005. Transient gene expression in HEK293 cells: Peptone addition posttransfection improves recombinant protein synthesis. *Biotechnol. Bioeng.* 90:332–344.

Pollack, A. 2009. Vaccine maker facing possible bankruptcy wins contract. *The New York Times*, June 24, 2009. http://www.proteinsciences.com/aboutus/pdf/news-6-24-09.pdf (accessed July 13, 2009).

Puck, TT. 1985. Development of the Chinese hamster ovary (CHO) cell. In: *Molecular Cell Genetics*, pp. 37–64. New York: John Wiley & Sons.

Richter, LJ, Y Thanavala, CJ Arntzen, and HS Mason. 2000. Production of hepatitis B surface antigen in transgenic plants for oral immunization. *Nat. Biotechnol.* 18:1167–1171.

Rigano, MM and AM Walmsley. 2005. Expression systems and developments in plant-made vaccines. *Immunol. Cell Biol.* 83:271–277.

Robertson, J. 1993. Clinical influenza virus and the embryonated hen's egg. *Rev. Med. Virol.* 3:97–106.

Robertson, J, G Bootman, C Nicholson, D Major, E Robertson, and J Wood. 1990. The hemagglutinin of influenza B virus present in clinical material is a single species identical to that of mammalian cell-grown virus. *Virology* 179:35–40.

Schild, G, J Oxford, J de Jong, and RG Webster. 1983. Evidence for host-cell selection of influenza virus antigenic variants. *Nature* 303:706–709.

Schirmbeck, R and J Reimann. 2001. Revealing the potential of DNA-based vaccination: Lessons learned from the hepatitis B virus surface antigen. *Biol. Chem.* 382(4):543–552.

Sharp, JM and PM Doran. 1999. Effect of bacitracin on growth and monoclonal antibody production by tobacco hairy roots and cell suspensions. *Biotechnol. Bioprocess. Eng.* 4:253–258.

Sharp, JM and PM Doran. 2000. Characterization of monoclonal antibody fragments produced by plant cells. *Biotechnol. Bioeng.* 73:338–346.

Solomon, JS, CP Nixon, ST McGarvey, LR Acosta, D Manalo, and JD Kurtis. 2004. Expression, purification, and human antibody response to a 67 kDa vaccine candidate for *Schistosomiasis japonica*. *Prot. Exp. Purif.* 36:226–231.

Spier RE. 1992. Prophylaxis: The foundation of our future progress. *Vaccine* 10(14):971–976.

Stern, AM and H Markel. 2005. The history of vaccines and immunization: Familiar patterns, new challenges. *Health Aff.* 24:611–621.

Streefland, M, B van de Waterbeemd, H Happé, LA van der Pol, EC Beuvery, J Tramper, and DE Martens. 2007. PAT for vaccines: The first stage for PAT implementation for development of a well-defined whole-cell vaccine against whooping cough disease. *Vaccine* 25:2994–3000.

Streefland, M, B van de Waterbeemd, J Kint, LA van der Pol, EC Beuvery, J Tramper, and DE Martens. 2009. Evaluation of a critical process parameter: Oxygen limitation during cultivation has a fully reversible effect on gene expression of *Bordetella pertussis*. *Biotechnol. Bioeng.* 102:161–167.

Taub, M, L Chuman, MH Saier Jr., and G Sato. 1979. Growth of Madin-Darby canine kidney epithelial cell (MDCK) line in hormone-supplemented, serum-free medium. *Proc. Natl. Acad. Sci.* 76:3338–3342.

Treanor, JJ, GM Schiff, FG Hayden, RC Brady, CM Hay, AL Meyer, J Holden-Wiltse, H Liang, A Gilbert, and M Cox. 2007. Safety and immunogenicity of a baculovirus-expressed hemagglutinin influenza vaccine: A randomized controlled trial. *JAMA* 297(14):1577–1582.

Treanor, JJ, BE Wilkinson, F Masseoud, J Hu-Primmer, R Battaglia, D O'Brien, M Wolff, G Rabinovich, W Blackwelder, and JM Katz. 2001. Safety and immunogenicity of a recombinant hemagglutinin vaccine for H5 influenza in humans. *Vaccine* 19:1732–1737.

Tsang, KH, NJ Samsatli, and N Shah. 2006. Modelling and planning optimisation of a complex flu vaccine facility. *Food. Bioprod. Process.* 84:123–134.

Ulmer, JB, U Valley, and R Rappuoli. 2006. Vaccine manufacturing: Challenges and solutions. *Nat. Biotechnol.* 24:1377–1383.

U.S. Food and Drug Administration. 2002. http://www.fda.gov/BiologicsBloodVaccines/SafetyAvailability/BloodSafety/ucm095107.htm (accessed October 15, 2010).

van Wezel, AL, G van Steenis, P van der Marel, and ADME Osterhaus. 1984. Inactivated polio virus vaccine: Current production and new methods. *Rev. Infect. Dis.* 6(Suppl. 2):S335–S340.

Walmsley, AM and CJ Arntsen. 2000. Plants for delivery of edible vaccines. *Curr. Opin. Biotechnol.* 22:126–129.

Wenger, MD, P DePhillips, CE Price, and DG Bracewell. 2007. An automated microscale chromatographic purification of virus-like particles as a strategy for process development. *Biotechnol. Appl. Biochem.* 47:131–139.

Witcher, DR, EE Hood, D Peterson, M Bailey, D Bond, A Kusnadi, R Evangelista et al. 1998. Commercial production of b-glucuronidase (GUS): A model system for the production of proteins in plants. *Mol. Breed.* 4:301–312.

Wolff, MW and U Reichl. 2008. Downstream processing: From egg to cell culture-derived influenza virus particles. *Chem. Eng. Technol.* 31:846–857.

Workman, J, M Koch, B Lavine, and R Crisman. 2009. Process analytical chemistry. *Anal. Chem.* 81:4623–4643.

World Health Organisation. 2005. Influenza vaccines. *Weekly Epidemiological Record* 80(33):277–288.

Wressnigg, N, D Voss, T Wolff, J Romanova, T Ruthsatz, I Mayerhofer, M Reiter et al. 2009. Development of a live-attenuated influenza B Delta NS1 intranasal vaccine candidate. *Vaccine* 27:2851–2857.

Wu, K, X Xue, Z Wang, Z Yan, J Shi, W Han, and Y Zhang. 2006. Construction, purification, and immunogenicity of recombinant cysteine–cysteine type chemokine receptor 5 vaccine. *Prot. Exp. Purif.* 49:108–113.

Yamagishi, Y, T Sadaoka, H Yoshii, P Sornboonthum, T Imazawa, K Nagaike, K Ozono, K Yarnanishi, and Y Mori. 2008. Varicella-zoster virus glycoprotein M homolog is glycosylated, is expressed on the viral envelope, and functions in virus cell-to-cell spread. *J. Virol.* 82:795–804.

Yasumura, Y and M Kawakita. 1963. The research for the SV40 by means of tissue culture technique. *Nippon Rinsho* 21:1201–1219.

Yuan, H, S You-en, Y Long-jiang, X Xiao-hua, LA Liu-zhe, M Cash, Z Lu, L Zhi, and S Deng-xin. 2007. Studies on the protective immunity of *Schistosoma japonicum* bivalent DNA vaccine encoding Sj23 and Sj14. *Exp. Parasitol.* 115:379–386.

28

Economic Implications of Preventive Care

George H. Avery
Purdue University

Kara E. Leonard
University of Texas Medical Branch

Steve P. McKenzie
Purdue University

Introduction 28-1
Need for Efficiency in Prevention: Problem of Limited Resources • Prevention: A Definition • Incentives for Prevention • Evaluation of Cost-Effectiveness
Examples of the Economic Implications of Prevention 28-6
Primary Prevention • Secondary Prevention • Tertiary Prevention • Rehabilitation
Discussion 28-11
References 28-11

Introduction

Need for Efficiency in Prevention: Problem of Limited Resources

The fundamental conflict in the search for optimal healthcare and public health systems is between our desire for perfect health and the reality of scarce resources. Far too often, as Fuchs notes in *Who Shall Live?*, health policy advocates ignore this conflict, taking either a romantic view that ignores resource constraints or a monotechnic view that acknowledges these constraints, but assumes that health is the only goal while ignoring competing wants (Fuchs, 1973). In reality, the infinite resources required to achieve all desires are unavailable, and every decision to allocate resources to health and healthcare creates an opportunity cost, in that those resources cannot then be used to attain other desirable ends. In reality, hard decisions need to be made as to whether programs, therapies, regulatory decisions, and so forth are wise and efficient uses of resources to advance welfare.

Although preventive medicine has a long history, predating much of modern clinical medicine, demand for preventive programs increased in recent decades. Since the 1960s, risk aversion, rising healthcare costs, and concerns over the quality brought a new emphasis to prevention and spurred greater interest in identifying efficient solutions to the problems of health and healthcare and in reducing the economic burden of healthcare through preventive programs. As the Health Project Consortium argued in 1993, "If there were no illness and no accidents, healthcare costs for a society would theoretically be zero" (Fries et al., 1993). This view is reflected in the widespread use of estimates of the economic burden of disease as an argument for programs to change risk behavior and mitigate risks.

Reducing healthcare demand is not without its own costs. In many, if not most, cases preventive care, while improving health, can increase net healthcare expenditures if all costs are accounted for (Russell, 1986, 1993). For example, disease management programs improve health by ensuring patient access to necessary preventive care, but significantly increase expenditures by increasing utilization of that care (Fireman et al., 2004). In fact, many preventive interventions are notoriously inefficient. For example, universal vaccination programs for Hepatitis B have been estimated to cost as much as $420,000 per quality-adjusted life-year (QALY) gained, while screening surgeons even once for HIV infection to prevent transmission to patients has been estimated to cost $4.1 million per QALY (Graham et al., 1998). Efficiency of prevention varies widely. A systematic review in 1995 found that the cost per life-year gained from prevention programs ranges from net savings (for programs to put smoke detectors in homes, mandatory motorcycle helmet laws, child sleepwear flammability standards, etc.) to $34 billion for control of radionuclide emissions at uranium fuel cycle facilities or sickle-cell screening of nonblack low-risk infants (Teng et al., 1995).

Over the course of the twentieth century, public health and other preventive measures demonstrated great success at improving morbidity and mortality rates, but the public health community perceives that prevention is chronically underfunded. For advocates of prevention, making the business case for investing in prevention has proven difficult to build and effectively communicate (Neumann et al., 2008). For example, the United States Preventive Services Task Force was explicitly forbidden from considering the cost-effectiveness of preventive services when it was created in 1984 to develop guidelines for such services (Woolf and Atkins, 2001). In healthcare organizations, an institutional reluctance to invest in programs to improve quality of care, derived from limited resources and competing priorities, hinders investment in efforts to develop efficient treatment modalities (Chao and Forum, 2008).

The use of cost-effectiveness assessments for regulatory interventions for the protection of human and environmental health is particularly controversial. Notably, in environmental risk regulation, advocacy groups strongly favor a decision approach based on the precautionary principle rather than the efficiency and effectiveness of the intervention. This preference has been described as taking the form "*If* there is (1) a threat, which is (2) uncertain, *then* (3) some kind of action (4) is mandatory." (Sandin, 1999) It is conspicuous for excluding concern over the efficiency or effectiveness of programs. Although groups such as the United States Environmental Protection Agency's (USEPA) Strategic Advisory Board recommend that regulatory decisions use assessment criteria (Table 28.1) that look at the efficiency and effectiveness of regulatory alternatives to best utilize resources (Strategic Advisory Board, 1990), regulation in the United States is often tied by cultural and legal constraints to a precautionary approach. For example, the Delaney Clause (regarding carcinogens) of the Food, Drug and Cosmetic Act; the Occupational Safety and Health Act; the Clean Air Act; the Resource Conservation and Recovery Act; the Safe Drinking Water Act; and the Comprehensive Environmental Response, Compensation, and Liability Act contain clauses that limit the use of cost-effectiveness analysis (Arrow et al., 1996). A similar attitude is seen in the public health community, where some leaders argue that health should be the overriding public value, taking precedence over *all* competing policy areas such as "transportation, economic development, and national security." (Gostin and Stone, 2007) Outside the United States, these views are entrenched in international environmental and health agreements as well as European Community policies (Foster et al., 2000). Fuchs describes this view as romantic, failing "to recognize the scarcity of resources relative to wants," denying "the inevitability of choice," and are coupled with

TABLE 28.1 USEPA Strategic Advisory Board Assessment Criteria

Annual cost of implementing a strategy
Social costs (public and private) of the strategy
Degree of assurance that the strategy will achieve the desired risk reduction
Speed of risk reduction following the implementation of the strategy
Ability to implement and enforce the strategy
Level of risk reduction from current risk levels
Cost-effectiveness
Short- and long-term desirability of the strategy

Source: Adapted from Strategic Advisory Board, *Reducing Risk: Setting Priorities and Strategies for Environmental Risk*. United States Environmental Protection Agency, Washington, DC, 1990.

authoritarian distinctions that dismiss competing desires as "'unnecessary' or 'inappropriate'" (Fuchs, 1973). This view denies any relevance to cost-effectiveness analysis of interventions by giving a privileged and unquestioned position to particular policy preferences.

The impact of this view can be tremendous. For example, it is estimated that the USEPA's listing of wood preservatives as hazardous materials costs over $6 trillion per life saved (Office of Management and Budget, 1993). The costs of healthcare regulation in the United States are believed to exceed benefits by $169 billion per year, more than the amount to purchase insurance for the estimated 44 million uninsured Americans (Conover, 2004). Skepticism exists over the economic impact of current food safety regulations, leading to a demand for more efficient programs (Henson and Caswell, 1999). Where agencies have attempted to report the cost-effectiveness of programs, criticism has risen over the underlying assumptions, crudity of the models, or examination of alternative strategies (Hahn, 1996). Failure to examine alternatives negates much of the utility of cost-effectiveness analysis in efficient resource allocation (Graham et al., 1998).

Prevention: A Definition

In public health, prevention consists of programs to prevent disease or injury at a population level, is initiated by health professionals rather than the patient, and is pervasive, affecting many facets of individual lives and liberty (Dawson and Verweij, 2007). Prevention is viewed as a four-tiered concept, with differences between levels derived from the point in the disease process that the preventive program addresses (Figure 28.1).

Primary prevention tries to minimize risk exposure, preventing the incidence of injury or disease. Secondary prevention seeks to minimize the impact of a disease or injury event once it has occurred, while tertiary preventive efforts focus on minimizing disability through appropriate and timely therapeutic (Schneider, 2006). Primary preventive programs include such efforts as health promotion campaigns, folic acid supplementation to prevent fetal neural tube defects, or vaccination programs. Secondary prevention efforts are represented by programs such as disease screening schedules, where the attempt is to identify a disease early enough to prevent or slow progression. Clinical guidelines identifying best therapeutic practices represent tertiary prevention, focusing on ensuring that the right treatment is obtained at the right time. Rehabilitation, or obtaining maximum functionality and quality of life after the state of active disease has passed, is the fourth level. The underlying philosophy of each is to maximize quality of life given the circumstances of the intervention. As a result, prevention encompasses all aspects of the health and public health system, including areas such as environmental and occupational safety regulation not typically considered part of the healthcare system.

Incentives for Prevention

Under the assumption that prevention reduces the cost of care, the United States has tried a number of efforts to change the incentive structures of the health system to encourage more efficient use

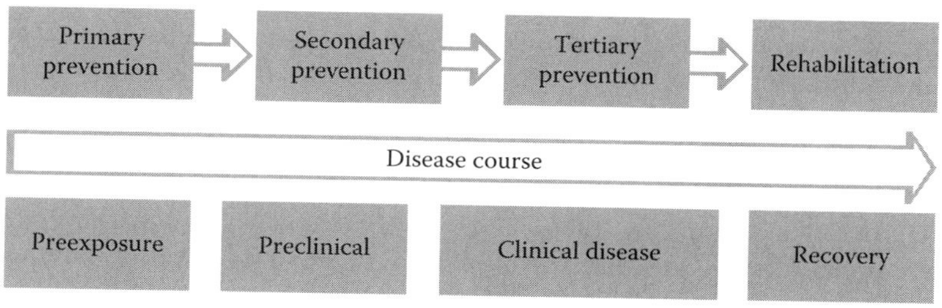

FIGURE 28.1 Levels of prevention as related to the course of a disease.

of resources. Many of these efforts are based on lessons learned from the traditional prepaid group practice (PGP) health maintenance organizations (HMOs). These organizations, such as the Kaiser Permanente plans, consist of a multispecialty group practice and affiliated hospitals that provide comprehensive healthcare to a voluntarily enrolled population on a capitated basis, with an ongoing relationship between the provider and insurance component organizations (Enthoven and Tollen, 2004). In traditional fee-for-service medicine, the provider receives additional revenue for additional services, creating an incentive to provide more services and a disincentive for prevention. With capitation, a provider maximizes revenue by delivering care in an efficient mix of preventive and remedial services. Evidence exists that this HMO model is better at providing preventive services than other organizational forms, including the single payer British National Health Service (Feacham et al., 2002; Miller and Luft, 2002; Casalino, 2003). As a result, this model significantly influenced proposals to improve the quality and efficiency of care, including the HMO Act of 1973, Medicare Managed Care programs, and the conversion of the military CHAMPUS system into the current TRICARE model (Christianson and Avery, 2004).

An alternative is to assess the cost-effectiveness of an intervention as a tool to make decisions on coverage and reimbursement levels. Beyond insurers, this information is needed to make a business case for interventions, required to overcome resistance from organizational chief executive officers (CEOs) and chief financial officers (CFOs) toward changes in care delivery methods (Chao and Forum, 2008). This can in theory be used to create incentives to use the most cost-effective treatment and prevention methods. Such technology evaluation is used in the private sector, most notably by the Blue Cross/Blue Shield organizations (Eddy, 2004). As a matter of public policy, significant political barriers exist in the public sector to explicit consideration of the healthcare cost-effectiveness. In the Medicare program, for example, the Center for Medicare and Medicaid Services tries to avoid explicit consideration of cost-effectiveness in these decisions (Foote, 2002; Jena and Philipson, 2008).

As a softer form of incentive, these evaluations can be integrated into educational efforts such as evidence-based care guidelines (Grimshaw and Hutchinson, 1995; Grimshaw et al., 1995). Current practices in producing guidelines identify a number of issues that distort the evaluation of cost-effectiveness. In particular, guidelines in general assume that findings from randomly controlled trials are reproducible in normal practice, which is manifested in a heavy weighing of evidence toward these trials and away from observational studies of the intervention in normal practice, and that the universal adoption of the guidelines produces optimal care in the population (Haycox et al., 1999). However, guidelines that yield the maximum population benefit often are not those that give the most benefit to the individual patient, raising the issue of how cost-effectiveness is to be measured—in terms of broad social goals or the individual patient welfare (Granata and Hillman, 1998). The production of guidelines also leaves much to be desired. One study of 279 published guidelines found mean adherence of only 43.1% with accepted standards for generating guidelines. Only 41.6% examined the cost impact of the intervention, and only 14.3% quantified the costs (Shaneyfelt et al., 1999).

Evaluation of Cost-Effectiveness

Three approaches (cost–benefit analysis, cost-effectiveness analysis, and cost–utility analysis) are used to assess the cost-effectiveness of an intervention. These can be contrasted to a typical cost analysis in that the three cost-effectiveness methodologies relate the cost of an intervention to differences between two intervention states in a measurable outcome, whereas cost analysis attempts only to determine the costs associated with a single outcome. Cost analysis is widely used to try to justify the need for an intervention. For example, this tactic has been used by advocates for anti-tobacco programs, as in the examples of Max (2001) and Rice et al. (1986). Rarely do these studies consider the cost of eliminating the problem. Programs designed to eliminate smoking and achieve the counterfactual state cannot be implemented without transaction costs, and so the actual cost of a nonsmoking population is higher than the baseline used to estimate these costs. Smokers can incur costs in two ways—through damage caused by smoking or through the programs used to change them from smoking to nonsmoking status. Thus, estimates based on cost differences between smokers and nonsmokers use an artificially low cost for nonsmokers. In fact, dependent on assumptions regarding the time frame and other modeling parameters, smoking cessation programs can actually result in net increases in healthcare expenditures and other costs, meaning that smoking may actually result in lower costs than the counterfactual (Barendregt et al., 1997). As a result, cost analysis alone does not allow managers or policy-makers to assess the efficient allocation of resources and identify welfare-maximizing preventive interventions.

Traditional cost–benefit analysis calculates the costs of an intervention and compares this to the resulting benefits, estimated in monetary terms. This is controversial in healthcare and public health because it places a monetary value on life and its quality, typically calculated based on willingness-to-pay measurements. This generates concern over social equity over and above the difficulty in measurement and assignment of a monetary value to quality of life. It has the advantage of directly comparing costs and benefits of interventions in terms of the same measurement units (Garber et al., 1996). This method has the broadest scope for evaluating the welfare implications of an intervention and the allocative efficiency of the intervention (Drummond et al., 1997). Cost-utility analysis compares the incremental cost of an intervention to the incremental benefits using natural units. For example, the units of benefit for a program to reduce hypertension might be mm Hg of improvement in blood pressure. It is limited because only final outcomes, typically measured is the QALYs gained or lost from the intervention, can be used to assess benefits. QALYs are calculated using utility weights that measure consumer preference for specific health states. This method is best suited to evaluation of the return to the patient of an intervention (Drummond et al., 1997).

Cost-effectiveness analysis, which also uses natural units, is a more generic form of the same class of analysis. It is distinguished by using units that may represent intermediate outcomes of policy significance that are not readily converted into final health outcomes such as lives saved or QALYs. Such an analysis might be used to evaluate a population screening and surveillance program where the critical policy issue is not the number of lives saved, but cases identified (Drummond et al., 1997).

Regardless of the form of the analysis, a significant number of technical issues become important. Assumptions concerning these issues can have a significant impact on the outcome of the analysis. The definition of costs can be a highly technical issue, with problems arising from the viewpoint from which costs are considered, the use of average or marginal costs, and allocation of expenditures spread across multiple interventions. The timescale can be critical, particularly when considering depreciation of capital expenditures (Drummond et al., 1997). Similar issues exist for the calculation of the benefits of an intervention, such as whether future benefits are discounted in the same way as costs (Drummond et al., 1997). Both of these need to be defined for the specific application and intervention rather than for a broad program to address risk. For example, significantly different cost-effectiveness results are obtained from a ban on asbestos usage when the impact is examined for different applications of the material (Van Houtven and Cropper, 1996).

The transaction costs of adoption of changes in practice are often neglected. As Coase notes, this occurs because of a fundamental flaw in the assumptions underlying the Pigouvian welfare model. Focused on a divergence between private and social costs, an analysis becomes biased toward the hypothesis that any corrective measure is desirable, with attention diverted from "other changes in the system…which may well produce more harm than the original deficiency." (Coase, 1960) Most cost-effectiveness studies, for example, focus on the direct intervention costs but neglect costs of changing practices to implement the interventions in place of current. As a result, many studies of cost-effectiveness do not capture the full costs of interventions, and hence give a biased view of the efficiency of a prevention program (Mason et al., 2001).

The issue of cost-effectiveness extends far beyond the social costs and benefits of prevention, but also to the individual level. Preventive measures that bring much to the community may have little benefit for individuals (Rose, 1992). The net benefit of a vaccination program, for example, lies more in the benefits of herd immunity than in the reduction of individual risk reduction for a disease. The costs are, therefore, a morally relevant consideration extending beyond the purely economic or health impact on the individual (van den Hoven, 2007). In general, cost-effectiveness analysis focuses on this level—evaluating the consumer surplus arising from preventive technology. This means that significant defects can exist in the measurement of the broader impact on social welfare, resulting in over- or underinvestment in preventive programs (Jena and Philipson, 2008). The implication of these issues is a need to examine both the individual and social welfare impacts of a program.

Transfer costs such as welfare or disability payments that redistribute income from one group to another may not be relevant from a societal perspective (Luce et al., 1996). From the frame of reference of an individual, these may be crucial. Nyman, for example, demonstrated that much of the purported moral hazard problem from health insurance is actually the welfare-enhancing income transfer effect that enhances access to costly care and motivates the consumer to buy insurance (Nyman, 2004).

A significant problem in the public health community is an unwillingness to assess the risk (defined as the probability of an event multiplied by the impact) in planning efforts. This has resulted in cases of poor risk communication that have distorted decision making regarding appropriate public health policies, because it often results in a distorted calculation of the potential benefits of an intervention. A classic example is the 1976–1977 swine flu fiasco, where communication of the occurrence of a 1918-type pandemic to President Ford as a certainty led to a series of catastrophic decisions that caused more harm than was prevented (Neustadt and Fineman, 1978). The same trend can be seen in recent impact assessments for scenarios such as a terrorist attack using biological weapons used to justify investing resources in preparedness programs (Kauffman et al., 1997). The accuracy of these assessments, however, is critically sensitive to the probability of exposure (Fowler et al., 2005). Such assessments have distorted policy-making with the effect of limiting the effectiveness of investments in the public health system (Avery, 2004). This unwillingness to estimate risk is often due to uncertainty resulting from incomplete information; however, Bayesian algorithms exist for estimating risk under such conditions of bounded rationality (Paté-Cornell, 2002).

Examples of the Economic Implications of Prevention

The use of cost-effectiveness analysis in the field of prevention can be illustrated by the following example from each level of prevention.

Primary Prevention

Vaccinations

Over 226,000 people in the United States are hospitalized and approximately 36,000 die each year from influenza and the complications that may result from such an infection (American Lung Association, 2008). Individuals are encouraged to get vaccinated not only to minimize their risk of infection but also to reduce the healthcare costs resulting from illness, estimated at \$71–\$167 billion annually in the United States (World Health Organization, 2003).

One study looked at the direct and indirect costs of the influenza vaccination in preschool children. This age bracket was chosen primarily because influenza generally infects more children than adults, and because of the high costs associated with childhood hospitalizations resulting from the flu. In this study, two vaccination settings were used: a restricted setting in which parents or guardians could only get their child vaccinated during normal work hours and a flexible setting that allowed the caregiver to chose when they wanted to bring their child in to get vaccinated. The cost of the vaccination was assumed to be \$10, which accounted for the vaccine, supplies, as well as personnel and administrative expenses. The direct costs that were studied were the costs incurred through physician visits for the infected child and secondarily infected adults (\$51), drugs (\$9.91), emergency room visits (~\$1242/visit), and the cost of hospitalization (roughly \$828/day). The indirect costs included in the analysis included wages lost by a parent who stayed home to care for an ill child or became ill after caring for their child and the time spent to obtain the vaccination. Net cost savings were seen in both settings. Vaccination in the restricted setting yielded a cost savings of $1.20 per patient and the flexible setting yielded a cost savings of $21.28 per patient (Cohen and Nettleman, 2000).

Despite these benefits, the CDC reported for the 2005–2006 flu season 76% of children remained unvaccinated (Santibanez et al., 2007). This raises the question of why, if the program generates savings, are children remaining unvaccinated? On one level, it can be noted that due to insurance coverage, the decision-makers (the parents) will rarely receive the measured benefit of the vaccination, while largely incurring the indirect costs. Other possible reasons include fear of autism, fear that vaccination will infect the child with the virus, and lack of time to obtain the immunization, indicating problems with identifying and measuring the utility value of costs relevant to the decision process.

Drinking Water Quality

Since the passage of the Clean Water Act in 1972 and the Safe Drinking Water Act (SDWA) in 1973, U.S. citizens have taken clean and safe potable water granted. The Clean Water Act established regulations for the discharge of pollutants into water and quality standards for surface waters. In March of 1993, a combination of ineffective chemicals, inadequate filtration, and poor weather conditions led to the largest cryptosporidium outbreak in Milwaukee, Minnesota (MacKenzie et al., 1994). Cryptosporidium is a protozoan parasite spread by the fecal–oral route that primarily affects the intestines in mammals and typically presents itself as a short-term diarrheal infection. During this month-long outbreak, over 403,000 residents became ill. The cost of the outbreak-associated illness was roughly $96.2 million with $31.7 million spent on medical costs and $64.6 in productivity losses. Individuals stricken with the illness were grouped into three categories: mild, moderate, and severe. The average cost of illness for individuals with a mild case was $116, $475 for those with moderate cases and $7808 for severe cases. A majority of the medical costs could be attributed to those with moderate and severe illnesses; however, those also infected with autoimmune diseases such as AIDS incurred medical costs as high as $18,000. The average ill person incurred $79 in medical costs and $160 in productivity losses. This outbreak not only negatively affected the health of thousands of individuals but had a profound impact on the economy as many people were out of work and many businesses were at a stand still. Following the outbreak, a new water purification system was installed costing $90 million, which was ultimately cheaper than the total cost of the outbreak ($96.2 million.) Even though the outbreak was a costly event that could have been prevented, some positive aspects did come from it (Corso et al., 2003). After this outbreak, changes were made around the world regarding water testing, treatment, and disease surveillance (Gradus et al., 1994). Since these changes have been enacted, there have not been any cryptosporidium outbreaks similar to the one that occurred in Milwaukee.

This is not to say that all preventive efforts designed to assure safe drinking water are effective. Proposals to reduce the maximum allowable levels of the volatile carcinogen trichloroethene in drinking water supplies from 11 to 2.2 μg/L, for example, were found to have a potential net cost of $34 million per life-year gained (Teng et al., 1995). In another example, a decision by voters in Pennsylvania to reject a tax increase to fund water treatment plant improvements in the aftermath of *Giardia* outbreak was found to be rational after the costs of alternative means of obtaining safe drinking water, such as boiling or purchase of bottle water, were calculated and found to be lower than the upgrades preferred by regulators (Laughland et al., 1993). The latter example is instructive as a reminder that what appears to be an optimal technical solution may in fact be less efficient than simple alternatives that are outside of the paradigmatic perspective of accepted experts.

Air Quality

The biggest problem currently affecting residents of California is air pollution. In one study, it was said that more individuals died in 2006 from respiratory related illnesses (3812) than vehicular deaths

(2521). Currently, San Joaquin Valley and the South Coast Air Basin are not meeting the standards for ozone and particulate matter. The cost of air pollution in these two regions is as much as $28 billion each year ($1600 per person in San Joaquin Valley and $1250 in the South Coast Air Basin) when medical costs, missed work days, lost income, school absences, and premature mortality were taken into account. If the current air standards were met in California, the state could prevent 13 premature deaths of infants, 1,950 cases of adult onset of chronic bronchitis, 3,860 premature deaths among individuals ages 30 years and older, 2,760 hospital admissions, 141,370 asthma attacks, 2,800 emergency room visits, 466,880 lost days of work, and two million cases of upper respiratory problems each year. Meeting current air standards however is not an easy task. To meet current standards, over 170,000 business owners would have to invest $5.5 billion dollars in order to reduce the emissions on their diesel trucks. If such an investment is made, the state could expect to see a savings in healthcare costs of $68 billion (Hall et al., 2008). A significant problem arises, however, in that the benefits of the regulations accrue to different parties than those who would bear the costs of compliance, resulting in little natural incentive to improve air quality.

Air quality regulation is an area where regulators have been notably resistant to the use of cost-effective alternatives. A classic case was observed in Yorktown, Virginia, where the Yorktown Prevention Project, a collaborative effort by environmental activists, Amoco, and state regulators, conducted a comprehensive study of emissions at a local Amoco refinery. The effort identified alternatives to EPA regulatory mandates that would result in greater reduction of air pollution at a savings of 80% of the cost of the EPA-mandated technology. The EPA Office of Air, which had refused to participate in the effort, attempted to block the negotiated regulatory change at the last minute because, as one participant noted, the organization "realized that their rules were going to look really stupid," with "damaging effects on its reputation" (Weber, 1998).

Physical Activity Promotion

Obesity is currently one of the main health concerns as seen by many healthcare workers as it has been linked to diabetes, hypertension, cardiovascular disease, and an array of other ailments. In an attempt to promote healthy living, there has been a recent push for exercise-based health promotion interventions. For years, physicians have been advocates in prescribing exercise as a preventative and rehabilitative therapy. Few studies of the effectiveness of these programs have included an economic evaluation; however, Kahn et al. (2002) assessed the economic and health implications of exercise in preventing coronary heart disease. Two cohorts consisting of 1000 men were followed for a 30-year period to detect the variance in the quality of life, the number of coronary heart disease events, and the life expectancy between the two groups. Through this intervention it was assumed that members of the exercise regimen cohort would have fewer coronary heart disease events, an increased life expectancy, and a better quality of life as compared to their counterparts. Costs associated with exercise included direct costs such as the cost of exercise equipment, exercise counseling, routine physical examinations, injuries resulting from exercise, and the indirect cost of the monetary value an individual places on time. For individuals who enjoyed exercise it was assumed that they did not place a monetary value on the time they spent working out, for individuals who were indifferent toward exercise it was assumed they valued their time at $4.50/hour, and for those individuals who disliked exercise they valued their time at $9/hour. The direct costs associated with CHD included emergency room visits, hospitalization, physician visits, medications, surgeries, and other treatments; and the indirect costs included loss of income due to morbidity, disability, or death. Through this study, participants in the exercise cohort experienced 78.1 fewer CHD events and gained 1138.3 QALYs. Exercise costs ($11,313/QALY) gained, which is favorable when compared to the QALY's of treating hypertension ($25,000–$60,000) or mild angina ($40,000). The study was sensitive to the time valuation placed on exercise. Where the opportunity cost of time spent on exercise was high, the relative efficiency of physical activity diminished (Hatziandreu et al., 1988).

Secondary Prevention

Colorectal Cancer

In 2008, over 50,000 individuals died from colorectal cancer, a decline from previous years (National Cancer Institute, 2009). Annual screening for men and women aged 50 years and older is strongly encouraged. Colorectal cancer screening, however, was among the eight preventive services with the lowest delivery rates (Maciosek et al., 2006). Screening procedures include fecal occult blood testing, colonoscopy, double-contrast barium enema, and flexible sigmoidoscopy. In recent years, there has been a shift in screening methods prescribed by physicians due to medical advancements and changes in cost-effectiveness. In 2001, screening with double-contrast barium enema examination every 3 years, or every 5 years with annual fecal occult blood testing, proved to be the most cost-effective method with an incremental cost-effectiveness ratio of less than $55,600/life-year saved. Colonoscopy proved to be the least cost-effective with an ICER of more than $100,000/life-year saved (McMahon et al., 2001). Five years later, in a study published in the *American Journal of Preventative Medicine*, colonoscopy was deemed the most cost-effective screening method at $8800/life-year saved, followed by annual fecal occult blood testing ($13300/life-year saved), and finally 5-year sigmoidoscopy ($18,900). Such changes can be attributed to the increased acceptance of colonoscopy as a reliable screening method among the medical community and changes in frequencies of utilization. Physicians choose colonoscopy and CT colonography over other methods as they can visualize both the rectum and colon at once and screenings only need to be preformed every 5–10 years. Although it is clear that colonoscopies can be beneficial, many individuals still fail to adhere to screening guidelines. Ten thousand additional deaths would be prevented each year if universal screening was offered, an over 12,000 deaths would be prevented if all individuals accepted screening (Maciosek et al., 2006). Barriers, representing unmeasured transaction costs in the analysis relevant to the decision to undergo screening, include poor doctor–patient communication, lack of patient knowledge of the procedure, fear of the examination and its risks, the opportunity cost of time, and costs of access to screening facilities.

Breast Cancer

Due to heavy funding for research, significant advances have been made in the treatment of breast cancer. For localized breast cancer the 5-year survival rate is 98% today, an increase of 18% since 1950. It is known that women who are carriers of the BRCA ½ mutations are at a greater risk for developing breast cancer. It is suggested that women begin mammography screenings once they reach the age of 40. Women whose breast cancer is first detected with a mammogram tend to live longer than those who find their breast cancer through other screening methods such as a self breast exam (Tabar et al., 2003). Although mammography is a great tool for detecting breast cancer in most women, it is not as beneficial for women with BRCA ½ mutations. Physicians have found that mammography is often unable to detect the cancer in these women; and many are using magnetic resonance imaging (MRI). MRI presents its own complications however. It is 10 times as expensive as mammography, and thus many insurance companies do not cover the costs of additional screenings. MRI also provides a better picture of the breast tissue, which results in a greater number of false positives compared to mammography. A comparison exist of the economic and health outcomes of BRCA ½ mutation carriers who did not participate in screening, those who obtained annual mammograms from ages 25–69, and those whom received annual mammography from ages 25–69 plus annual MRI for specific age groups. The cost of adding annual MRI from ages 25–69 is $88,651/QALY for BRCA 1 carriers and $188,034 for BRCA 2 carriers. Other than mammography alone, the strategy with the lowest cost per QALY gained adds annual MRI from ages 40–49 at a cost of $43,484/QALY for BRCA 1 carriers and $111,600/QALY for BRCA 2 carriers. Overall, it was determined that MRI screening was more cost-effective for BRCA 1 carriers than BRCA 2 carriers, as these carriers are at a greater risk for developing cancer, and their cancer tends to be more aggressive. Use of MRI was less cost-effective in women ages 25–34, who are less likely to develop breast cancer, and women over the age of 55, because of declining quality of life (Plevritis et al., 2006).

Tertiary Prevention

Specialist versus Primary Care Services

Specialist services are often believed to be a source of higher healthcare costs and inefficiency due to an increased number of diagnostic tests performed by these physicians. The reality is that they are often times able to provide more efficient and effective care than general practitioners. Northwestern University Medical School researchers evaluated the role of specialists in preventing the emergence of the "$100,000 Asthmatic," an individual whose asthma-induced expenditures exceed $100,000. Medical costs for most asthmatics range from $150 to $2500 each year. By increasing the number of patients managed by specialists, fewer asthmatics accumulated high medical expenditures. Specialist's patients were more likely to receive proper disease management, such as oral corticosteroids, inhaled corticosteroids, and daily medications, when compared to those managed by a primary care physician. Because specialists were more aggressive in their treatment, they were able to reduce unexpected doctor visits, emergency room visits, and hospital stays, resulting in lower medical expenditure (Greenberger, 1999). A similar study examined how hospital-care specialists affected clinical outcomes and costs. Hospital patients were either assigned to one of the 58 general internists or one of the two hospitalists. General internists devoted a smaller percentage of their time to hospital care than the hospitalists as there were more internists. The average adjusted costs per patient increased by $100 for the internists, and fell by $629 for the hospitalists. Although these changes seem relatively small, hospitalists produced savings of more than $600,000 over a 2-year period and had lower rates for emergency room visits (7.6%), 30-day readmission (10.8%), and in-hospital mortality (1.9%) than internists (8.2%, 12.2%, and 2.2%). Patients seen by hospitalists also had shorter hospital stays compared to internists, which also aided in reducing medical expenditures (Meltzer et al., 2002). Likewise, it has been found that while nominally more expensive, the use of orthopedic specialists as opposed to general practitioners to provide care for musculoskeletal problems is more efficient when outcome differences are considered (Nyman et al., 1998).

Rehabilitation

Stroke

Between 500,000 and 750,000 Americans suffer from a stroke each year, and over 160,000 will not survive their stroke. Strokes are one of the top causes of disability in the United States, leaving individuals facing significant functional impairment. The economic impact stokes is between $40 and $70 billion each year, largely associated with the care and rehabilitation needed following a stroke (St. John's Hospital, 2009). In the Copenhagen Stroke Study, 1197 acute stroke patients were followed. The average length of hospital stay was 27.1 days and the direct cost per patient was $12,150, which had included all rehabilitation and acute care. Individuals whose strokes were more severe incurred greater medical fees as their hospital stay was likely to be longer. All patients received daily therapy by physiotherapists, occupational therapists, and the nursing staff in the neurological ward of Bispebjerg Hospital. It was determined that social and medical factors such as age, gender, stroke type, hypertension, diabetes, and lifestyle factors did not influence the length of hospital stays for patients enrolled in the study. Based on their findings, it was concluded that the only way to reduce the direct costs associated to a stroke is to reduce the initial stroke severity or improve the rate of recovery (Jorgensen et al., 1997). A study was conducted in Denmark of two communities with programs for stroke patients. The first program was a dedicated stroke unit that provided both treatment and rehabilitation for patients in the region, the other program treated patients on general medical and neurological wards. Treatment on the stroke unit reduced the relative risk of discharge to a nursing home by 40% and almost doubled the chance of home discharge, and reduced the relative risk of death by 50%. Length of hospital stay among individuals in the stroke unit program was reduced by 30%, which resulted in a savings of 1313 bed days/100 stroke patients. Examining the cost of rehabilitative care when provided in a hospital setting versus a skilled nursing facility found that patients enrolled in a program where they received rehabilitative care at the hospital received twice as much care, making such a program more expensive. Costs for patients enrolled in the hospital program were $41,129 versus $18,129 for the skilled nursing facility. Charges per unit of functional status gain were $960 for hospital patients and $591 for patients in the nursing facility (Keith, 1996). Under this model, patient outcomes were significantly better from a rehabilitation program implemented in the hospital, but the overall efficiency was better for the nursing home option. This example highlights the potential gap between providing the best care for the patient and the best allocation of societal resources.

Discussion

Cost-effectiveness remains a crucial, if controversial and somewhat ill-defined, issue in preventive medicine and public health. Although advocates for preventive programs often argue that a program should be adopted because of the economic burden of disease, this does not mean that the prevention program will actually realize the savings implied by these costs. Understanding the economic implications of a preventive program requires careful attention to the assumptions underlying the calculations of the costs and net benefits of the intervention.

The techniques of cost-effectiveness are sensitive to assumptions and measurements, and debate remains over how to deal with the problems that these issues present. Despite these problems, no other realistic alternative exists to the use of cost-effectiveness analysis to assess the efficiency of resource use in preventive programs, whether in a healthcare organization operating in a relatively unconstrained market or by a government agency choosing to exert a command-and-control style regulatory program. Addressing the economic implications is necessary to build a business case for implementing an intervention and assuring that resources are best used for the program rather than alternative uses for resources. This, however, is controversial to those who consider the problem from a romantic viewpoint that does not acknowledge resource constraints or a monotechnic viewpoint wedded to a one-size-fits-all technical solution. Particularly in regulatory interventions, this tension between resource constraints and idealized solutions has become a problem in developing appropriate policy solutions to maximize individual and social welfare.

References

American Lung Association. 2008. Did you know? American Lung Association, Washington, DC. Available from http://www.facesofinfluenza.org/en/influenza-symptoms/ (cited January 12, 2009).

Arrow, K. J., M. L. Cropper, G. C. Eads, R. W. Hahn, L. B. Lave, R. G. Noll, P. R. Portney, M. Russell, R. Schmalensee, V. K. Smith, and R. N. Stavins. 1996. Is there a role for benefit-cost analysis in environmental, health, and safety regulation? *Science* 272:221–222.

Avery, G. 2004. Bioterrorism, fear, and public health reform: Matching a policy solution to the wrong window. *Public Administration Review* 64(3):275–288.

Barendregt, J. J., L. Bonneux, and P. J. van der Maas. 1997. The health care costs of smoking. *New England Journal of Medicine* 337(15):1052–1057.

Casalino, L. P. 2003. Benefits and barriers to large medical group practices in the United States. *Archives of Internal Medicine* 163(15):1958–1964.

Chao, S. and Forum on the Science of Health Care Quality Improvement and Implementation. 2008. *Creating a Business Case for Quality Improvement Research: Expert Views* (Workshop Summary). Washington, DC: National Academies Press.

Christianson, J. B. and G. Avery. 2004. Prepaid group practice and health care policy. In *Toward a 21st Century Health System: The Contributions and Promise of Prepaid Group Practice*, A. C. Enthoven and L. A. Tollen (eds.). San Francisco, CA: Jossey-Bass.

Coase, R. H. 1960. The problem of social cost. *Journal of Law and Economics* 3:1–44.

Cohen, G. M. and M. D. Nettleman. 2000. Economic impact of influenza vaccination in preschool children. *Pediatrics* 106(5):973.

Conover, C. J. 2004. Health care regulation: A $169 billion hidden tax. Washington, DC: The Cato Institute, p. 29.

Corso, P. S., M. H. Kramer, K. A. Blair, D. G. Addiss, J. P. Davis, and A. C. Haddix. 2003. Cost of Illness in the 1993 waterborne cryptosporidium outbreak, Milwaukee, Wisconsin. *Emerging Infectious Diseases* 9(4):426–431.

Dawson, A. and M. Verweij. 2007. Introduction: Ethics, prevention, and public health. In *Ethics, Prevention, and Public Health*, A. Dawson and M. Verweij (eds.). Oxford, U.K.: Oxford University Press.

Drummond, M. F., B. O'Brien, G. L. Stoddart, and G. W. Torrance. 1997. *Methods for the Economic Evaluation of Health Care Programmes*, 2nd edn. Oxford, U.K.: Oxford University Press.

Eddy, D. M. 2004. Technology assessment, deployment, and implementation in prepaid group practice. In *Toward a 21st Century Health System: The Contributions and Promise of Prepaid Group Practice*, A. C. Enthoven and L. A. Tollen (eds.). San Francisco, CA: Jossey-Bass.

Enthoven, A. C. and L. A. Tollen. 2004. Preface. In *Toward a 21st Century Health System: Contributions and Promise of Prepaid Group Practice*, A. C. Enthoven and L. A. Tollen (eds.). San Francisco, CA: Jossey-Bass.

Feacham, R. G. A., N. D. Sekhri, and K. L. White. 2002. Getting more for their dollar: A comparison of the NHS with California's Kaiser Permanente. *British Medical Journal* 324:135–141.

Fireman, B., J. Bartlett, and J. Selby. 2004. Can disease management reduce health care costs by improving quality? *Health Affairs* 23(6):63–75.

Foote, Susan. 2002. Why Medicare cannot promulgate a national coverage rule: A case of regula mortis. *Journal of Health Politics, Policy, and Law* 27 (5):707–730.

Foster, Kenneth R., Paolo Vecchia, and Michael H. Rapacholi. 2000. Risk management: Science and the precautionary principle. *Science* 288 (5468):979–981.

Fowler, R. A., G. D. Sanders, D. M. Bravata, B. Nouri, J. M. Gastwirth, D. Peterson, A. G. Broker, A. M. Garber, and D. K. Owens. 2005. Cost-effectiveness of defending against bioterrorism: A comparison of vaccination and antibiotic prophylaxis against anthrax. *Annals of Internal Medicine* 142 (8):601–610.

Fries, J. F., C. E. Koop, C. E. Beadle, P. B. Cooper, M. J. England, R. F. Greaves, J. J. Sokolov, and D. Wright. 1993. Reducing health care costs by reducing the need and demand for medical services. *New England Journal of Medicine* 329 (5):321–325.

Fuchs, V. 1973. *Who Shall Live? Health, Economics, and Social Choice*. New York: Basic Books, Inc.

Garber, A. M., M. C. Weinstein, G. W. Torrance, and M. S. Kamlet. 1996. Theoretical foundations of cost-effectiveness analysis. In *Cost Effectiveness in Health and Medicine*, M. M. Gold, J. E. Siegel, L. B. Russell, and M. C. Weinstein (eds.), Oxford, U.K.: Oxford University Press.

Gostin, L. O. and L. Stone. 2007. Health of the people: The highest law? In *Ethics, Prevention, and Public Health*, A. Dawson and M. Verweij (eds.), Oxford, U.K.: Oxford University Press.

Gradus, M. S., A. Singh, and G. V. Sedmak. 1994. The Milwaukee cryptosporidium outbreak: Its impact on drinking water standards, laboratory diagnosis, and public health surveillance *Clinical Microbiology Newsletter* 16 (8):57–60.

Graham, J. D., P. S. Corso, J. M. Morris, M. Segui-Gomez, and M. C. Weinstein. 1998. Evaluating the cost-effectiveness of clinical and public health measures. *Annual Review of Public Health* 19:125–152.

Granata, A. V. and A. L. Hillman. 1998. Competing practice guidelines: Using cost effectiveness analysis to make optimal decisions. *Annals of Internal Medicine* 128 (1):56–63.

Greenberger, P. A. 1999. Preventing the emergence of the $100,000 asthmatic. Review of Reviewed Item. *Medscape General Medicine* (3), http://www.medscape.com/viewarticle/408723.

Grimshaw, J., N. Freemantle, S. Wallace, I. Russell, B. Hurwitz, I. Watt, A. Long, and T. Sheldon. 1995. Developing and implementing clinical practice guidelines. *Quality in Healthcare* 4:55–64.

Grimshaw, J. M. and A. Hutchinson. 1995. Clinical practice guidelines—Do they enhance value for money in health care? *British Medical Bulletin* 51:927–940.

Hahn, R. W. 1996. *The EPA's True Cost*. Washington, DC: The American Enterprise Institute.

Hall, J. V., V. Brajer and F. W. Lurman. 2008. *The Benefits of Meeting Federal Clean Air Standards in the South Cost and San Joaquin Valley Air Basins*. Fullerton, CA: California State University.

Hatziandreu, E. J., J. P. Koplan, M. C. Weinstein, C. J. Caspersen, and K. E. Warner. 1988. A cost-effectiveness analysis of exercise as a health promotion activity. *American Journal of Public Health* 78 (11):1417–1421.

Haycox, A., A. Bagust, and T. Walley. 1999. Clinical guidelines—The hidden costs. *British Medical Journal* 318:391–393.

Henson, S. and J. Caswell. 1999. Food safety regulation: An overview of contemporary issues. *Food Policy* 24:589–603.

Jena, A. B. and T. Philipson. 2008. *Innovation and Technology Adoption in Healthcare Markets*. Washington, DC: The AEI Press.

Jorgensen, H. S., H. Nakayama, H. O. Raaschou, and T. S. Olsen. 1997. Acute stroke care and rehabilitation: An analysis of the direct cost and its clinical and social determinants. *Stroke* 28 (6):1138–1141.

Kahn, E. B., L. T. Ramsey, R. C. Brownson, G. W. Heath, E. H. Howze, K. E. Powell, E. J. Stone, M. W. Rajab, P. Corso, and the Task Force on Community Preventive Services. 2002. The effectiveness of interventions to increase physical activity. *American Journal of Preventive Medicine* 22 (Suppl 4): 73–107.

Kauffman, A. F., M. Meltzer, and G. P. Schmid. 1997. The economic impact of a bioterrorist attack: Are prevention and postattack intervention programs justifiable? *Emerging Infectious Diseases* 3 (2):83–94.

Keith, R. A. 1996. Rehabilitation after stroke: Cost-effectiveness analysis. *Journal of the Royal Society of Medicine* 89:631–633.

Laughland, A. S., L. M. Musser, W. N. Musser and J. S. Shortle. 1993. The opportunity cost of time and averting expenditures for safe drinking water. *Journal of the American Water Resources Association* 29 (2):291–299.

Luce, B. R., W. G. Manning, J. E. Siegel, and J. Lipscomb. 1996. Estimating costs in cost effectiveness analysis. In *Cost-Effectiveness in Health and Medicine*, M. M. Gold, J. E. Siegel, L. B. Russell, and M. C. Weinstein (eds.), Oxford, U.K.: Oxford University Press.

MacKenzie, W. R., N. J. Hoxie, M. E. Proctor, M. S. Gradus, K. A. Blair, D. E. Peterson, J. J. Kazmierczak, D. G. Addiss, K. R. Fox, J. B. Rose, and J. P. Davis. 1994. A massive outbreak in Milwaukee of cryptosporidium infection transmitted through the public water supply. *New England Journal of Medicine* 331 (3):161–167.

Maciosek, M. V., L. I. Solberg, A. B. Coffield, N. M. Edwards, and M. J. Goodman. 2006. Colorectal screening: Health impact and cost effectiveness. *American Journal of Preventative Medicine* 31 (1):80–87.

Mason, J., N. Freemantle, I. Nazareth, M. Eccles, A. Haines, and M. Drummond. 2001. When is it cost-effective to change the behavior of health professionals? *Journal of the American Medical Association* 286 (23):2988–2992.

Max, W. 2001. The financial impact of smoking on health-related costs: A review of the literature. *American Journal of Health Promotion* 15 (5):321–331.

McMahon, P. M., J. L. Bosch, S. Gleason, E. F. Halpern, J. S. Lester, and G. S. Gazelle. 2001. Cost-effectiveness of colorectal cancer screening. *Radiology* 219 (1):44–50.

Meltzer, D., W. G. Manning, J. Morrison, M. N. Shah, L. Jin, T. Guth, and W. Levinson. 2002. Effects of physician experience on costs and outcomes on an academic general medicine service: Results of a trial of hospitalists. *Annals of Internal Medicine* 137 (11):866–874.

Miller, R. H. and H. S. Luft. 2002. HMO plan performance update: An analysis of the literature, 1997–2001. *Health Affairs* 21 (4):63–86.

National Cancer Institute. 2009. Colorectal cancer screening. National Cancer Institute, Washington, DC, October 10, 2008. Available from Colorectal Cancer Screening (cited March 21, 2009).

Neumann, P. J., P. D. Jacobsen, and J. A. Palmer. 2008. Measuring the value of public health systems: The disconnect between health economists and public health practitioners. *American Journal of Public Health* 98 (12):2173–2180.

Neustadt, R. and H. Fineman. 1978. *The Swine Flu Affair: Decision-Making on a Slippery Slope*. Washington, DC: Department of Health, Education, and Welfare.

Nyman, J. A. 2004. Is 'Moral Hazard' inefficient? The policy implications of a new theory. *Health Affairs* 23 (5):194–199.

Nyman, J. A, W. G. Manning, S. Samuels, and B. F. Morrey. 1998. Can specialists reduce costs? The case of referrals to orthopaedic surgeons. *Clinical Orthopaedics and Related Research* 350:257–267.

Office of Management and Budget. 1993. Regulatory program of the United States government: April 1, 1992–March 31, 1993. Washington, DC: Government Printing Office.

Paté-Cornell, E. 2002. Risk and uncertainty analysis in government safety decisions. *Risk Analysis* 22 (3):633–646.

Plevritis, S. K., A. W. Kurian, B. M. Sigal, B. L. Daniel, D. M. Ikeda, F. E. Stockdale, and A. M. Garber. 2006. Cost-effectiveness of screening BRCA ½ mutation carriers with breast magnetic resonance imaging. *Journal of the American Medical Association* 295 (20):2374–2384.

Rice, D. P., T. A. Hodgson, P. Sinsheimer, W. Browner, and A. N. Kopstein. 1986. The economic costs of the health effects of smoking, 1984. *The Milbank Quarterly* 64 (4):489–547.

Rose, G. 1992. *The Strategy of Preventive Medicine*. Oxford, U.K.: Oxford University Press.

Russell, L. B. 1986. *Is Prevention Better than Cure?* Washington, DC: The Brookings Institution.

Russell, L. B. 1993. The role of prevention in health reform. *New England Journal of Medicine* 329 (5):352–354.

Sandin, P. 1999. Dimensions of the precautionary principle. *Human and Ecological Risk Assessment* 5 (5):889–907.

Santibanez, T. A, J. M. Santoli, G. Mootrey, G. L. Euler, and A. Fiore. 2007. Influenza vaccination coverage among children aged 6–23 months—United States, 2005–06 influenza season. *Morbidity and Mortality Weekly Report* 56 (37):959–963.

Schneider, M. 2006. *Introduction to Public Health*, 2nd edn. Sudbury, MA: Jones and Bartlett.

Shaneyfelt, T. M., M. F. Mayo-Smith, and J. Rothwangi. 1999. Are guidelines following guidelines? The methodological quality of clinical practice guidelines in the peer-reviewed medical literature. *Journal of the American Medical Association* 281 (20):1900–1905.

St. John's Hospital. 2009. Stroke facts 2009. St. John's Hospital, Springfield, IL. Available from http://www.st-johns.org/services/stroke_center/stroke_facts.aspx (cited February 24, 2009).

Strategic Advisory Board. 1990. *Reducing Risk: Setting Priorities and Strategies for Environmental Risk*. Washington, DC: United States Environmental Protection Agency.

Tabar, L., M. Yen, B. Vitak, H. T. Chen, R. A. Smith, and S. W. Duffy. 2003. Mammography service screening and mortality in breast cancer patients: 20-year follow-up before and after introduction of screening. *Lancet* 361 (9367):1405–1410.

Teng, T. O., M. E. Adams, J. S. Pliskin, D. G. Safran, J. E. Siegel, M. C. Weinstein, and J. D. Graham. 1995. Five-hundred life-saving interventions and their cost-effectiveness. *Risk Analysis* 15 (3):369–390.

United States Congress. 2004. Joint Economic Committee. The burden of health services regulation: Testimony before the joint economic committee of the United States congress. 108th Congress, Second Session. May 13, 2004.

van den Hoven, M. 2007. Reasonable limits to public health demands. In *Ethics, Prevention, and Public Health*, A. Dawson and M. Verweij (eds.), Oxford, U.K.: Oxford University Press.

Van, H., G. Cropper, and M. L. Cropper. 1996. When is a life too costly to save? The evidence from U.S. environmental regulation. *Journal of Environmental Economics and Regulation* 20:346–368.

Weber, E. P. 1998. *Pluralism by the Rules: Conflict and Cooperation in Environmental Regulation*, B. Rabe and J. Tierney (eds.), *American Governance and Public Policy*. Washington, DC: Georgetown University Press.

Woolf, S. H. and D. Atkins. 2001. The evolving role of prevention in health care: Contributions of the U.S. preventive services task force. *American Journal of Preventive Medicine* 20 (Suppl 1):13–20.

World Health Organization. 2003. Influenza. World Health Organization, Geneva, Switzerland, January 11, 2003. Available from http://www.who.int/mediacentre/factsheets/2003/fs211/en/ (cited January 11, 2009).

Design, Planning, Control, and Management of Healthcare Systems

IV.B Telemedicine

29 **Interactive Medicine** *Pamela Whitten, Samantha A. Nazione, and Jennifer Cornacchione* **29**-1
Defining Interactive Medicine • The Power to Communicate • Medical Fields Moving into the Future • Barriers and Nonbelievers • The Way Forward • Interactive Medicine in Action • Summary • References

29

Interactive Medicine

Pamela Whitten
Michigan State University

Samantha A. Nazione
Michigan State University

Jennifer Cornacchione
Michigan State University

Defining Interactive Medicine 29-1
The Power to Communicate 29-2
Medical Fields Moving into the Future 29-2
Diagnosis and Treatment • Management of Chronic Disease • Isolated Medicine
Barriers and Nonbelievers 29-7
The Way Forward 29-8
Interactive Medicine in Action 29-9
TeleKid Care • Telehospice • Home Monitoring for Congestive Heart Failure Patients
Summary 29-11
References 29-12

Defining Interactive Medicine

Eighteen-year-old Max wants nothing more than to keep a low profile during high school. However, Max's asthma makes this desire difficult. Max has to measure his peak flow everyday and take medication for his asthma. He is constantly forgetting to take these steps, which leads to the embarrassing result of his mom constantly nagging him. Recently, Dr. Monclave, Max's physician, connected Max's cell phone to an online computer system that can text message Max reminders. Max then text messages his peak flow to the system, which informs him and his physician of whether or not he is in good standing. Now when Max is managing his asthma, people might just think he is text messaging the cute redhead from chemistry class.

This is a true example of interactive medicine with the names changed to protect the participant's privacy (Holtz and Whitten 2009). Interactive medicine uses a variety of communication technologies to transmit health information between two or more parties. One of the advantages of interactive medicine is the freedom it allows its participants in terms of schedule and location. Individuals can choose the time and place that works best for them even if it does not work for others, depending on the needs of the interaction. As a result, interactive medicine can save time and money while providing services to those with limited access to care. Providing care through communication technologies also allows health facilities to share scarce resources such as specialists and subspecialists. For instance, only 9% of the country's physicians and 10% of the country's specialists practice in rural areas (Whitten and Sypher 2006). However, urban areas are often lacking resources as well. Urban telemedicine can improve patient management, general physician to specialist communication, provider education, timeliness, and the quality of care, especially for the uninsured (Grubaugh et al. 2008, Harrison et al. 1997, Maffei et al. 2008, Sheng et al. 1997). Interactive medicine is often referred to as telemedicine, telehealth, or e-health. Regardless of the rhetoric, the bottom line entails provision of health-related services using innovative telecommunication solutions. Furthermore, aiding patients in this format has been found to be effective in diagnosing, treating, and managing health issues across the globe (McConnochie et al. 2006).

This chapter will inform readers of the technologies used for performing interactive medicine, applications in the field of health, and challenges and needs associated with this practice. This chapter will conclude with three case studies that illustrate the potential impact of these solutions.

The Power to Communicate

In the broadest sense, there are two technologies that allow for interactive medicine, and both are defined by the timing of the interaction. The first kind of interactive technology is asynchronous, also known as store-and-forward. In asynchronous technologies, medical information is first captured by one party, then transmitted digitally to one or more other parties. Examples include the use of remote monitoring devices that can transmit patient information from distant locations, transmission of patient data via an electronic record, and a doctor text messaging a reminder to a patient on his/her cell phone. All of these technologies are not tied to a real-time interaction. The physician or patient can retrieve information when they have time rather than through a prescheduled appointment. Aside from this convenience, advantages of asynchronous technologies can include lower bandwidth requirements, lower costs, sharper images, and lighter equipment (Wootton 2006). The second type of interactive technology is synchronous, or real time, meaning the parties involved experience live communication. Examples include a child psychiatrist seeing students in their school via videoconferencing, a nurse checking in on an elderly patient at home via videophone, and an array of doctors learning about one another's cases via a tumor board. Instant feedback, incorporation of multiple elements simultaneously, ability to educate, and the ability to have the patient present during the consultation are some of the advantages of synchronous activities (Wootton 2006).

There is a trend for newer interactive technologies used for providing healthcare to be used for both asynchronous and synchronous communication (Wootton 2006). Mobile phones, for instance, can provide live feedback when used as a phone and convenient feedback when used as a short message system (SMS) for text messaging. The Internet is another instance where live video chats can take place, and e-mails can also be sent and retrieved freely. These types of technologies are used in a multitude of applications and locations.

Medical Fields Moving into the Future

Healthcare practice is no longer limited to healthcare facilities. Interactive medicine technologies are used in various locations and in nearly every field of medicine. These fields can be grouped into applications focused on diagnosis and treatment, management of chronic disease, and isolated medicine.

Diagnosis and Treatment

Interactive medicine is frequently used to diagnose and treat patients. Teleradiology is the most widespread and accepted form of interactive medicine (Mirza et al. 2008). The process of teleradiology requires a picture archiving system, a communication system, and a secure Internet network to transmit x-rays and diagnostic images (Kenny and Lau 2008). Teleradiology has many different uses including transmitting film for review by a radiologist at a convenient time, to receive a second opinion, and to gain access to a radiologist that would not otherwise be available (Kenny and Lau 2008). This application is successful because it is cost-effective, convenient, compatible, fast, and able to produce clear images (Dimmick and Ignatova 2006). Teleradiology allows for a quick response to cases, and can save time and money by avoiding unnecessary trips to a hospital by using a PC-based image transfer system (Kreutzer et al. 2008). Although store-and-forward technology is usually used for radiology purposes, real-time technology has also been used. Radiologists can use real-time technologies, such as videoconferencing equipment, for clinical discussions (Mort et al. 2009). Remote diagnosing is also used with synchronous technologies.

Telepsychiatry is one of the most frequently used clinical applications of telemedicine and is also one of the oldest forms of interactive medicine (Krupinski et al. 2008). In 1959, Wittson and his colleagues developed a two-way closed-circuit television system to deliver psychiatry consultations from the Nebraska Psychiatric Institute to the state's mental hospital (Grigsby 1997). With the use of telepsychiatry, individuals in underserved communities, such as prisons and rural areas, can have access to better behavioral healthcare. Videoconferencing is the preferred telepsychiatry channel (Maheu et al. 2001) because the synchronous technology enables interpersonal interactions between the clinician and patient (Krupinski et al. 2008). Research indicates that telepsychiatry is an effective way to provide better access to care for those suffering from post-traumatic stress disorder (PTSD), including war veterans (Frueh et al. 2007, Reger et al. 2009). Telepsychiatry is used with virtually every audience including children, adults, and the elderly, and within correctional facilities and schools (Hilty et al. 2004). Research suggests many benefits of telepsychiatry, such as improved access to care, chances for education, savings in time and money, and improved health (Pesamaa et al. 2004).

The use of interactive medicine for the treatment of dermatological issues is also widespread. Teledermatology is practiced with both real-time and store-and-forward technology (Mort et al. 2009, Whitten 2003). Practices include sending a digital image via e-mail to a specialist, using dermascopes or high-magnification video cameras (Wootton 2006). However, most of the evaluation studies in this field are done on store-and-forward technology and are concerned with the outcome of diagnosis accuracy (Eminovic et al. 2007). Mobile phones with cameras can also be used for dermatology, especially when individuals are away from home (Ebner et al. 2008). Patients capture and send an image of their skin lesion to a dermatologist. Overall, research indicates that store-and-forward technologies result in similar clinical outcomes as traditional care for dermatological issues (Ebner et al. 2008, Pak et al. 2007).

Oncologists are additional specialists often scarce in rural areas. The University of Kansas created the first teleoncology center in 1995 (Doolittle and Spaulding 2006). A television screen, video camera, speaker, and microphone were used to create an early videoconferencing system. Medical staff at the rural site also made use of an electronic stethoscope to allow the oncologist to listen to cardiac and breathing sounds of patients. Tomography scans and medical resonance images were also viewed online in real time. However, some patients expressed being uncomfortable with the nurse performing the inspection rather than the doctor. Another teleoncology intervention involved head and neck cancer patients. Individuals diagnosed with head and neck cancer are isolated because of physical debilitation and social limitations (Head et al. 2009). As a result, interactive medicine is used in Kentucky to provide support, education, and tools to better manage symptoms for head and neck cancer patients. Questions and information were programmed into a message device called Health Buddy, which plugs into an electrical outlet and telephone line. Both patients and physicians accepted the technology, and the patients found it easy to use.

Pathology has made use of real-time and store-and-forward technologies. Using interactive medicine in pathology helps when specialists are scarce (Horbinski and Wiley 2009). Whole slide imaging is one of the most common uses of telepathology today (Weinstein et al. 2009). Digital images of the slide are created, and then viewed using a virtual slide viewer. These virtual glass slides can be shared among pathologists via the Internet (Evans et al. 2009, Weinstein et al. 2009). Virtual microscopy is another type of technology used in pathology. This allows viewers to manipulate the virtual slides similar to the way they would using a traditional light microscope, such as positioning and brightness adjustments, while viewing the slide on a computer monitor (Weinstein et al. 2009). The Telehealth Rapid Breast Care Process in Arizona combined telepathology, telemammography, and teleoncology to avoid delays in services needed for breast cancer diagnosis and treatment plans by obtaining an immediate second opinion (Lopez et al. 2009). A virtual slide scanner was installed in the participating laboratory, and the glass slides of the breast tissue were scanned on the same day that they were produced to receive a timely second opinion. Overall, this program enhanced job satisfaction for pathologists who had not had training in breast pathology and prevented patients from having to travel to different locations to receive second opinions (Lopez et al. 2009).

Dentistry is another medical field that uses interactive medicine technologies. Park et al. (2009) tested three technologies for use in emergency dentistry: a special-purpose oral camera, a digital single lens reflex (DSLR) camera, and a mobile phone camera. Twenty participants were used to assess the connectivity, image quality, and usability of the devices. Each tool was found to have advantages and disadvantages for use in emergency situations. The DSLR had high image quality, but also a high cost; the oral camera was easy to use, but had poor image quality; and the mobile phone was easy to use but had unpredictable image quality. A project to provide early detection of cavities took place in six inner-city elementary schools and seven child care centers in New York where there was a shortage of dentists (Kopycka-Kedzierawski and Billings 2006). Dental assistants used intraoral cameras to take pictures of the children's teeth and sent the images to dentists for review. After recommendations had been made, the dental assistants called the parents to assist in setting up the proper dental care their child required. Over the first 9 months of the program, 123 patients were seen. However, this program did not require parents to follow through in seeking further care for their child, so care was not always sought. Once a health issue is diagnosed and treated, individuals must manage their condition.

Similarly, pediatrics, a growing field in telemedicine, uses various interactive medicine technologies to care for the newly born and adolescents. Synchronous technologies have been used to provide adolescent obesity consultations (Shaikh et al. 2008). Adolescents who met inclusion criteria went to a rural clinic to connect to a pediatric weight management specialist or endocrinologist via videoconferencing. Approximately 80% of patients who visited with the specialist displayed improvements with each visit related to lifestyle or weight (Shaikh et al. 2008). Tele-echocardiography is used to diagnose congenital health disease in newborn babies. One study used desktop videoconferencing computers to connect two community hospitals to a pediatric echocardiography laboratory (Sable et al. 2002). In 32 months, 500 telemedicine transactions took place. A total of 95% of the cases required transmission of an echocardiogram, and the largest condition represented in the cases was congenital heart disease. Asynchronous technology has also been useful in pediatrics (Callahan et al. 2005). ECHO-Pac, a store-and-forward system between pediatricians in the Western Pacific, was created because of the growing concerns amongst providers about the costs and scheduling needs of real-time telemedicine devices. ECHO-Pac used the Internet, a digital or video camera, and a scanner to send and receive pediatric subspecialty cases. A study taking place over 4 months found the system to save money and provide usable feedback regarding cases.

Interactive technologies are beneficial in caring for individuals at the end of their lives. Providing palliative care using interactive medicine is called telehospice. Benefits associated with telehospice include increased quality of care, decreased costs, and saved hospice worker time (Whitten et al. 2003). The majority of hospice practices (64.5%) were found to be eligible for telehospice during a content analysis of nurse notes (Doolittle et al. 2005). Videophones are frequently used in hospice care. These phones allow patients to be seen and heard by a nurse while they remain in their home. In an early videophone study, hospice patients and caregivers were excited about using the new technology, yet nurses were undecided regarding the quality of care it provided (Whitten et al. 2001). Videophones have also been tested regarding their usability among the elderly and hospice workers (Parker Oliver et al. 2005). Findings indicate that both parties perceived the phones to be easy to use and acceptable intervention tools. However, videophones have suffered from a lack of adoption in hospice care due to a lack of leadership, resources, and rewards to enforce uptake of the technology (Whitten et al. 2009a).

Management of Chronic Disease

Management of chronic disease is often aided by new technologies. Management through interactive medicine can be beneficial by increasing the amount of data collected. An increase in data collected can improve decision making, allow for more sensitive therapy adjustments, enable better patient–provider communication, and increase patient understanding of their health status (Hernando et al. 2006). Interactive medicine is often used at home to help individuals manage their chronic conditions. Home healthcare provides for individuals who are isolated, the elderly, and the chronically ill. For example, a system that monitors oxygen content can help those with asthma or chronic obstructive pulmonary diseases (COPD), and hand-held devices allow diabetic patients to transmit their glucose levels to a health practitioner (Botsis et al. 2008). One study used text messaging on cell phones to allow asthma patients to enter diary data regarding their health (Anhoj and Moldrup 2004). Participants were sent four messages a day including a medication reminder and questions regarding their peak flow, sleeping habits, and medication dosages. The majority of the 12 participants responded to most of the text messages they received. However, participants reported a desire to respond to only one message a day and to be able to view their diary data online (Anhoj and Moldrup 2004). Cell phones have also been used to attempt to overcome the barrier of noncompliance for HIV and AIDS patients undertaking therapy treatment (Puccion et al. 2006). Patients were given free cell phones for 6 months and were called regularly as a reminder. Most of the five patients found this process to be helpful rather than intrusive. However, the process did not appear to have long-term impacts.

Cardiovascular disease management has been performed using the Internet (Masucci et al. 2006). The system, Itsmyhealthfile, allowed individuals to submit data to their care provider. Participants were asked to enter data regarding their weight, blood pressure, number of cigarettes smoked, heart rate, and physical activity. Patients were also allowed to look online at educational materials and their health trends according to entered data. These types of online interventions can lead to better patient self-management skills and can track patient compliance. An Italian study documented chronic health failure (CHF) patients when they were treated by a physician with a telecardiology system compared to treatment with a home-based telecardiology system under medical supervision (Scalvini et al. 2006). The home patients used a portable electrocardiogram device that transferred ECG information to a nurse through a mobile phone or telephone. The physicians were given a portable electrocardiograph through a telephone that was connected to cardiologists who were available 24 hours a day to perform analyses. Both applications were found to work well and efficiently.

Elderly individuals are one specific population using interactive medicine for managing chronic diseases. Geriatrics is one of the less studied fields in this area despite relatively high patient acceptance (Brignell et al. 2007). This is unfortunate given the shortage of specialists in geriatric care. Additionally, a review of geriatric interactive medicine programs demonstrates that studies have shown to increase the effectiveness and efficiency of treatment for this group, but more studies are needed. A recent project using interactive medicine, IDEATel, was designed to enhance self-efficacy for an elderly population suffering from diabetes (Trief et al. 2009). Individuals were able to upload blood glucose and blood pressure readings over the Internet, videoconference with a nurse or dietitian, and to receive diabetes education. Increasing self-efficacy for older populations helped with controlling glycemic levels (Trief et al. 2009). Managing chronic disease using interactive medicine helps prevent unnecessary hospital visits and admission into long-term facilities (Darkins et al. 2008).

Isolated Medicine

Certain populations are cut off from the world's medical systems through geographical or institutional barriers. For these populations, interactive medicine provides one of the only means to receive care. The first astronauts in space in 1961 were measured using telemetry, which monitors life signs such as blood pressure (Williams et al. 2000). Videoconferencing and broadband Internet–based technologies have also been used. The first telemedicine instrumentation package (TIP) was a computer-based system that displayed video images of the eyes, ears, nose, throat, and skin. These tools have expanded over time as genitourinary ultrasounds can now be preformed in space (Jones et al. 2009). However, not all technology is able to function in space. Those flying closer to Earth also use interactive medicine (Ferrer-Roca et al. 2002). The average airplane is equipped with an emergency medical kit, a first-aid kit, and an automatic external defibrillator for en route medical problems. Additionally, some planes practice telemetry. Telephones or radios connected to medical establishments are used concurrently with these items to care for ill passengers. However, tools used on airplanes must withstand high cabin pressure levels and not interfere with aircraft signals (Ferrer-Roca et al. 2002). Additionally, it is important for emergency physicians to respond to in-flight emergencies because they can provide better medical advice compared to nonemergency physicians (Urwin et al. 2008). Interactive medicine can also be conducted on boats to provide care to individuals off-land (Telemedicine News 2007). A boat built to withstand harsh weather was used to service rural islands off the coast of Maine. The boat had a screening room, a videoconferencing system with ISDN lines connected to the nearest hospital, and a magnifying camera to give distant physicians a closer look at the patient's features. A present nurse conversed with a physician or psychiatrist to provide care.

Treatment information via interactive medicine is also sought by developing countries which are often cut off from robust medical care. An already-existing mobile surgery program in Ecuador was improved through the use of communication technologies (Cone et al. 2009). For patients in remote areas, an electronic health record was created and e-mailed to medical staff at a large hospital. The practitioner then assessed the situation, recommended further diagnostics tests, and scheduled surgery, if necessary. The surgery occurred in a truck that has an operating room, and videoconferencing was sometimes used for pre- and postoperative care. Dial-up modems were sufficient for the communication to occur between the rural and urban patients and practitioners (Cone et al. 2009). RetCams have been used to help diagnose and treat retinoblastoma in children in El Salvador, Guatemala, and Honduras (Wilimas et al. 2009). The RetCam was used to upload pictures onto the Web. Various Web sites allowed for consultations via the Internet between healthcare workers in these developing countries and specialists in developed countries, composed of a U.S.-trained pediatric ophthalmologist and a treatment team that included the International Outreach Program at the St. Jude Children's Hospital and the ocular oncology team at the University of Tennessee Hamilton Eye Institute. Children treated with this telemedicine service experienced significantly lower treatment abandonment and refusal rates, as well as an increase in salvaged eyes (Wilimas et al. 2009).

Correctional facilities are another isolated population using interactive medicine. Numerous prison systems have acquired interactive technologies to serve inmates. A 2004 survey of correctional facilities in all 50 United States found that approximately 40% of these sites were making use of interactive technology to provide care because of the access, safety, and cost savings it provided (Larsen et al. 2004). Those not using the services cited technology costs and faculty non-adoption as problems. Using interactive medicine in correctional facilities saves the time and money that is required to physically transport inmates to a health facility and reduces the danger of escape or assault (Maheu et al. 2001). In one study, adolescents in correctional facilities were referred to receive special healthcare via a videoconferencing system (Fox et al. 2007). Most of the cases involved mental healthcare provided by a pediatric psychiatrist. This allowed many of the misdiagnosed adolescents to receive proper care and treatment. Wait times from referral to treatment declined by almost 60% because the adolescents did not have to be transported, and the process of scheduling and rescheduling appointments was simplified. Furthermore, outpatient use increased by 40% and emergency visits decreased by 7% (Fox et al. 2007).

The Department of Corrections in Virginia and the Virginia Commonwealth University Health System collaborated to provide a surgical telemedicine clinic for 16 prisons (Lavrentyev et al. 2008). A preoperative consultation occurred between the surgeon and inmate via videoconferencing equipment. Additionally, a dermascope camera was used to examine potential conditions such as hernia protrusion, and electronic stethoscopes were used to assess breathing, heart, and bowel sounds. Patients signed consent forms electronically, and postoperative consultations also took place. Prison inmates have generally been satisfied with their telemedicine interactions, and research indicates that there is little difference between face-to-face encounters and telemedicine interactions, especially in telemental health (Morgan et al. 2008). Not only are prisoners satisfied, but healthcare providers like using technologies as well because many correctional facilities are located in rural areas, thus eliminating the need for health practitioners to travel long distances and be in dangerous situations (Maheu et al. 2001).

Interactive medicine technology has been incorporated in both rural and urban schools to care for their student populations. Many children do not receive heath care simply because their guardians are not aware of locations at which they could seek treatment, do not have transportation to take the child to receive treatment, or cannot take time off from work to take their child to receive treatment. However, children across the globe regularly attend schools, making these institutions excellent sites at which to create awareness of and treat health needs. One interactive medicine program used videoconferencing equipment with an electronic stethoscope, endoscope, and otoscope to provide care (Young and Ireson 2003). The program was implemented at one urban and two rural elementary schools based on financial need. The practice provided physical and mental healthcare. Over a 2-year period, 142 consultations were provided over the system, which represented 4.3% of all students coming to see the school nurse. Another telemedicine program was implemented in 12 schools to help children aged 5–14 manage their type 1 diabetes (Izquierdo et al. in press). Children were provided with a blood glucose–monitoring device to use every 4–6 hours. Additionally, videoconferencing equipment was used to connect the school to the diabetes center. Compared to the 13 control schools whose students received usual care, urgent visits for those in the intervention decreased significantly, and they had better health outcomes. Interactive technologies provide improved access to healthcare for school children.

This overview of interactive medicine technologies, applications, and locations has demonstrated the wide use of technology to provide health services to those in need. However, barriers and limitations regarding these applications have been noted throughout. Challenges in interactive medicine are highlighted next.

Barriers and Nonbelievers

Although the practice of interactive medicine is widespread, its applications are not as abundant as they could be. The primary reason for this limited growth is resistance to change. Non-adoption of interactive medical technology can take place within an entire organization or can be focused on one specific practitioner (Jones et al. 2005, Krupinski et al. 2008, Whitten and Mackert 2005). Reasons for declining to participate in interactive medicine include a dislike of technology, a dislike of change, perceived risks, lack of perceived benefits, time constraints, and inconvenient placement of equipment (Aas 2002, Edirippulige et al. 2009, Larsen et al. 2003, Mair et al. 2007). Ethical problems can also cause resistance. Some scholars perceive interactive medicine as defeating the goals it seeks to attain, believing the use of telemedicine may create more isolation, depersonalize the provider–patient relationship, and create more errors by providing a means to avoid face-to-face contact (Kaplan and Litewka 2008). Also of concern is the level of control the patient has during long-distance care, such as if they are informed of the advantages and disadvantages and are able to choose whether or not they would like to be seen over technology (Kaplan and Litewka 2008).

Interactive medicine experiences difficulties when seeking adoption by legal systems as well (Matusitz and Breen 2007). Original medical laws did not foresee the possibility of technology allowing medicine to be practiced with a doctor in one country and a patient in another. Hence, some countries have heavy restrictions on the practice of interactive medicine for this sole reason, while other countries are working to keep up with the speed of technology by creating safe laws that can bring those they serve improved healthcare. Another legal restraint for interactive medicine is the issue of reimbursement (Matusitz and Breen 2007, Nesbitt et al. 2006). Not all insurance companies are willing to reimburse doctors for their services when they are not provided in a face-to-face consult. Another issue is sustainability. For example, despite the fact that telepsychiatry is one of the oldest forms of telemedicine and considered to be one of the most successful types of telemedicine, it has yet to receive a place in routine care (Hailey et al. 2009). A possible factor in this, and the lack of adoption regarding other applications, is that many programs are developed to test the prospect of an interactive medicine program through grant funding. However, once the funding runs out, so do the resources for the projects to exist (Moahi 1999, Smith 2007). This often prevents evaluation of systems that can be used to learn best practices (Smith 2007). Unfortunately, when studies do take place for interactive medicine they usually contain methodological problems. Sample sizes are often small, blinded researchers are not used, and comparison groups are often absent (Jennett and Andruchuk 2001, Jennett and Wantanabe 2006, Nelson and Palsbo 2006).

Besides funding, other low resources can constrain interactive medicine implementation. Staff attitudes represent one such deficiency. For projects to be successful, interactive medicine programs need at least one project champion a current staff member who is interested in supporting the project and motivating other staff members to use the equipment. However, such an asset is not always easy to find. Additionally, although one of the benefits of interactive medicine is that it can work outside traditional healthcare settings, untraditional settings can be challenging. As described earlier, not all technology can work on boats, airplanes, spaceships, and RVs (Blanchet 2008, Ferrer-Roca et al. 2002, Telemedicine News 2007, Williams et al. 2000). Additionally, developing countries often lack the technical infrastructure that is conducive to the latest technology (Elder and Clarke 2007). Regardless of location, learning to work with technology can be a struggle as well (Nesbitt et al. 2006).

Keeping up with the most current technology can be another challenge (Jennett and Wantanabe 2006). Both implementing interactive medicine technology and updating current systems can be expensive for organizations (Wen and Tan 2002). Once an organization gets used to a particular set of technology, it may have to begin training for a newer system in order to keep pace with the continuous growth of the field. This training can be time consuming and frustrating to providers, especially when they are not getting paid an additional fee to learn. As the number of technologies used in the medical setting mount, compatibility of systems is a concern both within an organization and among an organization's partners (Jennett and Andruchuk 2001, Jones et al. 2005). Because communication between different locations is crucial to the practice of interactive medicine, systems must be able to transmit data successfully with compatible technologies.

With large amounts of private patient information being sent between locations, the trustworthiness of technology has been scrutinized (Kaplan and Litewka 2008, Stanberry 2000). In the age of computer hackers and viruses, patients need to know their information is being kept confidential. Additionally, with telemedicine the information is usually no longer kept between a patient and a physician. More players are often needed during interactive medicine interactions. Trustworthiness of e-health Web sites is also of particular interest as the number of these sites grows, yet medical professionals have little control over the correctness of the information they provide (Guler and Ubeyli 2002, Kaplan and Litewka 2008, Wen and Tan 2002). Therefore, the millions of Americans turning to the Internet for health information may be dangerously misinformed.

The Way Forward

These challenges provide a map of where the field of interactive medicine needs to travel. One necessary step for organizations seeking to invest in new technologies to provide healthcare is to actively prepare for this adoption (Jennett and Andruchuk 2001). There is abundant research on the changes that take place in organizations when adopting new technologies. Administrators at organizations should be aware of these changes prior to implementation in an effort to make smoother transitions. Education and training should take place on an organization-wide and individual basis. It would be preferable for such training to start during medical professionals' schooling and continue throughout their careers. This process may prove helpful in finding champions who are invested in using technology to provide care early on. Preparation for the use of interactive medicine should include models of sustainability. Prior to implementation, knowledge of the fact that grants are not permanent should be realized and addressed. Soliciting advice from successful applications and programs is one way to work on a sustainability plan, but tailoring one's plan to meet the specific characteristics of the organizations should also be practiced (Jannett and Wantanabe 2006).

Improvements in research are another need. To appease ethical worries, future research should always inform patients regarding the process of interactive medicine prior to providing services in this manner. Studies should also examine the psychosocial variables impacted by interactive medicine to better understand the effects of this process. All types of interactive medicine would benefit from the evidence of studies undertaking larger sample sizes and completing more thorough evaluations. Interactive medicine research would benefit from guidance by theoretical foundations as well. Scholars should always be building from the knowledge that has been laid out by colleagues in the past. Roger's diffusion of innovations theory (Rogers 1962) and the technology acceptance model (Davis 1989) have been used in an abundance of studies investigating technology adoption, but the majority of interactive medicine studies are still not guided by any type of theoretical framework. Using more theory in this field could illuminate future paths and avenues to overcome obstacles by highlighting key variables of interest.

Meetings with lawmakers could also improve the field of interactive medicine. Researchers and participants can only do so much to aid the implementation of health technologies. If the use of technology is not congruent with the legal and regulatory aspects of the health field, then a major barrier is formed (CTEL 2009a). Hence, interactive medicine requires advocates to argue for their ability to practice across distances when medical licensure is largely state based. Reimbursement for this practice is an additional issue (CTEL 2009b). Legislators could aid in passing laws that require health insurance companies to recognize interactive medicine as a legitimate method for providing care and thereby reimbursing for all associated costs of providing such care.

E-health, online interactive medicine, can also be enhanced, particularly in terms of health Web sites. Although these sites provide the public with access to a great deal of information that can be directly catered to their unique needs, this information may not always be beneficial. Studies to date have demonstrated that health Web sites are in possession of the proper design elements (Whitten et al. 2008). However, Web sites' possession of motivational content, tailoring capabilities, and comprehensive material are lacking (Whitten et al. 2008, 2009c). These disadvantages of health Web sites prevent them from reaching all audiences which seek their information in such a way as to promote healthy behaviors. Further investigations of these Web sites should be made, followed by guidelines, applications, and user testing.

Interactive Medicine in Action

The chapter thus far has provided an overview of applications and challenges for interactive medicine. In the final section of this chapter, we take an in-depth look at three applications: TeleKid Care, Telehospice, and Telemonitoring.

TeleKid Care

The TeleKid Care program provided access to mental healthcare for low-income minority children inside an urban middle school (Whitten et al. 2009d). This service was provided by a videoconferencing system in back of the nurse's office that was connected to a child psychiatrist's office at a large Midwestern university.

Children were recommended to participate in this program through a teacher, the school nurse, or a parent. Once this referral had been made the child was sent home with a packet of information containing information about the program, consent forms for the clinical and research part of the study, an assent form for the child, and clinical measures to fill out for the child. Parents, teachers, and children were all participants in this project. Parents participated by completing a Strengths and Difficulties Questionnaire prior to their child beginning the program and a perception survey regarding the use of telemedicine in school after their child had participated in the program. Teachers also gave consent to participate and filled out the Strength and Difficulties Questionnaire before and after their student participated in the project. Children were participants by giving assent and receiving telepsychiatry from their school. After receiving a consultation from the participating psychiatrist, parents were informed of their child's diagnoses and given recommendations for future care.

During the 2007–2008 school year, 11 children were seen using the TeleKid Care program, five females and six males. Teachers were found to look favorably on the program via the perception survey ($N = 33$). However, they were less certain regarding specifically how students would benefit. These findings almost mirrored parent perception responses ($N = 7$). Parents felt the program was convenient, gave them consistent information, and was overall beneficial for their child. However, they were less certain regarding how their child's health and schoolwork benefited.

Regarding clinical findings, the most common diagnoses were hyperactive attention deficit disorder (6), adjustment disorder of mixed mood and conduct (2), anxiety not otherwise specified (1), and two students were lost to follow up. Paired sample *t*-tests on the Strength and Difficulties Questionnaires filled out by the parents and teachers ($N = 9$) on the same student prior to project implementation found that parents and teachers did not significantly differ in their assessment of emotional symptoms, conduct problems, hyperactivity, and peer relationship problems. However, the two parties did significantly differ regarding the students' level of pro-social behavior, with parents seeing their child as more pro-social than did teachers.

Advantages of this project included an enthusiastic project champion. The school nurse was completely supportive in the project and was able to get other faculty members excited about participating. Nonetheless, this project still had a difficult time getting research participation on behalf of the teachers. This may be attributed to other nonrelated financial difficulties the school was facing, which caused worry to override excitement regarding the program. Additionally, teachers did not understand that the pretest and posttest needed to be completed by the same teacher; hence, pretests and posttests were unreliable.

Parents were also difficult to contact for perception surveys. Although at the beginning of the study they agreed to participate, at the end of the project many could not be contacted. One reason for this was participant attrition. For instance, one participant moved away and another participant was suspended from school during the project. A way to remedy this situation in the future might be to make use of incentives, because participants did not see receiving services as enough of a benefit. As is found in face-to-face consults, teachers and parents were also more likely to recommend individuals with externalizing disorders like ADHD, as opposed to internalizing disorders like depression despite the fact that both pose severe health threats. This could be remedied through teaching school staff and parents to recognize the symptoms of internalizing disorders. Still, this project recognized teachers and parents as great sources to recommend children with mental health disorders for treatment, and that schools are an appropriate and beneficial location for increasing access to underserved populations.

Telehospice

Telehospice allows patients in need of end of life care to receive this service directly in their homes through technology. Videophones were given to two hospice organizations in mid-Michigan for use with patients (Whitten et al. 2009b). Nurses were trained on how to use the videophones, and researchers assisted in setting up the videophones both in the hospice organization and in patients' homes. Nurses and patients could use the videophones to contact one another with health concerns while avoiding travel. Hospice management was initially excited about using the technology to reach patients at their homes, even helping the researchers in securing funding to implement the project. However, despite training and interest by the hospice staff, the videophones were only used with two patients.

To assess reasons for non-adoption of this technology, phone surveys were administered to hospice employees. Twenty-five employees were interviewed. These surveys were guided by constructs from the Unified Theory of Acceptance of Technology (UTAUT) instrument and the Organizational Readiness for Change (ORC) assessment. The UTAUT is used to predict adoption of technology, and the ORC is used to predict an organizations' willingness to experience change. Interestingly, the quantitative findings from this survey, as guided by these two theories, predicted that the hospice staff would have adopted the videophones; however, that was not the case. The surveys reported that the nurses felt they had enough resources, the phones were easy to use, and that their organization was ready to make the change. To investigate this matter further, focus groups were performed with 10 hospice workers. Using qualitative research methods, these focus groups demonstrated that workers were not as confident and enthusiastic regarding the videophones as the survey indicated. Using the ORC and the UTAUT to analyze these discussions, reasons for non-adoption were found including that the telehospice project lacked incentives and a project champion.

This telehospice program recognized both the importance and limitations of using theory to guide research. Although theories were ultimately able to identify key components in this implementation failure, two methodological approaches had to be taken to find these answers. This project also demonstrated the need to convince practitioners that the goal of telehospice is to assist in face-to-face care rather than to replace it.

Home Monitoring for Congestive Heart Failure Patients

In Indiana, 50 congestive heart failure (CHF) patients who had been released from the hospital and prescribed home-based care tested a home monitoring technology system for acceptance and clinical outcomes (Whitten et al. 2009a). Through this telehealth system, patients could employ remote monitoring to enable a home health nurse to manage their home healthcare. The OASIS, SF-12, and the Minnesota Living with Health Failure Questionnaire (MLHQ) were administered to document the impact of the program before and after patient participation in the program. The first two instruments measure a patient's general health status and issues, while the MLHQ is specifically for CHF patients' health statuses. Additionally, after participation, patients were interviewed to inquire how they felt about using the telehealth system to receive services.

The mean patient participation length was 48 days. An average of 39 telehealth visits took place per patient compared to 14 face-to-face visits and 3 telephone visits per patient. Health benefits were found to be statistically significant from pretest to posttest. The OASIS indicated a reduced number of patients with shortness of breath and improved patient management. The SF-12 indicated that participants felt they had more energy and ability to participate in moderate activity. Additionally, overall better health approached significance on this measure. The MLHQ indicated patients needed less time to rest, had more energy, encountered less swelling in their ankles, required less hospitalization, and were less worried. The patient interview indicated that participants felt the system was easy to use, a beneficial method for receiving care, enjoyable, and overall satisfying. Still, patients were slightly less likely to agree they would rather be seen by telehealth than face-to-face. Open-ended responses to the interview also demonstrated positive aspects of the program such as being reminded to watch one's weight, take one's medication, provide health information, and allowed them to stay in the comfort of their homes. However, the system was found somewhat repetitive by some participants. Patients also commented that they preferred certain procedures such as drawing blood to take place in-person.

This project displayed how telehealth can be accepted by patients as a beneficial system. The use of interactive medicine was an effective means of monitoring patients while they remained at home.

Summary

This chapter has discussed the applications and technologies involved with interactive medicine. Technologies to provide healthcare at a distance can be done in real-time or in store-and-forward fashion among almost every medical specialty across an array of locations. Interactive medicine can be employed to diagnose, treat, and manage numerous health issues. Although this field is clearly growing at a rapid pace, it still faces numerous challenges such as sustainability and acceptance. Hopefully, future research will address these challenges with creative and innovative solutions to promote interactive medicine's most basic goal of providing efficient access to healthcare services.

References

Aas, I. H. M. 2002. Changes in the job situation due to telemedicine. *J Telemed Telecare* 8(1):41–47.

Anhoj, J. and C. Moldrup. 2004. Feasibility of collecting diary data from asthma patients through mobile phones and SMS (short message service): Response rate analysis and focus group evaluation from a pilot. *J Med Internet Res* 6:e42.

Blanchet, K. D. 2008. Mobile health clinics and telemedicine. *Telemed J E Health* 14(5):407–412.

Botsis, T., G. Demiris, S. Pedersen et al. 2008. Home telecare technologies for the elderly. *J Telemed Telecare* 14(7):333–337.

Brignell, M., R. Wootton, and L. Gray. 2007. The application of telemedicine to geriatric medicine. *Age and Ageing* 10:1–6.

Callahan, C., W. F. Malone, D. Estroff et al. 2005. Effectiveness of an internet-based store-and-forward telemedicine system for pediatric subspecialty consultation. *Pediatrics* 159:380–393.

Cone, S., E. J. Rodas, and R. C. Merrell. 2009. Telemedical support for surgeons in Ecuador. In *Telehealth in the Developing World*, eds. R. Wootton, N. G. Patil, R. E. Scott, and K. Ho, pp. 193–202. Ottawa, ON: The Royal Society of Medicine Press Ltd.

CTEL 2009a. Licensure main page, CTEL, Washington, DC. http://www.telehealthlawcenter.org/?c=118 (accessed August 6, 2009).

CTEL 2009b. Reimbursement main page, CTEL, Washington, DC. http://www.telehealthlawcenter.org/?c=117 (accessed August 6, 2009).

Darkins, A., P. Ryan, R. Kobb et al. 2008. Care coordination/home telehealth: The systematic implementation of health informatics, home telehealth, and disease management to support the care of veteran patients with chronic conditions. *Telemed J E Health* 14(10):1118–1126.

Davis, F. D. 1989. Perceived usefulness, perceived ease of use, and user acceptance of information technology. *MIS Q* 13(3):319–340.

Dimmick, S. L. and K. D. Ignatova. 2006. The diffusion of a medical innovation: Where teleradiology is and where it is going. *J Telemed Telecare* 12(Suppl 2):51–58.

Doolittle, G. C. and A. O. Spaulding. 2006. Providing access to oncology care for rural patients via telemedicine. *J Oncol Pract* 2(5):228–230.

Doolittle, G. C., P. Whitten, M. McCartney et al. 2005. An empirical chart analysis of the suitability of telemedicine for hospice visits. *Telemed J E Health* 11:90–97.

Ebner, C., E. M. Wurm, B. Binder et al. 2008. Mobile teledermatology: A feasibility study of 58 subjects using mobile phones. *J Telemed Telecare* 14(1):2–7.

Edirippulige, S., R. B. Marasinghe, V. H. W. Dissanayake et al. 2009. Strategies to promote e-health and telemedicine in developing countries. In *Telehealth in the Developing World*, eds. R. Wootton, N. G. Patil, R. E. Scott, and K. Ho. Ottawa, ON: Royal Society of Medicine.

Elder, L. and M. Clarke. 2007. Past, present and future: Experiences and lessons from telehealth projects. *Open Med* 1(3):e166–e170. http://www.openmedicine.ca/article/viewArticle/191/98 (accessed June 26, 2009).

Eminovic, N., N. F. de Keizer, P. J. E. Bindels et al. 2007. Maturity of teledermatology evaluation research: A systematic literature review. *Br J Dermatol* 156:412–419.

Evans, A. J., R. Chetty, B. A. Clarke et al. 2009. Primary frozen section diagnosis by robotic microscopy and virtual slide telepathology: The University of Health Network experience. *Hum Pathol* 40(8):1070–1081.

Ferrer-Roca, O., R. Diaz de Leon, F. J. de Latorre et al. 2002. Aviation medicine: Challenges for telemedicine. *J Telemed Telecare* 8(1):1–4.

Fox, K. C., G. W. Somes, and T. M. Waters. 2007. Timeliness and access to healthcare services via telemedicine for adolescents in state correctional faculties. *J Adolesc Health* 41(2):161–167.

Frueh, B. C., J. Monnier, E. Yim et al. 2007. A randomized trial of telepsychiatry for post-traumatic stress disorder. *J Telemed Telecare* 13(3):142–147.

Grigsby, J. 1997. Telemedicine in the United States. In *Telemedicine: Theory and Practice*, eds. R. Bashushur, J. Sanders, and G. Shannon. Springfield, IL: Charles. C. Thomas Publisher.

Grubaugh, A. L., G. Cain, J. Elhai et al. 2008. Attitudes toward medical and mental health care delivered via telehealth applications among rural and urban primary care patients. *J Nerv Ment Dis* 196(2):166–170.

Guler, N. F. and E. D. Ubeyli. 2002. Theory and applications of telemedicine. *J Med Syst* 26(3):199–220.

Hailey, D., A. Ohinmaa, and R. Roine. 2009. Limitations in the routine use of telepsychiatry. *J Telemed Telecare* 15(1):29–31.

Harrison, R. M., W. Clayton, and P. Wallace. 1997. Is there a role for telemedicine in an urban environment? *J Telemed Telecare* 3(Suppl 1):15–17.

Head, B. A., J. L. Studts, J. M. Bumpous et al. 2009. Development of a telehealth intervention for health and cancer patients. *Telemed J E Health* 15(1):44–52.

Hernando, M. E., E. J. Gomez, A. Garcia-Olaya et al. 2006. A mobile telemedicine workspace for diabetes management. In *M-Health: Emerging Mobile Health Systems*, eds. R. S. H. Istepanian, S. Laximinarayan, and C. S. Pattichis. New York: Springer.

Hilty, D., S. L. Marks, D. Urness et al. 2004. Clinical and educational telepsychiatry applications: A review. *Can J Psychiatry* 49(1):12–23.

Holtz, B. and P. Whitten. 2009. Managing asthma with mobile phones: A feasibility study. *Telemed J E Health* 15(9):907–909.

Horbinski, C. and C. A. Wiley. 2009. Comparison of telepathology systems in neuropathological intropерative consultations. *Neuropathology* 29(6):665–663.

Izquierdo, R., P. C. Morin, K. Bratt et al. 2009. School-centered telemedicine for children with type 1 diabetes mellitus. *J Pediatr* 155(3):374–379.

Jennett, P. and K. Andruchuk. 2001. Telehealth: 'Real life' implementation issues. *Comput Methods Programs Biomed* 64:169–174.

Jennett, P. and M. Wantanabe. 2006. Healthcare and telemedicine: Ongoing and evolving challenges. *Dis Manage Health Outcomes* 14(Suppl. 1):9–13.

Jones, V., F. Incardona, C. Tristam et al. 2005. Future challenges and recommendations. In *M-Health Emobile Health Systems*, eds. R. S. H. Istepanian, S. Laximinarayan, and C. S. Pattichis. New York: Springer.

Jones, J. A., A. E. Sargsyan, Y. R. Barr et al. 2009. Diagnostic ultrasound at mach 20: Retroperitoneal and pelvic imaging in space. *Ultrasound Med Biol* 35(7):1059–1067.

Kaplan, B. and S. Litewka. 2008. Ethical challenges of telemedicine. *Camb Q Healthc Ethics* 17:401–416.

Kenny, L. M. and L. S. Lau. 2008. Clinical teleradiology—The purpose of principles. *Med J Aust* 188(4):197–198.

Kopycka-Kedzierawski, D. T. and R. J. Billings. 2006. Teledentistry in inner-city child-care centres. *J Telemed Telecare* 12(4):176–181.

Kreutzer, J., H. Akutsu, R. Fahlbusch et al. 2008. Teleradiology neurosurgery: Experience in 1024 cases. *J Telemed Telecare* 14(2):67–70.

Krupinski, E. A., N. Charness, G. Demiris et al. 2008. Roundtable discussion human factors in telemedicine. *Telemed J E Health* 14(10):1024–1030.

Krupinski, E. A., M. Nypaver, R. Poropatich et al. 2002. Clinical applications in telemedicine/telehealth. *Telemed J E Health* 8:13–34.

Larsen, F., E. Gjerdrum, A. Obstfelder et al. 2003. Implementing telemedicine services in northern Norway: Barriers and facilitators. *J Telemed Telecare* 9(Suppl. 1):17–18.

Larsen, D., B. H. Stamm, K. Davis et al. 2004. Prison telemedicine and telehealth utilization in the United States: State and federal perceptions of benefits and barriers. *Telemed J E Health* 10(2):81–90.

Lavrentyev, V., R. Seay, A. Rafiq et al. 2008. A surgical telemedicine clinic in a correctional setting. *Telemed J E Health* 14(4):385–388.

Lopez, A. M., A. R. Graham, G. P. Barker et al. 2009. Virtual slide telepathology enables an innovative telehealth rapid breast care clinic. *Hum Pathol* 40(8):1082–1091.

Maffei, R., Y. Hudson, and K. Dunn. 2008. Telemedicine for urban uninsured: A pilot framework for specialty care planning for sustainability. *Telemed J E Health* 14(9):925–931.

Maheu, M. M., P. Whitten, and A. Allen. 2001. *E-Health, Telehealth, and Telemedicine*. San Fransisco, CA: Jossey-Bass.

Mair, F., T. Finch, C. May et al. 2007. Perceptions of risk as a barrier to the use of telemedicine. *J Telemed Telecare* 13(Suppl. 1):38–39.

Masucci, M. M., C. Homko, W. P. Santamore et al. 2006. Cardiovascular disease prevention for underserved patients using the internet: Bridging he digital divide. *Telemed J E Health* 12(1):58–65.

Matusitz, J. and G. Breen. 2007. Telemedicine: It's effects on health communication. *Health Commun* 21(1):73–83.

McConnochie, K. M., G. P. Conners, A. F. Brayer et al. 2006. Effectiveness of telemedicine in replacing in-person evaluation for acute childhood illness in office settings. *Telemed J E Health* 12(3):308–316.

Mirza, M. K., Z. Sajjad, M. Yousuf et al. 2008. Teleradiology between Afghanistan and Pakistan: One year experience. *Pak J Radiol* 1(18):22–25.

Moahi, K. H. 1999. Health information network for telehealth in Africa—Challenging prospects: A review of the literature. *Int J Libr Inform Ser* 49(1):43–50.

Morgan, R. D., A. R. Patrick, and P. R. Magaletta. 2008. Does the use of telemental health alter the experience? Inmates' perceptions of telemental health versus face-to-face treatment modalities. *J Consult Clin Psychol* 76(1):158–162.

Mort, M., M. Finch, and C. May. 2009. Making and unmaking telepatients: Identity and governance in new health technologies. *Sci Technol Hum Val* 34(1):9–33.

Nelson, E. and S. Palsbo. 2006. Challenges in telemedicine equivalence. *Eval Program Plann* 29:419–425.

Nesbitt, T. S., S. L. Cole, L. Pellegrino et al. 2006. Rural outreach in home telehealth: Assessment challenges and reviewing successes. *Telemed J E Health* 12(2):107–113.

Pak, H., C. A. Triplett, J. H. Lindquist et al. 2007. Store-and-forward teledermatology results in similar clinical outcomes to conventional clinic-based care. *J Telemed Telecare* 13(1):26–30.

Park, W., D. Kim, J. Kim et al. 2009. A portable dental image viewer using mobile network to provide a teledental service. *J Telemed Telecare* 15(3):145–149.

Parker Oliver, D. R., G. Demiris, and D. Porock. 2005. The usability of videophones for seniors and hospice providers: A brief report of two studies. *Comput Biol Med* 35:782–790.

Pesamaa, L., H. Ebeling, M. Kuusimaki et al. 2004. Videoconferencing in child and adolescent telepsychiatry: A systematic review of the literature. *J Telemed Telecare* 10(4):187–192.

Puccion, J. A., M. Belzer, J. Olson et al. 2006. The use of cell phone reminder call for assisting HIV infected adolescents and young adults to adhere to highly active antiretroviral therapy: A pilot study. *AIDS Patient Care STDs* 20:438–444.

Reger, M. A., G. A. Gahm, A. A. Rizzo et al. 2009. Soldier evaluation of the virtual reality in Iraq. *Telemed J E Health* 15(1):101–104.

Rogers, E. M. 1962. *Diffusion of Innovations*. New York: Free Press.

Sable, C. A., S. D. Cummings, G. D. Pearson et al. 2002. Impact of ton the practice of pediatric cardiology in community hospitals. *Pediatrics* 109(1):e3.

Scalvini, S., E. Zanelli, L. Paletta et al. 2006. Chronic heart failure home-based management with a telecardiology system: A comparison between patients followed by general practitioners and by a cardiology department. *J Telemed Telecare* 12(Suppl. 1):46–48.

Shaikh, U., S. L. Cole, J. P. Marcin et al. 2008. Clinical management and patient outcomes among children and adolescents receiving telemedicine consultations for obesity. *Telemed J E Health* 14(5):434–440.

Sheng, O. R. L., P. J. Hu, G. Au et al. 1997. Urban teleradiology in Hong Kong. *J Telemed Telecare* 3(2):71–77.

Smith, A. C. 2007. Telemedicine: Challenges and opportunities. *Expert Rev Med Devices* 4(1):5–7.

Stanberry, B. 2000. Telemedicine: Barriers and opportunities in the 21st century. *J Intern Med* 247:615–628.

Telemedicine News. 2007. Coastal boat brings telemedicine to residents of Maine islands. *Telemed J E Health* 13(5):477–482.

Trief, P. M., J. A. Teresi, J. P. Eimicke et al. 2009. Improvement in diabetes self-efficacy and glycaemic control using telemedicine in a sample of older, ethnically diverse individuals who have diabetes: The IDEATel project. *Age Ageing* 38(2):219–225.

Urwin, A., J. Ferguson, R. McDonald et al. 2008. A five-year review of ground-to-air emergency medical advice. *J Telemed Telecare* 14(3):157–159.

Weinstein, R. S., A. R. Graham, L. C. Richter et al. 2009. Overview of telepathology, virtual microscopy, and whole slide imaging: Prospects for the future. *Hum Pathol* 40(8):1057–1069.

Wen, J. and J. Tan. 2002. The evolving face of telemedicine & e-health: Opening doors and gaps in e-health services opportunities and challenges In *The 36th Annual Hawaii International Conference on System Sciences*. The Big Island, HI.

Whitten, P. 2003. Teledermatology delivery modalities: Real-time versus store and forward. *Curr Probl Dermatol* 32:24–31.

Whitten, P., A. Bergman, M. A. Meese et al. 2009a. St. Vincent's home telehealth for congestive health failure patients. *Telemed J E Health* 15(2):148–153.

Whitten, P., G. Doolittle, and S. Hellmich. 2001. Telehospice: Using telecommunication technology for terminally ill patients. *J Comput Mediat Commun* 6(4):1–16. http://jcmc.indiana.edu/vol6/issue4/whitten2.html (accessed June 20, 2009).

Whitten, P., G. Doolittle, M. Mackert et al. 2003. Telehospice: End-of-life care over the lines. *Nurs Manag* 34:36–39.

Whitten, P., B. Holtz, E. Meyer et al. 2009b. Telehospice: Reasons for slow adoption in home hospice care. *J Telemed Telecare* 15:187–190.

Whitten, P. and M. Mackert. 2005. Addressing telehealth's foremost barrier: Provider as initial gatekeeper. *Int J Technol Assess Health Care* 21(4):517–521.

Whitten, P., S. Nazione, S. Smith, and C. LaPlante. May, 2009c. Utilization of evidence strategies by breast cancer websites targeting diverse audiences. In *2009 International Communication Association conference*, Chicago, IL.

Whitten, P., P. Quinlan, S. Nazione et al. 2009d. Caring for underserved children's mental health needs through telepsychiatry in schools. In *Annual CyberTherapy and CyberPsychology 2009 Conference*, Villa Caramora, Italy, June 2009.

Whitten, P., S. Smith, S. Nazione et al. 2008. Communication assessment of the most frequented breast cancer websites: Evaluation of design and theoretical criteria. *J Comput Mediat Commun* 13:880–911.

Whitten, P. and B. D. Sypher. 2006. Evolution of telemedicine from an applied communication perspective in the United States. *Telemed J E Health* 12(5):590–600.

Williams, D. R., R. L. Bashshur, S. L. Pool et al. 2000. A strategic vision for telemedicine and medical informatics in space flight. *Telemed J E Health* 6(4):441–448.

Wilimas, J. A., M. W. Wilson, B. G. Haik et al. 2009. Development of retinoblastoma programs in Central America. *Pediatr Blood Cancer* 53(1):42–46.

Wootton, R. 2006. Realtime telemedicine. *J Telemed Telecare* 12:328–336.

Young, T. and C. Ireson. 2003. Effectiveness of school-based telehealth in urban and rural elementary schools. *Pediatrics* 112(5):1088–1094.

Design, Planning, Control, and Management of Healthcare Systems

IV.C Transplant Services

30 **The U.S. Organ Transplant Network: History, Structure, and Functions** *Timothy L. Pruett and Joel D. Newman* **30**-1
Introduction • Background of the National Transplant Network • OPTN Structure and Processes • Conclusion • References

30

The U.S. Organ Transplant Network: History, Structure, and Functions

Timothy L. Pruett
University of Minnesota

Joel D. Newman
United Network for Organ Sharing Communications

Introduction 30-1
Background of the National Transplant Network 30-1
Early History of Transplantation in the United States • Federal Legislation and Regulation • Roles of the OPTN and Scientific Registry
OPTN Structure and Processes 30-3
OPTN Membership and Representation • Scope of Bylaws and Policies • Policy Development Process
Conclusion 30-14
References 30-14

Introduction

In slightly more than 50 years, organ transplantation has progressed from a rare and experimental medical procedure to a successful, wide-scale treatment for end-stage organ failure. Yet, it remains a form of medical treatment that is uniquely interdependent, both to obtain needed organs and to ensure that these organs are used effectively and efficiently for the greatest possible benefit.

In the United States, a national network known as the Organ Procurement and Transplantation Network (OPTN) performs key functions to ensure efficiency and equity in the transplant process. United Network for Organ Sharing (UNOS), a private, nonprofit organization, has operated the OPTN under federal contract since its inception. The OPTN also derives key support from the Scientific Registry of Transplant Recipients (SRTR) in data analysis.

This chapter briefly outlines the historical development of the national transplant network and discusses in some detail the issues of policy development and enforcement, organ placement, and data collection and analysis. Case studies in each section illustrate how these concepts and processes translate into practical application.

Background of the National Transplant Network

Early History of Transplantation in the United States

In the latter half of the twentieth century, almost daily advances were made in many areas of surgery, medicine, and immunology. These efforts combined to make possible a long-desired goal to replace an isolated, failing human organ with a functional organ from another person.

A number of experiments, trials, and procedures preceded the first viable, long-term kidney transplant in 1954. The earliest procedure involved a living donor who was an identical twin of the recipient, thus, circumventing the still imperfectly understood process of organ rejection (Petechuk, 2006). By the early 1960s, a small number of academic medical centers had success transplanting kidneys both from closely related living donors and deceased donors. By the late 1960s, successful liver, pancreas, and heart transplants were also performed (Wolf, 1991).

While the early procedures proved technically viable and many recipients enjoyed a few years of graft function, immunologic organ rejection remained a major barrier to routine, long-term success. As a result, until the early 1980s, there were only a few dozen transplant centers in the United States, performing a total of several hundred transplants nationwide. Many centers independently managed all aspects of care including organ recovery, selection of the recipient for a given organ offer, and post-transplant follow-up and data collection.

In the early 1980s, cyclosporine was introduced as the first of a series of immunosuppressant drugs that vastly decreased the risk of organ rejection (Norman and Laurence, 2001). With this advance, the success of transplantation and the demand for it grew exponentially. At the same time, various organ procurement organizations and multicenter transplant networks had emerged to assume supporting and coordinating roles for transplant hospitals.

Federal Legislation and Regulation

The U.S. Congress recognized that with the increasing demand, a national system should be created to develop consistent and equitable policies for organ recovery and allocation. Congress also recognized the need for a national registry of scientific data, both to inform transplant policymaking and to provide clinicians with detailed information to improve care of transplant patients.

The nature of the network and registry was debated, particularly in the spirit of deregulation in the early 1980s. Rather than having these functions entirely within the federal government at taxpayer expense, Congress reasoned that a nonprofit coordinating organization, while operating under federal contract and oversight, could leverage the expertise of practicing transplant clinicians and professionals and could respond rapidly to new developments in the field. In addition, Congress valued the independence of a private/public network that would be less subject to partisan political influence.

The resulting National Organ Transplant Act of 1984 (NOTA) established the OPTN and a Scientific Registry of Transplant Recipients (Public Law, 1984). These entities were to be operated under competitive bid contracts with the U.S. Department of Health and Human Services (HHS). The organizations who qualified to bid on these contracts must be nonprofit organizations with specific expertise in organ transplantation. UNOS, which had existed as an independent transplant network since 1984, applied for and received the initial OPTN contract in 1986 and the initial Scientific Registry contract in 1987.

Separate provisions of the Social Security Act specified that any hospital wishing to operate a transplant program, and any organization wishing to recover and transport organs from deceased donors, must be an organizational member of the OPTN and follow its policies. If a transplant center does not abide by the OPTN's rules and requirements, the entire hospital may be ruled ineligible to participate in the Medicare or Medicaid program in any way; the penalty is not limited to reimbursement for transplantation.

For a number of years, the OPTN operated under this legislative guidance, but there was no specific regulatory authority to enforce adverse actions should a member not comply with OPTN policy. The Health Resources and Services Administration (HRSA), the division within HHS that oversees the OPTN contract, issued federal regulation in 2000. This regulation is commonly called the OPTN Final Rule.* The Final Rule established that the Secretary of HHS is responsible for regulatory enforcement of OPTN requirements, with or without the recommendation of the Board of Directors of the OPTN.

* 42 C.F.R §121 et seq.

Roles of the OPTN and Scientific Registry

NOTA and the Final Rule together specify certain responsibilities for the OPTN, including the following:

- Developing consensus-based policies and procedures for organ recovery, distribution (allocation), and transportation
- Developing policies to minimize the risk of disease transmission through organ transplantation
- Establishing bylaws outlining the experience and training criteria for key surgical and medical transplant personnel and the other required resources for non-Medicare transplant programs
- Monitoring compliance with policies and bylaws
- Establishing patient-specific priority for the equitable allocation of organs on the basis of medical judgment
- Developing and maintaining a secure Web-based computer system that maintains the nation's organ transplant waiting list and recipient/donor organ characteristics
- Facilitating the organ matching and placement process through the use of the computer system and a fully staffed Organ Center operating 24 hours a day
- Collecting data relating to the performance of the transplantation efforts in the country, and providing data to the public, students, researchers, and the Scientific Registry to help improve the field
- Conducting reviews and evaluations as directed by the Secretary of HHS
- Providing professional and public education about donation and transplantation, the activities of the OPTN and the critical need for donation
- Developing policies about any additional issues designated by the Secretary of HHS

UNOS operated the Scientific Registry until 2000, when the contract was awarded to the Arbor Research Collaborative for Health. The Scientific Registry is charged with conducting scientific analysis of transplant data and providing these analyses to HHS, the OPTN, the transplant community, and the public for the monitoring and improvement of transplant care. Registry analyses are frequently used by OPTN committees to assess both the performance of current OPTN policy and the likely future impact of policy proposals under consideration.

OPTN Structure and Processes

OPTN Membership and Representation

OPTN membership primarily consists of institutions providing transplant services and organizations dedicated in whole or in part to advancing the field of transplantation. All U.S. Medicare-approved transplant centers and designated organ procurement organizations are OPTN members. Additional members include non-Medicare-approved transplant centers and histocompatibility laboratories providing transplant services (either hospital-based or serving multiple hospitals). Other member categories include professional societies, health and patient advocacy organizations, and transplant consortia. A few individuals serve as "general public" members; these individuals often have a personal experience with organ donation or transplantation. (For a current distribution of OPTN members, see Table 30.1.)

Each member in good standing participates in the OPTN in a number of ways. The member is able to vote on the annual slate of members of the OPTN/UNOS Board of Directors as well as organizational bylaws. The member is also solicited for public comment on policy and bylaw proposals, a process described below in more detail. Representatives drawn from the various categories of membership also serve on the Board of Directors and on more than 20 advisory committees. (For a list of current OPTN/UNOS committees, see Table 30.2.) To assure adequate membership representation, each standing committee has a representation from each region of the country as well at-large expert members.

TABLE 30.1 OPTN/UNOS Members as of February 2009

Transplant centers	254
Business members	1
Organ procurement organizations	58
Histocompatibility laboratories	154
General public members	9
Medical/scientific organizations	20
Individuals	7

TABLE 30.2 OPTN/UNOS Committees as of February 2009

(Ad Hoc) Disease Transmission Advisory	Operation
Ethics	Organ procurement organization
Executive	Organ availability
Finance	Pancreas transplantation
Histocompatibility	Patient affairs
(Ad Hoc) international relations	Pediatric transplantation
Kidney allocation	Policy oversight
Liver and intestinal organ allocation	Thoracic organ transplantation
Living donor	Transplant administrators
Memberships and professional standards	Transplant coordinators
Minority affairs	

Scope of Bylaws and Policies

Federal law and regulation, as well as specifications in the OPTN contract, generally, define the OPTN's scope of responsibility.

The OPTN bylaws address minimum qualification standards for OPTN membership. All OPTN member institutions, including organ procurement organizations and independent histocompatibility laboratories, must show that they have proper designation and/or licensing to perform their functions.

Individual transplant programs must have onsite at least one transplant physician and one transplant surgeon who meet certain training and experience qualifications. These standards, particularly the experience qualifications, have been reviewed and revised several times to reflect the currency of expertise in the transplant field. Other bylaws spell out certain staff positions that transplant centers must designate, such as clinical transplant coordinators and a transplant financial coordinator, and the general responsibilities such positions should entail.

The bylaws also address

- Processes for application, review, and approval of OPTN members
- Processes for member inactivation or withdrawal
- Circumstances where the OPTN may review programs for issues including policy noncompliance, survival rates significantly below expectation, or functional inactivity

If a member is found to be consistently substandard in performance or is in violation of OPTN requirements after peer review determination, the OPTN may take certain actions under due process and/or make recommendations to HHS regarding possible adverse actions at its disposal. In other instances, the OPTN may direct a confidential peer visit to assess the member's performance and give recommendations to help the member improve outcomes.

In general, OPTN bylaws set broad standards and parameters for members. They are always subject to change to address new and emerging issues, but as a rule they are not frequently amended. By contrast,

TABLE 30.3 Major Sections of OPTN Policy

Minimum procurement Standards for an Organ Procurement Organization
Organ acceptable criteria
Deceased donor kidney allocation
Liver allocation
Thoracic organ allocation
Pancreas allocation
Intestinal organ allocation
Acquired immune deficiency syndrome and human pituitary-derived growth hormone
Standardized packaging of human organs and tissue typing materials
Transplantation of nonresident aliens
Data submission requirements
Release of information to the public
Access to data

OPTN policies address specific processes and requirements. New policies can be developed within a few months to address an emergent issue, and once enacted, their effect is continually studied to determine whether they can be further improved. In an average year, dozens of new or amended policies are approved to respond to developments in transplant practice or science.

Most of the policies address activities related to the recovery and allocation of organs from deceased donors, although some policies (such as data submission and reporting) address the process of both living and deceased donor transplantation. (For a list of major sections of current OPTN policy, see Table 30.3.)

Policy Development Process

The OPTN policy development process is intended to be flexible, to incorporate objective evidence whenever possible, and to strive for consensus among all of the various disciplines and viewpoints in the field.

Figure 30.1 provides a broad visual overview of the process. An issue, concern, or question is discussed by one or more OPTN/UNOS committees. The committees may review scientific data

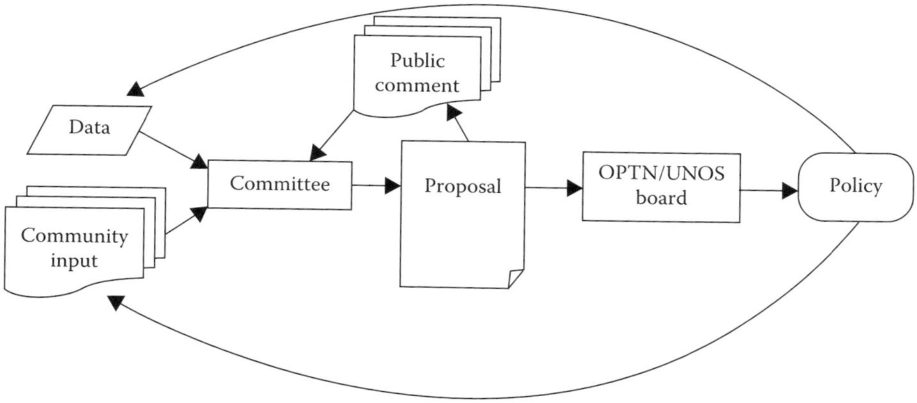

FIGURE 30.1 OPTN/UNOS policy development process.

or seek professional input to help them develop a proposal to revise an existing policy or develop a new policy.

Once a committee develops a proposal, the proposal is sent for public comment. Any interested party can indicate support or opposition or pose questions about the proposal. The sponsoring committee will review all comments and may amend the proposal and/or answer detailed questions about its intent or mechanics.

The reconsidered proposal would then be considered by the OPTN/UNOS Board of Directors. The Board may approve the proposal (with or without amending it), disapprove it, or direct that it go back through the process for further development before reconsideration.

Any policy, once implemented, is subject to ongoing data analysis and community discussion to determine if it is meeting stated goals and if additional improvements can be made. This will often generate the same processes to amend or add to existing policy.

Case Study: Development of MELD/PELD Liver Policy

Through the first several years of OPTN liver allocation policy, the assignment of medical urgency priority for liver transplant candidates was based on broad assumptions of their prognosis and current level of medical treatment. Patients who were hospitalized got more priority than those who were not. Those assessed by their transplant team to have less than 7 days to live without a transplant received the greatest priority.

While these concepts had ethical merit, the practical limitations became apparent. Hospital status was a poor surrogate for determining urgency, as some patients with more aggressive medical management and/or more lenient insurance coverage might stay long term in the hospital while others in similar health would not. It was difficult to monitor or objectively assess the transplant team's judgment that a candidate would not survive more than a week without a transplant.

The earlier policy was replaced by a formulaic scoring system that classified candidates based on diagnosis and the presence and severity of certain symptoms of end-stage liver failure. Again, in practice, this led to some difficulties. Points were given for some conditions (such as encephalopathy and ascites) that different clinicians might assess and treat differently. Some liver professionals were hesitant to share locally recovered organs with distant programs, who interpreted the candidate criteria in different ways.

During this same time, the OPTN Final Rule called for a review of liver allocation policy based on certain guiding principles, emphasizing the use of objective medical criteria and the goal of minimizing deaths among patients awaiting a transplant. Many new potential allocation systems were modeled prospectively, based on actual liver transplant data, and their likely effects were studied according to the desired metrics.

Eventually, the OPTN saw merit in an adaptation of a formula previously used to assess the utility of providing Transjugular Intrahepatic Portosystemic Shunt (TIPS) procedures for patients with advanced liver disease. With specific modifications and validation in a transplant setting, the model for end-stage liver disease (MELD) was shown to have considerable predictive power for a candidate's short-term risk of death without a liver transplant. It is based on commonly available and consistently interpreted laboratory tests, and it expresses an urgency score in a continuous range (6 as least urgent, 40 as most urgent) rather than a few broad and overlapping categories. A companion formula, the pediatric end-stage liver disease (PELD) model, addresses additional factors for liver candidates younger than age 11.

It was observed that while MELD/PELD accurately assesses the short-term mortality risk of most transplant candidates, it does not fully address all conditions (for example, early stage hepatocellular carcinoma). For this reason, regional review boards were established to review individual requests for higher exception scores on a confidential, blinded basis and determine whether such scores are medically justified.

As described in the policy development module, the OPTN/UNOS Liver and Intestinal Organ Transplantation Committee collaborated with several other committees and work groups to develop, validate, and model the MELD/PELD system. Extensive public comment was sought, including a public forum. After considerable review and discussion, the OPTN/UNOS Board of Directors approved the new policy in November 2001.

The MELD/PELD system, implemented in 2002, has been largely successful in meeting expectations. As with all policies, however, it is subject to ongoing review and improvement. Subsequent amendments have included the awarding of "standard exception" scores for some candidates who meet designated criteria and would not be well served with a calculated MELD/PELD, as well as broader (regional) liver allocation for candidates with a MELD/PELD score of 15 or higher.

EVALUATION OF POLICY COMPLIANCE AND PATIENT SAFETY

The OPTN Final Rule provides the mechanism for HHS enforcement of OPTN requirements and policies. It directs the OPTN to evaluate member compliance with bylaws and policies and to make recommendations to the Secretary of HHS for enforcement action when a member is found to be in violation or when a risk exists to the health of patients or to the public safety. The secretary is empowered to take action regardless of such recommendations.

UNOS staff routinely monitor all organ allocation matches to determine whether transplant candidates were considered in the proper sequence for organ offers and whether transplant programs have sufficiently documented a reason for refusing a given offer. Any significant alteration in the organ process would be further reviewed, such as when an organ with certain rare characteristics or risk factors is offered specifically to programs willing to accept it. This may be done to prevent wastage of a transplantable organ, a specific guideline of the Final Rule.

UNOS staff also review the criteria justifying a candidate's listing in a medically urgent status. This may involve a combination of reviews of electronic records submitted by transplant program and onsite visits conducted by reviewers. UNOS staff conduct periodic, scheduled routine site visits at all heart, liver, and lung transplant programs. Should particular questions or concerns arise, a special site visit may also occur independent of the routine schedule.

Should such reviews generate potential issues of noncompliance, or should a complaint be received that raises such concerns, UNOS will seek the guidance of the OPTN/UNOS Membership and Professional Standards Committee. This committee is empowered to investigate these issues under a confidential peer-review process. Peer review often involves correspondence or interviews with OPTN members and, for issues of greater concern, due process including formal hearings and the right for appeals.

Similar processes apply if evidence or complaints indicate that the health and safety of transplant patients or donors is at risk due to a member's actions. The review process may be prompted according to existing OPTN bylaws and policies, or HHS may request a special investigation for matters not directly within the purview of the OPTN.

A typical review of a potential policy violation or health/safety issue will focus on three primary issues:

- Is this a continuing/recurring situation or an isolated past event?
- Did (or does) it jeopardize patient safety and/or the equity of the transplant system?
- Has the issue been corrected already? If not, does the member pledge to take appropriate corrective action?

If the event is isolated and either has been or can be corrected, the presumptive approach is to allow the member to continue operations while addressing deficiencies. Potential disruptions in patients' access to care or continuity of care must be weighed against the nature of the infraction.

Should there be ongoing or egregious examples of noncompliance or compromised patient safety, the interests of patients and/or the public may be best served by member inactivation. In many instances, transplant programs have voluntarily inactivated before or during OPTN reviews. Of these, some have resumed operation after implementing corrective action, and others have closed permanently.

Table 30.4 lists the adverse actions the OPTN and UNOS have the ability to take in situations warranted by a member's poor or recalcitrant performance. The objective is performance improvement intended to bring the member into full compliance with OPTN policies or bylaws, rather than punitive enforcement action. Therefore, adverse actions for findings of lesser violations do not involve public notice.

The designations of probation and member not in good standing include notice to the public and a program's candidates and recipients about the adverse action. These two actions also require corrective action plans to regain regular membership status. Members understand that the policies may be "voluntary" with respect to enforcement under federal law and regulation, but failure to be in compliance can have serious consequences for a member.

TABLE 30.4 OPTN/UNOS Potential Adverse Actions against Members

Name of Action	What It Entails	Due Process Involved	Confidential or Public?
Letter of uncontested violation Letter of warning Letter of reprimand	Formal correspondence sent to member institution regarding a past incidence of policy noncompliance or potential health/safety issue. In general, letter of uncontested violation is for an action of least ongoing significance; letter of reprimand is for a more significant issue	Issued at the discretion of the OPTN/UNOS Membership and Professional Standards Committee (MPSC) after an interview with the member and consideration of any data or documentary evidence. MPSC may ask for a plan of corrective action to address specific deficiencies	Typically confidential. Action could be publicly acknowledged upon agreement of both the OPTN/UNOS and the member involved
Probation	Determination of a significant violation or deficiency requiring corrective action	Issued by the OPTN/UNOS Board of Directors upon MPSC recommendation. Member is entitled to a formal hearing before the MPSC and, if the member chooses, an appellate hearing before the entire OPTN/UNOS Board. MPSC will review the member's corrective action plan and make further recommendation to the Board regarding removal of either	Notice to public and to key state and/or federal agencies issued upon final Board determination. Member is also required to notify affected transplant candidates or recipients at the direction of the OPTN/UNOS Board
Member not in good standing	Finding of a critical violation or deficiency warranting corrective action and/or inactivation of the program involved. OPTN/UNOS member privileges, including voting and representation, are revoked		

ORGAN PLACEMENT ACTIVITIES

OPTN policies for deceased donor organ allocation are made operational in the process of organ placement. These activities include

- Gaining consent for deceased donation and obtaining needed medical information about the potential donor
- Accessing the computerized matching system and generating organ-specific match runs of suitable candidates
- Contacting transplant programs for named candidates and providing information to support their decision to accept or reject an organ offer
- Arranging the logistics of organ recovery, preservation, and transportation to the accepting transplant center(s)

For every organ allocation from a deceased donor in the United States, OPTN members will access the computerized match system operated by UNOS. This involves entering key data for a potential organ donor and accessing a ranked list of candidates who are to be offered a given organ in sequence. This list, unique for every organ offer, is called a "match run."

In many instances, the organ procurement organization where the donor originates (commonly called the "Host OPO") will handle all placement activities once the "match run" list of candidates is generated. Certain circumstances require the UNOS Organ Center (described in more detail below) to oversee the placement. The Organ Center can also assist in placement activities for the convenience of the Host OPO or to address unusual or emergent circumstances.

The Host OPO or the Organ Center will contact the transplant team for the highest-ranked candidate and provide detailed medical information about the potential donor's medical condition and history. The transplant team has 1 hour to decide whether to accept or refuse the organ offer for the candidate identified.

Medical judgment is paramount because the medical professionals providing direct patient care are in the best position to assess the candidate's current need and the amount of risk they are willing to assume for a given organ offer. An organ that may be entirely suitable for one candidate may have too much risk for another. Issues commonly weighed by the transplant team include

- The relative age of the donor and the candidate
- The donor's circumstances of death, treatment provided until death, and current measures of organ function
- The presence and severity of certain donor medical history such as hypertension, diabetes, hepatitis, cardiovascular disease, or cancer

Should the transplant team decline an organ offer, it will document a refusal reason to UNOS. The next team in sequence then has the right to accept or refuse, and so on until the organ is accepted or until circumstances no longer allow it to be used. Once all potential offers are accepted for a given donor, the Host OPO or the Organ Center will make logistical arrangements for surgical recovery of organs and transportation to the accepting center(s).

UNet℠ and DonorNet®

In the early history of the OPTN, transplant centers and OPOs entered and accessed candidate and donor data either by calling or faxing to UNOS' headquarters or by using a VAX computer system with a dedicated link to a terminal at the member institution. The organ offer process often involved a series of phone calls and faxes between the institutions involved, often conveying the same set of information multiple times if an organ offer was refused for more than one candidate. In addition, pre- and posttransplant data were managed in two separate applications that were not necessarily compatible with patient or donor data stored in the members' in-house computer network. As a result, pre- or posttransplant data often had to be reentered or converted between systems.

As Internet access became both more universal and more secure, UNOS began to develop an Internet-based system to enter and manage information on donors, candidates, and recipients. The UNet^{sm} application made its debut in 1999. This application links all pre- and posttransplant data in a single system that members can access from any computer with standard Internet capability. It also provides secure, user-specific access, and audit trails to determine precisely who has entered or modified any record. Many members have integrated UNet^{sm} data fields with their own donor and patient computer databases to reduce the need to reenter detailed information, thus saving time and reducing the potential for coding error.

Continuing advances in digital recordkeeping and electronic communication allowed UNOS to launch a separate application in 2007, DonorNet®, to facilitate the organ offer process and greatly reduce the need for the same information to be communicated serially via phone and fax. Through desktop computers or mobile devices such as PDAs, members can convey donor offer information simultaneously to multiple transplant teams for a single offer and the transplant program can review any electronically captured information, including text and images, to determine whether to accept the offer. Figure 30.2 shows an initial data entry screen from the DonorNet® application.

UNOS Organ Center

In 1982, years prior to the establishment of the OPTN, UNOS established a Kidney Center to assist with the placement of kidney transplants between distant OPOs and transplant centers. It was renamed the Organ Center in 1984 to reflect placement of additional organs, and it continues in operation today under an OPTN mandate to assist the transplant field in organ placement.

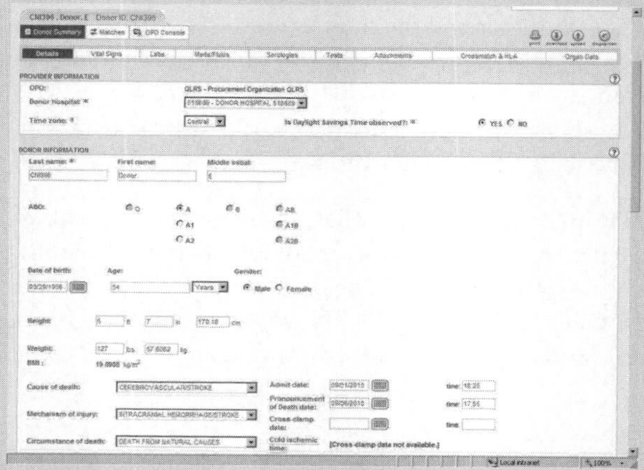

FIGURE 30.2 DonorNet® data entry screen.

The Organ Center is staffed 24 hours a day, 7 days a week, by organ placement specialists working 12-hour shifts and a manager either onsite or on call. The center's primary functions include

- Helping place donated organs for transplantation
- Helping record donor information and running the donor/recipient computer matching process
- Assisting with transportation of organs and tissues for the purposes of transplantation
- Serving as a resource to the transplant community regarding organ-sharing policies

Organ placement often occurs according to well-established procedures and expectations. However, given the immediate need to use available organs and the challenges posed by natural or technological disasters, transplant professionals must sometimes adapt quickly and creatively to emergent situations. In these circumstances, the preeminent goal is to prevent organ wastage, with the secondary goal of reestablishing routine activity as soon as possible.

Case Study: Organ Placement during September 11 Events

The tragic events of September 11, 2001, had many consequences far beyond the obvious effects on the American public. Of direct impact to the transplant field was the grounding of all air traffic other than military aircraft for nearly 24 hours. It is very common for deceased donor kidneys to be transported as cargo on commercial air flights. In addition, a number of donated hearts, lungs, and livers are transported by local charter flights, as are transplant teams sent to recover organs at donor hospitals.

The grounding of all private and commercial air traffic, and the uncertainty of when it would be allowed to resume, meant that organ placement would be very difficult for any candidates beyond a few hours' drive of the donor location. At the same time, while a few hospitals in the New York City area were temporarily unavailable for transplantation due to the need to provide trauma care, there were no other disruptions to medical care elsewhere in the United States. The transplant community had prior experience with temporary disruptions due to major snowstorms or hurricanes, but these are regional events and often affect the readiness of transplant institutions over a wide area.

As soon as it was clear that air restrictions were to be ordered, UNOS notified all OPOs and transplant centers of the issue. UNOS instructed that whenever possible, organ allocation should be made to the candidate most highly ranked on the match run. However, to prevent organ wastage, members were encouraged to place organs with local candidates as necessary and were given a special refusal code that UNOS could track to indicate when candidates were deferred because of transport restrictions.

Beginning September 12, some charter flights were allowed with special permission, and later commercial flights resumed on a limited schedule. UNOS continued to monitor these developments and conveyed this information rapidly to OPOs and transplant centers so that they could make needed arrangements. UNOS also worked closely with the U.S. Department of Health and Human Services to communicate with the Federal Aviation Administration on the vital need for organs to travel by air and offered guidance for airport security screeners to check for the legitimacy of packaged organs.

Of approximately 20 organs in transport or arranged for placement during the air shutdown, about half were able to be transplanted into the originally intended recipient. Despite the permission to place organs locally, if needed, some institutions found unique ways to ensure that the offer went to the intended candidate. OPO staff volunteered to drive a deceased donor kidney from Oklahoma to a transplant center in Nebraska, a distance of more than 400 miles. An Air National Guard flight conveyed a liver recovered in Tennessee for a 6-month-old candidate in Texas. UNOS is not aware of any candidate deaths awaiting transplantation that related directly to transportation difficulties during the shutdown.

DATA COLLECTION AND ANALYSIS

As mentioned previously, one of the key mandates of the OPTN is to collect and manage data on candidates listed for deceased donor transplantation, living and deceased organ donors, and recipients of living donor transplants. In addition to data collected at the time of transplantation, long-term follow-up data are collected on transplant recipients and living donors.

More data are publicly accessible about organ transplantation than any other medical discipline in the United States. The data can be used in many ways—at the macro level to discern general trends of donation and transplantation, or at the center-specific level to document whether a given transplant program or organ procurement organization is meeting the expectations.

Beyond the policy and clinical applications of data, transplantation is uniquely accountable to the public. This is in part because of the dramatic and life-saving nature of the field. But in a greater sense, transplantation depends on public trust and support. People look to transplant data to quantify the need for organ donation and to ensure that the transplant institutions are meeting public expectations of performance and integrity. Should these data not be available, mistrust may increase and many people would not consent to be organ donors either in their lifetime or upon their death. Transplant data are routinely accessed and commented upon by many nonclinical publics including potential transplant patients and donors, government agencies, students, and the news media.

Roles of the OPTN and SRTR

The OPTN collects all data provided by member institutions. As mentioned earlier, the UNet℠ and DonorNet® applications are the primary means of data entry. OPTN policies specify to members what data forms need to be completed at what intervals of time, as well as the specific fields that are required to consider a form complete. Some data fields are optional and may assist in placement or later analysis but are not necessary to close out a required form.

Many data fields are programmed to highlight inconsistencies that may indicate the data are incorrectly entered and allow the member to verify or correct the form before submission. UNOS staff also work with members to validate information and update or correct data submission.

OPTN data are made available in a variety of ways:

- Commonly requested summary data reports are available on the OPTN Web site (http://optn.transplant.hrsa.gov/).
- Individuals may request data, either as defined reports or a broad set of computerized data for analysis where individually identifying information has been removed.
- The OPTN provides descriptive data (counts or crosstabulated results) to OPTN/UNOS committees for policy analysis.

The OPTN also shares data with the SRTR, mentioned earlier, for its purposes. The SRTR is generally charged with data analysis to support policymaking and clinical advancement of transplantation. It makes these analyses available in a number of ways:

- Transplant center- and OPO-specific reports are available on the SRTR Web site (www.ustransplant.org).
- The SRTR conducts data analysis for OPTN/UNOS committees to review and consider policies.
- The SRTR and the OPTN jointly produce a statistical annual report that summarizes the most recent decade of data and analyses on transplant trends.

In addition, both the OPTN and SRTR frequently collaborate with transplant professionals to conduct studies for presentation and publication to advance the clinical understanding of good transplant practice. OPTN and SRTR research staff are frequently primary authors or coauthors of papers presented at leading transplant symposia and/or published in refereed medical journals.

Whether through committee support or individual studies, such research commonly identifies and promotes practices that may enhance access to transplantable organs, make more efficient use of the organs available, and/or enhance patient and graft survival while reducing the likelihood of serious complications associated with transplant care. Such practices may be at the level of national policy, such as modifying an allocation policy to better prioritize urgent transplant candidates. They may also be at an individual practice level, such as whether to accept or reject donors with a history of a certain cancer that has a risk of being transmitted to a recipient.

Case Study: Amendment to Heart Allocation Policy

Heart and lung allocation policy is affected by the relatively short preservation and travel time for optimal organ function. Most transplant professionals will not consider thoracic organ offers involving more than 6 hours of preservation time, with 4 hours or less preferable. For this reason, heart and lung candidates are stratified for available organ offers by their center's geographic distance from the donor location; candidates within the local donor service area are considered first, then more distant candidates in widening 500-mile concentric circles from the donor site.

This practical consideration is counterbalanced by the urgent need of many transplant candidates. Those in the two most urgent status categories (Status 1A and 1B) are at higher risk of dying awaiting an organ transplant than candidates in the other active category, Status 2. The longstanding heart allocation policy considered all eligible candidates, in descending urgency status, at one geographic level before proceeding to the next. This could mean that an urgent candidate just beyond the allocation boundary would have less allocation priority than a more local, less urgent Status 2 candidate.

Beginning in 2002, the OPTN/UNOS Thoracic Organ Transplantation Committee reviewed OPTN data and SRTR analyses of the relative risk of pretransplant and early posttransplant deaths by the status of heart transplant candidates. The committee focused specifically on the comparable risk of death awaiting transplantation and in the first 30 days following transplantation.

For Status 1A and 1B candidates, posttransplant survival was significantly better in the short term as compared to the risk of dying while awaiting a transplant. By contrast, Status 2 recipients had a significant risk of mortality within the first 30 days of a transplant as compared to Status

2 candidates who remained on the waiting list. This suggested the allocation policy could be changed to give greater priority to Status 1A and 1B candidates, who would receive greater benefit from timely transplantation than their Status 2 counterparts.

The committee began to consider a policy amendment that would prioritize heart offers available within 500 miles of the donor's location to all eligible Status 1A and 1B candidates before any Status 2 patients would be considered. As the committee continued to consider this policy change, the SRTR performed simulation modeling to compare the proposal's predicted effect to the results of the then-current system.

The simulation suggested that implementing the policy change would result in a 7% reduction in total deaths (including both pretransplant and early posttransplant deaths) among heart transplant patients. Some variations to the policy were also modeled, but the committee ultimately backed the initial proposal. After public comment and committee reconsideration, the proposal was approved by the OPTN/UNOS Board of Directors in November 2005.

Once the policy was implemented in July 2006, the committee, utilizing OPTN and SRTR data and analyses, examined the policy's actual effects to determine whether it was meeting expectations. Comparing the year before the policy implementation to the year after implementation, deaths as a function of time waited on the list (deaths per 100 patient-years) decreased threefold for the most urgent (Status 1A) candidates, from 96.3 before implementation to 30.3 afterward. Deaths among Status 1B candidates were cut nearly in half, from 20.3 to 11.8. Deaths among Status 2 patients also decreased slightly, from 5.8 to 3.7; this was a positive but somewhat unexpected finding, as the primary intent of the policy was to benefit the more urgent candidates. Longer term outcomes of the policy will continue to be studied to determine whether additional improvements can be made.

Conclusion

The nation's organ transplant system continues to develop and expand upon the framework established through federal legislation and regulation. It also depends vitally on the expertise of its members in developing standards and policies for the network, and in ensuring that they are met for the benefit of transplant candidates, living donors, and the loved ones of deceased donors.

A sophisticated, yet highly adaptable process exists to place available organs with candidates identified by policy to have the greatest need and the highest potential benefit. The use of modern communications technology is transforming organ placement in some ways, but is not intended to supplant the medical judgment of transplant teams who must ultimately determine which organ may be best for their patient.

The national system depends upon the collection and reporting of detailed data to advance clinical knowledge and to continually examine improvements to transplant policy. Such reporting is also vital to the public's understanding and trust of the transplant system, of unique importance because the public ultimately supports the transplant process through the life-giving act of organ donation.

References

Norman, J. D. and A.T. Laurence, eds. 2001. *Primer on Transplantation*, 2nd edn. Mt. Laurel, NJ: American Society of Transplantation, pp. 1–2.

Petechuk, D. 2006. *Organ Transplantation*. Westport, CT: Greenwood Press, pp. 11–13.

Public Law 98-507. 1984.

Wolf, J. S. 1991. Brief history of transplantation. In *Organ Procurement, Preservation and Distribution in Transplantation*, M. G. Phillips, ed. Richmond, VA: UNOS, p. 5.

Design, Planning, Control, and Management of Healthcare Systems

IV.D Pharmacy Operation

31 **Pharmacoeconomics and the Drug Development Process** *Stephanie R. Earnshaw, Thomas N. Taylor, and Cheryl McDade* **31**-1
Introduction • Drug Approval Process • Modeling within the Process and Guidelines • Model Analyses • References

31

Pharmacoeconomics and the Drug Development Process

Stephanie R. Earnshaw
RTI Health Solutions

Thomas N. Taylor
Wayne State University

Cheryl McDade
RTI Health Solutions

Introduction 31-1
Drug Approval Process 31-2
Modeling within the Process and Guidelines 31-3
Model Analyses 31-5
Cost-Effectiveness Analyses • Budget Impact Analyses • Threshold Analyses • Other Analyses
References 31-10

Introduction

The use of decision-analytic modeling in healthcare has increased dramatically over the years. It is a useful technique to logically outline and examine problems when data are limited, and to solve problems efficiently when the solution is unknown and/or difficult to determine. As seen in the previous chapters, these techniques have been particularly useful in supporting health-related topics such as vaccine production, hospital bed and equipment planning, surgical scheduling, and optimal radiation administration. In the past 15 years, the use of decision-analytic modeling has increased in supporting pharmaceutical preparation and planning.

Traditionally, the primary objective of getting a new pharmaceutical product to market has revolved around the examination of the product's clinical efficacy and safety. This is still the case in today's market. However, the added pressures of high medical costs and availability of limited funds to pay for these new technologies has become a major concern. Understanding the value of healthcare technologies, whether they are new or existing pharmaceuticals, medical devices/procedures, or diagnostics is important. Decision-makers seldom have sufficient monies to permit the use of all approved healthcare technologies for their population (i.e., country, region, healthcare system). However, controlling costs of these technologies is more complicated than choosing the cheapest technology. As in many industries, new technological approaches such as developing new ways to create energy or the development of new electronic devices take time to become cost efficient. We see similar effects in the pharmaceutical industry. In contrast to new approaches to energy production or the development of new electronic devices where the new and old approaches may be used interchangeably or even substituted with one another for some time; healthcare technologies must be examined more closely. Pharmaceuticals are more personal and prevent an adverse outcome for people. Thus, sometimes these new technologies cannot be substituted with other, older forms of pharmaceuticals because these new technologies may be the only available efficacious treatment for a particular condition or a patient with specific characteristics.

As a result, decision-makers need to make careful and informed judgments about the value (in terms of significance to patients and benefit for money) of new or existing technologies relative to other therapeutic technologies.

These issues have led to the formation of a field of research called pharmacoeconomics and outcomes research. This area of research examines the impact of new pharmaceutical products on quality of life and economic outcomes. This field has skyrocketed in visibility and in interest from decision-makers and patients because of its importance and personal impact. Overall, studies in this field examine the value of a specific pharmaceutical with respect to other technologies. In general, the technologies examined may be a form of pharmacotherapy compared with one or more pharmacotherapies (Rindress et al. 1998, Drummond et al. 2003). However, these technologies may be expanded to examine medical devices, which may represent "usual care" and/or examine the value of specific diagnostics used to identify medical conditions. All in all, these studies examine the impact that different healthcare technologies have on costs and outcomes such as quality of life within a therapeutic area and around the technology to be utilized within a therapeutic area. The purpose of these studies is to understand the potential value along with the safety and efficacy that the technology can provide.

Decision-analytic modeling is particularly important for examining the economic value of a technology. Economic modeling can be used to measure the overall cost impact of a technology against the level of achievable health benefit or the financial impact that having this technology in the market will have in general. Modeling is particularly important because it provides decision-makers with a systematic approach to examining the potential impact of a technology's attributes in the presence of limited data.

The economic value of healthcare technologies is important to examine at various points of the approval and marketing process. Value can be examined prior to a technologies approval for market and as early as in animal studies or in initial human studies. In this chapter, we focus on decision-analytic modeling to support the examination of the value of pharmaceutical products. Modeling has become well accepted in supporting the assessment of pharmaceutical products. The application of these methods is perhaps less defined when examining the value of medical devices and diagnostics. However, decision-makers can easily extrapolate these methods to support the assessments of these healthcare technologies. In the following sections, we present an overview of the drug approval, marketing, and reimbursement process and also discuss the points in the process where decision-analytical modeling becomes an important task. We also present an overview of the different types of analyses that are important to perform and a case study to demonstrate the type of model that may be beneficial to decision-makers.

Drug Approval Process

The process of getting a drug to market is a long, involved, and expensive process throughout the world. For brevity, we describe the drug approval process in the United States. There are five main stages in the drug approval process. These consist of drug discovery, preclinical testing, clinical development, regulatory review, and postmarketing safety surveillance. During the drug discovery process, the chemical or biological structure and key characteristics of the drug candidate (i.e., compound) are determined and methods for small scale production are developed. The preclinical phase involves testing the compound in the laboratory and in animals to determine whether the compound is likely to be safe when used in humans and in what ways it may be effective in addressing unmet medical needs (US FDA 2002). Before a new compound may be used in humans, the available preclinical data must be submitted to the Food and Drug Administration (FDA) in the form of an investigational new drug (IND) application.

Unless disapproved by the FDA, clinical trials in humans may begin shortly after filing the IND. Clinical testing of INDs consist of four phases. In Phase I studies, the drug is tested in healthy volunteers to ensure that it is safe enough to test in patients with disease. The drug is administered to patients with the targeted disease in Phase II where the objectives are to better understand the safety and potential efficacy of the drug. Data from Phase II clinical trials provide the basis for the design of the large scale, confirmatory trials in Phase III. Typically, at least two well-designed, randomized controlled trials are conducted in Phase III. This is the most expensive stage of the clinical development process as Phase III trials may involve recruiting and testing in thousands of patients (DiMasi et al. 2003).

Upon completion of the Phase III clinical trials, pharmaceutical companies submit an extensive new drug application (NDA) to the FDA for review. FDA staff review the NDA and meet with the companies, academic experts, and other key decision-makers to review the safety and efficacy evidence. The regulatory approval process takes approximately 18 months to complete. Overall, the process of clinical development and regulatory review typically lasts 7–8 years. From the early phases of drug discovery to approval by the FDA, the full drug development process takes an average of 12–13 years with an estimated capitalized cost per approved new molecular entity of $1.2 billion to $1.3 billion in 2005 dollars (DiMasi and Grabowski 2007). As a result, we observe that the development of new pharmaceuticals for market is quite costly.

Regulatory oversight does not end with the approval of the drug. Phase IV clinical studies may be performed to assess the long-term benefits and risks (Rados 2003). The limited clinical experience in the use of the drug generated during the clinical development period does not typically provide enough data to assess the potential for rare side-effects. For many new drugs, the FDA may require postmarketing, safety studies involving large numbers of patients to more fully evaluate the risk of rare side-effects.

As a drug progresses through the development pipeline, pharmaceutical companies continually assess its commercial prospects (e.g., clinical need, target patient populations, potential pricing, and associated reimbursement). The first reports of Phase II trial results become a major barometer of the drug's potential marketability. Compounds that fail to demonstrate adequate safety and differentiation from existing drugs in the market may be discontinued. The period just prior to the initiation of the Phase III development program becomes an important time for assessing commercial viability. One of the keys to determining commercial viability is the drug's prospects for reimbursement. Drugs with a better safety profile and improved efficacy or quality of life relative to existing market leaders for treating the condition of interest are likely to receive preferred status in terms of reimbursement, depending on the pricing of the product. Many new drugs, however, may come to market with some safety or efficacy advantages over existing competitors, but at a higher price. It is at this point where modeling has been typically used to evaluate whether these improved product features represent "value for money."

Modeling within the Process and Guidelines

Decision-analytic modeling is useful at various points of the drug approval process. In the early phases of clinical development, modeling can be used to determine the value of compounds for in-licensing (Stewart et al. 2001, Frei and Leleux 2004, Villiger and Bogdan 2005, Hartmann and Hassan 2006). Additionally, modeling can be useful to forecast the clinical benefit that is necessary for a new drug to be competitive with other drugs currently in the market. These tools help decision-makers make "go-no-go" drug development decisions. Modeling has also been used to examine the risk–benefit trade-offs associated with drugs that have been approved for marketing but have shown to have significant adverse effects only after they have entered the market (Lynd and O'Brien 2004, Wilson et al. 2008).

Perhaps the most common use of decision-analytic modeling in the drug approval and planning process is the use of models to support the reimbursement of new and existing drugs and healthcare technologies. Payers, whether they are managed-care organizations within the United States, government payer systems such as Medicare and Medicaid in the United States and the National Health Service in the United Kingdom, or even the patient, have limited monetary resources to pay for new and existing healthcare products. As a result, more and more payers are concentrating on these costs and are attempting to employ methods to efficiently assess and allocate medical resources among their covered populations. Thus, getting a drug approved for treating a condition is just one of the many battles that pharmaceutical companies face in the approval process. They also now must demonstrate the value for money so that payers are interested in covering these technologies. A healthcare technology that has been proven to be safe and effective is of little value if health insurers are not willing to pay for it. Thus, efficiently allocating medical resources is an important issue in today's market.

Decision-analytic modeling is certainly not a foreign concept to reimbursement agencies within various countries. A number of countries have made the assessment of a drug's value as a requirement for reimbursement (Tarn 2004). These countries or payer agencies recognize that the complete and perfect economic information about how a particular drug will compare to other already commonly used or to be used drugs in the respective therapy area limited. Thus, their guidelines for technology appraisal or health technology assessment submissions include sections that outline requirements for developing a decision-analytic model to examine the cost-effectiveness and sometimes the budget impact of a drug (Philips et al. 2004, 2006, AMCP 2005, Canadian Agency of Drugs and Technologies for Health 2006, Pharmaceutical Benefits Advisory Committee 2006, Scottish Medicines Consortium 2007, National Institute for Health and Clinical Excellence 2008).

The National Institute for Health and Clinical Excellence (NICE) (National Institute for Health and Clinical Excellence 2008), Scottish Medicines Consortium (SMC) of England and Wales (Scottish Medicines Consortium 2007), Canadian Agency for Drug and Technologies in Health (CADTH) (Canadian Agency of Drugs and Technologies for Health 2006), Pharmaceutical Benefits Advisory Committee (PBAC) of Australia (Pharmaceutical Benefits Advisory Committee 2006), and the Academy of Managed Care Pharmacy's (AMCP 2005) have been at the forefront of publishing guidelines for pharmacoeconomic evaluations. These agencies have formally recognized modeling as a valid and acceptable analytical approach to perform economic evaluations. In addition to the pharmacoeconomic guidelines for the above agencies, guidelines for pharmacoeconomic analyses for additional countries/payers can be found at the International Society for Pharmacoeconomics and Outcomes Research (ISPOR) website (Tarn 2004).

These guidelines outline a number of important issues to consider when developing or presenting a model to perform a specific evaluation. From the presentation of the analysis perspective, issues such as presenting the selection and justification for the type of analysis being performed along with the scope, perspective, comparators, target population, time horizon, and cycle times of a specific analysis are reviewed. From the model development perspective, the guidelines are careful to delineate specifics to the modeling approach (i.e., structure and assumptions around the structure) that should be presented in the model. Some guidelines may summarize the preferred approaches to collecting data, such as performing systematic literature reviews. In addition, the type of data (i.e., clinical efficacy, costs, and quality of life) and level of evidence preferences around specific data points used in the model may be discussed. For example, NICE requests that "changes in health-related quality of life be reported directly from patients and the value of changes" or utilities "should be based on public preferences" for estimating quality-adjusted life years (QALYs). Thus EQ-5D is the preferred measure for health-related quality of life (National Institute for Health and Clinical Excellence 2008). QALYs are discussed in more detail later in this chapter.

These guidelines describe different approaches to examine uncertainty around data inputs and model structure. To examine the uncertainty and impact of changes in one variable at a time can be seen in one-way or univariate sensitivity analysis. Recommendations for performing multivariate and/or probabilistic sensitivity analyses are often provided. Additional analyses such as variability, scenario, and subgroup analyses may also be outlined. Briggs et al. (2006) and Briggs (2000) detail the basics of many of these concepts.

Guidelines also recognize that validation is an important part of the economic evaluation process. Thus, the importance of assessing the consistency and quality of the model is typically addressed and model validation is recommended. While guidelines will touch upon these issues, a number of articles have been published to discuss these issues in greater detail (McCabe and Dixon 2000, Sculpher et al. 2000, Weinstein et al. 2003, Philips et al. 2004, 2006).

Model Analyses

Decision-analytic modeling has become a very useful tool in pharmacoeconomics because preapproval studies concentrate on examining the safety and efficacy of a particular drug, and not on the economic endpoints. These studies are developed and powered to evaluate changes in one to two clinical efficacy endpoints for a new drug compared with the minimally ethical standard treatment. In addition, these studies are structured such that they can be completed in a reasonably short-time frame. As a result, studies often do not examine economic endpoints such as costs and resource utilization and are often not powered to examine differences in safety endpoints. For drugs that may be used long-term, the preapproval clinical trials typically have treatment durations shorter than those observed in usual practice. These trials often examine the effects of treatment on intermediate endpoints such as blood concentrations rather than final outcomes such as death. For example, new hypertensive agents typically examine the impact on blood pressure levels and are performed over a period of 4–12 weeks in length. However, the true economic impact of these drugs is measured via their reduction of events such as myocardial infarction (MI), stroke, and death. These events are what impact the costs and outcomes. Because of the amount of time and high cost required to establish the link between treatment and final outcomes, decision-analytic modeling is an accepted tool to evaluate the impact of these drugs for chronic conditions. Thus, because of these and many other issues good practices in decision-analytic modeling in healthcare evaluations is important (Weinstein et al. 2003).

The types of analyses that tend to be performed during the drug development process are

- Cost-effectiveness analyses to examine the underlying value (i.e., costs while considering clinical outcome) of a drug
- Early cost-effectiveness threshold analyses to examine the impact that different drug pricing or clinical effectiveness assumptions have on a drug's potential value for money
- Budget-impact analyses to examine the financial impact that including a drug in a reimbursement agencies formulary would have
- Benefit–risk analyses to examine the overall potential benefits of a drug while considering all its potential risks
- Valuation analyses to examine the expected value that a new drug may bring to a company in terms of market and benefit for potential in-licensing and investment

We present each type of analysis below.

Cost-Effectiveness Analyses

Cost-effectiveness analyses is an economic evaluation that examines both the costs and health outcomes of alternative healthcare technologies. These analyses are used to determine if a healthcare technology is good value for money. Several publications present the formal requirements for performing these analyses (Gold et al. 1996, Siegel et al. 1997, Murray et al. 2000, Muennig 2002, Drummond et al. 2005).

In cost-effectiveness analyses, the incremental cost and incremental outcomes of one healthcare technology are compared to alternative healthcare technologies. These components are compiled into an incremental cost-effectiveness ratio (ICER) presented as

$$\text{ICER}=\frac{\text{Costs}_\text{A}-\text{Costs}_\text{B}}{\text{Outcome}_\text{A}-\text{Qutcome}_\text{B}},$$

where

$Costs_A$ are total costs incurred by patients on treatment A
$Costs_B$ are total costs incurred by patients on treatment B
$Outcome_A$ is total outcomes incurred by patients on treatment A
$Outcome_B$ is total outcomes incurred by patients on treatment B

Decision-analytic modeling can be used to simulate the care process according to a "status quo" healthcare technology. These models can generate costs and outcomes over a prespecified time horizon. By changing the care process to include the new healthcare technology, the effect on costs and outcomes can be generated. Given these two sets of results, the cost-effectiveness of the new healthcare technology compared with the "status quo" healthcare technology is estimated.

The ICER per some outcome of interest can be presented in a variety of ways. Some of the more common ICERs that are presented are incremental cost per life year gained, incremental cost per case of illness prevented, and incremental cost per outcome achieved. The ICER is generally chosen based on the costs and outcomes that are appropriate for the disease area and analysis perspective. The costs used in the ICER naturally depend upon the perspective of the analysis. For example, if the perspective is that of the hospital, then only costs that are relevant to the hospital should be considered. Whereas, the outcomes used in the ICER are dictated by the disease and impact that the new healthcare technology may have. For example, in a lifetime chronic disease in which the new healthcare technology may improve survival, an ICER such as the incremental cost per life year gained is appropriate. Whereas, in a short-term disease such as the use of an antibiotic to treat an ear infection, an ICER such as the incremental cost per clinical success is more appropriate. Detailed methods for conducting cost-effectiveness analyses have been published by a number of authors (Gold et al. 1996, Siegel et al. 1997, Drummond et al. 2005, Briggs et al. 2006).

The drawback of ICERs that define the denominator in natural units such as cost per clinical success or life years gained, is that they are not appropriate for making comparisons between different therapy areas. For example, a new healthcare technology in one therapy area may improve survival and have a better side-effect profile than the status quo versus a new healthcare technology in another therapy area, which may improve survival but have no additional benefits in side-effect profile than the status quo. The former new healthcare technology essentially not only improves survival, but it also improves quality of life. Thus, ICERs that use incremental life years saved as a measure of outcome will understate the benefits of interventions that improve the quality of life. Because of these limitations, researchers have developed methods for standardizing health outcomes into a measure that accounts for improvements in both the quantity and quality of life, thereby facilitating comparisons across therapeutic areas.

QALYs is the measure used to adjust survival time for subjective quality of life. In other words, it is the composite measure of length of life and quality of life (Muennig 2002, Drummond et al. 2005), where a year of life under certain conditions is assigned a value called a patient's "utility." This utility value is a person's subjective measurement of the desirability of a health state and is a value between 0.0 and 1.0, where 0.0 is the worst imaginable quality of life and 1.0 is perfect health (Gold et al. 1996, Siegel et al. 1997, Murray et al. 2000, Muennig 2002, Drummond et al. 2005). For example, a person who lives 10 years at a quality of life reflecting 0.8 is assigned a value of 8 QALYs.

The incremental cost per QALY is being used increasingly in cost-effectiveness analysis to facilitate comparisons across therapeutic areas. In the United States, the generally accepted threshold for an intervention being good value for money is $50,000 per QALY (Weinstein 1995, Hirth et al. 2000, Eichler et al. 2004). However, this value has not been adjusted over the years to account for issues such as inflation. In the United Kingdom, interventions with an ICER of £20,000 per QALY or less are generally considered cost-effective; interventions with an ICER of £30,000 or greater are generally considered not being cost-effective; and interventions with ICERS falling between £20,000 and £30,000 are generally subject to further discussion (National Institute for Health and Clinical Excellence 2008). This standard metric enables decision-makers to rank the importance of a broad set of healthcare interventions relative to each other. However, this ranking is not without flaws (Drummond et al. 1993).

Budget Impact Analyses

Given the growing cost of healthcare and the availability of limited resources, decision-makers at private health plans as well as public healthcare programs (e.g., the Veterans Administration, state Medicaid programs) find budget impact analyses useful for examining the financial impact that including a new healthcare technology would have on their budgets. Budget-impact analyses compare the current healthcare spending of a mix of pharmaceuticals for a particular condition to the financial demands for spending of a new mix of pharmaceuticals that includes the uptake of the new healthcare technology over time. These analyses can be used to plan budgets, forecast, and compute changes on health insurance premiums. For example, a managed-care organization may be interested in understanding how their current budgets for cholesterol-lowering medications will change if they include a new cholesterol-lowering medication on formulary, while continuing coverage of the other cholesterol-lowering medications (Mauskopf et al. 2005, 2007).

When constructing budget impact and cost-effectiveness analyses, we find that these analyses share many of the same data components when incorporating them into models. In both types of models, it is important to consider costs, clinical efficacy, safety, and impact on mortality and their impact on similar health states. Important differences in budget impact and cost-effectiveness analyses instead revolve around the method to compile the inputs and the output necessary for appropriate decision-making. Just as in cost-effectiveness analyses, it is important to not only consider pharmaceutical acquisition costs, but to also consider the impact on other medical costs such as cost of administering the pharmaceutical (if applicable) and costs associated with incident hospitalizations or outpatient visits. Considering these other medical costs is important because a healthcare technology could be priced lower than all other competing technologies. However, if it is ineffective, it could instead cause other healthcare resources to be incurred. Thus, the true overall impact to budgets would be underestimated if these medical costs were excluded.

Even though the main outcome of interest in budget impact analyses is costs, it is equally important to examine the overall financial impact associated with outcomes. Similar to cost-effectiveness analyses, these outcomes may include survival, symptom-free days, and successful resolution of the condition. Including these measurements of effectiveness provides decision-makers with a sense of the potential medical benefit that result from their potential financial investment. As an example, a new diabetes medication comes on the market at a higher price than the other diabetes medications. Patients using this medication, however, have been shown to have better control of their plasma glucose concentrations as measured by glycosylated hemoglobin (HbA1c)—a key clinical factor that drives future healthcare resource use in diabetes patients. So, within a mix of covered diabetes medications, we may observe an increase in budget, but we also observe an increase in better HbA1c control.

It is not uncommon that a cost-effectiveness analysis may indicate that a new healthcare technology is efficient and a good value for money, while the budget impact analysis may find that including the new healthcare technology is not affordable. To date, there is no formal guidance on what to do in this situation (Mauskopf et al. 2007).

Threshold Analyses

Early in the drug development process, pharmaceutical companies may examine the impact that different prices have on the potential value of a new drug. Threshold pricing models are developed early in the drug approval process to understand drug pricing necessary to gain reimbursement. Specifically, in these models, threshold analyses are a form of cost-effectiveness modeling that identifies combinations of price, efficacy, and safety parameters that would be acceptable from payer or reimbursement agency perspectives.

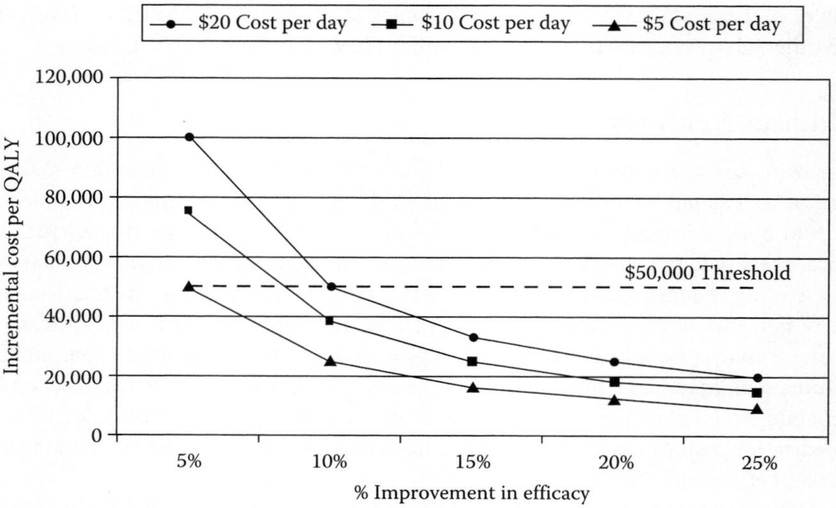

FIGURE 31.1 Threshold analysis: Impact of changes in drug price and drug efficacy on incremental cost per QALY.

For example, for a drug in development that has a similar safety profile to the leading drug on the market, a threshold analysis would provide estimates of the maximum price for an assumed improvement in efficacy that would meet a prespecified cost-effectiveness threshold. Thus, such a model might suggest that a drug with an expected 5% improvement in efficacy could be priced 15% higher than the leading marketed drug and still fall within the cost-effectiveness threshold. These models combine the early known or projected clinical efficacy, acceptable value threshold or incremental cost per QALY threshold (Weinstein 1995, Hirth et al. 2000, Eichler et al. 2004), and variable pricing levels to understand their synergies.

Threshold analyses examine the price and/or clinical efficacy that is necessary for a healthcare technology to achieve a prespecified cost-effectiveness threshold (i.e., $50,000) early in the drug development process. The perspective of the analysis should be specific to the reimbursement agency or payer as they are the ultimate decision-maker on reimbursement issues. Figure 31.1 presents a graphical view of the results of a threshold analysis. In this figure, we observe several lines representing an assumed price for the drug. As the efficacy of the drug increases along the horizontal axis, we observe that the incremental cost per QALY decreases. Thus, if the new compound is priced at $10 per day, it will have to have an incremental improvement in efficacy of approximately 7.5% over the comparator treatment to achieve a cost-effective threshold of $50,000 per QALY. These models provide information to decision-makers such that they can examine a number of assumptions with respect to price and efficacy early in the drug development process. These analyses can be expanded to examine the impact of price and efficacy on additional ICERs such as incremental cost per life year gained or incremental cost per symptom-free day gained.

Other Analyses

We have seen how decision-analytic modeling is typically used to support reimbursement activities and decision-maker "buy-in" to the use of these methods. But there are a variety of areas in which decision-analytic modeling is being discovered as a useful tool in the drug approval and planning process. Among these areas are in clinical planning, benefit–risk evaluation, and drug valuation.

In clinical planning, modeling can be used to project the potential long-term clinical outcomes of a drug based on short-term information in early development of compounds. This information can be compared to the potential marketplace competitors to understand the needs for clinical trial planning and "go/no-go" decisions on early compounds. For example, a diabetes drug may have shown to lower

HbA1c; however, it may have also shown the adverse effect of causing weight gain. Early clinical trials exist to demonstrate the impact that the drug had on HbA1c and weight gain in the first six months of therapy. Marketplace competitors may have similar information and perhaps even have some longer term data. The question to answer is how might the drug impact the patient's HbA1c and weight in subsequent years (i.e., beyond 6 months) and might its long-term benefits be meaningful to differentiate it from the other potential competitors.

An area of great interest is benefit–risk analyses (Lynd et al. 2004, Wilson et al. 2008). With today's drugs, fewer are coming on the market with clear cut improved efficacy over their potential competitors. Instead, we see drugs with similar efficacy and perhaps greater safety. In addition, we see more issues where drugs have a clear benefit but there may be a small, but significant risk. For example, a drug has been shown to clearly reduce the pain associated with rheumatoid arthritis; however, there is a small risk of cardiovascular death in some patients. Benefit–risk analyses can put these benefits and risks into perspective to examine whether the benefits of the drug outweigh the risks such that it is acceptable to patients to keep taking the drug. Current guidelines for examining the benefit–risk

Case Study

Statins are a common prescription medication for the reduction of total cholesterol and prevention of cardiovascular (CV) events (e.g., MI and stroke) in patients without a history of these events. Recent studies have shown that the use of low dose aspirin, an over-the-counter medication, has benefits in the prevention of coronary events. Although lower in price, aspirin has clinical benefits in terms of preventing MI whereas stroke benefits are more limited. However, aspirin can have adverse events such as gastrointestinal bleeding whereas the common adverse event for patients on statins is myopathy (i.e., a tightening of muscles such as the heart). Pignone et al. (2006, 2007) examine the trade-offs in terms of benefits, risks, and costs for prescribing low dose aspirin and the combination of both aspirin and statins in the primary prevention of CV events. This analysis enables physicians to better understand what prevention approach provides patients with the best value for money in the primary prevention of CV disease in male and female patients with various 10-year coronary heart disease (CHD) risks. The analysis performed by Pignone et al. (2006) estimated the costs and QALYs gained by prescribing aspirin alone or aspirin plus statins (combination) in males 45 years of age and with 10-year CHD risk of 2.5%, 5.0%, 7.5%, 10.0%, 15.0%, and 25.0%.

Compared with no therapy, the use of aspirin was found to be cost-savings (i.e., lower cost and greater benefit) in all 10-year CHD risk groups except in patients with low risk of CHD in which aspirin was found to be cost-effective (i.e., incremental cost per QALY <= $50,000). Results are presented in Table 31.1. One-way sensitivity analysis showed that the incremental cost per QALY was sensitivity to changes in gastrointestinal bleeding risks. As long as the patient's risk of bleeding was below 4.9%, aspirin remained effective in males with a moderate 10-year risk of CHD (7.5%).

Assumptions around the model's approach to considering ischemic versus hemorrhagic stroke as one or separate health states were tested, since aspirin can have a negative effect on hemorrhagic stroke. The analysis found that a model structure with combined stroke versus a model structure that separated the two types of stroke had a slight effect. Cost-effectiveness was relatively similar between the two approaches.

Probabilistic sensitivity analysis showed that 91.0% of the time, the use of aspirin was cost-savings in males with a moderate 10-year risk of CHD. As a result of this analysis, it was observed that physicians should be recommending the use of low dose aspirin as a cost-effective way to

TABLE 31.1 Incremental Cost per Quality-Adjusted Life Year for Different Preventative Treatments

	Incremental Cost per QALY	
10-Year CHD Risk	Aspirin vs. No Therapy	Combination Therapy vs. Aspirin Alone
Low CHD risk (2.5%)	$9800	$164,700
Low to moderate risk (5.0%)	Cost savings	$97,900
Moderate risk (7.5%)	Cost savings	$56,200
Moderate to high (10.0%)	Cost savings	$42,500
High risk (15.0%)	Cost savings	$33,600
Very high risk (25.0%)	Cost savings	$15,300

prevent CVD events in all male patients after the age of 45 years. The benefits outweigh the risks and the costs are minimal for this patient population.

In patients who were already on aspirin, combination therapy was found to be cost-effective in 45-year old, male patients with a 10-year CHD risk of 10% or higher (Table 31.1). Since men were already receiving benefits from low dose aspirin, the incremental benefits of adding a higher cost statin did not add value for lower risk patients.

Thus, given the evidence of clinical benefits that aspirin and statins provide when used for preventing CV events in male patients without a history of previous events, physician now have added information on the value for money with the use of these specific treatments. Overall, aspirin is a cost-effective if not cost-savings treatment for males when these patients are not previously on other preventive treatments. In males who are currently on aspirin, adding a statin has an incremental clinical benefit, but is only of value in higher risk patients.

trade-offs are limited and are a significant subject of discussion for regulatory agencies such as the FDA and European Medicines Evaluation Agency (EMEA).

Valuation modeling is another growing area for the use of decision-analytic modeling (Stewart et al. 2001, Frei and Leleux 2004, Villiger and Bogdan 2005, Hartmann and Hassan 2006). Often the development and discovery of new drug compounds is being performed by small startup/biotechnology companies rather than the major pharmaceutical companies. After a drug is discovered and taken to limited early trials, these smaller companies will seek candidates to license the drug for taking the drug to later clinical trials and eventual market. As a result, valuation of the new drug is important both from the licenser and licensee perspective to determine the price for licensing the drug and what the potential return on investment may be. Decision-analytic modeling is a useful technique to bring together potential success of and market for the compound to determine the net present value of a compound.

References

Briggs, A.H. 2000. Handling uncertainty in cost-effectiveness models. *Pharmacoeconomics* 17(5):479–500.

Briggs, A., K. Claxton, and M. Sculpher. 2006. *Decision Modelling for Health Economic Evaluation*. Oxford, U.K.: Oxford University Press.

Canadian Agency for Drugs and Technologies in Health. 2006. *Guidelines for the Economic Evaluation of Health Technologies,* 3rd edn., Ottawa, Canada.

DiMasi, J.A. and H.G. Grabowski. 2007. The cost of biopharmaceutical R & D: Is biotech different? *Manage Decis. Econ*. 28:469–479.

DiMasi, J.A., R.W. Hanson, and H.G. Grabowski. 2003. The price of innovation: New estimates of drug development costs. *J. Health Econ.* 22(3):141–185.

Drummond, M., R. Brown, A.M. Fendrick, P. Fullerton, P. Neumann, R. Taylor, M. Barbieri, and ISPOR Task Force. 2003. Use of pharmacoeconomics information—Report of the ISPOR Task Force on use of pharmacoeconomic/health economic information in health-care decision making. *Value Health* 6(4):407–416.

Drummond, M.F., M.J. Sculper, G.W. Torrance, B.J. O'Brien, and G.L. Stoddart. 2005. *Methods for the Economic Evaluation of Health Care Programmes*, 3rd edn. Oxford, U.K.: Oxford University Press.

Drummond, M.F., G.W. Torrance, and J.M. Mason. 1993. Cost-effectiveness league tables: More harm than good? *Social Sci. Med.* 37:33–40.

Eichler, H., S.X. Kong, W.C. Gerth, P. Mavros, and B. Jonsson. 2004. Use of cost-effectiveness analysis in health-care resource allocation decision-making: How are cost-effectiveness thresholds expected to emerge? *Value Health* 7(5):518–528.

Frei, P. and B. Leleux. 2004. Valuation-what you need to know. *Nat. Biotechnol.* 22(8):1049–1051.

Gold, M.R., J.E. Siegel, L.B. Russell, and W.C. Weinstein. 1996. *Cost-Effectiveness in Health and Medicine.* Oxford, U.K.: Oxford University Press.

Hartmann, M. and A. Hassan. 2006. Application of real options analysis for pharmaceutical R&D project valuation-empirical results from a survey. *Policy Res.* 35:343–354.

Hirth, R.A., M.E. Chernew, E. Miller, A.M. Frederick, and W.G. Weissart. 2000. Willingness to pay for a quality-adjusted life year: In search of a standard. *Med. Decis. Making* 20:332–342.

Lynd, L.D. and B.J. O'Brien. 2004. Advances in risk-benefit evaluation using probabilistic simulation methods: An application to the prophylaxis of deep vein thrombosis. *J. Clin. Epidemiol.* 57:795–803.

Mauskopf, J.A., S.R. Earnshaw, and C.D. Mullen. 2005. Budget impact model analysis: review of the state of the art. *Exp. Rev. Pharmacoecon. Out. Res.* 5(1):65–79.

Mauskopf, J.A., S.D. Sullivan, L. Annemans, J. Caro, C.D. Mullins, M. Nuijten, E. Orlewska, J. Watkins, and P. Trueman. 2007. Principles of good practice for budget impact analysis: Report of the ISPOR Task Force on good research practices—Budget impact analysis. *Value Health* 10(5):324–325.

McCabe, C. and S. Dixon. 2000. Testing the validity of cost-effectiveness models. *Pharmacoeconomics* 17(5):501–513.

Muennig, P. 2002. *Designing and Conducting Cost-Effectiveness Analyses in Medicine and Health Care.* San Francisco, CA: John Wiley and Sons, Inc.

Murray, C.J.L., D.B. Evans, A. Acharya, and R.M.P.M. Baltussen. 2000. Development of WHO guidelines on generalized cost-effectiveness analysis. *Health Econ.* 9:235–251.

National Institute for Health and Clinical Excellence. 2008. *Guide to the Methods of Technology Appraisal.* London, U.K.

Pharmaceutical Benefits Advisory Committee. December 2008. *Guidelines for Preparing Submissions to the Pharmaceutical Benefits Advisory Committee (PBAC)*. Version 4.3, Australian Government, Department of Health and Ageing, Canberra, ACT, Australia.

Philips, Z., L. Bojké, M. Sculpher, K. Claxton, and S. Golder 2006. Good practice guidelines for decision-analytic modelling in health technology assessment: A review and consolidation of quality assessment. *Pharmacoeconomics* 24(4):355–371.

Philips, Z., L. Ginnelly, M. Sculpher et al. 2004. Review of guidelines for good practice in decision-analytic modelling in health technology assessment. *Health Technol. Assess.* (36):iii–iv, ix–xi, 1–158.

Pignone, M.P., S.R. Earnshaw, J.A. Tice, and M.J. Pletcher. 2006. Aspirin, statins, or both drugs for the primary prevention of coronary heart disease events in men: A cost–utility analysis. *Ann. Int. Med.* 144:326–336.

Pignone, M.P., S.R. Earnshaw, J.A. Tice, and M.J. Pletcher. 2007. Aspirin for the primary prevention of cardiovascular disease in women: A cost-utility analysis. *Arch. Intern. Med.* 167:290–295.

Rados, C. 2003. Inside clinical trials: Testing medical products in people. *FDA Consumer Magazine*, September–October, 37(5). http://www.fda.gov/fdac/features/2003/503_trial.html (accessed on February 16, 2009).

Rindress, D., M.D. Smith, and Advisory Panel Chairs. 1998. International Society for Pharmacoeconomics and Outcomes Research: Pharmacoeconomics: Identifying the issues: Advisory Panel Reports.

Scottish Medicines Consortium. 2007. *Guidance to Manufacturers for Completion of New Product Assessment Form (NPAF)* (Revised June 2007). Scottish Medicines Consortium (SMC) of England and Wales.

Sculpher, M. et al. 2000. Assessing quality in decision analytic cost-effectiveness models. A suggested framework and example of application. *Pharmacoeconomics* 17(5):461–477.

Siegel, J.E., G.W. Torrance, L.B. Russell, B.R. Luce, M.C. Weinstein, and M.R. Gold. 1997. Guidelines for pharmacoeconomic studies. Recommendations from the panel on cost effectiveness in health and medicine. Panel on cost effectiveness in health and medicine. *Pharmacoeconomics* 11(2):159–168.

Stewart, J.J., P.N. Allison, and R.S. Johnson. 2001. Putting a price on biotechnology. *Nat. Biotechnol.* 19:813–817.

Tarn, T.Y.H. 2004. Pharmacoeconomic guidelines around the world. *ISPOR Connections* 10(4) (August): http://www.ispor.org/PEguidelines/index.asp (accessed on March 7, 2009).

The Academy of Managed Care Pharmacy (AMCP). 2005. *Format for Formulary Submissions: A Format for Submission of Clinical and Economic Data in Support of Formulary Consideration by Health Care Systems in the United States*. Version 2.1, Alexandria, VA.

United States Food and Drug Administration. 2002. The FDA's drug review process: Ensuring drugs are safe and effective. *FDA Consumer Magazine*, July–August. http://www.fda.gov/fdac/features/2002/402_drug.html (accessed on February 16, 2009).

Villiger, R. and B. Bogdan. 2005. Getting real about valuations in biotech. *Nat. Biotechnol.* 23(4):423–428.

Weinstein, M.C. 1995. From cost-effectiveness ratios to resource allocation: Where to draw the line. In: Sloan FA, ed. *Valuing Health Care: Costs, Benefits, and Effectiveness of Pharmaceuticals and Other Medical Technologies*. New York: Cambridge University Press.

Weinstein, M.C., B. O'Brien, J. Hornberger, J. Jackson, M. Johannesson, C. McCabe, and B.R. Luce. 2003. ISPOR Task Force on good research practices—Modeling studies. Principles of good practice for decision analytic modeling in health-care evaluation: Report of the ISPOR Task Force on good research practices—Modeling studies. *Value Health*. 6(1):9–17.

Wilson, D.P., P.M. Coplan, M.A. Walnberg, and S.M. Blower. 2008. The paradoxical effects of using antiretroviral-based microbicides to control HIV epidemics. *PNAS* 105(28):9835–9840.

Design, Planning, Control, and Management of Healthcare Systems

IV.E ED/ICU Operation

32 **Emergency Department Crowding** *Joshua A. Hilton and Jesse M. Pines* **32-1**
History • Epidemiology • Significance • Definitions of ED Crowding • Conceptual Framework • Measurement • Administrative and Policy Response to ED Crowding • Summary • References

33 **Emergency Department Throughput from a Healthcare Leader's Perspective** *Airica Steed* **33-1**
Background/Context • Emergency Department Throughput • Patient Reception Bottleneck • Mini-Registration and Mobile Bedside Registration • Rapid Triage • Diagnostic Procedure Area • Intradepartmental Flow Bottleneck • Diagnostic Imaging Improvement • Laboratory Services Improvement • Team-Based Approach to Transition of Care • Decompression Block and Inpatient Capacity Bottleneck • Inpatient "Pull" System • Housekeeping Room Turnover • 4-Tier High Census Alert Strategy • Lessons Learned and Sustainment Strategy • References

32

Emergency Department Crowding

History 32-1
Epidemiology 32-2
Significance 32-3
Definitions of ED Crowding 32-4
Conceptual Framework 32-4
Input • Throughput • Output
Measurement 32-11
Emergency Department Crowding Score • Emergency Department Work Index • National Emergency Department Overcrowding Study
Administrative and Policy Response to ED Crowding 32-14
Summary 32-16
References 32-16

Joshua A. Hilton
University of Pennsylvania

Jesse M. Pines
George Washington University

History

Over the past 30 years, hospital-based emergency departments (EDs) have evolved to provide not only acute care services for the critically ill, but a host of services: safety net care for indigent patients, public health surveillance, disaster preparedness, observation and procedural care, occupational services, employee health, and, in many cases, primary healthcare (Institute of Medicine, 2006). Despite this expansion of services, EDs have seen their resources decline relative to these demands. The overall number of ED beds, inpatient beds, and total number of U.S. hospitals has decreased considerably in the last 20 years (Nawar et al., 2007). According to the Institute of Medicine, this increase in demand and reduction in capacity has led to a national crisis of ED crowding (Institute of Medicine, 2006). ED crowding results when the demand for services exceeds resources (either personnel or capacity), and patients experience long waits for those services.

ED crowding has received considerable attention in the past few years; however, it is not a new phenomenon. ED crowding has been recognized in the medical literature for over 20 years (Gallagher and Lynn, 1990; Andrulis et al., 1991; Lynn and Kellermann, 1991). In the early 1990s, professional associations published position statements (American College of Emergency Physicians, 1990a,b), state and local governments appointed task forces to address the issue, and alarming stories appeared in the popular press (Will, 1990). By 1992, the problem had gained enough attention at the highest levels of government that the U.S. Senate Committee on Finance commissioned the General Accounting Office to do a national study of hospital-based EDs. At that time, they concluded that the problem was confined to large urban hospitals and was predominantly caused by patients seeking care for nonurgent conditions (General Accounting Office, 1993). ED utilization seemed to stabilize during the mid-1990s. The reasons for this are not entirely clear, but it is thought to be secondary to a number of factors: efforts by managed care organizations to reduce utilization, an increase in the number of emergency medicine training programs, and strategies devised by local communities and individual organizations to address ED crowding (Derlet and Richards, 2000). Many EDs continued to experience seasonal crowding problems throughout the remainder of the decade, but the national scrutiny had subsided. It appeared that ED crowding was being accepted as the status quo.

The new millennium brought renewed interest in ED crowding. A report published in 2001 showed that 91% of ED directors surveyed reported crowding as a problem. These directors represented large academic hospitals, community hospitals, and public hospitals. They all reported levels of crowding that were believed to impact the quality of patient care on a daily, if not weekly basis (Derlet et al., 2001).

Epidemiology

The United States is not alone in its struggle with ED crowding problems. Crowding in accident and emergency rooms across Canada has become a serious national issue as well (Kondro, 1998). Great Britain, Taiwan, Spain, and Australia have also accumulated a literature base describing their challenges with this complex problem (Hu, 1991, 1994; Bagust et al., 1999; Miro et al., 1999; Shih et al., 1999; Richardson, 2002; Sprivulis et al., 2005). Although ED crowding has been studied and described most intensively from a North American perspective, many of these international papers describe similar conditions and causes across the world—emergency care systems that are overwhelmed by a demand for services are unable to meet that demand largely because of difficulty moving admitted patients to inpatient beds, and are exhibiting adverse quality outcomes as a result.

In the United States, the most reliable data on ED visits is provided through the National Hospital Ambulatory Medical Care Survey (NHAMCS), which has been conducted annually since 1992 by the National Center for Health Statistics. The past 20 years have seen continued growth in the demand for ED services with a significant decrease in the number of healthcare facilities providing ED and inpatient care. From 1995 to 2005, annual ED visits in the United States increased by 20% (from 96.5 to 115.3 million), and the ED utilization rate increased by 7%, from 36.9 to 39.6 ED visits per 100 persons. Despite this increase in ED visits, the number of hospital EDs decreased by 381, the number of U.S. hospitals decreased by 535, and the number of hospital beds decreased by 134,000 during the same decade (see Figure 32.1).

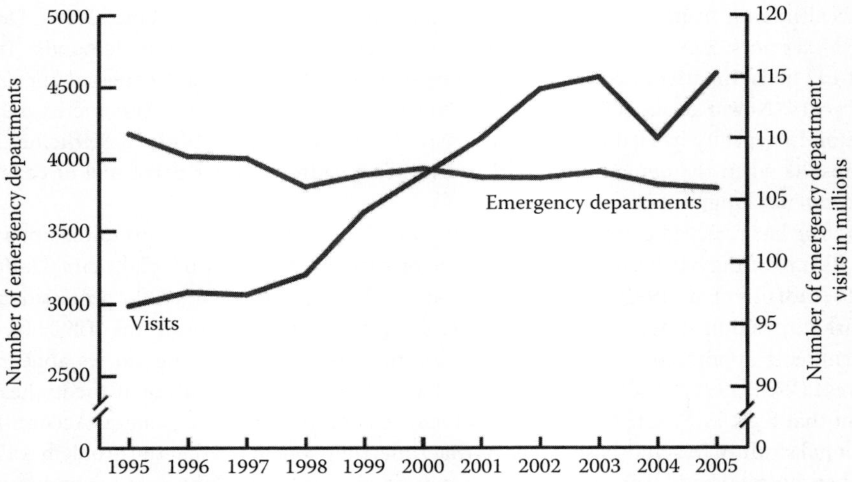

FIGURE 32.1 Emergency department visits/number of emergency departments: 1995–2005. (From Nawar, E.W. et al., *Adv. Data*, 386, 1, 2007.)

The bottom line is that higher ED volumes have been concentrated in few EDs. The response by many hospitals has been to increase ED capacity to meet this demand, but without a significant impact on the underlying crowding problem (Lambe et al., 2002).

Significance

The scope of ED crowding has been well described in the medical literature, but its causes and impact have just begun to be realized within the last decade. Crowding has been shown to have a significant impact on the safety and quality of patient care that is delivered in the ED: delays to definitive therapy and decreased adherence to published guidelines for patients with acute myocardial infarction (Schull et al., 2004; Diercks et al., 2007), delays in antibiotic administration to patients being admitted to the hospital for pneumonia (Fee et al., 2007), and perhaps most importantly, delays in the initial assessment and treatment of many urgent and potentially emergent conditions, causing patients pain and anxiety for prolonged periods (Pines and Hollander, 2008).

ED crowding has even been associated with the mortality of patients after they have been admitted to the hospital (Richardson, 2006; Sprivulis et al., 2006). In patients admitted to the hospital with chest pain, ED crowding is associated with a higher rate of adverse cardiovascular complications (Pines et al., 2009). These downstream effects may seem intuitive, that care and outcomes would be poorer when the ED is crowded. However, the impact of this problem is also felt upstream in the out-of-hospital setting. The process of signaling to out-of-hospital providers to direct ambulance patients to other hospitals during crowded periods (also known as ambulance diversion) is a considerable problem and one that is worsening. In 2003 alone, it was estimated that more than half a million ambulances were diverted from EDs, an average of one per minute (Burt et al., 2006). This "system gridlock," when ambulances circle a city in search of an open ED, occurs with alarming frequency and has a significant impact on both transportation time and the ability of a patient to receive care where their physicians and medical records are located (Adams and Biros, 2001; Pham et al., 2006). High levels of system-wide diversion are associated with delays in time-critical care for acute myocardial infarction (Schull et al., 2004). An unmeasured impact of ambulance diversion may be the morbidity of those patients who do not receive timely ambulance service because of the increased time spent transporting patients or waiting to unload a patient in a crowded ED with no open beds.

Although crowding manifests itself in the ED and out-of-hospital setting, the causes of this problem lie within the larger healthcare delivery system, most importantly, the ability of hospitals to handle surges in demand for inpatient beds (Richardson and Hwang, 2001a,b). There is a prevailing consensus opinion in the literature that ED crowding is a reflection or symptom of these larger supply and demand mismatches (Richardson et al., 2002). This in and of itself may seem simple, but ED crowding is more than a problem of numbers. Understanding these supply and demand relationships requires an understanding of the market forces that drive the supply of hospital beds and EDs, the demographic, socioeconomic, and health factors that affect demand for emergency care, and how regulation and reimbursement have constrained the inpatient hospital system (Asplin, 2001; Asplin and Knopp, 2001; Richardson and Hwang, 2001). EDs are not just a safety net for their local communities, but a safety net for the entire U.S. healthcare system (Adams and Biros, 2001). This safety net has been described as "unraveling" and the consequences have been described as "devastating" (Asplin, 2001; American Academy of Pediatrics, 2004). EDs are the only place that patients can go when all other medical care options are exhausted, and many times the only option for acute care. EDs are the only place in the U.S. healthcare system that anyone can receive care regardless of their ability to pay (Bitterman, 2006). To fix this system we must fully understand what crowding is and what its causes are, define and characterize its effects, and implement solutions that will improve patient-oriented outcomes and the delivery of emergency care.

Definitions of ED Crowding

ED crowding has received a growing amount of attention over the past 20 years, but there still remains a lack of consensus on the terminology used to identify it, define it, or measure it. "Overcrowding" has been used interchangeably with "crowding," both in the medical literature and in the more recent 2006 IOM report on hospital-based emergency care (Institute of Medicine, 2006). Both terms describe a condition in which there are too many patients and too few resources or treatment areas to care for them. Some authors have preferred to use the term "overcrowding" since it suggests a more extreme situation or crisis situation, but other authors have noted that the term "overcrowding" somehow implies that "crowding" is acceptable. It is now generally well accepted that both "crowding" and "overcrowding" pose significant risks to patients and that a consensus is emerging in favor of the term "crowding" (Moskop et al., 2009a,b).

Despite this emerging consensus in favor of its terminology, a concise definition of ED crowding is still lacking. Because of the absence of a universally accepted definition or criterion standard, researchers, policymakers, and administrators have experienced fundamental difficulties in studying and understanding ED crowding (Richardson et al., 2002; Schull et al., 2002; Hwang and Concato, 2004). Many proposed definitions may only be specific to a certain type of ED or only one ED system. Some definitions have focused only on the delays in transfer of an ED patient to an inpatient bed while ignoring other potential front-end measures that address time to initial care or delays in therapy. Some emergency physicians have attempted to define crowding in more practical terms: a situation in which demand for services exceeds the ability to provide care within reasonable time, causing physicians and nurses to feel that they cannot provide quality care (Derlet and Richards, 2000). Although ED crowding is clearly related to volume, EDs can be busy without being crowded. Crowding is in part a function of patient volume, patient acuity, physical space, and the on-duty staff (Bernstein and Asplin, 2006). The more recent and more rigorous approach by the emergency medicine community has been to identify the factors and determinants that are most likely to contribute to ED crowding at the patient, ED, hospital, and community level (Schull et al., 2002). By identifying these factors, measuring their contribution, and assessing their impact on patients, we can move closer to an operational definition for ED crowding: inadequate resources available to meet patient demands leading to a reduction in the quality of care provided (Pines, 2007).

Conceptual Framework

In 2003, Asplin et al. published "A Conceptual Model of Emergency Department Crowding" to help administrators, researchers, and policymakers understand the causes of ED crowding and develop potential solutions (Asplin et al., 2003). This model applies a set of 38 different consensus measures of ED and hospital workflow that contribute to ED crowding at varying points in the patient flow process (Solberg et al., 2003). These measures are then divided into three interdependent domains—input, throughput, and output—based on their corresponding sites of action. Although it is apparent that the factors identified originate in many different parts of the healthcare system, the model focuses on ED crowding from the perspective of the ED (Bernstein and Asplin, 2006). The input–output–throughput model is an effort to frame the acute care system and apply operations management concepts to patient flow among the various delivery components that provide unscheduled care. It explains ED crowding as a result of increased numbers or acuity of arriving patients, inefficient ED operational processes, and downstream obstacles to moving patients out of the ED. By providing this framework, it was the author's intention to guide research, operational, and policy solutions to ED crowding (Asplin et al., 2003) (see Figure 32.2).

Input

The input component of this model includes any condition, event, or system characteristic that contributes to the demand for ED services (Asplin et al., 2003). The ED serves many roles in the medical

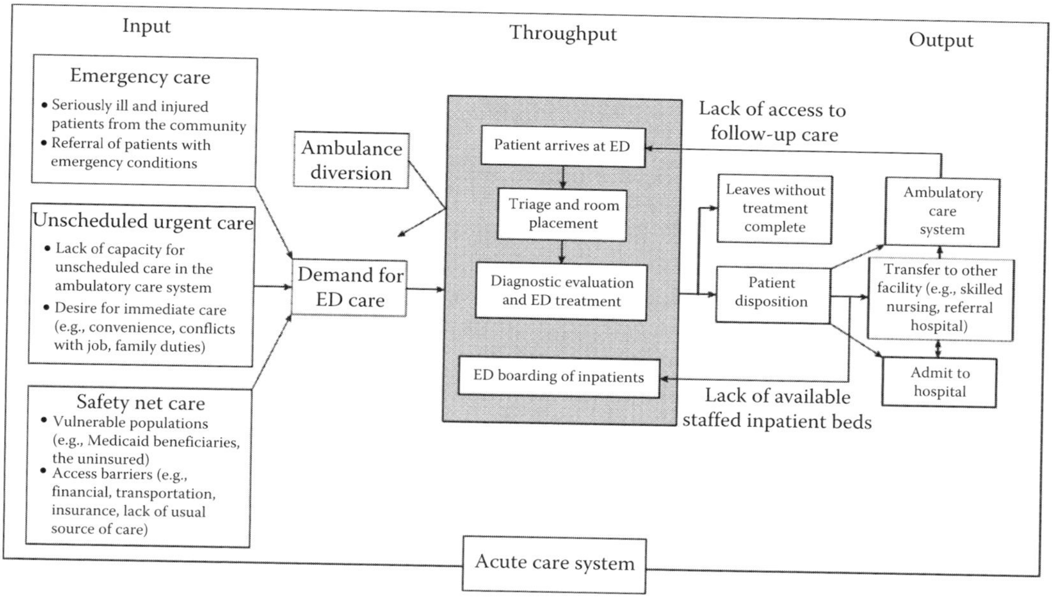

FIGURE 32.2 Input–throughput–output model of emergency department crowding. (Reprinted from Asplin, B.R. et al., *Ann. Emerg. Med.*, 42, 173, 2003. With permission from Elsevier.)

community, and provides many different types of care. These roles are most logically grouped by the type of care provided: emergency care, unscheduled urgent care, and safety net care.

First and foremost, the most visible and indispensable role of an ED is the treatment of seriously ill and injured patients (Kellermann, 1991). In addition to caring for the acutely ill, the ED serves as a referral site for other healthcare providers when they determine that patient stabilization, specialty consultation, or admission are required. These patients may be referred from ambulatory clinics, home healthcare providers, skilled nursing facilities, urgent care centers, hospitals, and other EDs. Although it is possible to directly admit patients with straightforward problems or needs to the hospital from an ambulatory clinic or out-of-hospital setting, patients with complex problems or time-dependent diagnoses are referred to the ED for stabilization, triage, and an initial diagnostic evaluation prior to admission. The concentration of diagnostic and therapeutic technologies available to the ED may contribute to referral patterns for ambulatory patients (Asplin et al., 2003).

The ED provides a significant amount of unscheduled urgent care. In many cases, patients are sent to the ED because their usual clinic cannot quickly diagnose or treat them for an acute problem, or an exacerbation of an existing chronic problem. This is often because there is inadequate capacity for this type of care in the acute care system, other sources of after-hours care are unavailable, or these systems lack immediate access to advanced services, such as specialists, radiology, or hospital laboratories (Kellermann, 1994). Although some ambulatory-care systems have had success providing same-day appointment scheduling with advanced scheduling systems, many patients have found that the delay for an acute appointment is often longer than they are willing to wait (Murray and Berwick, 2003; Murray et al., 2003). In many cases, despite access to same-day care in a clinic, the convenience of same-day after-hours care in the ED guides patients' decisions about where they will seek care. Although they may have to wait to be treated in the ED, the availability of after-hours care may create fewer conflicts with employment, educational, and family responsibilities (Rask et al., 1998).

The healthcare safety net is comprised of those providers that organize and deliver a significant level of healthcare and other health-related services to uninsured, Medicaid, and other vulnerable patients (Institute of Medicine, 2000). Although the ED shares this role with other safety net providers and clinics, it is often the only open door for patients that experience substantial barriers to accessing unscheduled care. Because of cost and access barriers, a disproportionate number of Medicaid beneficiaries and uninsured individuals rely on the ED as their usual source of care (Rask et al., 1994; Jones et al., 1999). It is this relationship between the ED and vulnerable populations that highlights the safety net role that EDs play in a community (Asplin, 2001).

EDs have seen a significant increase in volume over the past 15–20 years. National statistics reveal continuing strong growth in demand for ED care, coupled with a significant decrease in the number of healthcare facilities. From 1995 to 2005 alone, annual ED visits in the United States increased by 20% (from 96.5 to 115.3 million per year), and the ED utilization rate increased by 7%, from 36.9 to 39.6 ED visits per 100 persons. During the same period, number of inpatient hospital beds decreased by 134,000 (Nawar et al., 2007). It is hypothesized that many of these facility closures are likely due to financial pressures imposed by cuts in private and public insurance reimbursement and by treatment requirements imposed by the federal Emergency Medical Treatment and Active Labor Act (EMTALA) (Espinosa et al., 2002). EMTALA requires hospitals that participate in Medicare offer ED services and provide a medical screening examination when patients request care for an emergency condition. EMTALA applies regardless of the patient's ability to pay, and it is often described as an "unfunded mandate." Hospitals must provide stabilizing care for patients with emergency conditions, and if it cannot stabilize a patient within its capability, a transfer to another facility may be arranged.

Initial investigations into the causes of ED crowding and this uneven year after year growth in volume addressed input factors such as the demand for ED services and the use of the ED for nonemergent complaints. Early descriptions of ED crowding highlighted the growth in the number of substance abusers, homeless, AIDS patients, and mentally ill in urban areas (Gallagher and Lynn, 1990). A 1993 report by the U.S. General Accounting Office attributed the growing volume of ED visits to many of these same factors, noting that many of these patients either had Medicaid or were uninsured, and were using the ED for nonurgent conditions (General Accounting Office, 1993). This report, and the prevailing assumptions of the early 1990s, focused attention on nonurgent or unnecessary visits by uninsured and underinsured patients as the root cause of ED crowding. More recent research, however, strongly suggests that this is not the case, and that low-acuity patients with nonurgent conditions contribute little if at all to ED crowding and ambulance diversion (Emergency Medical Treatment and Active Labor Act, 1986; Trzeciak and Rivers, 2003; Sprivulis et al., 2005). In 2002, Canadian investigators examined over 4.2 million visits to 110 EDs in Ontario and concluded that the number of patients with minor illnesses and injuries in these EDs had a negligible effect on waiting times for care of other, more acutely ill, ED patients (Schull et al., 2007). A systematic review published in 2008 addressed many of the assumptions made about the uninsured population and their utilization of ED resources. Based on currently available data, there is no evidence that uninsured patients use the ED for nonurgent, nonemergent, or primary care complaints—deemed inappropriate care by some authors. There is also no evidence that uninsured patients are a leading cause of ED crowding or that they utilize ED services disproportionately to their insured counterparts (Newton et al., 2008). Conversely, a 2003 study noted that 66% of the increase in ED visits between 1997 and 2001 was accounted for by patients with private insurance or Medicare (Cunningham and May, 2003).

It is evident from the literature on this topic that the increase in demand for ED services over the past 20 years is not well understood. Many of the assumptions that are still perpetuated in the popular press and policy arguments are not supported by the currently available data. Much more work is needed in this area to determine more accurate drivers of demand so that solutions can be targeted appropriately. Currently, only a few approaches to demand management have been investigated in the literature: nonurgent referrals, ambulance diversion, and destination control (Hoot and Aronsky, 2008).

In an attempt to redirect nonurgent patients from the ED to other sources of appropriate care, several investigators have succeeded in arranging alternative appointments in primary care and community settings without adverse events (Derlet et al., 1992; Washington et al., 2002; Diesburg-Stanwood et al., 2004). When these patients were followed up, over 40% were able to receive same-day care in another healthcare setting (Derlet et al., 1992). In addition, a large percentage of these patients (38%) stated that they would be willing to trade their ED visit for a follow-up primary care visit in the next 72 hours (Grumbach et al., 1993). Triage of nonurgent patients away from the ED appears to be an appealing option at face value, but the amount of resources necessary to perform an appropriate medical screening examination and effective triage can be onerous, especially given the minimal impact this is projected to have on ED crowding. In addition, some clinics do not have the resources required to care for acutely ill patients, such as same-day access to radiography.

Ambulance diversion is an equally complex issue. Hospitals have traditionally used ambulance diversion to control demand when the capacity of the hospital or ED has reached levels that are thought to compromise patient care. The demand impact of turning ambulances away is variable. In one study, ambulance diversion decreased the rate of ambulance arrivals by 30%–50% (Lagoe et al., 2002), while a similar study found a reduced arrival rate of 0.4 hours (Scheulen et al., 2001). The significance of this reduction on an individual ED is dependent on the hourly arrival volume and the resources available, whereas the negative impact of routine ambulance diversion on a city- or county-wide healthcare system is much more dramatic and predictable (Pham et al., 2006). Many cities and EMS systems have put policies in place to limit or eliminate diversion completely, while others have initiated programs to redistribute ambulances within the system using internet-based operating information or physician-directed destination control (Vilke et al., 2004a,b; Sprivulis and Gerrard, 2005; Patel et al., 2006; Shah et al., 2006). Massachusetts completely eliminated ambulance diversion in 2009.

Throughput

ED throughput refers to the operational processes specific to the ED and identifies patient length of stay as a potential contributing factor to ED crowding. This segment of the model highlights the need to look internally at ED care processes and modify them to improve their efficiency and effectiveness (Asplin et al., 2003). The care of an ED patient is best conceptualized in two phases. The first phase comprises triage, placement into a care area, and the initial evaluation by a healthcare provider. The second phase of care typically constitutes the majority of the patient's length of stay in an ED with efficient front-end operations; it is comprised of diagnostic testing and treatment.

Within these phases of care, there are several factors that can affect throughput:

- Time to triage
- Time to bed placement
- Physical layout of the ED
- Nurse and physician staffing ratios
- Availability of medical information
- Efficiency and use of diagnostic testing
- Communication systems
- Availability of timely specialty consultation

Although this list is not exhaustive by any means, it highlights the complex and interdependent nature of ED operations. Effective patient care depends on the interaction of multiple care providers, laboratory and imaging services, inpatient units, and on-call specialists who are not immediately available in the ED. If any one of these components becomes overwhelmed or is performing poorly, delivery of ED care will suffer (Moskop et al., 2009). Since many of these components are controlled by stakeholders outside of the ED, operational inefficiencies resulting from poor performance may not receive the attention or priority necessary to make meaningful changes or reorganize delivery of services.

Given the complexity of care delivery in the ED, front-end operations, or the first phase of care, have been the focus of several emergency care researchers. It is the phase of care that is most dependent on the ED itself and few other outside influences. Triage of patients is the first step in this process and standardization of triage classification is recommended to facilitate a common understanding of ED patient workload (Wuerz et al., 2000). Some EDs can successfully complete triage and room placement within 10 minutes of patient arrival if there are open care spaces available (Hoffenberg et al., 2001), although some experts argue the need for any triage in this instance. By definition, triage is the sorting of patients to receive care in a setting of limited resources. If there are open care areas available (resources), then triage is an unnecessary step. Immediate bedding is the placement of patients directly into an available care space while simultaneously completing bedside registration and the nursing intake evaluation. This process can occur in parallel with the physician evaluation and has been shown to reduce patient wait times, decrease overall length of stay, and reduce the numbers of patients waiting to be seen (Chan et al., 2005). Once patients are triaged, low-acuity patients may be redirected to an area or service line where they are evaluated in a separate but parallel process from the patients with higher acuity (Meislin et al., 1988). Studies have reported that this "fast track" can decrease length of stay, shorten wait times for all ED patients, and reduce the number of patients that leave without being seen (Simon et al., 1997; O'Brien et al., 2006; Rodi et al., 2006; Sanchez et al., 2006).

Queuing theory and discrete event simulation are two operations management tools that have been applied to the ED in attempts to optimize throughput. Initially used to quantify the contribution of non-urgent visits to ED workload and waiting times, queuing theory has recently been used to assess variability in arrival patterns and determine the most effective allocation of staff to optimize time between patient arrival and provider evaluation (Siddharthan et al., 1996; Green et al., 2006). Discrete event simulation has been used to model ED operations, test proposed triage schemes, examine the utility of capacity increases, and evaluate the effects of physician utilization on patient waiting times (Chin and Fleisher, 1998; Connelly and Bair, 2004; Khare et al., 2009).

Output

Output refers to the ability to move patients from the ED after acute care has been provided. The inability to complete this process efficiently contributes to crowding for both admitted and discharged patients (Derlet et al., 2001). When patients are discharged after evaluation and treatment in the ED, follow-up evaluation, additional diagnostic testing, or therapeutic services are often required. The availability of timely follow-up appointments in the ambulatory-care setting, and the access barriers experienced by vulnerable populations, often create significant obstacles for emergency providers who are trying to arrange appropriate follow-up care. The time spent by ED providers arranging appropriate follow-up can undermine the efficiency of care and prolong ED length of stay. The process can be time-consuming and ultimately unsuccessful for many patients (Rask et al., 1994). In cases where adequate arrangements for outpatient follow-up care cannot be made, emergency physicians are more likely to admit patients to the hospital for their care (Pickert, 2009). This is possibly the most expensive alternative, and serves to demonstrate the lack of capacity in the ambulatory-care system. The impact of these costs on our healthcare system has not been studied. Ultimately, the inability to appropriately discharge patients from the ED impacts crowding in several ways. It increases the number of patients waiting for an inpatient bed (boarding), and it increases demand for services on the input side of the model. Patients who are unable to obtain follow-up care often return to the ED if their condition does not improve or deteriorates (Asplin et al., 2001).

Although the appropriate and timely disposition of discharged patients may prove challenging, it is the inability to move admitted patients from the ED to an inpatient bed that is the most frequently cited cause for ED crowding, and the most important determinant of ambulance diversion (Gallagher and Lynn, 1990; Andrulis et al., 1991; Espinosa et al., 2002; Forster et al., 2003; Schull et al., 2003; Olshaker and Rathlev, 2006; Rathlev et al., 2007). Australian investigators have termed this phenomenon "access block." It is a problem that forces the ED to board admitted patients until inpatient beds are available, and effectively reduces the ED's capacity to care for new patients (Henry, 2001; Richardson, 2002). In addition to causing delays in care, these "boarders" or inpatient holds require considerable amounts of nursing time, physician time, and medical resources that could be directed to toward the evaluation and stabilization of new patients (Bernstein and Asplin, 2006).

Many factors contribute to inpatient boarding in the ED (Asplin et al., 2001):

- A lack of physical inpatient beds
- A lack of inpatient bed availability because of inadequate or inflexible nurse to patient staffing ratios
- Isolation requirements and cohorting of patients with communicable diseases
- Delays in cleaning rooms after patient discharge
- An overreliance on intensive care or telemetry beds
- Inefficient diagnostic and ancillary services on inpatient units
- Delays in discharging hospitalized patients to post–acute care facilities

Although each of these representative factors demonstrates an operational problem that may appear solvable in isolation, it is the combination of these factors and the financial incentives behind hospital payment that have aligned to obstruct the development of sustainable solutions to ED crowding. The Institute of Medicine addressed this overarching financial barrier in their comprehensive 2006 report on hospital-based emergency care: "No major change in healthcare can take place without strong financial incentives, and today hospitals have almost no incentives to address the myriad problems associated with inefficient patient flow or ED crowding. Indeed … hospitals have a number of financial incentives to continue the practices that lead to these problems" (Institute of Medicine, 2006).

Hospitals maximize revenue by operating at high capacity and caring for insured patients. Insured patients provide higher reimbursement for virtually all procedures, diagnostic tests, and inpatient care. Operating near full capacity ensures the greatest utility of a hospital's employees and facilities (Institute of Medicine, 2006). ED crowding serves each of these aims indirectly. When a hospital is operating near full capacity, the ED acts as an escape valve that stores patients in a queue during periods of high demand while providing necessary care until a bed becomes available. Patients that are boarded in the ED compete for inpatient beds with patients who are awaiting elective admission to the hospital for surgery or other invasive procedures. Elective admission patients are usually insured, and the procedures they undergo are often well reimbursed, generating significant revenue for hospitals. Emergency admissions, in contrast, are more likely to be uninsured or underinsured, to have more severe illnesses, and to have lower rates of reimbursement (Munoz et al., 1985; Moskop et al., 2009). Hospitals thus have a financial incentive to prefer elective over emergency admissions, and no disincentive to allow ED boarding of patients.

In the United States, federal Emergency Medical Treatment and Active Labor Act (EMTALA) regulations require hospitals that have EDs to provide a screening examination and necessary emergency care for all patients, regardless of ability to pay (New Jersey Commission on Rationalizing Health Care Resources, 2008). When an ED is crowded, wait times are increased and access to emergency care is delayed; some patients may choose to leave the ED without being seen. If an ED is closed due to hospital diversion, access to care through the ED is temporarily denied to ambulance patients.

Given these circumstances, hospitals may have a financial incentive to permit ED crowding and closure because the conditions limit the hospital's legal duty to assume the care of uninsured and underinsured patients (Henry, 2001; Institute of Medicine, 2006; Moskop et al., 2009). Financial incentives that permit or encourage ED crowding are thought to be a function of market-based healthcare systems. Although market driven healthcare delivery is most prevalent in the United States, it has been shown that ED crowding is a global problem that affects nationalized healthcare systems and countries with universal health coverage as well (Hu, 1991, 1994; Kondro, 1998; Bagust et al., 1999; Miro et al., 1999; Shih et al., 1999; Richardson, 2002; Fatovich et al., 2005; Sprivulis et al., 2005). The underlying culprit in all of these systems is a shortage of available inpatient beds and resultant boarding in the ED. This shortage is thought to represent explicit or implicit rationing of scarce resources in virtually all healthcare systems (Moskop et al., 2009).

The number of inpatient hospital beds in the United States decreased by 134,000 between 1995 and 2005 (Nawar et al., 2007). This contraction of resources may be attributed to a variety of cost-containment measures, including prospective reimbursement systems, preadmission certification, and limits on length of stay. Debate continues regarding the optimal number of hospital beds necessary to serve the daily and disaster needs of the U.S. population. Despite documented widespread crowding, some state-initiated needs assessments have found capacity–demand mismatches and have recommended even further contraction of inpatient bed capacity in certain areas (New Jersey Commission on Rationalizing Health Care Resources, 2008). Although it may not be clear that increasing physical inpatient bed capacity is the solution to ED crowding, there is a growing body of evidence that correction of operational inefficiencies within the hospital may lead to improved patient flow and decrease the crowding burden in the ED.

The 2006 IOM Report on hospital-based emergency care highlighted several operational strategies that have been employed and tested to reduce ED crowding. Creation of multidisciplinary teams to address crowding from a systems standpoint increases understanding of the problem and accountability for addressing it among hospital leaders (Clark, 2005; McCarthy, 2005), while establishment of coordinated bed management programs to optimize the occupancy of inpatient beds directs increased attention, additional resources, and explicit procedures toward the most efficient use of those beds (Institute for Healthcare Improvement, 2004; Wilson and Nguyen, 2004). Efforts to disposition potential inpatient admissions more efficiently, or to queue patients awaiting admission or discharge from the hospital, has led to the creation of several hospital-based units to address crowding and flow problems. Clinical decision units have evolved to monitor patients with symptoms such as chest pain, abdominal pain, congestive heart failure, or shortness of breath who may or may not ultimately need hospitalization (Maag et al., 1997; Ross et al., 2003). Admission units queue patients in an area outside of the ED where dedicated staff and inpatient physicians can care for their needs while awaiting an open bed. In some hospitals, this has included inpatient hallways (Viccellio et al., 2009). Discharge units and lounges serve to hold patients who may be awaiting discharge, but no longer need the care and attention required of a hospital bed and nursing. Since many of the final components of a patient's stay are related to transportation, case management, and social services, moving these patients from their physical bed while coordinating discharge can create more capacity in the system (National Academy of Engineering and Institute of Medicine, 2005).

In 2005, the National Academy of Engineering and the Institute of Medicine published a joint report emphasizing the increase in safety and efficiency that could be realized through a stronger engineering/healthcare partnership. The authors referred to the U.S. healthcare system as a "cottage industry" structure, with physicians and other healthcare providers operating semiautonomously. The result has been hospitals, and other provider organizations, that lack the hierarchical control of the typical business enterprise, making it difficult to introduce efficiency principles to streamline flows in production, inputs, and inventory as in other industries. In addition, the prevalent payment structures in healthcare, which focus on individual encounters and practice settings, tend to reinforce silos, reward inefficient practices, and discourage investment in new technologies and process improvements (National Academy of Engineering and Institute of Medicine, 2005). Although operations management is much more mature in industries like banking, airlines, and manufacturing, healthcare has adopted a number of these strategies and tools. Their application to hospital flow has significant potential to streamline care and improve effective bed capacity (Institute of Medicine, 2006):

- Quality functional deployment
- Failure modes and effects analysis
- Root-cause analysis
- Human factors engineering
- Queuing theory
- Supply-chain management
- Statistical process control

For example, by smoothing the inherent peaks and valleys of patient flow and eliminating the artificial variability that impairs flow, hospitals can minimize the occurrence of queues and improve safety and quality while simultaneously reducing hospital waste and costs (Magid et al., 2004; Litvak, 2005; Institute of Medicine, 2006).

Measurement

An important but under recognized aspect of this complex issue involves the challenge of measuring ED crowding. As researchers in this area look to identify potential solutions, they have been confronted by lack of a criterion standard. The existing literature on ED crowding exhibits confusion among the causes of crowding, outcomes of crowding, and measures of crowding (Hwang and Concato, 2004). In an attempt to reconcile this problem, a panel of 74 experts convened and created a list of 38 potential measures using a modified Delphi process (Solberg et al., 2003). These measures were originally grouped into seven domains based on patient demand, patient complexity, ED capacity, ED workload, ED efficiency, hospital capacity, and hospital efficiency, but authors of the input–throughput–output model have reorganized these measures relative to their location within the model (see Tables 32.1 through 32.3).

TABLE 32.1 Input Measures

Input Measure	Concept	Operational Definition
1. ED patient volume, standardize for bed hours	Patient demand	Number of new patients registered within a defined period (hour, shift, day) ÷ number of ED bed hours within this period
2. ED patient volume, standardized for annual average	Patient demand	Number of new patients registered within a defined period ÷ annual mean number new patients registered within this period
3. ED ambulance patient volume, standardized for bed hours	Patient demand	Number of new ambulance patients registered within a defined period ÷ number ED bed hours within this period
4. ED ambulance patient volume, standardized for annual average	Patient demand	Number of new ambulance patients within a defined period ÷ annual average of new ambulance patients registered within this period
5. Patient source	Patient demand	Time, arrival mode, reason, referral source, and usual care for each patient registering at an ED in a defined period (hour/shift/day)
6. Percentage of open appointments	Patient demand	Percentage of open appointments at the beginning of a day in ambulatory care clinics that serve an ED's patient population
7. Percentage of patients who leave without treatment complete[a]	ED capacity	Number of registered patients who leave the ED without treatment complete ÷ total number of patients who register during this period
8. Leave without treatment complete severity[a]	ED capacity	Average severity of patients who leave the ED without treatment complete within a defined period (shift/day/week)
9. Ambulance diversion episodes	ED capacity	Number and duration of all diversion episodes at EDs within the EMS system within a defined period (week/month/year)
10. Ambulance diversion requests denied and forced openings	ED capacity	Number of diversion requests denied or forced openings within a defined period (week/month/year)
11. Diverted ambulance patient description	ED capacity	Chief complaints and final destination of diverted EMS patients within a defined period (week/month/year)
12. Average EMS waiting time	ED capacity	Total time at hospital for ambulances delivering patients to ED during a defined period (shift/day/week/month) ÷ number of ambulance deliveries within that period
13. Patient complexity as assessed at triage	Patient complexity	Mean complexity level as assessed at triage (using local criterial) for all patients triaged in a defined period (shift/day/week/month)
14. Patient complexity as the percentage of ambulance patients	Patient complexity	Percentage of patients registering at an ED in a defined period (shift/day/week/month) who arrived by ambulance
15. Patient complexity as assessed by coding	Patient complexity	Mean complexity level as coded at the end of the visit for all patients completed in a defined period (shift/day/week/month)

Source: Reprinted from Asplin, B.R. et al., *Ann. Emerg. Med.*, 42, 173, 2003. With permission from Elsevier.

[a] Leave without treatment complete includes those patients who leave without being seen, leave before being finished, and leave against medical advice.

TABLE 32.2 Throughput Measures

Throughput Measure	Concept	Operational Definition
1. ED throughput time	ED efficiency	Average time between patient sign-in and departure (separately for admitted vs. discharged patients) within a defined period (days/week/month)
2. Ed bed placement time	ED efficiency	Mean interval between patient sign-in and placement in a treatment area within a defined period (shift/day/week/month)
3. ED ancillary service turnaround time	ED efficiency	Average time between physician order and result report (separately for each service area) within a defined period (shift/day/week/month)
4. Summary workload, standardized for ED bed hours	ED workload	Summary of (patients treated × acuity) in a defined period (shift/day/ week) ÷ number of ED bed hours within this period
5. Summary workload, standardized for registered nurse staff hours	ED workload	Summary of (patients treated × acuity) in a defined period (shift/day/week) ÷ total Ed staff registered nurse hours within this period
6. Summary workload, standardized for physician staff hours	ED workload	Summary of (patients treated × acuity) in a defined period (shift/day/ week) ÷ total Ed staff physician hours within this period
7. ED occupancy rate	ED workload	Total number of ED patients registered at a defined time ÷ number of staffed treatment areas at that time
8. ED occupancy	ED workload	Total number of patients present in the ED at a defined time ÷ number of staffed treatment areas at that time
9. Patient disposition to physician staffing ratio	ED workload	Number of patients admitted or discharged per staff physician during a defined period (shift/day/week)

Source: Reprinted from Asplin, B.R. et al., *Ann. Emerg. Med.*, 42, 173, 2003. With permission from Elsevier.

An ideal measure of ED crowding is universal, reproducible, and consistently accurate across EDs of different sizes. It consists of data elements that are immediately available from existing sources or continuously monitored by existing information systems (Bernstein and Asplin, 2006). If this measure could be programmed into electronic patient tracking systems, it could be used in real time to provide updated information at the point of service while allowing researchers to study the relationships between ED crowding, quality of care, and adverse events (Magid et al., 2004).

Early attempts to measure the extent of ED crowding relied heavily on provider perceptions. In a 1999 survey of directors of U.S. EDs, 91% of respondents reported that crowding is a problem, and 39% reported that their EDs are crowded every day (Derlet et al., 2001). Later studies proposed multiple different scoring systems using empirical variables to determine the existence and extent of ED crowding. Comprehensive measures of ED crowding have developed. However, their lack of generalizability to varying practice settings, lack of sensitivity, or their focus on individual components of crowding has limited their usefulness. Three of the most widely cited measures are explained below. Comparative evaluations of these measures have not demonstrated clear superiority of one over the others in identifying or predicting ED crowding (Jones et al., 2006).

Emergency Department Crowding Score

This score was developed by fitting an ordinal logistic model to variables identified from the input–throughput–output model. It was created in a multicenter, prospective, time-series study that used physician and nurse assessment of crowding as the criterion standard (Asplin and Rhodes, 2004). In this model, variables found to be independently predictive of crowding were the number of boarders, the total number of ED patients, and the number of critical care patients (Bernstein and Asplin, 2006). The Emergency Department Crowding Score is scaled from 0 to 100. Higher scores are associated with ED length of stay, mean boarding time, patients that leave without being seen, and diversion of ambulances. At a threshold value of 65, diversion and patients leaving without being seen become more likely.

TABLE 32.3 Output Measures

Output Measure	Concept	Operational Definition
1. ED boarding time	Hospital efficiency	Mean time from inpatient bed request to physical departure of patients from the ED overall and by bed type within a defined period (shift/day/week)[a]
2. ED boarding time components	Hospital efficiency	Mean time from inpatient bed request to physical departure of patients from the ED by bed type by component (bed assignment, bed cleaning, transfer arrival) within a defined period[a]
3. Boarding burden	Hospital efficiency	Mean number of ED patients waiting for an inpatient bed within a defined period ÷ number of staffed ED treatment areas
4. Hospital admission source, standardized and adjusted	Hospital efficiency	Number of requests for admission within a defined period (shift/day) overall and by admission source ÷ annual mean requests for admission during that period and source and adjusted for day of week and season of year[b]
5. ED admission transfer rate	Hospital efficiency	Number of patients transferred from ED to another facility who would normally have been admitted within a defined period ÷ number of ED admissions within this period
6. Hospital discharge potential	Hospital efficiency	Number of inpatients ready for discharge at or within a defined period ÷ number of hospital inpatients at that time
7. Hospital discharge process interval	Hospital efficiency	Mean interval from discharge order to patient departure from a unit in a defined period (shift/day/week/month)
8. Inpatient cycling time	Hospital efficiency	Mean amount of time required to discharge an inpatient and admit a new patient to the same bed within this period
9. Hospital census	Hospital capacity	Mean number of inpatient beds available by bed type at a defined time ÷ number of staffed inpatient beds by bed type[a]
10. Hospital occupancy rate	Hospital capacity	Number of occupied inpatient beds overall and by bed type ÷ number of staffed inpatient beds overall and by bed type[a]
11. Hospital supply/demand status forecast	Hospital capacity	Forecast of expected hospital admissions and discharges as reported daily at 6 a.m. and compared with hospital census
12. Observation unit census	Hospital capacity	Mean number of available ED observation beds at a defined time ÷ number of staffed ED observation beds
13. ED volume/hospital capacity ratio	Hospital capacity	Number of new ED patients within a defined period (shift/day) ÷ number of available hospital beds at the beginning of analysis period overall and by bed type[a]
14. Agency nursing expenditures	Hospital capacity	Registered nurse agency nursing expenditures (ED/overall) within a defined period ÷ total nursing expenditures (ED/overall) within this period

Source: Reprinted from Asplin, B.R. et al., *Ann. Emerg. Med.*, 42, 173, 2003. With permission from Elsevier.

[a] Bed type = ICU/telemetry/psychiatry/ward.

[b] Admission source = ED/operating room/catheterization laboratory/outpatient/other.

Emergency Department Work Index

$$\text{EDWIN} = \sum \frac{n_{it} t_j}{N_t (B - B_t)}$$

The emergency department work index (EDWIN) is a composite index that incorporates components of the input–throughput–output model (Bernstein et al., 2003). In this equation, n_i is the number of patients present in the ED in triage category i at time t, t_j is the triage score (1–5) for the jth patient, N_t is the number of attending physicians on duty at time t, B is the total number of beds or treatment beds available in the ED, and B_t is the number of admitted patients (boarders) in the ED at time t. EDWIN was developed and tested at a single ED. It was a prospective, observational study that measured agreement between nurse and physician perceptions of ED crowding and EDWIN, and studied the strength of association between EDWIN and a composite index of clinical end points (Bernstein and Asplin, 2006). This composite index exhibited excellent correlation with nurse and physician assessment of crowding, and was strongly predictive of ambulance diversion. The data suggest that ED activity may be demarcated into three ordinal zones:

$$\text{Active/Manageable} = \text{EDWIN score} < 1.5$$

$$\text{Busy ED} = \text{EDWIN between 1.5 and 2}$$

$$\text{Crowded ED} = \text{EDWIN} > 2$$

National Emergency Department Overcrowding Study

The National Emergency Department Overcrowding Study (NEDOCS) score is a five-question instrument that was developed at eight academic EDs. The five data elements that comprise the score are

1. The number of ED patients divided by number of ED beds
2. The number of admitted patients in the ED divided by the number of hospital beds
3. The number of ED patients using a mechanical ventilator
4. The longest admit time for any patient
5. The waiting room time for the last patient placed in an ED bed

A nomogram is used to assign a point value based on the answer for each question. These points are then tallied and the final number is used to reference a separate nomogram that gives a score between 1 and 200 that correlates with a composite outcome variable consisting of nurse and physician perceptions. During development, the scores were validated against charge nurse and attending physician assessments of crowding (Weiss et al., 2004).

Multiple other measures and scores have been developed and tested at single institutions, but none of them have been validated, scaled for use at other institutions, or been applied as real-time measures of ED crowding (Bernstein and Asplin, 2006). A 2007 study evaluating the feasibility of using EDWIN and NEDOCS to monitor crowding in real time found that, in terms of forecasting, none of the measures showed a clear advantage over occupancy level alone (Jones et al., 2006; Hoot et al., 2007). There are new directions and techniques being pursued in this area, specifically the application of neural networks as a forecasting tool and a focus on better objective endpoints for crowding (Hoot et al., 2009). In addition, several authors have considered moving from complex measures to simpler ones, such as ED occupancy (McCarthy et al., 2008).

Administrative and Policy Response to ED Crowding

ED crowding is an administrative problem with important clinical consequences that has waxed and waned in severity for almost 20 years (Bernstein and Asplin, 2006). In the 1990s, the emergency medicine community seemed to be standing alone as it sounded the horn for action. Despite the growing body of evidence outlining the causes and extent of ED crowding, policymakers and administrators previously thought that this was merely a cyclical phenomenon that would not require a dedicated policy response (Tye, 2000). It was not until 2000 that the first dedicated administrative response by a state or federal entity was realized. In a letter to all hospital administrators, the state health commissioner of New York reported that "Emergency Department overcrowding is a hospital-wide problem and hospital administrators must continue to be proactive and accountable in addressing overcrowding situations." In this letter, Dr. Novello directed hospitals to use all available inpatient beds to move patients out of the

ED, designate an individual to monitor that all available beds are made available for admissions from the ED, and assure that ancillary services are available to the ED (Novello, 2000).

In 2002, the Robert Wood Johnson Foundation designed a national program to identify practical solutions to ED crowding and to assess its impact on the healthcare safety net. The program was named Urgent Matters, and it awarded grants to 10 healthcare systems to study and alleviate crowding. In 2004, Urgent Matters published the key lessons learned from the first learning network (Urgent Matters, 2004):

- Recognizing that ED crowding is a hospital-wide problem, not an ED problem
- Building multidisciplinary, hospital-wide teams to oversee and implement change
- Determining the presence of a "champion" for patient flow
- Guaranteeing management's support
- Using formal improvement methods
- Committing to rigorous metrics
- Making transparency an organizational value
- Finding the right balance between collaboration and competition

The results of this project suggest that a combination of hospital-wide policies are necessary to reduce diversion and improve ED throughput; some of these include greater attention to inpatient discharge planning, faster turnaround from radiology and laboratory services, and greater coordination of care among EDs in a geographic region (Bernstein and Asplin, 2006).

The year 2003 marked the first time that ED crowding was recognized as a national problem by an accrediting body. Although not a strong policy directive, the Joint Commission (accrediting agency for healthcare organizations) issued guidelines on crowding and recognized the link between crowding and quality. These guidelines call for hospitals to have plans in place to handle crowded EDs, and to provide a level of service to admitted patients boarding in the ED comparable with that which they would receive on inpatient units (Bernstein and Asplin, 2006). Although this level of awareness appeared promising, further progress has been slow and there continues to be some disconnect between institutional and national priorities, and those of the emergency medicine community. In a recent survey of members of the American College of Emergency Physicians, respondents ranked ED crowding caused by boarding of admitted patients as their most important patient safety concern (Sklar et al., 2008). By contrast, reduction of ED crowding is not one of the 12 target interventions included in the IHI 100,000 Lives and 5 Million Lives Campaigns for hospital quality improvement (Institute for Healthcare Improvement, 2006), nor is it one of the 2008 National Patient Safety Goals adopted by the Joint Commission (The Joint Commission, 2008).

In 2006, the Institute of Medicine published a series of reports on the future of emergency care in the United States. These reports focused on the state of pediatric emergency care, prehospital emergency care, and hospital-based emergency and trauma care (Institute of Medicine, 2006). The committee directly addressed many issues related to ED crowding, boarding, and ambulance diversion. Of their recommendations, the two most notable policy proposals involved federal oversight and assistance:

1. Congress should establish dedicated funding (initially $50 million) to reimburse hospitals that provide significant amounts of uncompensated emergency and trauma care for financial losses incurred by those services.
2. Hospitals should end the practices of boarding patients in the ED and ambulance diversion, except in the most extreme cases. The Centers for Medicare & Medicaid Services should convene a working group of experts to develop boarding and diversion standards, incentives, and enforcement.

Since the publication of this report, the American College of Emergency Physicians has proposed legislation that would provide for this oversight. The "Access to Emergency Medical Services Act" continues to gain the support of congressional sponsors while organizations like ACEP continue to educate policymakers about the dangers of crowding and boarding.

Summary

ED crowding is a pervasive and significant problem throughout the world. In the United States it has reached epidemic levels and threatens the ability of our healthcare system to handle not only daily emergencies, but national disasters as well (Institute of Medicine, 2006). Over the past 15 years, substantial progress has been made quantifying and measuring ED crowding. More recent work has begun to convincingly establish the effects of crowding on patient safety and quality of care (Bernstein and Asplin, 2006). Despite our improved understanding of crowding and its effects, there is significant work to be done, on many fronts, for sustainable solutions to be realized. ED crowding is a problem that will require the collaboration researchers, administrators, and policymakers at all levels of government and industry, public and private. Research and innovation in ED crowding continues to evolve. The future holds promise for new solutions, better measures, and increased awareness, but without the financial and operational incentives to drive flow through the system, the system will continue to fail those who need it the most.

References

Adams, J.G. and Biros, M.H. 2001. The endangered safety net: Establishing a measure of control. *Academic Emergency Medicine* 8(11):1013–1015.

American Academy of Pediatrics. 2004. Overcrowding crisis in our nation's emergency departments: Is our safety net unraveling? *Pediatrics* 114(3):878–888.

American College of Emergency Physicians. 1990a. Hospital and emergency department overcrowding. *Annals of Emergency Medicine* 19(3):336.

American College of Emergency Physicians. 1990b. Measures to deal with emergency department overcrowding. *Annals of Emergency Medicine* 19(8):944–945.

Andrulis, D.P., Kellermann, A., Hintz, A., Hackman, B., and Weslowski, V. 1991. Emergency departments and crowding in United States teaching hospitals. *Annals of Emergency Medicine* 20(9):980–986.

Asplin, B.R. 2001. Tying a knot in the unraveling health care safety net. *Academic Emergency Medicine* 8(11):1075–1079.

Asplin, B.R. and Knopp, R.K. 2001. A room with a view: On-call specialist panels and other health policy challenges in the emergency department. *Annals of Emergency Medicine* 37(5):500–503.

Asplin, B.R., Majid, D.J., Rhodes, K.J., Solberg, L.I., Lurie, N., and Camargo, C.A. Jr. 2003. A conceptual model of emergency department crowding. *Annals of Emergency Medicine* 42(2):173–180.

Asplin, B.R. and Rhodes, K.V. 2004. Is this emergency department crowded? A multicenter derivation and evaluation of an emergency department crowding scale (EDCS). *Academic Emergency Medicine* 11(5):484.

Bagust, A., Place, M., and Posnett, J.W. 1999. Dynamics of bed use in accommodating emergency admissions: Stochastic simulation model. *British Medical Journal* 319(7203):155–158.

Bernstein, S.L. and Asplin, B.R. 2006. Emergency department crowding: Old problem, new solutions. *Emergency Medical Clinics of North America* 24(4):821–837.

Bernstein, S.L., Verghese, V., Leung, W., Lunney, A.T., and Perez, I. 2003. Development and validation of a new index to measure emergency department crowding. *Academic Emergency Medicine* 10(9):938–942.

Bitterman, R.A. 2006. EMTALA and the ethical delivery of hospital emergency services. *Emergency Medical Clinics of North America* 24(3):557–577.

Burt, C.W., McCaig, L.F., and Valverde, R.H. 2006. Analysis of ambulance transports and diversions among U.S. emergency departments. *Annals of Emergency Medicine* 47(4):317–326.

Chan, T.C., Killeen, J.P., Kelly, D., and Guss, D.A. 2005. Impact of rapid entry and accelerated care at triage on reducing emergency department patient wait times, lengths of stay, and rate of left without being seen. *Annals of Emergency Medicine* 46(6):491–497.

Chin, L. and Fleisher, G. 1998. Planning model of resource utilization in an academic pediatric emergency department. *Pediatric Emergency Care* 14(1):4–9.

Clark, J.J. 2005. Unlocking hospital gridlock. *Healthcare Finance Management* 59(11):94–96, 98, 100–102 passim.

Connelly, L.G. and Bair, A.E. 2004. Discrete event simulation of emergency department activity: A platform for system-level operations research. *Academic Emergency Medicine* 11(11):1177–1185.

Cunningham, P. and J. May. 2003. Insured Americans drive surge in emergency department visits. *Issue Brief Centennnial Study of Health Systems Change* 70:1–6.

Derlet, R.W., Nishio, D., Cole, L.M., and Silva, J. Jr. 1992. Triage of patients out of the emergency department: Three-year experience. *American Journal of Emergency Medicine* 10(3):195–199.

Derlet, R.W. and Richards, J.R. 2000. Overcrowding in the nation's emergency departments: Complex causes and disturbing effects. *Annals of Emergency Medicine* 35(1):63–68.

Derlet, R., Richards, J., and Kravitz, R. 2001. Frequent overcrowding in U.S. emergency departments. *Academic Emergency Medicine* 8(2):151–155.

Diercks, D.B., Roe, M.T., Chen, A.Y., Peacock, W.F., Kirk, J.D., Pollack, C.V. Jr., Gibler, W.B., Smith, S.C. Jr., Ohman, M., and Peterson, E.D. 2007. Prolonged emergency department stays of non-ST-segment-elevation myocardial infarction patients are associated with worse adherence to the American College of Cardiology/American Heart Association guidelines for management and increased adverse events. *Annals of Emergency Medicine* 50(5):489–496.

Diesburg-Stanwood, A., Scott, J., Oman, K., and Whitehill, C. 2004. Nonemergent ED patients referred to community resources after medical screening examination: Characteristics, medical condition after 72 hours, and use of follow-up services. *Journal of Emergency Nursing* 30(4):312–317.

Emergency Medical Treatment and Active Labor Act (EMTALA). 1986. Examination and treatment for emergency medical conditions and women in labor, 42 USC 1395dd (United States Code Title 42, 1395dd).

Espinosa, G., Miro, O., Sanchez, M., Coll-Vinent, B., and Milla, J. 2002. Effects of external and internal factors on emergency department overcrowding. *Annals of Emergency Medicine* 39(6):693–695.

Fatovich, D.M., Nagree, Y., and Sprivulis, P. 2005. Access block causes emergency department overcrowding and ambulance diversion in Perth, Western Australia. *Emergency Medicine Journal* 22(5):351–354.

Fee, C., Weber, E.J., Maak, C.A., and Bacchetti, P. 2007. Effect of emergency department crowding on time to antibiotics in patients admitted with community-acquired pneumonia. *Annals of Emergency Medicine* 50(5):501–509, 509 e1.

Forster, A.J., Stiell, I., Wells, G., Lee, A., and van Walraven, C. 2003. The effect of hospital occupancy on emergency department length of stay and patient disposition. *Academic Emergency Medicine* 10(2):127–133.

Gallagher, E.J. and Lynn, S.G. 1990. The etiology of medical gridlock: Causes of emergency department overcrowding in New York City. *Journal of Emergency Medicine* 8(6):785–790.

General Accounting Office. 1993. Emergency Departments: Unevenly affected by growth and change in patient use. United States General Accounting Office: Washington, DC.

Green, L.V., Soares, J., Giglio, J.F., and Green, R.A. 2006. Using queueing theory to increase the effectiveness of emergency department provider staffing. *Academic Emergency Medicine* 13(1):61–68.

Grumbach, K., Keane, D., and Bindman, A. 1993. Primary care and public emergency department overcrowding. *American Journal of Public Health* 83(3):372–378.

Henry, M. 2001. Overcrowding in America's emergency departments: Inpatient wards replace emergency care. *Academic Emergency Medicine* 8(2):188–189.

Hoffenberg, S., Hill, M.B., and Houry, D. 2001. Does sharing process differences reduce patient length of stay in the emergency department? *Annals of Emergency Medicine* 38(5):533–540.

Hoot, N.R. and Aronsky, D. 2008. Systematic review of emergency department crowding: Causes, effects, and solutions. *Annals of Emergency Medicine* 52(2):126–136.

Hoot, N.R., Leblanc, L.J., Jones, I., Levin, S.R., Zhou, C., Gadd, C.S., and Aronsky, D. 2009. Forecasting emergency department crowding: A prospective, real-time evaluation. *Journal of the American Medical Informatics Association* 16(3):338–345.

Hoot, N.R., Zhou, C., Jones, I., and Aronsky, D. 2007. Measuring and forecasting emergency department crowding in real time. *Annals of Emergency Medicine* 49(6):747–755.

Hu, S.C. 1991. Clinical and demographic characteristics of 13,911 medical emergency patients. *Journal of the Formosan Medical Association* 90(7):675–680.

Hu, S.C. 1994. Clinical and demographic characteristics of adult emergency patients at the Taipei Veterans General Hospital. *Journal of the Formosan Medical Association* 93(1):61–65.

Hwang, U. and Concato, J. 2004. Care in the emergency department: How crowded is overcrowded? *Academic Emergency Medicine* 11(10):1097–1101.

Institute for Healthcare Improvement. 2004. Optimizing capacity in an acute care hospital. Lehigh Valley Hospital and Health Network: Allentown, PA.

Institute for Healthcare Improvement. 2006. Protecting 5 million lives from harm. http://www.ihi.org/IHI/Programs/Campaign (accessed April 16, 2009).

Institute of Medicine. 2000. America's Health Care Safety Net: Intact but Endangered. The National Academies Press: Washington, DC.

Institute of Medicine. 2006. *Hospital-Based Emergency Care: At the Breaking Point*. The National Academies Press: Washington, DC.

Jones, S.S., Allen, T.L., Flottemesch, T.J., and Welch, S.J. 2006. An independent evaluation of four quantitative emergency department crowding scales. *Academic Emergency Medicine* 13(11):1204–1211.

Jones, D.S., McNagny, S.E., Williams, M.V., Parker, R.M., Sawyer, M.F., and Rask, K.J. 1999. Lack of a regular source of care among children using a public hospital emergency department. *Pediatric Emergency Care* 15(1):13–16.

Kellermann, A.L. 1991. Too sick to wait. *Journal of the American Medical Association* 266(8):1123–1125.

Kellermann, A.L. 1994. Access of Medicaid recipients to outpatient care. *New England Journal of Medicine* 330(20):1426–1430.

Khare, R.K., Powell, E.S., Reinhardt, G., and Lucenti, M. 2009. Adding more beds to the emergency department or reducing admitted patient boarding times: Which has a more significant influence on emergency department congestion? *Annals of Emergency Medicine* 53(5):575–585.

Kondro, W. 1998. Relief at a price for emergency wards in Ontario. *The Lancet* 352:1451.

Lagoe, R.J., Hunt, R.C., Nadle, P.A., and Kohlbrenner, J.C. 2002. Utilization and impact of ambulance diversion at the community level. *Prehospital Emergency Care* 6(2):191–198.

Lambe, S., Washington, D.L., Fink, A., Herbst, K., Liu, H., Fosse, J.H., and Asch, S.M. 2002. Trends in the use and capacity of California's emergency departments, 1990–1999. *Annals of Emergency Medicine* 39(4):389–396.

Litvak, E. 2005. Optimizing patient flow by managing its variability, in: *From Front Office to Front Line: Essential Issues for Health Care Leaders*. Joint Commission Resources, Inc.: Oakbrook Terrace, IL, pp. 91–111.

Litvak, E. and Long, M.C. 2000. Cost and quality under managed care: Irreconcilable differences? *American Journal of Managed Care* 6(3):305–312.

Lynn, S.G. and Kellermann, A.L. 1991. Critical decision making: Managing the emergency department in an overcrowded hospital. *Annals of Emergency Medicine* 20(3):287–292.

Maag, R., Krivenko, C., Graff, L., Joseph, A., Klopfer, A.H., Donofrio, J., D'Andrea, R., and Salamone, M. 1997. Improving chest pain evaluation within a multihospital network by the use of emergency department observation units. *The Joint Commission Journal on Quality Improvement* 23(6):312–320.

Magid, D.J., Asplin, B.R., and Wears, R.L. 2004. The quality gap: Searching for the consequences of emergency department crowding. *Annals of Emergency Medicine* 44(6): 586–588.

McCarthy, L. 2005. Hospital crowding and ED delays: A case study. *Trustee* 58(7):30–1, 1.

McCarthy, M.L., Aronsky, D., Jones, I.D., Miner, J.R., Band, R.A., Baren, J.M., Desmond, J.S., Baumlin, K.M., Ding, R., and Shesser, R. 2008. The emergency department occupancy rate: A simple measure of emergency department crowding? *Annals of Emergency Medicine* 51(1):15–24, 24 e1–2.

Meislin, H.W., Coates, S.A., Cyr, J., and Valenzuela, T. 1988. Fast track: Urgent care within a teaching hospital emergency department: Can it work? *Annals of Emergency Medicine* 17(5):453–456.

Miro, O., Antonio, M.T., Jimenez, S., De Dios A., Sanchez, M., Boras A., and Milla, J. 1999. Decreased health care quality associated with emergency department overcrowding. *European Journal of Emergency Medicine* 6(2):105–107.

Moskop, J.C., Sklar, D., Geiderman, J., Schears, R., and Bookman, D. 2009a. Emergency department crowding, part 1: Concept, causes, and moral consequences. *Annals of Emergency Medicine* 53(5):605–611.

Moskop, J.C., Sklar, D.P., Geiderman, J.M., Schears, R.M., and Bookman, K.J. 2009b. Emergency department crowding, part 2: Barriers to reform and strategies to overcome them. *Annals of Emergency Medicine* 53(5):612–617.

Munoz, E., Laughlin, A., Regan, D.M., Teicher, I., Margolis, I.B., and Wise, L. 1985. The financial effects of emergency department-generated admissions under prospective payment systems. *Journal of the American Medical Association* 254(13):1763–1771.

Murray, M. and Berwick, D.M. 2003. Advanced access: Reducing waiting and delays in primary care. *Journal of the American Medical Association* 289(8):1035–1040.

Murray, M., Bodenheimer, T., Rittenhouse, D., and Grumback, K. 2003. Improving timely access to primary care: Case studies of the advanced access model. *Journal of the American Medical Association* 289(8):1042–1046.

National Academy of Engineering and Institute of Medicine. 2005. *Building a Better Delivery System: A New Engineering/Health Care Partnership*. The National Academies Press: Washington, DC.

Nawar, E.W., Niska, R.W., and Xu, J. 2007. National Hospital Ambulatory Medical Care Survey: 2005 emergency department summary. *Advance Data* 386:1–32.

New Jersey Commission on Rationalizing Health Care Resources. 2008. Final report. State of New Jersey: Trenton, NJ.

Newton, M.F., Keirns, C.C., Cunningham, R., Hayward, R.A., and Stanley, R. 2008. Uninsured adults presenting to U.S. emergency departments: Assumptions vs data. *Journal of the American Medical Association* 300(16):1914–1924.

Novello, A. 2000. Hospital ED Overcrowding. New York State Department of Health, editor: Albany, NY.

O'Brien, D., Williams, A., Blondell, K., and Jelinek, G.A. 2006. Impact of streaming "fast track" emergency department patients. *Australian Health Review* 30(4):525–532.

Olshaker, J.S. and Rathlev, N.K. 2006. Emergency Department overcrowding and ambulance diversion: The impact and potential solutions of extended boarding of admitted patients in the Emergency Department. *Journal of Emergency Medicine* 30(3):351–356.

Patel, P.B., Derlet, R.W., Vinson, D.R., Williams, M., and Wills, J. 2006. Ambulance diversion reduction: The Sacramento solution. *American Journal of Emergency Medicine* 24(2):206–213.

Pham, J.C., Patel, R., Millin, M.G., Kirsch, T.D., and Chanmugam, A. 2006. The effects of ambulance diversion: A comprehensive review. *Academic Emergency Medicine* 13(11):1220–1227.

Pickert, K. 2009. Starting health-care reform in the ER. *Time Magazine*. Time Inc.: New York.

Pines, J.M. 2007. Moving closer to an operational definition for ED crowding. *Academic Emergency Medicine* 14(4):382–383; author reply 383–384.

Pines, J.M. and Hollander, J.E. 2008. Emergency department crowding is associated with poor care for patients with severe pain. *Annals of Emergency Medicine* 51(1):1–5.

Pines, J.M., Pollack, C.V., Diercks, D.B., Chang, A.M., Shofer, F.S., and Hollander, J.E. 2009. The association between emergency department crowding and adverse cardiovascular outcomes in patients with chest pain. *Academic Emergency Medicine* 16(7):617–625.

Rask, K.J., Williams, M.V., McNagny, S.E., Parker, R.M., and Baker, D.W. 1998. Ambulatory health care use by patients in a public hospital emergency department. *Journal of General Internal Medicine* 13(9):614–620.

Rask, K.J., Williams, M.V., Parker, R.M., and McNagny, S.E. 1994. Obstacles predicting lack of a regular provider and delays in seeking care for patients at an urban public hospital. *Journal of the American Medical Association* 271(24):1931–1933.

Rathlev, N.K., Chessare, J., Olshaker, J., Obendorfer, D., Mehta, S.D., Rothenhaus, T., Crespo, S. et al. 2007. Time series analysis of variables associated with daily mean emergency department length of stay. *Annals of Emergency Medicine* 49(3):265–271.

Richardson, D.B. 2002. The access-block effect: Relationship between delay to reaching an inpatient bed and inpatient length of stay. *Medical Journal of Australia* 177(9):492–495.

Richardson, D.B. 2006. Increase in patient mortality at 10 days associated with emergency department overcrowding. *Medical Journal of Australia* 184(5):213–216.

Richardson, L.D., Asplin, B.R., and Lowe, R.A. 2002. Emergency department crowding as a health policy issue: Past development, future directions. *Annals of Emergency Medicine* 40(4):388–393.

Richardson, L.D. and Hwang, U. 2001a. Access to care: A review of the emergency medicine literature. *Academic Emergency Medicine* 8(11):1030–1036.

Richardson, L.D. and Hwang, U. 2001b. America's Health Care Safety Net: Intact or unraveling? *Academic Emergency Medicine* 8(11):1056–1063.

Rodi, S.W., Grau, M.V., and Orsini, C.M. 2006. Evaluation of a fast track unit: Alignment of resources and demand results in improved satisfaction and decreased length of stay for emergency department patients. *Quality Management in Health Care* 15(3):163–170.

Ross, M.A., Compton, S., Richardson, D., Jones, R., Nittis, T., and Wilson, T. 2003. The use and effectiveness of an emergency department observation unit for elderly patients. *Annals of Emergency Medicine* 41(5):668–677.

Sanchez, M., Smally, A.J., Grant, R.J., and Jacobs, L.M. 2006. Effects of a fast-track area on emergency department performance. *Journal of Emergency Medicine* 31(1):117–120.

Scheulen, J.J., Li, G., and Kelen, G.D. 2001. Impact of ambulance diversion policies in urban, suburban, and rural areas of Central Maryland. *Academic Emergency Medicine* 8(1):36–40.

Schull, M.J., Kiss, A., and Szalai, J.P. 2007. The effect of low-complexity patients on emergency department waiting times. *Annals of Emergency Medicine* 49(3):257–264, 264 e1.

Schull, M.J., Lazier, K., Vermeulen, M., Mawhinney, S., and Morrison, L. 2003. Emergency department contributors to ambulance diversion: A quantitative analysis. *Annals of Emergency Medicine* 41(4):467–476.

Schull, M.J., Slaughter, P.M., and Redelmeier, D.A. 2002. Urban emergency department overcrowding: Defining the problem and eliminating misconceptions. *Canadian Journal of Emergency Medicine* 4(2):76–83.

Schull, M.J., Vermeulen, M., Slaughter, G., Morrison, L., and Daly, P. 2004. Emergency department crowding and thrombolysis delays in acute myocardial infarction. *Annals of Emergency Medicine* 44(6):577–585.

Shah, M.N., Fairbanks, R.J., Maddow, C.L., Lerner, E.B., Syrett, J.I., Davis, E.A., and Schneider, S.M. 2006. Description and evaluation of a pilot physician-directed emergency medical services diversion control program. *Academic Emergency Medicine* 13(1):54–60.

Shih, F.Y., Ma, M.H., Chen, S.C., Wang, H.P., Fang, C.C., Shyu, R.S., Huang, G.T., and Wang, S.M. 1999. ED overcrowding in Taiwan: Facts and strategies. *American Journal of Emergency Medicine* 17(2):198–202.

Siddharthan, K., W.J. Jones, and Johnson, J.A. 1996. A priority queuing model to reduce waiting times in emergency care. *International Journal of Health Care Quality Assurance* 9(5):10–16.

Simon, H.K., Ledbetter, D.A., and Wright, J. 1997. Societal savings by "fast tracking" lower acuity patients in an urban pediatric emergency department. *American Journal of Emergency Medicine* 15(6):551–554.

Sklar, D., Crandall, C., and Zola, T. 2008. Emergency physician perceptions of patient safety risks [abstract]. *Annals of Emergency Medicine* 51:501.

Solberg, L.I., Asplin, B.R., Weinick, R.M., and Magid, D.J. 2003. Emergency department crowding: Consensus development of potential measures. *Annals of Emergency Medicine* 42(6):824–834.

Sprivulis, P.C., Da Silva, J.A., Jacobs, I.G., Frazer, A.R.L., and Jelinek, G.A. 2006. The association between hospital overcrowding and mortality among patients admitted via Western Australian emergency departments. *Medical Journal of Australia* 184(5):208–212.

Sprivulis, P. and Gerrard, B. 2005. Internet-accessible emergency department workload information reduces ambulance diversion. *Prehospital Emergency Care* 9(3):285–291.

Sprivulis, P., Grainger, S., and Nagree, Y. 2005. Ambulance diversion is not associated with low acuity patients attending Perth metropolitan emergency departments. *Emergency Medicine Australasia* 17(1):11–15.

The Joint Commission. 2008. National Patient Safety Goals. The Joint Commission: Oakbrook Terrace, IL. http://www.jointcommission.org/PatientSafety/NationalPatientSafetyGoals/ (accessed April 16, 2009).

Trzeciak, S. and Rivers, E.P. 2003. Emergency department overcrowding in the United States: An emerging threat to patient safety and public health. *Emergency Medical Journal* 20(5):402–405.

Tye, L. 2000. Officials offer little hope for emergency room diversion. *The Boston Globe*. Boston, MA. November 14, p. A12.

Urgent Matters. 2004. Bursting at the Seams: Improving patient flow to help America's Emergency Departments. The George Washington University Medical Center: Washington, DC.

Viccellio, A., Santoro, C., Singer, A.J., Thode, H.C. Jr., and Henry, M.C. 2009. The Association Between Transfer of Emergency Department Boarders to Inpatient Hallways and Mortality: A 4-year experience. *Annals of Emergency Medicine* 54(4):487–491.

Vilke, G.M., Brown, L., Skogland, P., Simmons, C., and Guss, D.A. 2004a. Approach to decreasing emergency department ambulance diversion hours. *Journal of Emergency Medicine* 26(2):189–192.

Vilke, G.M., Castillo, E.M., Metz, M.A., Ray, L.U., Murrin, P.A., Lev, R., and Chan, T.C. 2004b. Community trial to decrease ambulance diversion hours: The San Diego county patient destination trial. *Annals of Emergency Medicine* 44(4):295–303.

Washington, D.L., Stevens, C.D., Shekelle, P.G., Henneman, P.L. and Brrok, R.H. 2002. Next-day care for emergency department users with nonacute conditions. A randomized, controlled trial. *Annals of Internal Medicine* 137(9):707–714.

Weiss, S.J., Derlet, R., Arndahl, J., Ernst, A.A., Richards, J., Fernandez-Frackelton, M., Schwab, R. et al. 2004. Estimating the degree of emergency department overcrowding in academic medical centers: Results of the National ED Overcrowding Study (NEDOCS). *Academic Emergency Medicine* 11(1):38–50.

Will, G.F. 1990. The trauma in trauma care. *Newsweek* 115(11):98.

Wilson, M. and Nguyen, K. 2004. Bursting at the Seams: Improving patient flow to help America's Emergency Departments. The George Washington University Medical Center: Washington, DC.

Wuerz, R.C., Milne, L.W., Eitel, D.R., Travers, D., and Gilboy, N. 2000. Reliability and validity of a new five-level triage instrument. *Academic Emergency Medicine* 7(3):236–242.

33

Emergency Department Throughput from a Healthcare Leader's Perspective

Airica Steed
Advocate Health Care

Background/Context ... 33-1
Emergency Department Throughput ... 33-2
Patient Reception Bottleneck ... 33-2
Mini-Registration and Mobile Bedside Registration ... 33-3
Rapid Triage ... 33-4
Diagnostic Procedure Area ... 33-5
Intradepartmental Flow Bottleneck ... 33-6
Diagnostic Imaging Improvement ... 33-6
Laboratory Services Improvement ... 33-7
Order to Specimen Collection • Specimen Collection to Received • Received to Resulted
Team-Based Approach to Transition of Care ... 33-9
Decompression Block and Inpatient Capacity Bottleneck ... 33-10
Inpatient "Pull" System ... 33-10
Housekeeping Room Turnover ... 33-11
4-Tier High Census Alert Strategy ... 33-12
Lessons Learned and Sustainment Strategy ... 33-15
References ... 33-20

Background/Context

The emergency department (ED) serves as the "front door" to most hospitals and is the primary source of inpatient volumes and revenue. It is a well-known fact that the EDs of hospitals provide much-needed access to healthcare for many of the nation's insured, underinsured, and uninsured. In most hospital organizations, more than 50% of admissions originate in the ED. According to the Center for Disease Control, 12.8% of ED visits in 2006, or one in seven visits, resulted in a hospital admission. Needless to say, the ED contributes greatly to hospital financial performance, as well as patient's experience. EDs also deliver significant community benefits 24 hours a day, 7 days a week without regard for patients' ability to pay. To say the very least, hospital EDs are a critical part of our health system.

As the nation's uninsured and underinsured population grows, more and more Americans are seeking primary care or nonurgent care from EDs. Also, as the nation's population ages, EDs are seeing increased numbers of Medicare patients. Within a decade, ED visits increased by approximately

32% from 90.3 million visits in 1994 to 119.2 million visits in 2006. Increased ED utilization coupled with inappropriate ED usage has led to severe overcrowding. According to the American Hospital Association's (AHA) "The State of America's Hospitals—Taking the Pulse" released in 2006, half of the country's ED were "at" or "over" capacity. ED crowding at critical levels often lead to diversion of inbound ambulances.

Hospital EDs face major barriers that impede their ability to serve the needs of their surrounding communities and fill the huge gap in healthcare access. The foremost areas of concern stem from the triage process, availability of inpatient beds especially on critical care units, lab and radiology turnaround, and patient transportation. In addition, EDs are currently experiencing many challenges as it relates to an increased demand yet with no additional capacity.

Symptoms of this demand–capacity divergence include ED crowding, ambulance diversion and bypass, and holding admitted patients due to lack of hospital beds. Most patients experience very lengthy waits before receiving care, and some leave without being treated. Despite the many highlighted benefits denoted above, the ED has been a key target in many hospital organization quality improvement efforts due to many concerns related to poor throughput, poor patient satisfaction, lack of compliance with quality measures, and scant financial returns. As an integral part of the hospital's operations, the ED should be a major focus for hospital quality improvement and performance enhancement efforts. These efforts result not only in financial return on investment due to increased efficiency, but more importantly they produce immeasurable returns in the quality of care provided, safety, and satisfaction of hospital patients.

Emergency Department Throughput

Congested EDs continue to afflict the hospitals across the country, and the expense of poor service resulting from disproportionate impediments is a costly problem to have. Any effort to alleviate ED overcrowding, reduce treatment delays, and improve patient throughput can create a healthier environment for all concerned, including patients, staff, and physicians, and fundamentally bolster a hospital's financial position. ED throughput can be defined as the seamless and continuous flow of patients throughout the emergent value stream. Throughput truly occurs only when a patient actually leaves the ED. Despite the multitude of strategies available to improve ED throughput, applying a mixed methods approach, which includes a combination of lean thinking, six sigma, best practice fundamentals, and extensive industry knowledge, is a proven methodology that could produce breakthrough outcomes. The variability in the time to get a patient triaged, in a bed, assessed, orders written, orders entered, tests completed, consults consulted, diagnosis completed, bed assigned, and turnover report given, all combine for actual ED average length of stay (ALOS).

When analyzing the holistic ED experience from entrance to exit, otherwise known as the value stream, there are typically three primary throughput bottlenecks or restricted access points relevant to the ED: (1) patient reception, (2) intradepartmental flow obstruction, and (3) decompression block. These three areas that comprise the primary bottlenecks can be visualized in the diagram below of the ED value stream (see Figure 33.1).

Patient Reception Bottleneck

The patient reception bottleneck is a front-end obstruction to the efficient intake and triage of patients in the ED value stream. This typically encompasses patients who arrive by ambulance or on foot who are waiting to be positioned in an ED location. The patient reception traffic jam is often the cause of delays to triage, to a room, to treatment, and to see a physician, and is the patient's first perception of their ED visit. Reception difficulties are a likely root cause of extended waiting room times, poor

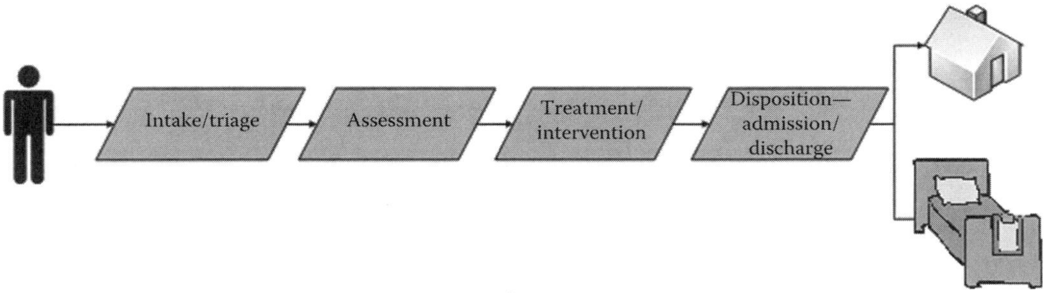

FIGURE 33.1 Emergency department value stream.

patient satisfaction, and high walkout rates. One key determining factor when you have a patient reception bottleneck is excessive patients in waiting room or waiting in line for triage with a high volume of patients who leave without treatment in parallel. In addition, many EDs that have a patient reception bottleneck are more than likely to have available ED beds and/or space to position patients; however, they lack the necessary movement to expedite the patient the appropriate location in a timely manner.

There have been many approaches to remedy the patient reception obstructions in the industry because this is the perception of the patient's first encounter. Most strategies are geared toward refining the triage capabilities in order to enhance the patient filtering and movement into the ED space. However, some evidence-based practices that have been successful consist of the implementation of the following best practice strategies: mini-registration and mobile bedside registration, rapid triage which includes the "triage is a process and not a place mentality," and the institution of a diagnostic procedure area.

Mini-Registration and Mobile Bedside Registration

In the ED, time is a critical element when expediting emergency care. Mini-registration otherwise known as "greet" in the industry is a modified function of access or registration in which minimal patient identification is received in order to quickly render treatment. The standard identifiers for mini-registration include the patient's name, date of birth, social security number, hospital visit history, reason for visit, and primary physician. When implemented, this process is initiated for both ambulance and walk-in patients, and is generally the first time stamp for ED throughput. In addition, institutionalizing the mini-registration process allows the clinical professionals the ability to proactively manage the patient movement on the basis of complaint and time of arrival once the mini-registration has been complete on a "just in time" system. This also allows for a more appropriate patient identification function to be in place immediately upon arrival by placing an armband at mini-registration.

Patients entering the ED have a dedicated greeter at the mini-registration desk who quickly initiates the process to receive treatment more efficiently. The workspace area typically has been redesigned and equipped with signage to appropriate direct patients to the greeter. The greeter function can also be interchangeable and be incorporated into existing business functions within an already functioning ED. For example, institutions that have a triage nurse as the first point of contact can incorporate the mini-registration task as a part of their standard work.

Once the mini-registration is completed in a timely manner, the remainder of the registration can be reconciled at any point in the treatment cycle. In this case scenario, the patient is more satisfied with the business practices of carrying out the registration process due to the function being rendered at the bedside versus at an unfriendly booth. Mobile bedside registration is a process that is carried out at

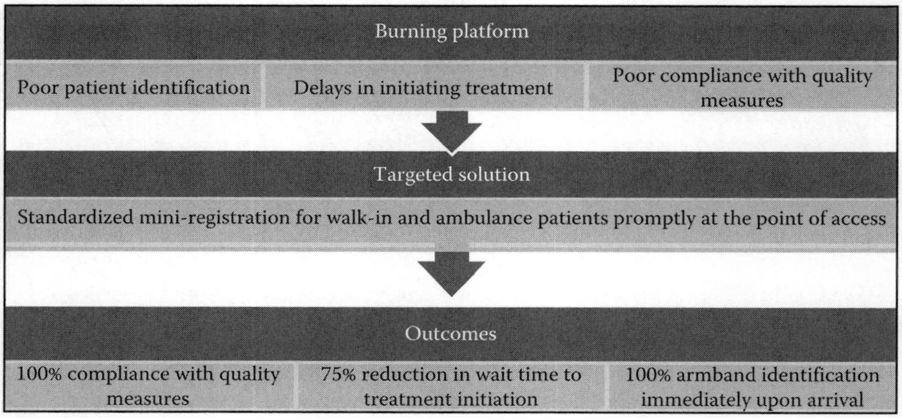

FIGURE 33.2 Mini-registration case study in a 24-bed ED in a community hospital setting.

the point-of-care (Figure 33.2). The intention of this design is to have a more "patient-focused" process versus "registration-focused" process.

Rapid Triage

Triage is one of the most critical rudiments of ED throughput. Some of the telltale signs of an inefficient triage system are overcrowded waiting areas, poor patient satisfaction scores, elongated overall ALOS, and lost revenue due to elevated walkout rates. The goal of the "rapid triage" process is to fill "all" empty space in the ED versus sending patients into the waiting area. Triage is often identified as location in the ED operational infrastructure versus as a process by which it operates. In the simplest of terms, triage is a quick evaluation rendered in order to filter and disseminate a patient to the appropriate area and allocate the correct type of service within the ED. Therefore, based on this definition, "triage is a process and not a place," and that mentality should also be instituted when implementing performance improvements within this setting.

Triage should be termed "rapid triage" in settings where throughput is a high priority. The target performance indicator for rapid triage should be 3 minutes or less in order to be most productive in expediting a seamless flow in the ED value stream. This process should encompass an evaluation of the need for treatment, brief historical basis, and determination of an appropriate acuity or severity level. Once the rapid triage is complete, the patient is then filtered to a specific location to continue the cycle of treatment until completion. The goal should be to have all available ED locations filled at all times in order to continue the efficient movement of patients. The ED is comparable to that of a revolving door that never stops. If there is space available, the objective should be to fill it immediately in order to prevent any downstream delays. It is counterproductive for an ED not to take advantage of the triage practices to be the initiating point in expediting patient flow and movement throughout the ED. In addition, it is extremely vital that specific operational roles and responsibilities be in place in order for the "rapid triage" to function as appropriate. These roles are inclusive of a dedicated greeter, triage nurse, and charge or lead nurse role. The greeter operates as the first point of contact for the ED.

The commonly developed process for all patients who meet the acuity description within the Emergency Severity Index (ESI) level 1 or 2 is to immediately be escorted into the main ED area upon arrival for mini-registration, triage, and mobile bedside registration. For patients who are less acute with the ESI levels 3–5, mini-registration and quick triage will take place on front end, and if ED space is available, patient will be escorted immediately to ED area for completion of treatment including full triage (see Figure 33.3).

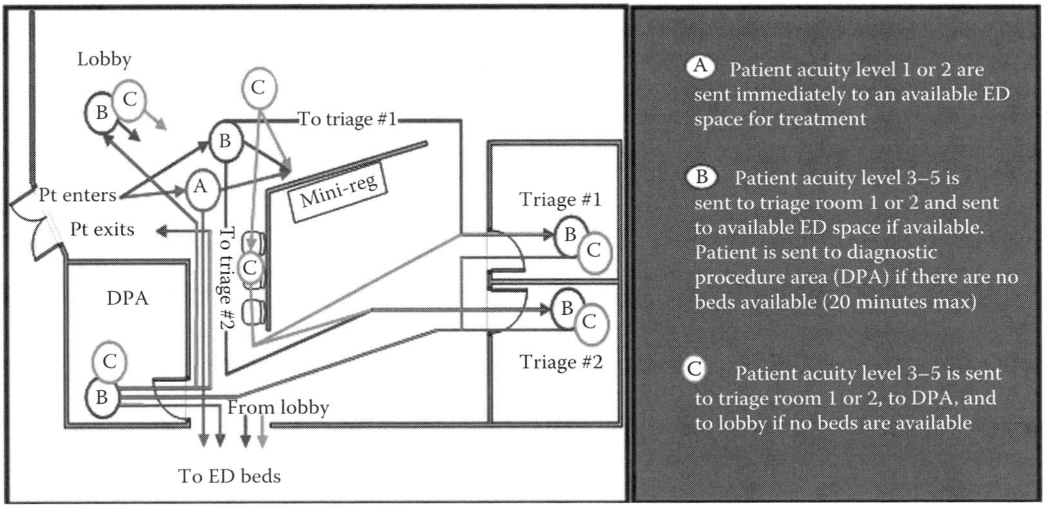

FIGURE 33.3 24-Bed ED triage improvement workflow.

Diagnostic Procedure Area

The diagnostic procedure area otherwise referred to as the DPA is a specialized intake location designed to accommodate treatment parameters when there are ED space limitations. The implementation of a DPA allows for a lack of dependence on and abuse of the waiting area to funnel patients who are in need of emergency services. This area allows for the specific services and regimes including the initiation of protocols and treatments when there is no or limited ED space available. The maximum time allotted to the DPA should be a maximum of 20 minutes and should be able to accommodate the rapid discharge of the less acute patients when needed (see Figure 33.4).

Case Study Example

It is 4 p.m. on a Tuesday in February in a 25-bed Level II ED. January and February are considered active months for this particular hospital. All existing ED space is occupied with four potential admissions and two soon-to-be discharges. The waiting room is beginning to crowd with a continued influx of patients who require treatment. Patient X arrives with a complaint of breathing difficulties that appears to be an Asthma exacerbation based on the rapid triage assessment. The triage nurse communicates to the team lead/charge nurse of the patient's need for an emergency bed; however, the lack of available logistics makes the decision to initiate treatment protocol on this patient following the asthma guidelines in the DPA. Due to the availability of this area, the nurse was able to immediately begin the treatment process following the predetermined protocol that included acquiring lab tests, obtaining appropriate diagnostics, and initiating respiratory treatment in a suitable manner. In this particular case, the patient was also able to be seen by a physician, treated, and discharged from this area without the need for an extended duration in the main ED. The patient's total ALOS was 2 hours and 17 minutes versus an average of 6 hours for a comparable acuity and condition. Furthermore, this ED has experienced greater than a 75% reduction in the patient walkout rate and 50% reduction in the overall ALOS based on this implementation of a DPA to expedite treatment parameters.

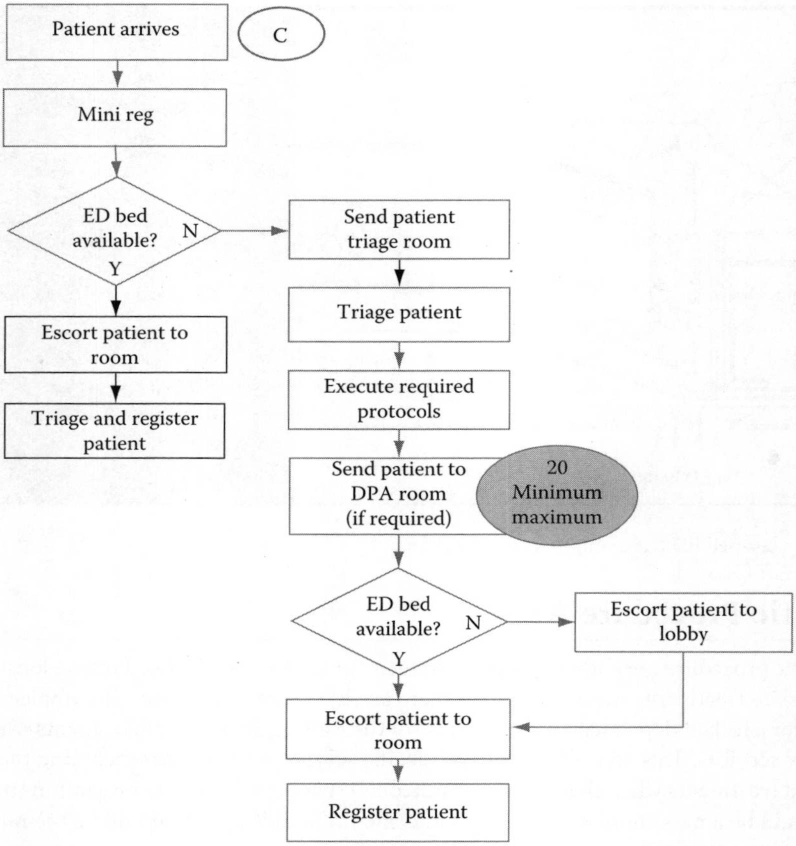

FIGURE 33.4 Diagnostic procedure area workflow.

Intradepartmental Flow Bottleneck

The intradepartmental flow bottleneck is a mid-flow roadblock that inhibits a timely disposition from the ED. These patients are typically pending a specific decision point relevant to qualifying for a disposition such as pertinent diagnostic result, test, or procedure outcomes. For example, patient X was admitted to the ED 7 hours ago with abdominal pain and tests have been initiated; however, the physician is pending specific results relevant to render a decision. In this particular example, there is no concern related to receiving the patient to have emergency services completed; however, there are issues relevant to discharging the patient from the space in order to welcome additional patients. When there is a perceived complexity moving the patient from the ED space, there is a throughput and intradepartmental flow issue that needs to become decompressed. While there is a multitude of processes that could make an impression on the progression of patients throughout the ED space, the improvement of diagnostic imaging and laboratory services within the emergency compound are the most prevalent.

Diagnostic Imaging Improvement

Diagnostic imaging barriers are commonly the root cause of many ED flow limitations. Getting diagnostic information in a timely manner has significant impact upon patient flow through the ED because a high proportion of emergent patients require some type of diagnostic service. Significant

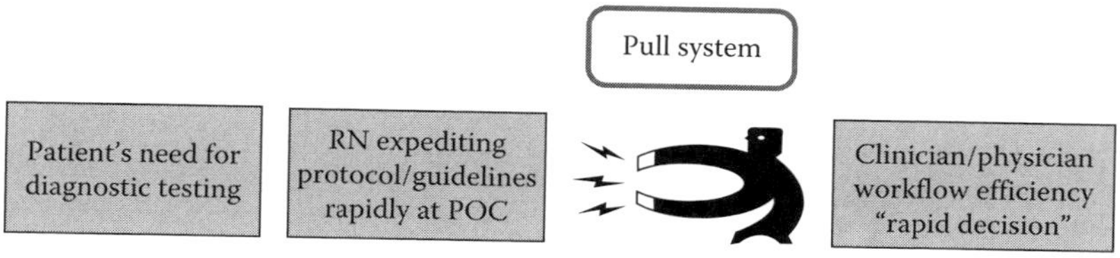

FIGURE 33.5 Intradepartmental pull system in a 24-bed ED.

improvements to diagnostic imaging services could enhance the movement of patients in the ED from an intradepartmental flow perspective because it assists the provider in making a rapid decision more quickly. Enhancing diagnostic imaging services creates what is known to be an "intradepartmental pull" because the demand for diagnostic treatment is triggered based on customer request; however, optimization of these processes could create a more worthwhile flow overall (see Figure 33.5).

Some evidence-based enhancements to diagnostic imaging in the ED include the following:

- Incorporating technological enablers to optimize flow and render the visualization of results in a timely fashion. This includes the implementation of PACS for viewing digital images and emergency department information systems (EDIS) that allows for timely viewing of preliminary results in order to make a rapid disposition decision.
- Developing a solid and collaborative partnership between the ED and diagnostic imaging versus fragmented workflow practices can definitely enhance the quality of emergent services more readily. It was found that if there is a shared vision with a shared goal, there will be shared results.
- Enhancing department logistics to support diagnostic imaging throughput. This includes having dedicated radiology services rooms located in a close proximity to the ED in order to prevent service delays, or considering dedicated ED transport during peak hours to decrease wait times from the overall diagnostic imaging transport process. This is especially apparent when there is an influx in demand for diagnostic imaging services and the service component is not logistically favorable to the ED.
- Implementing a standardized diagnostic imaging checklist to hardwire necessary process components into workflow and eliminate unnecessary and redundant phone calls. This will include incorporating a standard pregnancy verification procedure to improve the overall quality of radiology procedures performed on females who are within child-bearing years. Lastly, having hardwired "standard work" for the ED diagnostic imaging workflow has been found associated with improved overall throughput, decreased diagnostic imaging turnaround time, and improved quality of services provided (Figure 33.6).

Laboratory Services Improvement

Laboratory services play a vital role in the process of patient diagnosis, treatment, and monitoring of the emergent patient population. One of the key functions of the laboratory as it relates to the ED is to provide accurate and reliable data to providers in timely fashion in order to assist in rendering a medical decision. A basic process flow of the lab processes is primarily broken down into three distinct phases (Table 33.1).

Order to Specimen Collection

Order to specimen collection is defined as the time from when the order is placed within the ordering system until the specimen is collected. As it relates to the ED, this could be further identified as a part of the ED handling time or when the control is still geared toward ED stakeholders. In some instances, the flow of this process could be "specimen collection to order" due to the flow of the initiation of ED

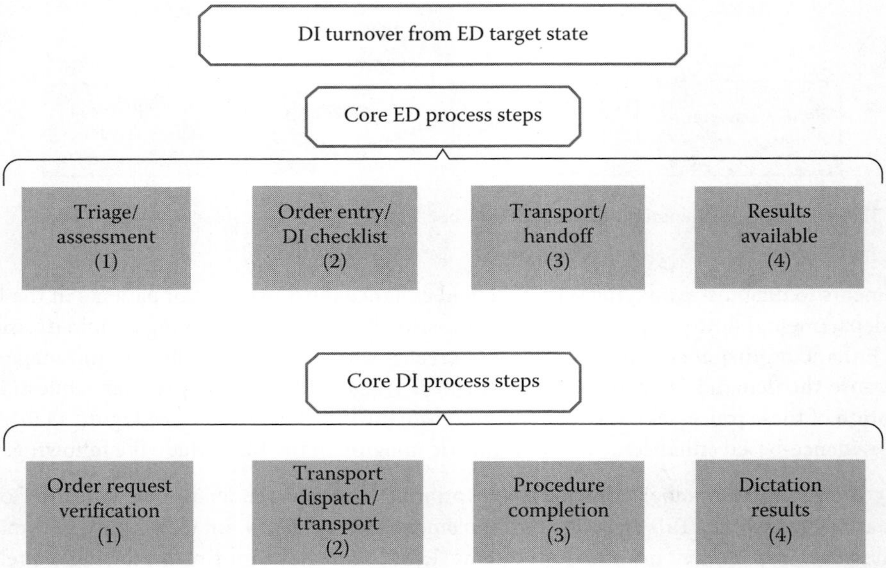

FIGURE 33.6 Diagnostic imaging turnover improvement diagram.

TABLE 33.1 Laboratory Improvement Scorecard Table

Measure	Current State	Target State
ED throughput		
Aggregate LOS (April)	222 minutes	>10% reduction
Door to Dr. Done (overall)	163 minutes	
Door to Dr. Done (admits)	224 minutes	
Overall lab TAT (collect → result)		
CBC	112 minutes	≤55 minutes
BMP	130 minutes	≤75 minutes
Troponin	118 minutes	≤75 minutes
CKMB	147 minutes	≤90 minutes
PT/PTT	114 minutes	≤70 minutes
ED workflow (collect → lab receipt)	60 minutes	<30 minutes (<15 stretch)
Lab workflow (lab receipt → result)		
CBC	36 minutes	≤25 minutes
BMP	52 minutes	≤45 minutes
Troponin	44 minutes	≤45 minutes
CKMB	69 minutes	≤60 minutes
PT/PTT	47 minutes	≤40 minutes
Hemolyzed %	1.5%	<1.25%
Contaminated %	3.04%	<2.3%
Total process steps	43	18
ED specific workflow steps	24	7
Lab-specific workflow steps	19	11

protocols and guidelines. In this case scenario, lab service collection is initiated by a clinician and the ordering process takes place after the specimen is drawn.

Specimen Collection to Received

Specimen collection to received is defined as the time from when the specimen is collected until the specimen is received in the lab. There are some instances where there are laboratories located specifically within an ED compound and others depend on technological enablers such as tube systems or other resources to deliver the specimen in a timely fashion.

Received to Resulted

Received to resulted is defined as the time from when the specimen is received in the lab until the result is verified and report returned to the ED physician. This process could also be deemed as "laboratory handling" time or when the turnaround is completely under the control of lab service professionals. This process includes lab specimen processing, resulting, and reporting.

Comprehensive emergency treatment requires that well-functioning laboratory services are in place to expedite the flow of care. Laboratory services can cause numerous delays and gaps in ED workflow practices and pose serious threats to the quality of patient-care services. These delays can include but are not limited to poor labeling practices; ineffective use of protocols and procedure guidelines to immediately accelerate treatment; lack of pull from physicians to expedite laboratory workflow; knowledge gaps with appropriate phlebotomy practices, which intensifies the number of contaminated and hemolyzed specimens coming from the ED; technological barriers; and generalized fragmentation in the ED and laboratory processes, which can be a major disconnect to clinicians and providers.

Some key examples of laboratory services enhancements relevant to the ED include the implementation of laboratory tests at the point of care to include cardiac markers, pregnancy screening, and drug toxicity analysis because these are common tests noted to cause delays in patient throughput. The implementation of lab tests at the point of service would not only provided efficiency benefits with a decreased wait time to turnover lab results, but also incorporate a cost reduction to the organization by decreasing the outsourcing or operational costs to man the laboratory.

In addition, instituting tighter controls on the key process elements can provide significant throughput benefits overall. Incorporating top lab services into treatment protocols has been a proven method to decrease order to specimen collection times because this practice can be initiated at the point of triage and results can be returned once the patient is placed in an emergency bed. Other significant improvements relevant to the lab include formalized education/training blitzes geared toward optimizing the quality of specimen collection, which will alleviate quality concerns such as hemolyzed specimens and contaminated blood cultures. It should also be denoted that blood culture collection should be minimized in the ED unless absolutely necessary to the fragmentation in care once ED services are delivered.

Team-Based Approach to Transition of Care

The team-based approach to the transition of care goes against the grain of a traditional ED staffing strategy. Most EDs are staffed based on the logistical layout of the department and based on the number of providers that you have on shift at certain times of the day. In addition, many ED managers are beginning to build their respective budgets based on the number of ED visits and the ALOS, respectively; however, they are typically behind the eight ball without even realizing that most budgets are built off of inefficient systems of work. Therefore, staff that manages the ED in the standard and traditional model always feel understaffed, and we are not even speaking of the acuity levels. Safe and effective staffing with qualified professional staff is needed to deliver optimal patient care, achieve an operationally efficient department, and maintain satisfied associates.

In the industry, there is an average nurse-to-patient ratio of 4:1 assuming that the level of care is even across all organizations. The team-based approach eradicates all of the traditional assumptions and provides staffing management not based on the operational layout, but based on the number of patients and the team requirements. This model assumes that all patients requiring emergent services will need to at least see a nurse, a physician, and a business office professional in order to be discharged in a rapid fashion. Based on the systematic rigor of attempting to understand the difference between value-added and non-value-added activities, the value for the patient is to see the physician and be released in a timely fashion. Therefore, in the team-based approach to the transition of care scenario, the team approaches the patient together to render all needed activities, and then the patient is released rather quickly. Everyone is on the same page the moment they walk in the patient's room. There is no rudimentary science to this approach because it is an art of patient flow. Now let's speak in terms of staffing models and plans: nurses in this model are typically assigned to more patients because they have a partner in collaboration with them. An example of a model of this nature coming to fruition in practice is dedicating 10 patients to a team of two nurses, a physician, business office associate, and a technician in order to enable a smooth and justifiable practice. In addition, this model will diminish the siloed effect and will help to enable a more seamless movement and decrease the feeling of being understaffed.

Decompression Block and Inpatient Capacity Bottleneck

The majority of the throughput trepidations applicable to the ED are related to issues stemming from areas outside of the ED itself. Decompression block is a condition otherwise known as an inpatient capacity bottleneck that is symptomatic of when there is no available capacity to mobilize patients on the inpatient side. Less common are decompression blocks based on discharging or transferring patients to an external discharge location. In addition, this is a high cause for ED "holds" or "boarders." This is otherwise known in industry as "patient access block."

Inpatient "Pull" System

A pull system is traditionally defined in manufacturing terms by where processes are designed and motivated on the basis of customer demand. A common visual depiction of a pull system is by imagining a treadmill machine that moves based on a person's stimulated movements that control the depth and speed in which the machine operates. The customer in this particular example is driving the equipment at a pace that proves to be beneficial to the operator. One of the key identifiers of a "pull" system comes from having visual mechanisms otherwise known as a kanban in manufacturing terms to trigger when more demand is necessary in order to complete the process. Some of the associated benefits of having a "pull" system relevant to specific processes is having the ability to reduce workflow times and costs associated with the process itself.

The inpatient pull system is a demand-based system designed in the healthcare realm in order to maximize capacity and demand relevant to the throughput to inpatient logistics. In other words, the inpatient pull system is a process designed based on the patient desire for an inpatient bed in which there is constant flow in order to supply the customer to their desired location in a timely fashion. The object of this system is to keep the bed flow cycle moving at all times. Therefore, if there is an "available" bed, the objective should be to fill it because that frame of thinking is what keeps the hospital operational at all times. The necessity for emergency services is always unpredictable, which makes planning for resources challenging. There are so many peaks and valleys with the influx of demand and at any moment in time, resources can be either maximized or minimized. Therefore, this situation places hospital leadership in a position to have to even out the resources more evenly (Figure 33.7).

Case Study Example: Patient Logistics Center (Inpatient Pull)—250-Bed Hospital

In one particular example of an inpatient pull system, a special department by the name of a patient logistics center was designed to be the central nucleus to the "inpatient pull system" in which all bed requests funnel through this area with the majority being ED patients. A centralized department focused on the patient placement and bed management cycle whose primary function is the ongoing management of an automated bed board (kanban) that monitors the bed status across the hospital. The department will perform the bed assignment for emergency admissions, admissions from surgery, and direct admissions from physician offices. In addition, the department will coordinate the bed assignment for all inter- and intra-unit transfers. The department is overseen by the clinical operations manager and house supervisors on the off-shifts, whose main functions are to manage operational throughput, collecting and evaluating data concerning room turnover times, patient placement and delays, and facilitating communications with environmental services, charge nurses, and other primary stakeholders. There is a 24/7 patient logistics coordinator who is centrally located in the clinical operations office, who is the focal point for bed assignments for emergency admits, surgical admits, and direct admissions from physician offices, as well as unit transfers. The patient logistics coordinator is able to know the exact status of each bed in the hospital and can anticipate when beds will become available for placement of patients.

Initial state condition: Significant inpatient bottlenecks, ED "holds," overdependence on bypass and diversion, patient placement and housekeeping delays, elongated ED ALOS, and patient access block.

Solutions approach: Implementation of inpatient pull system by way of a patient logistics control center.

Breakthrough outcomes: Reduced ED ALOS by 100 minutes in the first month of rollout, which encompassed mainly a reduction in bed placement time, housekeeping delays, and patient access block. Reduced holds or boarders in the ED greater than 4 hours to significantly reduce the ALOS overall.

Housekeeping Room Turnover

The most common impediment to ensuring that beds are "available" to receive an additional patient from the ED is environmental services setbacks. Available beds must be ready to move promptly in order to provide the most efficient care possible. Although many of the hospital rooms are housed outside the proximity of the ED, restricted access and traffic jams due to unavailable inpatient beds are one of the main causes of overcrowded EDs. There could be a multitude of reasons for why inpatient beds are not available. The most common reason is the fact that there is another patient holding up the space due the inpatient flow problems. However, one of the most prevalent, yet highly ignored cause for flow issues stems from delays in environmental services relevant to cleaning the room in a timely fashion.

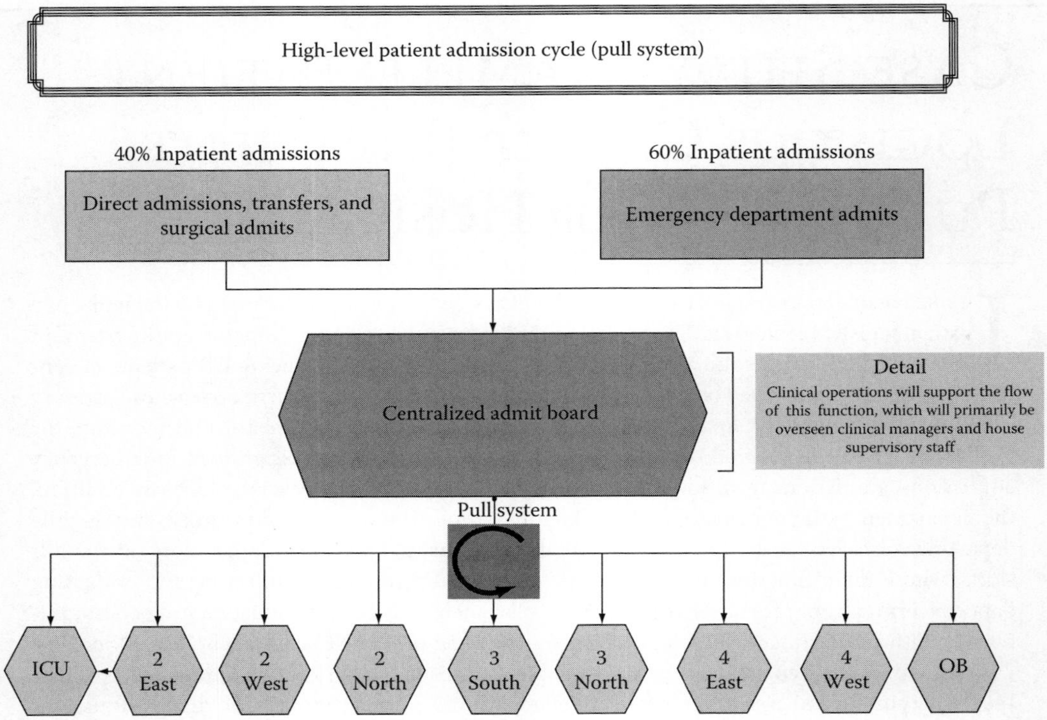

FIGURE 33.7 High-level patient admission pull system.

The matrix is a priority system for hospital housekeeping staff to help manage throughput in an environmental services type of way. The matrix is a proven system to adequately manage the multitude of housekeeping services, yet keep your eye on the prize at all times. The matrix is team-based system designed for environmental services staff to become an integral aspect of the ED throughput team. The priority system is designed as follows:

- Priority 1: Patient-flow and patient-care-related tasks, such as room turnover requests
- Priority 2: Patient care requests; however, there is no denoted impact on patient flow
- Priority 3: Request does not impact either patient flow or patient care

The environmental services management team administrates the assignments on a 24-hour basis based on this matrix priority system with the majority of the focus being concentrated on priority-one-related tasks. In this system, the unit-based housekeeping model is replaced by a constantly moving method to maximize associate productivity while placing the patient in the center. In addition, this method is directly tied to ED throughput because the level one task's main objective is to move the bed in a timely fashion. Based on this method, the environmental services staff is proactively managing the turnover of a room prior to the trigger being pulled. The trigger in this case can be a manual flag, a pager notification, a phone call, or other means of triggering the need for a room turnover (Table 33.2).

4-Tier High Census Alert Strategy

It sounds like a straightforward concept; however, the ED culture functions on the need to respond quickly to challenging and chaotic situations otherwise referred to in the ED world as "functional chaos." However, on the same notion, this is a more "reactive" mechanism of managing patient flow versus taking a more proactive angle. When the ED is sluggish, the sense of urgency to complete tasks

TABLE 33.2 Environmental Services Resource Allocation Matrix (265-Bed Hospital)

Shift	ADT	Dedicated	Patient Rooms	Tertiary	Trash	Special Projects	Total Resources	Total FTEs
7 a.m. to 3 p.m.	1	6	2	0	1	1	11	15.4
11 a.m. to 7 p.m.	1	0	1	0	0	0	2	2.8
3 p.m. to 11 p.m.	2	6	0	0	1	1	10	14
11 p.m. to 7 a.m.	0	2	0	3	0	0	5	7
Total resources	4	14	3	3	2	2	28	
Total FTEs	5.6	18.0	4.2	4.2	2.8	2.8	37.6	
Contingency staffing (10%)	6.2	19.8	4.6	4.6	3.1	3.1	41.4	

Assumptions

ADT refers to admissions, discharges, and transfers.

Staffing is based on function versus dedicated floor resources for workload leveling and balance.

Function staffing allocation is based on volume/productivity analysis minus dedicated areas.

This matrix assumes that there is a need for dedicated resources in the operating room, obstetrics, and the emergency room.

Productivity analysis indicator provides room to clean 2.5 rooms per hour (regular) and 1.5 rooms per hour for terminal cleans. (Target goal is room turnovers should be completed in less than 40 minutes.)

Operating rooms and ambulatory surgery centers do not operate on a 24 hours per day/7 day per week schedule.

This analysis did not trend the surgical schedule data as an indicator for dedicated ambulatory surgery center (ASC) and operating room (OR) staffing.

Tertiary functions will be allocated to the third shift with targeted productivity based on areas specified.

Those resources assigned to patient rooms are also responsible for daily patient rounding and spot cleaning.

Due to the minimal amount of discharges/transfer/terminal cleans on third shift, no resource will be allocated for ADT function; however, this role can be conducted by individuals conducting tertiary responsibilities and/or ED.

There is a 11 a.m. to 7 p.m. shift that has been implemented to even out the workload due to volume trends.

There is a 10% contingency staffing plan in place for replacements and paid time off (PTO).

There is no need to allocate an additional 6.0 FTEs based on this assessment as there is adequate staffing to support functions based on this model.

should not be altered because ED associates understand and believe in the revolving door theory that states that there is no true prediction of a patient's arrival regardless of historical demand.

The 4-tier high census alert strategy is a proactive model to manage throughput and flow from the ED to other key areas in the hospital. This is a practical management plan to decrease overdependence on bypass and diversion otherwise sending revenue to surrounding hospitals. In addition, this is a mechanism to complete tasks that could be done in preparation of surges of emergency demand. The high census alert strategy is a mechanism to proactively intercept and expedite patient flow when capacity exceeds the demand for beds. This type plan is generally put into place to enhance and sustain patient and staff satisfaction when high census challenges hospital resources because it helps to accommodate morale during high stressful situations. In addition, this procedure is especially useful

Case Study: 4-Tier High Census Strategy—276-Bed Hospital

Burning platform: The 4-tier high census alert strategy was implemented as a mechanism to expedite the seamless flow of patients regardless of demand. Prior to the implementation of this model, there was a high level of ED overcrowding, overdependence on bypass and diversion to decompress, high levels of cancelled surgical cases, poor staff morale and physician satisfaction, and lack of synergy and teamwork between the ED and inpatient units.

Solution vehicle: The organization rolled out an "all hands" initiative to properly manage capacity demand called the "4-tier high census alert." There are four levels that make up this strategy, each with a designed set of rules that helps to manage patient flow.

1. *Level 1 status*: This level is defined as a state of normalcy when there is adequate capacity to expedite the movement of patient to and from the ED and other source areas. In addition, there are adequate placement locations to accommodate the various modes of entry into the hospital environment such as emergent, surgical, and direct admissions. This level calls for daily huddles on each unit, which allows key constituents to be knowledgeable of the current capacity, forecast demand, and expedite discharges/admissions appropriately. In addition, at the first level there is a high level of integration with case management, physician partners, and leadership to mobilize the sense of urgency to institute prevention mechanisms to alleviate bottlenecks.
2. *Level 2 status:* This is the second tier in the high census level strategy in which flow constrictions are becoming readily apparent as defined by a limited amount of inpatient and emergent capacity. The high demand areas are more restricted in the ability to access from a patient placement perspective, and emergency waiting room utilization increases. All leadership is on alert and is notified immediately of the status. Key action strategies to prevent from moving up to the next level requires that an emergency "all-hands huddle" meeting take place in a central location in order for key stakeholders to strategize throughput parameters such as considering the utilization of nontraditional areas for additional capacity. These areas could include post-anesthesia recovery units, skilled nursing space, preadmission testing, and ambulatory services facilities. In addition, the inpatient pull system is enhanced by initiating mechanisms such as inpatient transporters and creating short-stay admission areas are considered options.

3. *Level 3 status:* This is the third tier in the high census strategy in which the capacity is at a proximity that is near full with no available beds to place patients. At this level, there are patients in ED waiting areas with no emergency space to mobilize the increasing demand. In addition, there is limited to no available high demand area capacity such as critical care space and monitored beds. There are increasing numbers of "ED holds" or "boarders" because of the patient access block limitations on the inpatient side. At this level comparable to Level 2, all leadership is notified and on an alert status until level is cleared. An emergency "all hands huddle meeting" is called to determine appropriate action strategy to prevent escalation to the next tier level. In addition, this level is considered "emergent" in terms of staffing levels for the organization, and a specialized staffing strategy is put into place to accommodate the additional volume of patients by utilizing internal registry pool, expediting the internal float plan, and increasing number of physician resources.
4. *Level 4 status:* This level is deemed house-wide disaster being that there is no capacity to position patients. At this level, last resort options such as bypass, diversion, and cancellation/deferment of surgical cases are considered as temporary options until capacity is decompressed and available to accommodate patient demand. All levels of leadership are notified and engaged to de-escalate to the next available tier.

Target outcomes: On the basis of instituting this proactive strategy, the ability to properly manage patient throughput became embedded within the fabric of this organization. The daily objective was to prevent escalating to the next tier which in turn was a "win-win" for all stakeholders involved. The organization was able to reduce the overall ALOS in both the ED and inpatient units. The hospital decreased the inpatient ALOS by over 1 day overall with increased patient and physician satisfaction. In addition, on the basis of the capacity/demand forecasting and management model, the hospital was able to exercise more appropriate staffing allocation patterns.

when high demand areas are bursting at the seams in terms of capacity, such as critical care and monitored beds (Table 33.3).

Lessons Learned and Sustainment Strategy

One of the fundamental lessons learned when discussing improvements related to ED throughput is having an awareness of how to sustain the changes instituted. The specific methodology utilized to gain breakthrough outcomes does not drive change to be permeated within an organizational compound. In fact, having a strong combination of transformational leadership with the ability to drive results, understanding how to imbed change within the fabric of the organizational culture, and knowing the control and monitoring mechanisms to keep outcomes consistent are key attributes of lasting change. In order to make change last, as a leader you need to learn how to lead by example. You have to ask yourself the hard questions related to how you would like to receive emergency services if you were sitting in the patient's shoes. In addition, having the support of physician champions and administrative buy-in is a critical component of cultural transformation. Other lessons learned include, but are not limited to the following:

- Change the knowledge paradigm of ED throughput to hospital throughput. Understand that issues with ED flow are not just a reflection of a localized bottleneck. Remember that there are two primary doors. One that is located in the front where the patient enters and one that is located in the back where the patient exits. In order to shift the paradigm that this is a hospital-wide concern, all constituents need to have a burning platform to change from the current state.

TABLE 33.3 4-Tier High Census Alert Strategy (Proactive Demand Management)

Level 1	Level 2	Level 3	Level 4
Remain on floors	Huddle up with managers/leader, clinical assistant managers, charge nurse, case manager, housekeeper on floor, and physicians available	Huddle up in clinical operations after evaluating opportunity for movement of patients on the floor within 15 minutes. Huddle up on floor first and discuss with staff discharges, transfers, status of bed availability, and potential for crisis	Bypass declared
Definition Beds are available, no patients waiting for ICU, telemetry, med/surg, and no patients waiting in ED for bed placement. This is considered a typical proactive day	**Definition** Patient placement is getting difficult as defined by any one of the following: • ICU has less than 5 beds • Telemetry has less than 5 beds • ED wait area >5 patients waiting who potentially need beds for admission • 2 or more units are affected and direct admissions are increasing • Patients are waiting in the ED >1 hour for bed placement	**Definition** Full occupancy is near as defined by the following: • 1 ICU bed • 1 telemetry bed and more than 3 units affected **-OR-** • Patients are waiting over 30 minutes for bed placement **-OR-** • ED wait has >10 patients waiting for admission **-OR-** • Hospital is >90% capacity	**Definition** • No ICU, telemetry, or med/surg beds are available • ED has >5 patients awaiting admission for critical beds • 2 or more patients waiting admission meet trauma team criteria in ED or are in shock
Action Identify patients for discharge and notify alpha pagers of current status—Level 1	**Action** **Do what it takes to stay off bypass** • House supervisor to deploy staff to retrieve patients admitted to identified beds • Housekeeping supervisors deploy staff expedite admissions and discharges • Housekeeping supervisors deploy staff to expedite admissions and discharges • Initiate ED surge plan (see ED surge plan) • Case manager rounding with ED and on unit as available • Open nontraditional inpatient/outpatient treatment areas: 1. Rehabilitation services 2. Outpatient 3. 2 south 4. 2 east • ED **considers calling** in additional physicians • Check PACU availability • Day surgery stay late for discharges	**Action** **Consider activations of internal disaster versus bypass** • House supervisor to deploy staff to expedite admissions and discharges • Consider cancellation of elective procedures schedule • Consider potential SNF admissions movement • Consider use of outpatient area for discharge holding area or admission holds i.e., ASC, PACU, rehabilitation services • Determine if disaster modality is needed, especially if staff is challenged	**Action** Insure IDPH criteria and reporting requirements are met bypass initiated (see IDPH Bypass Guidelines) • House supervisors deploy staff to retrieve patients admitted to identified beds • Housekeeping supervisors deploy staff to expedite admissions and discharges • Contact appropriate administrator for approval continue operations from Level 3 plus surgery manager, surgery director, ASC manager and cath. lab director, and SNF manager responds • ***STATUS FOR RED SHOULD BE UPDATED EVERY 2 hours!!***

TABLE 33.3 (continued) 4-Tier High Census Alert Strategy (Proactive Demand Management)

Level 1	Level 2	Level 3	Level 4
Expedite patient flow • Look for opportunity to discharge safely • Case managers rounding on units and assisting with all patient movement • Who has beds/placement elsewhere? For example, SNF • Send patients immediately to destination as appropriate • Automatically provide bed status update to clinical operations/house supervisor within 15 minutes after huddle up	**Status** for Level 2 should be updated at 7:00 and 15:00 via alpha pager	**Status** for Level 3 will be updated every 4 hours via alpha pagers. Vice president, directors, housekeeping, lab, and transport should be notified	**Contingency plan** **Beds** • 2 south rooms: 31, 32, 33, 34 • 2 east rooms: 284, 285, 286 • Open outpatient • Open cardiac rehab • Post anesthesia care with (PACU) • Skilled nursing facility (SNF) • Hospice **Staff** 1. ED Physicians 2. House fellows 3. Labor pool (staff units opened) 4. Physicians available in-house

Note: Debrief following each alert level with appropriate action plan.

- Adapt the saying, "It takes a village" to the improvement effort. Improving ED flow is a monster when approached as an individual leadership effort. The traditional leadership paradigms of "dictate and everyone will be on board with the change" is old news that does not inspire a great deal of creativity. Sustained improvements to ED flow requires innovative creativity inspired by informal frontline leaders who are intimately engaged in the daily activities.
- "You do not know what you do not know." This saying refers to incorporating a tracking mechanism to visualize what you need to improve and what you need to sustain. EDs must take advantage of reporting and tracking tools that will help manage throughput. Stakeholders must be able to see at a glance where the opportunity for improvement exists and it should always point to the root cause of why it exists in the first place. For example, if my daily target is to have an ALOS of 200 minutes and today's average looks more like 300 minutes, how can I understand where my opportunity exists and what to manage? A more appropriate example is to set up a daily monitoring system that breaks down the ALOS into components such as door to triage, door to nurse, door to doctor, triage to room, diagnostic turnover, lab turnover, disposition to admit, disposition to discharge, and fast track turnover, which will help to appropriately manage and control efficiency and to easily identify where the breakdown is occurring.
- Accountability is inevitable and is not an option. The golden rule of operational improvements is to engage constituents to a point in which everyone has a sense of ownership and acceptance to holding each other accountable. Sustainable change efforts require that all stakeholders keep their eye on the prize...which in most cases consist of customer safety and satisfaction. The only way that the ball does not get dropped is having an understanding of who is on the bus and who is not.
- The rule of thumb with process improvement is to "try it before you deny it." There is no such thing as a bad solution, unless it impacts quality and patient safety. All of the best evidence-based practices were developed with a brave soul being empowered to ask the question "why do we do this and why can't we try that instead?" (see Figure 33.8).

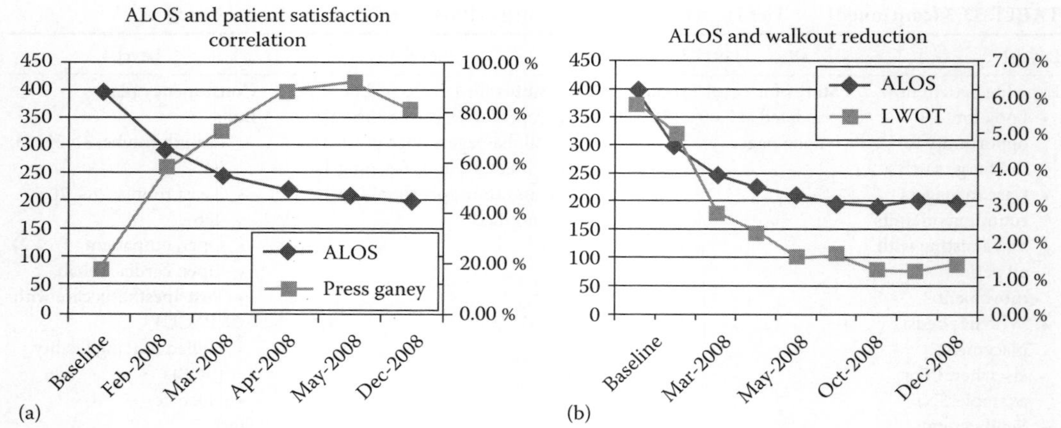

FIGURE 33.8 (a) ALOS and patient satisfaction correlation (12-month sample) and (b) ALOS and walkout rate comparison (12-month sample).

Case Study: Emergency Department Transformation Journey 24-Bed ED

Burning platform: Can you imagine having a medical emergency and going to your local hospital only to have waiting over 6 hours on average to receive the treatment that you deserve? Not only that, can you envision being circulated back and forth from the waiting area to a business office booth prior to seeing a physician? In the same scenario, can you imagine waiting over 6 hours for a 5-minute meeting with the physician? Can you imagine waiting another 3 hours to get your labs drawn when you felt that you could have had that done hours ago? Can you imagine repeating the same history to multiple providers only to be rewarded with another request to repeat the same repetitive information? Have you ever felt the urge to just leave to seek treatment elsewhere because the wait times were so long that you cannot tolerate another moment in agony? Can you imagine waiting over 3 hours for a minor cold? If you answered yes to any of these questions, this was an adequate description of a 24-bed Community Hospital in Illinois prior to starting their performance enhancement journey. In fact, below is a snapshot of this hospital's initial state condition.

- Overall ALOS: 393 minutes
- Overall ALOS—fast track: 203 minutes
- Door to triage (average): 120 minutes
- Patient walkout rate (average): 5.76%
- Patient satisfaction: 16th percentile
- Inpatient housekeeping room turnover time: 265 minutes

- Disposition to room time: 130 minutes
- Open full time equivalents (FTE): 13 open

Solution strategy: Instituted a house-wide performance enhancement transformation effort utilizing a combination of improvement methodologies including lean, change acceleration process (CAP), and six sigma geared toward revitalizing initial state practices. The ED was selected as a key target area due to the significance in the opportunities for improvement and the impact that this area has on the organization overall. The ED was denoted as an area to provide a regular pulse on the status of other organizational performance standards and is the patient's first perception of their entire experience. The deployment of performance enhancement was an effort fully supported and spearheaded by hospital executive leaders. The leadership team led through engaging and empowering frontline associates to learn different mechanisms to improve their practice. The improvement effort specifically geared toward the ED improvement was a *12 month initiative* consisting of a combined rigor of 2- to 5-day kaizen and/or rapid improvement activities holistically focused on the following areas:

- Triage and mobile registration
- Admission phase I: Bed placement
- Admission phase II: Housekeeping room turnover
- Admission phase III: Inpatient pull system and high census alert
- Treat and release: Fast track turnover
- Intradepartmental pull tier 1: Laboratory turnaround
- Intradepartmental pull tier 2: Diagnostic imaging turnaround
- Intradepartmental pull tier 3: Team-based approach to transition of care
- Physician workflow effectiveness
- Clinician workflow effectiveness
- 6S workspace efficiency (Sort, Scrub, Straighten, Standardize, Safety, Sustain)

Breakthrough outcomes: At the conclusion of this 12 month effort the results were beyond breakthrough. The ED experienced both a cultural and process-related transformation through the power of engagement and empowerment. The fabric of the department became a learning environment in order to envision workflow differently from a patient's perspective and begin to respect and appreciate the disparity between value-added and non–value added activities. It was a sense of enlightenment to understand that just because we have always done things a certain way does not make it the best mode for the customer. The outcomes were not localized specifically in the ED because as indicated previously, throughput is a reflection of downstream inconsistencies as well as internal bottlenecks. The organization as a whole began to function as a complete value stream delivering service to the patient. On the inpatient side, the availability of an inpatient bed is a trigger to "pull" more patients from the revolving door, hence the ED. Some outcomes relevant to these improvements are listed below in their target state:

- Overall ALOS: 191 minutes (50% reduction)
- Overall ALOS—fast track: 75 minutes (75% reduction)
- Patient walkout rate: 1.23%
- Patient satisfaction: >85th percentile
- Revenue enhancement: 1.2 million dollars (year end 2007 to year end 2008)
- Additional full time equivalents: 0!!

References

American Hospital Association. 2006. The State of America's hospitals—taking the pulse: Findings from the 2006 AHA Survey of Hospital Leaders, Chicago, IL, http://www.aha.org/aha/content/2006/PowerPoint/StateHospitalsChartPack2006.PPT (accessed on February 1, 2009).

National Center for Health Statistics. 2008. National hospital ambulatory medical care survey: 2006 emergency department summary. National Health Statistics Report, Hyattsville, MD, http://www.cdc.gov/nchs/data/nhsr/nhsr007.pdf (accessed on February 1, 2009).

Design, Planning, Control, and Management of Healthcare Systems

IV.F OR Management

34 **Capacity Planning in Operating Rooms** *John T. Blake* **34**-1
Introduction • Bed Planning • Frameworks for Understanding Tactical and Operational OR Capacity Planning • Tactical Planning: Allocating Operating Room Time • Operational Planning: Sequencing Cases • Conclusion • References

35 **Managing Critical Resources through an Improved Surgery Scheduling Process** *Erik Demeulemeester, Jeroen Beliën, and Brecht Cardoen* **35**-1
Introduction • Surgery Scheduling at the Tactical Level: Master Surgery Scheduling • Surgery Scheduling at the Operational Level: Patient Scheduling • Conclusion and Future Research • References

36 **Anesthesia Group Management and Strategies** *William H. Hass, Alex Macario, and Randal G. Garner* **36**-1
Introduction • A Brief History of Anesthesia Practice • Cultural Differences between Anesthesia Groups and Facility Management • The Evolution of Closed Staffs and Exclusive Contracts • Physician Practice Management Companies • Autonomy as a Core Value • The Urgency of Today • Change and Transitions in Anesthesia Groups • Macro-Level Transition Models • Impact of Transitions on People • Aligning Culture and Strategy • Leadership in an Anesthesia Group • At a Crossroads…Again • Conclusion • References

34

Capacity Planning in Operating Rooms

John T. Blake
Dalhousie University

Introduction 34-1
Capacity Planning in Healthcare
Bed Planning 34-2
Frameworks for Understanding Tactical and Operational OR Capacity Planning 34-3
Tactical Planning: Allocating Operating Room Time 34-4
Operational Planning: Sequencing Cases 34-6
Case Sequencing • Estimating Case Duration • Optimizing Patient Flow
Conclusion 34-10
References 34-10

Introduction

Capacity planning is a concept familiar to most students and practitioners of operations research and management science. Davis et al. (2005) define capacity planning as the process of specifying a level of capacity necessary to meet market demands in a cost-efficient way. Capacity planning activities are generally classified according to time frame: long-term (strategic), intermediate (tactical), or short-term (operational). In a traditional manufacturing environment, capacity planning is assumed to take place after a facility location decision has been made (Where should we place our factory?) and product forecasting has been completed (How many products or services do we anticipate selling or delivering over the planning horizon?), and serves as an important step in the creation of a production plan. At the strategic level, capacity planning decisions largely revolve around capacity expansion or capital equipment purchases, though decisions regarding out-sourcing and make-versus-buy are common. At the tactical level, capacity planning decisions are closely tied with the aggregate planning process. The function of aggregate planning is to assign resources to a product or service forecast to create a time-staged plan for meeting demand. Master production scheduling (MPS) and rough-cut capacity planning (RCCP) exercises are usual activities for medium-term capacity planning in a manufacturing environment. Tactical capacity decisions typically include decisions to modify capacity to meet demand through hiring or layoffs, subcontracting, or building to inventory. At the operational level, capacity planning decisions involve activities to formalize and finalize the production plan set by the tactical level plan. Short-term capacity planning activities include materials requirement planning (MRP), capacity requirements planning (CRP) or capacity scheduling, final assembly scheduling, input/output planning control, production activity control, and purchase planning and control (Davis et al., 2005).

Capacity Planning in Healthcare

Smith-Daniels et al. (1988) define capacity planning in healthcare as "decisions concerning the acquisition and allocation of three types of resources: work force, equipment, and facilities." They note that capacity planning decisions in healthcare are made according to the time frame: long-term planning involves the acquisition of facilities and major equipment; medium-term planning involves decisions concerning workforce, overtime, and subcontracting; and short-term planning involves scheduling activities to allocate capacity to tasks or patients.

Green (2004) notes the importance of right-sizing facilities to deploy resources effectively and argues that capacity planning for hospitals includes questions of determining the correct number of beds, identifying staffing requirements, setting operating room (OR) capacity, and calculating resource requirements for major diagnostic equipment. Green's review of the capacity planning literature is prescient. While ORs are described as a significant component of hospital capacity, Green is able to list only three references, none of which are actually strategic in nature.

A review of the available literature, thus, suggests that OR capacity planning differs from the general capacity planning since there are virtually no models for strategic OR capacity planning. The literature in OR capacity planning deals entirely with questions of medium- to short-term planning in which it is assumed that the physical resources in the OR are fixed. Capacity planning, in this context, largely revolves around methods for determining policies for making the best use of fixed resources. Thus, the vast majority of models within the context of OR capacity planning can be classified more specifically as resource allocation and/or scheduling decisions.

Bed Planning

The fundamental measure of hospital capacity has traditionally been assumed to be the number of inpatient beds available (Green, 2004). Thus, capacity decisions for hospitals are largely based on methods for identifying and achieving target occupancy (i.e., the percentage of beds occupied). Strategic planning decisions for OR planning are almost entirely subsumed in the overall context of bed planning, since inpatient beds are assumed to be the bottleneck factor constraining overall surgical patient throughput.

While there are very few models of strategic capacity planning for ORs, there is a long and established literature on bed planning in operational research. Bed planning can be defined as the process of identifying the minimum number of beds a hospital requires to meet demand (Hancock et al., 1978). The key issue in bed planning is, of course, to determine an appropriate trade-off between the requirements for meeting peak capacity and making efficient overall use of resources (utilization). In general, the more beds an institution has, the greater its ability to meet peak capacity demand. However, excess beds also result in higher capital and operating costs and lower overall bed utilization. Green notes that while an optimal occupancy rate in the United States has been considered to be 85%, actual utilization rates historically hovered around 64% (Green, 2004).

There are a substantial number of papers describing the use of queuing theory and simulation methodologies to determine the appropriate number of beds for an inpatient hospital. Hancock and associates authored several papers that describe the development and use of an inpatient bed planning model called the admissions scheduling and control system (ASCS). Because the number of patient arrivals to a hospital and patient lengths of stay are random, Hancock et al. argue that it is difficult to determine the ideal number of beds to ensure both adequate patient service and high bed utilization. They therefore divide patients into three groups (scheduled, emergency, and call-ins) and employ a simulation method to establish upper and lower bounds for hospital census. If the number of patients exceeds the upper bound, scheduled patients are cancelled; if census is below the lower bound, call-in patients are used to return the census to target values (Hancock et al., 1978). Hancock et al. show that higher overall utilization can be achieved with their model. OR capacity, however, is not explicitly considered.

Harper and Shahani (2002) adopt a similar methodology to Hancock et al. (1978) but employ a classification and regression tree analysis (CART) to construct homogenous patient groups that are then simulated to identify appropriate bed capacities. The Harper and Shahani model is based on a generic simulation shell that can be tailored to any hospital and is able to represent pooled (all beds belong to a common pool) or ring-fenced (beds are assigned for the use of a specific service) beds. OR capacity is not specifically included in the Harper and Shahani model, though Harper does provide an extension (Harper, 2002) in which ORs are included and rules for sequencing cases within a surgical block are simulated.

Utley et al. (2003), conversely, employ analytical techniques to determine the beds required to implement a policy in which all elective admissions to hospital are booked in advance. They use probability theory to identify the expected number of beds a patient admitted on a particular day will require some days into the future. From this information, an exact expression for the total demand for the number of beds required by both elective and emergency patient on a particular day is calculated.

Lapierre et al. (1999) derive a model in which the scale of bed planning is extended from daily to hourly. They note that most bed planning models are based on midnight census data, which may or may not represent the peak. Using only readily available administrative data supplemented with a sample of hour-by-hour census data, Lapierre et al. develop a model that includes an hourly mean, a week-to-week variance term, and an hour-to-hour autoregressive term. They then employ a discrete event model to simulate the hourly census over a longer planning horizon and apply the results to a decision problem experienced by an Atlanta-area hospital. Côté (2005) demonstrates in a later paper that equivalent results can be obtained without the computational effort of a simulation, if an appropriate forecast is fit to hourly data.

Frameworks for Understanding Tactical and Operational OR Capacity Planning

Unlike strategic planning for OR capacity, there is an enormous wealth of knowledge on OR planning at the tactical (medium-term) and operational (short-term) levels. The literature in these areas covers a broad range of topics and encompasses a wide variety of methods. Indeed, Blake and Carter (1997) note the need for a taxonomy for classifying the OR capacity planning literature at the tactical and operational level to foster understanding of the issues and to make sense of the broad range of solution techniques.

Magerlein and Martin (1978) argue that OR capacity encompasses two decisions: advance and allocation scheduling. They define advance scheduling as the process for determining which patients are to be scheduled into a surgical suite on a particular day; allocation scheduling is the process of determining the sequence of cases within an operating theatre on a particular date, given that a slate of patients has been identified. In the Magerlein and Martin framework, advance scheduling is a medium-term problem of matching patient demand to a previously defined OR capacity; allocation scheduling is as an operational problem of sequencing patients and determining case start times that is solved shortly before a schedule is executed in order to achieve a specified operational goal (i.e., minimizing overtime or maximizing surgeon utilization). Magerlein and Martin furthermore divide advance scheduling into two categories depending on whether or not OR time is considered to be the sole constraint on surgical throughput.

At the tactical planning level, decisions about how capacity is to be allocated to patients depend on the booking rules in force in an institution. In general, two major booking philosophies are employed to allocate OR capacity to patients (and hence by extension to their attending surgeons): block and non-block systems. In a block booking system, each surgeon (or service) is assigned a specific date and time interval into which he or she may freely book patients. In non-blocked systems, patients are assigned typically on a first-come, first-served basis into the first available OR. In practice, block systems are preferred to non-blocked scheduling arrangements and are more common. From a tactical standpoint, block booking systems allow institutions to better plan their surgical case mix by allocating specific quantities of capacities to surgeons or surgical services a priori. Such allocations may be made on the basis of equity (ensuring that every surgeon has an equal amount of OR time), the basis of need within a community (ensuring that sufficient capacity is available to meet an assumed volume of demand), maximizing profit for the hospital and/or surgeons, or any one of a number of other objectives. Operationally, blocked systems reduce friction between surgeons by minimizing the effect of case overruns in which one surgeon's case end time interferes with the start time of another's.

Blake and Carter (1997) extend the Magerlein and Martin taxonomy to include external resource scheduling. Arguing that surgery requires that a patient be matched with needed resources over the entire course of his or her journey through an institution, Blake and Carter note that the date, time, and resources needed for care must all be identified and reserved before surgery can take place. Thus, they suggest that resources external to the OR must be considered both when determining on which day a patient is to be scheduled and in what order cases are to be sequenced.

Gupta (2007) lists three issues that drive OR planning: allocating OR time to specialties, managing elective bookings, and selecting the sequence of cases within a surgeon's block. The allocation of surgical time to specialties, Gupta notes, may or may not require model-based reasoning—time may be allocated on the basis of strategic direction, clinical need, or financial contribution. Booking control is described as identifying trade-offs between access to care (i.e., a maximum wait for care) and costs (regular time, overtime, or penalty costs). Surgical case scheduling is described as the process of identifying the number of cases that can be booked into a block of surgical time. Estimating the durations of cases and thus the estimated start time of each procedure, as well as the likely end time of the surgical block, are important subcomponents of case sequencing.

Cardoen et al. (2010) differentiate between planning and scheduling for ORs. They describe planning as a process of reconciling supply and demand, while scheduling is defined as setting the sequence and time to be allocated to an activity. Focusing on surgical scheduling they develop a taxonomy for classifying the literature according to dimensions of patient characteristics (inpatient or outpatient), performance measures (waiting time, utilization, etc.), decision type (date, time, room) and scope (patient or provider), solution methodology (simulation, integer programming, heuristic), stochastic or deterministic case times, and potential for application. Using these six components to classify the literature, Cardoen et al. suggest a standard nomenclature for OR scheduling problems similar in nature to the Kendall–Lee notation for queuing problems.

Thus, while there is some variation in the literature on definitions, there is a relatively common understanding of OR planning as involving two stages and three problems: identifying how OR time should be allocated to surgeons or services in advance of patient scheduling a priori and determining how which patients should be allocated to what OR and identifying the sequence in which cases should be completed at the time of schedule execution.

Tactical Planning: Allocating Operating Room Time

The fundamental issue for OR planning at the tactical level is determining how an available block of resources, as specified by a strategic planning process, will be used. While it is natural to think of OR time as being allocated to patients for their care, in reality the allocation of resources is not made to patients but to the providers of care. In most jurisdictions, healthcare is delivered by independent physician-entrepreneurs, who are paid a fixed fee for each service. Surgeons, who are usually not formally employed by a hospital, use hospital resources to provide care and, thus, to generate income. Therefore, the allocation of resources has important financial, clinical, and educational considerations for surgeons as well as the hospital itself.

The primary way in which OR time is allocated in the medium term is through the master surgical schedule (MSS). The MSS is a cyclic timetable that defines the number and type of ORs available in an institution, the hours that rooms will be open, and the service or surgeons (if any) who are to be given priority for OR time (Blake and Donald, 2002). The MSS, under a block scheduling methodology, assigns a fixed amount of time on a given day and time to a particular surgeon or service. For example, every Monday Otolaryngology might be assigned 7.5 hours in OR A. The master schedule typically has a time horizon of 1 week, although many institutions define exceptions to the weekly schedule based on the number of calendar days in a month. Master schedules developed under non-block methodologies do not assign a priority for OR time to any particular service or surgeon; under such systems all surgeons compete for OR time on a first-come, first-served basis. Accordingly, the allocation of time to services is more random and thus medium-term planning and control is more difficult under non-blocked systems. While common in the 1960s and 1970s, pure first-come, first-served scheduling systems are now rarely seen in practice. Nevertheless, it is not uncommon to see hybrid environments in which some rooms are block booked, while others are set aside for use on a first-come, first-served basis. Non-blocked time is typically set aside to accommodate overflows or urgent cases (Gupta, 2007). Institutions may specifically reserve a block of time for open bookings or they may specify that any blocked time assigned to a surgeon or a service that is not allocated prior to a fixed deadline (i.e., 24–48 hours in advance) is available on a first-come, first-served basis for any surgeon.

Blake and Donald (2002) argue that the MSS is analogous to the aggregate production plan in a manufacturing environment. Because it defines the number and types of procedures that will be performed by a hospital over a medium-term horizon, the MSS implicitly defines aggregate resource requirements, such as the demand for nurses, drugs, diagnostic procedures, laboratory tests, and perioperative nurses. Conversely, the daily OR schedule, which lists cases to be performed, start times, end times, attending physician, and anesthetist, is an operational document that functions in a manner similar to the master production schedule in a manufacturing plant.

Blake and Donald (2002) develop a model for allocating OR time to surgical services on the basis of equity. As formulated in their model, tactical OR planning is a response to overall levels of resources that are set by the hospital on a periodic basis. Blake and Donald note that while the MSS is relatively constant over time, changes in budget, holiday schedules, and staff and equipment availability require that the schedule be modified from time to time. In the problem under study, the objective of the planning process was to ensure that the total amount of surgical time allocated to each surgical service (as measured as a percentage of the total amount available) remained constant, even as the total time available was adjusted in response to operational or budget constraints. Blake and Donald develop a mixed integer goal programming model to minimize weighted deviations from a target allocation of time, subject to constraints on the total number of rooms available and service-specific bounds on minimum and maximum numbers of rooms per day and per week. The goal programming model produces an MSS with a 1-week planning horizon. A post-process routine is also run to determine if improvements to equity can be made by modifying the weekly MSS over the course of a month or by splitting whole day blocks into two half-day blocks.

Kuo et al. (2003) employ a linear programming approach to adjust the allocation of surgical time among a group of surgeons. Their model maximizes physician revenues subject to constraints on allowable growth or decline in a particular surgeon's workload.

Beliën and Demeulemeester (2007) introduce a model for constructing a master schedule that accounts for inpatient bed usage. Under the assumption that the overall allocation of time has been determined, they propose a nonlinear programming model for constructing the MSS in such a way that the total expected bed shortage is minimized, subject to constraints on the number of blocks that must be assigned. They then develop a linearization of the problem in which the weighted combination of the mean number of beds occupied and the variance of beds occupied is minimized. They note, however, the difficulty of solving this model and suggest a number of heuristic solution techniques.

Van Oostrum et al. (2008) develop a methodology that builds the MSS from a daily surgical roster. They argue that many of the types of cases performed in a surgical suite tend to be common and suggest creating the MSS based on an aggregation of slots based on typical patient profiles. A two-phase approach is adopted. In the first phase, slots are assigned to OR days to minimize the number of rooms required. In the second phase, the OR days are arranged into a cyclic MSS, using a column generation technique, in such a way that the workload in inpatient units is leveled.

Dexter et al. (2006) present a case study for allocating OR time under the assumption of an increase in resource capacity. The objective of their model is to allocate additional time to maximize the financial contribution to the hospital. Dexter et al. describe the allocation process as a two-step process. The first step is a screening process; surgeons whose contribution margin is below average, who have a small practice, or whose throughput is constrained by resources outside of the OR are identified and eliminated from further consideration. Those surgeons remaining become candidates for expanded practice. Dexter et al., noting the importance and the difficulty of identifying demand distributions for individual surgeons, suggest the screening process as a means of maintaining problem tractability. In the case study presented, the first-stage screening process eliminated 85% of surgeons from further consideration. Once the candidate surgeons are identified, a simple demand distribution is generated and a nonlinear programming problem that maximizes the expected contribution margin is formulated. The resulting model has specific structural properties that allow an optimal solution to be identified with simple analytical techniques. O'Neill and Dexter (2007) describe a similar problem, but use data envelopment analysis to evaluate the potential for expanding practice.

McIntosh et al. (2006) also describe OR planning as a two-stage process involving allocation of time to specific services and case sequencing. They define OR time allocation as a process of determining how many ORs should be staffed by each service, for each day of the week, and the number of hours for which the room should be available. They suggest that, for small changes from an existing schedule, complete enumeration is possible and argue that the efficiency of the room utilization (including overtime costs and unused time) should be considered when comparing alternatives.

Operational Planning: Sequencing Cases

By far, the largest volume of work in the area of OR capacity planning has focused on operational issues of sequencing a set of cases. Magerlein and Martin (1978) define this process as determining the manner in which patients are assigned to ORs and given start times. In the operational planning problem, it is generally assumed that the list of cases to be scheduled is known and the objective is to sequence the cases in such a way to optimize some operational measure of performance (i.e., room utilization, completion time, patient time in system).

There is an obvious analogue between surgical case scheduling and machine scheduling, and thus it is not unsurprising that operational researchers have adapted methodologies from manufacturing to the healthcare environment. Blake and Carter (1997) note, however, that the engineering/operational research literature diverges from the health services administration literature. While operational researcher view case scheduling as a sequencing problem, healthcare administrators tend to think of OR scheduling as booking systems that capture, record, and report on activities within the surgical suite (Blake and Carter, 1997). There are three major subproblems that are addressed within the OR capacity planning problem: selecting the sequence of cases, estimating case durations, and allocating resources (both inside and outside of the OR) to optimize patient flow.

Case Sequencing

Some of the earliest work in OR capacity planning focused on the application of principles derived from manufacturing to healthcare to determine case sequences. Early work in this area focused primarily on sequencing, typically under the assumption that case times were known or could be accurately predicted before schedule execution.

Goldman et al. (1969), for instance, evaluate the effect of different queuing disciplines on OR performance. They compare shortest processing time (SPT) against longest processing time (LPT) via simulation and conclude that LPT produces higher room utilization, lower overtime, and increased operational flexibility. This result, although it differs from common machine dispatching heuristics, is not surprising. Scheduling longer cases earlier in a surgical block provides greater flexibility to juggle cases later in the day should unforeseen delays occur. Since surgeries cannot be pre-empted, once started, scheduling shorter cases later in the day provides a surgeon some flexibility to adjust the actual room completion time by canceling smaller (and presumably less urgent) cases should insufficient time remain at the end of the day.

Kwak et al. (1976) employ a simulation methodology to evaluate the effects of different queuing disciplines on a range of operational performance metrics including resource utilization, completion times, and in-process queues. Kwak et al. also conclude that a modified LPT discipline performs well. Like Goldman et al., the Kwak et al. model assumes that case times are known in advance.

Dexter et al. (2001) note that the bin-packing nature of OR scheduling makes it difficult to create a schedule that fully utilizes all available surgical time without incurring excess overtime or extended waits for surgery. Dexter et al. use a simulation model to evaluate the resulting changes in case volume and revenue. Their model shows that increasing the volume of cases completed in an already busy surgical suite does not always increase revenues and could, in fact, lead to reduced income. Furthermore, utilization does not always increase in proportion to increases in volume. They evaluate several potential care facility types (inpatient, ambulatory, and office) and conclude that because of the nature of bin-packing, institutions with longer case times (typically inpatient hospitals) necessarily have lower utilization than those with shorter cases. Another paper by Dexter et al. (1999) employs a similar methodology, but evaluates bin-packing heuristics against utilization and maximum acceptable patient wait.

Vargas et al. (2006) note the analogue between OR scheduling and the bin-packing problem, in which the objective is to maximize the number of objects in a container of a fixed capacity. In the case of OR scheduling, the objective may be either to minimize the number of ORs needed to complete a slate of procedures (Vargas et al., 2006) or to maximize the number of procedures that can be completed within a fixed set of ORs. Vargas et al. note that surgical scheduling may be online or off-line. Online scheduling is performed while the schedule is being executed in response to unexpected occurrences, such as cancellations, emergency add-ons, or case overruns. Off-line scheduling refers to the process of sequencing a predetermined slate of procedures a short time in advance of schedule execution.

In the simplest bin-packing approaches, it is assumed that procedure durations are deterministic and that room capacities are fixed. Bin-packing algorithms are well studied within the operational research literature, but are difficult problems to solve exactly. Nevertheless, a number of heuristic techniques have been evaluated, both in the context of manufacturing and healthcare, that are known to produce very good results (Vargas et al., 2006).

More sophisticated models relax the assumption of fixed OR capacity and are designed to trade off the costs of staff overtime against the fixed costs of opening another OR. Vargas et al. (2006) describe a model, labeled as a bin-packing problem with overtime costs (BPPwOC), in which the bins (ORs) are considered to be variably sized, with a target capacity and a maximum capacity that cannot be exceeded. In this model, case times are assumed to be deterministic and the problem is formulated as an integer programming problem, though the actual problem is solved using heuristic approaches.

Van Houdenhoven et al. (2007) also adopt a bin-packing analogue for case sequencing, but approach the problem from the standpoint of maximizing room utilization without using overtime. They describe a case study in which a First-Fit algorithm is applied to schedule cases into service-specific rooms and note that this leads to incomplete utilization of rooms, even after planned slack (allowance for variance) is discounted. They propose an algorithm to increase the utilization of OR time and to consolidate the number of rooms needed to complete a surgical roster. Their algorithm groups cases not by surgical service, but by variance. This grouping policy exploits the "portfolio effect" and ensures that, over the entire suite of rooms, total variance decreases. Once grouped, cases are sequenced according to a bin-packing heuristic suggested by Hans et al. (2006). Van Houdenhoven et al. compare this algorithm to the base method employed at the hospital and conclude that significant improvements can be achieved.

In addition to viewing OR sequencing as a bin-packing problem, a substantial number of authors have developed mathematical programming formulations. For instance, Guinet and Chaabane (2003) formulate the OR sequencing problem as a deterministic integer programming problem in which the objective is to minimize the total cost of assigning patients to OR slots. Their model, however, proved to be too large to be solved and so a heuristic solution methodology is adopted. Drawing on the similarity of their model to an assignment problem, Guinet and Chaabane solve a relaxed version of the problem as a pure assignment problem. They then evaluate the dual to the problem to evaluate infeasibilities in the full problem and apply a taboo-based heuristic to resolve any infeasibilities found.

Lamiri et al. (2008) also present an integer programming model for case sequencing that minimizes the regular and overtime costs of completing a slate of procedures. In their model, elective case must be sequenced into rooms while retaining an allowance for emergency case utilization. Elective procedure times are assumed to be deterministic and demand for OR time is determined from sampling a simulation model to generate a particular scenario, which is solved via IP methods. Lamiri et al. suggest that the resulting allocation of time derived from the solution to the IP model could then be used to determine short-term time allocations for surgical services.

In general, IP formulations for surgical sequencing, such as those developed by Guinet and Chaabane or Lamiri et al., produce problem instances that are too large and complex to be solved exactly. Problem scope is thus typically limited, and evidence of implementation is, to date, largely lacking.

Cardoen et al. (2010) have produced a survey paper with a focus on OR planning at an operational level. In this paper, the authors review the literature on OR planning and scheduling and classify it according to a six-dimensional taxonomy. The function of the taxonomy is to provide a compact means of representing problem instances and solution methodologies. As noted earlier, the Cardoen et al. taxonomy differs substantially from earlier review works, since it does not follow the traditional dimensions of time, scope, and problem subtype and instead employs dimensions based on six descriptive fields. The resulting taxonomy provides a compact means of classifying papers that is useful for researchers attempting to quickly parse the literature for a particular type or class of work. The taxonomy does not, however, neatly relate the literature to the problem structure, but the Cardoen et al. review of the literature is extensive and timely.

Estimating Case Duration

It is difficult to sequence cases into a surgical suite in both theory and practice. Packing surgical cases into a finite-sized OR bins is difficult even if the case times are assumed to be known ahead of time with certainty. If, as is the case of practical problems, the case time is not known prior to execution, sequencing cases becomes extremely complex and the problem becomes one of trading off over time costs against room underutilization and patient access (Pandit et al., 2007). Since case times are not known and overtime is typically more costly than underutilization, case sequencing is often a process of setting a probabilistic upper bound on completion time (i.e., being 95% certain that a particular room will have all of its cases completed by the planned room end time). In effect, the probabilistic upper bound requires that some scheduled OR time (slack) must be reserved for overruns or other unforeseen circumstances, in a manner analogous to holding safety stock in an inventory system to provide a service level to customers in the event of variable demand during order lead time. Since variance, by definition, gives rise to requirements for slack, improved methods of estimating case times, which would reduce variance, offers the potential to increase OR efficiency by allowing more cases to be sequenced into a given OR bin. Methods to estimate surgical case times, however, have emerged only recently after the wide-scale implementation of computerized surgical management systems to collect information on estimated and actual case durations.

Wright et al. (1996) provide a comparison of the accuracy of surgeons' estimates of case times against a moving average of the past 10 procedures completed. Their results suggest that neither surgeons, nor the moving average procedure used in popular commercial OR booking packages, are particularly good predictors of actual case time. Furthermore, the moving average was found to be less accurate than the manual estimate. Attempts to improve the accuracy of estimates by stratifying by patient gender, surgeon estimated level of difficulty, and experience of residents proved to be ineffective.

Strum et al. (2000), however, compare the accuracy of the normal distribution and a two-parameter lognormal distribution for estimating surgical case time completion. Their analysis includes somewhat over 40,000 records and considers both surgical procedure time (incision to close) and total procedure time (patient-in to patient-out). They hypothesize that the lognormal distribution, which models completion times with long right tails, should be a good model for surgery. The results of the analysis support this hypothesis: the lognormal distribution outperformed the normal distribution in most situations, except where the sample size for fitting the distribution was small. In a separate paper, Strum et al. (2000) presents an analysis of the same dataset in which an ANOVA is conducted to evaluate the sources of variability in case durations. The model includes surgeon, anesthesia type, risk class, patient gender, and age as explanatory variables and determines that, while many factors affect procedure completion time, surgeon and anesthesia type were the most significant. May et al. (2000) go on to present a methodology for fitting a three-parameter lognormal distribution to the dataset of Strum et al.

Macario and Dexter (1999) describe a method for estimating case completion times in the absence of data for a specific surgeon and procedure combination. They test several methods and conclude that, while none is perfect, using estimates based on simple averages from other surgeons performing similar cases works as well as, or better, than other more sophisticated methods. In a later paper, Dexter and Ledolter (2005) suggest a different methodology, arguing that procedures with no previous data may not be "new" so much as rare and thus no comparative data is likely to exist. Accordingly, they suggest a method based on determining the prediction interval using an estimate of new procedure's mean and variance and adjusting for errors in estimates derived from other cases. Included in their method is a procedure to generate an estimate given no historical data and a method for updating parameters as historical data becomes available.

Optimizing Patient Flow

ORs typically account for more than 40% of a hospital's revenues and a similar portion of their expenses (Denton et al., 2006). It is therefore critical to the overall function of a hospital that the surgical suite operate efficiently and effectively. There is a body of research in the operations research literature as well as the hospital management, industrial engineering, and quality literature that focuses on operational improvements in the surgical suite to smooth patient flow and eliminate delays and waste. While the literature is broad, it can be categorized into studies dealing with patient flow, turn over between surgical cases, and the first start of cases in a room.

Denton et al. (2006) describe a model to evaluate patient scheduling in an outpatient environment where surgical teams may be assigned more than one room. Under such a scenario, certain portions of the surgical cycle (setup, cleanup, and possibly induction) can take place in parallel with the main surgical activity. Performing activities in parallel increases the utilization of the surgical team, and thus potentially throughput, but at the cost of lower surgical room utilization and increased patient in-process wait. Denton et al. develop a model of an endoscopy suite that uses a simulated annealing algorithm along with a scenario-based simulation model to jointly evaluate patient schedules and resource utilization. Friedman et al. (2006) similarly discuss the potential advantages of parallel processing in an ambulatory care setting. Freidman et al. provide a pre–post observational study, which evaluates the impact of moving portions of the induction and cleanup activities for hernia operations to a parallel (or off-line) process. The results of the pre–post test suggested that throughput gains could be achieved while maintaining a positive experience for patients as measured by a qualitative satisfaction survey.

Although Dexter et al. note that the throughput improvements from decreasing case turn-around time are generally modest unless cases are frequent and short, there are a substantial number of studies that evaluate turn-around time (Dexter et al., 2003). Because of the bin-packing nature of surgical scheduling, reductions in turn-around time do not translate into an increased number of cases unless the sum of the gains in turn-around permits the scheduling of an integer number of extra cases. Nevertheless, increasing surgical suite efficiency by decreasing turn-around time is of perennial interest. Cendãn and Good (2006), for instance, present a case study in which work flow was redesigned at an academic teaching hospital to reduce the number of steps required to clean a room and set up for a new procedure. Cendãn and Good selectively apply their method to short, high-volume cases and note that increases in case throughput could be realized and that staff readily accepted the new work procedures. Overdyk et al. (1998) similarly present a pre–post case study in which surgical delays were classified, measured, and monitored in an effort to reduce delays in the start of the first case of the day as well as delays between successive surgical cases. In the pre-intervention study, Overdyk et al. noted that the vast majority of delay (67%) is related to elements under the control of surgeons. In their case study, delays were measured, graphed, and reported when necessary. The post-intervention arm of the study showed a significant decrease in both first-case tardiness and delay between cases. Overdyk et al. attribute much of the improvement to better attendance by surgeons resulting from the monitoring program.

McIntosh et al. (2006) also discuss the importance of measuring and monitoring turn-around times and first-case tardiness. They note that the impact of reducing turn-around time varies significantly by service, and argue that the overall effect on throughput of reducing case turn-around time is typically small. They note, however, that first-case tardiness can have a substantial impact on overall efficiency and throughput.

Berry et al. (2008) present the results of a regression study relating OR efficiency (as measured by the natural logarithm of total surgical time/total anesthetist salary) against hospital size, ownership, and management characteristics. Their analysis suggests rather interesting results. Only hospital size was found to be a significant predictor of surgical suite efficiency. Other factors, which include the diversity of surgical programs offered at a hospital, public/private ownership, and the functional organization of the surgical suite management, were, interestingly, not found to affect overall efficiency.

Conclusion

Capacity planning is a concept common to many industries. Capacity planning decisions are typically classified according to their scope and time frame: strategic (long term), tactical (intermediate), and operational (short term). The literature on capacity planning in ORs differs somewhat from the more general literature since models for strategic planning are largely absent. The literature instead focuses on tactical and operational issues of capacity planning. At the tactical level, OR capacity planning is a problem of determining how to allocate fixed resources a priori to surgeons or services, primarily through the design of the MSS. At the operational level, OR capacity planning consists of decisions regarding the allocation of cases to surgical suites and the determination of case start and end times. Aspects of efficiency and improving patient flow, as described in the clinical, industrial engineering, and quality literature, are complements to operational capacity planning.

References

Beliën, J. and Demeulemeester, E. 2007. Building cyclic master surgery schedules with leveled resulting bed occupancy. *European Journal of Operational Research* 176(2): 1185–1204.

Berry, M., Berry-Stolzle, T., and Schleppers, A. 2008. Operating room management and operating room productivity: The case of Germany. *Health Care Management Science* 11(3): 228–239.

Blake, J. T. and Carter, M. W. 1997. Surgical process scheduling: A structured review. *Journal of the Society for Health Systems* 5(3): 17–30.

Blake, J. and Donald, J. 2002. Using integer programming to allocate operating room time at Mount Sinai Hospital. *Interfaces* 32(2): 63–73.

Cardoen, B., Demeulemeester, E., and Belien, J. 2010. Operating room planning and scheduling: A literature review. *European Journal of Operational Research* 201(3): 921–932.

Cendan, J. C. and Good, M. 2006. Interdisciplinary work flow assessment and redesign decreases operating room turnover time and allows for additional caseload. *Archives of Surgery* 141(1): 63–69.

Côté, M. J. 2005. A note on bed allocation techniques based on census data. *Socio-Economic Planning Sciences* 39(2): 183–192.

Davis, M. M., Aquilano, N. D., Chase, R. B., and Balakrishnan, J. 2005. *Fundamentals of Operations Management (1st Canadian Edition)*. Toronto: McGraw-Hill Ryerson.

Denton, B. D., Rahman, A. S., Nelson, H., and Bailey, A. C. 2006. Simulation of a multiple operating room surgical suite. In *Proceedings of the 2006 Winter Simulation Conference*, eds. Peronne, L., Wieland, F., Liu, J., Lawson, B., Nicol, D. and Fujimoto, R., pp. 414–424. Monterey, CA: IEEE.

Dexter, F., Abouleish, A. E., Epstein, R. H., Whitten, C. W., and Lubarsky, D. A. 2003. Use of operating room information system data to predict the impact of reducing turnover times on staffing costs. *Anesthesia and Analgesia* 97(4): 1119–1126.

Dexter, F. and Ledolter, J. 2005. Bayesian prediction bounds and comparisons of operating room times even for procedures with few or no historic data. *Anesthesiology* 103(6): 1259–1267.

Dexter, F., Ledolter, J., and Wachtel, R. E. 2006. Tactical decision making for selective expansion of operating room resources incorporating financial criteria and uncertainty in subspecialties' future workloads. *Anesthesia and Analgesia* 100(5): 1425–1432.

Dexter, F., Maracio, A. and Lubarsky, D. 2001. The impact on revenue of increasing patient volume at surgical suites with relatively high operating room utilization. *Anesthesia and Analgesia* 92: 1215–1221.

Dexter, F., Macario, A., Traub, R., Hopwood, M., and Lubarsky, D. 1999. An operating room scheduling strategy to maximize the use of operating room block time: Computer simulation of patient scheduling and survey of patients' preferences for surgical wait time. *Anesthesia and Analgesia* 89: 7–20.

Friedman, D. M., Sokal, S. S., Chang, Y., and Berger, D. L. 2006. Increasing operating room efficiency through parallel processing. *Annals of Surgery* 243(1): 10–14.

Goldman, J., Knappenberger, H., and Moore, E. 1969. An evaluation of operating room scheduling policies. *Hospital Management* 12(3): 40–51.

Green, L. V. 2004. Capacity planning and management in hospitals. In *Operations Research and Health Care: A Handbook of Methods and Applications*, eds. Sainfort, F., Brandeau, M. L., and Pierskalla, W. P., pp. 15–41. Boston, MA: Kluwer.

Guinet, A. and Chaabane, S. 2003. Operating theatre planning. *International Journal of Production Economics* 85(1): 69–81.

Gupta, D. 2007. Surgical suites operations management. *Production and Operations Management* 16(6): 689–700.

Hancock, W. M., Magerlein, D. B., Storer, R. H., and Martin, J. B. 1978. Parameters affecting hospital occupancy and implications for facility sizing. *Health Services Research* 13(3): 276–289.

Hans, E., Wullink, G., Houdenhoven, M., and Kazemier, G. 2006. Robust surgery loading. *European Journal of Operational Research* 185(3): 1038–1050.

Harper, P. R. 2002. A framework for operational modelling of hospital resources. *Health Care Management Science* 5/3: 165–173.

Harper, P. R. and Shahani, A. K. 2002. Modelling for the planning and management of bed capacities in hospitals. *Journal of the Operational Research Society* 53(1): 11–18.

Kuo, P. C., Schroeder, R. A., Mahaffey, S., and Randall, R. B. 2003. Optimization of operating room allocation using linear programming techniques. *Journal of the American College of Surgeons* 197(6): 889–895.

Kwak, N., Kuzdrall, P., and Schmitz, H. 1976. The GPSS simulation of scheduling policies for surgical patients. *Management Science* 22(9): 982–989.

Lamiri, M., Xialoan, D., Xie, A., and Grimaud, F. 2008. A stochastic model for operating room planning with elective and emergency demand for surgery. *European Journal of Operational Research* 185(3): 1026–1037.

Lapierre, S. D., Goldman, D., Cochran, R., and Dubow, J. 1999. Bed allocation techniques based on census data. *Socio-Economic Planning Sciences* 33(1): 25–38.

Macario, A. and Dexter, F. 1999. Estimating the duration of a case when the surgeon has not recently scheduled the procedure at the surgical suite. *Anesthesia and Analgesia* 89(1): 1241–1245.

Magerlein, J. M. and Martin, J. B. 1978. Surgical demand scheduling: A review. *Health Services Research* 13(4): 418–433.

May, J. H., Strum, D. P., and Vargas, L. G. 2000. Fitting the lognormal distribution to surgical procedure times. *Decision Sciences* 11(1): 129–148.

McIntosh, C., Dexter, F., and Epstein, R. 2006. The impact of service-specific staffing, case scheduling, turnovers, and first case starts on anesthesia group and operating room productivity: A tutorial using data from an Australian hospital. *Anesthesia and Analgesia* 103(6): 1499–1516.

O'Neill, L. and Dexter, F. 2007. Tactical increases in operating room block time based on financial data and growth estimates from data envelopment analysis. *Anesthesia and Analgesia* 104(2): 355–368.

Overdyk, F., Harvey, R. L. F., and Shippey, F. 1998. Successful strategies for improving operating room efficiency at academic institutions. *Anesthesia and Analgesia* 86(1): 896–906.

Pandit, J., Westbury, S., and Pandit, M. 2007. The concept of surgical operating room "efficiency": A formula to describe the term. *Anesthesia* 62(9): 895–903.

Smith-Daniels, V. L., Schweikhart, S. B., and Smith-Daniels, D. E. 1988. Capacity management in health care services: Review and future research directions. *Decision Sciences* 19(4): 889–919.

Strum, D. P., May, J. H., and Vargas, L. G. 2000a. Modeling the uncertainty of surgical procedure times. *Anesthesiology* 92(4): 1160–1167.

Sturm, D. P., Sampson, A. R., May, J. H., and Vargas, L. G. 2000b. Surgeon and type of anaesthesia predict variability in surgical procedure times. *Anesthesiology* 92(5): 1454–1466.

Utley, M., Gallivan, S., Treasure, T., and Valencia, O. 2003. Analytical methods for calculating the capacity required to operate an effective booked admission policy for elective inpatient services. *Health Care Management Science* 6(2): 97–104.

Van Houdenhoven, M., van Oostrum, J. M., Hans, E. W., Wullink, G., and Kazemier, G. 2007. Improving operating room efficiency by applying bin-packing and portfolio techniques to case scheduling. *Anesthesia and Analgesia* 105(3): 707–714.

van Oostrum, J., van Houdenhoven, M., Hurkink, J., Hans, E., Wullink, G., and Kazemier, G. 2008. A master surgical scheduling approach for cyclic scheduling in operating rooms. *OR Spectrum* 30(2): 355–374.

Vargas, L. G., May, J. H., Spangler, W., Stanciu, A., and Strum, D. P. 2006. Operating room scheduling and capacity planning. In *Anesthesia Informatics*, eds. Jerry, S. and Keith, R., pp. 361–392. New York: Springer.

Wright, I. H., Kooperberg, C., Bonar, B., and Bashein, G. 1996. Statistical modeling to predict elective surgery time: Comparison with a computer scheduling system and surgeon-provided estimates. *Anesthesiology* 85(6): 1235–1245.

35

Managing Critical Resources through an Improved Surgery Scheduling Process

Erik Demeulemeester
Katholieke Universiteit Leuven

Jeroen Beliën
Hogeschool Universiteit Brussel

Brecht Cardoen
Vlerick Leuven Gent Management School

Introduction 35-1
Surgery Scheduling at the Tactical Level: Master Surgery Scheduling 35-2
Visualization of the Master Surgery Schedule • Optimization of the Master Surgery Schedule • Integrating Operating Room and Nurse Scheduling
Surgery Scheduling at the Operational Level: Patient Scheduling....... 35-7
Patient Scheduling Taxonomy
Conclusion and Future Research.. 35-10
References.. 35-11

Introduction

The costs of healthcare are rising up to 15% of the GDP in the United States and up to 10% in Europe (OECD, 2008). This is due to the increasing needs of an ageing population (Etzioni et al., 2003), but also due to technological and pharmacological innovations that are really widening the possibilities for diagnosis and treatment. Consequently, hospitals are confronted with a continuously growing demand. The available budget, however, often does not allow for an increase of the capacity at the same pace as demand, resulting in intolerably long waiting lists (Hurst and Siciliani, 2003). The only solution is a more efficient use of the scarce resources. Hospitals have to reduce costs and to improve their financial assets, but not at the price of a decreased quality of service. It becomes more and more obvious that it is not sufficient that health providers acknowledge the need to improve their quality of care; we should question how to structure the health delivery process and how to improve the major pitfalls such as the inefficient use of resources and the lack of communication and protocols. Hence, the managerial aspect of providing health services to patients in hospitals is becoming increasingly important. One unit that is of particular interest is the operating theater. Since this facility is the hospital's largest cost and revenue center (Macario et al., 1995; HCFMA, 2005), it has a major impact on the performance of the hospital as a whole. Managing the operating theater, however, is hard not only due to the conflicting priorities and the preferences of its stakeholders (Glauberman and Mintzberg, 2001) but also due to the scarcity of costly resources. These factors clearly stress the need for efficiency and necessitate the development of adequate planning and scheduling procedures.

In the past 60 years, a large body of literature on the management of operating theaters has evolved. Magerlein and Martin (1978) review the literature on surgical demand scheduling and distinguish between advance scheduling and allocation scheduling. Advance scheduling is the process of fixing a surgery date for a patient, whereas allocation scheduling determines the operating room (OR) and the starting time of the procedure on the specific day of surgery. Blake and Carter (1997) elaborate on this taxonomy in their literature review and add the domain of external resource scheduling, which they define as the process of identifying and reserving all resources external to the surgical suite necessary to ensure appropriate care for a patient before and after an instance of surgery. They furthermore divide each domain in a strategic, administrative, and operational level, although these boundaries may be vague and interrelated. Przasnyski (1986) structures the literature on OR scheduling based on general areas of concern, such as cost containment or scheduling of specific resources. Recently, Cardoen et al. (2010) studied contributions on OR planning and scheduling from multiple perspectives, such as performance measures, applied solution technique, uncertainty incorporation, or decision delineation, which they refer to as descriptive fields.

In general, we can distinguish between three levels of surgery scheduling. First, there is the strategic level in which one has to determine how much OR time will be assigned to the different surgeons or surgical groups. This level is often referred to as case mix planning (Blake and Carter, 2002). Second, there is a tactical level in which the master surgery schedule is developed. On the third and final level, individual patients or cases can be scheduled on a daily base. In this chapter, we will focus on the tactical and the operational level. "Surgery scheduling at the tactical level: Master surgery scheduling" presents a model for master surgery scheduling (tactical level), while "Surgery scheduling at the operational level: Patient scheduling" discusses a model for surgery case sequencing (operational level). Both models are illustrated with software tools and result from real-life case studies. "Conclusion and future research" concludes this chapter and states some directions for future research.

Surgery Scheduling at the Tactical Level: Master Surgery Scheduling

Basically, there exist two strategies for dividing the total available OR time between the different surgeons. In the first strategy, often referred to as "open scheduling," surgeons can submit requests for OR time during a certain time period (e.g., daily or weekly), after which the OR manager proposes a schedule that takes all OR and surgeon's availability constraints into account and optimizes some objectives. The main drawback of the open-scheduling strategy is that, after each period, a new schedule must be constructed, which is a time-consuming issue. In the second strategy, often referred to as "block scheduling," each surgeon or surgical group is "proprietor" of one of several OR blocks according to his or her availability and his or her needs (Kharraja et al., 2006). The schedule that defines the number and type of ORs available, the hours that rooms will be open, and the surgeon or surgical groups to whom the OR time is assigned is often referred to as the "master surgery schedule" (Blake et al., 2002). The main advantage of this strategy is that the OR manager does not have to build a new OR schedule daily or weekly. It suffices to evaluate the master surgery schedule, for instance, every 6 months, and change it if needed. This will be the case if the availability of surgeons has changed, the demand for surgery has altered (resulting in some surgeons having assigned too much OR time while others have too little), or the resource consumption patterns for one or more patient groups have changed, e.g., due to a new treatment, which might require for a new schedule in order to avoid resource usage peaks (see further). In the remainder of this section, we will assume a block scheduling strategy and describe some methodologies for building qualitative master surgery schedules. First, we present a system that visualizes the impact of the master surgery schedule on the use of different resources over time. The system allows identifying peaks in the resource usage before execution of the plan and helps in evaluating simple changes like the swap of two surgeon(s) (groups). Second, we enhance the visualization system with an optimization component that allows us to search for an "optimal" master surgery schedule, e.g., the one with the most leveled resulting bed occupancy. Both the visualization system and the optimization system are illustrated by means of a case study involving real-life data of two Belgian hospitals.

Visualization of the Master Surgery Schedule

The allocation of capacity and resources is not an isolated question and is related to the patients and the patient flow. The operating theater is generally considered as the most critical resource inside hospitals since it is one of the main cost drivers and many patients have to pass through it. Therefore, the OR schedule is an appropriate instrument to manage patient flow and, consequently, the timing and occupancy of other important resources like nursing staff, beds, anesthetists, specialized equipment, radiology, and so on. Indeed, what happens inside the OR dramatically influences the demand for resources throughout the rest of the hospital. In other words, the OR can be seen as the engine that drives the hospital (Litvak and Long, 2000). For instance, after surgery, a patient often occupies a bed and requires nursing services for recovery. Certain types of surgery require preceding tests (e.g., blood analysis) or post-surgery treatments that have to be carried out by correctly skilled staff. In the remainder of this section, we will hence limit the focus to the improvements that can be obtained through the organization of the operating theater. Some case studies will be introduced to highlight the practical value of this research.

Beliën et al. (2006) developed a model that, after implementation in a software system, visualizes the impact of the OR schedule on the demand for various resources throughout the entire hospital. It has been widely accepted that visualization is a simple yet powerful tool for managing complex systems like healthcare service units. The paper presents an example of a scheduling tool that visualizes the consumption of various resources as a function of the master surgery schedule. The system does not provide an online visualization of available and occupied resources during the daily working of a surgery hospital. It is neither a simulation package for analyzing the existing system and a limited number of alternative scenarios. The extremely intuitive graphical user interface (GUI) visualizes the impact on resource occupancy of modifications in the master surgery schedule. To this aim, schedulers can easily swap surgeon blocks and immediately see the consequences with respect to the expected use of various resources on a cyclic time axis.

The visualization tool serves two purposes. First, it eases the development of workable surgery schedules by visualizing possible resource conflicts. Second, it might be useful to convince surgeons during the master surgery schedule bargaining process to accept a surgeon block switch. Visualizing a resource conflict is often far more persuasive than hours of discussion with surgeons that are dissatisfied for not being scheduled by their preferences.

Beliën et al. (2006) describe a case study in a large Belgian surgery unit, hereby illustrating how the software can be used to assist in building better master surgery schedules. This case study concerns the surgical day-care center of the UZ Leuven Campus Gasthuisberg, situated in Leuven, Belgium. As the name suggests, this ambulatory center processes only outpatient admissions. To give an idea of the size of this surgical unit: in 2004, 12,778 surgical interventions have been performed, making up for more than 15,000 hours of total net operating time. The operating theatre consists of 8 rooms in which in total 27 different surgical groups, divided over 13 surgical and medical disciplines, have been assigned OR time. Each OR is open from Monday to Friday from 07:45 a.m. till 4:00 p.m. No elective surgery takes place during the weekends. Each OR is allocated for at least half a day to the same surgeon. The current master surgery schedule can be called cyclic since it basically repeats each week with the exception of three block allocations that alter each week between two surgeons.

In this case study, 12 critical resources have been identified that all share the following three properties: (1) expensive, (2) limited in capacity, and (3) the consumption pattern is directly linked to the OR schedule. These 12 resources can be distinguished into five groups. First of all, certain types of surgery require the patient to be lying and transported in a bed (1). Second, there are the human resources that consist of three skill-specific groups of nurses (2, 3, and 4), anesthetists (5), and anesthetist-supervisors (6). Third, some surgical interventions involve expensive material resources: laparoscopic towers (7), arthroscopic towers type 1 (8) and type 2 (9), and lasers type 1 (10) and type 2 (11). Finally, there is the radiology department (12).

Figure 35.1 shows a print screen of the GUI with the current surgery schedule for the odd weeks. The GUI visualizes the surgery schedule and the resulting resource use for a given master surgery schedule. Moreover, it allows the user to easily modify the existing schedule and view the impact of a change in the schedule on the use of the various resources. The main window is divided into two panes. In the left pane, the master surgery schedule is shown. The columns in the grid represent the time periods from Monday a.m. to Friday p.m. The eight rows represent the eight ORs, X1–X4 and Z1–Z4. Above the grid, a legend with the surgical groups is shown. Each surgical group has its own color and style. In this case, the style refers to the type of anesthetic. If the patients are completely anaesthetized during surgery, the surgeon block is colored solidly. Otherwise, when the patients are not fully anaesthetized, the block is arced. The schedule can easily be changed or built from scratch by dragging and dropping the surgeons to the timetable cells.

Each block assignment introduces a demand for resources in the system. The expected occupancies of these resources over time are represented in the right pane. A resource is visualized by a row that exists of different bars, each representing the resource consumption during a particular time instance (in Figure 35.1, six resources are visible). To accomplish this visualization, the system needs as input the resource usages over time corresponding to each surgeon block. Each resource has its own time horizon. The granularity does not necessarily coincide with that from the surgery cycle time horizon. As an illustration, consider the nursing resources for which on each day an extra time unit is added after

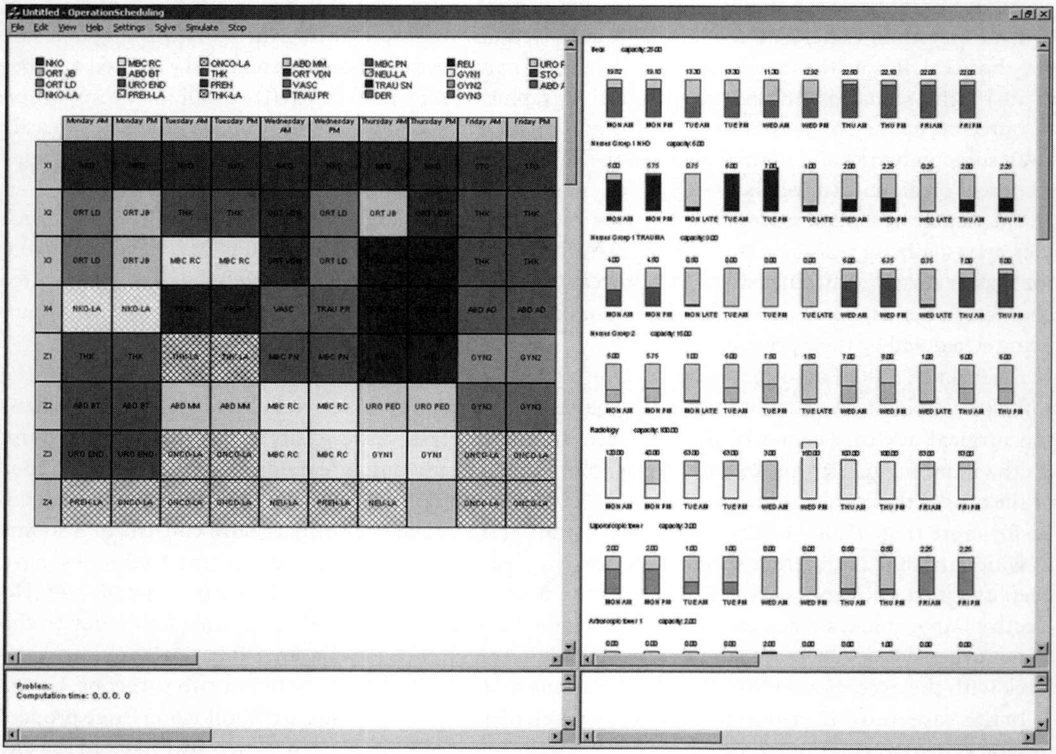

FIGURE 35.1 Print screen of the GUI showing the operating room schedule (left pane) and the impact on the usage of different resources (right pane).

the afternoon block. This extra resource unit represents the late shift. Furthermore, for each resource a capacity can be specified that is not necessarily fixed over the total time horizon.

Now that we are aware that the surgery schedule determines the resource utilization and the corresponding patient flow, we could determine how a qualitative surgery schedule should look like. In the next section, some algorithmic procedures will be presented for constructing an adequate master surgery schedule.

Optimization of the Master Surgery Schedule

The visualization system described in the preceding section could be complemented with an optimization component. An optimization component consists of one or more intelligent search procedures that can be applied to automatically generate a qualitative surgery schedule with certain favorable properties. Hence, the tool does not only visualize possible resource conflicts, but also actively searches for schedules that try to avoid these resource conflicts as much as possible. To this aim, the software searches a schedule in which the resulting resource occupancy is leveled as much as possible. In this way, the system is maximally protected against unexpected peaks in these occupancies. The optimization component can also prove to be useful for persuading hospital managers to invest in extra resource capacity. Insufficient resource capacities may not always be visible at first sight. It may, for instance, be the case that, although enough resource capacity is available for the individually summed needs for all resources over all surgeons, still no schedule can be found that provides enough capacity of each resource for each surgeon at each time instance.

In the model that supports the visualization tool described in the preceding section, all resources are assumed to have a deterministic utilization, that is, the load can be predicted accurately. In reality, however, the utilization of certain resources is subject to high uncertainty. The use of equipment is typically deterministic, whereas the bed occupancy is in many cases difficult to predict, due to the uncertainty in the patient's length of stay (LOS). Moreover, the model neglects no-shows. Therefore, Beliën and Demeulemeester (2006) propose an enhanced model that can be seen as a generalization, as well as a particularization, of the first model. It can be seen as a generalization, because it also takes uncertainty into account. The model is, however, also more specific, as beds are the only resource taken into consideration. The model starts from stochastic distributions for patient arrivals and a stochastic LOS associated with each type of surgery. The objective is to obtain a leveled bed occupancy distribution, and the master surgery schedule is again the main instrument to achieve this objective.

This new model has been tested using a case study in the Virga Jesse Hospital situated in Hasselt, Belgium (Beliën et al., 2009). Virga Jesse's central OR complex consists of 9 rooms in which a total of 46 surgeons have been assigned OR time. Each OR is open from Monday to Friday for 8.5 hours. The models applied in this study involve the development of a (cyclic) master surgery schedule with leveled bed occupancy in 10 major wards.

Figure 35.2 shows a print screen of the GUI of the scheduling tool. Although the GUI exhibits many similarities, there are three important differences with the previous system. First, the new model only focuses on the bed occupancy. The three rows that are shown at the right of Figure 35.2 each represent the weekly bed occupancy of a ward for which the bed occupancy on each day is predicted as a function of the master surgery schedule (shown left). Second, in contrast to the visualization model discussed earlier, the new model explicitly takes uncertainty in the arrival and LOS of patients into account. This uncertainty is translated into bed occupancy distributions characterized by a mean (reflected by the height of the color of the bars) and a standard deviation (reflected by the small T-ending bars at the top of each colored part). Third, the new system not only allows for the visualization of resource conflicts, but also incorporates an optimization component that can be used to automatically generate a surgery schedule for which the resulting bed occupancy at the wards is leveled as much as possible. In this way, the bed occupancy at the wards can be maximally protected against unexpected peaks caused by a sudden increase of urgency cases on a particular day.

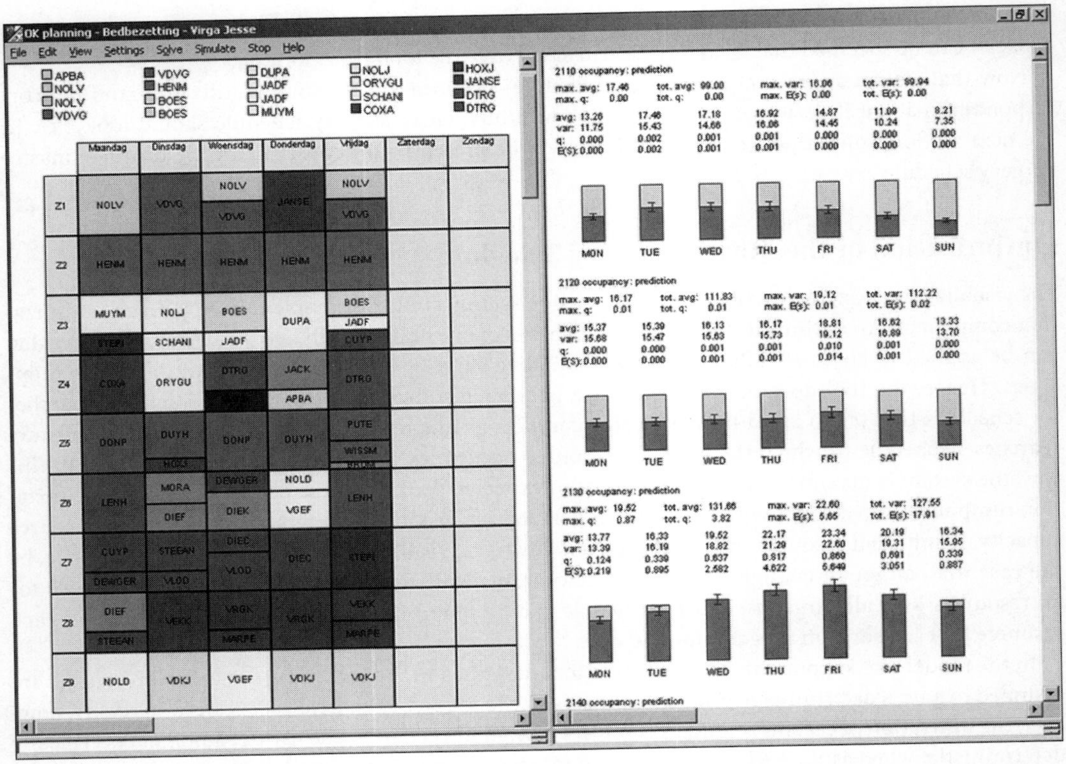

FIGURE 35.2 GUI of the software tool for building master surgery schedules with leveled resulting bed occupancy taking into account uncertainty in the arrival and LOS of patients.

Integrating Operating Room and Nurse Scheduling

As nursing services account for an important part of a hospital's annual operating budget, concentrating on this resource can lead to substantial savings. The situation is exacerbated by an acute shortage of nurses in all western countries, said to be 120,000 today and expected to grow to 808,000 by 2020 in the United States alone (USDHHS, 2002). Hence, it is of vital importance that nurses are used as much as possible at the right time and at the right place.

The second, third, and fourth resources in Figure 35.1 are groups of nurses, each having different skills. Observe that the need for nurses significantly varies over time. When the surgery schedule gives rise to peaks in the demand for nurses, it may be more difficult to schedule the nurses accordingly. Nurses have to be shifted from low demand shifts to peak shifts. Unfortunately, the nurse scheduling process is already constrained by itself. Indeed, when building the nurse schedule, different constraints have to be taken into account. These form an important hindrance for the flexibility with which nurses are scheduled. For instance, a nurse cannot be scheduled to work a morning shift when this same nurse is already scheduled to work an evening or night shift the preceding day. Another example includes the total number of shifts worked during weekends, which often must be equally divided among the different nurses. Taking into account these types of constraints that apply on the individual nurse schedules, a complete schedule (roster) including all nurses must be built that ensures the presence at the right time of the right number of nurses with the right skills. The timing of the requirement of nurses is determined by the number and type of patients present in the system, which on its turn is determined by the master surgery schedule, as mentioned in the previous two sections. Hence, to obtain an efficient

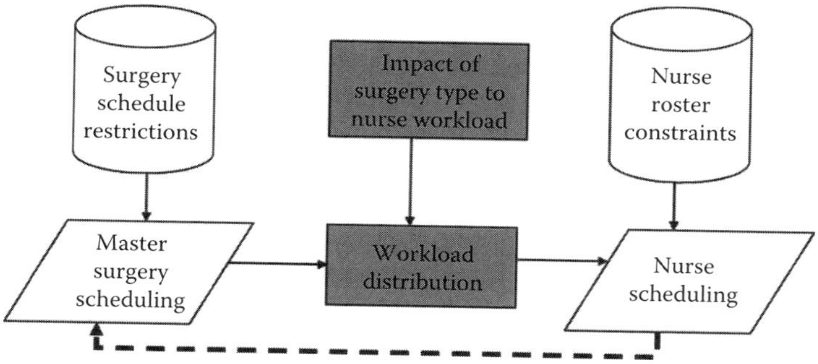

FIGURE 35.3 Integrating nurse and surgery scheduling.

system, it is very important to have a good integration between the nurse scheduling process and the master surgery scheduling process.

A specific model and algorithmic solution procedure to realize this integration is proposed by Beliën and Demeulemeester (2008). Figure 35.3 contains a schematic overview of the model developed in this work. The input for the nurse scheduling process (at the right) consists of the restrictions implied on the individual nurse roster lines (which are called the nurse roster constraints) on the one hand and the workload distribution over time on the other hand. The workload distribution itself depends on the master surgery schedule, since the timing of surgery determines which type of patients will be in the system at what time. In order to be able to deduce the workload from the surgery schedule, one also has to know the impact on the workload of each specific type of surgery. The dotted arrow at the bottom indicates the feedback that could be given from the nurse scheduling process to the surgery scheduling process in order to produce more favorable surgery schedules with respect to the resulting workloads and, as a consequence, more favorable nurse schedules. However, the freedom in modifying the surgery schedule is limited, since the master surgery schedule itself is restricted by a set of specific surgery constraints (e.g., capacity and demand constraints). The computational results presented in Beliën and Demeulemeester (2008) indicate that considerable savings could be achieved by integrating the nurse and surgery scheduling process.

Surgery Scheduling at the Operational Level: Patient Scheduling

The decisions that constitute the master surgery schedule and as such define the temporary assignment of OR capacity to medical disciplines, surgeons, or patient types depend on the average or expected population of patients that require surgery within the hospital of interest. The actual patient population of a specific surgery day, however, may substantially deviate from the expected population. This implies that next to the actual set of patients, also the resource consumption pattern that coincides with the population may deviate from the original prospects. Moreover, knowledge about the specific characteristics of the patients allows the introduction of new objectives and constraints compared to the master surgery schedule. Therefore, it seems necessary to have an adequate scheduling on the level of individual patients too, which we will refer to as *patient scheduling* or *case scheduling*. Since patient scheduling still covers a large set of possible configurations and scheduling problems, we introduce a simple taxonomy in the next section. Afterward, we report on one particular patient scheduling problem, namely a case sequencing problem, and this by means of a case study report.

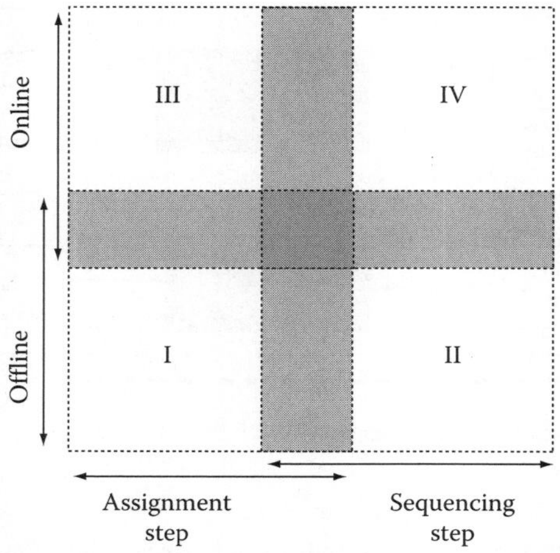

FIGURE 35.4 Two-dimensional classification matrix for patient scheduling problems.

Patient Scheduling Taxonomy

Within patient scheduling problems, one often distinguishes between an *assignment step* (Figure 35.4, I and III) and a *sequencing step* (Figure 35.4, II and IV). In the assignment step, individual patients are typically assigned to days and to surgery slots or ORs. The timing of the surgery on the specific day of surgery is determined by solving the sequencing step. When all surgeries have to be contiguously performed, this step boils down to determining the sequence of patients in the particular OR (slot). We refer to Jebali et al. (2006), Guinet and Chaabane (2003), Hsu et al. (2003), Marcon et al. (2003), Fei et al. (2008), or Cardoen et al. (2009a,b) for some studies that are structured by the two-step procedure. While many research efforts hierarchically solve both steps or focus on either the assignment step or the sequencing step, it should be clear that the quality of the sequencing step depends on the quality of the assignment step. Therefore, we encourage research efforts that simultaneously consider both optimization problems and that integrate the steps in one patient scheduling problem (vertical grey zone in Figure 35.4). Jebali et al. (2006), for instance, examine the sequencing step both with and without reconsidering the assignments made in the first step. The integration of both steps should definitively constitute an area for future research.

Next to the distinction between the assignment and the sequencing phase, we can also distinguish between approaches that optimize the patient scheduling problem from an *online* (Figure 35.4, III and IV) or *offline* (Figure 35.4, I and II) perspective. Equivalently, researchers may differentiate between a *static* or a *dynamic* phase. In contrast to the offline situation, online decisions have to be taken in real time. With respect to the assignment step, online decision making implies that a patient is immediately assigned to a day and possibly to an OR without knowing the entire population of patients that has to be divided over the time horizon (i.e., without exactly knowing the future entries of other patients). Online decision making may also prove useful when uncertainties materialize during the enrolment of the surgery schedule, so that rescheduling may be necessary. Marcon et al. (2003), for instance, construct an offline surgery schedule, but monitor and revise the schedule online when the risk of not realizing the original workload is substantial. Since most of the research efforts of the scientific community are currently directed toward offline patient scheduling, we encourage future research that examines the capabilities and the contributions of optimizing online decisions, especially when the developed policies are combined with or compared with offline procedures (horizontal grey zone in Figure 35.4).

In the next section, we address one particular patient scheduling problem in which patients of one particular surgery day are statically sequenced within their preassigned surgery slots.

Solving the Offline Sequencing Step: A Case Study

We recently examined how to optimize the surgery sequencing step at the surgical day-care (ambulatory) center of the UZ Leuven Campus Gasthuisberg, Belgium, by means of a case study (Cardoen, 2009). Note that this is the same unit that was addressed in the case study of Beliën et al. (2006) and that was discussed in the section on master surgery scheduling. The goal of the 10-day case study was to identify whether we are able to improve the surgery sequencing outcome on multiple levels. We aim, for instance, at scheduling children and prioritized patients as early as possible on the surgery day. This should result in a shorter period of soberness for the children and a reduced probability of being canceled due to unforeseen events for the prioritized patients. In order to increase the patient satisfaction and to reduce the arrival uncertainty, patients with a substantial travel distance to the center should be scheduled from a certain time along the day on. Overtime costs of unplanned hospitalizations are furthermore reduced by minimizing the recovery overtime. Finally, we aim at leveling the workload of the nursing personnel and at protecting the schedule against bed blocking by minimizing the peak use of beds in various recovery phases. Obviously, the optimization process is bounded by multiple constraints that are either patient-related or facility-related. The former category of constraints points at, for instance, the occurrence of incomplete presurgical tests for the specific patient or the additional cleaning obligations of the operating theater when the patient is MRSA-infected. The

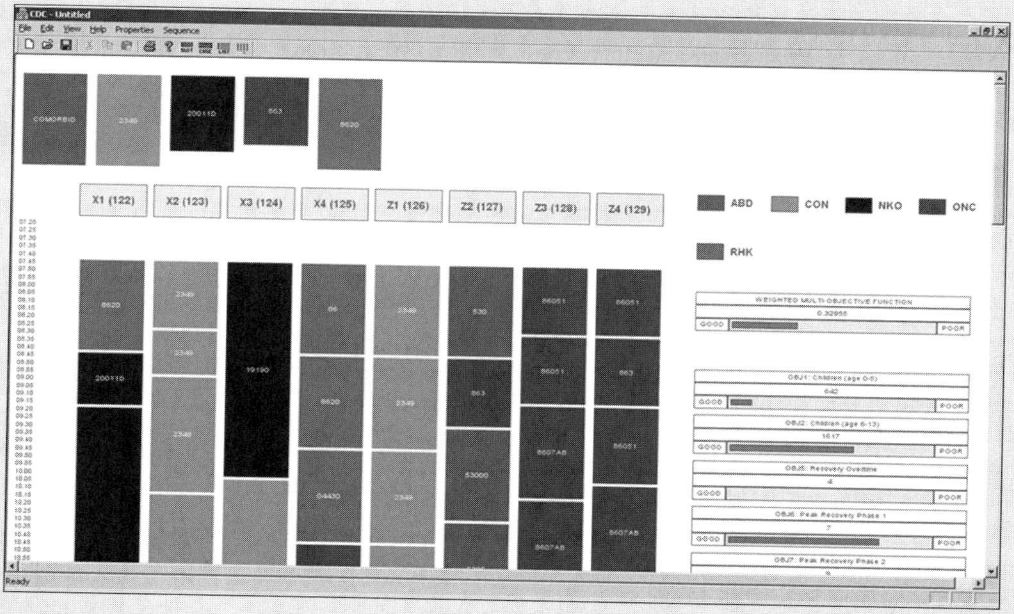

FIGURE 35.5 Print screen of the GUI for sequencing surgeries, showing the surgery schedule and the performance of the schedule with respect to the multiple objectives (dark gray bar indicates room for improvement).

latter category of constraints incorporates, for instance, the limited availability of recovery beds or medical instruments (including the sterilization requirements).

In the case study, we compared the original schedules, as proposed by the human planner of the day-care center, with the computerized schedules that are proposed by the mixed integer linear programming (MILP) procedures that were developed by Cardoen et al. (2009b). The daily number of surgeries over this 2-week horizon ranged from 44 to 64. Only 1 of the 10 original schedules was feasible with respect to all specified constraints, whereas the algorithm was able to identify even the optimal schedule in 7 out of 10 instances. For the remaining three instances, we were able to prove that no feasible schedule exists and showed how a GUI contributes to solving these troublesome situations. Figure 35.5 depicts a snapshot of the main pane of the software tool that was developed. Each rectangle represents a surgery. The sizes of the rectangles differ according to the required surgery time, whereas the color relates the specific surgeries to medical disciplines. The dark gray bars on the right-hand side of Figure 35.5 indicate whether some objectives can still be improved by re-sequencing the surgeries. The top dark gray bar indicates the overall quality of the surgery schedule. Other panes of the software tool inform the user about, for instance, the resource usage over time (and hence about possible resource conflicts) or about the underlying master surgery schedule. A comparison of the single feasible handmade schedule and the computerized optimal schedule indicated that the quality of the solution, as measured by the multi-objective function, improved by a factor 2. We obtained this optimal schedule in less than 3 seconds of computation time. The nonexistence of a feasible schedule was reported in less than 1 second.

Conclusion and Future Research

In this chapter, multiple procedures and software tools were presented in order to generate qualitative surgery schedules on the tactical and the operational level. We indicated that the efficient use of the operating theater improves the organizational efficacy of a hospital as a whole, since this facility is interrelated to many other departments or organizational problems (e.g., personnel scheduling, bed leveling, or instrument sterilization). We indicated that the advantages of an adequate surgery scheduling process do not only apply to the hospital, but also to the patients. In fact, the surgery schedule can contribute to the patient satisfaction by, for instance, equilibrating the patient flow or incorporating patient-specific information (e.g., age or travel distance). This quality of care could be further improved by integrating all processes described in *clinical pathways* or *care pathways*, since this concept focuses on both the medical and organizational issues. Such intensive integration, however, is complex for today's algorithms and constitutes an area for future research.

Embedding the algorithmic approaches in a flexible GUI augments the applicability of the solution approaches. On the one hand, visualization can provide additional insights to health managers and guide them through a process of trial and error for hypothesis testing or for triggering organizational discussions. On the other hand, they can present schedule outcomes that would surpass the experience of health managers due to the inherent complexity of the surgery scheduling process, specifically when it is related to other facilities.

Finally, intensive research should be performed on the strategic level of the surgery scheduling process, as these decisions mainly determine the financial revenues of the hospital. Since the provision of care is becoming increasingly competitive, strategic surgery decisions may lead to a specialization of the surgery type portfolio within a hospital and may hence provide a means to differentiate the care and to create a distinct hospital profile. Strategic surgery decisions will furthermore outline the general setting in which qualitative tactical and operational surgery schedules have to be developed and may lead to innovative OR scheduling approaches in which all decision levels can be well balanced.

References

Beliën, J. and Demeulemeester, E. 2006. Building cyclic master surgery schedules with leveled resulting bed occupancy. *European Journal of Operational Research* 176:1185–1204.

Beliën, J. and Demeulemeester, E. 2008. A branch-and-price approach for integrating nurse and surgery scheduling. *European Journal of Operational Research* 189(3):652–668.

Beliën, J., Demeulemeester, E., and Cardoen, B. 2006. Visualizing the demand for various resources as a function of the master surgery schedule: A case study. *Journal of Medical Systems* 30:343–350.

Beliën, J., Demeulemeester, E., and Cardoen, B. 2009. A decision support system for cyclic master surgery scheduling with multiple objectives. *Journal of Scheduling* 12(2):147–161.

Blake, J.T. and Carter, M.W. 1997. Surgical process scheduling: A structured review. *Journal of Health Systems* 5(3):17–30.

Blake, J.T. and Carter, M.W. 2002. A goal programming approach to strategic resource allocation in acute care hospitals. *European Journal of Operational Research* 140:541–561.

Blake, J., Dexter, F., and Donald, J. 2002. Operating room manager's use of integer programming for assigning block time to surgical groups: A case study. *Anesthesia and Analgesia* 94:143–148.

Cardoen, B. 2009. Operating room planning and scheduling: Solving a surgical case sequencing problem. Ph.D. dissertation, Katholieke Universiteit Leuven, Belgium.

Cardoen, B., Demeulemeester, E., and Beliën, J. 2009a. Sequencing surgical cases in a day-care environment: An exact branch-and-price approach. *Computers & Operations Research* 36(9):2660–2669.

Cardoen, B., Demeulemeester, E., and Beliën, J. 2009b. Optimizing a multiple objective surgical case sequencing problem. *International Journal of Production Economics* 119:354–366.

Cardoen, B., Demeulemeester, E., and Beliën, J. 2010. Operating room planning and scheduling: A literature review. *European Journal of Operational Research* 201(3):921–932.

Etzioni, D.A., Liu, J.H., Maggard, M.A., and Ko, C.Y. 2003. The aging population and its impact on the surgery workforce. *Annals of Surgery* 238(2):170–177.

Fei, H., Chu, C., Meskens, N., and Artiba, A. 2008. Solving surgical cases assignment problem by a branch-and-price approach. *International Journal of Production Economics* 112(1):96–108.

Glauberman, S. and Mintzberg, H. 2001. Managing the care of health and the cure of disease—Part I: Differentiation. *Health Care Management Review* 26:56–69.

Guinet, A. and Chaabane, S. 2003. Operating theatre planning. *International Journal of Production Economics* 85:69–81.

Health Care Financial Management Association (HCFMA). 2005. Achieving operating room efficiency through process integration. Technical report, Westchester, IL.

Hsu, V., de Matta, R., and Lee, C.-Y. 2003. Scheduling patients in an ambulatory surgical center. *Naval Research Logistics* 50:218–238.

Hurst, J. and Siciliani, L. 2003. Tackling excessive waiting times for elective surgery: A comparison of policies in twelve OECD countries. OECD Health Working Papers 6, Paris, France.

Jebali, A., Alouane, A., and Ladet, P. 2006. Operating rooms scheduling. *International Journal of Production Economics* 99:52–62.

Kharraja, S., Albert, P., and Chabaane, S. 2006. Block scheduling toward a master surgery schedule. *International Conference on Service Systems and Service Management* 1:429–435.

Litvak, E. and Long, M. 2000. Cost and quality under managed care: Irreconcilable differences? *The American Journal of Managed Care* 6:305–312.

Macario, A., Vitez, T.S., Dunn, B., and McDonald, T. 1995. Where are the costs in perioperative care?: Analysis of hospital costs and charges for inpatient surgical care. *Anesthesiology* 83(6):1138–1144.

Magerlein, J.M. and Martin, J.B. 1978. Surgical demand scheduling: A review. *Health Services Research* 13:418–433.

Marcon, E., Kharraja, S., and Simonnet, G. 2003. The operating theatre planning by the follow-up of the risk of no realization. *International Journal of Production Economics* 85:83–90.

Organization for Economic Co-operation and Development (OECD). 2008. OECD health data, Paris, France.

Przasnyski, Z. 1986. Operating room scheduling: A literature review. *AORN Journal* 44(1):67–79.

USDHHS. 2002. Projected supply, demand and shortages of registered nurses: 2000–2020. National Center for Health Workforce Analysis, US Department of Health and Human Services, Rockville, MD.

36

Anesthesia Group Management and Strategies

Introduction 36-1
A Brief History of Anesthesia Practice 36-2
Cultural Differences between Anesthesia Groups and Facility Management 36-3
Evolution of Closed Staffs and Exclusive Contracts 36-4
Physician Practice Management Companies 36-4
Autonomy as a Core Value 36-5
Urgency of Today 36-6
Change and Transitions in Anesthesia Groups 36-6
Macro-Level Transition Models 36-6
Impact of Transitions on People 36-6
Aligning Culture and Strategy 36-8
Leadership in an Anesthesia Group 36-9
At a Crossroads...Again 36-11
Conclusion 36-11
References 36-12

William H. Hass
Anesthesia Cooperative of the Panhandle

Alex Macario
Stanford University School of Medicine

Randal G. Garner
Medical Practice & Management Partners Inc.

Introduction

Despite the growing complexity of anesthesia services and the evolving healthcare environment, the fundamentals of anesthesia group management remain essentially unchanged since the origin of anesthesia groups. While drugs, equipment, and techniques have changed, anesthesia group management remains an exercise in human resources management. The goals of this chapter are to review the history of American anesthesia practice, its traditions of autonomy, the factors shaping anesthesia practice, the differences between medical facility and anesthesia group cultures, and to present ideas of how anesthesia groups should address organizational issues to meet the changing times. The main take home points are that the (1) disparity between the autonomy-based culture of physician groups and the positional authority–based culture of healthcare facility administration leads to ongoing conflict, (2) the field of anesthesiology is influenced by the search for recognition as a legitimate and innovative medical specialty, (3) community anesthesia groups are primarily operated by locally owned entities, (4) legal and regulatory factors (including exclusive contracting) have shaped the operation of anesthesia departments, (5) clinical anesthesia skills do not equate to business leadership or management skills, (6) human resource management is critical to an anesthesia group's long-term success, (7) change impacts anesthesia groups on a organizational and personal level, and (8) leadership education and involvement in the medical community will play an important role in the continued autonomy of the anesthesia group.

A Brief History of Anesthesia Practice

Similar to most physicians, American anesthesiologists place a high value on autonomy. Historically, anesthesia evolved from a technical function "that just about anyone available can do" (Lortie, 1946) to be ranked in 2007 as one of the top three medical breakthroughs since 1840 (Snow, 2008). Before the 1900s, nurses with varying amounts and types of training provided anesthesia to patients. Eventually, some general practice physicians began providing anesthesia to supplement their incomes, with some interesting exceptions. For example, when the general practitioner providing anesthesia became ill while William Worrell Mayo performed surgery, his 12-year-old son Charles Mayo administered his first anesthetic while his father operated (Lennon et al., 2009). Later and with significant difficulty, training programs for anesthesiologists were developed. Early anesthesiologists recognized that understanding of the scientific basis of anesthetics, not merely the facile application of techniques, was key to the growth of the specialty (Bunker, 1972).

Beyond technical skills and scientific advances, entrepreneurship was also a foundation of anesthesia practice. In 1919, Ralph Waters opened The Downtown Anesthesia Clinic in Sioux City, Iowa where surgeons and dentists were invited to bring their patients (Bunker, 1972). Similarly, in London, Robert Macintosh was a member of a dental anesthesia cartel that was chauffeured between nursing homes and dental surgeries. In a reference to the local utility, the Mayfair Gas, Light, and Coke Company, Macintosh's anesthesia group was jokingly referred to as the Mayfair, Fight, and Choke Company (Snow, 2008).

The history, evolution, and contributions of American nurses to anesthesia as well as the development and traditions of anesthesiology in other countries are beyond the scope of this review. It should also be noted that there has been and continues to be significant regional differences in anesthesia practice in the United States (Kumar, 2009). While some facilities are staffed exclusively by physician anesthesiologists, other areas employ the Anesthesia Care Team model (anesthesiologists medically directing nurse anesthetists and anesthesiologists' assistants). Some parts of the United States utilize collaborative relationships of anesthesia professionals (combinations of anesthesiologists and nurse anesthetists) to provide anesthesia services while other parts of the country rely exclusively on nurse anesthetists. These labor alternatives add to the complexity of the relationships between anesthesia professionals, medical staffs, and facility administrators. As a result, both nurse anesthetists and physician anesthesiologists have struggled for status in the medical community (Mueller and Evarts, 2002). Given these variations in thousands of anesthesia practices, it is difficult to generalize about the structure of American anesthesia groups during any era. Fundamentally, anesthesiologists maintained a long-standing effort to be perceived as a medical specialty and not as a hospital function with the characteristics of a commodity (Mueller and Evarts, 2002).

Anesthesia groups serving community hospitals started as cottage industries owned and operated by anesthesiologists imbued with independence, entrepreneurship, and seeking credibility. While some anesthesia groups were "Mom and Pop" operations with the day's anesthesia professional charges processed at the family kitchen table, others created formal businesses structures with large staffs, formal offices, and contracted billing services. This multitude of practice models, including homespun billing services, continues to this day (Morf, 2009). One of the main obstacles in the relationship of anesthesia professionals and healthcare facilities is the history of facilities considering anesthesia merely as a hospital service used to reap profits by employing low-cost nurse anesthetists and more recently, salaried anesthesiologists. This profit is used to balance the costs of most other hospital services, a strategy particularly common during periods of economic stress (Bunker, 1972). In response, community anesthesiologists sought the status of medical practitioner in open staff relationships to enable the coexistence of competing anesthesiologists and anesthesia groups (Bunker, 1972).

Cultural Differences between Anesthesia Groups and Facility Management

Hospitals are extremely complex organizations, combining many different professional groups within an intricate administrative structure. As medical facilities became more complex, conflicts developed between the anesthesiologists and the facilities. While the issue of economic control will probably always be present, an equally important conflict exists due to the dichotomy between the organization and culture of a medical facilities' leadership as compared to anesthesia groups. Physician culture is very different from that of healthcare facility. Medicine is driven by peer relationships and an effort to preserve autonomy while facilities' cultures are based on positional authority. For example, in a medical facility initiatives and operational plans pass down the organizational chart from the governing board through its administration to clinical and support employees. The essence of the problem becomes apparent as it is expected that hospital department directors reporting to the chief nursing officer will, more or less seamlessly, implement plans or initiatives from above. However, the chief medical officer, when interacting with the medical staff that is not employed by the medical facility about similar matters, may well get a response akin to "we'll talk about it." Implementation requires prolonged conversations and debates often without results.

When surveyed, nursing and administration attribute the highest power to the physicians, whereas physicians attribute the highest power to administration (Salvadores et al., 2001). Each group usually attributes the least power to itself. Power was defined as ability to execute decisions independently. The facility administrator sees the healthcare professional's autonomy as being unresponsive to the needs of the facility. This may be particularly true for anesthesia whose "loosey goosey" organizational structure of loosely affiliated independent anesthesiologists are considered difficult to influence by anyone. Managing anesthesiologists is compared to "herding cats" and is compounded by the view that anesthesiologists were "physicians without patients" (Lortine, 1946).

For anesthesiologists, the consequences of this perceived unresponsiveness or disorganization are seen first hand by administration: closed operating rooms (ORs) due to unavailability of anesthesia staff, delayed cases, wasted nursing resources, or an unhappy medical staff have real-time consequences in full view of the administration. These lapses in anesthesia services are reflected in short order on their financial and operational summaries or by complaints. In response, facilities may use a number of methods to gain more control over their anesthesia staffs including employment, exclusive contracts, and the use of management companies. Interestingly, hospitals increasingly ask clinicians to take management responsibility because hospitals realize they need the help of anesthesiologists to manage the surgical suite (Macario, 2006). This arrangement, however, needs to factor in that anesthesiologists typically focus on operational decisions on the day of surgery (short term) such as moving cases from one OR to another, assigning and relieving staff, prioritizing urgent cases, and scheduling add-on cases whereas upper management often focuses on longer term strategic decision making.

As noted, in some facilities, the governing body's solution to the physician management problem is the employment of anesthesiologists. In the past, this action created a complex mix of issues for community, academic, and entrepreneurial anesthesiologists (Bunker, 1972). The American Society of Anesthesiologists' strong objection to this practice was the subject of a Federal Trade Commission consent order in 1979 that "prohibited the association from restricting its members from rendering services in other than a fee of service basis."*

* 39FTC 101, 1979.

Evolution of Closed Staffs and Exclusive Contracts

Traditionally, physicians apply to a facility's medical staff for privileges to practice their specialty. The guiding principle was that a facility's bylaws constituted a contract and that the bylaws' provisions for suspension of privileges could be analogized to an employment contract requiring "for cause" termination (Biersten, 1996). As efficient operation of anesthesia departments became a greater concern, some facilities closed their staffs by not accepting new applicants. (Jefferson Parish involved events in 1977 and was decided in 1984.)* If properly done, the existing anesthesiologists encased in the closed department rarely raised objections. The situation escalated when a facility awarded an exclusive anesthesia contract and current medical staff members lost their privileges to practice anesthesia but remained on the medical staff (Mateo-Woodburn involved events of 1985 that was decided by the California Supreme Court in 1990).† From this point, the use of exclusive contracts expanded, often with unintended consequences.

Mateo-Woodburn influenced how hospitals managed their relationship with hospital-based doctors and how physicians interacted with each other. Prior to this decision, hospitals were limited in dealing with doctors with poor medical skills and often had to resort to revoking hospital privileges "for cause," which was difficult, expensive, and time consuming. This "quasi-judicial" process required evidence of malpractice. After Mateo-Woodburn, both doctors and hospitals realized that, by using a "quasi-legislative" process, a hospital could close an anesthesia department, and then contract with a physician charged with securing the anesthesia professionals of such numbers and quality that a stable clinical service and business entity was possible (Upton, 2009).

In this era, anesthesiologists' opinions of exclusive contracts varied from the idea that exclusive contracts circumvented due process rights of anesthesiologists, while others saw exclusive contracts as a medical facility's overt attempt to control medical professionals. More entrepreneurial anesthesiologists saw exclusive contracts' potential to promote efficient operations and to shorten the business development cycle. Soon, however, exclusive contracts were sought and granted for purely defensive purposes by well-positioned anesthesia groups. The contracts, unless a strong organizational structure and vision was in place, had the potential to enshrine the status quo. More important, with the advent of managed care that integrated the financing of care and the delivery of medical care under one organization, the increasingly complex business environment often overwhelmed the leadership and management skills of anesthesiologists. Selected for their clinical excellence, physician contract holders often did not have the business acumen or vision to respond to the complexities of running multimillion dollar companies in a changing environment. By June 1995, the *Harvard Business Review* published a case study on the discontinuity of clinical skill and business acumen in an anesthesia group managed by a local anesthesiologist (Peisch, 1995). This situation was not isolated and in response to the perceived poor performance of some community anesthesia groups, proprietary anesthesia practice management companies began to expand.

Physician Practice Management Companies

Physician practice management companies expanded rapidly in the 1990s. The concept was to combine experienced business people with physicians and medical groups promising superior business acumen, back-office experience, and economies of scale. The greater goal was to obtain capital and investors to grow larger businesses. The promise was that physicians could concentrate on practicing medicine while relinquishing the "business headaches of medicine," and eventually own a stake in the company. This approach seemed too slow for some companies competing for the interested physician pool so the concept was accelerated to use the available capital to buy medical practices. While a win–win strategy

* Jefferson Parish Hosp. Dist. No. 2 v. Hyde (466 U.S. 2, 104 S. Ct. 1551, 80 L. Ed. 2d 2, 52 U.S.L.W. 4385).

† Mateo-Woodburn et al. v, Fresno Community Hospital and Medical Center, Fresno, California.

was preached for all parties, market realities had each participant eventually making concessions. Many of these early physician practice companies failed.

Altered reimbursement for institutions and providers challenged the traditional anesthesia group. Anesthesia services became more important to facilities' increasing revenues goal through the expansion of services. As a result, more demands fell on anesthesia groups. Simultaneously, the supply of anesthesiologists and nurse anesthetists shrank, which, along with reduced reimbursement and increased service demands, negatively impacted physician's lifestyle and incomes. In turn, facilities, feeling like they were being held hostage by anesthesia-related issues, sought alternatives. This benefited anesthesia practice management companies.

Traditionally, anesthesia practice management companies were brought in by the hospital at the direction and insistence of powerful members of the medical staff. The objective was to generate more available OR time, better coverage in the labor and delivery suite, improved quality and staff management, and operational efficiencies. The print marketing of anesthesia practice management companies focused on these factors. Of greater concern, one advertisement in particular raised concerns among anesthesiologists about the true motive of anesthesia practice management companies when it stated that "...put control of your anesthesia department back where it belongs...in the hands of hospital administration" (Modern Healthcare, 1991).

In those early years and to some degree today, anesthesia practice management companies did not quite live up to their claims. The value added from the additional costs of proprietary anesthesia management companies was often marginal and sometimes illusionary. The sales pitch often exceeded the management company's ability to execute. An anesthesia group will not recover or retain core competence or credibility in the eyes of hospital leadership and the medical staff as a result of failed, absent, or arrogant leadership.

Autonomy as a Core Value

Despite the potential advantages of anesthesia practice management companies, they have a relatively small market penetration. This is because these organizations do not fully account for the philosophical and psychological makeup of physicians. Proprietary anesthesia practice management companies, as business people, do understand hospital executives who are typically their first contact and with whom they have little problem developing business relationships. Anesthesiologists, given the travails in development of their specialty, are highly sensitive to issues related to autonomy. In fact, autonomy is a core value to all physicians and is zealously guarded in times of change as it is perceived to impact physicians' control of the practice of medicine.

The low penetration of proprietary anesthesia practice management companies and the wide variations in management skills of the local anesthesia groups has spawned a large number of consultants for both anesthesia practices and facilities. Billing services have been present for many years and have become more important in an era of increasing regulation, multiple third-party payers, and technological requirements. Frequently, these services either provide or are associated with organizations that provide financial and benefits administration. Facilities are often interested in operational consultants in areas ranging from turnover analysis to supply cost control. As subsidies and other support arrangements become more prevalent between facilities and anesthesia groups, consultations about the fair market value of anesthesia professionals and the need for financial support has become more prevalent (Dexter and Epstein, 2008).

The employment of anesthesia professionals by facilities is a growing trend (Sermo, 2008), possibly as an effort to replace a physician's autonomy with the positional authority found in larger operations. While some states prohibit the employment of physicians, the number is small (4), the laws are poorly enforced, and there are growing pressures to end these prohibitions. The final scorecard on employment is not available, but this format may become more prevalent based on the generational changes in physicians.

Urgency of Today

Under normal circumstances, the market for community-based anesthesia services would be determined by the equilibrium between locally owned and operated services, proprietary anesthesia practice management companies, and employment models. Since the inception of anesthesiology as a specialty, the locally owned anesthesia practice has been the predominant community anesthesia practice format. Now, with the potential for major changes in healthcare in the next few years, new strategies are needed in anesthesia group management.

Change and Transitions in Anesthesia Groups

Change is inevitable and can be traumatic because people are the predominate asset of any anesthesia group. Even small changes in staffing and coverage obligations can significantly affect a group (Dexter and Epstein, 2006). Facilities lose insurance contracts, arbitrarily add or demand services inconsistent with the incumbent anesthesia group's skills or staffing, terminate long established services, and/or make financial decisions contrary to the short-term best interests of the anesthesia group. Whatever the cause, it may be difficult for an anesthesia group to respond to even small changes in service requirements. The bigger problem arises when the anesthesia group in an effort to maintain the status quo is seen as being unresponsive or irresponsible. A hospital's governing board, when facing financial or operational consequences, will become increasingly intolerant of an obstructionist anesthesia group. Replacement of contracted groups, affiliation with a proprietary anesthesia management organization, or employment will become increasingly acceptable. Survival of an anesthesia group does not depend on how many years they have worked in the facility, but rather on the ability to perform in short order the changes needed to the align with strategic initiatives of the facility. For this reason, anesthesia groups need to embrace and understand transitions and change. The business literature is a rich source of information on this process, but for anesthesia groups a few generalizations are possible.

Macro-Level Transition Models

Similar to other business organizations, anesthesia groups should see macro-level transitions in four categories:

- Start-ups
- Turnarounds
- Reorganizations
- Sustaining success

Each category has related tactics that can be reviewed in greater depth (Watkins, 2003). In practice, it may be very difficult for an anesthesia group to determine the type of transition required. An internally focused group might see itself as an ongoing success when others see it in turnaround status. Managing a transition in an anesthesia group is a delicate operation and requires detailed understanding of the psychosocial structure of the group. Unfortunately, there is a fifth type of transition that rarely gets mentioned: the failed transition which follows a poorly conceived and badly implemented transition plan.

Impact of Transitions on People

Beyond the macro-level organizational changes, each transition impacts people. In general, in an anesthesia group the following pattern occurs:

- The existing steady state
- Change demands

- Impact
- Disorganization
- Recovery
- Reorganization (Kraines, 2009)

Change places demands on the organization at several levels (Kraines, 2001). Each phase has characteristic factors. The leadership has special obligations to communicate and provide information, clarify implications, model behavior, and seek input and advice. In anesthesia groups where the leadership positions often rotate among those inexperienced or untrained, change at any level can be problematic. If there is a cautionary tale in anesthesia group management, it is the belief that clinical excellence also equates with organizational or business skills.

Anesthesia groups need to develop an internal structure that facilitates change. The management of an anesthesia group is essentially a human resources exercise in team building similar to any other business organization. Given its 24 × 7 role in high acuity circumstances, the urgency for high-quality human resources management in anesthesia department is greater than for many other services. Anesthesiologists often select potential associates and partners with only the most basic information and would benefit from more sophisticated hiring processes.

The success of an anesthesia service and its ORs requires teamwork and includes many other facility employees: nurses, advanced practice nurses, schedulers, transporters, central sterile workers, billers, etc. Even 90 years ago, when publishing about the Downtown Anesthesia Clinic in Sioux City in 1929, Waters made extensive reference to the importance of his office staff (Waters, 1919). Operation of an anesthesia service requires its professional staff to work in parallel and in close proximity. This pattern places emphasis on teamwork and teambuilding. Interestingly, and in contrast, emergency room physicians work primarily in series, in small numbers, and in separate shifts. Possibly, as a result of this clinical structure where group member interactions are more restricted, proprietary emergency room management organizations have much greater market penetration than anesthesia practice management companies.

The essence of internal group management is to enhance working effectiveness:

$$E = \int (\text{CMC}, \text{K/S}, \text{C/V}, -\text{X})$$

where

E = Working effectiveness
CMC = Current maximum capacity
= (Our intellectual horsepower)
K/S = Knowledge and skills
= (about the job and the organizations business)
= (about people and communication)
= (about practices, processes, and systems)
C/V = Commitment to and valuing of work
= (how much we value work)
= (are committed to applying ourselves)
–X = Absence of dysfunctional behavior
= (The absence of maladaptive coping mechanism) (Kraines, 2009)

Note the nullifying effect that dysfunctional behavior has on effectiveness. A small dose of arrogance, cynicism, and/or narcissism will trump affability, availability, and ability, which are the traditional determinants of a successful anesthesia practice.

Equally important is an understanding of what "makes you tick" as a leader. Eugene A. Stead, chairman of the Department of Medicine at Duke University, offered his chief residents the opportunity to undergo psychoanalysis understanding of the general concept that one cannot lead without knowing themselves (Neelon). His program has produced more directors of American academic medicine programs than any other. This does not necessarily mean that we all need to be psychoanalyzed, but it is important that we be self-aware (Drucker, 2005).

Aligning Culture and Strategy

There is a widely held belief that "When culture and strategy are not aligned, culture eats strategy for lunch every time." Many noble plans, headquarters' directives, and products of expensive consultations have been nullified by a group's culture. While it is possible that an anesthesia group will not match the positional authority model of facility management, it is important that anesthesia group members are held accountable to performance expectations and to be consistent with the culture of their group. This is the most fertile ground for anesthesia department management, but it is also the most difficult. A group's culture has several dimensions, organizational, professional, and geographic (Watkins, 2003), all of which ultimately impact operations and transitions.

Long-term success is more likely if a group can align its culture with these factors. For example, if an anesthesia group serves a regional medical center with sophisticated specialized services, specialization in the anesthesia services rather than egalitarian rotation of the staff through all services would be a better model. In the process of aligning cultures, the role of vision and perspective is important. Traditional business school thinking would have most, if not all, organizations develop formal vision and mission statements as well as a formal method of implementation and results testing. Understanding what an anesthesia group's business really is, who its customers are (McIntosh and Macario, 2009), how to maintain professional standards, and how to define success, require formal processes that are foreign to many anesthesiologists. To some degree, there are disincentives for clinicians to become service and system leaders (Mountford and Webb, 2009) Clinicians have important things to do, like taking care of patients who are quite anxious and fearful of their surgery. Medical schools and training programs never told physicians that they were actually in a very difficult and competitive business in which success may require the unthinkable: explicit goals, results testing, and consequences for nonperformance.

A common problem is that, if there is an explicit vision for the facility or the anesthesia group, there may be many different perspectives on that vision. The governing board or facility administrators may do things that seem irrational (Everett, 2009) or outright destructive to an anesthesia group, not because they are illogical or unintelligent, but because they have a different perspective on the acute problem or long-term viability of the facility. Although trying at times, an anesthesia group is best served by strong, not weak, institutional leadership. A healthcare facility is an intensely politico-economic entity. If an anesthesia group and its members are not participating in the facility's political life by attending medical staff meetings and other opportunities to interface with the governing board and administration, the group's economics may suffer and even its survival is at risk.

Just as there is a generational change in anesthesiologists, there is also a generational change in anesthesia organizations. Many anesthesia groups need to better prepare for the challenges ahead. For most anesthesia practices, the reality is manage or be managed and be politically active or be disenfranchised. Some anesthesia groups are fortunate to have capable managers and leaders with vision and spirit. Other groups need education on either general medical group operations, OR management and issues, or other anesthesia department management specific programs provided by the American Society of Anesthesiologists on Practice Management,* Medical Group Management Association's

* ASA Conference on Practice Management, Park Ridge, Illinois (www.ASAhq.org).

Anesthesia Administration Assembly,* or other organizations with experience and interest in anesthesia management.†,‡,§,¶,**

Leadership in an Anesthesia Group

The essence of leadership in an anesthesia group includes

- Understand what makes you, your associates, and your facility "tick."
- Forge psychological contracts at all levels based on fairness and trust.
- Determine performance expectations at all levels.
- Recruit, retain, and reward based on these expectations.
- Demand that staff "do what they say" and "earn their keep."
- Constantly review your psychological contracts (Kraines, 2009).

An important advantage of the psychological contract is in transitions at the personal level. If the validity of change is accepted in the recovery phase of the critical change sequence, a multilevel change may take a year or more (Figures 36.1 and 36.2).

Seen as a behavioral issue, all change is loss and coping with loss consumes physical, intellectual, and emotional energy. People in general go through some lengthy phases in this process from impact through disorganization and recovery, finally ending in reorganization. Without active leadership, this process can take years in a large organization because each level will go through these phases in sequence with each subsequent level not starting their process until the level above is in the recovery phase. If the change sequence can be accelerated to start in the impact phase and not the recovery phase, a change of similar complexity can be made over in months, not years.

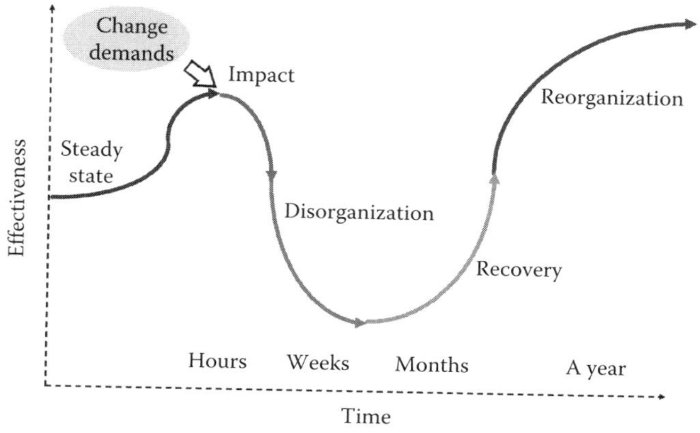

FIGURE 36.1 Critical change sequence.

* Medical Group Management Association Anesthesia Administration Assembly, Englewood, Colorado (www.mgma.com).
† American Association of Clinical Directors, Columbia, Maryland.
‡ American College of Physician Executives, Tampa, Florida.
§ The Greeley Company, Marblehead, Massachusetts.
¶ Operation Research for Surgical Service, Department of Anesthesia, University of Iowa, Iowa City, Iowa.
** The Levinson Institute, Boston, Massachusetts.

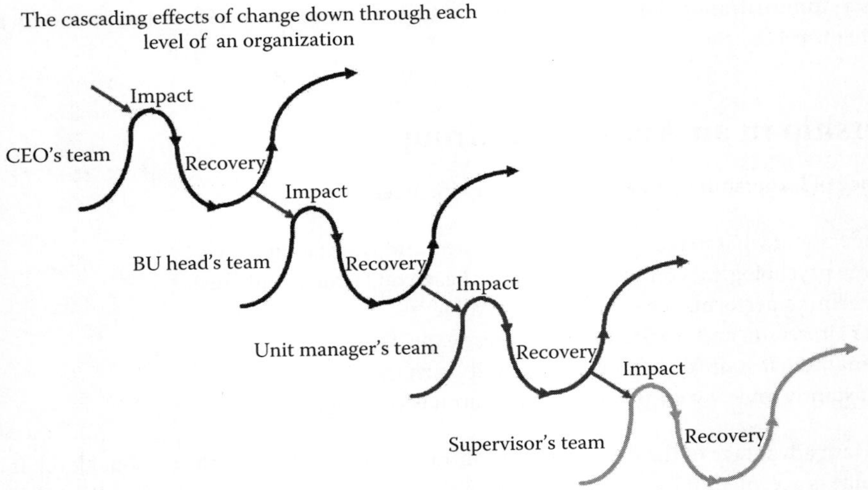

FIGURE 36.2 Critical factors in leading organizational change; cascading changes. (From Kraines, G.A. et al., Managing stress and leading change, in *Leadership for Physician Executives*, presented at the Harvard Medical School–Levinson Institute seminar, Boston, MA. With permission.)

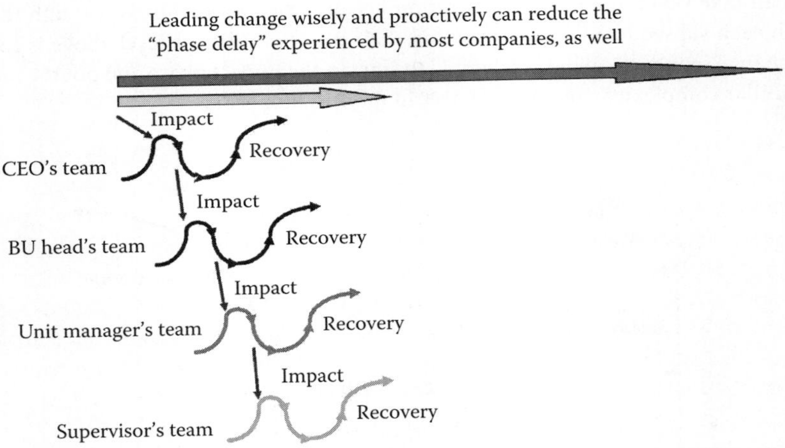

FIGURE 36.3 Critical factors in leading organizational change; aligning peoples' hearts and minds around change. (From Kraines, G.A. et al., Managing stress and leading change, in *Leadership for Physician Executives*, presented at the Harvard Medical School–Levinson Institute seminar, Boston, MA. With permission.)

The ability to accept change sooner rather later in the personal change sequence has the potential to yield results consistent with or better than positional authority.* Leadership, by gaining the "hearts and minds" of the staff, can reduce the intensity and duration of the dysfunction associated with change (Figures 36.3 and 36.4).

Remember, business skills are different than clinical skills (Desai et al., 2009). Advanced business skills education, including a master's degree in business administrations, could be a wise investment. Business education is not about interpreting contracts and reading balance sheets. Lawyers and accountants can be hired for these purposes. Team and accountability building as well as giving and

* The Levinson Institute, Boston, Massachusetts, Kraines et al. (2009).

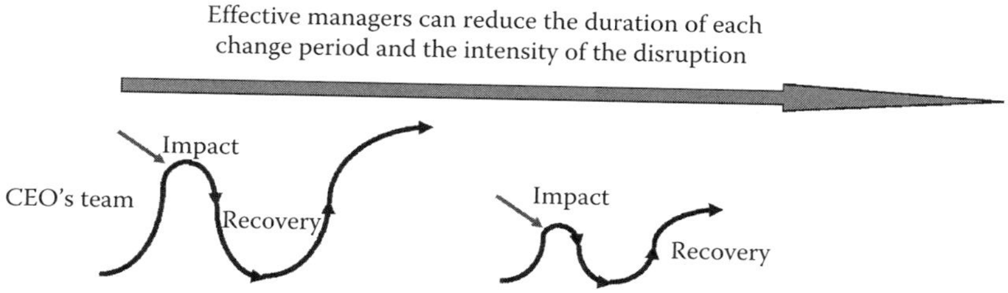

FIGURE 36.4 Critical factors in leading organizational change; aligning peoples' hearts and minds around change. (From Kraines, G.A. et al., Managing stress and leading change, in *Leadership for Physician Executives*, presented at the Harvard Medical School–Levinson Institute seminar, Boston, MA. With permission.)

taking feedback are the critical skills for the practicing anesthesiologist leader. Communication is critical at all levels as perception is reality until is either confirmed or corrected (Lockhart, 2009). Likewise, "get involved" leads to being members, and possibly actively, involved in national and state anesthesia organizations and local, state, and national medical organizations.

At a Crossroads...Again

Anesthesia is at crossroads. It has been suggested that there is conceptual evidence that the medical professions, including anesthesiology, are moving from professional status to that of a trade union. In this concept, a trade union is defined as a group of skilled individuals that delivers a product or service, while a profession not only provides a product or service, but also develops it through research and determines how it is delivered. As external pressures have increased, professional autonomy has been seen as a limitation to economic stability and responsiveness in healthcare. Attempts to control autonomy have come from a number of sources, including governmental and corporate entities, and in a number of different formats including safety initiatives (Miller, 2009).

From the perspective of the academic anesthesiologists, continued focus on excellence and innovation in research is considered to be fundamentally important. This is a vital component to the advancement of medicine and our profession that is as true today as it was in the past. Training in operations, teamwork, and team building, and giving and taking feedback may be critical to retention of our autonomy in the future.

Conclusion

- The disparity between the autonomy-based medical culture and positional authority–based medical facility administration culture leads to conflict.
- Anesthesia's history is influenced by the search for recognition as a medical specialty.
- Community anesthesia groups are primarily operated by locally owned entities.
- Legal and regulatory factors, including exclusive contracting, shape the operation of anesthesia departments.
- Clinical anesthesia skills do not equate to business leadership or management skills.
- Human resource management is critical to an anesthesia group.
- Change impacts anesthesia groups on an organizational and personal level.
- Effective leadership in anesthesia groups can replace the positional authority model of medical facilities.
- Leadership education and involvement in the medical community will play an important role in the continued autonomy of anesthesia practitioners.

References

Biersten, K. 1996. Loss of hospital privileges and the protection of the medical staff bylaws. *ASA Newsletter*, 60(7), www.asahq.org/Newsletters/1996/07_96/practice.htm

Bunker, J.P. 1972. *The Anesthesiologist and the Surgeon: Partners in the Operating Room*. Little and Brown, Boston, MA, pp. 2, 4, 55–56, 56–57.

Desai, A.M., R.A. Trillo, and A. Macario Jr. 2009. Should I get a master of business administration? The anesthesiologist with education training: Training options and professional opportunities. *Curr. Opin. Anaesthesiol.*, 22(2):191–198.

Dexter, F. and R.H. Epstein. 2006. Holiday and weekend operating room on-call staffing requirements. *Anesth. Analg.*, 103(6):1494–1498.

Dexter, F. and R.H. Epstein. 2008. Calculating institutional support that benefits both the anesthesia group and hospital. *Anesth. Analg.*, 106(2):544–553.

Drucker, P.R. 2005. Managing oneself. *Harvard Business Review*, January 2005, pp. 100–109.

Everett, P.C. 2009. Practice management M&M-lessons learned as an administrator turned consultant. In *American Society of Anesthesiologists, 2009 Conference on Practice Management*, Tampa, FL, p. 61.

Kraines, G. 2001. *Accountability Leadership*, Career Press, Franklin Lakes, NJ, p. 159.

Kraines, G. 2009. The practice of leading. In *Leadership for Physician Executives*, presented at the Harvard Medical School–Levinson Institute seminar, Boston, MA.

Kraines, G.A., T. Havens et al. 2009. Managing stress and leading change. In *Leadership for Physician Executives*, presented at the Harvard Medical School–Levinson Institute seminar, Boston, MA.

Kumar, K. 2009. Results of the RAND survey of ASA members. In *American Society of Anesthesiologists, Conference on Practice Management*, Tampa, FL, p. 111.

Lennon, R., R.L. Lennon, and D.R. Bacon. 2009. The anaesthetists' travel club: An example of professionalism. *J. Clin. Anesth.*, 20(2):140.

Lockhart, ASA. 2009. Lessons from bad situations. In *American Society of Anesthesiologists, 2009 Conference on Practice Management*, Tampa, FL, p. 67.

Lortie, D.C. 1946. Doctors without patients: The anesthesiologist—A new medical specialist. Master dissertation, The University of Chicago, Chicago, IL.

Macario, A. 2006. Are your hospital operating rooms "efficient"? A scoring system with eight performance indicators. *Anesthesiology*, 105(2):237–240.

McIntosh, C.A. and A. Macario. 2009. Managing quality in an anesthesia department. *Curr. Opin. Anaesthesiol.*, 22(2):223–231.

Miller, R. 2009. The pursuit of excellence. *Anesthesiology*, 110(4):714–715.

Modern Healthcare, September 23, 1991, p. 29.

Morf, C. 2009. Personal Communication.

Mountford, J. and C. Webb. 2009. When clinicians lead. *The McKinsey Quarterly*, http://www.mckinseyquarterly.com/When_clinicians_lead_2293

Mueller, C.B. and G.A. Evarts. 2002. *The Life, Lives and Times of the Surgical Spirit of St. Louis*, BC Decker, Inc., Hamilton, Ontario, Canada.

Neelon, F. "Contributor: Frank Neelon Chief Resident: 1969–1970", Eugene A. Stead Jr. A life of chasing what I did not understand, http://easteadjr.org/frank_neelon.html

Peisch, R. 1995. When outsourcing goes awry. *Harvard Business Review*, May–June, pp. 24–37.

Salvadores, P., J. Schneider, and I. Zubero. 2001. Theoretical and perceived balance of power inside Spanish public hospitals. *BMC Health Serv. Res.* 1(1):9.

Sermo, J.J. 2008. Our hospital wants to employ us: Now what? In *American Society of Anesthesiologists, 2008 Conference on Practice Management*, Tampa, FL.
Snow, S.J. 2008. *Blessed Days of Anesthesia*. Oxford University Press, New York, pp. xiv, 179.
Upton, J. 2009. Wallace Personal Correspondence.
Waters, R.M. 1919. The down town anesthesia clinic. *Am. J. Surg. Anesth.*, 33(Suppl.):71–72.
Watkins, M. 2003. *The First 90 Days*, Harvard Business School Press, Boston, MA, pp. 52–55, 66.

Design, Planning, Control, and Management of Healthcare Systems

IV.G Decontamination Service

37 **Turnovers and Turnarounds in the Healthcare System** *June M. Worley and Toni L. Doolen*......37-1
Introduction • Task Overview • Conclusion • References

38 **Decontamination Service** *Peter F. Hooper*......38-1
Introduction • Definitions • Where Should Decontamination Be Performed? • Instrument Life Cycle • Cleaning • Disinfection • Sterilization • Monitoring • Summary

37

Turnovers and Turnarounds in the Healthcare System

June M. Worley
Oregon State University

Toni L. Doolen
Oregon State University

Introduction 37-1
Task Overview 37-2
Operating Room Turnover • Hospital Bed Turnaround
Conclusion 37-6
References 37-7

Introduction

The medical field, though familiar to most people from a patient perspective, is an industry unto itself, with many characteristics shared with non-medical environments. The necessary support functions that are performed on a daily basis provide examples of tasks that, though performed within the context of medicine, are very similar to tasks in a variety of other industries. One of those important functions is the cleaning and setup of rooms.

In the medical field, the cleaning and setup functions of the operating room are commonly referred to as a turnover. The cleaning and setup functions of a hospital bed and/or room, however, are most commonly referred to as a turnaround. (A hospital bed turnover is usually associated with a broader hospital performance measurement that incorporates the average number of patients each hospital bed contains in a given time period (Osborn 2007).) Though the terminology may be different, both turnarounds and turnovers have been cited as key factors in patient throughput and bed capacity and are subsequently important to hospital operations.

During the 1990s, most hospitals saw a declining demand for beds. More recently, however, population growth, aging baby boomers, staffing shortages, and general inefficiencies within the medical system itself have found hospitals struggling with a lack of bed space (Kirby and Kjesbo 2003). More than 90% of hospitals with 300 or more beds have reported being at or over capacity (Mitchell 2009).

The bed capacity of a hospital impacts many areas within the hospital. Overcrowding in the emergency department is often attributed to lack of bed capacity (Kirby and Kjesbo 2003; Healthcare Excellence Institute). An overcrowded emergency department in turn can lead to patients being diverted to other hospitals (Healthcare Excellence Institute 2009; Kirby and Kjesbo 2003; Scalise 2006; WOWT 6 News 2005). In addition, some patients may leave without receiving needed care (Meditech 2008; O'Hare and McElroy 2007; Scalise 2006). Hospitals may also need to defer referrals or direct admissions from physicians (Kirby and Kjesbo 2003). All of these factors may combine to significantly influence revenue streams. One study estimated that ambulance diversions and patients leaving without being seen may have resulted in a yearly revenue loss of $3.8 million for one hospital (Falvo et al. 2007).

In the operating room, the lack of bed capacity in the hospital system often requires surgeries to be postponed or canceled (American Health Consultants 2002). Such practices can have significant financial impact as the operating room is estimated to generate 42% of hospital revenue (Lange-Kuitse and Meadows 2002). At times, patients may be held in the operating room, recovery room, or intensive care unit until a bed is available (Cendan and Good 2006; Healthcare Excellence Institute; Kirby and Kjesbo 2003; McGowan et al. 2007). Lack of bed capacity, in addition to other factors, was cited in a recent study that estimated approximately five working days a month may be lost in operating room utilization (Cendan and Good 2006). It is estimated that adding just one case per week to an operating room schedule could increase hospital profit by $100,000 per year per operating room (Maleki and Kram 2005).

With bed space at a premium, hospitals have been forced to look for solutions. Physically adding hospital beds is expensive, with an average cost of $1 million per bed (Kirby and Kjesbo 2003; McKesson Information Solutions 2006). Instead, some hospitals have chosen to review processes and manage patient throughput and bed capacity. Often, hospital bed turnaround is a focus of improvement efforts, with particular focus placed on the communication of bed status and the efficient dispatching of resources (Awarix 2006; Conger 2004; Hospital of the University of Pennsylvania 2006; Kirby and Kjesbo 2003; McGowan et al. 2007; McKesson Information Solutions 2006; Meditech 2008; Mitchell 2009; Pellicone and Martocci 2006; VanEssen and Reese 2008; WOWT 6 News 2005). Likewise, many hospitals have also focused on operating room turnaround as one factor that could be improved to ensure better utilization of the operating rooms (Cendan and Good 2006; Friedman et al. 2006; Maleki and Kram 2005).

Bed turnarounds and operating room turnovers have both been cited as factors in patient throughput. Though the two processes share common tasks related to cleaning and setup, each also possess characteristics that are unique to their environments. An overview of the tasks illustrates these differences.

Task Overview

Operating Room Turnover

The turnover of an operating room is defined as all processes that occur between the time a patient exits the room until the room is ready to receive the next patient (Dexter 2003; de Deyne and Heylen 2004). This time period includes all cleaning tasks associated with a completed surgery as well as all setup tasks for the next surgical procedure. The operating room turnover is completed by personnel with defined roles: the scrub person, the circulator, and, in some organizations, housekeeping.

The scrub person is either a registered nurse (RN) or a surgical technologist. The primary duty of a surgical technologist is to act as a scrub person and maintain the sterile field (the area immediately surrounding the patient) during the surgical procedure as well as other related duties during the surgery. During the turnover process, the scrub person is responsible, with the circulator, for managing the cleaning and setting up of the room. The circulator is either a circulating nurse or a surgical technologist who is under the supervision of an RN. During the surgery, the circulator is responsible for monitoring and coordinating all activities within the room and managing the care of the patient. In some organizations, housekeeping personnel are also utilized in the turnover of an operating room.

The division of duties between the scrub person and the circulator is defined in nursing textbooks (Atkinson and Fortunato 1996), but these roles may not be as clearly defined or standardized in actual operating room environments (Mormann et al. 2002; Shumpert et al. 1995). The procedures, however, are very clearly defined, and while the person(s) completing these tasks may vary, the tasks are fairly standardized for hospitals in the United States.

After the patient has exited the room, the turnover begins with the dismantling of the sterile field, usually by a scrub person. All contaminated, disposable equipment is discarded in appropriate containers. Reusable equipment and surgical instruments are placed in an area for sterilization after removal of all bodily wastes (such as blood, tissue, and bone). Equipment that is too large to be sterilized in standard sterilization equipment is placed in plastic bags and transported to a decontamination area. All solutions are also disposed of in a designated area. All used, disposable table drapes are placed in plastic bags. Fabric drapes, even if unused, are placed in a designated area to be laundered. After the sterile field has been dismantled, the scrub person discards his/her gown, gloves, cap, mask, and shoe covers before helping with the remainder of the cleaning. These cleaning tasks include decontamination of furniture and/or walls, disinfection of operating lights, collection and sorting of waste, and wet-vacuuming of the floor.

Once the room has been cleaned and all surfaces are dry, the setup for the next surgery can begin. All personnel involved with the turnover work together to ensure that the operating table is readied and positioned. All trash bins, laundry bins, and hazardous waste containers are put into place. Furniture and equipment are properly positioned. After these duties are completed, the scrub person dons gown and gloves and begins to construct the sterile field by draping the tables, preparing and arranging instruments and accessory items, and counting sponges, surgical needles, and other sharp objects with another member of the turnover team (Figure 37.1).

The tasks associated with an operating room turnover are detailed, and the order of tasks is specific to the environment. Most tasks are performed by nursing personnel. In contrast, many tasks associated with a hospital bed turnaround are performed by housekeeping staff.

Hospital Bed Turnaround

One definition of a hospital bed turnaround includes all activities that occur from the time discharge instructions are given to a patient until the time the admitting RN is made aware of a clean and ready bed (Pellicone and Martocci 2006). For the purposes of this review, the tasks involved in the actual discharge of the patient and all subsequent communications related to bed management have been excluded as these procedures can vary greatly depending on the technology employed by the hospital.

As with an operating room turnover, though documentation exists as to roles and tasks, the specifics may vary between organizations. For example, in some organizations, nurses may be responsible for making the beds, while in other organizations, this may be completed by housekeeping staff (College of Knowledge ISSA Hospital Housekeeping Training Manual 2009; Pellicone and Martocci 2006). It should also be noted that the cleaning procedures for a room containing a patient infected with a highly contagious or dangerous disease would be different. At one hospital, in cases such as this, housekeeping is directed to consult with the hospital epidemiologist prior to cleaning (University of Connecticut Health Center 2008).

Before housekeeping begins cleaning a room, nursing personnel are to contain and discard all blood or other bodily fluids. Nursing personnel are to place all nondisposable items in the appropriate bin for later sterilization. All used disposable items associated with patient care, such as IV tubings, are also to be discarded by nursing staff.

Housekeeping is responsible for dusting, cleaning all surfaces, and disinfecting any items that may have come in direct contact with the patient. Wastebaskets are emptied and disinfected. Likewise, all furniture, including drawers, telephone, tables, chairs, light switches, and door knobs are disinfected. After removal of the linen, the patient bed itself is disinfected by damp wiping all surfaces, including the exposed springs under the mattress. The clean bed linen is placed on the bed. The walls are inspected and spot cleaned as required. As a last step, the floor is mopped (Figure 37.2).

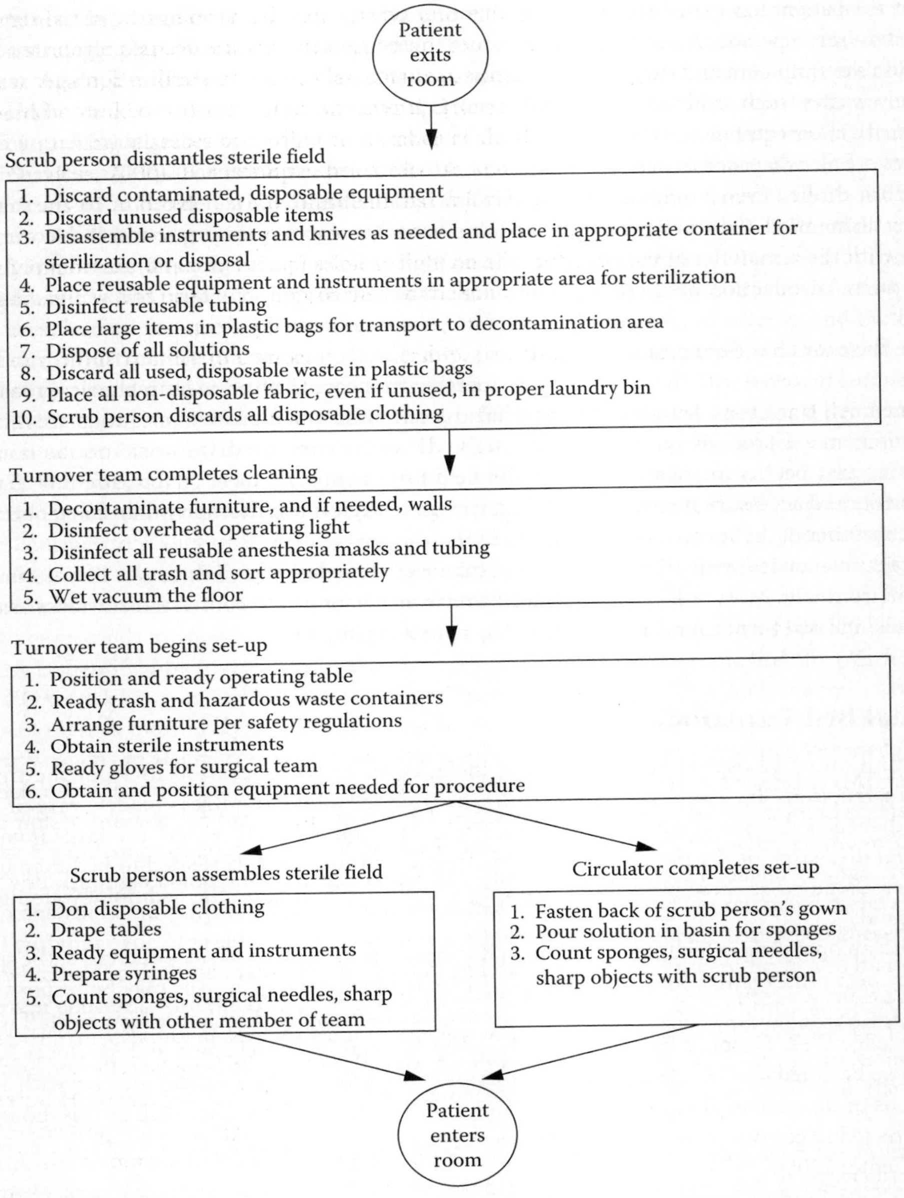

FIGURE 37.1 High-level flow diagram of an operating room turnover.

Though both bed turnarounds and operating room turnovers would appear to essentially accomplish the same tasks, it is clear that the environment dictates different processes for each. The staffing roles are also different, with nursing staff primarily responsible for the operating room turnover, while most of the tasks in a bed turnaround are the domain of housekeeping personnel. Though the cleaning tasks are very similar, the setup tasks are necessarily different. It is also interesting to note that during an operating room turnover, a clear distinction is made between cleaning and setup activities. The hospital bed turnaround, however, has setup activities occurring as cleaning activities are completed.

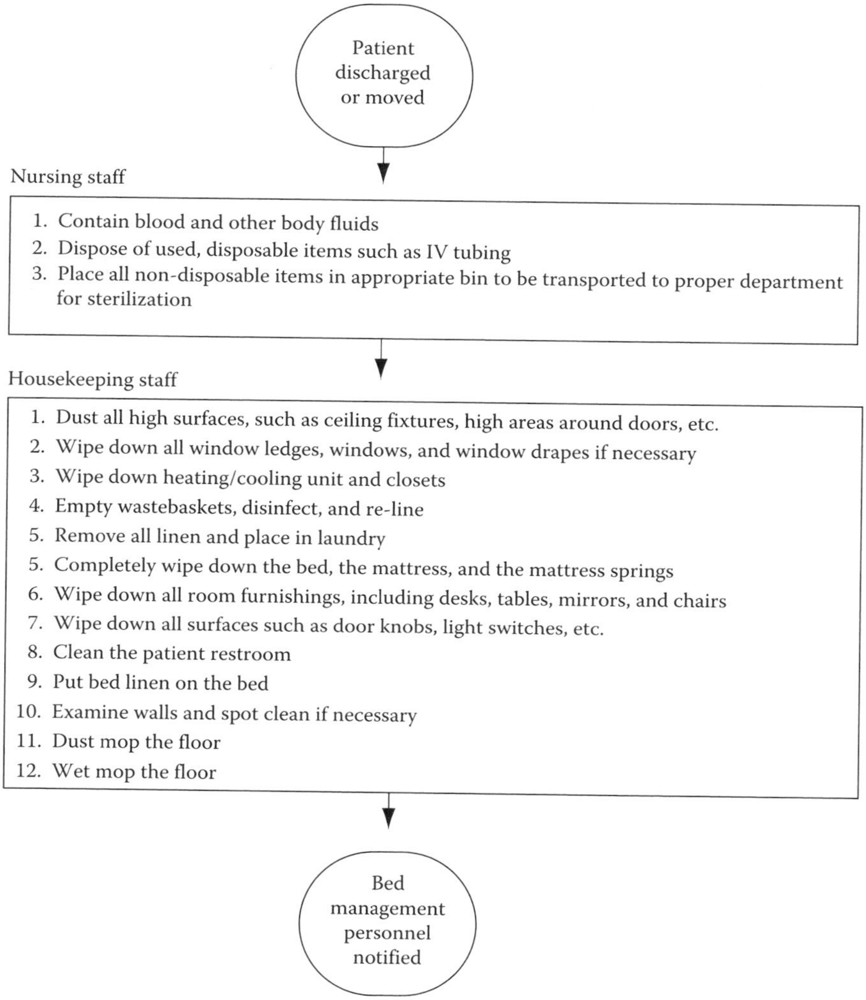
Patient discharged or moved
Nursing staff
1. Contain blood and other body fluids
2. Dispose of used, disposable items such as IV tubing
3. Place all non-disposable items in appropriate bin to be transported to proper department for sterilization
Housekeeping staff
1. Dust all high surfaces, such as ceiling fixtures, high areas around doors, etc.
2. Wipe down all window ledges, windows, and window drapes if necessary
3. Wipe down heating/cooling unit and closets
4. Empty wastebaskets, disinfect, and re-line
5. Remove all linen and place in laundry
5. Completely wipe down the bed, the mattress, and the mattress springs
6. Wipe down all room furnishings, including desks, tables, mirrors, and chairs
7. Wipe down all surfaces such as door knobs, light switches, etc.
8. Clean the patient restroom
9. Put bed linen on the bed
10. Examine walls and spot clean if necessary
11. Dust mop the floor
12. Wet mop the floor
Bed management personnel notified

FIGURE 37.2 High-level flow diagram for a hospital bed turnaround.

Case Study of an Operating Room Turnover

In an effort to better understand the turnover process, observations were conducted at an ambulatory surgery center. Ambulatory surgery centers, also known as out-patient surgery centers, typically have much shorter turnover times when compared to hospital environments. Some of this may be attributed to the lack of in-patient facilities and the corresponding lack of bed capacity that has been previously noted to significantly impact operating room flow. Another factor is the ability of the surgery center to schedule similar specialties for the same day, facilitating equipment flow. For example, a surgical suite may have only orthopedic surgeries scheduled on a particular day or during a particular block of time on one day.

The observed surgery center typically utilizes two surgical suites that operate simultaneously. This surgery center has a turnover goal of 8 minutes. For all observed turnovers, surgical personnel began the cleaning tasks 3–5 minutes prior to the patient leaving the surgical suite. These cleaning tasks included bringing out the equipment to be sterilized and the fluids and trash that required disposal. Typically, by the time the patient left the room, breakdown of the sterile field had been completed and decontamination had already begun. This differs from guidelines documented in the literature but does not appear to violate safety standards.

Setup of the operating room, after completion of cleaning and disinfection activities, did occur as documented in the literature, with careful attention paid to construction of the sterile field. As soon as setup was completed, the patient was wheeled into the room.

After the last surgery of the day, the surgical team removed all trash and equipment that did not belong in the surgical suite and re-stocked the room with supplies for the next day. All further cleaning was left to housekeeping. At the end of each day, housekeeping was responsible for wiping down every surface in the suite, including lamps, walls, and floors. This function was performed daily.

During most observations, the surgical team members quickly shifted into turnover mode and completed the cleaning and setup tasks within 20 minutes. Sometimes, if the surgeon had scheduled subsequent procedures, the patient was in the room before the surgeon had finished dictation on the previous patient. Teamwork clearly played a large part in the efficiency of the turnover process. One of the RNs acted as a float on one observation day, filling in as needed. On another occasion, one of the surgeons helped with the cleaning of the room to facilitate the process. Though the circulator and scrub person roles were observed to maintain sterility, the team worked together in whatever capacity was needed to complete the turnovers quickly.

During the observations of the turnovers at the ambulatory surgery center, the difference in teamwork observed at the surgery center and a typical hospital operating room was discussed with the staff. The turnovers were not considered to be typical of most operating room turnovers, especially those occurring in hospital environments. In particular, the ambulatory surgery center personnel noted that the team's ability to initiate the turnover processes at the end of the procedure and the surgeon's role in facilitating and even helping with the turnover were not considered to be the norm in most hospital settings. Though some previous researchers have linked a reduction in operating room turnover time and effective teamwork (Friedman et al. 2006), it has been noted that healthcare professionals are not usually provided training in teamwork (Hyer et al. 2000) and may be reluctant to adopt aspects of it (Powell and Hill 2006). The outcome from the teamwork of this turnover team was apparent, however, and appeared to be a key factor in enabling more efficient processes and in improving patient throughput.

Conclusion

The tasks related to an operating room turnover and a bed turnaround are similar in nature, but in actual practice, the associated specifics are quite unique. The environments dictate different roles and different setup procedures, especially in the operating room where the processes must be followed in a specific order to avoid contamination or re-contamination of sterile areas. Both processes also play an important role in patient safety. Poor disinfection or management of bodily fluids can result in serious infection and other medical complications. Though very practical and seemingly straightforward in nature, the consequences of an inadequate cleaning and/or setup can have devastating consequences for a patient or a member of the healthcare staff. Bed turnarounds and operating room turnovers may appear to be mundane processes but are, nonetheless, critical to the efficient and safe operation of any hospital.

References

American Health Consultants, Inc. 2002. Hospital bed utilization management team tackles 'Bed Crunch' problem. *Hospital Case Management* 10(11):161–176.

Atkinson, L. J. and N. Fortunato. 1996. *Operating Room Technique*. 8th edn. St. Louis, MO: Mosby.

Awarix. 2006. Hospital Bed Management System Adds RFID [cited July 29, 2009]. Available from www.usingrfid.com/news/read.asp?lc=t86719kx79zi

Cendan, J. C. and M. Good. 2006. Interdisciplinary work flow assessment and redesign decreases operating room turnover time and allows for additional caseload. *Archives of Surgery* 141(1):65–70.

College of Knowledge ISSA Hospital Housekeeping Training Manual. 2009. *Health Care Cleaning and Sanitation Procedures Module* [cited July 29, 2009]. Available from www.huskybrand.com/documents/pdfs/h12.pdf

Conger, K. 2009. Packard's new 'Bed Board' program boosts efficiency. Stanford Report, Standford University: Stanford, CA [cited July 29, 2009]. Available from http://news.stanford.edu/news/medical/2004/february11/bed.html

de Deyne, C. and R. Heylen. 2004. Introduction of an operating room information management system improved overall operating room efficiency. *Studies in Health Technology and Informatics* 110:61–67.

Dexter, F. 2003. Operating room utilization: Information management systems. *Current Opinion in Anaesthesiology* 16(6):619–622.

Falvo, T., L. Grove, R. Stachura, D. Vega, R. Stike, M. Schlenker, and W. Zirkin. 2007. The opportunity loss of boarding admitted patients in the emergency department. *Academic Emergency Medicine* 14(4):333–337.

Friedman, D. M., S. M. Sokal, Y. Chang, and D. L. Berger. 2006. Increasing operating room efficiency through parallel processing. *Annals of Surgery* 243(1):10–14.

Healthcare Excellence Institute, Inc. 2009. *Bed Management: Decreasing Bed Turn Around Times by 30%*. Overland Park, KS/Phoenix, AZ [cited July 29, 2009]. Available from www.sixsigmasystems.com/healthcare/casestudy-bed-management.htm

Hospital of the University of Pennsylvania. 2006. Patient flow project: Achieving top utilization for all our resources. *HUP* 17(2). www.uphs.upenn.edu/news/publications/HUPdate/files/HUPdate_2006_01_20.pdf

Hyer, K., S. Fairchild, I. Abraham, M. Mezey, and T. Fulmer. 2000. Measuring attitudes related to interdisciplinary training: Revisiting the Heinemann, Schmitt and Farrell 'attitudes toward health care teams' scale. *Journal of Interprofessional Care* 14(3):249–258.

Kirby, A. and A. Kjesbo. 2003. Tapping into hidden hospital bed capacity. *Healthcare Financial Management* 57(11):38–41.

Lange-Kuitse, D. and G. Meadows. 2002. Applying information technologies to pump up operating room efficiency. *Information Systems & Technology* 20(5):249–251.

Maleki, R. and M. Kram. 2005. Operating Room Turnover Analysis and Improvement. Paper read at Institute of Industrial Engineering Society for Health Systems.

McGowan, J. E., J. D. Truwit, P. Cipriano, E. Howell, M. VanBree Jr., G. Arthur, and J. B. Hanks. 2007. Operating room efficiency and hospital capacity: Factors affecting operating room use during maximum hospital census. *Journal of the American College of Surgeons* 204(5):865–871.

McKesson Information Solutions. 2009. Tackling the capacity crisis: Successful bed management strategies [cited July 29, 2009]. Available from www.hfma.org/NR/rdonlyres/E581803B-4E58-4E41-8E5A-DE4F4E262322/0/hfma_bedmgmt.pdf

Meditech. 2008. *MEDITECH and Forward Advantage Boost Greenwich Hospital's Bed Turnover Rates*. Medical Information Technology, Inc.: Westwood, MA [cited July 29, 2009]. Available from www.meditech.com/aboutmeditech.pages/customerachievegreenwichbedboard.htm

Mitchell, R. N. 2009. Bed tracking improves productivity, staff morale. *Advance for Health Information Executives* [cited July 29, 2009]. Available from http://health-care-it.advanceweb.com/Editorial/Content/PrintFriendly.aspx?CC=42473

Mormann, L. H., L. Nowel, P. Sponberg, P. G. F. Meckes, P. Giblin, J. A. Kidd, M. O'Connor, and J. Gray. 2002. *DACUM Research Chart for Operating Room Circulating Nurse*. Grossmont College Leadership and Economic Development Institute: El Cajon, CA.

O'Hare, D. and L. McElroy. 2007. Collaborative model leads to improved patient flow. *Patient Safety and Quality Healthcare*. Lionheart Publishing, Inc.: Marietta, GA [cited July 29, 2009]. Available from www.psqh.com/novdec07/flow.html

Osborn, C. E. 2007. *Essentials of Statistics in Health Information Technology*. 1st edn. Jones & Bartlett: Boston, MA.

Pellicone, A. and M. Martocci. 2006. Faster turnaround time. *Quality Progress*, March, 31–36. www.asq.org/healthcaresixsigma/pdf/qp0306pellicone.pdf

Powell, S. M. and R. K. Hill. 2006. My copilot is a nurse: Using crew resource management in the OR. *AORN Journal* 83(1):179–206.

Scalise, D. 2006. Improving patient throughput. *Hospitals and Health Networks* 80(11):49–54.

Shumpert, A., H. Smith, M. Voorhees, T. Buick, D. Keray, J. Robertson, R. Amaro, D. Bell, C. Bowsky, J. Gray, and J. Demos. 1995. *DACUM Competency Profile for Surgical Technologist*. Saddleback College: Mission Viejo, CA.

University of Connecticut Health Center. 2008. *Cleaning of Patient Rooms: Inpatient and Temporary*. John Dempsey Hospital, Infection Control Manual: Farmington, CT [cited July 29, 2009]. Available from http://nursing.uchc.edu/infection_control/manual/docus/ICM%202.5.pdf

VanEssen, D. and J. Reese. 2008. *Patient Progression: Connecting the Dots for Seamless Patient Care*. The Children's Hospital [cited July 29, 2009]. Available from www.thechildrenshospital.org/news/publications/tchnews/2008/Patient-Progression.aspx

WOWT 6 News. 2005. *Emergency Room Overcrowding*. Gray Television Group, Inc.: Atlanta, GA [cited July 29, 2009]. Available from www.wowt.com/news/features/2/1492392.html

38

Decontamination Service

Introduction 38-1
Definitions 38-2
Decontamination • Cleaning • Disinfection • Sterilization
Where Should Decontamination Be Performed? 38-3
Instrument Life Cycle 38-4
Instrument Purchase • Introduction into Use • Point of Use • Collection and Return to CSSD • Cleaning • Preparation for Sterilization • Sterilization • Storage • Delivery to Point of Use
Cleaning 38-6
Manual Cleaning • Automated Cleaning: Ultrasonic Cleaners • Automated Cleaning: Thermal Washer Disinfectors
Disinfection 38-6
Sterilization 38-7
Sterilization Kinetics • Steam: Properties • Steam: Sterilizers • Dry Heat Sterilizers • Low-Temperature Sterilizers • Choice of Sterilizing Process
Monitoring 38-10
Summary 38-11

Peter F. Hooper
Central Sterilising Club

Introduction

While many countries throughout the world have particular infection problems, the task of infection prevention and control is surely global. The basic principles are applicable on a worldwide basis. This is no more relevant than to the decontamination of medical devices used in surgical procedures. Instruments that are not decontaminated properly can act as a vector of transmission for minor and, unfortunately, fatal conditions. There is thus a need for a set of decontamination procedures that are universal in the sense that the type and degree of possible contamination on a reusable instrument need not be known prior to reprocessing. This universal—or standard—set of precautions must therefore be based on the worst-case scenario, so that if patients are protected from that situation then all other conditions will be suitably treated.

Such a set of procedures are naturally resource-hungry and require a great deal of input from that most difficult-to-control resource: human beings. Assessments of decontamination practice uncover a wide variety of procedures and practices that respond to local, national, or regional constraints as well as to widely differing resource availability within healthcare facilities. Decontamination is required in every type of facility from the largest general hospital to the smallest local clinic, but the complexities of the task remain the same.

It is tempting to suggest that the sole purpose of decontamination is patient safety, but it must be remembered that healthcare workers will be handling instruments throughout their use and reuse, and thus decontamination is also important for the protection of healthcare workers. Just as the use of instruments in theater is a job for qualified surgeons, it is suggested that the decontamination of instruments is a task that should be performed by decontamination professionals. While resources may require those healthcare providers to decontaminate instruments at the point of use, experience indicates that the complexities of decontamination, the retention of its records and documentation, and the management of staff undertaking the task is best performed within a department dedicated to decontamination performed by staff who are employed full time in that duty.

There is a wide variety of regulation to be applied to decontamination. Some countries have national legislation that require decontamination to be performed to certain defined standards, and some regions of the world similarly define a level of performance not only to be achieved but also to be evidenced by documentation and paperwork traceable for a lengthy period after any surgical procedure. Those performing decontamination must therefore be aware of any such constraints, be they local, national, or regional before they commence the task. Regulation may appear as legislation or guidance, but reference to standards—regional or international—will aid those manufacturing decontamination equipment as well as those using the equipment to achieve the required levels of performance. National government bodies or agencies may also provide policy statements or additional requirements to meet particular national difficulties. Clearly, where such problems could have wide-reaching consequences or cause concern on a global scale, the universality of decontamination procedures may be affected. As the community of decontamination achieves a global status, the networking of national associations and the World Wide Web has enabled greater discussion on these topics.

While local responses to these problems may differ, this chapter discusses the general principles of decontamination and accepts that their application will differ from hospital to hospital.

Definitions

It is difficult to discuss decontamination without using some precision in the meanings of the terms used. Such precision will enable equipment to be manufactured and tested and will also allow practitioners to produce method statements and operating procedures so that everyone involved in the decontamination process can be monitored and checked and relevant improvements made from time to time.

The following definitions are useful.

Decontamination

Decontamination is a set of procedures applied to reusable surgical instruments or medical devices to make them safe between use on one patient and reuse on another patient. The set of procedures may include a combination of cleaning, disinfection, and sterilization. The combination will depend upon many aspects of the instrument's design, construction and use, and instructions for decontamination of a particular device should be provided by the manufacturer/supplier at the time of purchase.

Cleaning

Cleaning is the act of removing visible soil from a surgical instrument. This may be performed manually or automatically. It should be noted that cleaning is unlikely to remove all soil, hence the need for further treatment. It should also be noted that cleaning is essential to the success of any later stage in the decontamination process.

Disinfection

Disinfection is the reduction of bioburden on a surgical instrument. This is often performed either thermally or chemically but will not necessarily destroy spores. The level of bioburden reduction is not universally defined, and thus it may be necessary to state the required log reduction in order for a particular process to be defined, validated, and tested.

Sterilization

Sterilization is a process that destroys or removes all living material. This definition is ideal for dictionaries but is not really practical for the purpose of designing and validating sterilization processes. As will be seen below sterilization processes, work in a statistical and probabilistic manner and thus the practical definition of sterilization will involve a probability of survival and a defined sterility assurance level.

Where Should Decontamination Be Performed?

The ubiquity of sterilization has been discussed in "Introduction" section. Wherever reusable surgical instruments are employed, there will be a need for decontamination. However, in order to perform the task in the safest and most efficient manner, a degree of specialization will be required. The question of location effectively reduces to a choice of two locations:

- At the point of use
- In a specialized decontamination unit

The former option benefits from the proximity of the decontamination site while the latter option benefits from the function of a dedicated unit. As the complexity of decontamination increases, areas designed for patient treatment may not necessarily have the space, utilities, and engineering services required. Conversely, the difficulties of collection, transportation, and distribution to and from a dedicated unit present their own difficulties. It is possible, however, to guide planners in the right direction when the requirements of decontamination are listed. An ideal decontamination unit, wherever it is placed, should achieve a number of conditions including the following:

- Segregate dirty instruments and clean instruments.
- Have restricted access only to those performing decontamination.
- Have a linear flow through the department.
- Provide controlled environmental condition in two areas the dirty area should be controlled so that contamination will not "leak" to the clean area, and the clean area should be controlled so that adventitious recontamination during packing or preparation for sterilization does not occur.
- Indication should be provided if these environmental controls fail so that, if necessary, decontamination can be stopped.
- Reprocessed surgical instruments, where packaged prior to sterilization, can be stored safely in conditions that maintain the pack's sterility during storage.

These conditions imply that the decontamination unit should be specifically designed and requires a high degree of engineering input. The economy of scale suggests, therefore, that some centralization is beneficial to the healthcare organization, its staff and, of course, its patients. Where local constraints inhibit this centralization, the principles applied above should equally apply. If this is not possible, then the organization should perform a risk assessment of the shortfalls and determine whether it can carry the subsequent responsibilities. This does not mean that local or "point-of-use" decontamination is not possible. Clearly, a great degree of healthcare provision would cease if this were so. However, any increase in patient risk owing to the performance of decontamination in unsuitable areas or facilities should be considered.

A large hospital/medical facility would thus be expected to centralize the reprocessing of its medical devices in a dedicated department, usually called a central sterile supply department (CSSD). There may, however, be some exceptions to this centralization. The major exception would be the decontamination of flexible endoscopes. Because of the materials of their construction, flexible endoscopes may not be compatible with the sterilization processes used in the CSSD, particularly steam sterilization. For this reason, these devices will commonly be cleaned and disinfected only in dedicated endoscope washer disinfectors (EWDs). These machines will usually be sited in the department where flexible endoscopes are used. A large medical facility may well contain a number of such units and thus there may be an option to centralize the decontamination of flexible endoscopes within a centralized unit dedicated to this task. Alternatively, new technologies have led to new low-temperature sterilization processes to which flexible endoscopes may be compatible. Such sterilizers could be sited locally or within a CSSD, but it must be remembered that the flow paths and requirements for flexible endoscopes may differ from that of stainless steel instruments. Specific centralization of local decontamination of flexible endoscopes may thus be considered, but the operating principles of the CSSD should equally apply.

Other exceptions that form the consideration of centralization could include the decontamination of instruments used in mortuary prosection or for tissue retrieval. Opinions differ regarding the problems of mixing such instruments with those used directly with patients and thus an option appraisal considering the advantages and disadvantages of mixing instrument streams should be considered.

Instrument Life Cycle

The decontamination of surgical instruments is a sequential process including a combination of cleaning, disinfection, and sterilization. The method of implementing these stages should consider the stages of the life cycle of the instruments themselves so that the decontamination stages are performed at the correct place in the correct manner.

The life-cycle stages are as follows.

Instrument Purchase

It is tempting to imagine that decontamination plays no part in the procurement of medical devices but it is, in fact, extremely relevant to the first stage of the instrument life cycle. It is pointless purchasing an instrument for which the relevant decontamination process is not available on site. Thus prepurchase consideration should be given to the prospective manufacturer's decontamination recommendations and instructions and checking that such processes are currently in place. If they are not, then the organization may consider purchasing the relevant process or, alternatively, utilizing an alternative provider where the required equipment is already on site. The use of prepurchase questionnaires and the perusal of decontamination instructions prior to purchase are essential. In some parts of the world, manufacturers are obliged to provide such instructions. Where this is not a requirement, some research and liaison may be required. By definition, those medical devices that are designated as "single use" are not designed to be reprocessed although resource issues may lead to their reuse and subsequent reprocessing. Differing regulations can be found worldwide on the reuse of single-use devices, but where allowed it should be performed with care. Absence of decontamination instructions for single-use devices may place the responsibility for the safety of reprocessed single-use devices with the reprocessing organization.

Introduction into Use

Devices should be fully decontaminated in accordance with manufacturer instructions prior to use.

Point of Use

The responsibility for unwrapping and using decontaminated medical devices lies with the user, but they do have a part to play in their life cycle. Packaging may include advice and instructions that should be followed. Additionally information from packaging providing traceability information should be utilized either automatically via dataloggers or scanners or manually in a longhand fashion. After use, local instructions regarding rewrapping and preparation for collection should be employed. Where a dedicated CSSD is used initial decontamination at the point of use may not be necessary.

Collection and Return to CSSD

Used instruments should be placed at an agreed position for collection. Transportation to the CSSD should be performed in such a way that contamination of surroundings, staff, and visitors does not occur. Similarly, instruments should be delivered to the CSSD dirty returns without penetrating the controlled dirty area.

Cleaning

Returned instruments should be transferred by washroom staff from the returns lobby to the washroom where they will be inspected and separated for the differing cleaning processes defined below. This stage should also include drying.

Preparation for Sterilization

Instruments should now be in a controlled clean room/area where they should be inspected for cleanliness. Any instrument not fully cleaned should be returned for re-cleaning. Functionality should also be checked. Instruments may be combined with new raw materials and packaged for sterilization.

Sterilization

The sterilization process may be one of a number of types including steam, dry heat, hydrogen peroxide gas plasma, ethylene oxide, low-temperature steam, and formaldehyde. The process used shall be chosen for compatibility and efficiency and the local definition of log reduction must be met. The process chosen should also be compatible with the packaging (or lack of it) utilized.

Storage

Theoretically, only instruments that have been sterilized in packaging may be stored before use. Such packaging should be inspected for dryness and viability after sterilization and then stored in suitable conditions for the relevant maximum period of time. Instruments sterilized in an unwrapped condition should, theoretically, be used immediately without storage. Any contravention of these conditions should, if approved, be risk assessed.

Delivery to Point of Use

Transportation should occur without impairing the validity of the packaging.

Traceability information and any other relevant documentation may be required at each of the stages above. Such traceability will enable a product release decision to be made at each stage and any instruments or sets not meeting requirements should be returned for reprocessing. This may well require return to the cleaning stage. The traceability will also enable the organization to validate instrument safety at the point of use and will also enable the organization to identify instruments and patients where instrument recall or known risk situations need to be met.

Cleaning

Cleaning requires the provision of three types of energy:

- Mechanical energy
- Thermal energy
- Chemical energy

Ideally, the provision of these three types of energy will be controlled, repeatable, and recorded.

Manual Cleaning

This is usually performed in a sink where human energy provides the requisite mechanical energy. The thermal energy is provided by the temperature of the water and the detergent will provide the chemical energy. Such a human process is not capable of validation but some variables can be controlled. A level line on the sink together with a defined amount of detergent will control the detergent concentration and a thermal control on the supply tap would control the thermal energy. Only the mechanical energy will not necessarily be repeatable although good training and management will be helpful.

Automated Cleaning: Ultrasonic Cleaners

This simple technology is particularly useful for cleaning those devices that are difficult to clean manually or where cannulations and internal lumens are included. Internal irrigation will be required for lumen devices. As with manual cleaning, instruments may require manual drying after this stage.

Automated Cleaning: Thermal Washer Disinfectors

With these machines, all stages of cleaning and thermal disinfection can be validated and repeatable. Cleaning is performed with a mixture of water and detergent and spray arms should ensure that all corners of the chamber are affected equally. Cleaning may be performed in two stages: a cool initial wash to remove gross soiling and a hot wash to complete the stage. Thermal disinfection can then be performed with purified water if necessary either by a specific time/temperature relationship or via a calculated thermal input. These machines may be single-or double-ended, where the latter will probably be sited in a barrier separating the dirty and clean areas. Such machines may also be single- or multichamber versions. In the former, all stages cleaning, disinfection, and drying will take place in the same chamber. In the latter, each stage may be performed in a separate chamber. This type will be able to simultaneously process different loads thus increasing decontamination capacity.

As stated above, this cleaning stage is vital to the whole decontamination process. Obviously, for those devices that are terminally disinfected, the cleaning/disinfection stage will be the complete process and thus its efficiency will directly define instrument quality and safety. For the majority of items that will be terminally sterilized, the cleaning/disinfection stage will perform a number of functions:

- Making items safe to handle in the packing stage
- Enabling full sterilant/device contact allowing sterilization to occur
- Performing initial bioburden reduction to ensure the complete log reduction will be met

Disinfection

Thermal disinfection within the automated washer disinfector has been described above. The relevant time/temperature control will be set to achieve a particular bioburden reduction. Recent changes to standards have introduced the Ao concept where a variety of times and temperatures with equivalent lethality are provided. These may include a temperature of 80°C for 10 minutes but other relationships are possible.

Such temperatures will be clearly too high for the heat-labile materials used in the construction of flexible endoscopes. Thus, the use of chemical disinfection at ambient or low temperatures will be employed. As stated above, the parameters used for cleaning and disinfection should be controlled and repeatable and thus automated washer disinfectors are advised. While manufacturer instructions will inevitably include prior manual cleaning, these automated machines can be validated to provide efficient cleaning both internally and externally. The user should choose the detergent and chemical disinfectant with care bearing in mind any compatibility issues raised by the manufacturer of the machine and the manufacturer of the flexible endoscope. There is no single ideal chemical disinfectant and all have their relevant advantages and disadvantages.

Liaison with both manufacturers at the time of procurements should ensure all compatibility measures are met. Unlike thermal disinfection, it is not possible to monitor chemical disinfection parametrically, and thus validation will include a determination of the log reduction required for chemical disinfection.

Opinions will differ on the amount of time that flexible endoscopes can be stored between reprocessing and use, but the use of storage cabinets may enable this storage time to be increased to cater for out-of-hours and emergency periods. Such increases, however, will require full validation and periodic verification.

Sterilization

Sterilization Kinetics

Before considering the different sterilization processes available, it is necessary to understand the mechanism by which any process achieves its aims. It should be noted that sterilization is not an instantaneous effect but that time and a combination of parameters are required. The method of operation can be shown by exposing a known number of spores (worst-case contaminant) to varying sterilization periods. While the details will be different for different spores, different sterilants, and different conditions, the principles will apply equally.

The number of survivors will be shown an asymptotic reduction as exposure time increases. These data can be better assessed if redrawn logarithmically whence the data will demonstrate a straight line. Clearly, this line will never meet a value of zero as the survivor number is decreasing by powers of 10. The graph is thus displaying logarithmic (log-) reductions for a given set of spore/sterilant conditions. Such data can be used to determine the parameter values required to meet the local/national/regional definition of the required log reduction for the process to be termed "sterilization." With an initial sample of 10^6 organisms and a sterility assurance level of, say, 10^{-6}, a 12-log reduction will be required before the process can be termed "sterilization."

Thus, the statistical microbiological basis of sterilization will enable the critical parameters for a particular process to be defined. Repeated assessments for different combinations of spore, sterilant, and critical parameter can be similarly repeated thus defining operational characteristics of all sterilization methods and processes.

Once the kinetics is understood, then the sterilizer manufacturer can then design the machine to achieve the required conditions. It is likely that the sterilization period will only occupy a minority of the sterilization cycle because a degree of prior preparation and later conditioning will be required as part of the whole cycle.

Steam: Properties

Steam was the sterilant in Chamberland's sterilizer, the first commercially produced in France in 1880. It remains the predominant sterilant today because of its efficiency, predictability, and relative ease of use. It is in daily use throughout the world. Steam is a highly complex compound, but its use in sterilization is extremely simple. It is used as a conveyor of energy from the point of generation to the load in the sterilizer chamber. However, some fundamental properties of steam should be understood.

Water is the obvious source for steam and is turned from liquid to vapor by the addition of thermal energy—heat. What appears to be a simple process is, however, rather complex. While in liquid form, H_2O demonstrates an increase in temperature when heat is added. This is so until the boiling point is reached. Once boiling temperature is reached, however, further heat is required to change the liquid into the vapor phase, but this change occurs without a change in temperature. Thus, boiling water and steam emanating from its surface are at the same temperature, but a typical water sample requires approximately four times the amount of energy to change it from boiling water to steam (latent energy) than the energy required to raise it from room temperature to boiling point (sensible energy). This is true for the wide range of temperatures at which water will boil. There is a fixed, repeatable relationship between the temperature at which water boils and the pressure acting on the surface of the water. As this pressure is increased, the boiling temperature is increased. Conversely, if the pressure is reduced the boiling temperature is reduced. Boiling temperature and pressure are called saturation conditions and if one is varied and controlled, the other will automatically follow. Steam sterilization utilizes boiling at both high and low temperatures for the process to occur.

Additionally, when steam is created it occupies a much greater volume than the water it originated from. Conversely, when it condenses in a sealed system or chamber, a vacuum is created.

Once steam is delivered to a sterilizer chamber it will meet a load at a lower temperature. The steam will condense on the load and deliver its latent energy to the load raising it to steam temperature. The condensate thus created will contain the sensible energy but is no longer required for the sterilization process. This water—a necessary by-product of steam sterilization—is redundant and should be removed from the chamber as quickly as possible or wet loads may occur. The condensation process must occur over the whole surface area of the load and thus all air contained within the chamber at the cycle start must be removed to allow this complete intimate contact to occur.

After sterilization, the steam must be removed from the chamber and any residual water removed in order for a dry load to be removed. For this final stage of the process, the steam supply is stopped and a vacuum is created in the chamber. While the vacuum creation system may well remove the steam, if the vacuum is low enough, the subsequent low saturation pressure thus created will enable the water to regain some energy from the load, be turned into the vapor phase and be removed by the vacuum system. As long as the drying vacuum is low enough and long enough, all residual water can be removed and thus after a short air-equalization period the door may be opened to reveal a dry, sterile load. Cleverly, the sterilizer has utilized saturation conditions both above and below atmospheric pressure to achieve the cycle's aim.

Steam: Sterilizers

In order to achieve the cycle described above, a steam sterilization cycle can be split into four phases:

- Air removal
- Heat-up and sterilization
- Vacuuming and drying
- Pressure equalization by filtered air inlet

It should be noted that there are different types of steam sterilizer that are dedicated to certain load types and the user must be aware of the (in)compatibilities between load and sterilizer. The main difference is in the method employed for the first cycle stage, air removal.

The simplest steam sterilizer will use the inflow of steam to remove residual air in the chamber. This process can be efficient as long as load items do not have any entrained air (via wrapping, lumens, etc.) and that the loading pattern does not inhibit this stage. The air removal may be by downward or upward flow of steam and sterilizers of this type are commonly referred to as "gravity displacement," "downward (upward) displacement," or by definition of typical load types such as unwrapped bowls and instrument. Because the air removal is relatively passive, it may not be possible to remove air from wrapped, hollow, or lumened instruments.

Such loads will require an active air removal system prior to sterilization where a variety of methods are used to physically drag the residual air from difficult areas. Evolution of this type of sterilizer has produced a machine where the vacuum creation system can be used for both air removal at cycle start and steam/water removal at cycle end. The vacuum system can be used to create a series of steam pulses alternating vacuum and steam introduction to mix with any residual air and to dilute the air remaining at each vacuum stage of the pulse. This pulsing air removal is now considered the norm for sterilizers described as "high vacuum" or "porous load" although different manufacturers will use different formats for the pulsing stage. As the efficiency of a single pulse is dependent upon the difference in pressure at the peak and trough, the deeper each pulse the better. However, it should be noted that any sterilizer chamber has a definite but hopefully small natural leakage, pulse at negative pressures will allow air to be drawn in through these leaks. Pulses at positive pressure will not. It is now common for sterilization cycles to include pulses at both negative and positive pressures. As long as residual air is removed before the cycle proceeds to sterilization, the method of removal is thus merely a factor of cycle time and hence departmental productivity.

Critical parameters are time, temperature, presence of moisture, and complete air removal. Typical time–temperature relationships for steam sterilization are as follows:

- 134°C for 3 minutes
- 126°C for 10 minutes
- 121°C for 15 minutes

Dry Heat Sterilizers

Steam sterilization is described as a moist heat process. The presence of moisture from the generation source as well as that from condensation allows the outer surface of spores to be broken down. If the sterilant were dry, then the efficiency of the process would be reduced and much longer exposure times would be required. Such a process would, however, be useful for those items that would be destroyed or damaged by becoming wet. Use of air heated to high temperatures may thus be used for load items such as nonaqueous powders. In this process, air removal is not required, but the free movement of heated air throughout the chamber and load is required. Energy transfer is by convection and conduction rather than condensation and any restriction to airflow of heat conduction will inhibit the process. Heat-up and cool-down are exceptionally long, and thus while there may be a need for this process, the number of possible cycles per day is low. It should also be noted that sterilization temperature is much higher than for steam sterilization.

Critical parameters are time, temperature, and complete air circulation. Typical relationships are as follows:

- 160°C for 120 minutes
- 170°C for 60 minutes
- 180°C for 30 minutes

Low-Temperature Sterilizers

Both steam sterilization and dry-heat sterilization are performed at high temperatures. There will always be a need for sterilization at low temperature for those items that are heat labile. A variety of techniques are available and innovative low-temperature processes may continue to occur. Most utilize a chemical effect, sometimes combined with thermal energy and humidity/moisture in order to achieve the required log reduction. Some examples are as follows.

Ethylene Oxide

The sterilant effects of ethylene oxide gas combined with thermal energy and humidity at the right values will achieve sterilization.

Low-Temperature Steam and Formaldehyde

Chemical effects of formaldehyde with thermal energy from steam at low temperature (and hence low pressure) may achieve sterilization.

Hydrogen Peroxide Gas Plasma

This relatively new process combines the chemical effect of hydrogen peroxide vapor with the effects of a plasma generated around the load to achieve sterilization.

Hydrogen Peroxide Vapor

The chemical effect of hydrogen peroxide vapor is often used for large volume fumigation and can be controlled in sterilizer chambers to meet the needs of sterilization.

Liquid Chemical Sterilization

Certain liquid chemical disinfectants may achieve sterilization if the exposure times are long enough. As in other processes, full surface-area contact will be required.

Irradiation

Many single-use or presterilized items used within healthcare facilities are sterilized by irradiation. This process is best used in large-scale decontamination facilities and is particularly relevant to large-scale manufacture. For this reason, it is unlikely that irradiation sterilization will be found in healthcare facilities.

These processes can be used at a variety of temperatures from ambient to 70°C.

Choice of Sterilizing Process

While steam remains the process of choice, practitioners may also choose from the list shown above. How is this choice made? Initially manufacturer instructions will be the main reference for the required sterilization process. Processes should always be chosen for compatibility between the process and the load taking into account all materials of construction of the devices, their configuration, and susceptibility to wide variations in temperature and pressure as well as any further susceptibility to moisture, chemicals, and corrosive environments. The cost of the sterilizer should be the final factor to be considered.

Monitoring

The whole purpose of the decontamination process is to make instruments and devices safe for reuse and it is a major item of infection prevention and control. Thus, not only should decontamination practitioners be fully aware of the process requirements, they should also be able to determine whether each and every stage of the decontamination process has met its requirements. This will enable a product release decision to be made at every stage and to define to the patient where necessary that the reprocessing was efficient.

Quality system standards define decontamination as a "special process," one which cannot be observed by monitoring the end product. Such a method would render all products non-sterile. The process can be monitored by a parallel system as follows:

- Define what must happen at each stage for the process to be acceptable.
- Monitor all critical variables for each stage.
- Determine whether any deviation is acceptable.
- Document all data and decision making.

For this monitoring procedure to be available, certain conditions must be met. These are as follows:

- Monitoring of all critical variables via an independent system, not the control system
- Provision of these data to the operator at the unloading door
- Knowledge by the operator of the values required
- Knowledge by the operator of the acceptable deviations
- Documentation of the decision

These requirements are reiterated in standards for sterilizers and washer disinfectors although they do not list the relevant critical parameters. It is suggested that the following parameters are critical:

- *Cleaning* (automated): water temperature, water pressure, water flowrate, water quality, detergent delivery, time
- *Disinfection* (thermal): temperature, time, water quality
- *Drying* (automated): air temperature, time, air quality
- *Sterilization* (steam): time, temperature, air removal, moisture presence

Most modern items of decontamination equipment will be capable of monitoring most of these parameters, but it is the responsibility of the purchaser to ensure at the procurement stage that the equipment will meet these requirements. However, two of these critical parameters—air quality and presence of moisture—are difficult to monitor and are invariably not monitored. It must therefore be accepted that even at the very best, decontamination contains certain assumptions regarding its efficacy.

In order to demonstrate continuing good practice, all items of decontamination equipment should be fully validated prior to use and, once in use, regularly maintained and periodically tested. The combination of this work will indicate that the operation continues to be acceptable and should be performed in addition to product release and process monitoring. All these data should be fully recorded and records should be retained for the period of time required by local requirements, standards, or legal requirements.

Summary

Decontamination is an essential part of infection prevention and control and is the process by which reusable medical devices are made safe for reuse. While the common problems are global, local and regional differences have led to differences in the implementation of universal precautions throughout the world.

In order to understand decontamination, precise definitions must be used in order for manufacturers to design and build suitable equipment and for users and operators to monitor and periodically test equipment.

Decontamination is performed in a variety of places, but there are common principles that should apply whether decontamination is centralized or performed locally.

The complete life cycle of reusable instruments should be understood in order for inspection at all stages of the decontamination process to be made.

The stages of the process—cleaning, disinfection, drying, and sterilization—are described and explained.

In order to demonstrate good practice, each and every stage and cycle should be monitored and all decontamination equipment should be regularly maintained and periodically tested.

Design, Planning, Control, and Management of Healthcare Systems

IV.H Laboratories

39 **Quality Control in Hospital Clinical Laboratories: A System Approach** *George G. Klee* **39**-1
Introduction • System Analysis and Flowcharting • Establishing Performance Limits • Error Budget • Assessment of Medical Needs for Accuracy and Precision • QC Systems for Assuring Production Meets Expectations • References

39

Quality Control in Hospital Clinical Laboratories: A System Approach

Introduction 39-1
System Analysis and Flowcharting 39-2
Establishing Performance Limits 39-4
Error Budget 39-4
Assessment of Medical Needs for Accuracy and Precision 39-5
Accuracy Limits • Imprecision Limits
QC Systems for Assuring Production Meets Expectations 39-6
References 39-6

George G. Klee
Mayo Clinic

Introduction

Most hospital clinical laboratories provide blood and urine testing services that require integration across to multiple areas. The processing of these test requests involves numerous tasks: ordering of the tests by health practitioners, the collection of specimens, the analytic measurements using equipment and reagents from multiple vendors, employment of well-trained laboratory technologists, reporting of the test results to the medical records (both electronic and paper reporting), and billing for the services using some accounting system. In most hospitals, no one person and not even any single group of individuals understand all these processes. However, this complete laboratory testing process can be considered as an integrated system and the principles of systems process control can be used to manage this process.

System analyses can help break complex systems into smaller, more self-contained processes.[7,11,18] In analyzing systems, there often is debate about what is the "center" of the system. As a laboratorian, it is tempting to consider the clinical laboratory as the center of the universe, with all other functions rotating around the laboratory. At the Mayo Clinic, we have our primary value statement that "the needs of the patient come first" and try to keep the patient at the center of everything we do. Figure 39.1 presents laboratory services as functions surrounding the patient. Each service box has defined inputs and outputs relating to the other boxes. Each of these surrounding boxes can be further exploded into subprocesses. As the process is more fully defined, key performance variables can be defined and quality control management systems can be developed to assure satisfactory performance. This chapter focuses on mechanisms to define and control the integration of these subsystems.

System Analysis and Flowcharting

Process control should consider both materials flow and information flow, since both are important. Formal flowcharting is a useful procedure for defining and documenting each of these processes.[18] For clinical laboratory testing procedures, material flow would include processes such as assigning patients to examining rooms, collection of specimens, transport of specimens, shipping of reagents, storage of reagents and specimens, and transporting reports if paper reports are utilized. Information flow would include processes such as registering patients, scheduling of patients, scheduling of healthcare workers (including phlebotomists), ordering of laboratory tests, entry of clinical information into medical records, billing for services, ordering reagents and supplies, payment for reagents and supplies, documentation of quality controls, and reporting of test results. These flowcharts often are interdependent, so the outputs from one chart may serve as the inputs to several other charts. Well-documented processes help to define the expectations and deliverables of each process.[11] A new term called "lean management" has been coined for the optimization of workflow processes.[4,5,12,21] Combining lean processes with improved technology such as bar codes and computerized data entry can substantially improve quality.[23]

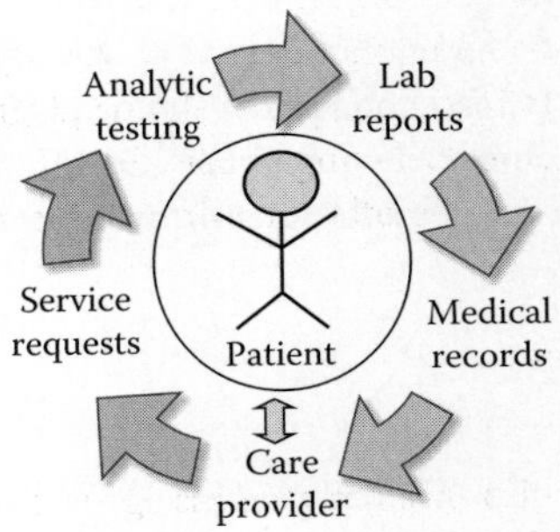

FIGURE 39.1 Laboratory services in a health system.

Quality control systems generally are directly linked to these material and/or information flow processes. Key variables and acceptable performance parameters need to be defined in order to develop reliable quality control systems. Some of these key variables can be identified as rate limiting steps in the flow diagrams and/or variables that are likely to have significant adverse outcomes if variation occurs. In addition to these flow diagrams, another source for identifying key QC variables is a historical "problem database."[6] Mapping of the historical problems onto the flow diagrams may help to further identify important variables to monitor. In many clinical laboratories problems often occur at the "hand-off" points between subsystems, especially when the different subsystems are in different locations and under different management. Good quality control systems should strive to identify changes in critical variables prior to the occurrence of critical problems, so that preemptive modifications can be made to prevent these problems.

A simplified flow diagram for the blood collection process is illustrated in Figure 39.2. The input and output quantities are depicted as ovals, the processes are depicted as rectangles, and the decision questions are diamonds. This is a combination of material flow (blood specimen, patient, and phlebotomist) and information flow (ordering of tests and scheduling of phlebotomy). Each of the boxes in this diagram could be expanded into more complex processes, such as expansion for the "Lab measurement system" box in this diagram with the more complete flow diagram illustrated in Figure 39.3. In Figure 39.3, the inputs are the analytic reagents, the analytic calibrator, the control materials, and the patient specimen. The outputs are the test report and the service bill. The decisions relate to evaluation of the assay calibration and evaluation of the testing quality control—each of which need to have specified QC performance criteria and specified QC evaluation rules. Two areas where problems often occur are mistakes in the ordering of the laboratory tests and the turnaround time (TAT) it takes between the ordering of the test and the final reporting.

The measurements of blood samples usually are performed on automated instruments using commercial reagents and commercial quality control materials. Before patient samples are measured, the instruments are calibrated by establishing a dose–response curve using reference materials with assigned concentrations (this process is called analytic calibration). The reliability of these calibration curves is evaluated by measuring stable control materials with assigned values. These assigned values may be provided by the control manufacturer or may be established by the laboratory. Once the calibration is accepted, the patient samples are measured; however, the measurements on patients generally are not reported until further

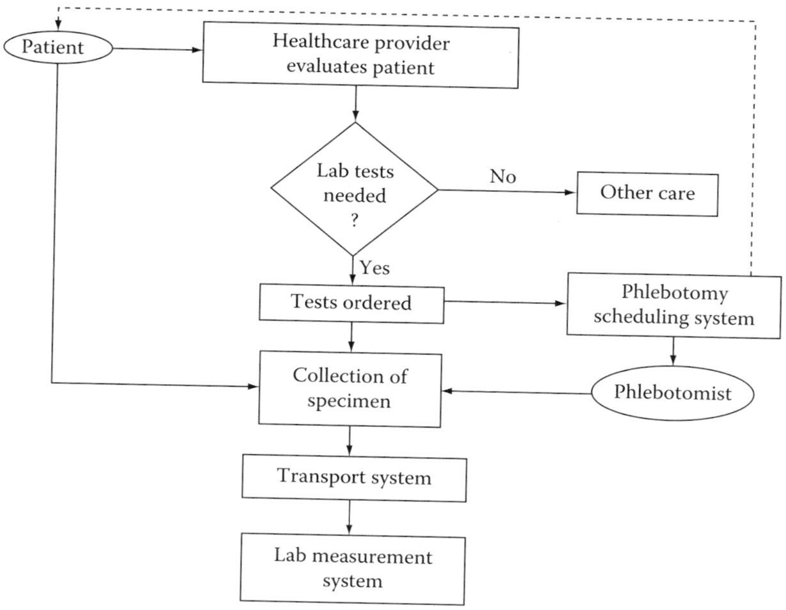

FIGURE 39.2 Simplified flow diagram for blood collection.

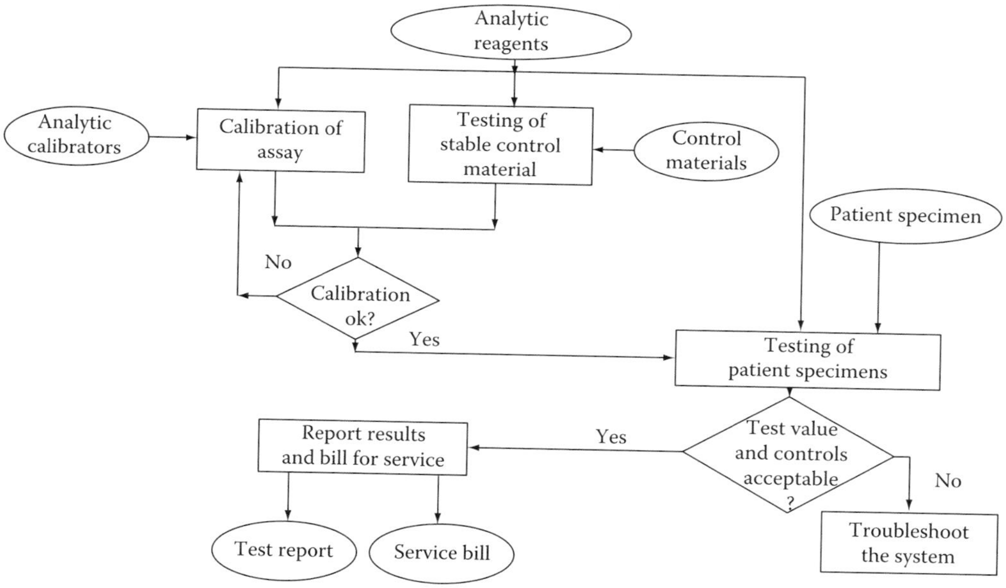

FIGURE 39.3 Simplified materials flow diagram for analytic test measurement system.

quality control specimens are analyzed and approved. The quality control criteria for approving the testing may involve limit checks to assure that the test value is within the analytic reporting range and specimen integrity checks to assure that there is no interference from hemolysis, lipemia, or icterus.[15]

Currently, there is considerable interest in the deployment of computerized physician order entry systems.[9] This technology not only reduces errors caused by illegible handwriting, but also helps to standardize the ordering processes. It can substantially decrease overuse, underuse, and misuse of healthcare resources, especially when linked to practice guidelines.[9] On the other hand, there often is a learning curve for implementing these systems and there may be adverse healthcare effects and increased costs during the first few years of adoption.[3]

The TATs for laboratory tests are affected by many factors including the test ordering procedure, the specimen transport systems, the measurement processes, and the reporting systems. The College of American Pathologists has monitored TAT for blood counts, chemistry profiles, and thyrotropin tests.[17] They found TATs of up to 3h for blood counts, 1–4h for chemistry profiles, and 1–24h for thyrotropin. Reports are considered "late" only when the expectations exceed the deliverables. Therefore, it is important to define performance criteria that are acceptable to all parties involved. Some areas such as the hospital emergency department may require shorter TATs.[16] Computerized provider entry has been shown to reduce TAT for medications[8] and laboratory services.[19] Computerized order entry systems also help improve both documentation and patient safety.[14,20]

Establishing Performance Limits

A fundamental requirement of all quality control systems is the formulation of well-defined performance limits for each of the critical variables. These performance limits are needed to establish acceptable quality control characteristics for false positive and false negative detection rates. In the manufacturing industry, the design engineer generally provides these performance limits to assure that the products meet the design specifications. However, in medicine, the laboratory performance limits often are less well defined. Quality control rules and quality control action limits often are set to minimize false positive signals, while very little attention is paid to false negative issues. For example, one can measure the variation of a quality control specimen (by calculating the mean and SD using 20 measurements) and use statistical quality control rules to assure that the false positive rate is low (say less than 1 per 1000). However, the statistical performance of these QC rules may be very low for detecting medically important assay changes and therefore the QC system would have a high false negative rate.

Performance limits for most clinical laboratory tests represent a trade-off between what is feasible with current technology and what is needed for optimal medical care. Feasibility of current technology can be determined either by measuring the performance of the current system or by a "system analysis" to integrate the tolerance limits defined for the components of the system. A disadvantage of only measuring the current system is that some components may be underestimated. For example, if the baseline measurements are made with only one lot of reagents and one technologist, the system may have larger variation when it is implemented in actual production. A better approach for defining assay performance involves collecting estimates for each of the components and statistically combining them.[1,2] These estimates of component variations can come from the manufacturer of the components, the published literature, or from specially designed experiments. Utilization of the integrated statistics combining all the components may overestimate the total error, but the performance of the total system should stay within specifications if the individual components are maintained within specifications, and it often is easier to manage the performance of subsystems as compared to managing the complex integrated system.

Error Budget

The statistical variances of the components identified in the system analysis can be mathematically combined into an error budget. Separate budgets can be determined for both systematic error (bias) and random error (imprecision) and these two budgets can be combined for a total error budget. The systematic errors add linearly, while the random errors add by the sum of squares:

$$\text{Systematic Error Budget} = \theta_{\text{collection}} + \theta_{\text{instability}} + \theta_{\text{calibration}} + \theta_{\text{pipetting}} + \theta_{\text{data reduction}}$$

$$\text{Random Error Budget} = \sqrt{SD^2_{\text{preanalyte}} + SD^2_{\text{instrument}} + SD^2_{\text{reagent}} + SD^2_{\text{measurement}} + SD^2_{\text{biologic}}}$$

The various components of the integrated system may be managed by separate production units; therefore, it is advantageous to have specific error budgets for each component. The overall performance is the statistical combination of the component errors as shown above.

Assessment of Medical Needs for Accuracy and Precision

Analytic test accuracy is most important for diagnostic tests, whereas analytic precision is important for tests used for monitoring.

Accuracy Limits

The medical diagnostic process involves comparison of a specific patient with representative reference groups of patients who either have the disease in question or are free of that disease. The absolute accuracy of a laboratory test used to facilitate diagnoses is not as important as the assurance that the patient's test results are standardized the same as the results from the reference populations. The best way to assure harmonization is to minimize systematic error from well-established reference standards and/or reference methods. If reference standards do not exist, "selected" materials can be used as working standards to harmonize the test results across the reference groups. The effects of analytic accuracy of laboratory tests is particularly important when medical practice guidelines use decision levels at fixed concentrations. Table 39.1 illustrates that for a medical decision based on the guideline action limit of 200 mg/dL of cholesterol, the error tolerance depends on how far a value is from that decision level. The further a test value is from this action limit, the more error that can be tolerated without altering the decision. This emphasizes why quality control monitors should be targeted at critical decision points.

Imprecision Limits

Performance limits for analytic precision are buffered by the effects of biologic variation. Clinicians see the combined effects of the biologic variation and the analytic variation when evaluating a test result. These two components of variation generally are statistically independent and add by the square root of the sum of squares.

$$\text{Total SD} = \sqrt{(SD_{\text{Biologic}})^2 + (SD_{\text{Analytic}})^2}$$

TABLE 39.1 Allowable Bias Error Depends on Test Value and Decision Level

True Value (mg/dL)	Max Allowable Error (mg/dL)	Allowable Error (%)
180	+20	+11.1
190	+10	+5.3
195	+5	+2.6
Decision level → 200	0	0.0
205	−5	−2.4
210	−10	−4.8
220	−20	−9.1

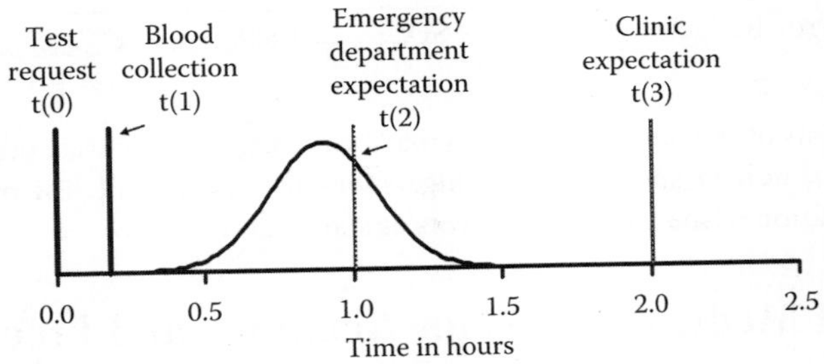

FIGURE 39.4 TAT expectations.

If the analytic SD is less than 25% of the biologic SD, the total error SD only increases by less than 3% (i.e., $\sqrt{1.0^2 + (0.25)^2} = 1.03$). Therefore, analytic limits for imprecision often are based on biologic variations. There are two types of biologic variation: (1) within subject changes over time and (2) differences between subjects. When a test is used for monitoring a patient over time, the within person biologic variation is the appropriate biologic reference. A good publication for finding biologic variations is the 1999 paper by Ricos et al.[13] A 2008 update of these data is available on the Westgard.com web site.[22]

QC Systems for Assuring Production Meets Expectations

Consider the process illustrated in Figure 39.2 for the ordering of a laboratory test, collection and transport of the sample, and measurement of the test values. A critical variable for this process is the TAT, which is the time interval from when the test is ordered until the result is available for the healthcare provider. Each of the processes in this system takes a defined amount of time that can be modeled using statistical distributions. These times can be combined together to estimate the total TAT. Quality control systems can be set up to monitor TAT. Ideally, one would want a "six sigma" performance to assure that all patient test results would be delivered within the expected TAT. This would require that the average TAT would be six SDs shorter than the expected test delivery time.[10] In practice, most clinical laboratories are not that good and laboratories often only perform at the one-sigma level, where only about 85% of the results are delivered on time.

This concept of TAT versus expectation is illustrated in Figure 39.4. The TAT for the combined ordering-collection-testing-reporting process has an average of 0.9 h with a SD of about 0.2 h. If the emergency department is expecting test results within 1 h, they will not be pleased when only about 70% of the patients have the tests delivered on time (t_2); whereas if the clinics are expecting results within 2 h (t_3) they would be well pleased with the 5.5 sigma performance almost always assuring test results on time. This difference between emergency department expectations and clinical laboratory TATs often causes dissatisfaction.[16] Defining clinical expectations consistent with systems performance is key to user satisfaction. Systems modeling and QC monitoring, as illustrated in this chapter, can help assure that these expectations are consistently met.

References

1. Anonymous. Quantifying uncertainty in analytical measurement. http://www.measurementuncertainty.org/ (accessed August 2009).
2. Anonymous. Statistical methods of uncertainty analysis: ISO 7C69/SC6/WG7 Draft 2. http://www.itl.nist.gov/div898/carroll/u.htm (accessed August 2009).
3. Berger, RG, Kichak, JP. Computerized physician order entry: Helpful or harmful? *J Am Med Inform Assoc* 2004;11:100–103.

4. Brown, T, Duthe, R. Getting "Lean": Hardwiring process excellence into Northeast Health. *J Health Inf Manag* 2009;23:34–38.
5. Casey, JT, Brinton, TS, Gonzalez, CM. Utilization of lean management principles in the ambulatory clinic setting. *Nat Clin Pract Urol* 2009;6:146–153.
6. Elston, DM. Opportunities to improve quality in laboratory medicine. *Clin Lab Med* 2008;28:173–177, v.
7. Hoffmann, GE. Concepts for the third generation of laboratory systems. *Clin Chim Acta* 1998;278:203–216.
8. Jensen, JR. The effects of computerized provider order entry on medication turn-around time: A time-to-first dose study at the Providence Portland Medical Center. *AMIA Annu Symp Proc* 2006:384–388.
9. Kuperman, GJ, Gibson, RF. Computer physician order entry: Benefits, costs, and issues. *Ann Intern Med* 2003;139:31–39.
10. Moidu, K, Margolis, S, Pandey, R. Improving the patient experience by improving performance: The Six Sigma Way. *AMIA Annu Symp Proc* 2008:1246.
11. Pansini, N, Di Serio, F, Tampoia, M. Total testing process: Appropriateness in laboratory medicine. *Clin Chim Acta* 2003;333:141–145.
12. Persoon, TJ, Zaleski, S, Frerichs, J. Improving preanalytic processes using the principles of lean production (Toyota Production System). *Am J Clin Pathol* 2006;125:16–25.
13. Ricós, C, Alvarez, V, Cava, F, García-Lario, JV, Hernández, A, Jiménez, CV, Minchinela, J, Perich, C, Simón, M. Current databases on biological variation: Pros, cons and progress. *Scand J Clin Lab Invest* 1999;59:491–500.
14. Rikli, J, Huizinga, B, Schafer, D, Atwater, A, Coker, K, Sikora, C. Implementation of an electronic documentation system using microsystem and quality improvement concepts. *Adv Neonatal Care* 2009;9:53–60.
15. Ryder, KW, Glick, MR. Erroneous laboratory results from hemolyzed, icteric, and lipemic specimens. *Clin Chem* 1993;39:175–176.
16. Steindel, SJ, Howanitz, PJ. Physician satisfaction and emergency department laboratory test turnaround time. *Arch Pathol Lab Med* 2001;125:863–871.
17. Steindel, SJ, Jones, BA. Routine outpatient laboratory test turnaround times and practice patterns: A College of American Pathologists Q-Probes study. *Arch Pathol Lab Med* 2002;126:11–18.
18. Truchaud, A, Le Neel, T, Brochard, H, Malvaux, S, Moyon, M, Cazaubiel, M. New tools for laboratory design and management. *Clin Chem* 1997;43:1709–1715.
19. Veltri, G. Transforming healthcare. A top U.S. hospital implements CPOE and improves patient safety while dramatically reducing turn-around time. *Health Manag Technol* 2008;29:14:18–19.
20. Wang, SJ, Blumenfeld, BH, Roche, SE, Greim, JA, Burk, KE, Gandhi, TK, Bates, DW, Kuperman, GJ. End of visit: Design considerations for an ambulatory order entry module. *Proc AMIA Annu Symp* 2002:864–868.
21. Weinstock, D. Lean healthcare. *J Med Pract Manage* 2008;23:339–341.
22. Westgard, J. Desirable specifications for total error, imprecision, and bias, derived from intra- and inter-individual biologic variation. http://www.westgard.com/guest32/index.php?option=com_content&view=article&id=238:biodatabase1&catid=37:quality-requirements&Itemid=66 (accessed August 2009).
23. Zarbo, RJ, Tuthill, JM, D'Angelo, R, Varney, R, Mahar, B, Neuman, C, Ormsby, A. The Henry Ford Production System: Reduction of surgical pathology in-process misidentification defects by bar code-specified work process standardization. *Am J Clin Pathol* 2009;131:468–477.

Design, Planning, Control, and Management of Healthcare Systems

IV.I Emergency Response and Pandemics Planning

40 **Emergency Planning Model for Pandemics** *J. Eric Dietz, David R. Black, Julia E. Drifmeyer and Jennifer A. Smock* **40**-1
Introduction • What Can Be Learned from the Past? • How Was the Current Model Developed? • How Does Epidemiology Relate to Strategic Planning? • What Are the Benefits of Planning? • Historical Background: Can Military Tactics Be Applied to Public Health Operations? • Pandemic Influenza: How Are These Strategies Applied? • Why Is Workplace Planning Important for Pandemic Prevention? • How Are Constraints on Resources Addressed during Strategic Planning? • How Can Situational Uncertainties Be Accounted for in the Strategic Plan? • Strategy Illustrations: How Are Strategies Applied during a Pandemic? • Acknowledgment • References

41 Public Health and Medical Preparedness *Eva K. Lee, Anna Yang Yang, Ferdinand Pietz, and Bernard Benecke* **41**-1
Introduction • Medical Surge • Population Protection: Medical Countermeasures Dispensing and Large-Scale Disaster Relief Efforts • Communication System • Emergency Evacuation • Summary • References

40

Emergency Planning Model for Pandemics

Introduction ... 40-1
What Can Be Learned from the Past? ... 40-2
How Was the Current Model Developed? ... 40-2
How Does Epidemiology Relate to Strategic Planning? ... 40-2
What Are the Benefits of Planning? ... 40-2
Historical Background: Can Military Tactics Be Applied to Public Health Operations? ... 40-3
Pandemic Influenza: How Are These Strategies Applied? ... 40-5
Why Is Workplace Planning Important for Pandemic Prevention? ... 40-6
How Are Constraints on Resources Addressed during Strategic Planning? ... 40-6
How Can Situational Uncertainties Be Accounted for in the Strategic Plan? ... 40-7
Strategy Illustrations: How Are Strategies Applied during a Pandemic? ... 40-8
What Is the National Strategy for Influenza Prevention? • What Are the Individual Strategies for Prevention? • What Strategy Should Be Used for Incident Command Selection? • What Are Strategies for Staffing Hospitals? • How Are Strategic Plans Developed and Implemented? • How Can the Hospital Plan Be Implemented? • What Emerging Lessons Were Learned?
Acknowledgment ... 40-15
References ... 40-15

J. Eric Dietz
Purdue University

David R. Black
Purdue University

Julia E. Drifmeyer
Purdue University

Jennifer A. Smock
National Association of County and City Health Officials (NACCHO)

Action springs not from thoughts, but a readiness for responsibility

—Dietrich Bonhoeffer

Introduction

This chapter introduces the reader to the historical development of strategic planning by military tacticians, application of military strategic plans to public health, key elements of strategic plans, and further understanding of how strategic planning can provide useful and necessary guidelines for healthcare providers during a pandemic. A model of strategic planning is introduced and explained in order to most effectively and efficiently serve the public's health needs and concerns. Evaluation methods to test hospitals and clinics are described and they must have an established and thoroughly tested plan in place. Uncertainty about the occurrence of a pandemic should be no excuse for not developing a plan, but rather should be a reason for doing so.

What Can Be Learned from the Past?

Centuries of military operations have shaped the planning and staff development concepts used in a number of fields today. Novel military planning concepts proposed by such historical figures as Sun Tzu, Clausewitz, and Frederick the Great continue to shape doctrine, tactics, and planning in military conceptual studies and organizational development (Clausewitz, 1984; Giles, 2007; Luvaas, 1999). The same operational planning foundations from the military have shaped public safety fields including law enforcement, fire services, and emergency management. Healthcare delivery also has benefited from military experience including learning ways to manage serious medical problems under highly stressful conditions and how to operate in "mass casualty" situations. Many American companies are modeled after military infrastructure and "lines of authority." All four authors have military experiences and this chapter is based on command positions, and receiving training in strategic planning and operations. The lessons learned from strategic planning and tactics were reinforced through exercises to make the points taught a reality. The first author also was former Indiana Director of Homeland Security and was in charge of developing and implementing plans, strategies, and tactics. The second author was graduate of the U.S. Army War College Class of 1999.

How Was the Current Model Developed?

The model in this chapter was developed using military theoretical concepts taught at the U.S. Army War College, throughout the military, and blended with other constructs of strategy, planning, and tactics. Validation has been a process based on "tabletop exercises" (TTXs) with clearly defined goals and objectives. Evaluation of "readiness" was based on the quality of the current strategic plan. This evaluation introduced necessary planning modifications as part of a continuous improvement process for Emergency Planning for Pandemics for 60 county governments and hospital preparedness programs throughout Indiana. These hospital TTXs were then used as a heuristic illustration for developing practical useable plans that could be applied in vitro.

How Does Epidemiology Relate to Strategic Planning?

Epidemiology is central because the field focuses on pandemics and prevention and control (EPI). Recent guidance and recommendations provided on the Web sites of the World Health Organization (WHO), the Centers for Disease Control and Prevention (CDC), and the Health Resources and Service Administration (HRSA) on the emergence of a novel strain of Type A influenza supports the need for continued development of thorough and complete strategic plans for healthcare providers. The continued presence of a pandemic can threaten abilities of hospitals and clinics to provide care at their normal operating levels, while undergoing stress to expand capacity to meet the demands of a pandemic. The development and implementation of systematic plans that carefully considers a variety of potential pandemic scenarios can provide a prior experience in hopes of easing the burden of coordinating and delivering healthcare services while a pandemic occurs. Evaluation of what should be considered "essential healthcare services" prior to a pandemic provides healthcare personnel the opportunity to devote resources to these priorities, while making adjustments to other services.

What Are the Benefits of Planning?

While the act of planning for a very uncertain events may be met with some resistance, hospital administrators and staff should understand that a comprehensive review of their process, policies, and services can be beneficial beyond improving their daily preparedness including the occurrence of a pandemic. By prioritizing and streamlining daily operations, healthcare providers can develop policies that increase their efficiency in delivery of services. Knowledge about hospital operations is especially necessary during a period of healthcare reform.

Historical Background: Can Military Tactics Be Applied to Public Health Operations?

Much of what is discussed below is based on a "scholar of the year" presented by the second author, titled "A Strategic Planning for Winning the War in Public Health" (Black, 2002). There is no organization in the twentieth century that has managed large-scale, worldwide threats as well as our modern-day military. The modern-day examples include World War I and World War II, but the advances in the Iraq War has further reduced the time and improved the methods available for trauma cases. The military has a long proud reputation for managing complex operations in an analytical way that is based on knowledge and past experience, as does the field of public health.

There are several similarities between the military and the public health. Alluded to above, both deal with people and large-scale operations in order to meet important national objectives. They both operate within large geographic areas and have multiple points of focus and concentration to accomplish their missions. The military and the Office of the Surgeon General (OSG) have the same commander-in-chief, the president of the United States. The OSG is commanded by a 4-star general officer. It is interesting that the word "General" appears in the title of this agency and as such acknowledges a military connection and is another branch of the military, which is often forgotten. The OSG is connected with a variety of other federal public health agencies (e.g., CDC and HRSA). There is probably less of a direct connection or awareness about military influence, but their structures and methods of operation model the military with tight security, and careful review and restrictions as to what is made available to the public.

Structure and organization are essential for a highly organized, efficient operation to protect Americans whether the enemy is human and wears a uniform or is an infectious agent. The translation of military principles to public health is readily applicable, especially to public health problems of major magnitude. The principles discussed below are from the U.S. Army War College located at Carlisle Barracks, Carlisle, PA. The War College has a rich tradition; faculty and students representing some of the most brilliant military strategists in the world. Some prestigious graduates from the War College include Generals Dwight D. Eisenhower, Omar Bradley, and Norman Schwarzkopf.

One very important principle is introduced by Carl von Clausewitz (1873). Clausewitz indicates that war is an extension of policy and policy leads to passion. Passion is essential among the people themselves, the commanders, and the government. No passion, no victory. If there is no passion or if existing passion diminishes, the war will be lost or millions of lives will unnecessarily be sacrificed to the pandemic. If the public is nonchalant, disinterested, or feels invincible, then it is likely that great effort and expense will be extended for naught. There are new procedures out of the field of informatics that might be very helpful in scientifically determining passion and predicting disease occurrence related to outbreaks, epidemics, or pandemics. Eysenbach (2009) described two tactics: infodemiology and infoveillance. These activities are based on monitoring activities on the Internet. He describes a number of practices using the Internet, such as analyses of queries from search engines, to predict disease magnitude. Increased communication via the Internet predicts disease outbreak and monitoring status updates on microblogs such as Twitter for disease surveillance communication.

We have witnessed several examples of the effects of the lack of public passion, with the Vietnam War being among the most well known. For victory, passion of the people has to be maintained. World War II is an example where the country's passion never waned and everyone was involved, wanted to join the military, and was willing to do what was necessary for victory to occur. This same type of positive response and population-wide involvement would likely diminish the effects of a pandemic. There are many public health examples of illnesses that never occurred, but were given high publicity, such as the Swine flu of 1976. An attitude that "government authorities" have created an incident is developed, and public trust is diminished. This shift in public attitude can lead to disastrous effects when futures crises occur.

No organization, large or small, can survive and efficiently and effectively accomplish its mission without a strategic plan. A military strategic plan is adaptable to a public health war (and to survival of species). Again, a military strategic plan entails passion, ends, ways, and means. Ends are objectives and should be ranked ordered based on several criteria. *Healthy People 2010* represents an example of ends by ranking diseases according to number of deaths caused (U.S. Department of Health and Human Services, 2000). For example, heart disease and cancer are the number one and two killers for Americans 65 and older, while unintentional injuries are the leading cause of death for those 1 to 44 years old. Gathering epidemiologic information about the next most likely epidemics would be extremely important. It is simply impossible to fight on all fronts concurrently. Objectives for the mostly likely pandemic would need to be approached in the same way, taking into account such factors as geographic area, human resources, physical resources, and the overall impact of success, and the engagement of our infrastructure to combat it. Leadership, personnel roles, resources, and plans, strategies, and objectives would need to be developed and refined.

Prioritizing ends also involves many other thoughtful processes. One is to develop a deliberate plan to assess situations thoroughly and accurately. The CDC surveillance system, which can be found on the CDC's Web site, might be an invaluable resource under these circumstances. Also, there should be crisis action plans for events such as a H1N1 pandemic. A plan is what we think will happen, which may be quite contrary to reality or something major that was overlooked in the initial planning processes. Preparedness and contingency plans should theoretically lead to fewer implementations of crisis plans and more opportunities to focus on prophylaxes versus treatment.

Ways are methods to apply force or what is known as courses of action (COA). In public health, the best COA is identified by investigating efficacious practices based on scientific literature or historical events. COA are known as instruments of power. The utilization of one or a combination of the most effective of these is most likely to aid in winning the war and diminishing the disease. Instruments of power or weapons in the behavioral arsenal that might include understanding how knowledge, facts, and beliefs relate to individual behavior change. Occam's razor or minimal intervention (MI) is known as the simplest intervention that works with a rich history of application and efficacy and seems appropriate for a pandemic situation (Last, 2000). The longer the list and more complicated the recommendation, will diminish compliance. Target is the sine qua non concepts of behavior change. These are generic constructs and skills appropriate for many different problems and not restricted or developed to be used with one type of problem only. One such method is problem solving that meets these requirements, which aid in decision making by leadership and the public alike (Frauenknecht and Black, 2004). The current concerns with the H1N1 pandemic appear to be reasonable, given the easy spread between humans. The uncertainty of severity led our strategy and tactics in our planning to question the vaccination and overall strategy. Using Occam's razor, we should proceed with vaccination processes, policy, and tactics. However, just as important is our public communication process conveying the need to reinforce the simplest strategy and tactics.

Means are resources to include budget and personnel. America can often be long on Ends, but short on Means. It is important to concentrate resources where they will have the greatest impact; some sickness will always occur because of the inability to interdict or save each individual, but the overall group should be well served. The idea is that triage must be accepted as an appropriate response. While the military reluctantly accepts the need for triage, the American public generally does not like this notion. However, if a pandemic characterized by high rates of morbidity and mortality occurs, limiting the abilities of hospitals to provide services, many may see and accept its necessity. It is projected, for example, there are insufficient vaccinations for the novel Type A strains of H1N1 or H5N1 influenza, and it has been noted that production will never catch up with demand (Fedson, 2003). Consequently, the only way to win a war of such nature is to focus on the center of gravity (CG) or in this case, with a virus, to concentrate on prioritizing Ends, applying instruments of power that are efficacious and graduated according to Means. Perhaps one priority would be to administer the vaccine to those at highest risk who might be pregnant women or who have the longest to live (e.g., 6 rather than 24-year olds). The criteria would need to be specified and communicated to the public by government officials.

In developing a strategic plan, CGs must be identified. CGs are objects where all energies must be directed. CGs are more than strengths and might; they are fixed centers on which all power hinges. Sometimes CGs cannot be attacked directly. In these instances, a main vulnerability or artery of the CG becomes the target that leads to toppling the enemy or disease agent. The key is determining the CGs of the pandemic being faced. In the case of H1N1, the CG is morbidity and mortality in excess of the endemic state. Perhaps the CGs, in this case, are primary and possibly secondary prevention methods and not operating out a crisis mode (i.e., tertiary prevention) or triaging people who cannot be saved. The two main issues that will need to be confronted with H1N1 are as follows: (a) assessing the will of the people and their commitment; and (b) apathy about health consequences, and invincibleness to disease.

Two additional principles are important: theater of war and the end state. The theater of war in public health is the community or the area within the jurisdiction of the command team. It is important to know the capabilities within a particular theater of war. It is essential to know what the response team can provide in the way of services. Surveillance can be used to identify where incubation is occurring, duration is longest, highest mortality exists, and where the most people are becoming disabled. The command post might be located right in the heart of the battle, but cannot be remote so current tracking is meaningless and observation is impossible. As noted earlier, the End state is reaching the ultimate objective and having plans as to what to do and how long to stay after the pandemic is on the decline and nearing the endemic state.

Pandemic Influenza: How Are These Strategies Applied?

In this section, military theories and tactics will be applied to the development and testing of strategic plans for healthcare settings. Though a number of pandemics have shaped human history (see Table 40.1), planning considerations associated with the threat of a novel strain of the influenza virus will be addressed.

In the last century, the United States has faced three distinct influenza pandemics: the 1918–1919 "Spanish flu," the 1956–1958 "Asian flu," and the 1968–1969 "Hong Kong flu." The 1918 pandemic was extremely deadly, killing approximately 675,000 Americans in just 8 months, and was ultimately responsible for an estimated 50–100 million deaths worldwide (Taubenberger and Morens, 2006). According to Potter (2001), it is considered the "greatest medical holocaust in history." The Asian flu was responsible for nearly 70,000 deaths in the United States, and over 1 million worldwide (U.S. Dept of Health and Human Services, 2009a). A vaccine was developed in 1957 that helped limit the impact of the virus. Last, the Hong Kong flu killed approximately 1 million people worldwide and over 33,000 in the United States (U.S. Dept. of Health and Human Services, 2009a). Improvements in detection mechanisms, vaccination development, and treatments are responsible for some of the differences in fatality rates between these pandemics. Distinct characteristics of each influenza strain also affect the spread and severity of the disease.

TABLE 40.1 Pandemics throughout Human History

Year	Pandemic
540–542	Bubonic plague
1300s	Black death/the plague (bubonic, pneumonic, and septicemic)
1816–1820s	Cholera
1918–1919	The Spanish influenza
1882	Tuberculosis
1957–1958	The Asian influenza

Though great progress has been made in terms of detection, prevention, and treatment of influenza over the past century, the fact still remains that emergence of a novel strain of influenza can be extremely unpredictable. Projections about the nature of future pandemics include estimates of 79,000 to 207,000 deaths in the United States, with a projected economic burden anywhere from $71 to $166 billion (Haber et al., 2007). Which portions of the population will be most affected (in terms of age group), specific symptoms, and the geographic spread of an influenza virus cannot be predicted with great certainty until the virus has already emerged (Brundage, 2006; Taubenberger et al., 2007). Uncertainty about the specifics of a potential pandemic should not be viewed as a reason not to plan for the future. In fact, the opposite is true: because there is such a high degree of uncertainty, this calls for considering and preparing for a variety of situations.

Seasonal influenza infects approximately 5%–20% of the United States population, and is responsible 30,000–40,000 deaths annually, according to the CDC (2009a). On average, more than 200,000 individuals/year are admitted to the hospital for complications related to influenza in the United States (CDC, 2009b). In addition, it is estimated that seasonal flu is responsible for 200 million days of diminished productivity, 100 million days of bed disability, and 75 million days of work absence in the United States alone (Greenbaum, 2006). The total economic burden related to seasonal influenza is estimated to be over $87 billion (Greenbaum, 2006).

As a respiratory illness, the flu is primarily spread through aerosol droplets (expelled during a cough or sneeze), and by transmission of those droplets by the hand to the mouth or nose (Collignon and Carnie, 2006). Because seasonal influenza has the most severe impact on the very old and very young, these tend to be the age groups who are viewed as a priority for receipt of a vaccination. Pandemic influenza differs in this regard because infection rate among different age groups depends on the particular strain of influenza (Heymann, 2004).

Why Is Workplace Planning Important for Pandemic Prevention?

There are a variety of community-wide behaviors that can be encouraged by healthcare providers and implemented by policy officials in order to reduce the spread of illness. Guidelines from the CDC for community action closely reflect lessons learned from past pandemics, emphasizing the "timeless and universal importance of public health" (Morens et al., 2009). "Because influenza pandemics cannot be predicted as to timing and antigenic type, community mitigation strategies will remain a key component of influenza pandemic responses insofar as they attempt to counter known mechanisms of transmission and can be broadly applied by ordinary citizens without specialized medical knowledge" (Morens et al., 2009). These mitigation strategies should include measures that can be undertaken at the workplace.

According to the U.S. Bureau of Labor Statistics (2006), the average American working full-time spends approximately 9.2 h at work, 7.5 h sleeping, 0.9 h doing household activities, 3.0 h doing leisure or sports activities, and 3.4 h doing other activities, such as eating and drinking, attending school, and shopping. The large amount of time spent outside the home should be considered in the development of prevention and control techniques and delivery strategies.

In a business or a healthcare facility, strategic plans need to account for not only the treatment of patients, but also aggressive implementation of prevention strategies for the benefit of their staff and their operations.

How Are Constraints on Resources Addressed during Strategic Planning?

An important consideration in pandemic planning is the constraints imposed upon Means. Means can be discussed in three major categories: (1) manpower, (2) supplies, and (3) funding.

During a pandemic influenza, all businesses and hospitals should have contingency plans available for operation with fewer than normal staff. Though it is impossible to predict exactly how much of the population will be infected by any particular pandemic virus, it is likely a fairly safe assumption that healthcare workers will be infected at similar rates as the rest of the population. Though personal prevention techniques and improved hygiene may be seen among healthcare workers, they also are more likely to be exposed to greater numbers of sick and infectious individuals, thus increasing their own risk of becoming ill. Also to be considered are those individuals who are not yet sick, but resist coming to work during the time of pandemic out of fear of infecting themselves or their families. Open communication between the hospital administration and staff is a key to allaying these fears and conveying expectations about employee conduct.

Most hospitals and clinics likely have a very clear leadership structure for day-to-day operations. For pandemic planning, the possibility of interruptions to normal operations and changes in personnel roles and responsibilities must be expected. For example, who communicates information about vaccination availability to the public? Who is in charge of managing staff operating on an abnormal schedule? Who is in charge of maintaining supplies and resources? What occurs if key decision-makers are too sick to work? What services might be changed or reduced under the demands of responding to pandemic needs including the constraints of staff with influenza? A thorough pandemic plan should account for at least a minimum of these uncertainties.

Healthcare providers also could find themselves limited in terms of supplies available during an influenza pandemic. Depending on reordering supplies in this scenario is not a reliable solution, as during a particularly severe pandemic, highway travel and delivery from supply companies may be limited or even nonexistent. Stockpiling supplies such as gloves, face masks, and sanitizer solutions should be considered. Relying on existing stockpiles of antiviral medication, such as Tamiflu, should also be done with caution. If your geographic area is hit with less severity than neighboring areas, you may be called upon to share and assist in distribution of your stockpile.

Last, the issue of funding cannot be ignored. With unlimited funding, there are fewer limitations in terms of manpower or physical resources. Of course, unlimited funding is never a reality, and many healthcare providers find themselves in a scenario in which their funding is the driving force behind the services provided. Rather than determining which services should be provided, based on their effectiveness in promoting good health of the population, providers are forced to choose services based on the efficiency and economics of their delivery. The goal should be to find a balance between the affordability and quality of services.

How Can Situational Uncertainties Be Accounted for in the Strategic Plan?

Pandemic planning must deal with uncertainty at many levels, but with the certainty that a pandemic will occur eventually (Lipsitch et al., 2009). The variable issues that planning must address include assembly of situational awareness that provides early warning of events that require initial response measures to commence. Planning measures must be relatively simple to implement, with the end effect of limiting or slowing the spread of disease (Centers for Disease Control and Prevention, 2007; Longini et al., 2005). The communication of the pandemic situation must be clear at all levels to ensure that individual actions are understandable and reasonable. Finally, response activities must be ready to accelerate counter measures that reestablish baseline conditions.

While we might not have a clear idea of the specific pandemic threat or knowledge of the pandemic time of onset, we do know that the dread of pandemic comes from knowledge that once this event occurs, it will likely be unstoppable. The problem in establishing situational awareness lies in the characteristics of the virus being monitored. The factors adding to the potential for viruses to change that impact the attack rates, severity, previous immunity, ability to propagate, and so on (Ferguson et al., 2006; Germann et al., 2006; Glass et al., 2006; Longini et al., 2004).

Strategy Illustrations: How Are Strategies Applied during a Pandemic?

What Is the National Strategy for Influenza Prevention?

The normal seasonal flu preparations are a good example of deliberate planning that involves the selection of serum for use in the seasonal flu shots. There is a panel that analyzes the global influenza situation as well as the recent influenza cases before determining a strategy or policy for the next flu season. The strategic plan is executed at a number of levels from international and national to state and local then finally at the business or hospital levels. The overall plan for determining the best serum is useless without a solid execution strategy at the local level with hospitals and doctors strongly believing in the system and the need. The last part of the system is the public communication needed to ensure that the public has the passion and will, especially by those at highest risk (Black, 2002).

What Are the Individual Strategies for Prevention?

At the tactical level, we need to reinforce the individual responsibility to wash well and stay home when sick. The strategic level for this same example is the communication programs needed by government to promote as well as the policy program within a specific business. The strength of this simple approach would be in the expectation that simple hand-washing and hygiene policies have been proven to reduce the rate of influenza infections by over 30% (Dyer et al., 2000). The resulting costs for implementing this strategy should actually result in savings in the overall business sick leave use.

What Strategy Should Be Used for Incident Command Selection?

One important component of the strategic and tactical planning is the understanding of the leadership available and the community issues in a particular area. For instance, a community must select the incident command structure for the pandemic response. The National Incident Management System (NIMS) allows the area to select the best command structure based on local knowledge of the individuals and situation. At the local government level, the incident command could include placing the local health office in charge, but variations like placing the emergency manager in charge or by using a Unified Command structure could be equally effective. Unified Command is a concept that provides a number of leaders to remain in control of resources but under a structure that provides a unified direction. Other considerations within NIMS can include the selection of deputy commanders and segregation of duties. For instance, when the health officer is the incident commander, the emergency manager who routinely manages a number of logistical assets needed to handle security, emergency power generation, or shelter issues would make this individual the logical deputy for the health officer. If the emergency manager is the incident commander then reinforcing the health aspects of a pandemic would make the health officer a logical deputy.

What Are Strategies for Staffing Hospitals?

Much planning and preparation has to be done prior to a pandemic to ensure adequate staffing throughout the event. Three staffing strategies include looking internally by increasing current staff capabilities, looking externally for volunteers within the community, or by alternatively decreasing the surge capacity.

The scope of practice, workload, and duration of work can be increased to enhance staffing capabilities. Cross training staff on multiple jobs before a pandemic will make an easier transition when compared to "just-in-time" training after the event occurs. Educating staff on the emergency situations and what is expected from them will create less confusion and staff refusal. Improving staff capabilities also can be done by increasing the workload/shift and the duration of work/week. This strategy will help fill the gaps of the absent employees and the rising need of inpatient care. Increasing part-time staff to full-time status may especially be a key strategy. However, increasing the workload and duration too fast too soon can lead to exhaustion and low staff morale.

The volume of staff can be increased by utilizing retired healthcare workers, students currently being trained in their future healthcare discipline, and other professional or nonprofessional volunteers. Prior to a pandemic, it is very important to create an extensive list of volunteers that would be willing to support the healthcare facility. A volunteer list has to be updated frequently to provide the most up-to-date contact information and credentials. Just-in-time training and a quick credentialing system should be in place to adapt the volunteers to their tasks and responsibilities during a pandemic. Important considerations must be taken regarding how committed they are to serving the healthcare facility, the responsibilities they will have, and how they will be compensated for their work.

Finally, the total amount of work placed upon the healthcare facility has to be evaluated. Although hospitals may want to increase the number of beds to their fullest capacity, having too many patients will drastically reduce the quality of care. The patients within such a facility will have greater risk of injury and the staff working within will have a greater risk of exhaustion. An optimum level between the available number of staff and consequently the number of patients that can be supported by the hospital needs to be evaluated prior to and routinely throughout a pandemic event.

Hearing the voice of the staff and providing staff support throughout a pandemic will help ensure good morale. It is highly recommended that staff is surveyed before a pandemic to evaluate the number of hours they would be willing to work, the scope of work they would be willing to perform, and their perceived ability to voice concerns. Strong staff support throughout a pandemic also will help to increase staff morale. This may include staff housing facilities, providing food, and offering free child care services. Staff commitment to increased expectations preceding a pandemic is essential. Therefore, much planning and preparation needs to be in place before a pandemic to ensure the staff will be able to support the community need.

How Are Strategic Plans Developed and Implemented?

It is important to emphasize again that planning used for the county-level and hospital exercises began a continuous planning process requiring distinct steps (see Figure 40.1 as a graphic representation of our planning process). The inner ring includes the four phases of emergency management: prepare,

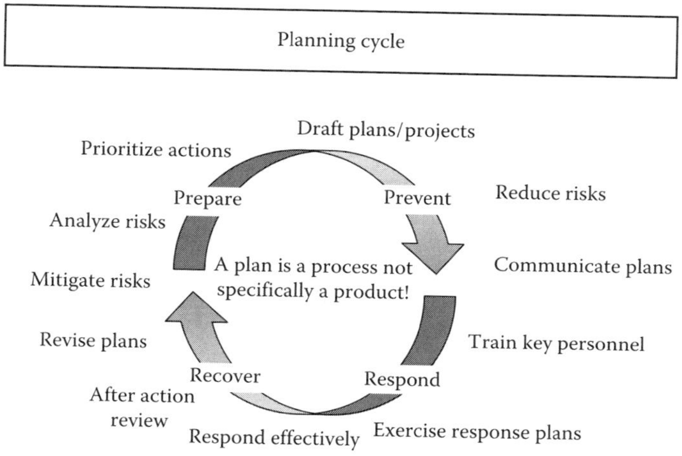

FIGURE 40.1 Planning cycle for implementing pandemic preparedness.

prevent, respond, and recover. "Prepare" and "prevent" occur before the pandemic influenza disaster. "Respond" includes the actions taken during the disaster followed by the "recovery" phase that includes reestablishment of the endemic state that existed before the influenza or other disaster. The outer ring provides the steps needed to develop plans consistent with the four phases of emergency management.

First step in implementation, the clear reason or requirements for the planning including urgency and passion are needed to ensure adequate stakeholder involvement. In the case of the H1N1 virus concerns in 2009, the need and urgency are quite clear, but the challenge to analyze the risks or to meet the requirements in a way that are achievable in human, financial, and material shortages that are present are not. The risks and requirements analyses are necessary to ensure that the strategy is prioritized to ensure a deliberate process for trading the most urgent planning task for the more routine and to monitor the passion of the people and Means at disposal to adequately fund it.

With the prioritized objectives, the business or hospital will use the strategies as a guide toward the development of tactical plans comprising feasible COA. These high-priority tactical plans must be well communicated to the public, taught to the workforce, and coordinated with key partners to ensure expectation management is maintained. The next planning step involves research and stakeholder buy-in that anticipates the problem, the support, and the partners involved in not only developing the draft plan, but also building the team needed to implement the plan. The planning process must be completed in a way that reduces the risks identified at the beginning of the planning process and is consistent with the research, prioritization, and team-building efforts.

Next, the planning needs to shift from actual development to the communication and training among stakeholders. The conclusion of this step yields the draft plan ready for validation testing through exercise. The validation testing is accomplished through an exercise designed to test key plan components such as planning assumptions, sequencing of key planning steps, overarching overall complexity, resource adequacy, training, and readiness to implement. The validation exercises may take many forms including seminars, TTXs, functional exercises, and full-scale exercises depending on the time and resources available. The seminars are essentially group meetings that are conducted to discuss planning problems and issues needed to effectively perform in an emergency. The TTXs are leadership events that take place in a classroom or conference facility where scenario-based situations are presented for discussion based on the planning. The functional exercises are intended for a single functional group like emergency medical services, emergency room, respiratory therapy, or an ancillary service where the functional group actually mobilizes the capability and response mission. This exercise level is usually significantly more expensive and complicated than previous exercise levels. The planning time is also much more extensive to accommodate the more complicated exercises. The full-scale exercise is the most complicated and expensive validation test of a planned capability. The time needed to prepare for a full-scale exercise is significant and in most cases will not be possible to conduct a full-scale pandemic preparedness exercise for a hospital, while maintaining normal operations.

For each exercise, a critical evaluation of strengths and areas requiring improvement are needed. This is the real value in exercise. The military equivalent to the TTX exercise is the command post exercise or exercise without troops which allows the leaders to test reaction and decision-making skills. Just as a military organization would not forego the concept of preparedness or "train as you fight" neither should healthcare providers. The pandemic plan for a hospital must be exercised in order to effectively mobilize for a pandemic response. The exercises help identify planning improvements and test the thoroughness of training. Exercises can clearly show problem areas and provide the ability to improve on these before they are actually needed by the community served. The exercise actions should be formally documented, including improvement plans that lead to revisions, and the return to the beginning of the planning cycle.

The final step is to determine the need for repeating the cycle with updates to the plan to improve on exercise weaknesses, perform further training or exercises, and finally the needs for sustaining the capability. The plan cannot be a binder that sits on the shelf without leadership attention to keep it current and ready to implement. The process is as important as the plan because the continuous improvement leads toward the needed capability while allowing for new information and adjustment of the planning needs. The process is the most important part of the planning activities.

How Can the Hospital Plan Be Implemented?

The best hospital plan will follow the planning cycle or an adaptation of the cycle based on specific needs of the hospital team. The planning should systematically follow the planning cycle in a way that the stakeholders understand. A number of resources, such as the U.S. Department of Health and Human Services' "Hospital Pandemic Influenza Planning Checklist" and "Pandemic Influenza Plan Supplement," are available to help guide a hospital's planning (U.S. Dept. of Health and Human Services, 2009b,c). A hospital must develop a systematic process that combines requirements or needs in a way that may be understood by executives, hospital workers, and patients as justifiable in a situation where long waits and differences in standards of care will likely occur. The planning also must be flexible to ensure that the unplanned or unexpected needs are addressed adequately while managing a number of other competing demands for resources. Two of the most important aspects of hospital planning are the availability to scale the mobilization to the actual event to ensure conservation of personnel, supplies, and funding for events that are less than a full pandemic. The second is the ability to build a plan that works in the most robust pandemic event possible. The public, government, and hospital workers must be convinced that the response can be sustained to ensure that a crisis in confidence does not occur.

The incident command plan is an important overview consideration for hospital planning. This is essentially the management cell that will interface with the government and manage the internal and external healthcare. The interfaces in the incident command team will include the information about the specific event once known as well as policy interfaces with government.

The triage, admission, and hospital access plan will be one of the most challenging aspects of a pandemic. Special considerations must include aspects of the patient population including children, families, elderly, pregnant women, young adults, physically or mentally challenged, patients with chronic conditions, and other special needs groups. The plan also must consider physical limitations such as available space, equipment, and transportation systems in place that might allow for a separate waiting area, additional screening space, and hospital admittance. The space limitations and conditions of patients also may impact the admittance process in a way that requires supervision oversight or additional nursing to accommodate care at home.

Once admitted, an essential healthcare services plan will be needed to ensure that essential services are maintained. Likewise, the nonessential operations or altered standards of care will need to be implemented and maintained dynamically according to the new standards. The trigger points for these adjustments may need to be modified according to the specific situation, but having a priority list on services and standards will allow for a more rapid and well-staffed decision process. Beyond altered standards of care, other plans may require changes, for example, the visitation policy, mortuary plan, pharmaceuticals plan, communication plan, palliative care/psychosocial support, security plan, laboratory plan, and maintenance procedures. Each of these may alter the staffing needs of the hospital, but also the patient acceptance and communication with the public will be needed for successful implementation.

The ideal staffing levels and patient ratios might be difficult to provide during a pandemic. A clear written contingency staffing plan for 8–12 weeks will be needed and this must be coordinated with neighboring facilities to ensure that temporary staff and volunteers have not committed to multiple facilities. The staffing levels must be identified to determine additional staff required to reach a specific surge level but also to identify the trigger points for reducing services. The surge personnel also may have a different level of credentialing, or volunteer staff might require further staffing modifications that must be considered. The numbers of additional staff and volunteers will likely require a surge in personnel screening and the vetting in place including background checks, credential checks with licensing agencies, and increase in payroll actions. The hospital is the likely site for uncoordinated and unsolicited volunteer surges that must be considered. The increase of ill and the additional hospital traffic will increase the need for an effective infection control plan.

The ancillary services plan including supplemental services such as laboratory, radiology, physical therapy, and inhalation therapy need to be provided in conjunction with medical or hospital care. The limitations for hospital surge and capacity will be different for each facility and in each set of specifics requiring the incident control team's composition to include knowledgeable staff across the healthcare service spectrum.

During a pandemic characterized by high morbidity and low mortality (as being faced in the United States during the H1N1 pandemic of 2009), healthcare providers may find themselves faced with large staffing shortages. Though the long-term effects of the disease may not be severe for the average previously healthy individual, the short-term effects would cause more than a minor disruption to home and work life. However, with just a few simple, efficient personal health measures implemented, the number of individuals exposed to and infected by a communicable disease can be greatly decreased.

Using a model developed to further understand the spread of influenza through a school, it was estimated that implementing a twofold flu prevention plan could reduce the numbers of those exposed and infected by the disease, and delay the peak of both exposure and infection rates, allowing more time for vaccine and antiviral development and distribution. In this model, the prevention techniques include (1) an aggressive hand-washing program and (2) a symptom-recognition program. The suggested hand-washing program would include educational elements (to explain the importance of hand washing as well as to demonstrate proper hand-washing techniques) as well as active components (consisting of reminders to engage in hand washing at key points throughout the day). The simulated effects of the symptom-recognition program demonstrate the importance of early detection of sick individuals, and distancing those individuals from others not yet exposed to the disease (Dietz et al., 2010).

Figure 40.2 shows the drastic difference in the number of infected individuals when these two health interventions were implemented in the simulation. The dotted line represents the number of infected students without the two health interventions, while the solid line represents the number of infected students expected when these health interventions are implemented thoroughly.

Though the simulation represents the spread of influenza through a school, rather than a healthcare setting, the implications are clear. With complete implementation and cooperation, even simple, inexpensive public and personal health tactics or an MI can be an effective method for preventing the spread of a contagious illness.

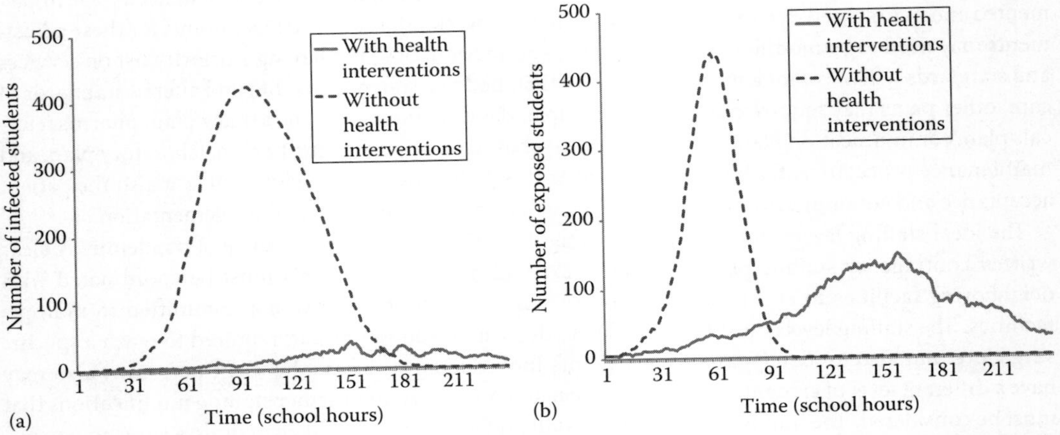

FIGURE 40.2 (a) Influenza infections and (b) influenza exposure during a pandemic wave (as estimated by simulation) illustrating the effects of two health interventions.

What Emerging Lessons Were Learned?

TTXs performed in the summer of 2009 gave significant insight toward the gaps within pandemic influenza hospital and county plans. Feedback was gained by surveying attendees on the "Top Three Lessons Learned" after the TTX was complete. Of the 108 surveys completed, Table 40.2 lists the top identified lessons learned listed by participants, observers, and evaluators that attended the TTX. As Table 40.2 shows, the attendees recognize the importance of having a well-developed plan that is exercised and reviewed regularly.

Communication, whether internal or external, also is seen as an essential component of pandemic planning and response. Educating the public, staff, and stakeholders concerning the rationale for altering services prior and throughout a pandemic is crucial. Last, attendees discovered the importance of the community involvement in a pandemic event. Such involvement may include gaining food supply from closed schools, looking within the community for volunteers, or developing mutual agreements with outside security agencies that could offer support during a pandemic.

Prior to the TTX, evaluators were chosen to examine specific objectives in which they have experience. Evaluators gave their feedback by noting strengths and weaknesses that they observed during the TTX. Table 40.3 shows the significant "areas for improvement" observed by these evaluators during the county exercises. Most of the healthcare facilities within the counties did not have clear trigger points

TABLE 40.2 Most Significant "Lessons Learned" Identified by TTX Attendee Surveys

Lessons Learned
Plan
Need to review, evaluate, and exercise plans regularly
Include surrounding areas and agencies in planning
Communication
Improve internal communication with staff and stakeholders
Need to develop community education and communication strategies
Develop public messages on how and why surge triage will be implemented
Community
Need to look for supply and personnel resources within the community
Develop mutual agreements between agencies that would provide support
Plan and prepare for a localized effort within the community
Staff
Survey staff on the roles and capabilities that can be expected (i.e., increased hours per week, broader job responsibilities)
Need to ensure good staff communication prior and throughout the event
Develop just-in-time training strategies to expand staff capacity
Supplies
Review current resources and stockpile necessary equipment
Evaluate the amount of beds that can be supported and increase beds if needed
Consider the ethical issues regarding supply allocation and altered standards of care
Security and emergency services
Develop just-in-time training for security and identify potential security issues
Need to develop altered standards of care for emergency services (i.e., 911, EMS)
Leadership
Evaluate the leadership model (i.e., too large of a command staff or chiefs)
Need to use (or improve upon) application of an incident command system

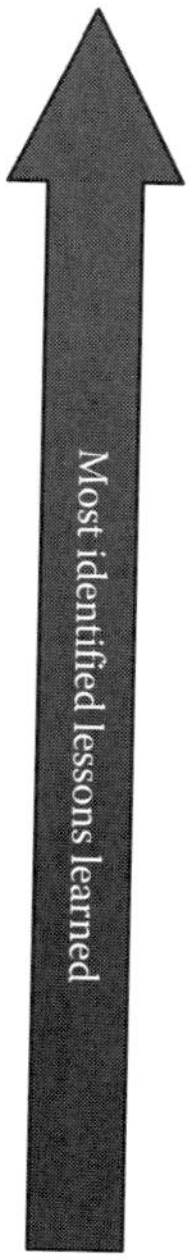

Note: The table expands from the most identified lessons learned (red) to the least identified lessons learned.

TABLE 40.3 The Significant Areas for Improvement Identified by Evaluators during the TTXs

Areas for Improvement	
Define clear trigger points for surge triage implementation	↑ Most identified improvement areas
Develop just-in-time training for staff and volunteers	
Improve supply strategies (i.e., consider a reuse policy)	
Reevaluate staff sustainment strategies	
Review and add details to current plans	
Develop mutual agreements between agencies that will provide support	
Need to gain input on the roles and capabilities that can be expected	
Reevaluate the number of beds that can be supported by staff	
Better identify how and when essential healthcare services will alter	

Notes: The table expands from the areas of improvement most consistently identified across counties to the least consistently identified areas of improvement across the counties.

on when and how they would increase triage and alter their normal healthcare services. To solve the identified problem, most of the healthcare facilities planned to formulate expert groups that regularly meet to discuss when a "trigger" would be pulled during a pandemic. Second, just-in-time training and efficient means of credentialing needs to be established in order for a quick utilization of staff and volunteers. Last, evaluators noted that supply strategies need to be reevaluated and used. Using a reuse policy may be effective in extending supplies, but much consideration needs to be given to the risks versus the benefits of doing so.

During the TTXs, many similarities were found between healthcare facilities regarding their pandemic preparation. The similarities are exemplified by both the consistency between the "lessons learned" identified on surveys completed by exercise attendees (Table 40.2), and the "areas for improvement" noted by TTX evaluators that were consistent throughout the counties (Table 40.3). The TTX found gaps within the pandemic influenza plans and the healthcare facilities have developed improvement plans in response to the findings summarized in Tables 40.2 and 40.3.

Our lessons learned from over 68 pandemic flu exercises at the county level proved that the incident command structure does have an impact on the general performance of tasks. The performance of health-related tasks for a pandemic exercise must meet expected standards without distinction between a health incident commander, an emergency management incident commander, or unified command. We did learn that the logistics-related tasks were performed best by the emergency management commander followed by the unified command and the health officer. This observation reinforces the expected strength of the emergency manager with logistics tasks. The unified command performed logistics tasks well, but generally required more time to execute leading to the observation that unified command. This also reinforces the need to ensure that unified command develops methods for making timely decisions. The health officer without the support of the emergency manager did not effectively demonstrate management of logistics functions. Our analyses do not suggest a best incident command structure but provides some considerations for selection of an incident command team. For instance, the emergency manager could be an effective choice if supported with a health officer as a deputy. Likewise, the health officer is a sound decision for incident commander if supported with a logistics deputy from an emergency management background. The unified command needs the addition of a chief of staff or equivalent to maintain a timely decision-making process. Based on the emerging data at this time, the specific selection needs to be based on local considerations as much as technical skills of the commander. The incident must have the technical skills, but also the leadership, communication and political skills judged to be needed for success.

Preparedness and simplicity of actions will be important in combating a pandemic. A strategic plan and tactics based on military constructs and concepts may have many practical examples for integrating public health and fighting the war related to Type A influenza virus or other diseases that influence masses. As noted, these concepts make practical sense for establishing strategic plans and tactics and the process has been tested over centuries of military conflict. A pandemic has the same uncertainties as to what the military might face and equivalent amounts of chaos. While lessons learned for pandemic response are still being developed, our initial findings are provided as observations discovered in the preparedness for pandemic influenza and are provided for consideration as the H1N1 pandemic situation unfolding in the fall of 2009. Precise lessons learned and actions will likely emerge after urgent needs pass. The military model for that overcomes uncertainty while seeking effective and timely response may be among the best response strategies developed for pandemic response.

Acknowledgment

The authors gratefully acknowledge the contributions of Alok Chaturvedi and Chih-hui Hsieh in the development and interpretation of the model of influenza transmission.

References

Black, D.R. 2002. A strategic plan for winning the war in public health. *American Journal of Health Education*. 33(5):267–275.

Brundage, J.F. 2006. Cases and deaths during influenza pandemics in the United States. *American Journal of Preventive Medicine*. 31(3):252–256.

Centers for Disease Control and Prevention (US). 2007. Interim pre-pandemic planning guidance: Community strategy for pandemic influenza mitigation in the United States—Early, targeted, layered use of nonpharmaceutical interventions. Available from: http://www.pandemicflu.gov/plan/community/community_mitigation.pdf

Centers for Disease Control and Prevention. 2009a. Influenza: The disease. Available from: http://www.cdc.gov/flu/about/disease/index.htm

Centers for Disease Control and Prevention. 2009b. Seasonal influenza-associated hospitalizations in the United States. 2009. Available from: http://www.cdc.gov/flu/about/qa/hospital.htm

Clausewitz, C.V. 1984. *On War* (trans. and eds. M. Howard and P. Paret). Princeton, NJ: Princeton University Press.

Collignon, P.J. and J.A Carnie. 2006. Infection control and pandemic influenza. *Medical Journal of Australia*. 185(10):S54–S57.

Dietz, J.E., J.E. Drifmeyer, K.E. Leonard, C. Hsieh, S. Dunlop, D. Braun, J. Burr, A. Chaturvedi, and D.R. Black. 2010, April 6–7. Pandemic preparedness training for schools (PTS). In *3rd Annual International Conference on Computer Games Multimedia & Allied Technology* (CGAT 2010), Singapore.

Dyer D.L., A. Shinder, and F. Shinder. 2000. Alcohol-free instant hand sanitizer reduces elementary school illness absenteeism. *Clinical Research and Methods*. 32(9):633–638.

Eysenbach, G. 2009. Infodemiology and infoveillance: Framework for an emerging set of public health informatics methods to analyze search, communication and publication behavior on the internet. *Journal of Medical Internet Research*. 11(1):11.

Fedson, D.S. 2003. Pandemic influenza and the global vaccine supply. *Clinical Infectious Diseases*. 36(12):1552–1561.

Ferguson, N., D. Cummings, C. Fraser, J. Cajka, P. Cooley, and D. Burke. 2006. Strategies for mitigating an influenza pandemic. *Nature*. 442(27):448–452.

Frauenknecht, M. and D.R. Black. 2004. Problem-solving training for children and adolescents. In E.C. Chang, T.J. D'Zurilla, and L.J. Sanna (Eds.), *Social Problem Solving: Theory, Research, and Training* (pp. 153–170). Washington, DC: American Psychological Association.

Germann, T., K. Kadau, I. Longini, and C. Macken. 2006. Mitigation strategies for pandemic influenza in the United States. *PNAS*. 103:5935–5940.

Giles, L. 2007. *Sun Tzu: The Art of War*. Ann Arbor, MI: Borders Classics.

Glass, R., W. Beyeler, and H. Min. 2006. Targeted social distancing design for pandemic influenza. *Emerging Infectious Diseases*. 12(11):1671–1681.

Greenbaum, E. 2006. Seasonal influenza: the economics of vaccination. Center for Prevention and Health Services. Issue Brief.

Haber, M.J., D.K. Shay, X.M. Davis, R. Patel, X. Jin, E. Weintrabuc, E. Orenstein, and W.W. Thompson. 2007. Effectiveness of interventions to reduce contact rates during a simulated influenza pandemic. *Emerging Infectious Diseases*. 13(4):581–589.

Heymann, D.L., ed. 2004. *Control of Communicable Diseases Manual*. Washington, DC: American Public Health Assoc.

Last, J.M. 2000. *A Dictionary of Epidemiology*. New York: Oxford University Press.

Lipsitch, M., S. Riley, S. Cauchemez, A.C. Ghani, N.M. Ferguson. 2009. Managing and reducing uncertainty in an emerging influenza pandemic. *New England Journal of Medicine*. 361(2):112–115.

Longini, I.M., M.E. Halloran, A. Nizam, and Y. Yang. 2004. Containing pandemic influenza with antiviral agents. *American Journal of Epidemiology*. 159(7):623–633.

Longini, I.M., A. Nizam, X. Shufu, K. Ungchusak, W. Hanshaoworakul, D. Cummings, and M.E. Halloran. 2005. Containing pandemic influenza at the source. *Science*. 309:1083–1087.

Luvaas, J. 1999. *Frederick the Great on The Art of War*. New York: Da Capo.

Morens, D.M., J.K. Taugengerger, G.K. Folkers, and A.S. Fauci. 2009. An historical antecedent of modern guidelines for community pandemic influenza mitigation. *Public Health Reports*. 124:22–25.

Potter, C.W. 2001. A history of influenza. *Journal of Applied Microbiology*. 91(4):572–579.

Taubenberger, J.K. and D.M. Morens. 2006. 1918 Influenza: the mother of all pandemics. *Emerging Infectious Diseases*. 12(1):13–22.

Taubenberger J.K., D.M. Morens, and A.S. Fauci. 2007. The next influenza pandemic: Can it be predicted? *Journal of the American Medical Association*. 297:2025–2027.

U.S. Bureau of Labor Statistics. 2006. The average day in 2004. Retrieved July 2008, from MLR: The Editor's Desk: http://www.bls.gov/opub/ted/2005/sept/wk3/art03.htm

U.S. Department of Health and Human Services. 2000. Healthy people 2010. 2nd edn. With understanding and improving health and objectives for improving health. 2 vols. Washington, DC: U.S. Government Printing Office.

U.S. Department of Health and Human Services. 2009a. Flu.gov: Pandemics and pandemic threats since 1900. Available from: http://www.pandemicflu.gov/general/historicaloverview.html

U.S. Department of Health and Human Services. 2009b. Hospital pandemic influenza planning checklist. Available from: http://www.flu.gov/professional/hospital/hospitalchecklist.html

U.S. Department of Health and Human Services. 2009c. HHS Pandemic Influenza Plan Supplement 3 Healthcare Planning. Available from http://www.hhs.gov/pandemicflu/plan/sup3.html#process

41

Public Health and Medical Preparedness

Eva K. Lee
Georgia Institute of Technology

Anna Yang Yang
Georgia Institute of Technology

Ferdinand Pietz
Centers for Disease Control and Prevention

Bernard Benecke
Centers for Disease Control and Prevention

Introduction 41-1
Medical Surge 41-2
Surge Patterns • Components of Surge Capacity • Balancing Daily Operational Efficiency and Maintaining Appropriate Surge Capacity • International Collaboration
Population Protection: Medical Countermeasures Dispensing and Large-Scale Disaster Relief Efforts 41-8
A Systems View of Mass Dispensing Operations: Integrating All the Elements • Mode of Dispensing and POD Placement • Resource Allocation and POD Layout Design • Disease-Propagation Analysis: Mitigation Strategies and Choice of Dispensing Modalities • Supply Chain Management: Demand, Supply, Fulfillment, and Partnership • Communication and Public Information • Lessons Learned and Continued Challenges • Large-Scale Disaster Relief Efforts
Communication System 41-20
Physical Infrastructure for Emergency Communication • Communication Facilitation Programs • Organizational Factors in Emergency Communication • Sociological Factors and Linkage to Human Behavior
Emergency Evacuation 41-26
Factors That Affect Emergency Evacuation Planning • Issues in Hospital Evacuation • Evacuation Behavior
Summary 41-30
Optimization, Simulation, and Dynamical Systems Methodologies • Integrated Approaches and Information and Decision Support Systems • Challenges
References 41-34

Introduction

A catastrophic health event, such as a terrorist attack with a biological agent, a naturally occurring pandemic, or a calamitous meteorological or geological event, could cause tens or hundreds of thousands of casualties or more, weaken the economy, damage public morale and confidence, create panic and civil unrest, and threaten national security. It is therefore critical to establish a strategic vision that will enable a level of public health and medical preparedness sufficient to address a range of possible disasters. Although present public health and medical preparedness plans incorporate the concept of "surging" existing medical and public-health capabilities in response to an event that threatens a large number of lives, the assumption that conventional public-health and medical systems can function effectively in catastrophic health events has proven to be incorrect in real-world situations. Therefore, it is necessary to transform the approach to healthcare in the context of a catastrophic health event in order to enable public-health and medical systems to respond effectively to a broad range of incidents.

According to the United States Department of Homeland Security Presidential Directive 21 2007 (The White House, 2007), public health and medical preparedness refers to "the existence of plans, procedures, policies, training, and equipment necessary to maximize the ability to prevent, respond to, and recover from major events, including efforts that result in the capability to render an appropriate public-health and medical response that will mitigate the effects of illness and injury, limit morbidity and mortality to the maximum extent possible, and sustain societal, economic, and political infrastructure."

Planning for a catastrophe involving a disease outbreak or mass casualties is an ongoing challenge for first responders and emergency managers. They must make critical decisions on treatment distribution points, staffing levels, impacted populations, and potential impact in a compressed window of time when seconds could mean life or death. Although extensive resources have been devoted to planning for a worse-case scenario on the local, regional, and national scale, the U.S. Government Accountability Office (GAO) found gaps still exist. While many states have made progress in planning for mass casualty events, many noted continued concerns related to maintaining adequate staffing levels and accessing other resources necessary to effectively respond.

This chapter reviews some key areas of public health and medical preparedness. "Medical Surge" reviews some of the literature on hospital surge capacity. "Population protection: Medical countermeasures dispensing and large-scale disaster relief efforts" highlights our own experience on projects with the Centers for Disease Control and Prevention and various public-health jurisdictions in emergency response and medical preparedness for mass dispensing for disease prevention and treatment, and large-scale disaster relief efforts. "Communication system" overviews communication infrastructure needs and findings from our recent study and evaluation of state-wide emergency communication systems in Georgia. "Emergency evacuation" describes issues pertinent to emergency evacuation. In the "Summary," we summarize some methodologies that are commonly employed in emergency responses. These techniques include optimization, stochastic processes, information technology, and an integrated framework of decision systems. The chapter concludes with some challenges for future research.

Medical Surge

As stated by the U.S. Department of Health and Human Services (HHS), the concept of medical surge forms the cornerstone of preparedness planning efforts for major medical incidents. Medical surge refers to the ability to provide adequate medical evaluation and care during events that exceed the limits of the normal medical infrastructure of an affected community. It encompasses the ability of healthcare organizations to survive a hazard impact and maintain or rapidly recover operations that were compromised (a concept known as medical system resiliency).

HHS makes a distinction between medical surge capacity and medical surge capability. Capacity relates to the ability to handle an overall increase in volume of patients, whereas capability refers to the ability to handle patients who are presenting with problems (e.g., a highly contagious disease) that are not normally handled at the location, as well as patient populations who are not normally handled (e.g., pediatric patients at a non-pediatric facility).

During a disaster, three categories of "players" must be ready to act: public-health, individual facilities, and the community at large. Therefore, it is important to consider surge capacity as it relates to each of these players. Table 41.1 summarizes the definitions of surge capacities at each of these levels.

Surge capacity plans should be scalable and flexible to cope with the many types and varied timelines of disasters. Improving surge capacity involves a multidisciplinary approach that includes all relevant partners and functions, from each of the community's healthcare facilities to local, state, and federal agencies. Facility-based or "surge-in-place" solutions maximize healthcare facility capacity for patients during a disaster. When these resources are exceeded, community-based solutions, including the establishment of off-site hospital facilities, may be implemented (Hick et al., 2004).

TABLE 41.1 Definition

Terms	Definitions
Surge capacity	Ability to manage a sudden, unexpected increase in patient volume that would otherwise severely challenge or exceed the current capacity of the healthcare system
Surge capability	Ability to manage patients who require specialized evaluation or interventions that are not normally provided at the facility/location (e.g., contaminated, highly contagious, or burn patients)
Public-health surge capacity	Ability of the public-health system to increase capacity not only for patient care but also for epidemiologic investigation, risk communication, mass prophylaxis or vaccination, mass fatality management, mental health support, laboratory services, and other activities
Facility-based surge capacity	Actions taken at the healthcare facility level that augment services within the response structure of the healthcare facility; may include responses that are external to the actual structure of the facility but are proximate to it (e.g., medical care provided in tenting on the hospital grounds). These responses are under the control of the facility's incident management system and primarily depend on the facility's emergency operations plans
Community-based surge capacity	Actions taken at a community level to supplement healthcare facility responses. These may provide for triage and initial treatment, non-ambulatory care overflow, or isolation (e.g., off-site "hospital" facility). These responses are under the control of the jurisdictional response (e.g., public health, emergency management) and represent a public effort to support and augment the healthcare system

This section focuses primarily on approaches for hospital surge capacity planning. The "Population protection: Medical countermeasures dispensing and large-scale disaster relief efforts" section will discuss related issues on hospital and community-based surge capacity for population health protection and large-scale prophylactic dispensing for disease and medical protection, and on general disaster relief efforts.

Surge Patterns

In order to better plan for hospital surge capacity during emergency events, researchers have studied data from various disaster events in the past decade to obtain a glimpse of the impact on the healthcare facilities from these events.

Okumura et al. (1996) investigated the case of 640 victims of the 1995 Tokyo gas attack, focusing on their symptoms and treatment. Case studies were given to describe the symptoms of patients upon arrival and the associated treatment provided. Emergency department (ED) treatment consisted mostly of administration of atropine sulfate and dosage with 2-PAM within a few hours of the initial exposure to sarin gas for severe and moderate cases. A few clinical management issues were raised. These included poor ventilation in the ED area; inadequate decontamination due to privacy provision and the large number of affected population; required patient follow up; and monitoring for long-term health effects.

Hogan et al. (1999) studied the pattern in epidemiologic injury data on patients who suffered acute injuries after the 1999 Oklahoma City bombing and concluded that more seriously injured patients tend to arrive in a second wave at emergency departments since they are less mobile and often require on-site treatment. It is understandable that the closest hospitals received the greatest number of victims by all transportation methods initially. There are lessons learned for EDs in terms of preparing for such phenomenon and to prepare and allocate/mobilize resources accordingly. Disaster response planning should avoid overloading hospitals in the vicinity of disasters. Rapid arrival of patients with non-life-threatening injuries may overwhelm the EDs. In this case, EDs must equip themselves with clinical personnel who can perform rapid assessment and stabilization, instead of staffing with specialty doctors who generally lack such skills.

Roccaforte (2001) reviewed various aspects of response by Bellevue Hospital Center to the 2001 World Trade Center attack, including challenges faced with communication, organization, staffing, and logistics. The hospital is 2.5 miles from the site of the attack. When the news just arrived, communication channels were overloaded. Poor communication hindered adequate response planning and therefore wasted resources. Fortunately, the response was well supported by full staffing on the day of the event. Obviously, full staffing would likely not be in place if an emergency event occurred at night or on a weekend or holiday. In any event, the on-hand workforce should be allocated to control and preserve important resources for likely more serious cases in the second wave. Upon arrival of patients, they were triaged based on injury conditions. Out of the 90 patients that arrived during the first 5 hours, 56 had minor injuries and most of them had respiratory complaints. Five of the 90 patients suffered a mixture of fractures and burns. Three patients were seriously injured.

Schull et al. (2006) investigated the surge capacity associated with restrictions on nonurgent hospital utilization and expected admissions during the Toronto Severe Acute Respiratory Syndrome outbreak. The study compared expected influenza-related hospitalization with the actual reduction in hospital admission for 8 weeks for three different pandemic severity levels: mild, moderate, and severe. It was found that influenza-related admissions generally exceed the reduction in admissions of nonurgent cases. Thus, simply reducing hospital admissions may not be sufficient for handling an influenza-related medical surge. Other strategies should be explored.

Gavagan et al. (2006) examined medical response in the aftermath of Hurricane Katrina at the Houston Astrodome/Reliant Center Complex. During the 2 weeks of operation, the center provided shelter to 27,000 evacuees, over 11,000 of whom sought some form of medical care. Common health problems with the patients included uncontrolled hypertension, respiratory infection, and acute gastroenteritis. At the medical center, five levels of care characterized treatment, from immediate triage upon arrival to the use of community resources. Most of the adult visits to the Katrina clinic were related to chronic disease or medication refills. Another major health condition found in adults related to skin problems as a result of exposure to tainted water. Over 3500 children and infants were seen at the medical center during the 2 week span.

People 65 or older accounted for 56% of the total patients seen, and 62% of the 37 total deaths. Other problems that were addressed include mental health, obstetrics, and gynecology. In terms of personnel management, instances were found where noncredentialed people set up medical clinics within the center, raising the critical issue of careful verification of staff qualification.

Stratton and Tyler (2006) studied characteristics of medical surge capacity demand data based on existing databases and literature and concluded that the earliest outside assistance for a community subject to a sudden-impact disaster arrived in roughly 24 hours, with a range that reached to 96 hours. After sudden-impact disasters, 84%–96% of healthcare demand was managed by ambulatory care. Emergency departments were the access point for care, with peak demand time occurring within 24 hours. The author also suggested that lack of standards for reporting disaster data and limited depth of the current disaster literature are limitations for surge capacity–related research.

Components of Surge Capacity

Surge capacity encompasses multidimensional aspects such as potential patient beds; available space in which patients may be triaged, managed, vaccinated, decontaminated, or simply located; available care personnel of all types; necessary medications, supplies and equipment; and even the legal capacity to deliver healthcare under situations that exceed authorized capacity. Further, close collaboration between public-health and healthcare facilities are very important to effective disaster response.

Surge capacity is tight in the nation's hospitals, as hospitals have undergone years of budget tightening and consequent efforts to control costs, resulting in diminished patient capacity. Another factor that affects rapid response to surges includes an overall shortage of nurses. In a 2006 nationwide blue-ribbon panel of healthcare experts, led by Dr. Kelen, head of emergency medicine at The Johns Hopkins Hospital and director of the Johns Hopkins Office of Critical Event Preparedness and Response, it was recommended that hospital plans for a surge of disaster victims should begin with a strategy to empty their beds of relatively healthier patients. Preliminary data suggest that such a strategy could safely empty 70% of a hospital's inpatient population within 72 hours.

There is consensus among healthcare officials that, whether dealing with a natural disaster like Hurricane Katrina, a possible terrorist attack like September 11, or epidemics like SARS or avian flu, affected hospitals have few means of making room for large numbers of incoming casualties.

In one common disaster response, medical centers would set up additional beds wherever they can (in hallways, cafeterias, etc.). But, there is serious concern that staffing levels could not expand to care for so many new patients, and "disposition classification" is being recommended as a must. Such an approach is important as it ensures that both the disaster victims as well as those patients who are already hospitalized, all would receive adequate treatment.

Disposition classification puts patients in one of five categories, based on their considered risk of a life-threatening or life-impairing medical problem within 72 hours of hospital discharge. Patients classified as "minimum" risk could go home upon being discharged. Those in the "low-risk" group could also be transferred home depending on the severity and scope of the disaster. Those in the "moderate" category could not go home but could be transferred to a facility offering basic medical resources. "High-risk" patients could only be transferred to an acute-care facility and "very high-risk" patients could only be served in a critical care facility.

The decision-making process is complex and the logistics behind transferring such a large number of patients to other facilities are hardly trivial. However, it offers an ethical and non-emotional approach, and could be implemented outside of a disaster situation as a tool to manage even routine, everyday overloads of hospital resources (Kelen et al., 2006).

The four critical areas comprising hospital surge capacity identified by various investigators are personnel, facility, equipment and supply, and management (Schultz and Koenig, 2006). Generally, hospitals have a concept on the amount of resources required for each category above a given number of patients. Therefore, improving surge capacity centers around the problem of determining how much a hospital could expand their capacity, how quickly the expansion can be implemented, and how long it can be sustained. For example, an arbitrary amount of 20% on top of normal capacity has been set for Israeli hospitals. In the United States, the Health Resource and Service Administration provides a surge guideline of 500 beds per 1 million population for patients with symptoms of acute infectious disease and 50 beds per 1 million population for noninfectious disease and injury (Barbisch and Koenig, 2006). It is also noted that a hospital will be unable to further increase surge capacity once its saturation point has been reached. Strategies for determining when hospitals will reach this position currently do not exist (Schultz and Koenig, 2006).

We discuss each of these four areas in more detail.

Care Personnel and Staff

When disaster happens, it is natural for hospitals to increase the number of staff by maximizing the use of their own personnel. This requires established protocol for revision of staff work hours (e.g., a 12-hour shift is standard in disaster events), call-back of off-duty personnel, use of nonclinical staff (e.g., nurse administration) in clinical roles as appropriate, and reallocation of outpatient staff resources (Hick et al., 2004).

One possibility to further support hospital staffing requirements is by providing emergency credentialing to volunteer healthcare professionals. However, many issues relating to this practice need to be addressed, for example, an institution's willingness to permit such individuals to work in their facility, credibility and confidentiality issues, and retention of such workers if they are needed for a time period that goes beyond expectation. Schultz and Stratton (2007) suggested a solution to credential issues by sharing a database of credentialed healthcare workers among mutually acceptable organizations, which will then assist in staff planning during disasters. In addition, family members could also assist in taking care of patients.

As discussed, the least serious casualties usually arrive at the hospital first during a disaster. Healthcare personnel may not be aware that more serious patients are yet to arrive. Careful planning must take this factor into consideration to avoid filling existing beds with minor injuries (Kaji et al., 2007). The "disposition classification" scheme can be used to help with proper resource allocation (Kelen et al., 2006).

Research was conducted on healthcare workers' ability and willingness to report to duty during catastrophic disasters (Qureshi et al., 2005). It was reported that one-fourth to one-third of the workforce may be deliberately absent for some period when the use of weapons of mass exposure was involved. Therefore, staffing during disaster will be a serious problem. In our own work, we focus on optimal (minimizing) resource allocation and staffing assignment for mass population protection, and improving system throughput via maximizing operations efficiency, optimal clinic layout design, and process workflow (Lee et al., 2006a,b, 2009a,b).

Facility

Expanding bed capacity during an emergency can be accomplished by multiple strategies. These include

- Reducing current bed occupancy such as canceling elective procedures, early discharge of inpatients (Kelen et al., 2009), and clearing patients with minor injuries.
- Expanding capacity within hospital including converting single rooms to double occupancy, using flat space as patient care wards, and using alternative sites in the parking lot.
- Collaboration with other hospitals and community facilities, including transferring patients to nearby hospitals or healthcare facilities and collaborating with other community organizations such as schools and churches for patient treatment and storage of supplies.

Some of the issues associated with facility expansion include

- Nature of disaster and effected areas—For example, in times of natural disasters such as hurricanes or earthquakes, large areas may be affected at the same time, thus making the transfer between hospitals or nearby community centers impossible.
- Security issues with temporary healthcare facilities—For example, setting up temporary hospitals in tents is a common practice after earthquake events. These facilities are often open to the public, thus making it difficult to control access and prevent theft of equipment and supplies.
- Local practicality—The practicality of the site is influenced by the climate and infrastructure support (e.g., water, electricity, and other utilities).

Equipment and Supplies

Building surge capacity must also take into consideration the requirement on equipment, supplies, and pharmaceuticals on top of availability of wards, spaces, and medical staff. In the United States, the Strategic National Stockpile (SNS) is a program developed by the federal Centers for Disease Control and Prevention (CDC) Bioterrorism Preparedness and Response Initiative that assists states and communities in responding to extreme public-health emergencies from terrorist attacks or natural disasters. SNS has large quantities of medicine and medical supplies to protect the public in a health emergency. The SNS is operated as a collaborative effort between local, state, and federal officials. The SNS contains medicines, vaccines, medical and surgical supplies, life-support medications, and breathing supplies. It is not a first-response tool. Rather, it is designed to supplement and resupply a local and/or state response to an emergency within the United States or its territories. The two major components of the stockpile are 12-hour push packages and the managed inventory. The push packages contain 50 tons of pharmaceuticals, antidotes, and medical supplies that will treat a variety of illnesses. Managed inventory can either replenish the push package or be tailored with specific medical supplies to respond to a defined agent or other specific public-health threat. The 12-hour push packages arrive within 12 hours once deployed at the federal level. Supplies are distributed to local communities as quickly as possible. Managed inventory is shipped to arrive within 24–36 hours after deployment.

Major issues with medical supplies and equipment held are

- Speed of delivery: Hanfling (2006) argues that it is necessary for each local community to create a local cache for these items. He further explored the funding requirements for this approach.
- Amount of supplies to stockpile: It is possible that stockpiled supplies that are very expensive are no longer functional when a disaster outbreak happens (for example, ventilators used for pandemic influenza). Whether we should stockpile for worst-case scenario or most likely scenario is another issue to be discussed.
- Strategies for effective dispensing: For example, in the event of an infectious disease outbreak or a biological attack, operational and strategic plans must be designed and put in place to dispense the medical supplies (e.g., vaccines, antiobiotics) to the affected population effectively and efficiently (Lee et al., 2006a,b, 2009a,b).

Incident Management System

Incident management systems and cooperative planning processes will facilitate maximal use of available resources. However, resource limitations may require implementation of triage strategies.

In building surge capacity, Burkle (2006) investigated a population-based bioevent triage management with the goal of identifying the population requiring immediate care, preventing secondary transmission, and building surge capacities that are population specific. In this management method, population self-identify into one of five categories: susceptible but not exposed, exposed but not yet infectious, infectious, removed by death or recovery, and vaccination or prophylactic medication.

One of the most important issues of surge capacity is the ability to implement an incident management system. In the United States, one of the most conflicted issues with incident management is that the healthcare system includes many private entities. Private hospitals have no jurisdictional boundaries and are not under any governmental or municipal operational authority or control. Successful implementation of an incident management system for effective disaster response requires careful planning and close collaboration between public-health and (private) healthcare facilities, and organizations from the local level to the federal government level.

Balancing Daily Operational Efficiency and Maintaining Appropriate Surge Capacity

With the need to balance budgets, hospital administrators often look toward closures and downsizing to reduce costs, and toward process optimization to improve efficiency. These efforts to decrease costs and increase efficiency often run counter to simultaneous efforts to enhancing or maintaining surge capacity, as staffing and usage of resources are maintained at very high utilization rates, leaving very little room for medical surge. There is also a serious gap between daily surge capacity versus rapid large-scale surge requirements for catastrophic events.

Among the many issues that the U.S. Congress needs to address for public health and medical preparedness and response, medical surge capacity has been identified as inadequate. The Government Accountability Office (GAO) issued an updated report in January 2010, "State Efforts to Plan for Medical Surge Could Benefit from Shared Guidance for Allocating Scarce Medical Resources" (Bascetta, 2010). The report states that many hospitals in the United States are unprepared for treating the overwhelming "surge" of victims from a large scale mass casualty event. GAO said that "based on a review of state emergency preparedness documents and interviews with 20 state emergency preparedness officials, many states had made efforts related to three of the four key components of medical surge that GAO had identified—increasing hospital capacity, identifying alternate care sites, and registering medical volunteers, but fewer had implemented the fourth: planning for altering established standards of care. More than half of the 50 states had met or were close to meeting the criteria for the five medical surge-related sentinel indicators for hospital capacity reported in the Hospital Preparedness Program's 2006 midyear progress reports. In a 20-state review, GAO found the following: "All 20 were developing bed reporting systems and most were coordinating with military and veterans hospitals to expand hospital capacity. Eighteen were selecting various facilities for alternate care sites. Fifteen had begun electronic registering of medical volunteers, and fewer of the states—7 of the 20—were planning for altered standards of medical care to be used in response to a mass casualty event."

International Collaboration

As illustrated vividly by the recent tsunamis and the 2010 Haiti earthquake, surge capacity remains critical when catastrophic events elsewhere in the world demands it. Research has been done internationally on improving healthcare surge capacity in the face of a high-consequence event. Peleg and Kellermann (2009) summarized 14 principles developed by Israel's Ministry of Health on enhancing system surge capacity. Shih and Koenig (2006) also discussed Taiwan's experience in managing surge needs through sending doctors to the scene of an event, immediately recalling off-duty hospital personnel, managing volunteers, designating specialty hospitals, and use of incident management systems.

In the recent Haiti situation, the destruction of the local healthcare infrastructure required reaching out to hospitals outside the country, as well as immediate establishment of a network of on-site healthcare facilities. In this case, the United States naval ship USS Comfort served as an acute treatment site, whereas temporary makeshift hospital tents were set up to provide medical care for the mass injured. This illustrates the intimate and critical interplay between hospital surge capacity and the urgent need for setting up (temporary) facility-based and community-based solutions to manage medical surges.

Population Protection: Medical Countermeasures Dispensing and Large-Scale Disaster Relief Efforts

Public-health emergencies, such as bioterrorist attacks or pandemics, demand fast, efficient, large-scale dispensing of critical medical countermeasures (i.e., vaccines, drugs, and therapeutics). Such dispensing is complex and requires careful planning and coordination from multiple federal, state, and local agencies, and the potential involvement of the private sector. Dispensing medications quickly (within 48 hours for anthrax prophylactic) to large population centers (with tens of thousands or even millions of people) is urgent; moreover, the multifaceted nature of dispensing (e.g., sending federal stockpiles to local points of dispensing (PODs), coordination at the local level to manage the transportation of citizens to PODs, and the POD operations) makes the process highly unpredictable. Thus, emergency managers and public-health administrators must be able to quickly investigate alternative response strategies as an emergency unfolds.

The focus of this section is on *mass dispensing* of medical countermeasures for protection of the general population. Other issues pertinent to large-scale disaster relief efforts will also be highlighted. Much of the writing below are excerpts from our recent work with the Centers for Disease Control and Prevention on modeling and optimizing public-health emergency response infrastructure and the development of a large-scale simulation-optimization decision support system, RealOpt (Lee et al., 2005, 2006a,b, 2009a,b; Lee, 2008).

Large-scale public-health emergencies may involve thousands of sick or injured people who will require various levels of medical care, ranging from patient evacuation (see "Emergency Evacuation"), hospital care, and sustainable and potentially long-term health-recovery procedures. Thus, such emergencies present a daunting set of challenges, including the surge capacity and flexibility of our existing medical systems (see "Medical surge"), federal and state emergency capacity for rapid medical dispatching, and the resolve and resilience of healthcare workers and emergency responders to perform under critical timelines and exceedingly stressful conditions.

In the wake of the 2001 anthrax attacks, the Department of Health and Human Services (HHS) increased its order for smallpox vaccine, accelerated production, and began working to develop a detailed plan for the public-health response to an outbreak of smallpox. By January 2003, the United States had sufficient quantities of the vaccine for every person in the country in an emergency situation (Gerberding, 2003). Subsequently, HHS required each state to submit a mass-vaccination plan for administering smallpox vaccine. Further, states are charged with developing city-readiness programs that deal with establishing regional treatment and dispensing centers, and developing procedures, policies, and a planning framework for efficient allocation of staff and resources in response to these events.

The importance of such population protection has been carefully studied for human, social, and economic benefits. Kaplan et al. (2002) argued that immediate mass vaccination after a smallpox bioterrorist attack would result in fewer deaths and faster eradication of the potential epidemic; Wein et al. (2003) concluded that immediate and aggressive dispersion of oral antibiotics and the full use of available resources (local nonemergency care workers, federal and military resources, and nationwide medical volunteers) are extremely important.

A Systems View of Mass Dispensing Operations: Integrating All the Elements

Public health and medical preparedness involves three phases: (1) preparedness and prevention, (2) detection and response, and (3) recovery and mitigation.

Modeling and optimizing public-health infrastructure involve elements of resource allocation under risk, uncertainty, and time pressure; large-scale supply-chain management; transportation and operational logistics; and medical treatment and population protection. The operations must be supported by an effective communication infrastructure. There is a necessity for vertical and horizontal integration and communication, where federal, state, local, tribal, territorial, private, and business stakeholders work toward a common goal of a resilient public-health system. The infrastructure must be *flexible*, *scalable*, *sustainable*, and *elastic* to support an effective and timely response, and to mount rapid recovery and mitigation operations (Lee, 2009, Lee et al., 2009a,b).

The global integration plan for population protection in the event of medical and emergency response includes multiple interconnected components: strategic planning; management command and control with key leaders working cohesively together as a team; requesting supplies and equipment from strategic national stockpiles; tactical communication and information technology; public information and risk communication; security; regional and local distribution sites (for receiving, staging, and storing of supplies, as well as transportation and routing); inventory control and management; distribution—supply and resupply; dispensing; treatment centers; and planning, training and evaluation (Lee, 2009). The ultimate goal is to *dispense* the medical countermeasures to the affected regional population.

Mode of Dispensing and POD Placement

Mass dispensing requires the rapid establishment of a network of dispensing sites and health facilities that are *flexible, scalable,* and *sustainable* for medical prophylaxis and treatment of the general population. Moreover, each POD must be capable of serving the affected local population within a specified short time frame. Clearly, for very large-scale dispensing, the sophisticated logistical expertise needed to deal with the complexities of selecting an adequate number of strategically well-placed POD locations, and of designing and staffing each POD, is beyond the capability of any human planner or public-health administrator. The limited availability of trained critical staff, such as public-health professionals, further compounds the inherent complexities.

The CDC and public-health administrators work closely with one another to prepare for and document the steps required to administer medication in the event that mass dispensing is needed. The goal and objectives of a dispensing facility, POD, are to deliver appropriate emergency services (e.g., vaccine, medical service, and education/training) to high-risk populations in an orderly, expeditious, and safe manner. Within the POD facility (e.g., Figure 41.1), the potential tasks and objectives may include

1. Assess health status of clients
2. Assess eligibility of clients to receive service
3. Assess implications of each case and refer case for further investigation if necessary
4. Counsel clients regarding service and associated risks
5. Administer service
6. Educate regarding adverse events
7. Document services
8. Monitor vaccine take rates
9. Monitor adverse reactions
10. Monitor development of disease

Mode of Dispensing

The *key* to mass dispensing is to protect the general population efficiently and effectively under time pressure. For example, in an anthrax attack, the goal is for citizens to receive antibiotic prophylaxis within 48 hours of the determination that an attack has occurred, as the mortality rate for persons demonstrating symptoms of inhalation anthrax is extremely high (Lawler and Mecher, 2007). Thus, it is recognized that multiple dispensing modalities often must be employed in order to *serve* (*cover*) the entire regional population. For example, special dispensing services will be utilized to serve homebound, disabled, and special need populations. In some instances, it is unreasonable to expect residents to travel to a designated POD facility. For example, nursing homes, assisted living facilities, homeless shelters, hospitals, and prisons house many residents for whom it would be inconvenient or inadvisable to travel

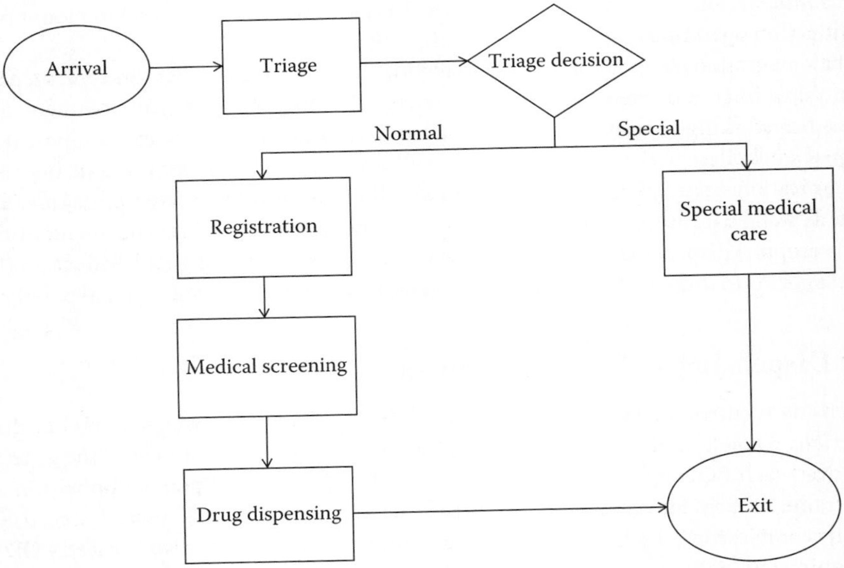

FIGURE 41.1 The flowchart shows a POD that was set up in a national drill exercise to dispense anthrax antibiotics.

to a public dispensing facility. Moreover, in many of these instances, there are already medical personnel on site who can assist in the dispensing process. In such cases, it would be more efficient to set up a *closed* POD inside these locations for dispensing, or to have medication dispensed by a mobile POD facility near the site. In this case, the POD is *closed* as it provides services only to the residents on-site, and is not open to walk-ins from the general public. Corporate offices that staff a large number of employees could be served in a similar manner. Once these sites receive prophylactic supplies, they could set up a closed POD within their building, with their own healthcare staff and volunteers, or with public-health staff supplemented by the state. Several factors suggest that such closed PODs will have fewer security concerns and will be easier to manage than public PODs. These factors include familiarity with the environment and people (e.g., fellow residents/employees), existing security measures including established checkpoints, and previously authenticated identification badges with photo and/or biometric markers, and less stress than having to commute to a public POD.

Airports and hotels, where a large number of nonresident travelers can be found, are also candidates for setting up PODs to service specific vulnerable populations. Universities can use their own health facilities (and if necessary, additional mobile on-campus PODs provided by the state) to provide prophylaxis to on-campus students, staff, and faculty. Clearly, if large employers and medical facilities provide prophylaxis to their own employees, families, and patients, it will eliminate a high percentage of the population (may be as high as 40% in some large cities) from visiting public PODs, thus reducing the load on those facilities.

Public PODs are *open* facilities that are set up to serve the general public.

In the literature (Lee et al., 2006a,b, 2009a,b), public PODs have generally been described as being set up inside existing facilities, or in outdoor tents, with areas set aside for various activities in the dispensing process, including assembly/intake, triage, orientation, registration, screening, service, education, and discharge. Public PODs can be mobile or stationary, and in the latter case, they can be set up as *facility-based* or *drive-through*.

A facility-based POD operates within physical locations, such as buildings, warehouses, open fields, or large parking lots. Citizens are asked to arrive at the POD location and then *walk through* the POD to receive their medication or other treatment. Facility-based PODS may be scaled to operate within a setting as large as a professional sports stadium or as small as a volunteer fire house within a rural community.

These walk-through PODs are suitable for relatively large-capacity facilities, where the possibility of traffic jams preclude the use of the drive-throughs. Because parking is typically limited, individuals may be directed to arrive at designated points, and they are bused to the POD. Examples of pickup points include bus stations, subway stations, and parking lots of large shopping malls, where sufficient parking is available.

High schools are often selected as potential POD locations. The fact that they are government-owned makes logistics easier. Other considerations include existence of offices, computer communications, cafeterias, storage, etc. Shopping malls, churches, and stadiums are also suitable, and in some cases, PODs are set up outdoors using tents and temporary constructs.

Drive-through PODs are suitable to serve a spread-out population. Ideally, government-owned properties are preferred over privately owned ones for logistics reasons. Locations for setting up drive-through facilities should have enough space for multiple dispensing lanes; surrounding access roads; and room for command tent, employee rest area, and medication storage.

POD (Facility) Placement

Facility location problems are classical optimization problems, and have been a critical element in strategic planning for a wide range of private and public organizations. The earliest facility location problems incorporating emergency response related to location of emergency facilities (Swain et al., 1971; Larson, 1975; Aly and White, 1978). Chaiken and Larson (1972) provided a survey on urban emergency unit allocation. Some researchers (Hogan and Revelle, 1986; Pirkul and Schilling, 1988; Narasimhan et al., 1992) explicitly took the need for backup facilities (in case the main facility is overloaded) into account. More recently, Jia et al. (2002) provided a modeling framework for location of medical services for large-scale emergencies. Berman and Gavious (2007) took a game-theoretic approach toward location of terror response facilities. Church et al. (Church et al., 2004; Church and Scaparra, 2007) studied the problem of identifying and protecting critical infrastructure. A comprehensive review of facility location research can be found in Brandeau and Chiu (1989), where the authors presented a survey of over 50 representative problems in location research. Most of the problems reviewed have been formulated as optimization problems. Owen and Daskin (1998) provided another review of the strategic facility location problem. They considered a wide range of model formulations across numerous industries, including stochastic formulations, and discuss solution approaches.

While many of the facility location problems involve permanent construction and establishment of service facilities, facility location problem for mass dispensing concerns the placement of PODs (mobile or stationary) in existing facilities (e.g., high schools, stadiums, shopping malls, open parking lots) in a region to provide the necessary services to the population within a designated period of time.

Various objectives can be incorporated within the models. In the event of catastrophic incidents, it is critical that PODs are strategically located so as to allow easy access by the affected public. Hence, minimizing transportation time can be one critical objective. Further, the setup and operating costs of PODs cannot be neglected. A POD must be accessible by service workers, it should include a good communication infrastructure, it must be easily protected by law-enforcement personnel, and the facility must be capable of handling a large flow of people. Physical constraints on the facility must be modeled properly, e.g., capacity of a facility cannot be violated (e.g., POD parking capacity is limited, and fire codes limit the number of individuals who can be inside a facility simultaneously).

For operational purposes, there is also a desire to ensure that the number of PODs in each jurisdiction is at least two. This is due to the concern that if a catastrophic event at one site necessitates shutting down a POD, emergency dispensing can still be carried out in the remaining location. In this case, the response manager can reroute populations to the remaining site, while reestablishing a new POD, if deemed necessary.

Modeling of the POD placement problems involves the traditional facility location characteristics, as well as the incorporation of spatial, geographical, and demographics information. The problem can be modeled using a two-stage integer programming approach. For a large metropolitan area with a population over 5 million, such a POD placement problem can result in optimization (integer programming) instances involving millions of variables and constraints, for each jurisdiction that consists of hundreds of thousands of people in the region. The challenge is to determine the tradeoffs between the quality of solution, the practicality of planning, and real-time optimization. Exact algorithms and heuristics must be developed and advanced to address such computational challenges (Lee et al., 2009a,b).

Resource Allocation and POD Layout Design

Resource Allocation

Mason and Washington (2003) at the CDC investigated optimal staffing arrangements for dispensing sites (PODs) in the face of limited resources via a simulation/optimization system "Maxi-Vac" that they developed. Their study offered insight into the practicality of such a system as a planning tool for emergency situations, but revealed critical bottlenecks between the commercial simulation software and the optimization software: over 10 hours were needed to obtain a usable feasible solution in each scenario with about 25–30 staff. This initiated our collaboration with CDC and the development of RealOpt, a large-scale real-time simulation-optimization decision support system.

Given a staff assignment (obtained from an initial optimization step) and input of service distributions at each station, we can model and simulate the movement of individuals inside a POD. The simulation output is a set of parameters (including statistics of average flow time, queue length, wait time, utilization rate, etc.) that enable evaluation of the objective function being optimized (e.g., the resulting throughput).

The optimization of labor resources involves placement of staff at various stations in the POD to maximize throughput or minimize the staffing needs to satisfy a preset throughput population. The cost at each station depends on the type and number of workers who are assigned to that station and have the required skills, and on the average wait time, queue length, and utilization rate of the station. The total system cost depends on the cost at each station, and on system parameters, such as cycle time and throughput. These cost functions are not necessarily expressible in closed form.

Constraints in the model include maximum limits on average wait time and queue length, range of utilization desired at each station, and upper and lower bounds on the number of workers with the required skills who are needed to perform various tasks at the POD. Constraining the average cycle time to be less than a prespecified upper bound is critical for emergency response because individuals must move through the system as quickly as possible to facilitate crowd control, reduce sources of human frustration and potential disorderly outbursts, and reduce the potential spread of disease or contamination. The resulting nonlinear mixed-integer program poses unique challenges for existing optimization engines.

POD Layout Design

Designing the appropriate POD for various medical dispensing is critical. Further, POD layout will affect the overall staffing and efficiency of the dispensing operations.

Figure 41.2 contrasts two POD designs that were employed in a Hepatitis A booster shot event for 10,000 citizens (The Buffalo News, 2008). The left shows the drive-through POD design used in the morning, and the right shows the redesign in the afternoon after real-time reconfiguration (based on service times collected on site) was performed. The redesign offers 10% improved throughput, 18% improved utilization, and a range of 10%–85% reduction in wait time and queue length at various stations. This illustrates the paramount importance of POD design to any emergency operation where resources are scare, time is precious, and there is a large affected population to serve.

Disease-Propagation Analysis: Mitigation Strategies and Choice of Dispensing Modalities

Large-scale dispensing clinics could facilitate the spread of disease because of their high-volume population flow. The field of dynamical systems (mostly differential equation systems) provides the principle methods of modeling in classical mathematical epidemiology (Anderson et al., 1992; Diekmann and Heesterbeek, 2000). Despite their simplicity when compared to recent complex simulation studies (Ferguson et al., 2005, 2006; Longini et al., 2005; Germann et al., 2006), these methods have helped generate functional insights, such as the transmission threshold for the start of an epidemic and the vaccination threshold for containment of an outbreak. As modelers attempt to incorporate more realistic dynamics into their models (such as stochasticity, nonexponential waiting times, sample-path dependent events, demographical and geographical data, etc.), more flexible tools, such as individual-based stochastic simulations, are preferable. Although simulation is a powerful approach, it is less mathematically tractable (i.e., it requires intensive computing time) than the classical methods.

RealOpt opens up an opportunity to explore disease-propagation studies in which stochasticity of systems can be incorporated readily. It includes a disease-propagation module that aids users in understanding facility design and flow strategies that mitigate the spread of disease. The module incorporates the standard four-stage SEIR (susceptible, exposed, infectious, and recovered) model (Kermack and McKendrick, 1991), and a novel six-stage SEPAIR model to capture the disease

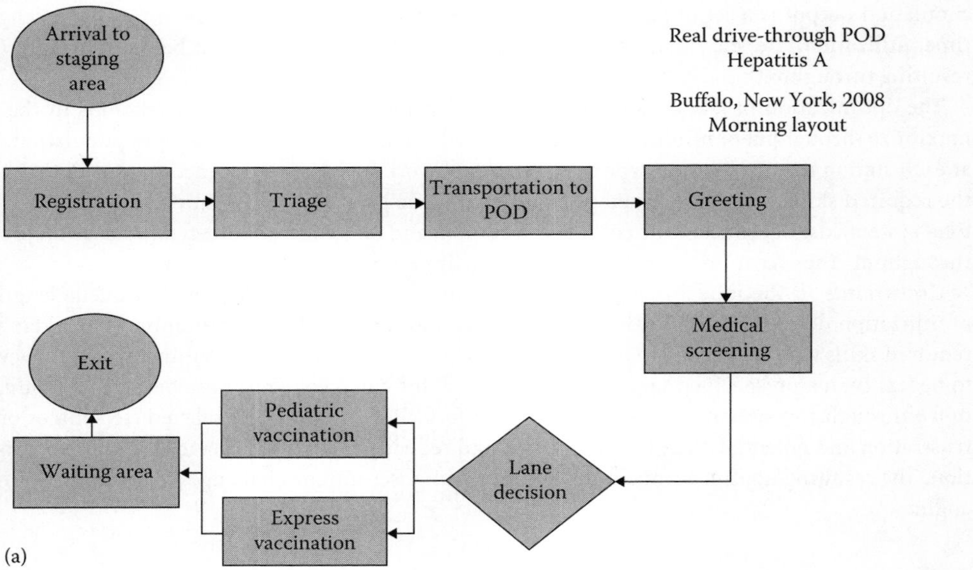

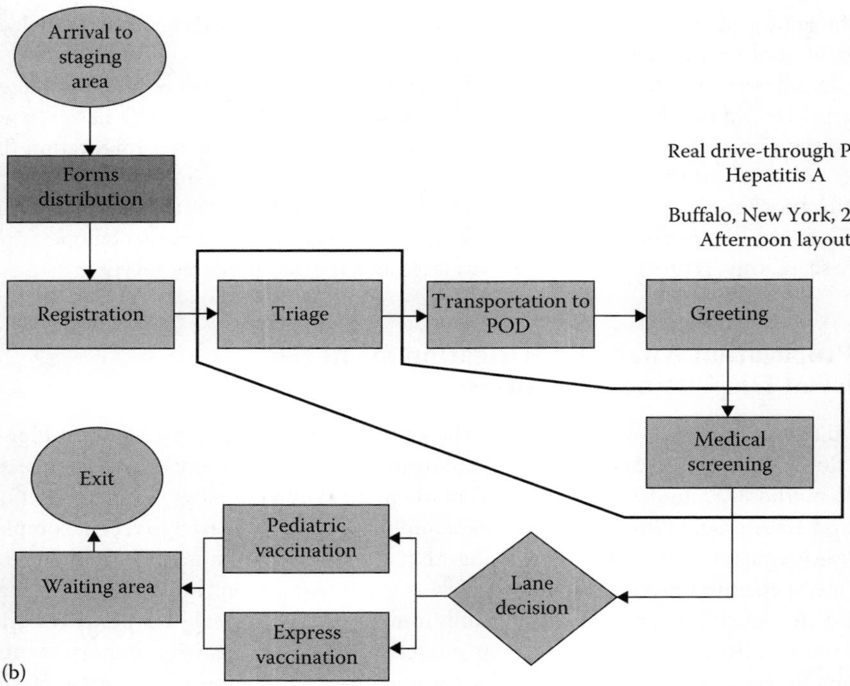

FIGURE 41.2 Two POD layouts used during a 2008 Hepatitis vaccination event.

development (i.e., asymptomatic or symptomatic). By distinguishing the symptomatic stage from the asymptomatic stage, this model allows one to examine the effect of triage accuracy in POD facility design.

Lee et al. (2009a, 2010) gave a detailed theoretical and computational analysis of disease propagation and strategies for mitigation during biological or pandemic outbreaks and mass dispensing. In addition to the incorporation of stochasticity of client arrival and service distribution into the model, it also accommodates the following factors:

- The clinic model can be represented as an n-server system with queuing; transmission can occur between clients or between clients and staff. (In a real emergency, staff members will be given medical countermeasures to protect them from the disease prior to their assignment to POD services. However, a medical countermeasure does not guarantee 100% protection; each staff member still has a small probability of being infected by clients.)
- The intra-clinic infectivity between clients and staff can vary.
- If symptomatic individuals are not triaged out properly during the initial screening, they could infect other people inside the POD. The system allows users to observe the effect of triage and screening errors, determine improved strategies for triage and screening, and establish guidelines for mitigating the spread of disease because of such errors.
- Inhomogeneous mixing within the community is possible.
- The infectious, asymptomatic, and symptomatic individuals can infect at various rates.

Figure 41.3 contrasts the triage accuracy with respect to the symptomatic proportion, when simple mass-action incidence infection is considered (Lee et al., 2009a, 2010). This analysis assesses errors in triage and their infection consequences. It provides estimates for POD planners and epidemiologists to help determine the level and expertise of triage that should be in place with respect to the transmission coefficient.

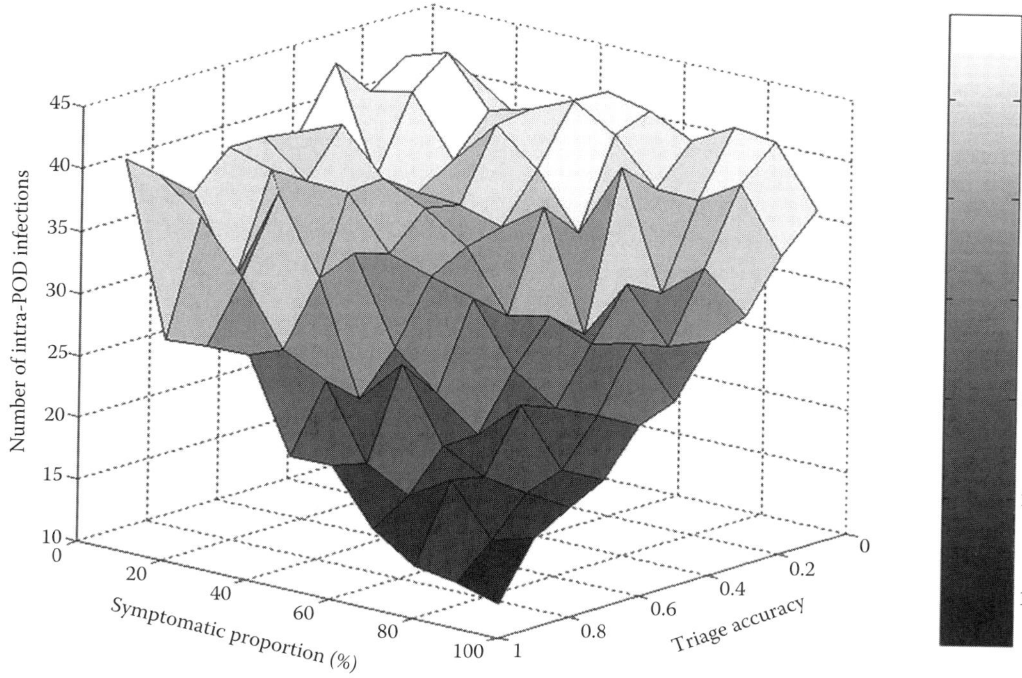

FIGURE 41.3 The graph shows the triage accuracy versus symptomatic proportion and the importance of using the SEPAIR six-stage propagation model, because it allows us to examine the effect of implementing triage accuracy. The graph shows the number of intra POD infections under different triage accuracy and symptomatic proportions. The throughput is 36,000 over a period of 36 hours. The contact number is 193 (for outer-POD disease propagation), and the transmission coefficient is 0.18E-5/minutes. The incoming percentage for susceptible is 95%, and for infectious is 5%. The mean dwell time is 1 day for both exposed and infectious and 3 days for asymptomatic and symptomatic.

Such analyses may influence the selection of dispensing modalities. Specifically, over the past few years, we have observed more use of drive-through PODs for infectious-disease prophylaxic dispensing (e.g., seasonal flu vaccination for communities). In January 2008, a Hepatitis A confirmation of a grocery worker triggered the prophylaxic vaccination of 10,000 residents in Erie County in New York who were potentially exposed to the disease, costing the county's public-health agency at least $500,000. The health department dispensed the first vaccination in February when it set up a stationary clinic (walk-through POD). Because of the medical logistics and infectious nature of the disease, some people had to wait for hours in frigid temperatures. In September 2008, the health department used a Hepatitis A follow-up drive-through POD to provide a second round of vaccinations to individuals potentially exposed to the disease. The POD was also the first test of the county's "drive-through" plan. The drive-through process is quick, efficient, and convenient, and minimizes the potential of intra-infectivity (The Buffalo News, 2008).

Supply Chain Management: Demand, Supply, Fulfillment, and Partnership

Although supply chain management during a disaster response mirrors that of business supply chain management, damaged or destroyed infrastructure force the use of ad hoc solutions that limit the effectiveness and efficiency of the operation.

Demand management can be extremely difficult due to the fluidity of the population and the collapse of the supporting infrastructure. Problems vary depending on the nature of the disaster. In the event of an infectious disease outbreak, as in the recent H1N1 event, when there is not a sufficient supply of medical countermeasures for the affected populations, predicting and allocating the proper distribution across the nation becomes critical, but is highly stochastic and uncertain. Decisions can have a major impact on overall infectivity and mortality rates. In the same manner, demand within an earthquake zone fluctuates rapidly due to the movement of people fleeing from one site to another. And the time it takes to implement an effective response can be critical to the survivors of the affected population.

In disasters, suppliers and stakeholders can be very diverse, and there is usually no unifying business and operating theme to manage them. Further, unsolicited and unwanted donations can burden the management team, causing overload of arrivals at sea or airports, or congesting the warehouses (Cassidy, 2003; Chomilier et al., 2003; Murray, 2005).

Routing of available and necessary goods from entry ports (sea or air) to affected sites can pose daunting challenges. Efficient usage of potentially limited sea/air space and landing sites, available roads, vehicles, fuels, drivers, and materiel handling equipment at the receiving ends are all uncertain and unreliable. Food safety, sanitation hygiene, and opportunistic looting further complicate the process.

Effective coordination of multiple humanitarian agencies, in addition to military, government, and private entities, is of great importance in response to disasters. This is both a challenge and an opportunity given the differing missions, histories, and expertise of these institutions.

In our work on modeling and optimization of public-health infrastructure and mass dispensing strategies (Lee et al., 2009a,b), we describe the importance of collaboration among federal, state, local, and private sectors for successful response to large-scale emergency scenarios, and report public/private solutions for meeting the Strategic National Stockpile dispensing requirements, as prescribed within the Cities Readiness Initiative program. Van Wassenhove (2006) described how business and relief organizations can partner and learn from each other, and included a successful and effective business–humanitarian partnership between a major global logistics company and the World Food Program.

Communication and Public Information

Communication and Information Technology

Communication programs and infrastructure for emergency response are discussed in detail in "Communication System" section. Communication efforts should be coordinated, planned, and tested. Regular training on usage should be performed.

Public Information and Risk Communication

Risk communication plays a crucial role to any successful emergency response. The social challenges that arise as a result of human behavioral patterns cannot be overemphasized. During the high concern and high stress situation, the messages to the public must be concise, unified, and coordinated. Getting correct and credible information out quickly assures the public that they can trust the authority in protecting themselves and their families. The public needs to know in timely manner that there is a problem and the nature of the problem. Appropriate measures must be performed to curtail rumors that may cause unnecessary panic and fear, and potential unrest. Hotlines should be established to share factual information and timely updates. Educational information pertinent to the medical countermeasures and dispensing sites should be clearly stated. Finally, care must be taken to ensure that vulnerable and special need populations are served appropriately.

Lessons Learned and Continued Challenges

Our Experience through Anthrax Drills and Actual Vaccination Events

Our experience illustrates that by combining mathematical modeling, large-scale simulation, and powerful optimization engines, and coupling these with automatic graph-drawing tools and a user-friendly interface, we can design and implement a fast and practical emergency response decision support tool that can run on a wide range of computing platforms, including PDAs for real-time usage. The system offers public-health emergency coordinators the following capabilities:

1. Determine strategically most effective locations for POD facilities to best serve the affected population.
2. Design customized and efficient POD floor plans via an automatic graph-drawing tool. Users can design and compare various floor plans to determine the trade-offs in personnel usage as well as operations efficiency.
3. Determine optimal labor resources required and provide the most efficient placement of staff at individual stations within the POD. The resulting staffing plans maximize the number of individuals who can be treated, minimize the average time patients spend in the clinic, and equalize utilization across clinic stations.
4. Perform disease propagation analysis, understand and monitor the intra-POD disease dilemma, and help to derive dynamic response strategies to mitigate casualties. The what-if analysis and worst-case scenarios can also equip epidemiologists with knowledge that may assist emergency planners in testing alternative POD facility layouts, assess batch size for patient orientation, and analyze the trade-offs between POD throughput operations and degree of infectiousness.
5. Assess current resources and determine minimum needs to prepare for readiness in emergency situations for their regional population.
6. Carry out large-scale virtual drills and performance analyses, and investigate alternative strategies.
7. Train personnel, and design emergency exercises with a variety of dispensing scenarios. Such training exercises could be used to quickly get new emergency preparedness planners up to speed and to keep existing planners sharp.

The computational advances also provide flexibility to quickly analyze design strategies and decisions, and can generate a feasible regional dispensing plan (with a network of cost-effective PODs, each operating at various throughput rates and utilizing various dispensing modalities) based on the best estimates and analyses available, and then allow for reconfiguration of various PODs as the event unfolds. Some of the regional planning and operational analysis reveal that

1. Sharing labor resources across counties and districts within the same jurisdiction is important.
2. The most cost-effective dispensing plan across a region consists of a combination of drive-through, walk-through, and closed PODs, each operating at a throughput rate that depends on the surrounding population density, facility type, and labor availability.

3. The optimal combination of POD modalities changes according to various facility capacity restrictions, and the availability of critical public-health personnel.
4. An increase in the number of PODs in operation does not necessarily increase the total number of core public-health personnel needed.
5. Optimal staffing is nonlinear with respect to throughput; thus we cannot estimate the optimal staffing and throughput by simply using an average estimate.
6. Depending on the population, an "optimal" capacity that provides the most effective staffing exists for each POD location. If a POD is operating above its optimal capacity, reduction in capacity (and thus hourly throughput) eases the crowd-control tasks of law-enforcement personnel and helps to minimize potential operational problems inside the POD.

RealOpt has been used successfully by over 1900 public-health and emergency directors and coordinators in planning for biodefense drills (e.g., anthrax, smallpox) and pandemic response events in various locations in the United States since 2005. It has also been used for dispensing clinic design and staff allocation for the recent H1N1 mass vaccination campaign. Users have tested various POD layouts, including drive-through, walk-through, and closed-PODs. Because of the system's rapid speed, it facilitates analysis of "what-if" scenarios, and serves not only as a decision tool for operational planning, actual drill preparation, and personnel training, but also allows dynamic reconfigurations as an emergency event unfolds. In addition, it supports performing "virtual field exercises," offering insight into operation flows and bottlenecks when mass dispensing is required.

Continued Challenges and the Need for Multilayer Protection

The ability to analyze planning strategies, compare the various options, and determine the most cost-effective combination dispensing strategy are critical to the ultimate success of mass dispensing.

The federal government continues to seek advances in this challenging area. In the recent Executive Order, signed on December 30, 2009 by the President of the United States, a policy was set up to plan and prepare for the timely provision of medical countermeasures to the American people in the event of a biological attack in the United States through a rapid federal response in coordination with state, local, territorial, and tribal governments. The policy seeks to (1) mitigate illness and prevent death; (2) sustain critical infrastructure; and (3) complement and supplement state, local, territorial, and tribal government medical countermeasure distribution capacity.

Specifically, the executive order stipulates that the federal government shall pursue the establishment of a national U.S. Postal Service medical countermeasures dispensing model to respond to a large-scale biological attack with anthrax as the primary threat consideration. Further, the federal government must develop the capacity to anticipate and immediately supplement the capabilities of affected jurisdictions to rapidly distribute medical countermeasures following a biological attack by establishment of a federal rapid response capability. The executive order also asks for Continuity of Operations where the federal government must establish mechanisms for the provision of medical countermeasures to personnel performing mission essential functions to ensure that mission-essential functions of federal agencies continue to be performed following a biological attack.

Postal delivery of medical countermeasures has been discussed in detail in Wein (2008). Because postal workers deliver mail service to all households on a regular basis, the possibility of their usage for the first 12-hour initial dispensing is appealing. This will allow time for the establishment of PODs for continued dispensing service. The availability of personnel during crisis can be volatile, as articulated in "Medical Surge" section. However, such a multilayer dispensing plan allows flexibility in response as well as leveraging and integration of heterogeneous resources for maximum coverage and outcome. Postal and POD distribution strategies require different levels of security; their trade-offs and complimentary characteristics should be carefully analyzed.

Large-Scale Disaster Relief Efforts

Large-scale disaster (humanitarian) relief efforts (e.g., in response to earthquakes, hurricanes, forest fires) where homes are destroyed, critical infrastructures are damaged, and tens of thousands or millions of people's lives are affected, require rapid establishment of "*service constructs*." These service constructs serve as home shelters for the population being displaced; as distribution nodes for receiving supplies for on-the-ground responders; as dispensing sites for handing out food and water to the affected population; and as hospital tents for medical care of the sick. In the aftermath of such an event, the medical surge requirement is acute (see "Medical surge"), evacuation orders are highly probable (see "Emergency evacuation"), and the need for effective communication and coordination for humanitarian relief effort is crucial (see "Communication system").

The scope and complexity of establishing such service constructs are very similar with those for large-scale mass dispensing efforts. Past disaster relief efforts such as in the aftermath of the recent earthquake in Haiti highlight the daunting challenges as the regional response must rapidly establish (in an ad hoc manner) dispensing and distribution networks. Many elements discussed in this section on mass dispensing and population protection come into play. Further, the lack of water, electricity, shelters, poor sanitation, and the existence of at most a barebones critical infrastructure present enormous challenges.

The following issues are pertinent to mass dispensing, but are more prominent within disaster relief efforts.

Coordination among Different Stakeholders

Humanitarian operations often have a large number and variety of stakeholders and multiple organizations operating in the same place simultaneously but without (formal) coordination. A loosely coupled coordination of different aid agencies, suppliers, and local and regional actors, each has their own way of operating and own organizational structures, can work charmingly, yet it can also pose discord (Long and Wood, 1995). The different political agendas, ideologies, and religious beliefs, and the need for appeal to public for donations and media attention complicate the work. Perhaps, the greatest challenge here lies in aligning these organizations properly without compromising their mandates and beliefs. Further, people from different cultural background may have different traditions that may hinder the communication and coordination between organizations (Van Wassenhove, 2006). As seen in the recent Haiti event, operational and organizational differences can also create frictions and misunderstanding among various responding nations, thus masking the effectiveness of the operations.

Sometimes, affected areas may not be reachable due to political reasons. For example, after the 2005 South Asian Tsunami, the Indonesian Government felt compelled to allow free entry in a region that had been very restricted for a long time. This caused a huge influx of personnel from humanitarian organizations, ad hoc organizations and volunteers on sites, overcrowding the sites.

Risk and Uncertainty

Personnel working within a disaster response environment are often exposed to destabilized infrastructure (Cassidy, 2003; Murray, 2005). Not only do they need to work in facilities or areas that are physically damaged, the social effect taking place after a disaster could often become overwhelming. Many disasters such as tsunamis and earthquakes have after-effects that could further cause panic or disruption to response operations. Uncertainty in risk, in when the suppliers will arrive and where, in the amount of supplies that are available, in the overwhelming demand needed by the affected population, add layers of anxiety and stress to these on-the-ground workers. The section "Disaster relief supply chain" shows the extremes of a trend toward more uncertainty and risk prevalent in today's global business supply chain.

Media Exposure

Disaster events often have high exposure to the media. However, their relationship is described by some as a love–hate one (Van Wassenhove, 2006). On the positive side, high exposure to the media means more public attention on the affected areas. This often translates into more donations and general support. However, mass media is shortsighted and tends to be more interested in catastrophic events while putting less focus on long-term humanitarian and relief effort. There is a need to educate and collaborate with news media personnel on disseminating long-term challenges and efforts to the general public. In recent years, some improvement has been seen as news media and public have been made aware of response failures in the emergency responses related to Katrina and other natural disasters, and the high-profile public scrutiny of the federal and local response effort. In general, appropriate media usage can educate the public and help spread word of the situation so as to garner financial donations that are much needed in any disaster response scenario.

Communication System

Multifaceted communication infrastructures are needed for effective medical and emergency response. Two-way communication lines must be kept open between emergency/medical responders and commanders for coordination and facilitation of the response effort; broadcast communication lines must be available to inform the general public about medical precautions and available services; and phone service and call answering stations must be maintained to allow the public to report critical emergency situations. In this section, we focus on the communication infrastructure of hospitals and related medical care entities.

Developing and maintaining a robust communication infrastructure among hospitals, emergency medical services and other healthcare facilities, as well as private medical transport companies and medical supplies vendors, is vital to providing relief operations and services during emergency situations. Such infrastructure provides the core foundation for basic knowledge sharing such as patient volume and severity, emergency room capacity, hospital bed availability; special wards availability; medical personnel specialties; transport vehicle availability; and blood, medicine, and medical supplies inventories. During an emergency situation, such critical information can be communicated to a regional coordinating control center, which can assess available resources, identify surpluses and shortages, and coordinate distribution efforts. In fact, building capacity for an interoperable communication system for emergency response is identified as one of the areas that must be prioritized according to The Hospital Preparedness Program established by the U.S. Department of Health and Human Services.

Previous instances of emergency situations such as the 9/11 terrorist incident and the Rhode Island night club fire incident have brought forth the challenges and necessity in establishing and sustaining a redundant emergency communication network. Kapucu (2006) examined the importance and challenges in establishing a coordinated interagency communication network and the role information technology serves to enhance such communication and decision-making, as in the context of the 9/11 terrorist incident. Challenges include interoperability among the various communication tools, reliability of the tools during emergency situations, technical limitations, barriers in interagency communication and related aspects.

Physical Infrastructure for Emergency Communication

Studies have been done in analyzing the requirement for effective hospital communication systems. Becker (2004) discussed the effectiveness of focus groups and tabletop exercises involving key stakeholders in the public-health community for initial structuring of the emergency communication infrastructure. Such exercises serve as a platform for discussing the functional and performance requirements for redundant communication and the type of information to be delivered. Manoj and Baker (2007) identified three categories of communication challenges from literature review: technological, sociological, and organizational. Recently, we have completed an evaluation of emergency communication infrastructure among a network of hospitals in Georgia. Below, we summarize some of our findings, and discuss the status quo and challenges faced by the health systems (Lee et al., 2009c).

Communication Tools

A wide range of communication tools are used in the healthcare facilities. They can be classified into three main categories: phones (such as landline, mobile phones, satellite, dedicated, VoIP), radios (such as 700, 800 MHz, UHF, VHF, microwave, HAM) and computer-based tools (such as email and Web-based collaborating platforms). When comparing the effectiveness of the tools, some of the metrics to take into consideration are medium of communication, security, emergency reliability factors, emergency response services, cost of installation and usage, general application in public and private domain, and technological limitation. Tables 41.2 and 41.3 compare telephones used in healthcare facilities.

Among all the hospitals in the State of Georgia, 800 MHz radio, VHF, UHF, and HAM radio are more commonly seen in the hospitals than other radio technologies. (Lee et al., 2009c). The percentage of hospitals possessing these tools ranges from 36% to 50%. Microwave radios, in particular, offer a wide range of features for emergency communication but are currently not used for hospital emergency communications. Adoption of new technology can be slow due to the lack of financial resource as well as potential training cost in equipment usage.

Researchers continue to examine the functionality and effectiveness of some novel tools with hybrid technologies. Ammenwerth et al. (2000) examined the usability of a multifunctional mobile

TABLE 41.2 Telephony Networks Comparison

Features	Landline	Cellular	Satellite	Dedicated	VoIP
Medium of communication	• Metal wire • Optical fiber • Airwaves	Airwaves	Airwaves	• Metal wire • Optical fiber	• Metal wire • Optical fiber • Airwaves
Security	Secure	Insecure	Secure	Secure	Insecure
Emergency reliability factors	Network congestion	• Network congestion • Infrastructure reliability	Satellite congestion	Infrastructure reliability	• Network congestion • Infrastructure reliability • Transmission system crash
Emergency applications	Text messaging	• Push to talk • Text messaging • E-mail	• Text messaging • Calling services	Seamless connectivity between terminals	• E911 services • Text messaging • Calling services
Cost of installation and usage	• Installation: $50–$75 • Usage: around $40/month	• Installation: $25–$50 • Usage: Ranges from $30 to $100/month	• Installation: $200–$2600 (handset cost) • Usage: Prepaid cards ranging from $200 to $5000	• Requires specialized cable installation • Applicable for high priority communication services, e.g., military applications	• Free installation • Usage depends on subscription and Internet connection
Strength	Ease of usage and subscription	• Easy of usage and subscription • Mobility	• Seamless connectivity • High mobility	• Dedicated connection between terminals • No network congestion	• Wide range of applications • Ease of usage and subscription • Mobile connectivity

Source: Lee, E.K. et al., Survey & analysis of emergency communication infrastructure among Georgia State Hospitals. Georgia Division of Public Health, Atlanta, GA, 2009c.

TABLE 41.3 Radio Networks Comparison

Features	700 MHz	800 MHz	VHF	UHF	Microwave	HAM
Frequency	700–800 MHz	800–900 MHz	30–300 MHz	300–3000 MHz	7–38 GHz	1.6–27 MHz
Security	• Digital encryption • Local IP address	• Digital encryption • Privacy plus • Private conversation	• Analog direct • Unintercepted communication	• Digital encryption	• Highest link reliability • IP/data transmission protocols	• Digital encryption • Dual/round table transmission
Emergency networks range	Block D: 758–763 and 788–793 MHz	Public safety 21–824 866–869 MHz	156.8, 164.4 MHz	450–470, 800 MHz subband, 2500 MHz subband	7–38 GHz	148.8 MHz
Usage features	• VoIP services • High-speed broadband access • Video for surveillance • High speed in built access for MTU/MDU	• Trunked radio service • Computer controlled network assignment • Call monitoring • Interference reduction • Frequency allocation	• Voice operations in repeaters and voice links • Link with computer controlled equipment • Reliable telemetry link in place of expensive phone lines	• Trunked frequency radio communication • Computerized call/data monitoring	• Cellular networks for high speed links between stations • Wireless local loop systems • Broadband internet • Voice/data application and emergency restoration	• Automatic dialer • Node terminal operation • Multiple scan • Computer interface
Cost	Handset:$99–$1000	Handset: $80–$1000	Handset: $75–$500	Handset: $100–$3000	System: $2000 and above	Handset: $50–$2500
Pros	• Direct operation with other 700–800 MHz users • No infrastructure needed for field communications • Non-repeated system • Simple reliable system • No audio delays	• Wide area coverage • Digital signaling • Features • Interoperability • Talk group creation	• No special infrastructure requirements for field communications • Non repeated systems • Simple reliable systems • No audio delays	• Physical barrier penetration • Less interference from other bands • High data transmission efficiencies • Widely used	• More signal transmission than wired systems • Immediate spread spectrum • Microwave link setup for disaster situations • Military use • Wide ranging frequencies for transmission	• Networking for amateur usage • Used in emergency communication during/after disasters

Cons	• Frequencies not available in all areas • Units keying up • Simultaneously • Audio quality least preferred • No warning of fading	• Complex infrastructure • Noticeable audio delays • Loss of system • Coverage required in building • Inconsistent interior communication	• System must meet FCC narrow banding requirements by 2013 • Limited interoperability with other agencies on 700–800 MHz • Systems not seamless • Analog equipment may not be available due to digital transition	• Commercial licensing underway • Digital transmission lessens bands for emergency/amateur usage • Requires advances in equipment • Battery requirements for sustained communication	• Free space loss • Transmitter sensitivity • Infrastructure requirements • Multipath interference • Signal to noise ratio considerations	Amateur licensing requirements
Application	• Public safety • Government entities • Logistics • Property management • Hotel • Port	• Public safety • Amateur radio communication • Closed network communication	• Airband (aircraft) radio • Amateur radio • FM radio broadcasts • Marine VHF radio	• Emergency response in public networks • Private closed circle data transmission • Amateur radio	• Low power radio for wireless networking within a building • Long distance telephone signal transmission	• Amateur radio • Emergency response systems
Special features	• Communication range alert • Programmable frequencies • CTCSS/CDCSS work group authorization	• Interoperability • Interference control through computerized network traffic monitoring	• IP switch frequency allocation • Noise synthesizer • Commercial grade TCXO for tight frequency accuracy	• Programmable frequencies • Interference reduction techniques	• Digital data transmission • Superior technology for 100% data transmission capabilities • Interfaced with computer	High frequency stability with built in TCXO grade modules

Source: Lee, E.K. et al., Survey & analysis of emergency communication infrastructure among Georgia State Hospitals. Georgia Division of Public Health, Atlanta, GA, 2009c.

information and communication system through a simulation study conducted in a model hospital environment. Holzman (1999) proposed the design of a computer-based communication device that can be used for on-site patient information retrieval during traumatic situations. The purpose of this user interface is to facilitate a common platform for patient data collection and transmission so that the medical facilities can be prepared for the proper medical procedure immediately upon the patient's arrival rather than spending time on information retrieval and diagnosis. Among the various information technology applications for out-of-hospital response phase, Arnold and Levine (2004) analyzed the usage of P2P wireless communication application in a hospital setting and concluded that it provides superior performance than related applications by integrating reliability, flexibility, and information security.

Communication Infrastructure

Building a reliable communication infrastructure requires not only the use of the right tool, but also using the tool right. Jennex (2007) proposed a model for emergency response system and discussed the imperative need for a dynamic integrated collaborative method to communicate between users and data sources and the necessity for establishing protocols to facilitate communication and to improve decision making. Related work by Jan et al. (1993) included optimizing the topological layers of links within the design of a communication network that simultaneously minimizes cost while satisfying reliability constraints over the links.

Communication during a disaster involves the connection between multiple agents, such as a regional coordinating hospital, community emergency operations center, local EMS services, county health department, and local police and fire. A reliable system also requires multiple layers of communication systems. According to our analysis of hospitals in the state of Georgia (Lee et al., 2009c), most hospitals have two levels of communication infrastructure built with tools that are commonly seen but are subject to damage/congestion during emergency (such as cell phones and landlines). Manoj and Baker (2007) identified the multi-organizational radio interoperability issue as an important obstacle to overcome.

Communication Facilitation Programs

Within the United States, the Federal Communications Commission's and the National Communication System have established various emergency communication restoration systems and protocols that facilitate public as well as hospital communications during emergency situations. Below we compare three existing programs, namely, Telecommunications Service Priority (TSP) Program, Government Emergency Telecommunications Services (GETS), and Wireless Priority Service (WPS) Program.

In Table 41.4, we first analyze the operational attributes of each of these facilitation systems and then compare their effectiveness. Although the three existing facilitating programs that are sanctioned and run by the federal government and dedicated for emergency communications restoration offer some valuable features for emergency response, they are not fully utilized as our findings show low enrollment among the hospital networks. Such communication facilitation programs can be invaluable during an emergency situation and should be encouraged at a national level.

Organizational Factors in Emergency Communication

Organizational factors in emergency communication involve managerial attitude toward building healthy communication systems as well as the flexibility and adaptability of an organization in terms of hierarchical reporting structure in the event of a disaster.

Adapting to novel technologies could involve a somewhat steep learning curve. It is therefore important that training and testing of emergency communication tools are emphasized from the managerial level.

TABLE 41.4 Comparison between the TSP, GETS, and WPS

Features	TSP	GETS	WPS
Objective	Prioritize communication of wireline and wireless subscriber	• Prioritize communication of wireline subscriber • Communication restoration through usage of GETS card	Wireless priority and communication restoration for authorized personnel's
Controlling authority	Federal Communication Commission and National Communications Systems	National Communication Systems	Federal communication Commission and private wireless carriers
Enrolling requirements	• Enrollment in one of the National Security/ Emergency preparedness program • Pay the required dues and submit requisition form • After scrutiny, notify authorities for emergency restoration protocols	• Enrollment in National Security/Emergency preparedness program • Public health, safety and maintenance of law and order	• Key federal, state, local and tribal government and critical infrastructure • Personnel requirements: • Executive leaderships • Disaster response/Military command • Public health/safety/law enforcement command • Public services/utilities
Cost of enrolling	• Enrollment fee: $100 • Monthly charge per line: $3	• No enrollment charge • Call charge: 10¢/minute for calls within US	• Activation charge: $10 • Monthly charge: $4.50
Benefits	Restoration of services in essential disaster communication centers such as 911 call centers, police, fire, etc.	• Essential program for unrestricted emergency operations • Around 90% call completion rates when congestion factor is 8 • No additional software requirements	• High call completion probability • Originating radio channel priority • Terminating radio channel priority by call queuing
Limitations	• Monthly payment for service restoration • Revalidation of TSP authorization every 3 years • Entire restoration structure pertains to subscribed telephone company and needs to be modified in case of phone change	• Usage charge and tariff based on wireline provider • Requires calls to be placed in landline for priority treatment • Federal thresholds based on tariff, usage • Private entities require further scrutiny	• Monthly payment for service restoration and program enrollment • Cannot be provisioned on prepaid cell phones • Service not available on TDMA technology
Special features	Prioritizing serves as a source of National Security/Emergency preparedness	• Toll-free access number • PIN Number Access control • Failsafe access • Enhanced/alternative carrier routing • Interoperability with other networks • International calling/Number translation	• Computerized cellular prioritizing and priority ranking • Service availability is carrier dependant • High availability throughout the country • Software enhancements are provided for priority restoration of services

Source: Lee, E.K. et al., Survey & analysis of emergency communication infrastructure among Georgia State Hospitals. Georgia Division of Public Health, Atlanta, GA, 2009c.

It is also not practical to assume that operations will function properly in a crisis. A regular testing of the communication system will improve the organization's responsiveness to crisis in the following ways:

- Test the effectiveness of training.
- Familiarize staff and workers with emergency procedures.
- Identify further problems existing with the system as well as organization policies.

Another important factor in emergency communication is the reporting hierarchy and decision making. Response to emergencies may require decision making to take place as they might in a flatter, more dynamic, ad hoc organization. While hierarchical organizations can lead to wider information gaps across the organizations, flat organizations are not easily scalable. (A hierarchical organization refers to one with more structured pyramid-like organization where one person is in charge of a functional area with one of more subordinates handling the sub-functions. Flat organization refers to an organization structure with few or no levels of intervening management between staff and managers.) Therefore, a hybrid organizational model needs to be developed to best utilize the two organizational approaches (Manoj and Baker, 2007; Lee, 2009; Lee et al., 2009a,b).

Sociological Factors and Linkage to Human Behavior

The social challenges that arise with communication as a result of human behavioral pattern must be considered when designing a communication system.

Confidentiality and information security are always legitimate concerns in the dissemination of medical information. These concerns are escalated in emergency situations since the setting is unfamiliar and emergency response usually involves multiple agencies and stakeholders, some of whom may use volunteers who may not understand the sensitivity of information and the need to protect patient privacy.

Emergency situations can also cause volatile emotions which may hinder communication. Fear, stress, and other emotions can be aggravated by the lack of information. Therefore, periodic information updates are important. Hegde et al. (2006) presented a technological solution that provides differentiated services for an agitated caller by detecting the emotional content in speech packets over a wireless network.

The lack of common vocabulary between response agencies and between organizations and victim populations makes communication even more difficult. While concerted effort has been made to improve the communication between organizations through common vocabulary, efficiency is still lacking. Social science research has been conducted to investigate common languages and principles such as icon languages for use between response organizations and the affected population. Social networks such as Twitter and Facebook are common meeting places nowadays. Such communication infrastructure can be very effective in message dissemination. However, its full effect relies on users' capability to differentiate facts from rumors, and to perform measures according to instruction upon receiving the information.

Emergency Evacuation

The early work by Quarantelli (1980) provides a comprehensive report on evacuation behavior based on existing literature and evacuation data available at the Disaster Research Center at the Ohio State University. Evacuation is defined as "…the mass physical movement of people, of a temporary nature, that collectively emerges in coping with community threats, damages or disruptions." It involves movement of people and equipment from unsafe areas to relatively safe places.

The scope of an evacuation refers to the general number of people affected. The scope could grow over time depending on the nature of the event. Some examples of escalating scope of evacuations are as follows (Continuum, 2006):

- Defense in place: minor adjustments are made to accommodate the event, but essentially no one is moved
- Single department/floor/unit in a venue
- Section—multiple floors/units within a single building
- Entire building to another location on campus
- Entire campus evacuation
- Citywide evacuation

In this section, we examine evacuation at both a healthcare facility level and a community level. The discussion will be limited to evacuation caused by emergency scenarios, excluding war-time evacuation.

Factors That Affect Emergency Evacuation Planning

The first factor affecting evacuation planning is the nature of the threat itself. Depending on the geographic location and/or time of year, communities may have a different probability for facing different natural or man-made threats. While cities located close to the coast might be mostly concerned with seasonal hurricanes, those located on or near tectonic faults must be prepared at all times for a possible earthquake. And in high-density population areas, major concerns may involve fire, hazardous material spills, or even terrorist attacks.

A second factor concerns the potential extensiveness for damage. In the case of a fire or chemical spill, the affected area is generally smaller than natural disasters that hit an entire geographical region. In the latter case, various facilities in the region may all be affected, and thus a large-scale evacuation is triggered (for example, citywide evacuation). Thus, this factor has a direct impact on the scope of evacuation.

In the event of a healthcare facility evacuation, a third factor to consider is the risk to patients. Risk to patients varies depending on patients' conditions, acuity, and nature of the event. For example, in an emergency involving loss of electric power, patients in need of ventilators are more vulnerable compared to patients with mobility issues; whereas an event involving structural damage to the building may require allocating more resources to transferring patients with less mobility.

Overall, the resources demanded for evacuation is a critical issue. Indeed, evacuation requires resources of types and levels very different from routine operations. Further, structural damage (for example to airports and roads) or severe conditions may prohibit the transportation of much needed supplies to the affected population or in a timely manner.

Issues in Hospital Evacuation

Traditional hospital evacuation plans involve horizontal (moving to a safer location on the same floor) and vertical (moving to another floor that is unaffected by the event) evacuations. However, full hospital evacuation requires moving patients and staff and others to a safe haven in preparation for a move to another facility.

According to Continuum (2006), a comprehensive evacuation plan addresses three basic elements: *facility, people,* and *support services*. Facility involves rapidly identifying areas of the hospital that require a high priority for evacuation, areas of vulnerability and areas that have potential risk. People involves assessing, triaging, tracking and reconciling patients, staff, visitors and others as they move throughout the evacuation, which is the single most important aspect of a hospital evacuation plan. Support service addresses areas such as systematic shutdown of medical gases, support of utilities and generators, telecommunication systems (see "Communication system"), and operations logistics (see "Population protection: Medical countermeasures dispensing and large-scale disaster relief efforts").

Facility

Facility issues involve rapidly identifying areas of the hospital that require a high priority for evacuation, areas of vulnerability, and areas that have potential risk.

Collaboration between nearby hospitals and healthcare facilities are important in identifying facility problems and solutions. In the United States, many counties have their own emergency operation center to help facilitate communication, coordination, and transportation between facilities. However, it was reported in one study that hospitals are capable of communicating among themselves during emergency events and can successfully transfer a large number of patients into safe facilities (Schultz et al., 2003).

People

Accounting for people, including patients, staff, visitors, and other personnel, is a core component of hospital evacuation planning.

Emergency situations present many difficulties that are not faced during regular operations. For example, in the event of electric power outage, basic tracking and updating of patient records may be difficult without availability of the computer system. Cases have been reported as early as the mid-1980s where patient records were not updated until days after the event, resulting in confusion among caretakers (Blaser and Ellison, 1985). This problem can become very acute when electronic medical records are in use throughout the facility. It is recommended that a paper record system be in place to record patient information, their attending physician information, accepting facility and accepting physician as well as discharges, diagnostic tests, procedures, equipment needed, mode of transport, time of departure, and arrival for transferring (Cocanour et al., 2002; Continnum, 2006).

It is also necessary to identify and prepare patients for evacuation of the inpatient unit by preparing necessary medical information, medical records, and medications for accepting facility to carry on continuous care when patients are transferred (Continnum, 2006).

Based on the patient record, a triage system must be in place to determine the urgency of each patient case and prioritize transferring of inpatients, and to facilitate the evacuation process. To achieve the maximum number of evacuated patients in the shortest time, it is common practice that hospitals evacuate the most mobile patients first. However, when faced with limited resources, hospitals tend to transfer the most care-intensive patients first.

In terms of staff, research has suggested that each evacuation area should designate a unit evacuation leader who should coordinate the evacuation of the entire area. The role of volunteers in emergency evacuation has been mentioned.

Support Service

Support service addresses processes such as systematic shutdown of medical gases, assessing and maintaining utilities, emergency generators, telecommunication systems, and emergency logistics.

It is possible that an emergency event arises from nonstructural damage scenarios such as a water or power outage. In this case, hospitals should have backup power system that can operate until patients can be transferred safely. (All business-critical computer systems, including financial and clinical systems, should of course have offsite backup.)

Normal communications could be disrupted with structural damage of the landline or cellular towers. Emergency communication infrastructure should be put in place to plan for unforeseeable events (see "Communication system").

A variety of transportation modes can be deployed. These include helicopters, buses, trains, ambulances, or family vehicles. The choice of different transportation modes largely depends on the condition of the patients. Decisions have to be made based on an assessment of the potential benefit of transport versus the potential risks.

Evacuation on this scale is expensive, as it entails extra staffing, EMS utilization, and overnight housing. In the decision making process, a cost-benefit analysis is often used in evaluating different evacuation plans. However, it is difficult to put a monetary value on patients' lives. Just as with many events within an emergency response, the key lies in optimizing the operations under limited resources.

Evacuation Behavior

For general community evacuation, one critical element concerns evacuation behavior, including factors that affect decision making and traffic pattern of evacuees.

There has been mounting interest in gaining a better knowledge of how individuals in emergency situations behave when evacuating from a venue. One study suggests that a person's total evacuation process can be divided into four phases: assessment of the situation, movement, pathfinding, and evacuation (Notake et al., 2001). The variations with respect to time of individuals' progression through different phases of evacuation were observed in a study of the 1993 bombing of the World Trade Center (Fahy and Proulx, 1997). People in a panic-causing emergency typically show stubborn and suboptimal behavior, such as overcrowding and congestion (Helbing et al., 2000). Their research shows that panic may cause people to become oblivious to alternative (preferable) evacuation routes as their instincts are to follow the crowd and get to the head of the pack. The effect of structural parameters on individuals' ability to successfully egress has also been studied. Research shows that egression time increases as corridor complexity increases, and decreases if clear signage is provided (Notake et al., 2001).

Much research has been done on evaluating evacuation decision making. Fischer et al. (1995) investigated the factors and circumstances in which citizens would actually evacuate when receiving a warning from the authority. Based on survey data collected after a fire incident at Hamilton Distributing Company in Ephrata, Pennsylvania on May 1, 1990, it was found that residents are most likely to evacuate if they are ordered to do so, if they are contacted frequently by authority, if past warnings were accurate, and if dependent children were at home.

Lindell et al. (2005) collected survey data from 2002 Hurricane Lili evacuation from some counties in Louisiana and Texas to investigate factors that affect evacuation decision for households. Some of the major findings are

- Local news media is the most extensive source of information for hurricane development.
- The environmental cue is the most important factor in making an evacuation decision, followed by personal experience and social cues.
- Evacuation impediments include job requirement and traffic congestion.

Drabek (1992) looked at the difference between public response versus response made by business executives of tourist firms when making a disaster evacuation decision. It was found that most business executives have evacuation plans although they may vary greatly in term of preparedness. Managerial decision making is parallel to public response. Five key differences between public response and business response are influence and planning, firm versus family priorities, shelter selection, looting concerns, and media contacts.

Cohn et al. (2006) interviewed both residents and public officials from western United States on the issues and problems they are facing when dealing with wildfire evacuation. A contrast of interests was found between the two parties when making evacuation decisions through stages. For example, during anticipation stage, the public officials' greatest interest lies in ensuring safety of the entire community. Residents tend to gauge the seriousness of the threat, preparing appropriately and at the same time maintaining a normal life. This contrast in interest pertains throughout all stages of evacuation: anticipation, warning, displacement, notification, and return and recovery. Keeping these differences in mind may better assist authorities for designing effective evacuation planning.

Aguirre (1991) surveyed the population in Cancun, Mexico during Hurricane Gilbert in 1988 and identified factors that affected their evacuation behavior. A post-disaster survey was conducted 1 week after the impact and collected responses from 431 individuals, among whom 25% of them were evacuated during the impact. Family and friends tended to be the first-stop shelter evacuees sought. The survey result also demonstrated that environmental context and physical characteristics of residence greatly impacted the perception of risk, which subsequently influenced the evacuation behavior. Other factors such as socioeconomical factors have also been studied.

Other researchers have been concerned with the logistics aspects of evacuation, such as cost and transportation. Dow and Cutter (2002) examined the demand of transportation infrastructure during the 1999's Hurricane Floyd evacuation. It was found that about 65% of South Carolina residents decided to evacuate. The study revealed three factors that contributed to the traffic congestion on interstate highways: (1) 25% of families took two or more cars for evacuation; (2) only half of those with a map made an effort to find alternative routes instead of staying on the interstate; and (3) the majority of evacuees made extra trips that were unnecessary in order to get away from the hurricane.

Evacuation without guidance on timeline and traffic routes often proves to be deficient. Even in well-planned scenarios, as in the September 2005 evacuation of Texas citizens from Hurricane Rita, major problems can ensue. Although the governor had announced a staggered schedule of evacuation for various districts and population zones within a 24-hour period well in advance of the storm's possible landfall later in the week, it was still not early enough to ensure that all residents could evacuate safely in advance of the storm. This reinforces the key elements of emergency response—that careful planning with procedural and policy guidelines must be in place, and that improvised and dynamic reconfiguration must be executed as the event unfolds.

Summary

Optimization, Simulation, and Dynamical Systems Methodologies

Operations research, with its roots in defense and military operations, has a natural place in emergency response planning and execution. Optimization, stochastic, simulation, systems modeling, and decision analysis approaches are routinely used to plan for and/or aid in analyzing a broad spectrum of emergency responses as a result of natural or man-made disaster (Larson, 1975; Green and Kolesar, 2004; Larson et al., 2006; Lee et al. 2006a, 2009b). Specifically, Green and Kolesar (2004) traced the history of operations research and management science applications in emergency response, with a particular focus on the work done in New York City between 1969 and 1989. Many projects were undertaken by a group of researchers as part of the New York City-RAND Institute (NYCRI) initiative. These included applications to ambulance, fire, and police car location and deployment.

Resource allocation, scheduling, facility location, vehicle routing, inventory control, and transportation logistics in emergency response have all been formulated into optimization models. Among the resource allocation models, Fiedrich et al. (2000) used dynamic optimization model for the initial search-and-rescue period after a strong earthquake. Branas et al. (2000) used a trauma resource allocation model for ambulances and hospitals. Tzeng et al. (2007) presented a multi-objective optimal planning model for designing relief delivery systems. The three goals are minimizing the total cost, minimizing the total travel time, and maximizing the minimal satisfaction during the planning period. Yan and Shih (2007) used a time-space network model (based on an integer network flow problem with side constraints) to minimize the length of time needed for emergency repair, with related operating constraints for emergency repair work team scheduling.

Lee et al (2006a, 2009a) investigated resource allocation, staffing, facility location, and multimodality mass dispensing strategies and emergency response for biodefense and infectious disease outbreaks. Some of the integer programming instances include on the order of 10 million variables, and the authors provided rapid solution engines to arrive within 5% to optimality under 3 minutes. Zhang and Yang (2007) presented an optimization model and algorithm of a facility location problem in a perishable commodities emergency system. Doerner et al. (2009) presented a model for multi-objective decision analysis with respect to the location of public facilities such as schools in areas near coasts, taking risk of inundation by tsunamis into account. Coskun and Erol (2010) used an integer optimization model to decide locations and types of service stations, and regions covered by these stations under service constraints in order to minimize the total cost of the overall system. The model can produce optimal solutions within a reasonable time for large cities having up to 130 districts or regions.

Many authors present routing and transportation studies. Harewood (2002) used a multi-objective version of the maximum availability location problem to determine emergency ambulance deployment. Wang et al. (2009) analyzed and proposed the concept of post-earthquake road safety, dividing emergency vehicle routing choice and optimization problem into two decision-making stages: pre-trip and en-route. Sheu (2007) used a hybrid fuzzy clustering-optimization approach to study the operation of emergency logistics co-distribution when responding to urgent relief demands in the crucial rescue period. Yi and Kumar (2007) presented a meta-heuristic of ant colony optimization for solving a logistics problem arising in disaster relief activities. Yuan and Wang (2009) presented two mathematical models for path selection in emergency logistics management. The models include actual factors in time of disaster. Liu and Zhao (2009) modeled an emergency materials distribution problem in an anti-bioterrorism system as a multiple traveling salesman problem.

Simulation has been used in numerous public health and medical preparedness topics, including evacuation, resource allocation and patient flow, routing in emergency medical services and surge planning, and disease propagation analysis.

Models have been developed in the area of evacuation (Bakuli and Smith, 1996; Pidd et al., 1996; Graat et al., 1999; Papamichail and French, 1999; Wong and Fong, 2005; Chen et al., 2006; Saadatseresht et al., 2009; Shi et al., 2009; Zheng et al., 2009). The article by Hobeika and Kim (1998) described a software tool, MASSVAC 4.0, developed to model the evacuation of an area near a nuclear power plant. A crowd simulation system, MACES (Pelechano et al., 2005), was developed by researchers at the University of Pennsylvania that integrates a psychological model that models emergency behaviors. Shendarkar et al. (2006) presented a novel virtual reality trained belief, desire, intention software agent used to construct crowd simulations for emergency response. Samuelson et al. (2007) described real-time models that simulate mass egress of a stadium and a subway station. Luo et al. (2008) developed a model that adopts an agent-based approach and employs a layered framework to reflect the natural pattern of human-like decision making process, which generally involves a person's awareness of the situation and consequent changes on the internal attributes.

Simulation has also been used in resource allocation and patient flow (Rossetti et al., 1999; Hupert et al., 2002, 2003; Mason and Washington, 2003; Lee et al., 2006a,b; Saleh and Othman, 2008; Wang et al., 2008), and in the area of pandemic response strategies and mitigation (Meltzer et al., 2001; Hupert et al., 2002; Aaby et al., 2006; Lee et al. 2006a,b, 2009a–c, 2010; Das et al., 2007; Wang et al., 2008; Barnes et al., 2009; Wu et al., 2009). It has found many applications in routing in emergency medical services and surge planning (Goldberg and Paz, 1991; Su and Shih 2003; Haghani et al., 2004; Barnes et al., 2009).

As modelers attempt to incorporate more realistic dynamics into epidemiology and disease propagation models (such as stochasticity, nonexponential waiting times, sample-path dependent events, demographical and geographical data, etc.), more flexible tools, such as individual-based stochastic simulations, are preferable. Although simulation is a powerful approach, the resulting models are often mathematically intractable, and require advances in computational strategies (Gani and Leach, 2001; Eubank, 2002; Epstein et al., 2004; Ferguson et al., 2005; Longini et al., 2005; Ferguson et al., 2006; Germann et al., 2006; Lee et al., 2009b, 2010).

The discipline of dynamical systems, mostly differential equation systems, provides the principle methods of modeling in classical mathematical epidemiology (Anderson et al., 1992; Diekmann and Heesterbeek, 2000). It has also been used to analyze strategies and policies. Wein et al. (2003) used a system of differential equations to model the effects of different policies in response to an anthrax bioterror attack. The system includes an atmospheric dispersion model for the spread of the bacterium causing anthrax, an age-dependent dose-response model for the impact of treatment on an individual, a disease progression model to capture the stages through which an infected individual goes, and a set of two-stage queueing systems for antibiotic distribution and hospital care. Kaplan et al. (2002) imbeded the evaluation of vaccination logistics policy within a disease propagation model and compares strategies of traced vaccination, mass vaccination, and the mixed response advocated by the Centers for Disease Control. Eichner et al. (2007) developed a deterministic model for evaluating impact of different intervention strategies during pandemic influenza. The model is based on over 1000 differential equations which extend the classic SEIR model by clinical and demographic parameters relevant for pandemic preparedness planning. The model aims to operate with an optimal combination of precision, realism and generality. Wu et al. (2007) developed models to demonstrate that a pre-pandemic vaccine allocation policy that allocates vaccine to each state in proportion to the population size is not the most efficient. In fact, an inequitable strategy that allows no allocation to some regions while the sufficient vaccines being allocated to other regions demonstrates larger benefit. However, if considering other strategy selection criteria such as simplicity, robustness, and equity, the current pro-rata policy is a good compromise.

Integrated Approaches and Information and Decision Support Systems

The burden of responding to a public-health or medical disaster is multifaceted and a genuine test to the sustainability of critical infrastructure. Negotiating emergency operations is especially difficult due to interagency goal conflicts, differences in organizational culture and bureaucratic constraints, discrepancies in situation assessment, scarcity of resources and organizational complexity. Nevertheless, interplay among many agencies is critical, and consequently, integrated approaches, and information and decision support systems prove to be very beneficial as part of the solution strategies (Kananen et al., 1990; Subramaniam and Kerpedjiev, 1998; Rotz and Hughes, 2004; Kwan and Lee, 2005; Nguyen et al., 2005; Raghu et al., 2005).

Iakovou and Douligeris (2001) presented the development of IMASH, an information management system for hurricane disasters. IMASH is an intelligent integrated dynamic information management tool, capable of providing comprehensive data pertaining to emergency planning and response for hurricane disasters. Popp et al. (2004) developed information-analysis tools for an effective multiagency information-sharing effort.

Zografos et al. (1998) described an integrated framework consisting of a data management module, a vehicle monitoring and communication module, and a modeling module, for managing emergency response of the electric utility companies. The framework integrates a GIS system with a decision-making modeling module to deliver solutions in real time that optimize deployment of the available emergency resources. El-Anwar et al. 2009 presented the development of an automated system to support decision makers in optimizing post-disaster temporary housing arrangements. The system has been integrated in MAEviz and provides the capability of optimizing a number of important objectives, including minimizing negative socioeconomic impacts, maximizing housing safety, minimizing negative environmental impacts, and minimizing public expenditures.

Bui et al. (2000) proposes a framework for developing a global information network (GIN). The application would incorporate four factors that affect the design of a GIN: nature of disaster relief operations, negotiation styles of participants, social/cultural/organizational characteristics of participants, and resource availability. Such a framework could provide a set of basic metrics/factors to characterize any disaster situation. GIN would use high-speed Internet as backbone, it includes a command center where the disaster management team would be, and telecommunication channels that connect to expert advice groups from around the world. The GIN would also be linked to an array of data and knowledge base warehouses.

NYU's PLAN C is an innovative tool for emergency managers, urban planners, and public-health officials to prepare and evaluate Pareto-optimal plans to respond to urban catastrophic situations. Doheny and Fraser (1996) described a software tool for modeling the decisions that people make in emergency situations in offshore environments. It can be used to predict the likely behaviors of a population in hazardous situations and help evaluate the effectiveness of emergency procedures and training.

Mondschein (1994) reviewed the use of spatial data by environmental managers and emergency responders who are charged with the responsibility to perform hazard assessments, identify the location of toxic and hazardous materials, deploy emergency resources, and review demographic data to ensure the safety of the public, and the surrounding communities.

In our own work, the decision support system RealOpt combines OR modeling techniques, novel and large-scale computational engines, sophisticated graph-drawing tools, 3D geographical spatial information with federal census data, and demographic and socioeconomic data for operational and strategic planning, and policy analysis. RealOpt allows public-health emergency coordinators to (1) determine locations for service facilities setup; (2) design customized, efficient floor plans for each facility via an automatic graph-drawing tool; (3) determine (in real time) optimal resource allocation through advanced computational techniques in simulation and optimization; (4) monitor intra-facility disease propagation through a novel disease propagation model, and derive dynamic response strategies to reduce the spread of disease and mitigate the risk of casualties; (5) assess resources and determine minimum needs to prepare for treating regional populations; (6) carry out large-scale virtual drills and performance analyses, and investigate alternative dispensing strategies; and (7) design a variety of dispensing scenarios and emergency-event exercises to train personnel (Lee, 2009; Lee et al., 2006a,b, 2009a,b, 2010).

Challenges

Modeling and optimizing public-health infrastructure involve elements of resource allocation under risk, uncertainty, and time pressure; large-scale supply-chain management; transportation and operational logistics; and medical treatment and population protection. The operations must be supported by an effective communication infrastructure. There is a necessity for vertical and horizontal integration and communication, where federal, state, local, tribal, territorial, private, and business stakeholders work toward a common goal of a resilient public-health system. The infrastructure must be *flexible, scalable, sustainable, and elastic* to support an effective and timely response, and to mount rapid recovery and mitigation operations.

The 2007 Homeland Security Presidential Directive-21 (HSPD-21) established a National Strategy for Public Health and Medical Preparedness, which builds upon a four pillar framework: threat awareness, prevention and protection, surveillance and detection, and response and recovery. It aims to transform our national approach to protecting the health of the citizens against all disasters. Although the four pillars were developed initially to guide the efforts to defend against a bioterrorist attack, they are applicable to a broad array of natural and man-made public-health and medical challenges, and are appropriate to serve as the core functions of the strategy for public health and medical preparedness.

Public health and medical preparedness continue to shower challenges to the scientific community. Some critical issues include (a) realistic systems modeling; (b) intractability of large-scale instances; (c) interdependencies among multiple critical components/agencies; and (d) the importance and necessity for end-to-end systems modeling and design. Technological advances are needed to allow for complex realistic modeling while providing users with affordable computational power that result in decision systems that are practical for actual scenario-based analysis. The effective integration and alignment of care personnel, facilities, and equipment and supply for optimal outcome remains essential. Capability to solve large-scale resource allocation and location problems is a must. Tracking of disease and designing and implementing dynamic mitigation strategies will have a tremendous impact on population protection. Supply chain management needs to be dynamic, and multi-agency partnership models should be developed. Information sharing and management, and risk and communication strategies continue to evolve. Multi-modality integration of technologies and reliable platforms for communication and public dissemination are critical. Policy and coordination among different stakeholders across country borders need to be studied and potentially streamlined. While many issues relate to operational and strategic planning, many others involve policies, risk management, security, public communication, and cultural and human behavior.

> The key to success is flexibility and adaptability—in staffing, in operations strategies, in coordinating and communications strategies, and in the willingness (for multiple agencies) to collaborate. Initial plans must be put in place and executed rapidly, and yet allow reconfiguration on the fly as an event unfolds (Lee et al., 2006a).

References

Aaby, K., J. W. Herrmann, C. S. Jordan, M. Treadwell, and K. Wood. 2006. Montgomery county's public health service uses operations research to plan emergency mass dispensing and vaccination clinics. *Interfaces, 36*(6), 569–579.

Aguirre, B. E. 1991. Evacuation in Cancun during Hurricane Gilbert. *International Journal of Mass Emergencies and Disasters, 9*, 31–45.

Aly, A. A. and J. A. White. 1978. Probabilistic formulation of the emergency service location problem. *The Journal of the Operational Research Society, 29*(12), 1167–1179.

Ammenwerth, E., A. Buchauer, B. Bludau, and R. Haux. 2000. Mobile information and communication tools in the hospital. *International Journal of Medical Informatics, Elsevier Science Ireland Ltd., 57*, 21–40.

Anderson, R. M., R. M. May, and E. Anderson. 1992. *Infectious Disease of Human: Dynamics and Control.* Oxford, U.K.: Oxford University Press.

Arnold, J. L. and B. N. M. R. Levine. 2004. Information-sharing in out-of-hospital disaster response: The future role of information technology. *Prehospital and Disaster Medicine, 19*, 201–207.

Bakuli, D. L. and J. M. Smith. 1996. Resource allocation in state-dependent emergency evacuation networks. *European Journal of Operational Research, 89*, 543–555.

Barbisch, D. F. and K. L. Koenig. 2006. Understanding surge capacity: Essential elements. *Academic Emergency Medicine, 13*, 1098–1102.

Barnes, A. J., J. O. Jacobson, M. D. Solomon, H. Kun, and I. J. Eugene Grigsby. 2009. Los Angeles county pandemic flu hospital surge planning model, National Health Foundation, Los Angeles, CA.

Bascetta, C. A. 2010. Emergency preparedness: State efforts to plan for medical surge could benefit from shared guidance for allocating scarce medical resources. United States Government Accountability Office, Danville, PA. http://www.gao.gov/new.items/d10381t.pdf

Becker, S. M. 2004. Emergency communication and information issues in terrorist events involving radioactive materials. *Biosecurity and Bioterrorism, 2*, 195–207.

Berman, O. and A. Gavious. 2007. Location of terror response facilities: A game between state and terrorist. *European Journal of Operational Research, 177*(2), 1113–1133.

Blaser, M. J. and R. T. I. Ellison. 1985. Rapid nighttime evacuation of a veterans hospital. *Journal of Emergency Medicine, 3*, 387–394.

Branas, C. C., E. J. MacKenzie, and C. S. ReVelle. 2000. A trauma resource allocation model for ambulances and hospitals. (Managerial and Policy Impact). *Health Services Research, 35*(2), 489–507.

Brandeau, M. L. and S. S. Chiu. 1989. An overview of representative problems in location research. *Management Science*, 35(6), 645–674.

Bui, T., S. Cho, S. Sankaran, and M. Sovereign. 2000. A framework for designing a global information network for multinational humanitarian assistance/disaster relief. *Information Systems Frontiers, 1*, 427–442.

Burkle, J. F. M. 2006. Population-based triage management in response to surge-capacity requirements during a large-scale bioevent disaster. *Academic Emergency Medicine, 13*, 1118–1129.

Cassidy, W. 2003. A logistics lifeline. *Traffic World, 27*, 1.

Chaiken, J. M. and R. C. Larson. 1972. Methods for allocation urban emergency units: A survey. *Management Science, 19*(4), P110–P130.

Chen, X., J. W. Meaker, and F. B. Zhan. 2006. Agent-based modeling and analysis of hurricane evacuation procedures for the Florida Keys. *Natural Hazards, 38*, 321–338.

Chomilier, B., R. Samii, and L. N. V. Wassenhove. 2003. The central role of supply chain management at IFRC. *Forced Migration Review, 18*, iii.

Church, R. L. and M. P. Scaparra. 2007. Protecting critical assets: The R-interdiction median problem with fortification. *Geographical Analysis, 39*(2), 129–146.

Church, R. L., M. P. Scaparra, and R. S. Middleton. 2004. Identifying critical infrastructure: The median and covering facility interdiction problems. *Annals of the Association of American Geographers, 94*(3), 491–502.

Cocanour, C. S., S. J. Allen, J. Mazabob, J. W. Sparks, C. P. Fischer et al. 2002. Lessons learned from the evacuation of an urban teaching hospital. *Archives of Surgery, 137*, 1141–1145.

Cohn, P. J., M. S. Carroll, and Y. Kumagai. 2006. Evacuation behavior during wildfires: Results of three case studies. *Western Journal of Applied Forestry, 21*(10), 39–48.

Continuum Health Partners. 2006. Evacuation planning for hospitals (draft document). Center for Bioterrorism Preparedness and Planning, New York.

Coskun, N. and R. Erol. 2010. An optimization model for locating and sizing emergency medical service stations. *Journal of Medical Systems, 34*, 43–49.

Das, T. K., A. A. Savachkin, and Y. Zhu. 2007. A large scale simulation model of pandemic influenza outbreaks for development of dynamic mitigation strategies. Tampa, FL: Department of Industrial and Management Systems Engineering, University of South Florida.

Diekmann, O. and J. Heesterbeek. 2000. *Mathematical Epidemiology of Infectious Diseases: Model Building.* New York: Wiley.

Doerner, K. F., W. J. Gutjahr, and P. C. Nolz. 2009. Multi-criteria location planning for public facilities in tsunami-prone coastal areas. *OR Spectrum, 31*, 651–678.

Doheny, J. G. and J. L. Fraser. 1996. MOBEDIC—A decision modelling tool for emergency situations. *Expert Systems with Applications, 10*, 17–27.

Dow, K. and S. L. Cutter. 2002. Emerging hurricane evacuation issues: Hurricane Floyd and South Carolina. *Natural Hazards Review, ASCE, 3*, 12–18.

Drabek, T. E. 1992. Variations in disaster evacuation behavior: Public responses versus private sector executive decision-making processes. *Disasters, 16*(2), 104–118.

Eichner, M., M. Schwehm, H. P. Duerr, and S. O. Brockmann. 2007. The influenza pandemic preparedness planning tool InfluSim. *BMC Infectious Diseases, 7*, 7–17.

El-Anwar, O., K. El-Rayes, and A. Elnashai. 2009. An automated system for optimizing post-disaster temporary housing allocation. *Automation in Construction, 18*, 983–993.

Epstein, J., D. A. T. Cummings, S. Chakravarty, R. Singa, D. S. Burke, J. D. Cummings. 2004. *Toward a Containment Strategy for Smallpox Bioterror: An Individual-Based Computational Approach.* Washington, DC: The Brookings Institution Press.

Eubank, S. 2002. Scalable, efficient epidemiological simulation. In *SAC '02: Proc. 2002 ACM Sympos. Appl. Comput.* New York: ACM Press, pp. 139–145.

Fahy, R. F. and G. Proulx. 1997. Human behavior in the world trade center evacuation. *Fire Safety Science, 5*, 713–724.

Ferguson, N. M., D. A. Cummings, S. Cauchemez, C. Fraser, S. Riley et al. 2005. Strategies for containing an emerging influenza pandemic in Southeast Asia. *Nature, 437*, 209–214.

Ferguson, N. M., D. A. T. Cummings, C. Fraser, J. C. Cajka, P. C. Cooley et al. 2006. Strategies for mitigating an influenza pandemic. *Nature, 442*, 448–452.

Fiedrich, F., F. Gehbauer, and U. Rickers. 2000. Optimized resource allocation for emergency response after earthquake disasters. *Safety Science, 35*, 41—57.

Fischer, H. W., G. F. Stine, B. L. Stoker, M. L. Trowbridge, and E. M. Drain. 1995. Evacuation behaviour: Why do some evacuate, while others do not? A case study of the Ephrata, Pennsylvania (USA) evacuation. *Disaster Prevention and Management, 4*(4), 30–36.

Gani, R. and S. Leach. 2001. Transmission potential of smallpox in contemporary populations. *Nature, 414*(6865), 748–751.

Gavagan, T. F., K. Smart, H. Palacio, C. Dyer, S. Greenberg et al. 2006. Hurricane Katrina: Medical response at the Houston Astrodome/Reliant Center complex. *Southern Medical Journals, 99,* 933–939.

Gerberding, J. L. 2003. Testimony, United States Department of Health and Human Service, Washington, DC (January 30).

Germann, T. C., K. Kadau, I. M. Longini, and C. A. Macken. 2006. Mitigation strategies for pandemic influenza in the United States. *Proceedings of National Academy of Sciences, 103,* 5935–5940.

Goldberg, J. and L. Paz. 1991. Locating emergency vehicle bases when service time depends on call location. *Transportation Science, 25*(4), 264–280.

Graat, E., C. Midden, and P. Bockholts. 1999. Complex evacuation; effects of motivation level and slope of stairs on emergency egress time in a sports stadium. *Safety Science, 31,* 127–141.

Green, L. V. and P. J. Kolesar. 2004. Anniversary article: Improving emergency responsiveness with management science. *Management Science, 50,* 1001–1014.

Haghani, A., Q. Tian, and H. Hu. 2004. Simulation model for real-time emergency vehicle dispatching and routing. *Transportation Research Record: Journal of the Transportation Research Board, 1882,* 176–183.

Hanfling, D. 2006. Equipment, supplies, and pharmaceuticals: How much might it cost to achieve basic surge capacity? *Academic Emergency Medicine, 13,* 1232–1237.

Harewood, S. 2002. Emergency ambulance deployment in Barbados: A multi-objective approach. *Journal of the Operational Research Society, 53,* 185–192.

Hegde, R., B. S. Manoj, B. D. Rao, and R. R. Rao. 2006. Emotion detection from speech signals and its applications in supporting enhanced QoS in emergency response. In *Proceedings of the 3rd International ISCRAM Conference,* Newark, NJ, May 2006.

Helbing, D., I. Farkas, and T. Vicsek. 2000. Simulating dynamical features of escape panic. *Nature, Nature Publishing Group, 407,* 487–490.

Hick, J. L., D. Hanfling, J. L. Burstein, C. Deatley, D. Barbisch et al. 2004. Health care facility and community strategies for patient care surge capacity. *Annals of Emergency Medicine, 44,* 253–261.

Hobeika, A. G. and C. Kim. 1998. Comparison of traffic assignments in evacuation modeling. *IEEE Transactions on Engineering Management, 45,* 192–198.

Hogan, K. and C. Revelle. 1986. Concepts and applications of backup coverage. *Management Science, 32*(11), 1434–1444.

Hogan, D. E., J. F. Waeckerle, D. J. Dire, and S. R. Lillibridge. 1999. Emergency department impact of the Oklahoma City terrorist bombing. *Annals of Emergency Medicine, Mosby, 34,* 160–167.

Holzman, T. G. 1999. Computer–human interface solutions for emergency medical care. *Interactions, ACM, 6,* 13–24.

Hupert, N., G. M. L. Bearman, A. I. Mushlin, and M. A. Callahan. 2003. Accuracy of screening for inhalational anthrax after a bioterrorist attack. *Annals of Internal Medicine, 139*(5), 337–345.

Hupert, N., A. J. Mushlin, and M. A. Callahan. 2002. Modeling the public health response to bioterrorism: Using discrete event simulation to design antibiotic distribution centers. *Medical Decision Making, 22*(5, Suppl.), S17–S25.

Iakovou, E. and C. Douligeris. 2001. An information management system for the emergency management of hurricane disasters. *International Journal of Risk Assessment and Management, 2,* 243–262.

Jan, R.H., F. J. Hwang, and S. T. Cheng. 1993. Topological optimization of a communication network subject to a reliability constraint. *Reliability, IEEE Transactions, 42,* 63–70.

Jennex, M. E. 2007. Modeling emergency response systems. In *HICSS '07: Proceedings of the 40th Annual Hawaii International Conference on System Sciences, IEEE Computer Society, 22,* Big Island, Hawaii.

Jia, H., F. Ordonez, and M. Dessouky. 2002. A modeling framework for facility location of medical services for large-scale emergencies. *IIE Transactions, 39*(1), 41–55.

Kaji, A. H., K. L. Koenig, and R. J. Lewis. 2007. Current hospital disaster preparedness. *JAMA*, *298*, 2188–2190.

Kananen, I., P. Korhonen, J. Wallenius, and H. Wallenius. 1990. Multiple objective analysis of input-output models for emergency management. *Operations Research*, *38*, 193–201.

Kaplan, E. H., D. L. Craft, and L. M. Wein. 2002. Emergency response to a smallpox attack: The case for mass vaccination. *Proceedings of National Academy of Sciences*, *99*, 10935–10940.

Kapucu, N. 2006. Interagency communication networks during emergencies: Boundary spanners in multiagency coordination. *The American Review of Public Administration*, *36*, 207–225.

Kelen, G. D., C. K. Kraus, M. L. McCarthy, E. Bass, E. B. Hsu et al. 2006. Inpatient disposition classification for the creation of hospital surge capacity: A multiphase study. *The Lancet*, *368*, 1984–1990.

Kelen, G. D., M. L. McCarthy, C. K. Kraus, R. Ding, E. B. Hsu et al. 2009. Creation of surge capacity by early discharge of hospitalized patients at low risk for untoward events. *Disaster Medicine and Public Health Preparedness*, *3*, S10–S16.

Kermack, W. O. and A. G. McKendrick. 1991. Contributions to the mathematical theory of epidemics—III. Further studies of the problem of endemicity. *Bulletin of Mathematical Biology*, *53*, 89–118.

Kwan, M.P. and J. Lee. 2005. Emergency response after 9/11: The potential of real-time 3D GIS for quick emergency response in micro-spatial environments. *Computers, Environment and Urban Systems*, *29*, 93–113.

Larson, R. C. 1975. Approximating the performance of urban emergency service systems. *Operations Research*, 23(5):845–868, September–October.

Larson, R. C., M. D. Metzger, and M. F. Cahn. 2006. Responding to emergencies: Lessons learned and the need for analysis. *Interfaces*, *36*(6), 486–501.

Lawler, J. V. and C. E. Mecher. 2007, Homeland Security Council, private communication.

Lee, E. K. 2008. Doing good with good O.R O.R.s do-gooders. National biodefense—In case of emergency. *OR/MS Today*, *35*(1), 28–34.

Lee, E. K. 2009. A systems view of POD operations: Integrating all the elements. Institute of Medicine Workhop "Medical Countermeausres Dispensing: Emergency Use Authorization". Washington, DC, November 2009.

Lee, E. K., C. H. Chen, F. Pietz, and B. Benecke. 2009a. Modeling and optimizing the public health infrastructure for emergency response. Interfaces—The Daniel H. Wagner Prize for Excellence. *Operations Research Practice*, *39*(5), 476–490.

Lee, E. K., C. H. Chen, F. Pietz, and B. Benecke. 2010. Disease propagation analysis and mitigation strategies for effective mass dispensing. *Proceedings of the American Medical Informatics Association 2010 Conference* (accepted for publication).

Lee, E. K., S. Maheshwary, and J. Mason. 2005. Real-time staff allocation for emergency treatment response of biologic threats and infectious disease outbreak. INFORMS William Pierskalla Best Paper Award on Healthcare and Management Science.

Lee, E. K., S. Maheshwary, J. Mason, and W. Glisson. 2006a. Large-scale dispensing for emergency response to bioterrorism and infectious disease outbreak. *Interfaces*, *36*(6), 591–607.

Lee, E. K., S. Maheshwary, J. Mason, and W. Glisson. 2006b. Decision support system for mass dispensing of medications for infectious disease outbreaks and bioterrorist attacks. *Annals of Operation Research Computing and Optimization in Medicine Life Science*, *148*, 25–53.

Lee, E. K., H. K. Smalley, Y. Zhang, F. Pietz, and B. Benecke. 2009b. Facility location and multi-modality mass dispensing strategies and emergency response for biodefense and infectious disease outbreaks. Biosecurity assurance in a threatening world: Challenges, explorations, and breakthroughs. *International Journal on Risk Assessment and Management*, *12*(2/3/4), 311–351.

Lee, E. K., A. Y. Yang, S. G. Chinnappan, and T. W. Guilford. 2009c. *Survey & Analysis of Emergency Communication Infrastructure among Georgia State Hospitals*. Atlanta, GA: Georgia Division of Public Health.

Lindell, M. K., Lu, J.-C., Prater, C. S. 2005. Household decision making and evacuation in response to Hurricane Lili. *Natural Hazards Review, ASCE, 6*(4), 171–179.

Liu, M. and L. Zhao. 2009. Optimization of the emergency materials distribution network with time windows in anti-bioterrorism system. *International Journal of Innovative Computing, Information and Control, 5*, 1349–4198.

Long, D. C. and D. F. Wood. 1995. The logistics of famine relief. *Journal of Business Logistics, 16*, 213–229.

Longini, I. M., A. Nizam, S. Xu, K. Ungchusak, W. Hanshaoworakul, D. A. T. Cummings, and M. E. Halloran. 2005. Containing pandemic influenza at the source. *Science, 309*, 1083–1087.

Luo, L., S. Zhou, W. Cai, Y. H. F. Malcolm, F. Tian, Y. Wang, X. Xiao, and D. Chen. 2008. Agent-based human behavior modeling for crowd simulation. *Computer Animation Virtual Worlds, John Wiley and Sons Ltd., 19*, 271–281.

Manoj, B. and A. H. Baker. 2007. Communication challenges in emergency response. *Communication of the ACM, 50*, 51–53.

Mason, J. and M. Washington. 2003. Optimizing staff allocation in large-scale dispensing centers. CDC report, Atlanta, GA.

Meltzer, M., I. Damon, J. W. LeDunc, and D. J. Miller. 2001. Modeling potential responses to smallpox as a bioterrorist weapon. *Emerging Infectious Diseases, 7*(6), 959–969.

Mondschein, L. G. 1994. The role of spatial information systems in environmental emergency management. *Journal of the American Society for Information Science, 45*, 678–685.

Murray, S. 2005. How to deliver on the promises: supply chain logistics: Humanitarian agencies are learning lessons from business in bringing essential supplies to regions hit by the tsunami. *Financial Times*.

Narasimhan, S., H. Pirkul, and D. A. Schilling. 1992. Capacitated emergency facility siting with multiple levels of backup. *Annals of Operations Research, 40*(1), 323–337.

Notake, H., M. Ebiharaa, and Y. Yashirob. 2001. Assessment of legibility of egress route in a building from the viewpoint of evacuation behavior. *Safety Science, 38*, 127–138.

Nguyen, S., J. Rosen, and C. Koop. 2005. Emerging technologies for bioweapons defense. *Studies In Health Technology And Informatics, 111*, 356–361.

Okumura, T., N. Takasu, S. Ishimatsu, S. Miyanoki, A. Mitsuhashi, K. Kumada, K. Tanaka, and S. Hinohara. 1996. Report on 640 victims of the Tokyo sarin attack subway. *Annals of Emergency Medicine, 28*, 129–135.

Owen, S. H. and M. S. Daskin. 1998. Strategic facility location: A review. *European Journal of Operational Research, 111*(3), 423–447.

Papamichail, K. N. and S. French. 1999. Generating feasible strategies in nuclear emergencies-a constraint satisfaction problem. *The Journal of the Operational Research Society, Palgrave Macmillan Journals on behalf of the Operational Research Society, 50*, 617–626.

Pelechano, N., K. O'Brien, B. Silverman, and N. Badler. 2005. *Crowd Simulation Incorporating Agent Psychological Models, Roles and Communication*. Philadelphia, PA: Center for Human Modeling and Simulation, University of Pennsylvania.

Peleg, K. and A. L. Kellermann. 2009. Enhancing hospital surge capacity for mass casualty events. *JAMA, 302*, 565–567.

Pidd, M., F. N. de Silva, and R. W. Eglese. 1996. A simulation model for emergency evacuation. *European Journal of Operational Research, 90*, 413–419.

Pirkul, H. and D. A. Schilling. 1988. The siting of emergency service facilities with workload capacities and backup service. *Management Science, 34*(7), 896–908.

Popp, R., T. Armour, T. Senator, and K. Numrych. 2004. Countering terrorism through information technology. *Communications of ACM, 47*, 36–43.

Quarantelli, E. L. 1980. *Evacuation Behavior and Problems: Findings and Implications from the Research Literature*. Columbus, OH: Disaster Research Center, Ohio State University.

Qureshi, K., R. R. Gershon, M. F. Sherman et al. 2005. Health care workers' ability and willingness to report to duty during catastrophic disasters. *Journal of Urban Health: Bulletin of the New York Academy of Medicine, 82*, 378–388.

Raghu, T. S., R. Ramesh, and A. B. Whinston. 2005. Addressing the homeland security problem: A collaborative decision-making framework. *Journal of the American Society for Information Science and Technology, 56*(3), 310–324.

Roccaforte, J. D. 2001. The world trade center attack observations from New York's Bellevue Hospital. *Critical Care, 5*, 307–309.

Rossetti, M. D., G. F. Trzcinski, S. A. Syverud, P. A. Farrington, H. B. Nembhard, D. T. S., and G. W. Evans, (eds.) 1999. Emergency department simulation and determination of optimal attending physician staffing schedules. In *Proceedings of the 1999 Winter Simulation Conference,* Phoenix, AZ.

Rotz, L. D. and J. M. Hughes. 2004. Advances in detecting and responding to threats from bioterrorism and emerging infectious disease. *Nature Medicine, 10*, S130–S136.

Saadatseresht, M., A. Mansourian, and M. Taleai. 2009. Evacuation planning using multiobjective evolutionary optimization approach. *European Journal of Operational Research, 198*, 305–314.

Saleh, M.S. and Z. Z. A. Othman. 2008. ASRTS: An agent-based simulator for real-time schedulers. *AICMS 08. Second Asia International Conference on Modeling & Simulation, 2008*, Kuala Lampur, Malayasia, pp. 7–12.

Samuelson, D. A., A. Zimmerman, J. Thorp, P. McCormick, M. Parker et al. 2007. Panel: Agent-based modeling of mass egress and evacuations. In *Proceedings of the 2007 Winter Simulation Conference*, Washington, DC.

Schull, M. J., T. A. Stukel, M. J. Vermeulen, A. Guttmann, and M. Zwarenstein. 2006. Surge capacity associated with restrictions on nonurgent hospital utilization and expected admissions during an influenza pandemic: Lessons from the Toronto severe acute respiratory syndrome outbreak. *Academic Emergency Medicine, 13*, 1228–1231.

Schultz, C. H. and K. L. Koenig. 2006. State of research in high-consequence hospital surge capacity. *Academic Emergency Medicine, 13*, 1153–1156.

Schultz, C. H., K. L. Koenig, and R. J. Lewis. 2003. Implications of hospital evacuation after the Northridge, California, earthquake. *The New England Journal of Medicine, 348*, 1349–1355.

Schultz, C. H. and S. J. Stratton. 2007. Improving hospital surge capacity: A new concept for emergency credentialing of volunteers. *Annals of Emergency Medicine, Mosby, 49*, 602–609.

Shendarkar, A., K. Vasudevan, S. Lee, and Y. J. Son. 2006. Crowd simulation for emergency response using BDI agent based on virtual reality. In *WSC '06: Proceedings of the 38th conference on Winter simulation, Winter Simulation Conference*, Monterey, CA, pp. 545–553.

Sheu, J. B. 2007. An emergency logistics distribution approach for quick response to urgent relief demand in disasters. *Transportation Research Part E: Logistics and Transportation Review, 43*, 687–709.

Shi, L., Q. Xie, X. Cheng, L. Chen, Y. Zhou, and R. Zhang. 2009. Developing a database for emergency evacuation model. *Building and Environment, 44*, 1724–1729.

Shih, F. Y. and K. L. Koenig. 2006. Improving surge capacity for biothreats: Experience from Taiwan. *Academic Emergency Medicine, 13*, 1114–1117.

Stratton, S. J. and R. D. Tyler. 2006. Characteristics of medical surge capacity demand for sudden-impact disasters. *Academic Emergency Medicine, 13*, 1193–1197.

Su, S. and C. L. Shih. 2003. Modeling an emergency medical services system using computer simulation. *International Journal of Medical Informatics, 72*, 57–72.

Subramaniam, C. and S. Kerpedjiev.1998. Dissemination of weather information to emergency managers: A decision support tool. *Engineering Management, IEEE Transactions on, 45*, 106–114.

Swain, R., C. ReVelle, C. Toregas, and L. Bergman. 1971. The location of emergency service facilities. *Operations Research, 19*(6), 1363–1373.

The Buffalo News. 2008. Drive-through vaccination effort a success in Amherst: 1,385 people receive hepatitis A booster (September 22).

The White House. 2007. Homeland security presidential directive 21 [HSPD-21]: Public Health and Medical Preparedness. Accessed February 27, 2010. http://www.fas.org/irp/offdocs/nspd/hspd-21.htm

Tzeng, G. H., H. J. Cheng, and T. D. Huang. 2007. Multi-objective optimal planning for designing relief delivery systems. *Transportation Research Part E: Logistics and Transportation Review, 43*, 673–686.

Van Wassenhove, L. 2006. Blackett Memorial Lecture Humanitarian aid logistics: Supply chain management in high gear. *Journal of the Operational Research Society*, *57*, 475–489.

Wang, J., X. Hu, and B. Xie. 2009. Emergency vehicle routing problem in post-earthquake city road network. In *International Conference on Transportation Engineering 2009*, Chengdu, China.

Wang, J., H. Yu, J. Luo, and J. Sui. 2008. Medical treatment capability analysis using queuing theory in a biochemical terrorist attack. In *The 7th International Symposium on Operations Research and Its Applications* (*ISORA'08*), Lijiang, China, pp. 2415–2424.

Wein, L. M. 2008. Neither snow, nor rain, nor anthrax. *The New York Times*, October 13, 2008. Accessed February 22, 2010 http://www.nytimes.com/2008/10/13/opinion/13wein.html?_r=1

Wein, L. M., D. L. Craft, and E. H. Kaplan. 2003. Emergency response to an anthrax attack. *Proceedings of National Academy of Sciences*, *100*, 4346–4351.

Wong, L. and N. Fong. 2005. Risk analysis of escape time from buildings. *Facilities*, *23*, 487–495.

Wu, J. T., G. M. Leung, M. Lipsitch, B. S. Cooper, and S. Riley. 2009. Hedging against antiviral resistance during the next influenza pandemic using small stockpiles of an alternative chemotherapy. *PLoS Medicine*, *6*, 1–11.

Wu, J. T., S. Riley, and G. M. Leung. 2007. Spatial considerations for the allocation of pre-pandemic influenza vaccination in the United States. *Proceedings of the Royal Society B: Biological Sciences*, *274*, 2811–2817.

Yan, S. and Y. L. Shih. 2007. A time-space network model for work team scheduling after a major disaster. *Journal of the Chinese Institute of Engineers*, *30*, 63–75.

Yi, W. and A. Kumar. 2007. Ant colony optimization for disaster relief operations. *Transportation Research Part E: Logistics and Transportation Review*, *43*, 660–672.

Yuan, Y. and D. Wang. 2009. Path selection model and algorithm for emergency logistics management. *Computers & Industrial Engineering*, *56*, 1081–1094.

Zhang, M. and J. Yang. 2007. Optimization modeling and algorithm of facility location problem in perishable commodities emergency system. In *ICNC '07: Proceedings of the 3rd International Conference on Natural Computation*, IEEE Computer Society, Haikou, China, pp. 246–250.

Zheng, X., T. Zhong, and M. Liu. 2009. Modeling crowd evacuation of a building based on seven methodological approaches. *Building and Environment*, *44*, 437–445.

Zografos, K. G., C. Douligeris, and P. Tsoumpas. 1998. An integrated framework for managing emergency-response logistics: The case of the electric utility companies. *IEEE Transaction on Engineering Management*, *45*, 115–126.

Design, Planning, Control, and Management of Healthcare Systems

IV.J Mental Health

42 **Mental Health Allocation and Planning Simulation Model** *H. Stephen Leff, David R. Hughes, Clifton M. Chow, Steven Noyes, and Laysha Ostrow* 42-1
Introduction: Type of Operations Research Models Used in Behavioral Health • HSRI Mental Health Allocation and Planning Simulation • Summary and Conclusions • References

43 **Correlation with Social and Medical Factors** *Kathleen Abrahamson, Karis Pressler, and Melissa Grabner-Hagen* 43-1
Introduction • Defining Psychosocial Distress • Psychosocial Distress and Disease Outcomes • Influence of Psychosocial Distress on Caregiving and Healthcare Delivery • Risk Factors for Illness-Related Psychosocial Distress • Assessment of Distress • Interventions to Manage Distress • Geography • Barriers to the Management of Distress • Issues in Researching Psychosocial Distress • Conclusion • References

42

Mental Health Allocation and Planning Simulation Model

H. Stephen Leff
Human Services Research Institute

David R. Hughes
Human Services Research Institute

Clifton M. Chow
Human Services Research Institute

Steven Noyes
Human Services Research Institute

Laysha Ostrow
Human Services Research Institute

Introduction: Type of Operations Research Models Used in Behavioral Health 42-1
HSRI Mental Health Allocation and Planning Simulation 42-3
Theoretical and Conceptual Framework • Mathematical Formulation • Functional Level Groups and Estimating Persons in Need of Service • Planning Service Packages • Assigning Unit Costs and Revenues • Estimating Outcomes • Web-Based Implementation of HSRI MHAPS
Summary and Conclusions 42-16
Criminal Justice • Quebec Planning Study
References 42-17

Introduction: Type of Operations Research Models Used in Behavioral Health

Operations research (OR) is a scientific extension of mathematics that attempts to explain the behavior of systems based on an understanding or knowledge about the behavior of the system's components (Sacolick, 1980). It utilizes diverse methods such as mathematical modeling, statistics, and algorithms to arrive at optimal (or near optimal) solutions to intricate problems. It is typically concerned with maximizing or minimizing some goal stated as an "objective function."

OR as a paradigm has the potential for aiding decision makers in improving the planning, management, and operations of the mental health service system and its interactions with other systems. Problems and issues are approached by understanding the system being studied, that is, defining the objectives or goals of concern, the flows of people, the facilities and processes within and outside the system, the inputs to and outputs from the system, and the data needed to develop OR models of the system (Pierskalla, 1981).

OR models—conceptual frameworks and mathematical formulations of systems—have been used for capacity planning, resource allocation, and systems management in general health and in mental health

(Pierskalla, 1981). Applied in a planning process, OR models can be used to project* the consequences of particular courses of action which suggest how to improve the plan (Nutt, 1984). As used in health systems planning, OR employs interdisciplinary methods and expertise, such as that from mathematics, statistics, psychology, sociology, and economics.

There is a great need for quantitative planning models in mental health. Since the beginning of "deinstitutionalization"—the move to treat persons with serious mental illness in community programs rather than large state institutions—mental health system planning has been governed by overly optimistic and simplistic plans with respect to amounts of services and resources required (Levin and Roberts, 1976; Foley and Sharfstein, 1983; Rochefort, 1997; Frank and Glied, 2006; Grob and Goldman, 2006). As a result, flawed plans have resulted in persons with serious mental illness failing to progress in their recovery, and in the worst instances, becoming homeless or incarcerated (Rochefort, 1997). In many cases, careful modeling of system functioning could have foreseen these unintended consequences (Levin, 1977). However, more typically, systems planning, has been in the form of repeated commissions at the federal and state levels designed to enlist public opinion rather than specify needed amounts of services and resources (Lippmann, 2004; Frank and Glied, 2006; Grob and Goldman, 2006).

Certain aspects of OR models make them particularly useful in mental health planning, such as

1. Most mental health problems are complex and require knowledge from multiple disciplines for their solution. OR models lend themselves to development by multidisciplinary teams (Pierskalla, 1981).
2. By manipulation of model variables, OR models can project the performance of innovative systems that differ substantially from existing ones (Pierskalla, 1981).
3. OR models can be used to make system projections "just in time." Evaluation and applied research studies generally take extended periods of time. As Levin and Roberts (1976) note "If many studies ranging over a long period of time are needed to build a good scientific account of some social phenomenon, the social practitioner will probably not have time to wait (p. 7)."

A variety of different types of models have been described as OR models. These include linear programming models, network flow models, integer programming models, nonlinear programming models, dynamic programming models, stochastic programming models, combinatorial optimization models, stochastic process models, discrete time Markov chain models, continuous time Markov chain models, queuing models, and simulation models (Jensen and Bard, 2003; Sainfort et al., 2004). It is beyond the scope of this chapter to describe these various models; however, the texts cited above are good examples of the many that do so.

The Human Services Research Institute mental health allocation and planning simulation (HSRI MHAPS) model, discussed here, is a deterministic first-order Markov simulation model. This model is an offshoot of a mental health allocation and planning linear programming model (HSRI MHAPLP) developed by Leff and Graves (Leff, 1981; Leff et al., 1985, 1986).

Planning models generally, and simulation models in particular, require specific steps as listed below (Levin and Roberts, 1976; Pierskalla, 1981; Hargreaves, 1986).

1. Development of a conceptual framework or theory describing key elements of the system to be modeled
2. Mathematical formulation of the model

* Note that "a *projection* specifically allows for significant changes in the set of 'boundary conditions' that might influence [a] prediction, creating 'if this, then that' types of statements. Thus, a *projection is... statement that it is possible that something will happen in the future if certain conditions develop.* The set of boundary conditions that is used in conjunction with making a projection is often called a scenario, and each scenario is based on assumptions about how the future will develop...For a decision maker, a projection is an indication of a possibility, and normally of one that could be influenced by the actions of the decision maker" (MacCracken, 2009).

3. Collection of data necessary to populate model variables
4. Scenario review and selection
5. Presentation of "user-friendly" results to different audiences

HSRI Mental Health Allocation and Planning Simulation

Theoretical and Conceptual Framework

Figure 42.1, below, depicts the framework we developed for both HSRI MHAPS and MHAPLP. At regular intervals, mental health systems take into consideration current service users that continue in care, as well as recent arrivals from outside the system. Arrivals occur under a number of circumstances. They may be persons who have just been diagnosed or evaluated for a serious mental illness (treated incidence). They may also be persons who have had a serious mental illness for some time but who are participating in services for the first time, either under the prevailing service system or due to service system changes (latent demand becoming expressed). Arrivals may also be previously served persons who have left the system but are returning for service. Persons are assigned to combinations of different services (service packages) based on their service needs, judgments as to the effectiveness of candidate service packages, and on the availability of new and existing resources to meet service package resource requirements. During the delivery of services, resources are consumed. Following the delivery of service packages, service recipients either improve, worsen, or remain the same in terms of one or more system objective(s). They may also disappear from the system or die. The number of persons still in need of service and continuing in a system influence the future number of persons to be served. The amount of resources consumed influences the future resources supply, and so on (Leff et al., 1985, 1986).

Given this conceptual framework, we postulated that, with respect to the need for services, the most salient characteristics of persons with serious mental illness would be reflected in their overall level of functioning. Level of functioning is not a fixed trait but a state that changes with the natural course of the mental disorder and the receipt of services. For that reason, when discussing functioning we will typically speak of persons in terms of "when they are at specific functional levels." We further postulated that persons in need of service would require different types and amounts (packages) of services depending on their level of functioning. Finally, we postulated that service recipient outcomes could be most relevantly measured in terms of functional level changes. System level outcomes would be most meaningfully expressed as aggregate changes in levels of functioning and system performance would be best articulated as some ratio of outcomes to total resources expended.

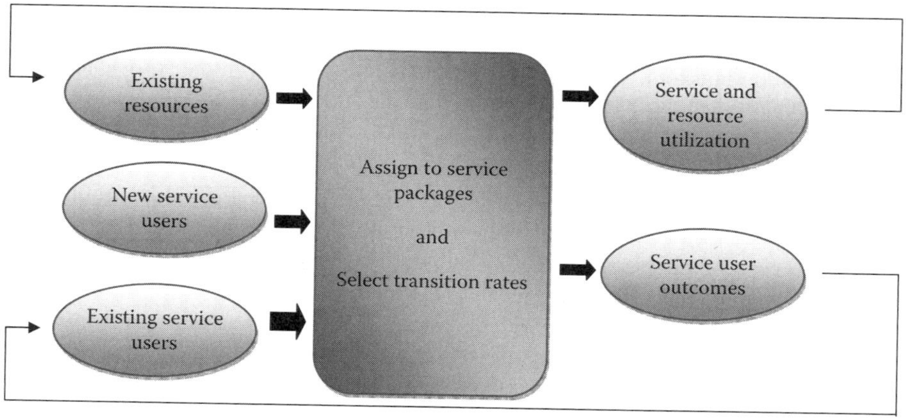

FIGURE 42.1 HSRI MHAPS conceptual framework.

We selected 1 month as the planning unit of time for our model based on the rates at which persons with a serious mental illness who were very low and mid-range functioning transition. Persons when they are very low functioning typically are suffering from acute psychiatric symptoms. In many instances, these symptoms can be ameliorated fairly rapidly by psychoactive medications. Hence, persons when they are low functioning often improve in functioning in days or weeks. Persons with a serious mental illness when they are mid-range functioning are typically engaged in learning community living skills, such as how to find and retain employment or how to deal with the stresses of everyday life. It can take periods of 1 year or more to learn skills like these. Given a range of transition times—from days and weeks to years—we chose 1 month as a plausible unit of time for our model. We do note that since persons when they are low functioning may transition in days or weeks, our use of a month period may overestimate service needs for these groups. However, we believe this bias is somewhat mitigated by the fact that service systems probably lag to some degree in responding to rapid functional level changes.

At this point, it is instructive to note why we went from using MHAPLP to HSRI MHAPS. In its initial formulation, for each month in the planning time frame, MHAPLP was allowed to assign monthly service packages differing in types and amounts of service to functional level groups (functional level groups and service packages are discussed further below). Planning time frames typically ranged from 12 to 60 months. As we experimented with MHAPLP, we found that it made a number of decisions that would not be acceptable in real systems. For example, it made different service package assignments within functional level groups with no justification other than optimizing long-term system outcomes, given resource constraints. As another example, MHAPLP would change service packages from month to month, sometimes substituting "poorer" service packages for "richer" ones, again to maximize long-term system outcomes. As a final example, toward the end of a planning period, MHAPLP would myopically tend to assign "poorer" service packages to some groups because there was insufficient time for favorable outcomes and associated cost savings to occur. These decisions would have the appearance of inequities and arbitrary rationing to providers, service users, and other stakeholders in mental health systems. While real systems may engage in such behaviors as unintended consequences of resource constraints (Levin and Roberts, 1976; Levin, 1977) more often than we would like to admit, we found that systems planners could not choose plans that had these characteristics. As a result, we increasingly constrained MHAPLP so that it would not make these decisions. Eventually, it seemed more straightforward to employ a simulation model than a severely constrained MHAPLP that, in many ways, was functioning like a simulator.

Mathematical Formulation

As noted above, we mathematically formulated HSRI MHAPS as a deterministic first-order Markov simulation model. Markov models have been and are being used in mental health planning (Sweillam and Tardiff, 1978; Hargreaves, 1986; Perry et al., 1987; Korte, 1990; Liu et al., 1992; Shumway et al., 1994; Patten, 2005; Bala and Mauskopf, 2006; James et al., 2006; Norton et al., 2006; Heeg et al., 2008; Miller et al., 2009b). Markov transitions have been proposed as a useful way to think about mental health outcomes for mental health evaluation and planning (Pierskalla, 1981; Hargreaves, 1986). These outcomes can be the number of individuals who enter, remain, or leave a mental health service system. Markov transitions for most health settings have been calculated to describe the progression of phases from the onset of illness to recovery. Two great attractions of Markov models for planning are (1) their basis in states for which services can be planned and (2) their ability, given that even the most effective services do not have favorable outcomes for all persons at all times, to describe backward as well as forward movement or change.

In the HSRI MHAPS model, planners assign service packages to functional level groups. Functional level groups describe states through which persons pass (although not necessarily linearly) in the course of mental illness. Service packages start as menus of multiple services. For each functional level, planners "prescribe" the *services* that persons in the functional level group should receive, the *percents of persons* in the functional group who should receive the services, and the *average amounts of service* that persons in need should receive. The percent of persons prescribed a service multiplied by the average amount of service prescribed is the utilization rate for that service. Each service is associated with a unit cost (or any other resource requirement, e.g., staffing) and can also be associated with revenues realized.

Additionally, for each service package, planners estimate a set of monthly Markov transition probabilities reflecting the effectiveness of the service package in improving service recipients' level of functioning (discussed below). Simply put, for each month in the planning time frame, the model multiplies the number of new and arriving persons in each functional level group by the service utilization rates and uses these numbers to estimate service costs and revenues. It also uses the Markov transition probabilities to distribute persons to functional levels to set the stage for the next month.

Functional Level Groups and Estimating Persons in Need of Service

Given our theory that functional level is the most useful way to think about persons with serious mental illness for system planning purposes, we developed a functional level framework for use with MHAPLP that we also use with HSRI MAHPS. To develop this functional level framework, the first author interviewed psychiatric case managers specializing in treatment planning and care management for persons with serious mental illness (Leff et al., 1986). These case managers typically placed persons into three to six groups. The first author also observed that many multi-item and multi-scale measures often were reduced for planning and evaluation purposes to only one score consisting of no more than 10 levels (Weissman, 1975). Given these observations and the need for a framework that could be translated into minimally burdensome measures for assessing functional levels repeatedly and system-wide, a global and resource associated level of functioning framework with seven levels was developed.

This framework is described in Table 42.1. The framework is "global" because the levels are meant to describe functional areas such as activities of daily living and community living skills, rather than individual skills. Other frameworks break down functioning into multiple individual skills, although, as stated above, they often combine them into a global measure (The Evaluation Center@HSRI, 2004). The framework is "resource associated" because the functional areas it focuses on have implications for service needs. In fact, planners using these levels prescribe service packages that focus on services that control symptoms of persons at the lower functional levels, and prescribe services packages that focus on rehabilitation and community integration for persons at the higher levels. Resource requirements decrease as functional level increases (Leff et al., 1985).

Following this, we developed a functional level scale to measure functioning according to this framework, the Resource Associated Functional Level Scale (RAFLS). The RAFLS is a global measure of functioning with seven levels paralleling the levels in the global, resource associated functional level framework. This scale has proved to have acceptable reliability (Leff et al., 2004). Other scales are available for measuring level of functioning (Goldman et al., 1992). One scale that is typical of others, and for which data is frequently available, is the Global Assessment of Functioning (GAF) Scale used to measure Axis V in the Diagnostic and Statistical Manual of Mental Disorders (DSM) (Goldman et al., 1992). We have been able to cross-walk scores on the GAF (and on a number of other scales) to our functional level framework, although without some collapsing of items and rearrangement of resulting levels, these scales may not be ideal for planning services (Moos et al., 2002).

HSRI MHAPS requires information on the number and functional level distribution of persons in the mental health system at the start of a planning period (snapshot data) and the average number and functional levels of persons arriving monthly (arrival rates). We can estimate the numbers of persons in, and arriving, to systems either through the use of administrative data or sample surveys. However, estimating functional level distributions is more difficult when using administrative data. Administrative data systems do not necessarily measure level of functioning. Those that do, do not measure it monthly. Instead, information systems that measure functional level take varied approaches: some measure it at the initiation of service, and some at initiation and termination. Others measure it at the time of service

TABLE 42.1 Resource Associated Functional Level Scale (RAFLS)

Level	Level Name	Level Description
1	At risk	At risk to self or others, or to property of value. Unable or unwilling to participate in one's own care or to cooperate in control of violent or aggressive behavior. May require continuous (24 hours) supervision, high staff/consumer ratio.
2	Unable to function, current, acute psychiatric symptoms	Acute symptoms may result in behavior that is seriously disruptive or at risk to self or others, but if so, is able/willing to control impulses with assistance and willing to participate in own care. Alternatively, acute symptoms seriously impair role functioning. Examples of acute symptoms: lack of reality testing, hallucinations or delusions, impaired judgment, impaired communication, or manic behavior. Nonetheless, may be able to carry out *some* activities of daily living. May require continuous supervision, or moderate staff/consumer ratio.
3	Lacks ADL/personal care skills	Lacks ADL due to active symptoms that do not result in behavior that is seriously disruptive or dangerous. Unable or unwilling to make use of sufficient ADL and/or personal care skills to carry out basic role functions. May require continuous (24 hours) prompting, skill training, and encouragement.
4	Lacks community living skills	Able to carry out ADL personal care skills. Role functioning impaired by lack of community living skills or motivation to perform. Community living skills include money management, ability to engage in competitive employment, maintaining interpersonal contacts. May require regular and substantial but not necessarily continuous training, prompting, and encouragement.
5	Community living skills but vulnerable to stresses of everyday life	Can perform role functions, at least minimally, in familiar settings and with frequent support to deal with the ordinary stresses of everyday life; although may need the regular assistance of a roommate, homemaker-aide, etc., or can work outside of sheltered situations with on-site support or counseling. Requires support under the stresses associated with the frustrations of everyday life and novel situations. May require frequent (e.g., weekly) information, encouragement, and instrumental assistance.
6	Community living skills and only needs support/treatment to cope with extreme stress or seeks treatment to maintain or enhance personal development	Can perform role functions adequately except under extreme or unusual stress. At these times, the support of natural or generic helpers such as family, friends, or clergy is not sufficient. Mental health services are required for the duration of stress; or performs role functions adequately, but seeks mental health services because of feelings of persistent dissatisfaction with self or personal relationships. Intensity and duration of treatment can vary.
7	System independent	Can obtain support from natural helpers or generic services. Does not require or seek mental health services.

changes, and others quarterly. Additionally, management information systems do not tend to use functional level measures designed to relate directly to service need. Therefore, although it is possible to estimate functional level changes from management information system data, we prefer to measure it using sample surveys and a functional level measure.

It is possible for persons to vary in functioning within months. Since we use monthly planning periods, some error is unavoidable. Our rule for these situations is to "code to or take the lowest." For clinical and safety reasons we believe it is better to overestimate system needs than to underestimate them.

Planning Service Packages

A population of persons with serious mental illness can require between 20 and 40 services in the service domains of medical inpatient and outpatient treatment, mental health inpatient and outpatient treatment, case management, housing, rehabilitation, and social support (Leff et al., 2004). Table 42.2 contains an illustrative list of services and their definitions. Depending on level of functioning and other considerations (e.g., family supports) individuals with serious mental illness typically receive four to six services. For a desired service system, HSRI MHAPS planners prescribe the percentage of persons

TABLE 42.2 Service Variables, Component Services, and Service Definitions

Service Domain	Component Services	Definition
Inpatient	Specialty inpatient	Provides continuous treatment that includes general psychiatric care, medical detoxification, and/or forensic services in a general hospital, a general hospital with a distinct part, or a freestanding psychiatric facility.
Emergency	Crisis intervention services	Crisis intervention services for the purpose of stabilizing or preventing a sudden episode or behavior.
	Crisis respite	24-hour services for individuals in crisis in homelike settings.
Residential treatment	Short-term and long-term residential	Residential services that are provided by a behavioral health agency. These agencies provide a structured treatment setting with 24-hour supervision and counseling or other therapeutic activities for persons who do not require on-site medical care.
Community treatment	Assessment	Evaluation for the purposes of intake, treatment planning, eligibility determination.
	Individual counseling	Scheduled outpatient mental health services provided on an individual basis in a clinic or similar facility.
	Group counseling	Psychotherapy to multiple clients in same session.
	Family counseling	Psychotherapy to a family or couples to improve insight, decision-making, and to reduce stress.
	Medication evaluation/management	Services provided by physician or other qualified medical provider to evaluate, prescribe, and monitor psychiatric medications.
	Substance abuse treatment	Programs for persons with both mental illness and substance abuse.
	Assertive community treatment	ACT is a multidisciplinary approach to providing an inclusive array of community-based rehabilitation services following SAMHSA EBP guidelines.
Rehabilitation	Supported employment	Job finding and retention services following SAMHSA EBP guidelines.
	Skills training	Individual or group training in activities of daily and community living skills.
Support	Case management	Assistance in accessing services and making choices about opportunities and services in the community.
	Peer support	Self-help/peer services are provided by persons or family members who are or have been consumers of the behavioral health system. This may involve assistance with more effectively utilizing the service delivery system or understanding and coping with the stressors coaching, role modeling, and mentoring.
	Supported housing	Supported housing services are provided to assist individuals or families to obtain and maintain housing in an independent community setting including the person's own home or apartments and homes that are owned or leased by a subcontracted provider.

in each functional level group who are in need of a service and the average amount of service persons in need should receive. If the purpose of a plan is to change the service system, the services available and the percentages and amounts prescribed for the desired system will always differ from those available and utilized in the current system. In some cases services will be added or increased.

However, an important part of service planning is removing or reducing ineffective or inefficient services, a process Frank and Glied (2006) have described as exnovation. We refer to the resultant multi-service prescriptions for each functional group as "service packages." The group process by which these prescriptions are made is described in the "Prescribe percents and amounts of services for persons with serious mental illnesses at different functional levels" section.

Initially, we developed service packages (and estimated outcomes) by convening diverse mental health system stakeholders from the locales for which we were planning. We would then engage them in a consensus process for assigning services to functional groups (Leff et al., 1985). Recently, we have modified this approach, although we still convene planning workgroups of diverse mental health system stakeholders. These stakeholders include service users, service providers, advocates, policy makers, and planners. However, given findings from social-psychological research, we no longer have the workgroups reach consensus. Bringing together groups to plan services is based on the idea that individuals, by virtue of their unique life experiences and expertise, make more informed decisions than single individuals (Gustafson et al., 1973; Reuter and Gustafson, 1981; Sunstein, 2006). However, social-psychological research has shown that when groups are asked to seek consensus they can be heavily influenced by factors such as the dominance of a few individuals, or the predisposition of others to withhold their ideas because they are shy or concerned about alienating other group members (Sunstein, 2006). Consequently, we now use an evidence-based method described by Reuter and Gustafson (1981) as "estimate-talk-estimate." In this approach, individuals first make service recommendations privately. These recommendations are averaged and fed back to the workgroup. If the members' recommendations vary widely, we may transform the estimates to minimize the influence of extreme ratings (Charemza, 2002). The workgroup then talks about the recommendations. Prior to the discussion, workgroup members are asked to discuss general principles for making recommendations and not the specific percents and amounts they prescribed. They then privately re-recommend services. The second round of service recommendations becomes the primary service prescriptions for the modeling effort.

When we first began modeling mental health systems in the late 1970s, administrative data sets with monthly data on service utilization were rarely available. When they were available, they were expensive to access. Monthly service utilization data that could be organized by level of functioning was even more rare. Consequently, we either used sample surveys to collect data on utilization and functioning, or planned without current system information. However, service utilization data that can be organized by month and by functional level has become much more accessible in administrative data sets. Consequently, we are usually able to present our planning workgroups with data for their systems showing current service packages for functional groups. The planning task then becomes modifying the current service packages to make them more effective or efficient.

Assigning Unit Costs and Revenues

We also assign a unit cost and revenue generated to each service. Units differ as a function of service. For example, hospital units of service are typically days and outpatient therapy units of treatment are typically hours. Unit cost and revenue data for existing services are usually available from system financial divisions. It should be noted that the unit cost data available is more accurately unit price data. If new services are being planned, unit cost data may have to be obtained from outside the system. In some cases it may have to be estimated based on staffing and other resource requirements.

Estimating Outcomes

MHAPLP and HSRI MHAPS are unique among mental health planning approaches in the way they incorporate outcomes. Under our theory, persons with serious mental illness improve or regress in functioning depending on their current level of functioning and the service packages they receive. Our models assume that a Markov property applies to these transitions. More specifically, we assume that a person in FL i, depending on the service package received, makes a transition (improves, regresses, or does not change) to FL j within a certain period of time. For HSRI MHAPS, this is 1 month. Additionally, for planning purposes, we assume that these transitions occur exactly at their expected value despite the probabilistic nature of individual service recipient movements. For example, suppose the probability of improvement is 0.3 for each person in FL i that receives service package k. If there are 100 persons in FL i receiving service package k, exactly 30 of these persons will improve in the immediate time period. As noted in Leff et al. (1986), we believe that ignoring transition randomness is appropriate for, and consistent with, the development of an aggregate resource-planning model. A number of studies

TABLE 42.3 Transition Probability Matrix for Functional Levels

Initial Functional Level	Destination									
	1	2	3	4	5	6	7	Death	Disappearance	Total
1	FL *11*	FL *12*	FL *13*	FL *14*	FL *15*	FL *16*	FL *17*	1 De	1 Dis	1.00
2	FL *21*	FL *22*	FL *23*	FL *24*	FL *25*	FL *26*	FL *27*	2 De	2 Dis	1.00
3	FL *31*	FL 32	FL 33	FL 34	FL 35	FL 36	FL 37	3 De	3 Dis	1.00
4	FL *41*	FL *42*	FL *43*	FL *44*	FL *45*	FL *46*	FL *47*	4 De	4 Dis	1.00
5	FL *51*	FL *52*	FL *53*	FL *54*	FL *55*	FL *56*	FL *57*	5 De	5 Dis	1.00
6	FL *61*	FL *62*	FL *63*	FL *64*	FL *65*	FL *66*	FL *67*	6 De	6 Dis	1.00

Note: Values in italics represent transitions per period in functioning.

demonstrate how Markov transitions can be used to estimate forward and backward transition of mental health clients (Pierskalla, 1981; Hargreaves, 1986; Liu et al., 1992; Sonnenberg and Beck, 1993; Bala and Mauskopf, 2006; Norton et al., 2006; Miller et al., 2009a).

Given our 7-level functioning conceptual framework, in model applications we develop a 6×9 transition probability matrix to represent outcomes for functional groups given defined service packages. Table 42.3 presents an example of such a matrix. There are only 6 rows for initial functional groups since persons at functional level 7 are, by definition, not in need of service. There are nine outcome states, one for each functional group, one for persons transitioning to death, and one for persons transitioning to disappearance. Many persons with serious mental illness leave the mental health system in unplanned ways. Under these circumstances little is known about their levels of functioning at the time (Olfson et al., 2009). Some may have become system independent (i.e., reached functional level 7). Others may have regressed and become involved with the criminal justice system, homeless, or hospitalized on some other system (Rochefort, 1997).

After we complete the service planning process, as described above, we use the planning workgroups to estimate Markov transition probabilities for the planned service packages. Once again, because administrative data sets with functional level data have become more available, we are able to provide planning workgroups with matrices showing transition probabilities for their systems given current service packages. However, since the functional level data available to us are not monthly, we have to make assumptions about functional level changes occurring between measurements. This allows us to translate the differing time intervals between functional level measures we have into monthly functional level ratings and monthly changes. For this reason, we still prefer to collect level of functioning data using sample surveys that ask for functional level ratings for the current and the previous month. These ratings allow us to estimate transitions based on monthly data.

We also follow an estimate-talk-estimate approach for transition probabilities. After presenting the planning workgroup with current transition rates we have members privately estimate what they think transition probabilities will be under the planned system. We then average the members' estimates (making some modifications, if necessary, to make the row totals equal to 1.00), enter them into HSRI MHAPS, and implement a simulation with the new plan's data elements. Next, we present the simulation results to the planning workgroup and allow them to discuss the findings. As in the service planning component, workgroup members are asked to discuss general principles and not their specific estimates. After a discussion period, we ask the workgroup members to reestimate transition probabilities for the new service packages. The averages of these estimates (again modified to sum to 1.00) becomes the transition probabilities for the new plan.

Web-Based Implementation of HSRI MHAPS

Following the development of our simulator we have spent over two decades using the model to assist states, counties, and local entities to explore mental health system options. During this time, we identified several barriers to widespread model use. The first was the lack of "desktop" model accessibility to state planners. Another was a lack of experience among state planners with model-based planning. A third was our desire to be constantly enhancing and improving our model. A fourth was the relative isolation of state mental health planners from other planners and scientists working on planning problems. Last but not least, was the lack of empirical data for the model.

Motivated by these practical experiences, we decided to develop a Web-implemented version of the model. This version has screens and instructions for entering all the model inputs described above. It is programmed in…and located on a server operated by HSRI. The enhancement enables us to make the model accessible to local planners and to provide technical assistance on appropriate uses of the model. Further, Web dissemination of our model allows us to fix model problems and disseminate new model versions. Finally, a version of the model, situated on a Web site along with community building and information sharing mechanisms such as shared databases, bulletin boards, and list serves, seemed to us a way to overcome the isolation of state planners and of increasing the available data for modeling efforts.

The second enhancement we made to the current model also addressed the lack of empirical data for model inputs. This enhancement involved developing a model component for generating different inputs for the model in a particularly important and data-sparse area (estimates of treatment outcomes) to be used in sensitivity analysis.

Case Study: *Arnold v. Sarn* Service Capacity Plan

BACKGROUND

Arnold v. Sarn is a class action suit that was brought by advocates on behalf of persons with mental illness in 1981, alleging that the Division of Behavioral Health Services of the state of Arizona (ADBHS) was not providing adequate or comprehensive mental health services in Maricopa County. In 1986, the court found that the mental health system was in violation of state statutes. To provide support in the resolution of this suit, the plaintiffs, representatives of the Court, and the ADBHS retained HSRI in 1991 to conduct a study to develop a mental health system plan for Maricopa County that would be acceptable to all parties. In 1996, the parties negotiated an exit stipulation to the suit to determine when the state had sufficiently implemented a system that satisfied these criteria. The exit stipulation included requirements on the Arizona State Hospital, service planning and quality improvement efforts, and obligations to case management, rehabilitation, and housing services. In 1998, a supplemental agreement was reached between the parties to avoid further litigation against the ADHAS for not being in compliance with the exit stipulation. There has been continuing action taken in regard to the suit, with the Court's Office of the Monitor conducting independent assessments of progress to determine compliance. HSRI completed the service capacity plan for ADBHAS in 1999.

STEPS IN AND RESULTS OF THE PLANNING PROCESS

To develop the plan, a planning workgroup representing all parties to the suit was formed. The steps taken in the planning process and the findings of those steps are presented below.

Estimate Functional Level Distribution

We used ADBHS Colorado Client Assessment Record (CCAR) (Ellis et al., 1984) data for 1998 to estimate the functional levels of persons in the planning population. Several algorithms

TABLE 42.4 Estimated Snapshot and Arrival Functional Level Distribution: Numbers and Percents in Planning Population

	Snapshot		Monthly Arrivals	
MAHPS Level	Number	%	Number	%
1 At risk	840	7	224	9
2 Acute symptoms	1,428	12	527	21
3 Lacks ADL/personal care skills	3,516	29	734	30
4 Lacks community living skills	1,536	13	389	16
5 Needs role support and training	2,124	18	347	14
6 Needs support/ treatment to cope with extreme stress	2,556	21	239	10
Total	12,000	100	2463	100

were developed for crosswalking CCAR data to the MHAPS functional level framework. Representatives of parties to the suit acted as a planning committee and agreed on a crosswalk that yielded the distribution shown in Table 42.4. Distributions were developed for service users who received assessments prior to 1998 (the "snapshot population") and for persons who received intakes in 1998 (the "arrival population"). Note that arriving service users are at a lower level of functioning than persons who have been in the system, indicating some degree of improvement associated with the current system in Arizona.

Determine and Define Services

In consultation with the planning participants, we developed a list of services and service definitions judged necessary for persons in the planning population. These services were suggested by reviews of services provided in Arizona and other states, consideration of the scientific literature on evidenced-based mental health services, and the literature on service user and family preferences. The service domains covered included residential, emergency services, hospital and crisis services, treatment, outpatient treatment, rehabilitation, and support. Services that were consistent with the scientific evidence and the clinical principles cited above were selected, which are that services should ensure service user and community safety, be least restrictive, respond flexibly to changes in need, promote functioning, empowerment, and recovery, and be cost-effective. The final list of 35 services, organized by domain, is presented below in Table 42.5.

Estimate Service Unit Costs Based on Data from Arizona and Other States

Unit service costs for 18 states were examined. For data prior to 1998, an inflation rate equation was utilized to provide updated costs. This equation was based on data from the Bureau of Labor Statistics' Consumer Price Index for Medical Care Services. For some services, unit costs were calculated using information provided and reviewed by the planning process participants relating to staffing patterns and assumptions about amounts of service to be delivered. In addition, whenever possible, unit cost estimates were compared with unit cost estimates in the published literature on services for persons with severe mental illness. Table 42.6 also shows the final service unit costs estimated by HSRI and the planning participants organized by service domains.

Prescribe Percents and Amounts of Services for Persons with Serious Mental Illnesses at Different Functional Levels

For each functional group, the planning workgroup generated service prescriptions (percentages of persons to receive a service and average amount of service per recipient) for each of the services in Table 42.5. These prescriptions were based on prescriptions from a previous Arizona study, other state prescriptions from earlier studies, expert judgment, information about the current Arizona system, and the scientific literature.

Table 42.6 below shows service package costs by service domain and functional level. Patterns of costs indicate that the planning workgroup prescribed services according to the logic of the functional level framework. Total service package costs and all but two costs per domain decreased as level of functioning increased. The only exceptions to this were the treatment and rehabilitation domains. Treatment costs did not vary, but types of treatment did. Treatments for persons who were at lower functional levels were primarily intensive clinical services and medication, treatments for persons at higher functional levels included individual and group psychotherapy. Rehabilitation costs increased as functional level increased. Rehabilitation costs were highest for functional levels 3 and 4, but decreased for functional levels 5 and 6. This reflects the fact that many persons at functional level 1 may have symptoms that are too severe to benefit from intensive rehabilitation, while many at functional levels 5 and 6 do not need it. Persons at functional levels 2 through 4 are typically both in need of rehabilitation and in a position to take advantage of it.

ESTIMATE TRANSITION PROBABILITIES

After service packages were planned, the planning workgroup was presented with monthly transition probabilities from various other planning or evaluation efforts including ones in Arizona (Leff et al., 1985; Hargreaves, 1986; Leff et al., 1996). The planning workgroup discussed these estimates and recommended modifications based on differences between the newly planned service packages and the ones used in previous studies. These monthly transition rates are shown in Table 42.7, below.

One important aspect of this table is that most persons at each of the functional levels stay at the same functional level from month to month. Another important aspect is that even under the newly planned services, estimated to be more effective than current services, the planning workgroup estimated some regression (or backward transitions) for all levels of functioning. Additionally, consistent with our theory that persons at lower levels of functioning tend to progress in shorter periods of time, persons at functional levels 1 and 2 are estimated to progress more in 1 month than persons at other functional levels. Persons at functional level 3 are also estimated to change somewhat rapidly, but a part of that change is estimated to be regression. Finally, note that although some persons from functional levels 5 and 6 transition to functional level 7, the proportions that do are very small.

Estimate Annual Service System Costs, Taking into Account Estimated Service Needs, Unit Costs, and Service User Outcomes

After the workgroup had estimated the information described above, HSRI entered this information into HSRI MHAPS and explored a variety of planning options with the planning workgroup. The final model selected estimated service system costs for a fully funded and implemented plan serving 14,258 persons with serious mental illness at $435,943,267, yielding a per person cost of $30,576. The cost estimated administrative costs and costs of medication separately. These estimates were expected to apply to the system for the year 2002.

TABLE 42.5 Unit Costs Estimated for Services in Needs Assessment

Service	Unit	Cost
Hospital and crisis		
1. Inpatient—specialty/state	Days	$285.00
2. Inpatient—general	Days	$440.00
3. Inpatient—forensic	Days	$285.00
4. Inpatient—detoxification	Days	$150.00
5. Crisis outreach	Hours	$115.00
6. Crisis residential	Days	$285.00
Emergency		
7. Respite care	Days	$132.00
8. Crisis emergency walk-in	Hours	$166.00
Residential		
9. Intensive staff/supervision	Days	$250.00
10. Moderate staff/supervision	Days	$200.00
11. Minimum staff/supervision	Days	$90.00
12. Independent living w/housing subsidy	Days	$11.51
13. Independent living w/o housing subsidy[a]	Days	
14. Specialized residential	Days	$275.00
Treatment		
15. Evaluation (diagnosis)	Hours	$110.00
16. Court ordered evaluation	Hours	$110.00
17. Medication management	Hours	$64.00
18. Intensive clinical services	Hours	$90.00
19. Individual psychotherapy	Hours	$85.00
20. Group psychotherapy	Hours	$20.00
21. Family psychotherapy	Hours	$80.00
22. Therapeutic supervision	Hours	$25.00
23. Outpatient detoxification	Hours	$75.00
24. Substance abuse counseling	Hours	$75.00
25. Methadone maintenance clinic	Week	$75.00
Rehabilitation		
26. Psychosocial rehabilitation	Hours	$11.00
27. Consumer operated services	Hours	$5.00
28. Vocational assessment	Hours	$60.00
Support		
29. Assertive community treatment	Hours	$123.00
30. Supported employment	Hours	$60.00
31. Supported education and other educational services	Hours	$30.00
32. Protection and advocacy	Hours	$22.50
33. Client transportation	Hours	$10.00
34. Family psycho-education	Hours	$60.00
35. Friend advocacy	Per person	$83.00

[a] Independent Living w/o Housing Subsidy does not have an associated cost because the assumption is that housing costs are paid by other sources.

TABLE 42.6 Service Package Option Costs by Domain, Functional Level, and Total

Service Domains	Functional Levels 1	2	3	4	5	6
Hospital and crisis	$2,087	$647	$71	$156	$20	$0
Emergency	$880	$467	$208	$165	$82	$27
Residential	$8,556	$8,122	$6,753	$6,204	$5,573	$4,791
Treatment	$175	$222	$219	$245	$246	$156
Rehabilitation	$2,040	$2,924	$3,038	$2,155	$1,349	$733
Support	$1,650	$1,454	$568	$732	$276	$75
Total	$15,388	$13,835	$10,856	$9,657	$7,546	$5,782

TABLE 42.7 Revised Arizona Transition Probability Matrix

Initial Functional Level	Destinations 1	2	3	4	5	6	7	Disappearance	Death	Total
1	**0.624**	0.118	0.050	0.154	0.007	0.005	0.000	0.037	0.005	1.000
2	0.099	**0.624**	0.129	0.037	0.068	0.002	0.000	0.037	0.004	1.000
3	0.006	0.031	**0.716**	0.184	0.022	0.001	0.000	0.037	0.003	1.000
4	0.014	0.019	0.069	**0.734**	0.111	0.013	0.000	0.037	0.003	1.000
5	0.004	0.007	0.015	0.073	**0.747**	0.103	0.013	0.036	0.002	1.000
6	0.000	0.008	0.000	0.008	0.050	**0.879**	0.017	0.037	0.001	1.000

Note: Values in bold represent probability of groups on average within a given functional level remaining in their respective functional level from one period to another.

Figure 42.2 shows the projected distribution of year 1 expenditures for the fully implemented simulation by major service domains. This figure shows that the bulk of expenditures are directed at housing, rehabilitation, and support. This expenditure distribution is reflective of the clinical principles that informed the planning process. These principles emphasized service user and community safety, least restrictive environment, flexible services, and service user recovery and independence. Note that residential care was a substantial portion of estimated service costs and that rehabilitation cost exceeded treatment costs.

CASE STUDY DISCUSSION

This plan for a comprehensive, full capacity mental health system for Arizona was based on the best information and planning technology currently available. The plan was very explicit about the types of persons to be served, the types and amounts of services needed, the outcomes to be expected, and the probable costs of the services.

The Department of Health Services (the umbrella agency for the ADBHS) presented this plan to the Judge in *Arnold v. Sarn* (Charles, 1999). The presentation described the planning methods used and the plan in all its detail. The scientific underpinnings of the planning process and the detailed plan allowed the Arizona Department of Health to orally testify to the Judge:

> In particular, the Department of Health Services is, I think, pleased with the Arizona Service Capacity Planning Project...The project represents many months of work analyzing data, developing program models and costs and refining a cost-efficient approach for developing a

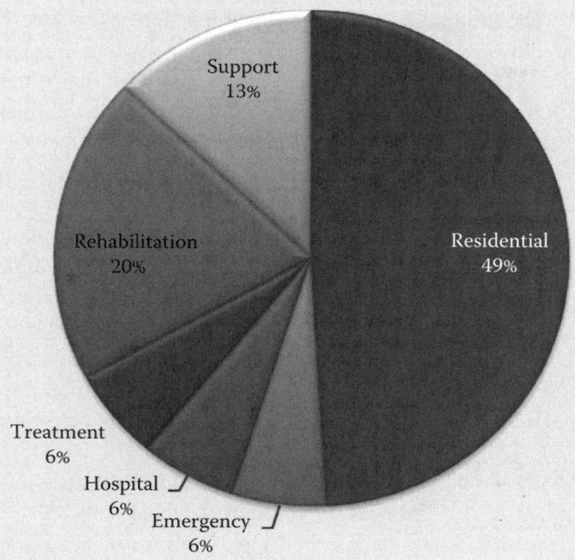

FIGURE 42.2 Year 1 distribution of expenditures by service domains.

> comprehensive mental health system for seriously mentally ill people in Maricopa County... The Department concurs with the client movement model presented by HSRI, the contractor, and believes that its conclusion represents a reliable estimate of what is required in order to have an opportunity to meet the State's requirements in this case. (Charles, 1999)

Although the Judge expressed that he lacked the expertise to fully evaluate the plan, he recognized the work that had gone into the planning process, and accepted it as a basis for going forward, illustrating the usefulness of HSRI MHAPS in the setting of mental health policy:

> I feel optimistic by the fact that the parties have worked together diligently over many months to develop the remedial strategic plans, including service gap analysis...Consequently, it is my belief that the Department should go forward... (Charles, 1999)

The ADBHS has been implementing the plan since 1999. The specificity of model estimates allows for testing of the model's accuracy as the plan is implemented. Recently, we received system cost and number of persons for the served information on the performance of the Maricopa County mental health system for the years 1999–2008 (Franczak, 2009). We had estimated that 2001 would be the earliest the Maricopa County mental health system might approach full implementation of the plan developed. Our HSRI MHAPS estimate for the number of persons to be served in the first full year of system implementation was 14,257 persons. Our estimate of system costs for that year was $435,943,267 or $30,844 per person. The number of persons served in 2002 was 13,407 and the total system cost was $413,523,978, or $30,843 per person. These observed data points are satisfyingly close to our projections. However, it is not clear that more detailed data would be equally consistent with model projections. More detailed findings are not available to us. However, they could be very useful. To the extent that there are variances from our projections, the plan could be revised using the new information.

The total system cost was substantially more than the ADBHS was currently spending. The court suit caused the ADBHS to receive more dollars to meet the models requirements. This will not be the case in most localities and simulations in these settings will have to be used to "back into" available dollars. However, one bright spot is that simulations for more extended periods of time suggest system costs might level off or even decrease as persons improve in functioning and some reach the point that they no longer need regular services from the public mental health system. One danger in backing into affordable system changes is that planners will dilute service packages without correspondingly making transition probabilities less positive and ignoring the fact that this will increase backward transitions. Probably the best options for reducing system costs involve maintaining service package integrity, but implementing plans only incrementally in selected geographic localities. However, this is a difficult option for public officials because it results in inequalities.

It is important to note that the projections presented assumed a "frictionless" system in which services could be changed rapidly in response to changes in service user needs. Real systems experience friction and should be expected to change more slowly than our model projects and Arizona exhibited, particularly when a judge and court monitor are overseeing the system's changes.

Additionally, the Arizona plan addressed only the monetary resources required by the new and expanded services. It is also important to note that implementing the plan required well-trained and skilled "front-line" staff to deliver the planned services with fidelity to the service models identified in Arizona's service definitions. The Arizona data we were recently given suggest ADBHS has so far been able to recruit, train, and retain staff for the services planned. If service fidelity drifts away from desired models, refresher training will be necessary. Other states planning new service systems need to attend to staff recruitment, training, and retention issues as well.

Summary and Conclusions

We have described a simulation model for mental health system planning and we provide an illustrative case study of an actual implementation. We have implemented the model in over two dozen States and counties. The model conceptual framework has been accepted as a plausible and useful theory of how mental health systems function. The model has been mathematically formulated and a computer-implemented, Web-based version of the model has also been developed. Over time, more administrative data have become available to estimate model parameters; nevertheless, in the absence of survey data, estimating monthly service needs by functional level and estimating functional level changes continues to be a challenge. However, we have developed evidence-based methods for using groups comprised of mental health system stakeholders for estimating these data.

Currently, we are continuing to implement our model in additional states. We hope that in some of these states we will obtain data to further assess the accuracy of our model. We are also attempting to extend our modeling in two ways.

Criminal Justice

One goal identified for additional model development identifed by The Ad Hoc Advisory Group on Operations Research and the Mental Health System was building models that can represent the flow or transfers between mental health and other systems (Pierskalla, 1981). Given concerns about the flow of persons with mental illness into criminal justice systems, we have developed and are continuing to extend versions of HSRI MHAPS to describe how this flow occurs and to plan and evaluate service options to divert persons into mental health systems (Norton et al., 2006). The HSRI MHAPS Mental

Health/Jail Diversion Cost Simulation was developed to help communities as they plan and budget for programs that divert persons from the criminal justice system into community-based mental health services. The model projects the costs, effectiveness, and potential cost offsets of implementing a jail diversion program for persons with mental illness. The model is a strategic planning tool intended to provide program stakeholder groups with information for planning resource allocation strategies and prioritizing and choosing options for jail diversion programs.

This model compares the service utilization, consumer outcomes, and costs for a group of individuals who are diverted into community-based services and supports to the costs for the same group of individuals in the absence of a jail diversion program. Program planners can use the model to explore the fiscal and outcome implications of implementing different jail diversion strategies, providing different services, and choosing different target populations. The model has been tested in two counties and is currently being used by one state.

Quebec Planning Study

It is our theory, and the theory of others, that the use of planning models like HSRI MHAPS should result in plans that meet service needs more adequately and efficiently than planning not based on models (Pierskalla, 1981). However, this theory remains to be empirically verified by comparing planning efforts with and without models. We are currently engaged in a project to do this with colleagues in Quebec, Canada including McGill University, the Quebec Mental Health Directorate, and the Quebec Health and Social Service Centers. We will compare a simple approach to planning (systematic enumeration of anticipated costs and benefits associated with each option) with the dynamic modeling approach to system and services planning described above.

References

Bala, M. V. and J. A. Mauskopf. 2006. Optimal assignment of treatments to health states using a Markov Decision Model: An introduction to basic concepts. *PharmacoEconomics* 24(4):345–354.

Charemza, W. W. 2002. Guesstimation. *Journal of Forecasting* 21(6):417–433.

Charles, L. Arnold et al. Plaintiffs vs. James Sarn et al., Defendents. 1999. In *Fredrick Gaio III*: Superior Court of the State of Arizona in and for the County of Maricopa.

Ellis, R., N. Wilson, and F. Foster. 1984. Statewide treatment outcome assessment in Colorado: The Colorado Client Assessment Record (CCAR). *Community Mental Health Journal* 20(1):72–89.

Foley, H. A. and S. S. Sharfstein. 1983. *Madness and Government: Who Cares for the Mentally Ill?* Washington, DC: American Psychiatric Press.

Franczak, M. 2009. Personal communication, June 18, 2009.

Frank, R. G. and S. Glied. 2006. *Better But Not Well: Mental Health Policy in the United States Since 1950.* Baltimore, MD: Johns Hopkins University Press.

Goldman, H. H., A. E. Skodol, and T. R. Lave. 1992. Revising axis V for DSM-IV: A review of measures of social functioning. *American Journal of Psychiatry* 149(9):1148–1156.

Grob, G. N. and H. H. Goldman. 2006. *The Dilemma of Federal Mental Health Policy: Radical Reform or Incremental Change?* (*Critical Issues in Health and Medicine*). New Brunswick, NJ: Rutgers University Press.

Gustafson, D. H., R. K. Shukla, A. Delbecq, and G. W. Walster. 1973. A comparative study of differences in subjective likelihood estimates made by individuals, interacting groups, Delphi groups, and nominal groups. *Organizational Behavior and Human Performance* 9(2):280–291.

Hargreaves, W. A. 1986. Theory of psychiatric treatment systems. An approach. *Archives of General Psychiatry* 43(7):701–705.

Heeg, B. M. S., J. Damen, E. Buskens, S. Caleo, F. De Charro, and B. A. Van Hout. 2008. Modelling approaches: The case of schizophrenia. *PharmacoEconomics* 26(8):633–648.

James, G. M., C. A. Sugar, R. Desai, and R. A. Rosenheck. 2006. A comparison of outcomes among patients with schizophrenia in two mental health systems: A health state approach. *Schizophrenia Research* 86(1):309–320.

Jensen, P. A. and J. F. Bard. 2003. *Operations Research: Models and Methods*. Hoboken, NJ [Great Britain]: Wiley.

Korte, A. O. 1990. A first order Markov model for use in the human services. *Computers in Human Services* 6(4):299–312.

Leff, H. S. 1981. Apartments or houses in community support systems: A computer modeling approach. In *American Psychological Association Convention*. Los Angeles, CA.

Leff, H. S., M. Dada, and S. Graves. 1986. An LP planning model for a mental health community support system. *Management Science* 32(2(Feb)):139–155.

Leff, H. S., S. Graves, J. Natkins, and J. Bryan. 1985. A system for allocating mental health resources. *Administration in Mental Health* 13(1(Fall)):43–68.

Leff, H. S., M. Lieberman, V. Mulkern, and B. Raab. 1996. Outcome trends for severely mentally ill persons in capitated and case managed mental health programs. *Administration and Policy in Mental Health* 24(1):3–11.

Leff, H. S., J. C. McPartland, S. Banks, B. Dembling, W. Fisher, and I. E. Allen. 2004. Service quality as measured by service fit and mortality among public mental health system service recipients. *Mental Health Services Research* 6(2):93–107.

Levin, G. 1977. Point of view: Poor quality is the solution, not the problem. *Health Care Management Review* 2(3):69–72.

Levin, G. and E. B. Roberts. 1976. *The Dynamics of Human Service Delivery*. Cambridge, MA: Ballinger Pub. Co.

Lippmann, W. 2004. *Public Opinion*. Mineola, NY: Dover Publications.

Liu, C. Y., T. W. Hu, and J. Jerrell. 1992. A Markov analysis of the service system for severe mental illness. *Biometrical Journal* 34(4):443–457.

MacCracken, M. 2009. Prediction versus projection: Forecast versus possibility. *Weatherzine* edition number 26 [cited June 22, 2009].

Miller, L., T. Brown, D. Pilon, R. Scheffler, and M. Davis. 2009a. Measuring Recovery from Severe Mental Illness: A Pilot Study Estimating the Outcomes Possible from California's 2004 Mental Health Services Act.

Miller, L., T. Brown, D. Pilon, R. Scheffler, and M. Davis. 2009b. Patterns of recovery from severe mental illness: A pilot study of outcomes. *Community Mental Health Journal* 46(2):177–187.

Moos, R. H., A. C. Nichol, and B. S. Moos. 2002. Global assessment of functioning ratings and the allocation and outcomes of mental health services. *Psychiatric Services* 53(6):730–737.

Norton, E. C., J. Yoon, M. E. Domino, and J. P. Morrissey. 2006. Transitions between the public mental health system and jail for persons with severe mental illness: A Markov analysis. *Health Economics* 15(7):719–733.

Nutt, P. A. 1984. *Planning Methods for Health and Related Organizations*. New York: John Wiley & Sons.

Olfson, M., R. Mojtabai, N. A. Sampson, I. Hwang, B. Druss, P. S. Wang, K. B. Wells, H. A. Pincus, and R. C. Kessler. 2009. Dropout from outpatient mental health care in the United States. *Psychiatric Services* 60(7):898–907.

Patten, S. 2005. Markov models of major depression for linking psychiatric epidemiology to clinical practice. *Clinical Practice and Epidemiology in Mental Health* 1(1):2.

Perry, J. C., P. W. Lavori, and L. Hoke. 1987. A Markov model for predicting levels of psychiatric service use in borderline and antisocial personality disorders and bipolar type II affective disorder. *Journal of Psychiatric Research* 21(3):215–232.

Pierskalla, W. P. 1981. *Operations Research and the Mental Health Service System*. Washington, DC: National Institute of Mental Health.

Reuter, J. and D. H. Gustafson. 1981. Need, demand, and utilization models for the mental health system. In *Operations Research and the Mental Health Service System, Volume 1: Report of Ad Hoc Advisory Group*, edited by L. G. Kessler. Washington, DC: Superintendent of Documents, U.S. Government Printing Office.

Rochefort, D. A. 1997. *From Poorhouses to Homelessness: Policy Analysis and Mental Health Care*, 2nd edn. Westport, CT: Auburn House.

Sacolick, J. 1980. The role of operations research in systems analysis. *Interfaces* 10(5):49–54.

Sainfort, F., M. L. Brandeau, and W. P. Pierskalla. 2004. *Operations Research and Health Care: A Handbook of Methods and Applications, International Series in Operations Research & Management Science 70*. Boston, MA: Kluwer Academic.

Shumway, M., T. L. Chouljian, and W. A. Hargreaves. 1994. Patterns of substance use in schizophrenia: A Markov modeling approach. *Journal of Psychiatric Research* 28(3):277–287.

Sonnenberg, F. A. and J. R. Beck. 1993. Markov models in medical decision making: A practical guide. *Medical Decision Making* 13(4):322–338.

Sunstein, C. R. 2006. *Infotopia: How Many Minds Produce Knowledge*. New York: Oxford University Press.

Sweillam, A. and K. Tardiff. 1978. Prediction of psychiatric inpatient utilization: A Markov chain model. *Administration in Mental Health* 6(2):161–173.

The Evaluation Center@HSRI. 2004. *Level of Care Instruments*. Cambridge, MA: The Evaluation Center@ HSRI.

Weissman, M. M. 1975. The assessment of social adjustment: A review of techniques. *Archives of General Psychiatry* 32(3):357–365.

43

Correlation with Social and Medical Factors

Kathleen Abrahamson
Western Kentucky University

Karis Pressler
Purdue University

Melissa Grabner-Hagen
Indiana University

Introduction 43-1
Defining Psychosocial Distress 43-1
Psychosocial Distress and Disease Outcomes 43-2
Influence of Psychosocial Distress on Caregiving and Healthcare Delivery 43-3
Risk Factors for Illness-Related Psychosocial Distress 43-4
Assessment of Distress 43-5
Interventions to Manage Distress 43-6
Spirituality and Psychosocial Distress • Race and Psychosocial Distress
Geography 43-9
Barriers to the Management of Distress 43-9
Issues in Researching Psychosocial Distress 43-10
Conclusion 43-11
References 43-11

Introduction

Few would dispute that physical illness is an unpleasant experience. Not only does a person face the possibility of physical discomfort and disability, the uncertainty and lifestyle disruption that surrounds illness has a potentially negative influence on patient quality of life. The totality of this negative influence is referred to as illness-related psychosocial distress. Psychosocial distress is common among individuals facing illness (Cohen and Rodriguez 1995, Sobel 1995, Schrader et al. 2004, Astin et al. 2003, Cukor et al. 2007, Hodges et al. 2009). It is estimated that among individuals seeking medical attention, one-third of bodily symptoms are artifacts of this distress (Sobel 1995). This chapter provides an overview of illness-related psychosocial distress, including the effects of distress on disease outcomes, the influence of health status and social resources on levels of psychosocial distress, and the effectiveness of psychosocial intervention. Specific issues related to research pertaining to psychosocial distress and healthcare conclude this chapter.

Defining Psychosocial Distress

Definitions of psychosocial distress vary within the literature. Broadly defined, psychosocial distress is a multidimensional concept, representing a negative emotional, psychological, social, spiritual, economic, and/or practical influence on an individual's quality of life (Bean and Wagner 2006, National Comprehensive Care Network 2008). Within the medical literature, psychosocial distress is defined through a variety of methods, most commonly utilizing a combination of established scales addressing psychological status (depression, anxiety), social resources/support, and patient perceived quality of life (Kojima et al. 2009).

There is debate among social scientists as to whether psychosocial distress is conceptually distinct from psychological disorders, or if distress and mental disorder exist on a continuum with distress being a milder form of psychological disorder. By assessing the relationships between distress, disorder, and mental health, Payton (2009) concludes it is inappropriate to view distress and disorder as varying degrees of a single concept. Though the definition and measurement of psychosocial distress is similar to that of disorders such as depression and general anxiety disorder, psychosocial distress appears to be an experience separate from that of having a diagnosed mental disorder (Payton 2009). The importance of this differentiation is noted by Schleifer et al. (1989), who highlight the need to separate those patients experiencing situational distress from patients with clinical depression.

Psychosocial Distress and Disease Outcomes

Given the difficulties presented by illness, a certain amount of distress is normal. However, extreme mood alterations, excessive worry, decreased social function, and a decline in quality of life that is persistent or disruptive to the healing process must be addressed by healthcare delivery systems if positive outcomes are to be maintained (Vachon 2006). The consequences of unresolved psychosocial distress on patient outcomes are well documented, but the mechanism of influence remains largely unclear.

Distress influences disease outcomes through a combination of behavioral, cognitive, and physiological pathways (Cohen and Rodriguez 1995, Kojima et al. 2009). Some research suggests a pathway from physical illness to distress that is mediated by a biological stress response, a process highly dependent on individual perception of illness effects and, therefore, highly variable (Everson-Rose and Lewis 2005, Cukor et al. 2007). Symptoms of distress may stem from the physiological effects of disease on neurological function, which at times results in "sickness syndrome," a biological tendency toward anxious or depressive states. The effects of distress on health are complex, as distress affects health/lifestyle behaviors and treatment compliance, which in turn creates additional physical consequences. Biological pathways to distress are strongly influenced by an individual's social environment, economic opportunity, and access to healthcare, further complicating our understanding of the mechanism from psychosocial distress to disease outcomes (Vachon 2006). An example of multiple influences on disease outcomes is seen in a study of female osteoarthritis patients whose levels of disability and pain were correlated with depression and anxiety more so than the degree of damage and osteoarthritis observed in the knee (Salaffi et al. 1991).

Researchers have demonstrated a relationship between psychosocial distress, diagnosis of disease, and disease outcomes for a number of varying disease states. Among diabetic patients, psychosocial distress negatively influences patient compliance, quality of life, and glycemic control. Having a diagnosis of diabetes doubles the odds of depressive symptoms (Anderson et al. 2001). There is literature linking distress to poor physical outcomes, including mortality, among patients diagnosed with congestive heart failure and other cardiovascular disease (CVD) (Schleifer et al. 1989, Moser and Dracup 2004, Everson-Rose and Lewis 2005, Chung et al. 2009). Up to one-third of patients suffer from emotional distress post-myocardial infarction (MI) (Broadbent et al. 2009, Saab et al. 2009). The influence of depression and negative mood state on post-MI mortality is strong. Frasure-Smith and Lespérance (2003) determined that depression is independently predictive of mortality in post-MI patients, even when accounting for overall health and cardiac history. The dimension of hopelessness appears to have a particularly detrimental effect on outcomes among patients with CVD (Everson-Rose and Lewis 2005). In addition, depression and anxiety are common post-stroke, and rehab potential is limited when levels of distress are high (Sagen et al. 2009).

Approximately, 40% of cancer patients suffer from diagnosable levels of psychosocial distress (Carlson and Bultz 2003). Self-reported poor quality of life and negative psychosocial status are prognostic for survival in cancer patients, though the mechanism of influence is unclear (Fawnzy et al. 1993, Cameron et al. 2005, Lis et al. 2006, Efficace et al. 2008). In a review of literature addressing breast cancer patients, 80% of identified studies showed a significant relationship between distress, disease reoccurrence, and survival (Falagas et al. 2007).

End-stage disease presents a unique psychosocial challenge. Patients with advanced and worsening cancer have demonstrated high levels of psychosocial distress (Botti et al. 2006, Simon et al. 2007). Cukor et al. (2007) found that psychosocial distress influences outcomes, including mortality in patients with end-stage kidney disease. Though a poor prognosis is generally associated with high levels of psychosocial distress (Clark 2001, Vachon 2006), Cameron et al. (2005) found stronger feelings of personal control in women with cancer and a poor prognosis, perhaps as a means of emotional defense or acceptance of the final disease stage. Illness that requires a patient to face the potential of death allows for both the possibility of existential crisis, which increases distress levels, and self-transcendence, a spiritual maturity, which allows a patient to look beyond personal boundaries for meaning and actually increases quality of life in patients facing terminal illness (Bean and Wagner 2006). Thus, providing support to a patient dealing with potentially life-threatening illnesses can have an important effect on the patient's experience. Unfortunately, healthcare professionals have noted that times of worsening prognosis are among the most difficult for them to provide psychosocial support (Botti et al. 2006).

Chronic illnesses, such as arthritis and chronic pain syndrome, have high potential to both be a cause of distress as well as have outcomes that are negatively affected by imbalances in patient mood, treatment noncompliance, and decreased social function (Astin et al. 2003, Kojima et al. 2009). Chronic illness is by nature ongoing and incurable, a difficult situation for both patients and caregivers. It is crucial that psychosocial distress be properly managed in patients facing chronic illness so that social functioning is not limited, negatively influencing patient quality of life for the lifelong duration of the chronic condition (D'Antono et al. 2009).

Diseases for which there is no clear causation or which have unexplained mechanisms of action may be especially stressful to patients. D'Antono et al. (2009) found that depression is common in patients with recurrent, unexplained syncope, most likely because of the uncertainty surrounding causation, treatment, and disease course. Patient attribution of disease causality has an important influence on the level of psychosocial distress for those suffering from illnesses of ambiguous etiology. Patients diagnosed with irritable bowel syndrome (IBS) who attribute the cause of their symptoms to stress/distress are more likely to experience high levels of illness-related distress, causing perhaps a vicious cycle between IBS exacerbations and symptoms of psychosocial distress (Riedl et al. 2009).

Influence of Psychosocial Distress on Caregiving and Healthcare Delivery

Family members play an important role in healthcare delivery, providing a considerable amount of informal caregiving services (Pyke and Bengtson 1996). Illness-related psychosocial distress negatively influences family member quality of life. Family members are at risk of psychosocial distress both from interaction with a loved one who may be experiencing distress and because of their own transition into the demanding role of caregiver (Broadbent et al. 2009). Wartella et al. (2009) finds families of critically ill patients have the highest distress immediately after diagnosis. However, for conditions that require long-term caregiving and community integration, family member distress may be ongoing and even increase over time (Wartella et al. 2009). Family members who provide long-term care for persons with chronic conditions tend to have poorer health and lower reported life satisfaction than non-caregivers (Hoyert and Seltzer 1992, Pavalko and Woodbury 2000). As the majority of intervention and attention is directed at the patient, the distress experienced by family members often goes unnoticed. Family members play an important role in the patient recovery process, and interventions aimed at improving spousal quality of life may improve quality of life for the patient as well (Moser and Dracup 2004). Therefore, it is important for family to be included in the design of interventions to reduce the distressful aspects of the illness experience (Chung et al. 2009).

In circumstances where treatment is difficult, disruptive, or has uncertain outcomes, psychosocial distress can have a strong influence on patient compliance and decision making (Clark 2001, Sloan et al.

2007). Issues of access, such as economic disadvantage, transportation, or childcare needs, can influence both level of psychosocial distress and disease outcomes (Kogan et al. 2009). Kroenke et al. (2006) found women with breast cancer who lacked close friends, relatives, or living children had significantly greater mortality, which the authors attribute to a lack of instrumental caregiving and access to care. Patients with physical disabilities may experience distress not only as a result of barriers within the environment but also barriers within the medical system (Neri and Kroll 2003, Scheer et al. 2003). In Scheer et al.'s (2003) qualitative study, a female respondent with Cerebral Palsy mentioned how mammogram machines and exam tables are too high for wheelchair-bound individuals. In another example, a man with multiple sclerosis (MS) who injured his knee when he slipped while using his walker could not get a doctor's recommendation for physical therapy because the doctor mistook his knee injury as a symptom of MS and claimed that insurance would not cover therapy related to the disease (Scheer et al. 2003). Respondents relayed that barriers to healthcare placed strain on social relationships, thus prompting depression, devaluation, and unnecessary stress (Neri and Kroll 2003).

Unresolved patient distress is challenging for professional caregivers as well as patients. Patients who are distressed may overutilize emergency medical services, fail to adhere to the prescribed treatment regimen, or displace illness-related anxiety on to healthcare providers (Clark 2001). Patient education is difficult when patients and family members are overwhelmed (Sharma et al. 2007). Nurses have expressed a need to maintain a protective distance from patients in order to protect their own emotional well-being, a situation that further contributes to the under-management of psychosocial distress (Botti et al. 2006).

Risk Factors for Illness-Related Psychosocial Distress

Low socioeconomic status (SES) is a well-established risk factor for a variety of health conditions and appears to increase the risk of significant psychosocial distress as well (Anderson and Armstead 1995, Simon et al. 2008). SES is generally defined as a mix of education, occupation, and income. SES influences distress both through increasing the prevalence of stressors, such as inadequate housing, poor access to care, economic difficulties, and difficult work environments, and decreasing the resources available to cope with such stressors (Anderson and Armstead 1995, Everson-Rose and Lewis 2005, Kogan et al. 2009). Low education and economic stress have been shown to have an effect on the level of glycemic control among rural African-American elders with diabetes, both directly and indirectly through the influence of depression (Kogan et al. 2009). Levels of psychosocial distress have been found to be influenced by gender (higher distress levels in women), age (higher distress among the young and the very old), marital status (higher distress among unmarried), low income, low education, hospitalization, poor prognosis, low social support, and history of emotional or functional difficulties (Mirowsky and Ross 1986, Clark 2001, Vachon 2006, Simon et al. 2008). However, in their study examining the predictive power of psychological distress to understand mortality disparities, Fiscella and Franks (1997) found that even though distress levels were higher among African-Americans and those earning lower incomes, distress does little to explain the mortality disparities observed between racial and SES groups. These findings beg the question, what mechanisms work to link SES to levels of distress?

In an examination of predictors of depression after cardiac illness, Schrader et al. (2004) found that scommon demographic variables such as gender, income, household size, level of education, and occupation are not as predictive of illness-related depression as history of depression, depression at admission, and history of previous bouts of cardiac illness. This is consistent with the previous work of Schleifer et al. (1989) who found that severity of cardiac disease has less influence on psychosocial distress than previous history of distress and other lifestyle factors. There is a vicious cycle effect for some aspects of distress-related outcomes. For example, the failure to return to work post-illness and resulting economic disability contributes to patient distress (Broadbent et al. 2009). However, psychosocial distress contributes to an inability to return to work (Schleifer et al. 1989). Cause and effect in the relationship between illness and distress are at times unclear. Gupta et al. (2007) found that depression at baseline was predictive of a future diagnosis of chronic widespread pain, confirming that psychosocial distress may cause as well as be affected by physical illness.

The negative connotations of some diagnoses, for example, cancer, can evoke fear and anxiety. Patients may experience anticipatory distress prior to the initiation of treatment (Arantzamedi et al. 2006). It is important that the distress be evaluated continually as psychosocial needs change over the course of disease and treatment. Distress may actually be highest at the end or discontinuation of treatment when the patient has a sudden decrease in contact with healthcare professionals (Botti et al. 2006).

Assessment of Distress

A broad spectrum of measures reflects the breadth and depth of research that examines psychosocial distress. In quantitative research, single distress measures can utilize simple and direct questions such as that found in the study by Ellis et al. (2009). In this study, the authors examined distress experienced by spouses of MI patients by asking spouses to rate on a five-item scale the level of distress they felt as a result of their spouse's symptoms. Similarly, in a study measuring patient perceptions of distress management by primary care physicians, the authors quantified patient distress by asking respondents to rate the effect that emotional distress has on everyday function (Brody et al. 1997). On the other end of the spectrum, other measures have used items housed within questionnaires and scales to measure distress. These include the General Health Questionnaire (Goldberg 1972, Frasure-Smith et al. 1997); the General Well-Being (GWB) Schedule (Fiscella and Franks 1997); the Hospital Anxiety and Depression Scale (HADS) (Zigmond and Snaith 1983, Holland and Reznick 2005); the distress thermometer (Holland and Reznick 2005), the Medical Outcomes Health Study health distress scale (Lorig et al. 2001). The tendency for researchers to use a variety of measures to assess distress instead of moving toward a single, valid, and reliable distress measure is a shortcoming of the evaluations of psychosocial distress interventions among cancer patients (Manne and Andrykowski 2006).

Researchers frequently utilize a combination of established depression, anxiety, and quality of life scales for measurement, yet these scales are often impractical for busy nurses and physicians, having not been designed specifically for clinical use (Everson-Rose and Lewis 2005, Gupta et al. 2007, Hodges et al. 2009). Because of limitations on staff time, there is a need for effective and usable short-form assessment tools to measure patient distress (D'Antono et al. 2009, Sagen et al. 2009). In cancer care, a short-form assessment tool known as a distress thermometer with problem list has been shown to be both effective and manageable for busy clinicians (NCCN 2008). When using the distress thermometer, patients are asked to subjectively rate their level of distress. It is followed by a form listing objective problems such as housing, finances, and relationships, and patients are asked to indicate if they are currently experiencing problems in any of these areas (Jacobsen 2007, Sloan et al. 2007).

Psychosocial distress is a complex concept and one that healthcare providers admit is not routinely assessed among patients, perhaps because patients do not always convey psychological need in the clinical setting (Arantzamendi and Kearney 2004). Because of this complexity and medical providers realization of patients psychosocial needs, measures such as the distress thermometer that include both objective and subjective segments may be needed to fully capture the patient experience (Arantzamendi and Kearney 2004, Honea et al. 2008). In the current healthcare delivery system, the assessment of psychosocial distress is often left to the informal, subjective view of the busy clinician. Though clinical practice guidelines recommend the use of a systematic tool to allow for uniform assessment and the ability to document improvement or decline, this is frequently not common practice (Arantzamendi and Kearney 2004, NCCN 2008). For example, Pirl et al. (2007) found only 3% of surveyed oncologists used a systematic distress assessment tool in their practice. Tools that rely upon patient self ratings of distress, an evaluation method consistent with the person-centered care focus called for by the Institute of Medicine (2001), have been found to be valid in clinical practice and may provide insight to the patient condition not attainable through traditional provider-directed instruments (Efficace et al. 2008). For example, self-report measures of distress indicate higher levels of depressive symptoms than provider-report measures in studies of diabetic patients (Anderson et al. 2001). Patient self-report measures need to be clearly interpretable to clinicians for the information to be useful. For example, asking a patient to rate distress on a scale from 1 to 10 can present a challenge for clinicians. The clinician must interpret the qualitative difference between distress rated at a 2 and distress rated at a 4 and then act accordingly (Sloan et al. 2007).

One study finds that distress is so common among patients presenting with syncope that authors recommend assessing all patients presenting with syncope for psychosocial distress (D'Antono et al. 2009). Kogen et al. (2009), noting the particular toxicity of depression in combination with diabetes, also recommends assessing and treating all patients for distress symptoms. Schrader et al. (2004) notes that predictors of distress in patients with cardiac illness are included in most routine admission assessments. It may be that the information needed to assess for psychosocial distress is already being collected but the identification of these aspects by clinicians as risk factors for distress may be the missing component.

Interventions to Manage Distress

Interventions implemented to alleviate psychosocial distress are multifarious and use a host of settings, measures, and study designs to determine intervention effectiveness. In their meta-analysis of experiments testing the effectiveness of psychosocial interventions for cancer patients, Meyer and Mark (1995) identified five intervention types including cognitive-behavioral, informational and educational, nonbehavioral counseling/psychotherapy, social support, and unusual treatments. While there is no consensus on common intervention types among evaluations focused on interventions aiming to alleviate distress, it appears that intervention types are closely related to those outlined by Meyer and Mark (1995). It is important to realize that, while experiments testing distress intervention effectiveness are usually patient-centered, the experiments test a variety of programs that occur in an array of settings ranging from individual to group therapy settings. These interventions also extend beyond the patient-centered focus to include the effectiveness of interventions on spouses (Broadbent et al. 2009). Distress research also considers healthcare provider's perceptions of patient distress (Arantzamendi and Kearney 2004).

The most common psychosocial interventions that aim to minimize distress among patients facing chronic conditions, such as cancer, include support group therapy, patient education, and coping skills (Telch and Telch 1985, Rustaøen and Hanestad 1998). Participants for interventions are usually recruited from clinics and hospitals (Frasure-Smith et al. 1997, Hosaka et al. 2000, Shaw et al. 2007, Ellis et al. 2009). Occasionally, patients are recruited through public service announcements and community groups (Lorig et al. 2001, Yanek et al. 2001).

Research testing the effectiveness of psychosocial interventions occurs mostly among cancer patients (e.g., Classen et al. 2001, Coyne et al. 2006). Other studies have focused on patient populations experiencing MI, heart disease, HIV/AIDS, lung disease, stroke, and arthritis (Frasure-Smith et al. 1997, Lorig et al. 2001, Prado et al. 2004). Rarely do studies examine the effect of an intervention on psychosocial distress among relatively healthy community-based samples (a noted exception is a faith-based intervention that occurred in inner-city churches by Yanek et al. 2001. See below). It has been argued that, as long as the patients are not near death, a psychosocial intervention that has positive effects among one group of patients suffering a specific condition should translate to another patient group and garner similar effects (Coyne et al. 2006). Patients in the palliative care context may benefit more from interventions that focus on spirituality and on minimizing distress and fear related to death and dying (Breitbart et al. 2004, Miller et al. 2005). Almost inherent in research measuring distress levels prior to and following an intervention are measures of self-efficacy as an additional means to test an intervention's effect.

There is limited evidence that interventions addressing psychosocial distress save money. Lorig et al. (2001) randomized patients with a host of chronic conditions including but not limited to heart disease and lung disease into a 7-week Chronic Disease Self-Management Program (CDSMP). Patients were followed for 2 years and at the study's conclusion, they experienced a decrease in distress and an increase in self-efficacy. Patients also experienced fewer ER and physician visits, thereby decreasing healthcare costs. However, these results must be interpreted with caution because the study did not have a control group. In a follow-up study, Lorig et al. (2003) found that even with a control group in place, 4 months following the intervention, treatment group participants had greater self-efficacy and lower healthcare utilization compared to control group participants.

Manne and Andrykowski (2006) note the freedoms researchers have used to cast and recast research findings, which may be inherently negative, in a more positive light. This "best foot forward approach" has been criticized as "endemic in randomized controlled trails (RCTs) for psychosocial interventions in cancer care," suggesting that the positive findings associated with intervention research may be an artifact of having to present positive outcomes in order to be published (Coyne et al. 2006). Psychosocial intervention research is further complicated by the difficulty associated with studying terminal populations, such as cancer patients who may die or be too ill to participate in endpoint measures and the fact that those who choose to participate in interventions may not be as distressed as those who chose not to participate (Classen et al. 2001, Coyne et al. 2006). Taken together, the findings associated with psychosocial intervention trials must be read, analyzed, and applied with caution. However, despite the difficulties associated with these interventions and research to test their effectiveness, it appears that factors outside an intervention's control such as doctor–patient communication, spirituality, social support, and geography play important roles in determining whether psychosocial interventions can assuage distress when individuals are faced with chronic, disabling, and potentially terminal conditions.

Healthcare practitioners have great clout in affecting patients' levels of psychosocial distress. A study of oncology patients found that the patients' opinion of physicians' attentiveness and empathy during their initial consultation were related to lower levels of patient distress following the consultation even after controlling for baseline distress (Zachariae et al. 2003). Likewise, in a review of published and unpublished research focused on patient–physician relations, Stewart (1995) linked good communication between physicians and their patients with better emotional health among patients. Despite the rising realization that psychological distress occurs in patients experiencing adverse health conditions, patients want to have open and honest communication with their doctors about distress (Meryn 1998), no psychological assessment tool has been identified as a standard measure that can be used by healthcare professionals to quantify patients' distress (MacMahon and Lip 2002). One area and tool that may allow healthcare providers to examine patient distress and provide a more holistic approach to medicine is through a discussion of spirituality (Anandarajah and Hight 2001).

Spirituality and Psychosocial Distress

Spirituality is described as "multidimensional" by Anandariajah and Hight (2001). While it is difficult to define spirituality, concepts such as hope, prayer, and self-transcendence along with religion and religious practice are used as measures of spirituality in research that also analyzes psychosocial distress (Rustaøen and Hanestad 1998, Rustaøen et al. 1998, Yanek et al. 2001, Robinson-Smith 2002, Coward 2003). Studies sometimes distinguish between vertical and horizontal spirituality with vertical spirituality relating to the respondent's feelings toward God, and horizontal spirituality relating to well-being with respect to the individual's purpose and meaning in life (Hill and Hood 1999, Miller et al. 2005). It has been suggested that interventions with a spiritual focus may help with coping for those experiencing chronic and life-threatening conditions. Studies focused on helping those with these conditions grapple with spiritual matters sometimes take place in faith-based settings (Yanek et al. 2001), cancer centers (Coward 2003, Kristeller et al. 1999), outpatient clinics (Miller et al. 2005), hospitals (Rustaøen et al. 1998), and palliative care centers (McClain et al. 2003).

In their study of HIV-positive African-American mothers, Prado et al. (2004) found that while there was no direct significant relationship between religious involvement and distress, distress was indirectly mediated by religion that lessens avoidant coping and boosts social support that then decreases distress. This supports research that has found religious participation and religious expression to increase social interaction, buffer against stress, and lessen psychosocial distress (Williams et al. 1982, Shaw et al 2007). Religious belief and spirituality have also been shown to help patients come to terms with death and other end-of-life issues. Among those enrolled in a computer support group for breast cancer patients, participants who demonstrated higher levels of religious expression had less fear about what happens after death and the possibility of an afterlife while also showing higher levels of health self-efficacy and better functional status (Shaw et al. 2007).

The concept of spirituality and its relationship to distress during end-of-life care is a growing topic of interest and one that is becoming a priority in end-of-life care (MacMahon and Lip 2002, Breibart et al. 2004). Research has noted the link between spirituality and death distress. Among a sample of patients experiencing potentially life-threatening conditions including but not limited to HIV/AIDS, cancer, kidney disease, and frailty, death distress was more frequent among those who were living alone, and those who experienced multiple life-threatening diseases, depression symptoms, low levels of patient–physician communication, and among those who expressed less spiritual well-being (Chibnall et al. 2002). Similarly, among palliative care patients in another study, spiritual well-being was significantly and negatively related to end-of-life despair, hopelessness, desire for hastened death, and suicidal ideation (McClain et al. 2003). The authors suggest that measures of spirituality may be more effective in predicting these latter three measures in palliative care patients, more so than measures of depression. In light of these findings, McClain et al. (2003) point to the importance of interventions that could help boost spirituality in terminal patients, but note the lack of intervention research that could support or refute the claim that spirituality may buffer against adverse feelings of despair and hopelessness in those nearing death. However, the research that tests the effect of interventions with a spiritual component are few and far between (Miller et al. 2005), perhaps because religious participation, praying, and other actions associated with spirituality are personal and voluntary.

Race and Psychosocial Distress

To our knowledge, no study to date has identified which psychosocial interventions are optimal for patients of different racial backgrounds. Previous population-based research suggests distress across the life course is experienced differently by persons of varying racial/ethnic backgrounds. In their analysis of teens between 1995 and 2001 using the National Longitudinal Study of Adolescent Health (Add Health), Brown et al. (2007) examined baseline depressive symptoms and found that among females, Hispanics had the highest levels of baseline depression followed by African-Americans and Whites. Male adolescents demonstrated a similar tendency with depressive symptoms being highest among Hispanics. Six years later, depressive symptoms converged; however, Whites continued to experience lower levels of depression compared to minority young adults. Research suggests that depression in adolescent and young adulthood is predictive of future mental health disorders (Weissman et al. 1999).

While studies highlighting distress interventions do not directly discuss health disparities with regard to race and distress, an issue related to race was raised in one intervention. In their study of LTI-SAGE intervention, Miller et al. (2005) noted that minorities felt their needs were not being met if they were placed in predominantly Caucasian support groups. Literature supports the notion that racial concordance is important in the healthcare setting with patients having higher levels of patient participation if the race between the patient and physician is concordant (Cooper-Patrick et al. 1999). Compared to White patients, patient participation was markedly lower among African-American patients who were paired with a non-African-American physician during a routine visit (Cooper-Patrick et al. 1999).

Studies that have directly considered race generally focus on a specific racial group for their intervention. For instance, Yanek et al. (2001) examined the effect of a spiritual intervention on health and distress outcomes among African-American women, Prado et al. (2004) considered religious involvement and distress among HIV-positive African-American females, while Lorig et al. (2003) focused the effect of a peer-led self-management program among Hispanics. All of these programs suggest that the intervention had a positive effect on its participants, but it is impossible to conclude whether these programs are optimal for the racial/ethnic group they studied without including a variety of people from different racial backgrounds in the study (Gonzalez et al. 2009).

It is worth noting that racial differences in distress intervention research may be scant because of the small sample sizes generally used in these interventions. In addition to small sample sizes, attrition due to death may mask effects that could be due to race unless mortality selection within the study population is controlled.

Geography

Intervention studies rarely identify whether their programs occurred in a rural or urban setting, but some have described their setting as urban or in an area surrounding an urban center (Frasure-Smith et al. 1997, Yanek et al. 2001). Psychosocial intervention research is usually localized and focuses on a patient population within a particular hospital. There is no research to our knowledge that determines whether interventions that work in an urban area could be equally effective in a rural area.

Population studies suggest that psychological distress is different across neighborhoods, rural verses urban areas, and even across states. Between 1996–2001 and 2003–2006, distress levels were especially concentrated in the southern and Midwestern corridors of the United States, and increases in distress between 1993 and 2006 were observed in many states including West Virginia, Mississippi, and Oklahoma (Moriarty et al. 2009). Distress levels are shown to be different in rural versus urban areas, partly due to the different types of stressors encountered in the areas. For instance, farmers in a rural area experience stressors related to their occupation that are rarely encountered by those in an urban area. Iowa residents were surveyed in 1991 and again in 1992 to assess changes in depression and attitudes toward mental healthcare (Hoyt et al. 1997). Results reveal that men living in rural villages and small towns had greater increase in depressive symptoms compared to those living on farms or more densely populated areas, while size of place had no effect on women's depressive symptoms. However, size of place was linked to attitudes of mental healthcare with rural residents holding more negative attitudes toward mental healthcare and being less likely to seek mental healthcare than urban residents (Hoyt et al. 1997). On a more microscale, neighborhood disorder, which is measured by greater socioeconomic disadvantage, incidences of victimization, and alienation, is linked to psychological distress that then negatively influences health (Hill et al. 2005). Clearly, geography and the size of one's community can influence distress levels regardless of a chronic or terminal condition.

Barriers to the Management of Distress

A primary barrier to the management of psychosocial distress is under-identification of patient needs (D'Antono et al. 2009). As was discussed in the previous section, organizational processes frequently fail to allow the time or resources for psychosocial assessment (Jacobsen 2007). Lack of proper assessment is complicated by the difficulty in differentiating the signs and symptoms of psychosocial distress from manifestations of illness or side-effects of treatment. Fatigue, lack of concentration, poor appetite, and sleep disturbance are examples of symptoms that could be caused by either disease states or distress (Ryan et al. 2005). There is evidence that underlying anxiety is especially under-recognized (Schleifer et al. 1989).

Physicians receive little training regarding the management of psychosocial distress (D'Antono et al. 2009). Patients often perceive the M.D. to be either too busy to discuss emotional issues or disinterested in discussion that moves beyond the physical manifestations of illness. The literature shows that physicians share this discomfort surrounding distress management (Ryan et al. 2005). A stigma still exists regarding mental health services. Patients may fear becoming labeled as "crazy" if they ask for help with psychosocial issues, adding to the discomfort surrounding communicating psychosocial needs (Madden 2006). Interestingly, the term "distress" has been viewed as an accurate and less stigmatizing term to capture what is referred to as "an unpleasant emotional experience" that includes a range of emotions and feelings including but not limited to anxiety and depression (NCCN 2008).

Lack of reimbursement for social services presents a significant barrier to service provision (Clark 2001). There is little economic incentive for facilities to bear the cost-burden of resource-intensive psychosocial services (Astin et al. 2003). Reimbursement is especially poor for survivor or posttreatment services, which can result in long-term distress for the patient that goes unmanaged (Holland and Resnick 2005). Distress management often falls to clinic staff and direct care nurses who provide informal emotional support and active listening, but often lack the time, training, and information to adequately meet patient needs (Arantzamedi and Kearney 2004, Botti et al. 2006).

Additionally, the management of psychosocial distress is complicated by the heterogeneous histories and needs of patients (Berkman 2009). Interventions need to address the complexity of the patient population; differing disease states, stages of illness, and life situations require different interventional techniques (Vachon 2006). An intervention may be effective for only one subset of a population. For example, a peer-support group may be an effective intervention environment for cancer patients who are parents of young children, but completely ineffective for patients of advanced age. Interventions should be targeted to the patient populations that will be served most effectively by the intervention, which is a challenge given the resource limitations of most healthcare delivery environments (Wengstrom et al. 2001).

Time and workload are significant barriers to the ability of healthcare professionals to address the psychosocial needs of patients (Astin et al. 2003, Madden 2006, Fulcher and Gosselin-Acomb 2007, D'Antono et al. 2009). The complicated nature of many assessment tools makes them unrealistic for use in busy clinical settings where patients may present with significant physical needs as well (Sagan et al. 2009). As more and more care is delivered in busy outpatient settings and hospital stays become shorter, issues of time will become even more pressing (Clark 2001).

Issues in Researching Psychosocial Distress

The literature addressing illness-related distress contains a variety of operational definitions of key concepts, measurement tools, sampling strategies, and intervention techniques, making it difficult to draw conclusions (Iacovino and Reesor 1997, Lepore and Coyne 2006, Falagas et al. 2007, Berkman 2009). Psychosocial distress is complex and difficult to capture quantitatively. Perhaps, it is due to complexity and methodological difficulties in the study of psychosocial distress that there remains skepticism regarding the influence of distress on outcomes (Falagas et al. 2007).

There is little research addressing the effectiveness of psychosocial intervention (Vachon 2006). Primarily because of methodological difficulties such as the use of small, convenience samples, poorly differentiated samples, and nonrandomized designs, there is little evidence that psychosocial interventions are effective enough to justify their costs (Coyne et al. 2006, Lepore and Coyne 2006). It is challenging to clearly differentiate between the influences of the multiple dimensions of the distress concept; emotional aspects tend to become highly confounded with practical concerns such as employment, transportation, and access to care (Meyer and Mark 1995, Ross et al. 2002, Vachon 2006). There are few RCTs dealing with the outcomes of psychosocial distress. However, RCTs may not be the appropriate research method given the complexity of distress (Everson-Rose and Lewis 2005).

Despite the research challenges mentioned above, there exists evidence that psychosocial interventions are helping at least some patients. It is assumed that many patients are being helped but, given the difficulties inherent in research addressing psychosocial distress, the evaluation of interventions is missing the measurement of these positive outcomes due to methodological difficulties (Meyer and Mark 1995, Ross et al. 2002). Additional research is needed that includes low-income populations and ethnic and racial minorities (Everson-Rose and Lewis 2005, Manne and Andrykowski 2006). More research is needed that moves beyond the domains of cardiovascular illness and cancer to address a wider variety of illness experiences. It has been suggested that in the future, recipients of psychosocial care may benefit by being grouped according to underlying attitudes, beliefs, values, and psychosocial needs as opposed to clinical diagnosis (Sobel 1995). Additionally, it would be beneficial for future research to focus upon the implementation of programming or the translation of findings into cost-effective practices (Stanton 2005, Sloan et al. 2007).

Conclusion

Though unresolved distress has a negative influence on physical outcomes as well as patient quality of life, the current healthcare delivery system fails to adequately address psychosocial needs (D'Antono et al. 2009). Distress is under-addressed clinically and often overlooked or under-prioritized in medical education (Astin et al. 2003). Clinical practice guidelines exist for the management of psychosocial distress in cancer patients (NCCN 2008), yet research shows that these guidelines are rarely followed in practice (Fulcher and Gosselin-Acomb 2007).

Intervention effectiveness is difficult to measure (Astin et al. 2003, Manne and Andrykowski 2006). Health outcomes and the effectiveness of medical treatment need to be viewed within the social context, as it is likely that this context is what partially accounts for the currently unmeasured and unexplained variations in disease outcomes (Berkman 2009).

When distress is properly addressed and an intervention is implemented, the results can be positive (D'Antono et al. 2009). Fulcher and Gosselin-Acomb (2007) found overall patient satisfaction increased when cancer care nurses followed the established distress management guidelines. Despite the increase in work time, nurses voluntarily agreed to continue following guidelines in order to receive the benefit of more satisfied patients. Adequate management of psychosocial distress positively influences professional caregivers such as physicians and nurses as well as interacting with less distressed patients makes emotional caregiving, patient teaching, and encouraging compliance less difficult (Clark 2001, Sharma et al. 2007). Perhaps most importantly, quality-of-life issues are a priority to patients (Bean and Wagner 2006), and therefore must be properly addressed if the goal of patient-centered care is to be achieved (Institute of Medicine 2001).

References

Anandarajah, G. and E. Hight. 2001. Spirituality and medical practice: Use the HOPE questions as a practical tool for spiritual assessment. *American Family Physician*, 63(1): 81–88.

Anderson, N.B. and C.A. Armstead. 1995. Toward understanding the association of socioeconomic status and health: A new challenge for the biopsychosocial approach. *Psychosomatic Medicine*, 57: 213–225.

Anderson, R.J., K.E. Freedland, R.E. Clouse, and P.J. Lustman. 2001. The prevalence of comorbid depression in adults with diabetes. *Diabetes Care*, 24(6): 1069–1078.

Arantzamendi, M. and N. Kearney. 2004. The psychological needs of patients receiving chemotherapy: An exploration of nurse perceptions. *European Journal of Cancer Care*, 13: 23–31.

Astin, J.A., S.L. Shapiro, D.M. Eisenber, and K.L. Forys. 2003. Mind-body medicine: State of science, implications for practice. *Journal of the American Board of Family Practice*, 16: 131–147.

Bean, K.B. and K. Wagner. 2006. Self-transcendence, illness distress, and quality of life among liver transplant recipients. *The Journal of Theory Construction and Testing*, 10(2): 47–53.

Berkman, L.F. 2009. Social epidemiology: Social determinants of health in the United States: Are we losing ground? *Annual Review of Public Health*, 30: 27–41.

Botti, M., R. Endacott, R. Watts, J. Cairns, K. Lewis, A. Kenny. 2006. Barriers to providing psychosocial support for patients with cancer. *Cancer Nursing*, 29(4): 309–316.

Breitbart, W., C. Gibson, S.R. Poppito, and A. Berg. 2004. Psychotherapeutic interventions at the end of life: A focus on meaning and spirituality. *Canadian Journal of Psychiatry*, 49(6): 366–372.

Broadbent, E., C.J. Ellis, J. Thomas, G. Gamble, and K.J. Petrie. 2009. Can an illness perception intervention reduce illness anxiety in spouse of myocardial infarction patients? A randomized controlled trial. *Journal of Psychosomatic Research*, 67(1): 11–15.

Brown, J.S., S.O. Meadows, and G.H. Elder. 2007. Race-ethnic inequality and psychological distress: Depressive symptoms from adolescence to young adulthood. *Developmental Psychology*, 43(6): 1295–1311.

Cameron, L.D., R.J. Booth, M. Schlatter, D. Ziginskas, J.E. Harman, and S.R.C. Benson. 2005. Cognitive and affective determinants of decisions to attend a group psychosocial support program for women with breast cancer. *Psychosomatic Medicine*, 67: 584–589.

Carlson, L. and B. Bultz. 2003. Cancer distress screening: Needs, models and methods. *Journal of Psychosomatic Research*, 55: 403–409.

Chibnall, J.T., S.D. Videen, P.N. Duckro, and D.K. Miller. 2002. Psychosocial-spiritual correlates of death distress in patients with life-threatening medical conditions. *Palliative Medicine*, 16(4): 331–338.

Chung, M.L., D.K. Moser, T.A. Lennie, and M.K. Rayens. 2009. The effects of depressive symptoms and anxiety on quality of life in patients with heart failure and their spouses: Testing dyadic dynamics using actor-partner interdependence model. *Journal of Psychosomatic Research*, 67(1): 29–35.

Clark, P.M. 2001. Treating distress: Working toward psychosocial standards for oncology care. In *Proceedings of the 26th Congress of the Oncology Nursing Society*, http://www.medscape.com (accessed June 26, 2008).

Classen, C., L.D. Butler, C. Koopman, E. Miller, S. DiMiceli, J. Giese-Davis, P. Fobair, R.W. Carlson, H.C. Kraemer, and D. Spiegel. 2001. Supportive-expressive group therapy and distress in patients with metastatic breast cancer. *Archives of General Psychiatry*, 58: 494–501.

Cohen, S. and M.S. Rodriguez. 1995. Pathways linking affective disturbances and physical disorders. *Health Psychology*, 14(5): 374–380.

Cooper-Patrick, L., J.J. Gallo, J.J. Gonzales, H.T. Vu, N.R. Powe, C. Nelson, and D.E. Ford. 1999. Race, gender, and partnership in the patient-physician relationship. *Journal of the American Medical Association*, 282(6): 583–589.

Coward, D.D. 2003. Facilitation or self-transcendence in a breast cancer support group: II. *Oncology Nursing Forum*, 30(2): 291–300.

Coyne, J.C., S.J. Lepore, and S.C. Palmer. 2006. Efficacy of psychosocial interventions in cancer care: Evidence is weaker than it first looks. *Annals of Behavioral Medicine*, 32(2): 104–110.

Cukor, D., S.D. Cohen, R.A. Peterson, and P.L. Kimmel. 2007. Psychosocial aspects of chronic disease: ESRD as a paradigmatic illness. *Journal of the American Society of Nephrology*, 18: 3042–3055.

D'Antono, B., G. Dupuis, K. St-Jean, K. Levesque, R. Nadeau, P. Guerra, B. Thibault, and T. Kus. 2009. Prospective evaluation of psychological distress and psychiatric morbidity in recurrent vasovagal and unexplained syncope. *Journal of Psychosomatic Research*, 67(3): 213–222.

Efficace, F., P.F. Innominato, G. Bjarnason, C. Coens, Y. Humblet, S. Tumolo, D. Genet, M. Tampellini, A. Bottomley, C. Garufi, C. Focan, S. Giacchetti, and F. Levi. 2008. Validation of patient's self-reported social functioning as an independent prognostic factor for survival in metastatic colorectal cancer patients: Results of an international study by the Chronotherapy Group of the European Organisation for Research and Treatment of Cancer. *Journal of Clinical Oncology*, 26(12): 2020–2026.

Ellis, J., J. Lin, A. Walsh, C. Lo, F.A. Shepard, M. Moore, M. Li, L. Gagliese, C. Zimmermann, and G. Rodin. 2009. Predictors of referral for specialized psychosocial oncology care in patients with metastatic cancer: The contributions of age, distress, and marital status. *Journal of Clinical Oncology*, 27(5): 699–705.

Everson-Rose, S.A. and T.T. Lewis. 2005. Psychosocial factors and cardiovascular diseases. *Annual Review of Public Health*, 26: 469–500.

Falagas, M.E., E.A. Zarkadoulia, E.N. Ioannidou, G. Peppas, C. Christodoulou, and P.I. Rafailidis. 2007. The effect of psychosocial factors on breast cancer outcome: A systematic review. *Breast Cancer Research*, 9(4): R44.

Fawnzy, F.I., N.W. Fawnzy, C.S. Hyun, R. Elashoff, D. Guthrie, J.L. Fahey, and D.L. Morton. 1993. Effects of an early structured psychiatric intervention, coping, and affective state on recurrence and survival 6 years later. *Archives of General Psychiatry*, 50(9): 681–689.

Fiscella, K. and P. Franks. 1997. Does psychological distress contribute to racial and socioeconomic disparities in mortality? *Social Science and Medicine*, 45(12): 1805–1809.

Frasure-Smith, N. and F. Lesperance. 2003. Depression and other psychological risks following myocardial infarction. *Archives of General Psychiatry*, 60: 627–636.

Frasure-Smith, N., F. Lespérance, R.H. Prince, P. Verrier, R.A. Garber, M. Juneau, C. Wolfson, and M.G. Bourassa. 1997. Randomised trial of home-based psychosocial nursing intervention for patients recovering from myocardial infarction. *The Lancet*, 350(9076): 473–479.

Fulcher, C.D. and T.K. Gosselin-Acomb. 2007. Distress assessment: Practice change through guideline implementation. *Clinical Journal of Oncology Nursing*, 11(6): 817–821.

Goldberg, D.P. 1972. *The Assessment of Psychiatric Illness by Questionnaire*. Oxford University Press: London, U.K.

Gonzalez, J.S., E.S. Hendriksen, E.M. Collins, and R.E. Durán. 2009. Latinos and HIV/AIDS: Examining factors related to disparity and identifying opportunities for psychosocial intervention research. *AIDS Behavior*, 13(3): 582–602.

Gupta, A., A.J. Silman, R. Morriss, C. Dickens, G.J. MacFarlane, Y.H. Chiu, B. Nicholl, and J. McBeth. 2007. The role of psychosocial factors in predicting the onset of chronic widespread pain: Results from a prospective population-based study. *Rheumatology*, 46: 666–671.

Hill, P.D. and R.W. Hood. 1999. *Measures of Religiosity*. Religious Education Press, Birmingham, AL.

Hill, T.D., C.E. Ross, and R.J. Angles. 2005. Neighborhood disorder, psychophysiological distress, and health. *Journal of Health and Social Behavior*, 46: 170–186.

Hodges, L., I. Butcher, A. Kleiboer, G. McHugh, G. Murray, J. Walker, R. Wilson, and M. Sharpe. 2009. Patient and general practitioner preferences for the treatment of depression in patients with cancer: How, who and where? *Journal of Psychosomatic Research*, 67(5): 399–402.

Holland, J.C. and I. Resnick. 2005. Pathways for psychosocial care of cancer survivors. *Cancer*, 104(11): 2624–2637.

Honea, N.J., R.A. Brintnall, B. Given, P. Sherwood, D.B. Colao, S.C. Somers, and L.L. Northouse. 2008. Putting evidence into practice: Nursing assessments and interventions to reduce family caregiver strain and burden. *Clinical Journal of Oncology Nursing*, 12(3): 507–517.

Hosaka, T., Y. Tokuda, and Y. Sugiyama. 2000. Effects of a structured psychiatric intervention on cancer patients' emotions and coping styles. *International Journal of Clinical Oncology*, 5(3): 188–191.

Hoyert, D.L. and M.M. Seltzer. 1992. Factors related to the well-being and life activities of family caregivers. *Family Relations*, 41(1): 74–81.

Hoyt, D.R., R.D. Conger, J.G. Valde., and K. Weihs. 1997. Psychological distress and help seeking in rural America. *American Journal of Community Psychology*, 25(4): 449–470.

Iacovino, V. and K. Ressor. 1997. Literature on interventions to address cancer patients' psychosocial needs: What does it tell us? *Journal of Psychosocial Oncology*, 15(2): 47–71.

Institute of Medicine. 2001. *Crossing the Quality Chasm: A New Health System for the 21st Century*. National Academies Press, Washington, DC.

Jacobsen, P.B. 2007. Screening for psychological distress in cancer patients: Challenges and opportunities. *Journal of Clinical Oncology*, 25(29): 4526–4527.

Kogan, S.M., G.H. Brody, and Y. Chen. 2009. Depressive symptomatology mediates the effect of socioeconomic disadvantage on HbA_{1c} among rural African Americans with Type 2 diabetes. *Journal of Psychosomatic Research*, 67(4): 289–296.

Kojima, M., T. Kojima, N. Ishiguro, T. Oguchi, M. Oba, H. Tsuchiya, S. Fumiaki, T.A. Furukawa, S. Suzuki, and S. Tokudome. 2009. Psychosocial factors, disease status, and quality of life in patients with rheumatoid arthritis. *Journal of Psychosomatic Research*, 67(5): 425–431.

Kristeller, J.L., C.S. Sumbrun, and R.F. Schilling. 1999. 'I would if I could': How oncologists and oncology nurses address spiritual distress in cancer patients. *Psycho-Oncology*, 8(5): 451–458.

Kroenke, C.H., L.D. Kubzansky, E.S. Schernhanner, M.D. Holmes, and I. Kawachi. 2006. Social networks, social support, and survival after breast cancer diagnosis. *Journal of Clinical Oncology*, 24(7): 1105–1110.

Lepore, S.J. and J.C. Coyne. 2006. Psychological interventions for distress in cancer patients: A review of reviews. *Annals of Behavioral Medicine*, 32(2): 85–92.

Lis, C.G., D. Gupta, and J.F. Grutsch. 2006. Patient satisfaction with quality of life as a predictor of survival in pancreatic cancer. *International Journal of Gastrointestinal Cancer*, 37(1): 35–44.

Lorig, K.R., R.L. Ritter, and V.M. González. 2003. Hispanic chronic disease self-management. *Nursing Research*, 52(6): 361–369.

Lorig, K.R., P. Ritter, A.L. Stewart, D.S. Sobel, B.W. Brown, A. Bandura, V.A. Gonzalez, D.D. Laurent, and H.R. Holman. 2001. Chronic disease self-management program: 2-year health status and health care utilization outcomes. *Medical Care*, 39(11): 1217–1223.

MacMahon, K.M. and G.Y.H. Lip. 2002. Psychological factors in heart failure. *Archives of Internal Medicine*, 162(2): 509–516.

Madden, J. 2006. The problem of distress in patients with cancer: More effective assessment. *Clinical Journal of Oncology Nursing*, 10(5): 615–619.

Manne, S.I. and M.A. Andrykowski. 2006. Seeing the forest for the trees: A rebuttal. *Annals of Behavioral Medicine*, 32(2): 111–114.

McClain, C.S., B. Rosenfeld, and W. Breitbart. 2003. Effect of spiritual well-being on end-of-life despair in terminally-ill cancer patients. *The Lancet*, 361(9369): 1603–1607.

Meryn, S. 1998. Improving doctor-patient communication; Not an opinion, but a necessity. *British Medical Journal*, 316(7149): 1922–1930.

Meyer, T.J. and M.M. Mark. 1995. Effects of psychosocial interventions with adult cancer patients: A meta-analysis of randomized experiments. *Health Psychology*, 14(2): 101–108.

Miller, D.K., J.T. Chibnall, S.D. Videen, and R.N. Duckro. 2005. Supportive-affective group experience for persons with life-threatening illness: Reducing spiritual, psychological, and death-related distress in dying patients. *Journal of Palliative Medicine*, 8(2): 333–343.

Mirowsky, J. and C.E. Ross. 1986. Social patterns of distress. *Annual Review of Sociology*, 12: 23–45.

Moriarty, D.G., M.M. Zack, J.P. Holt, D.P. Chapman, and M.A. Safran. 2009. Geographic patterns of frequent mental distress; U.S. adults, 1993–2001 and 2003–2006. *American Journal of Preventive Medicine*, 36(6): 497–505.

Moser, D.K. and K. Dracup. 2004. Role of spousal anxiety and depression in patient's psychosocial recovery. *Psychosomatic Medicine*, 66: 527–532.

National Comprehensive Cancer Network (NCCN). 2008. Clinical practice guidelines in oncology: Distress management. http://www.nccn.org (accessed on November 20, 2008).

Neri, M.T. and T. Kroll. 2003. Understanding the consequences of access barriers to health care: Experiences of adults with disabilities. *Disability and Rehabilitation*, 25(2): 85–96.

Pavalko, E.K. and S. Woodbury. 2000. Social roles as process: Caregiving careers and women's health. *Journal of Health and Social Behavior*, 41: 91–105.

Payton, A.R. 2009. Mental health, mental illness, and psychological distress: Same continuum or distinct phenomena? *Journal of Health and Social Behavior*, 50(2): 213–227.

Pirl, W.F., A. Muriel, V. Hwang, A. Kornblith, J. Greer, K. Donelan, D.B. Greenberg, J. Temel, and L. Schapira. 2007. Screening for psychosocial distress: A national survey of oncologists. *The Journal of Supportive Oncology*, 5(10): 499–504.

Prado, G., D.J. Feaster, S.J. Schwartz, I. Abraham Pratt, L. Smith, and J. Szapocznik. 2004. Religious involvement, coping, social support, and psychological distress in HIV-seropositive African American mothers. *AIDS and Behavior*, 8(3): 221–235.

Pyke, K. and V.L. Bengtson. 1996. Caring more or less: Individualistic and collectivist systems of family eldercare. *Journal of Marriage and Family*, 58: 379–382.

Riedl, A., J. Maass, H. Fliege, A. Stengel, M. Schmidtmann, B.F. Klapp, and H. Monnikes. 2009. Subjective theories of illness and clinical and psychological outcomes in patients with irritable bowel syndrome. *Journal of Psychosomatic Research*, 67(5): 449–455.

Ross, L., E.H. Boesen, S.O. Dalton, and C. Johansen. 2002. Mind and cancer: Does psychosocial intervention improve survival and psychological well-being? *European Journal of Cancer*, 38(11): 1447–1457.

Rustaøen, T. and B.R. Hanestad. 1998. Nursing intervention to increase hope in cancer patients. *Journal of Clinical Nursing*, 7(1): 19–27.

Rustaøen, T., I. Wiklund, B.R. Hanestad, B. Rokne, and M. Torbjørn. 1998. Nursing intervention to increase hope and quality of life in newly diagnosed cancer patients. *Cancer Nursing*, 21(4): 235–245.

Ryan, H., P. Schofield, J. Cockburn, P. Butow, M. Tattersall, J. Turner, A. Girgis, D. Bandaranayake, and D. Bowman. 2005. How to recognize and manage psychological distress in cancer patients. *European Journal of Cancer Care*, 14(1): 7–15.

Saab, P.G., H. Bang, R.B. Williams, L.H. Powell, N. Schneiderman, C. Thoresen, M. Burg, and F. Keefe. 2009. The impact of cognitive behavioral group training on event-free survival in patients with myocardial infarction. *Journal of Psychosomatic Research*, 67(1): 45–56.

Sagen, U., T.G. Vik, T. Moum, T. Morland, A. Finset, and T. Dammen. 2009. Screening for anxiety and depression after stroke: Comparison of the Hospital Anxiety and Depression Scale and the Montgomery and Asberg Depression Rating Scale. *Journal of Psychosomatic Research*, 67(4): 325–332.

Salaffi, F., F. Cavalieri, M. Nolli, and G. Ferraccioli. 1991. Analysis of disability in knee osteoarthritis. Relationship with age and psychological variables but not with radiographic score. *Journal of Rheumatology*, 18(10): 1581–1586.

Scheer, J., T. Kroll, M.T. Neri, and P. Beatty. 2003. Access barriers for persons with disabilities: The consumer's perspective. *Journal of Disability Policy Studies*, 13 (4): 221–230.

Schleifer, S.J., M.M. Macari-Hinson, D.A. Coyle, W.R. Slater, M. Kahn, R. Gorlin, and H.D. Zucker. 1989. The nature and course of depression following myocardial infarction. *Archives of Internal Medicine*, 149: 1785–1789.

Schrader, G., F. Cheok, A. Hordacre, and N. Guiver. 2004. Predictors of depression three months after cardiac hospitalization. *Psychosomatic Medicine*, 66: 514–520.

Sharma, A., D.M. Sharp, L.G. Walker, and J.R.T. Monsoon. 2007. Stress and burnout among colorectal nurse specialists working in the National Health Service. *Colorectal Disease*, 10: 397–406.

Shaw, B., J.Y. Han, E. Kim, D. Gustafson, R. Hawkins, J. Cleary, F. McTavish, S. Pingree, P. Eliason, and C. Lumpkins. 2007. Effects of prayer and religious expression within computer support groups on women with breast cancer. *Psycho-Oncology*, 16(7): 676–687.

Simon, A.E., M.R. Thompson, K. Flashman, and J. Wardle. 2009. Disease stage and psychosocial outcomes in colorectal cancer. *Colorectal Disease*, 11(1): 19–25.

Sloan, J.A., M.H. Frost, R. Berzon, A. Dueck, G. Guyatt, C. Moinpour, M. Sprangers, C. Ferrans, and D. Cella. 2007. The clinical significance of quality of life assessments in oncology: A summary for clinicians. *Support Care Cancer*, 14 (10): 988–998.

Sobel, D.S. 1995. Rethinking medicine: Improving health outcomes with cost-effective psychosocial interventions. *Psychosomatic Medicine*, 57(3): 234–244.

Stanton, A.L. 2006. Psychosocial concerns and interventions for cancer survivors. *Journal of Clinical Oncology*, 24(32): 5132–5137.

Stewart, M. 1995. Effective physician-patient communication and health outcomes: A review. *Canadian Medical Association Journal*, 152(9): 1423–1433.

Telch, C.F. and M.J. Telch. 1985. Psychological approaches for enhancing coping among cancer patients: A review. *Clinical Psychology Review*, 5(4): 325–344.

Vachon, M. 2006. Psychosocial distress and coping after cancer treatment. *American Journal of Nursing*, 106(3): 26–31.

Wartella, J.E., S.M. Auerbach, and K.R. Ward. 2009. Emotional distress, coping, and adjustment in family members of neuroscience intensive care unit patients. *Journal of Psychosomatic Research*, 66(6): 503–509.

Weissman, M.M., S. Wolk, R.B. Goldstein, D. Moreau, P. Adams, S. Greenwald, C.M. Klier, N.D. Ryan, R.E. Dahl, and P. Wickramaratne. 1999. Depressed adolescents grow up. *Journal of the American Medical Association*, 281(18): 1707–1713.

Wengstrom, Y., C. Haggmark, and C. Forsberg. 2001. Coping with radiation therapy: Effects of a nursing intervention on coping ability for women with breast cancer. *International Journal of Nursing Practice*, 7: 8–15.

Yanek, L.R., D.M. Becker, T.F. Moy, J. Gittelsohn, and D.M. Koffman. 2001. Project joy: Faith based cardiovascular health promotion for African American women. *Public Health Reports*, 116(1): 68–81.

Zachariae, R., C.G. Pedersen, A.B. Jensen, E. Ehrnrooth, P.B. Rossen, and H. von der Masse. 2003. Association of perceived physician communication style with patient satisfaction, distress, cancer-related self-efficacy, and perceived control over the disease. *British Journal of Cancer*, 88(5): 658–665.

Zigmond, A.S. and R.P. Snaith. 1983. The hospital anxiety and depression scale. *Acta Psychiatric Scandinavia*, 67: 361–370.

Design, Planning, Control, and Management of Healthcare Systems

IV.K Food and Supplies

44 **Healthcare Foodservice** *L. Charnette Norton* **44**-1
History of Segments • Management of Foodservice Departments • Nutrition Therapy • Retail Operations • Catering • Layout and Design • Receiving and Storage • Production • Patient Feeding • Cafés • Offices • Patient Service Centers/Call Centers • Food Safety and Security • Emergency and Disaster Preparedness • References

45 **Healthcare-Product Supply Chains: Medical–Surgical Supplies, Pharmaceuticals, and Orthopedic Devices: Flows of Product, Information, and Dollars** *Leroy B. Schwarz* **45**-1
Organizations Involved in Healthcare-Product Supply Chains • Products in Healthcare-Product Supply Chains • Product-, Information-, and Dollar-Flow for Medical-Surgical Products • Product-, Information-, and Dollar-Flow for Pharmaceutical Products • Product-, Information-, and Dollar-Flow for Orthopedic Devices • References

44

Healthcare Foodservice

History of Segments.....44-1
Acute Care • Long-Term Care • Hospices • Systems • Current Trends in Healthcare Foodservice
Management of Foodservice Departments.....44-3
Self-Operated versus Contracted Managed • Patient/Resident Feeding
Nutrition Therapy.....44-5
Retail Operations.....44-6
Catering.....44-6
Layout and Design.....44-7
Receiving and Storage.....44-7
Production.....44-8
Patient Feeding.....44-8
Cafés.....44-9
Offices.....44-9
Patient Service Centers/Call Centers.....44-10
Food Safety and Security.....44-10
Emergency and Disaster Preparedness.....44-10
References.....44-11

L. Charnette Norton
The Norton Group, Inc.

History of Segments

Acute Care

The first acute care hospital, Pennsylvania Hospital, was founded in 1751 by Benjamin Franklin and Dr. Thomas Bond. The web site for Pennsylvania Hospital does not mention foodservice. Most likely, the food was prepared in the traditional manner of earlier colonial days over an open fire in large kettles or cooked on the hearth (University of Pennsylvania Health System, 2009). The menus were boring and offered a basic mush and molasses menu featuring items like ox tail soup and brown bread (Lawn, 1997a).

Moving fast forward to the 1900s, hospital foodservice transitioned to food prepared in ovens and large steam-jacketed kettles. The kitchens were sizeable requiring large numbers of employees to prepare the food from raw products for the patients and staff. The kitchens included areas not found in modern kitchens such as a butcher shop and a root cellar. Some hospitals served meals to staff and visitors while others restricted visitors.

Healthcare foodservice remained the same until the introduction in the 1970s of pre-plated meals followed by cook chill using rethermalization systems. The cafeterias transition from straight line lock step lines into scramble and scatter systems to improve throughput and efficiencies as healthcare workers were limited to 30-minute meal breaks.

Long-Term Care

Long-term care facilities sometimes known as holding hospitals or home for the aged or retirement homes experienced a major resurgence as women began to work outside of the home during World War II. With women working, they could no longer care for aged parents. The need for 24/7 care made it impossible for the critically ill/aged to be cared for in the home. In the 1960s, foodservice provided to long-term care residents consisted of bland, low-sodium, low-fat, and texture-modified consistency foods. Much of the food was ground and colorless, presenting a very unappetizing meal. In recent years, the American Dietetic Association has supported a liberalized diet for long-term care facilities. The decision was made to encourage the residents to consume their food, treating their medical conditions by other means such as medication, exercise, etc.

Hospices

The term hospice is credited to Dame Cicely Saunders, a British physician, and Dr. Elizabeth Kuebler Ross who brought the subject of dying into the open. "Today the hospice care provides humane and compassionate care for people in the last phases of incurable disease so that they may live as fully and comfortable as possible" (Hospice of Michigan, 2009). The first hospice in America, the Connecticut Hospice opened in 1974 followed shortly by an inpatient hospice at the Yale Medical Center and a hospice program in Marin County California (Hospice of Michigan, 2009; Puckett and Lucas, 2009).

Not all hospices are institutional base. Some families choose to provide family-centered care in the home for the patient. Other hospice care can be provided in the hospital, nursing home, or a private hospice facility. The foodservice requirements for a hospice patient are usually based upon what the patient can tolerate in the end stage of their life. The physician's order can prescribe the diet as tolerated, leaving the decision for feeding the patient up to the family and the caregiver. The ultimate goal is to make the patient and the family as comfortable as possible.

Systems

In the 1970s, hospitals began to seek opportunities for remote clinics, physician's office buildings, and other opportunities outside their four walls. Government intervention in the methodology of reimbursement for Medicare and Medicaid patients changed the face of healthcare forever. Hospitals began to investigate the potential of becoming part of a system. Across the United States, hospitals began to form organizations of like-minded healthcare organizations. With early systems, the individual hospitals retained their individual boards and ownerships. Some of the systems began as group purchasing organizations and morphed into the systems that we know today. Foodservice was one of the first areas to support the group purchasing endeavors. Other hospitals were quick to realize that they would gain leverages if they had a single ownership with a single board of directors. With the development of hospital systems, individual departments within each hospital began a transition into a centralized department across the system. Foodservice was no exception.

Coupled with cook chill as a method of preparing food, centralized production facilities that would satellite food to all hospitals within a system were built. The Veterans Administration became a leader in this type of services with centralized production facilities serving a Vison. Kaiser Permanente on the West Coast chose to outsource their meal preparation to other organizations that could provide the complete tray ready for rethermalization by the nursing staff and then service to the patient.

As the 2009 legislative initiatives for healthcare reform are developed, systems as well as individual healthcare facilities will change. Foodservice will be impacted to become more efficient and reduce all costs with a changed service model as the initiatives mature and stabilize.

Current Trends in Healthcare Foodservice

In today's fast-moving world, one would agree that foodservice is a trendy business. Healthcare foodservice is no exception. "The most challenging trend in healthcare foodservice is the move to bring higher-quality, fresh foods into the system...moving away from the traditional institutional food preparation" (Peterson, 2009).

Several trends identified in *Dietary Manager's* February 2009 issue (Kopp, 2009) were

- Utilizing local farm grown food to reduce the carbon footprint
- Bite-size desserts
- Ethnic foods to include Chinese, Mexican, Italian, Greek, and Thai with Cuban and Ecuadorian complementing Mexican, Vietnamese blurring the line with Chinese, and Italian evolving to Tuscan and Sicilian
- Room service
- Finger foods
- Dining with dignity
- Unique theme meals

Even the Army has embraced a trend by developing the "Making It Fresh-Your Choice for Performance" program intended to bring a new and innovative concept to Army hospital foodservice including patient and cafeteria seating" (Spielman et al., 2008).

Health food in healthcare is a trend promoted by Health Care Without Harm. Several healthcare facilities are supporting "healthy food that is defined not only by nutritional quality but equally by a food system that is economically viable, environmentally sustainable, and supportive of human dignity and justice" (Harvie, 2008).

Management of Foodservice Departments

Self-Operated versus Contracted Managed

Foodservice departments in healthcare facilities were self-operated until the early 1960s. The foodservice facilities were managed by a chef or a home economist, as nutrition was not considered important until Florence Nightingale's efforts in the Crimean war pioneered dietetics as well as the nursing profession. In 1917, healthcare foodservice experienced a turning point with the formation of the American Dietetic Association (Lawn, 1997b).

As the profession of dietetics grew, dietitians began managing the departments. Because of their education and their ability to communicate with the physicians regarding nutritional issues and the increased importance of nutrition, dietitians, while not always educated in management and finance, became the healthcare foodservice director. Some hospitals' foodservice departments were managed by chefs and others with degrees in home economics or hotel and foodservice hospitality.

Contract management in foodservice began in 1897 at industrial facilities. The early contract service pioneers were Fred W. Profit Co., Automated Canteen Company of America, and Hot Shops Inc. These companies transitioned into Restaura, Inc., Compass and Marriott. Another company, The Wood Company, was the first that expanded into the healthcare foodservice in 1961 (Lawn, 1997b).

Statistics on the number of hospitals foodservice departments that are self-operated is difficult to determine. Contract companies for a number of years have touted that their penetration has increased annually. The contract companies have not been forthcoming in publishing their accounts lost to other contractors or hospitals' foodservice operations that converted to self-operated.

The contract-managed foodservice department has numerous ways of managing the department. Contract companies usually prefer to have all employees work for them, both management and hourly. Other options include only the department head, part of the management staff, or all of the management staff. The clinical nutrition staff may work for the hospital, or the clinical nutrition manager may be the only clinical nutrition staff person on the contractor's payroll.

Pros and cons exist for a healthcare administrator to determine feasibility of being contract or self-operated for foodservice. Either approach of contracted or self-operated can yield dramatic results. Many times, the deciding factors are political in nature or related to a personal risk for the decision-makers. The overriding consideration must be the coherence of the management and its capacity to meet the stated needs. The management team is the key to long-term success regardless of the decision. The self-operated foodservice operation cannot succeed without a strong, qualified director. On the other hand, the effectiveness of a contract operation is also dependent on the same strong, qualified individual. The leadership essential to the true success for the department and for the facility can be either contract or self-operated. The healthcare administrator must understand that the hidden agenda of the contractor is profitability at the expense of the client.

Patient/Resident Feeding

Acute Care

The feeding of acute-care patients for many years has followed two primary scenarios. Patients were served a nonselect meal with opportunities for limited alternate choices. The nonselect menu was usually a cycle menu repeating itself every 4–6 weeks. The second option was for a select menu cycling 5 days to 2 weeks depending upon the length of stay of the patients. A third option used in a small number of healthcare facilities was a restaurant style menu. Complaints of the repetitiveness of this menu resulted in most facilities returning to a nonselect or selective cycle menu.

Today, approximately 50% of acute-care healthcare facilities have transition to a room service model or have one under consideration (Norton, 2006). The room service model is foodservice "on-demand" for the hospitalized patient. The room service model does increase labor costs while reducing food and supply cost. The primary reason given for using the room service model is the increase in patient satisfaction.

A room service model requires specific software components that enable a call center to communicate with the tray assembly area. Without software, the standard 30–45 minutes for tray delivery to the patient is difficult or impossible to achieve for medium- or large-size hospitals. Other important components are the ability to communicate with the tray passers and dedicated elevators to the patient floors.

Traditionally, acute-care hospitals utilized specific diets for every disease state. The low-sodium diet would have 6–8 levels ranging from 500 to 3000 mg of sodium. The diabetic calorie-restricted diet would have numerous calorie counts ranging from a low of 500 cal to 3000+ cal. Some acute-care facilities reported they had up to 100 combinations of diets available for nutrition therapy. The vast number of diet types made it almost impossible for every patient to receive their specific order. In recent years, acute care has begun the transition to a liberalized diet plan with the exception of specific diets needed for research protocols and those for patients with unique dietary needs.

Most patients receive three meals a day at designated times. Those requiring in-between feedings receive them at 10 a.m., 2 p.m., and 8 p.m. In the past, some hospitals eliminated the requirement for snacks utilizing a five-meal plan. With the requirements to reduce labor, a five-meal plan is now seldom used in the acute-care setting.

Long-Term Care

Long-term care foodservice serves their residents in many venues depending upon the individual facility's preference in the types of residents. For the aging baby boomers utilizing long-term care, tray service is no longer acceptable as the boomers demand increased foodservice options and are not accepting of a traditional tray service. Many are sociable, well traveled, and want various congregate dining options. As residents aged in place, buffet lines were eliminated from some establishments. An alternate service model for congregate dining has occurred with the buffet being brought tableside to the resident. An upscale cart with two compartments, one for hot food and one for refrigerated items, is used. The hot food is appropriately garnished in upscale, colorful serving dishes. The cold items can be preportioned or also served in homelike, bulk containers. The resident can make their choices, increasing their nutritional intake by seeing the appealing foods before making their selections.

Congregate dining does have certain advantages for the resident (Norton, 2007):

- Residents are not required to make selections in advance with patients being offered a choice at the point of service.
- The amount of wasted food is reduced.
- The service is perceived as being upscale.
- Resident satisfaction increases.
- Menus can be tailored for specific populations.
- Any adjustment to diet preferences can be made immediately.

The current model for long-term care is promoting a cultural change, which focuses on outcomes. This social versus medical model of care improves quality of care, offering choices and control to the resident. The shift is to thinking about all aspects resulting in the outcomes. With the increased emphasis on making the long-term care facility more homelike, changes have occurred in the delivery of foodservice.

One change for the foodservice is to provide a liberalized diet plan. The residents are entitled to a personalized eating schedule with a personalized eating plan considering their individual preferences. This means increased flavor profiles and ethnic offerings. One size does not fit all with changes in the portion size for the resident. Many selections are offered with the alternate selection not always being baked chicken. Any substitution provided must have the same nutritional value as the original meal (Norton, 2009).

Current trends in long-term care are the addition of coffee shops, ice cream parlors, flexible menus, extended hours, high tea, and catering. The delivery systems are also changing to restaurant style service, buffet dining, family style, hotel/room service, and cooked to order (Norton, 2009).

Hospice

Because hospice care is at the end stage of life, foodservice in most hospice facilities have the ultimate goal of providing favorites for the patient that make them comfortable. The food offered is what is tolerated based on the order of the physician. While some hospice physicians still wish to have the patient follow a strict dietary regime, others consider that at the end of the life, the foodservice should be what the patient enjoys or what makes a family feel that their loved one is getting the best care available to make them comfortable.

Institutionalized hospice care foodservice is presented as near homelike as possible. While some hospices still opt for tray service at designated times, others follow the room service model with food served to the patient on demand.

Nutrition Therapy

In 1917, when the American Dietetic Association was formed, nutrition therapy began its formal recognition as instrumental in the recovery of patients with various diseases. Since those early years, nutrition therapy has become more scientific based with research supporting the delivery of nutrition therapy. Early diets for nutrition therapy were many times based on what the physician believed appropriate for their patients. Healthcare foodservice administrators found that the diets varied by hospital. The American Dietetic Association was instrumental in developing nationwide standards for nutrition therapy. The American Dietetic Association teamed with associations such as the American Heart Association and the American Diabetic Association in developing standardized protocols for patients with cardiac and diabetic diseases.

In early years, many hospitals had their own diet manual, even if they were not part of a university teaching hospital. This was necessary to meet the needs of the physicians practicing in their hospital. Because of the cost of maintaining an individual hospital-based diet manual, several hospitals joined together in cities and then states to have a citywide or statewide diet manual. Currently, most hospitals and healthcare foodservice contract companies use the diet manual published by the American Dietetic Association with an errata page for special dietary requirements of their individual medical staffs.

Nutrition therapy has changed to promote the liberalized diet for all residents and patients. In 2005, the American Dietetic Association developed the position stating "quality of life in nutritional status of older residents and long-term-care facilities may be enhanced by liberalization of the diet prescription" (American Dietetic Association, 2005a). In 2003, ADA designated aging as its second emerging area. Nutrition care in long-term settings must meet two goals: maintenance of health and promotion of quality of life (American Dietetic Association, 2005b).

When residents enter long-term care facilities, a lifetime of poor dietary habits were difficult to change. The decisions were made that it was more important to encourage the elder to eat what they wanted and treat their diseases by other means. Physicians and dietitians soon found that to deprive a senior of their favorite foods with an unacceptable or unpalatable diet would only accelerate their demise. Because of the success of a liberalized diet in the long-term care arena, nutrition therapy is changing in the acute-care setting to a liberalized diet for nutrition therapy.

The American Dietetic Association has promoted medical nutrition therapy "to maintain independence functional ability, chronic disease management and quality of life" (American Dietetic Association, 2005b). Dietitians are encouraged to take the lead in research and develop "national state and local collaborative networks to incorporate effectively the food nutrition services across a spectrum of aging" (American Dietetic Association, 2005b).

"A liberalized diet reduces food restrictions and promotes client preferences [in order to] provide a meal that is palatable and well received" (Puckett and Lucas, 2009). Using a liberalized diet plan usually reduces the number of diets offered. Diets are combined—for instance, a number of low-sodium diets become one with the notation, "no added salt." The diabetic diet has changed from calorie counting to carb counting with sugar restrictions. Texture modification is combined with the diets offered. If a facility is using a room service model, all diets are usually placed on one menu. A selection is even offered to the liquid diets with notations stating that when the physician progresses their diet, they will be able to have items other than liquids. The nutritional status of the patient/resident can be greatly improved when they have a selection on a liquid diet for tea or coffee, plus the flavor of gelatin or broth.

Retail Operations

For a number of years, the retail operations in healthcare facilities were just an extension of patient's selections. The food offered was bland and served in a lockstep line similar to that seen in some military and school foodservice facilities. The seating areas in the cafeterias were rows of tables with little or no ambience.

As Corporate America began to offer improved foodservice to office workers and executives, healthcare administrators wanted the same level of foodservice in their cafés. When the administrator was served a luncheon at a local business, healthcare foodservice directors found that they were asked why they could not serve the same types of food that the administrator had just consumed. The astute healthcare foodservice director visited the business and industry foodservice operation for ideas to upscale their café.

Grab and go meal have become big business in hospitals. A recent survey by Healthcare Foodservice Management found that 53% of respondents facilities offer made on-site meals for takeout (White, 2008).

Catering

In the 1950s and 1960s, catering in healthcare was limited to coffee service and a few sandwiches served to the administrative suite provided at no cost to the user but considered part of the foodservice expense.

As hospital departments began to have more meetings required by licensing and accreditation agencies, the requests for catering increased. The increased requirement to compete for physicians also increased in-house catering. The foodservice department was required to produce gourmet banquets complete in some instances with numerous courses plus a bar and wine service. Many healthcare facilities have the ability to produce five-star catering events ranging from a simple coffee and doughnuts to formal sit-down dinners with trained wait staff. The reemergence of chefs in healthcare as part of the foodservice team has helped raise the level of the on-site catering.

As hospitals have looked for increased opportunities for additional revenues, foodservice has the potential of becoming revenue producing rather than cost basis with off-site catering. While some hospital administrators choose not to compete with local businesses, the lack of catering services plus the request to have the local hospitals chefs provide off-site catering may promote the business.

Opportunities exist ranging from cakes to holiday meals to formal meals at medical staff and administrator's residences. If local service organizations meet regularly at the hospital and are provided catering, they may request that the hospital provide catering to their annual parties off-site with invited community guest and spouses.

Most food production systems can accommodate the demands of catering with minor adjustments based on their equipment and types in capacity of their prep and storage areas. If the catering increases to daily multiple events, including weekends, a separate catering kitchen with dedicated staff may become a necessity.

Layout and Design

Whether building a new facility or renovating an existing kitchen, independent designers or consultants are recommended to develop the overall design of the foodservice department. "Since they do not work for distributors or manufacturers, their advice on what equipment to buy should be less influenced by other considerations" (Boyan, 2007). The general architect will most likely not have the skill set to adequately design a foodservice department as foodservice design is considered a highly specialized area.

Receiving and Storage

The receiving for foodservice will depend upon the materials management policies of the healthcare facility. Some facilities have all food purchases handled by materials management including purchasing, receiving, and storage. Others will have the functions performed by the foodservice department. A third option is to have a combination of the two departments being responsible for the functions.

Regardless of who is responsible for the purchase, receiving, and storage of food, it is important that the traffic flow surrounding the facility allows for space for parking of the delivery trucks. The receiving should be as close to the storage areas as possible to prevent the deterioration of refrigerated and frozen products before entering the refrigerator and freezers. In new facilities, it is appropriate to have a receiving dock for incoming products and a second dock area for handling waste, to prevent cross contamination of food stuffs.

When designing dry storage areas, the walls should extend from floor-to-ceiling, preventing entrance from adjoining rooms. The dry storage areas should not be placed under overhead plumbing. A secure area in the dry storage area should be available for chemicals and combustible materials.

Space requirements for refrigerators and freezers will vary depending upon the foodservice operation. The spatial requirements will depend upon the menu and the type of finish for the products received. As example, if all produce is received, washed, cut, and diced, ready for utilization, the space requirements will be less than if product is purchased as boxed in the field or orchard. Refrigeration space for raw products will be decreased if many convenience entrées are purchase frozen, thus increasing the need for additional freezer space.

Traditionally, healthcare facilities were only required to keep a 3-day emergency supply of food, water, and disposables. CMS, TJC, and local governments are recommending the supplies be increased to 7–14 days. The recommendation for pandemic supplies is recommended for 28 days by some. The storage of this volume of food and disposables drastically increases the storage space requirements. Some cities, counties, and states are recommending that the supplies be meals ready to eat, which increase the storage requirements even more due to their low density. Coupled with increased storage are the increase of trash and the problem of disposal. Water storage must be planned for emergency use as foodservice is usually assigned this responsibility.

Production

The design of the production facility will depend upon the menu and the population served by the healthcare facility. The production facility should be close to the dry and refrigerated storage areas to improve the efficiency of operations. "The size and shape allocated for production facility will influence the equipment arrangement and workflow patterns" (Puckett, 2004).

The hot cooking component of the production facility's equipment will be a combination of major pieces of equipment such as steam-jacketed kettles, ranges, fryers, ovens, broilers, steamers, etc., arranged to promote an efficient workflow supported with tables, sinks, and roll-in or reach-in refrigerators and freezers. The cold component for vegetable and salad preparation should be adjacent to the hot cooking area with appropriate tables for the equipment for dicing, slicing, chopping, and dish up.

A bake shop will usually be separated from the hot cooking component because of the contamination caused by flour and yeast, thus reducing the shelf life for vegetables and meat items. The bakeshop equipment and layout will depend upon the volume and types of items produced.

When designing the production area it is crucial that "aisles between equipment should be wide enough to park carts, turn them around and permit employees to use them without blocking traffic" (Puckett, 2004). Adequate handwashing sinks must also be incorporated within the production facility.

Patient Feeding

The design of the patient feeding components of healthcare foodservice has seen many reiterations throughout the years. The original designs included steam tables where food was plated, covered, and placed on trays, then put in carts for delivery to the patient without a temperature maintenance system. The trays were assembled on a skate wheel or motorized line with hot and cold supporting equipment in an assembly line fashion. Another option for large healthcare facilities was to place the food in bulk in steamtables that were transported to the patient floors with accompanying carts with service ware and cold items. In the 1960s, hot and cold carts were introduced for patient feeding where the food was plated and placed on trays with hot items on one side and cold items on the other side of the tray. The tray was then placed in the cart with a gasket separating the hot and cold side of the tray. Once assembled, the cart was delivered to the patient areas for service. In the 1970s, insulated trays and heated pellets were followed by unitized bases for temperature maintenance. For approximately 20 years, the method/design of patient feeding remained unchanged.

In the mid-1990s, the room service model was introduced in the cancer hospitals of New York's Sloan-Kettering and Houston's M.D. Anderson plus an acute-care hospital—Swedish Hospital in Seattle. Although more labor intensive, numerous hospitals have moved or are moving to the room service model for patient feeding due to the requirement for increased patient satisfaction. The design of a room service kitchen is similar to that of a hotel room service kitchen with trays being assembled when the patients, families, or nursing staff order the patient selections. The unitized base is used for a temperature maintenance system. Six to eight trays are placed into small carts and delivered to patients every 10–15 minutes.

Cafés

In 1961, Kotschevar and Terrell stated that for cafeterias the "counter shape should be based on volume and type of service. Shape of the room and traffic patterns should also be considered. Counters are straight-line, L, or U shaped. Parallel straight counters may be used" (Kotschevar and Terrell, 1961).

In the 1970s, the designs for healthcare employee feeding began to change with the introduction of the scramble system. The 1980s brought additional changes with courtyards and scatter systems being popular designs. In the 1990s, to serve staffs at large medical centers, roving carts were introduced, followed by kiosks whose explosion can be credited to the popularity of the Starbucks concept.

Courtyard designs became popular in the late 1990s. As branding became popular, the design of the cafés changed as the multiple concepts became part of the courtyard design. Brands were either in-house brands or corporate brands such as Starbucks, Dunkin Donuts, McDonald's, Burger King, etc.

The design for in-house brands for retail spaces requires the equipment to support the brand concept such as display cases and marketing logos. For corporate brands, the brand's corporate policy dictates the design requirements for their venue. Most have stringent guidelines on their logo size, location, and use. Some require their own cashier while others allow for the operation to have all sales using a single cash system. The retail software determines the allocation of revenues to each brand. Storage and refrigeration requirements may change with some brands requiring separate spaces while others are willing to share spaces.

Regardless of the design concept chosen for a retail operation "overall space requirements for the employee's dining area must be carefully analyzed to ensure efficient movement of customers and service workers" (Puckett, 2004). Current designs emphasis self-service stations to reduce labor requirements and give customers control over choices of the items selected and the portion size.

The dining area of healthcare cafés resembles commercial restaurants rather than the institutional design of prior years. The tables are of varying size and shape allowing for single seating or larger groups wanting an impromptu meeting during their meal period. The healthcare interior designer works with the foodservice design team to coordinate the ambiance to be in concert with the other public spaces in the facility.

Offices

Offices are an integral part of any foodservice healthcare operation. It is imperative that offices be provided for supervisory oversight of the production and patient meal service areas and staff. The most desirable location for these offices is in or adjacent to the production and service line areas. A management person should be available to answer employee questions and provide oversight to prevent the potential of slippage.

The foodservice director in large facilities can be located in a suite of offices with the support staff for finance and other clerical functions. Some healthcare facilities choose to keep all offices including the dietitians in a centralized location. Depending upon the size of the healthcare facility, it may be more efficient to have the clinical staff located near the patients with adequate space for counseling the patient. With a large outpatient population, office space should be provided for the clinical nutrition staff in the outpatient area.

Offices are needed for the retail and catering operations area. The catering office should be easily accessible for those wishing to book catered events. The retail office should be close to the main café and have an area available for secure cash handling.

The number of offices and locations will depend upon the size, the operation, and the number of management staff requiring office space.

Patient Service Centers/Call Centers

Patient service centers have been traditionally called diet offices. The diet office function is to communicate with nursing, ensuring each patient receives the tray of food adhering to the diet as prescribed by the physician. The diet office manages communication between the kitchen, the clinical staff, and nursing staff for patient request and physician orders for nutrition intervention and education. The location of the diet office has traditionally been placed adjacent to the patient tray line.

With a room service model, the diet office transitioned into a call center. The call center is similar to a call center in any type of business, with the staff receiving the order from the patient, nursing staff, or the family, and sending the order electronically to the production area for assembly for delivery to patients at multiple sites within 30–45 minutes. Because of the software available, call centers no longer need to be adjacent to the tray assembly area. In fact, the call center does not even have to be in the building where the kitchen is located. Hospital systems have enjoyed economies of scale by having one call center for multiple hospitals or multiple departments.

Food Safety and Security

Although hazard analysis critical control process (HACCP) began in the 1960s with NASA, healthcare foodservice was slow to adopt the HACCP principles. In 1982, when the American Dietetic Association sponsored seminars throughout the United States to present HACCP to the dietitians, many attendees thought that this was just another flavor of the year. With the *E. coli* disaster at Jack in the Box, food safety became more important to all of foodservice including healthcare. Subsequent food safety events such as peanut butter, spinach, etc., indicated the awareness and the need to have a sound foodservice safety program. Food safety is crucial in healthcare foodservice because of serving food to the elderly, the young, and the immune compromised. Until HACCP, a system did not exist to ensure, if followed, all components were utilizing appropriate food safety practices. While a HACCP program is not a requirement, it is an organized methodology for food safety and security required by TJC. Many local health departments encourage healthcare to adopt all or part of the HACCP program.

Since 9/11, food security throughout the country as well as in healthcare has received scrutiny. What better way to contaminate the food supply in the terrorist attacks and render inoperable first responders and eliminate caregivers with a food borne illness outbreak in a healthcare facility.

Manufacturers have developed equipment and tools to assist the healthcare foodservice provider in delivering safe wholesome food to their clientele. Refrigeration equipment performs better, more efficiently, and maintains consistent temperatures. Alarms are built-in to notify the user of variances in the danger zone. Antimicrobial surfaces are available for tables and counters, plus are impregnated into cutting boards and utensils. Other smallwares to rapidly chill products as well as antimicrobial wipes are just some of the additional products available to foodservice operators.

Emergency and Disaster Preparedness

Traditionally, healthcare foodservice departments were required to have components in a disaster manual. The plans usually included what to do in the case of a fire, internal flood, and an electrical outage. "Most likely the plan paid little attention to the dangers of microbial, chemical, or communicable diseases are terrorism. After 9/11, however disaster planning forever changed" (Puckett and Norton, 2003). The responsibility of the foodservice department's plan was usually stated to provide beverages, sandwiches, and cookies to staff operating the command center. Some healthcare facilities even put in their plans that the departments would provide the same items to families for a mass casualty such as a bus accident, train derailment, or plane crash.

With the increase of national disasters in the 1990s plus the 9/11 disaster, healthcare facilities determined that the disaster emergency and preparedness plans were inadequate. In fact, the single plan for federal response to the disaster did not exist until 1987 when the plan for a federal response to a catastrophic earthquake was adopted. Prior to then, multiple federal agencies had separate plans. Healthcare followed what the federal government was doing in relation to disasters. This changed with Hurricane Hugo in 1989 with FEMA recognizing that a single focus on a single event was not practical. The federal government developed 15 emergency support function plans addressing the requirements for numerous disasters. Documents #8 Public Health and Medical Service and #11 Agricultural and Natural Resources serve as the basis for the federal plan to identify the requirements for foodservice. Healthcare facilities now are required by CMS to have an expanded Emergency and Disaster Preparedness Plan to include an operational plan for the disruption of normal operations for food and water to patients and staff. Without food and water, the best medical care to patients will not be successful.

The most important event for healthcare foodservice "is to be part of the disaster planning process. Being part of the process ensures that all foodservice are included in the hospital overall plan. Too often food and water are not considered with foodservice taking a back seat to the needs for nursing and physicians" (Norton, 2003). Disaster plans for healthcare foodservice should be developed by dividing disasters into categories. The categories are classified as, technological, natural, and man-made. Pandemic is considered a separate type of disaster. The foodservice disaster plan is developed for each of the four types with appendices identifying unique characteristics regarding each disaster. The plan does not need to be longer than approximately two pages, listing communications protocol, chain of command, the description of the scenario, and a specific plan for planning tasks for short-term, intermediate, and long-term contingency plans. The continuity form identifies the responsible person for each one of the planning tasks.

References

American Dietetic Association. 2005a. Position of the American Dietetic Association: Liberalization of the diet prescription improves quality of life for older adults in long-term care. *Journal of the American Dietetic Association*. 105(12):1955–1965.

American Dietetic Association. 2005b. Position of the American Dietetic Association: Nutrition across the spectrum of aging. *Journal of the American Dietetic Association*. 105(4):616–633.

Boyan, C. 2007. Cafeteria/kitchen renovations. *Trends*. 9(3):22–23.

Harvie, J. 2008. Menu of Change, Health Food in Health Care, A 2008 Survey of Healthy Foods and Healthcare Pledge Hospitals. Arlington, VA: Health Care without Harm. Institute of Sustainable Future: 4.

Hospice of Michigan. Brief History of the Hospice Movement. Detroit, MI. http://www.hom//movement.asp (accessed March 20, 2009).

Kopp, T. 2009. Trends and theme dining. *Dietary Manager*. February:32–34.

Kotschevar, L. and Terrell, M. 1961. *Foodservice Layout and Equipment Planning*. New York: John Wiley & Sons, Inc.

Lawn, J. 1997a. Healthcare and elder care. *Food Management*. October:74–81

Lawn, J. 1997b. Contract management. *Food Management*. October:84–91.

Norton, C. 2003. Part II: Contingency plan: Emergency preparedness avian influenza. *Trends*. 9(3):20–21.

Norton, C. 2006. Room service… The nuts and bolts (Part I), *Trends*. 8(2):6–19.

Norton, C. 2007. Congregate dining, an alternate service model. *Trends*. 9(3):18–19.

Norton, C. 2009. Transforming the long term care culture. *American Society of Healthcare Foodservice Administrators National Conference Presentation*, Clearwater, FL.

Peterson, R. D. 2009. Current trends in health care Foodservice. Culinary Cooking Schools Institute. http://www.foodnet.com.writers.html (accessed May 9, 2009).

Puckett, R. P. 2004. *Foodservice Manual for Health Care Institutions*. 3rd edn., San Francisco, CA/Chicago, IL: Jossey-Bass, A Wiley Imprint, Health Forum, Inc. An American Hospital Association Company, AHA Chicago Press.

Puckett, R. P. and Lucas, R. A. 2009. *Food, Nutrition and Medical Nutrition Therapy through the Lifecycle*. Dubuque, IA: Kendall Hunt Publishing Company.

Puckett, R. P. and Norton, L. C. 2003. *Disaster Emergency Preparedness in Foodservice Operations*, Chicago, IL: The American Dietetic Association.

Spielmann, S., Worley, M., and Harris, R. 2008. Making it fresh: Your choice for performance, the army's foodservice program. *Journal of the American Dietetic Association*. 102(9 Supplement):A71.

University of Pennsylvania Health System. 2009. Historical timeline, 1751–1800. http://www.uphs.upen.edu/paharc/timeline/ (accessed March 20, 2009).

White, L. 2008. Hospital food goes high-end. *Food Service Equipment and Supplies*. September. http://www.fesmag.com/article/CA658321.html. (accessed May 9, 2009).

45

Healthcare-Product Supply Chains: Medical–Surgical Supplies, Pharmaceuticals, and Orthopedic Devices: Flows of Product, Information, and Dollars

Leroy B. Schwarz
Purdue University

Organizations Involved in Healthcare-Product Supply Chains **45**-1
Manufacturers • Providers • Distributors • Group Purchasing Organizations • Pharmacy Benefits Managers
Products in Healthcare-Product Supply Chains **45**-4
Product-, Information-, and Dollar-Flow for Medical-Surgical Products **45**-5
Product-Flow • Information-Flow • Dollar-Flow
Product-, Information-, and Dollar-Flow for Pharmaceutical Products **45**-8
Product-Flow in the Provider Supply Chain • Information-Flow in the Provider Supply Chain • Dollar-Flow in the Provider Supply Chain • Product-Flow in the Retail/Mail-Order Supply Chain • Information-Flow in the Retail/Mail-Order Supply Chain • Dollar-Flow in the Retail/Mail-Order Supply Chain
Product-, Information-, and Dollar-Flow for Orthopedic Devices **45**-13
Product-Flow • Information-Flow • Dollar-Flow
References **45**-15

Organizations Involved in Healthcare-Product Supply Chains

Five organizations are to be found in the supply chains we examine: (1) manufacturers, (2) providers, (3) distributors, (4) pharmacy benefits managers (PBMs), and (5) group purchasing organizations (GPOs). The role of each organization is briefly described below. Table 45.1 identifies examples of some of the "major players." It should be noted that although their functions are distinct, the ownership of these

TABLE 45.1 The Major Players in Healthcare-Product Supply Chains

	Pharmaceutical	Orthopedic Devices	Medical-Surgical
Manufacturers	Pfizer	Zimmer	Johnson & Johnson
	GSK	Stryker	Becton Dickinson
	Johnson & Johnson	Biomet	
Providers	*Healthcare systems*	*Healthcare systems*	*Healthcare systems*
	• HCA	• HCA	• HCA
	• Ascension Health	• Ascension Health	• Ascension Health
	• Tenet Healthcare	• Tenet Healthcare	• Tenet Healthcare
	Retailers		
	• Walgreens		
	• CVS Caremark Corporation		
	• Rite Aid Corporation		
Distributors	McKesson	Typically, orthopedic devices are distributed regionally under exclusive contract with the manufacturer	McKesson
	Cardinal Health		Owens & Minor
	AmerisourceBergen		Medline Industries
			Cardinal Health
GPOs	Novation	(GPOs are not typically involved in the supply chains for orthopedic devices)	Novation
	Premier		Premier
	MedAssets		MedAssets
PBMs	Caremark	—	—
	Medco Health Solutions		
	ACS State Healthcare		

organizations is sometimes the same. For example, a given company may be both a manufacturer and a distributor (e.g., Cardinal), or a provider and a GPO (e.g., Tenet, HCA).

Manufacturers

For our purposes, a "manufacturer" is the source for the products involved in the supply chains described. A given company may manufacture both branded and nonbranded (i.e., generic) products. It is not unusual for manufacturers to outsource some or all of the manufacturing process to contract manufacturers. A given contract manufacturer may produce similar products for different manufacturers.

Providers

For our purposes, a "provider" is the organization that administers or uses a healthcare product in the treatment of a patient. Providers are typically clinics, hospitals, groups of hospitals, or networks of providers (e.g., integrated delivery networks, or IDNs). We also describe the pharmaceutical supply chains in which retail and mail-order pharmacies are the providers. Individual physicians or small-group practices are not included in our description.

Distributors

Distributors purchase products from manufacturers and sell them to providers. These products may be purchased by the provider "on contract" (i.e., "under contract") or "off contract." Pharmaceutical distributors are often called "wholesalers." For simplicity's sake, we will call them "distributors."

Group Purchasing Organizations

A GPO negotiates the prices that its "provider-members" pay for the manufacturer's products purchased "on contract." GPOs may also negotiate the "margin" their members pay to distributors (see below) and/or the logistics charges associated with the delivery of products to them.

These contracts are negotiated between each GPO and each manufacturer. For the provider-member, the apparent rationale for belonging to a GPO is that the provider-member will get lower prices through the GPO than it might obtain for itself (by purchasing "off contract," either directly from the manufacturer or through a distributor), because of the combined purchasing power of the GPO* (Schneller, 2009).

According to a GAO report (2003),† GPO "key contracting strategies" include: (1) sole-source contracts, which give one of several manufacturers of comparable products an exclusive right to sell a particular product on contract; (2) commitment, which refers to a specified percentage of purchasing volume that, when met by the GPO's provider-member, will result in a lower price; (3) bundling, which links prices to purchases of a specified group of products; and (4) contracts of long duration (e.g., 3–5 years).

Burns (2002) reports that "the majority or near majority of products purchased by hospitals and healthcare systems are on national GPO contracts." Burns (2002) also reports that membership of the top four national GPOs accounts for approximately 4300 of the approximately 6000 hospitals in the United States.

Three important characteristics about these GPO contracts are important to understand:

1. Despite the "contract" terminology, GPO provider-members are not necessarily‡ under an obligation to purchase products under the terms of the GPO-negotiated contract. (The manufacturer is obligated to sell at the on-contract price, given that the provider purchases through an authorized distributor.) Such purchases are called "off contract." To illustrate: Suppose provider P is a member of GPO G that has an arrangement with distributor D to sell a particular product, XYZ, to P "on contract." Many "off-contract" scenarios are possible. For example, P might choose to purchase XYZ from a different distributor. Alternatively, P might choose to purchase, ABC, the nominal equivalent of XYZ "off contract" from D, from another distributor, or directly from ABC's manufacturer.
2. The GPO-negotiated contract price paid by a given provider-member typically depends on the volume of product/s that the provider-member purchases on contract. GPOs use the term "tier" to describe the volume/price categories at which provider-members purchase products.§

   Using the example from (1) above, it is in the interest of management at the provider (e.g., hospital managers) to purchase as much of any given product "on contract" as possible, in order to qualify for a lower (tier) price. However, individual physicians may specify alternatives to the contracted product (so-called "physician preference") or a distributor may offer a lower, off-contract price for that product or its equivalent to the provider.

   The extent to which a provider-member purchases a contracted product is called "compliance." GPOs and their provider-members benefit from high levels of compliance, since higher

---

* Testimony by William J. Scanlon, Director, Health Care Issues, before the Subcommittee on Antitrust, Competition, and Business and Consumer Rights, Committee on the Judiciary, U.S. Senate, suggests that GPO members do not always get the lowest possible price through on-contract purchases. GAO-02-690T, released April 30, 2002.

† "Group Purchasing Organizations: Use of Contracting Processes and Strategies to Award Contracts for Medical-Surgical Products," GAO-03-998T.

‡ Some GPOs prohibit members from purchasing contracted items "off contract."

§ "Volume" can either be based on market share (e.g., 80% of purchases qualify for tier 1) or dollar thresholds.

compliance means higher volumes, more purchasing power for the GPO, and lower prices for the provider-members.

3. Manufacturers are not obliged to have any individual product "on contract," and, hence, the manufacturer is the final arbiter of the "on contract," GPO-negotiated price.

In order to obtain the GPO-negotiated price, the provider-member must purchase the product from a distributor authorized by both the GPO and the manufacturer.

A given distributor may be authorized to sell products on contract for several different GPOs. In a given market area, a given GPO may have more than one distributor authorized to sell products on contract. A provider may be a member of more than one GPO* and purchase a given product from more than one distributor.

It should be noted that GPOs typically provide other noncontracting services to their provider-members, including, but not limited to technology assessment and spend analysis. According to Schneller (2009) and Burns and Lee (2008), these services are valued by members; however, the information- and dollar-flows associated with these services are not included here.

Pharmacy Benefits Managers

A PBM works with its clients—typically third-party payers (e.g., insurance companies, public-health programs)—to plan and supervise the dispensing of pharmaceuticals to patients that are covered by the client's pharmacy benefit plan.

More specifically, PBMs help their clients to determine what pharmaceuticals will be covered by the benefit plan (i.e., the "formulary"), the patients' co-pays, deductibles, etc. PBMs also supervise the dispensing of pharmaceuticals by contracting with "authorized" retail and mail-order pharmacies.

Products in Healthcare-Product Supply Chains

According to Burns (2002), providers purchase products in eight different categories: pharmaceuticals, medical-surgical supplies (i.e., disposables), radiology and laboratory supplies, medical devices (e.g., stents and implants), capital equipment, food and dietary supplies and services, office forms and supplies, and cleaning supplies and services.† The combined cost of these products is typically a given hospital's second-largest operating cost (after labor).

These products are sold to a provider in two different ways: (1) direct from the manufacturer; or (2) through a distributor. The price the provider pays may or may not have been negotiated by a GPO. This yields the 2 × 2 classification provided by Burns (2002), reproduced in Table 45.2.

Note that low-value, high-volume products (e.g., generic pharmaceutical and medical-surgical supplies) typically flow through distributors. High-value, low-volume products (e.g., orthopedic devices) typically flow direct from the manufacturer to the provider (or through the manufacturer's representative)‡ (Burns, 2002).

It is estimated that U.S. expenditures for medical-surgical supplies, pharmaceuticals, and (all) devices was $275 billion in 2006, or 13% of total U.S. expenditures for healthcare (Projections, 2006).

* There are two types of GPOs: national and regional. Membership in a national GPO may prohibit membership in a second national GPO but may permit membership in regional GPOs.

† Burns (2002, p. 43): "Across these broad areas, providers order at least 30,000–50,000 items from their suppliers in a given year, and maybe as many as 100,000 different items for large IDNs with physician networks."

‡ Burns (2002) provides three reasons: (1) the manufacturer desires direct contact with the clinicians who use its products (indeed, clinicians are often involved in product development for the manufacturer); (2) use of the product may require the special knowledge of the manufacturer or its representative; and (3) low profit margins for the distributor.

TABLE 45.2 GPO-Contracted vs. Distributor-Mediated Products

	Suppliers Contract with GPOs	Suppliers Do Not Contract with GPOs
Suppliers use wholesale or distributor	Medical-surgical products of low value and high volume Generic drugs	Some branded drugs (oncology, cardiovascular) Small-volume arcane items Generic drugs
Suppliers use direct delivery	Lower-end implants and medical devices Branded drugs	Higher-end implants and medical devices, specialty items of high value and low volume

Source: Burns, L.R., Wharton school colleagues. *The Health Care Value Chain*, Jossey-Bass, San Francisco, CA, 2002.

Product-, Information-, and Dollar-Flow for Medical-Surgical Products

We define medical-surgical supplies as any product that is used in the diagnosis and treatment of patients.* The product-flow and information-flow for medical-surgical products are diagrammed in Figure 45.1. Product-flow is represented by heavy solid lines.

Product-Flow

The vast majority of medical-surgical products (estimated 70%–75%) flow to providers through distributors.† The frequency, size, and packaging of deliveries from the distributor to the provider

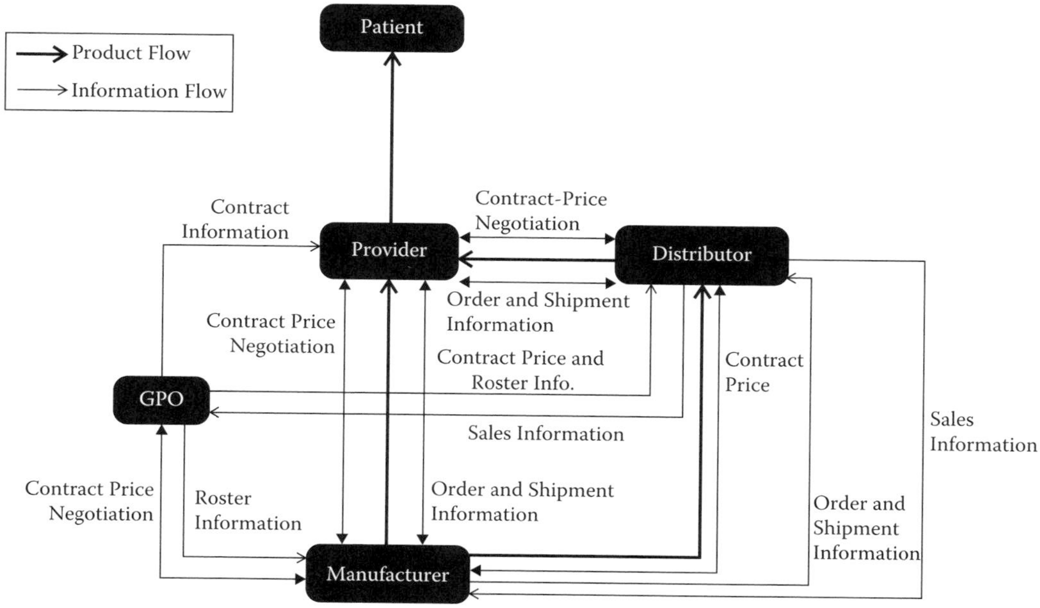

FIGURE 45.1 Product- and information-flows in medical-surgical product supply chains.

* Some providers distinguish between "medical" supplies, which are used in the patient's room and "surgical" supplies, which are generally used only in surgical procedures.

† According to Burns (2002, p. 135), Goldman Sachs analysts estimate that only 16% of medical-surgical products are shipped directly by manufacturers.

depend on the type of product and on the type of service requested (e.g., daily, weekly) and paid for by the provider.

Information-Flow

Order-information flows from the provider to the distributor (by phone, fax, Web-based catalog, etc.) or to the manufacturer. Distributors replenish their inventories by ordering from the manufacturer.

Distributors are obligated to provide information (tracing) about on-contract product sales (e.g., by provider, sales territory) to the manufacturer and to the GPO. Distributors may also provide off-contract sales information to the GPO and/or the manufacturers. Depending on the information technology being used, this sales information might be detailed to specific stock-keeping units (SKUs) and the specific units (i.e., departments) at the provider.

Another set of information flows is related to the role that GPOs play in these supply chains. As part of the process of negotiating prices with manufacturers on behalf of their provider-members, GPOs share their membership rosters with manufacturers. Contract-price information is exchanged between manufacturers and GPOs as new products are introduced, new prices are negotiated, etc. Both the manufacturer and the GPO inform the distributor about the contract price—i.e., what price should be paid for which product by which provider. The GPO communicates contract information (e.g., products, pricing) to its provider-members.

For noncontract items, the provider negotiates directly with the manufacturer and/or distributor.

Dollar-Flow

The dollar-flow for medical-surgical products is diagrammed in Figure 45.2. Table 45.3 describes these flows in tabular form. Burns (2002, pp. 49–51) suggests several possible reasons for this complexity.

For products that providers order directly from manufacturers, providers pay the manufacturer the GPO-negotiated contract price if the product is on contract. If not, then the provider pays the

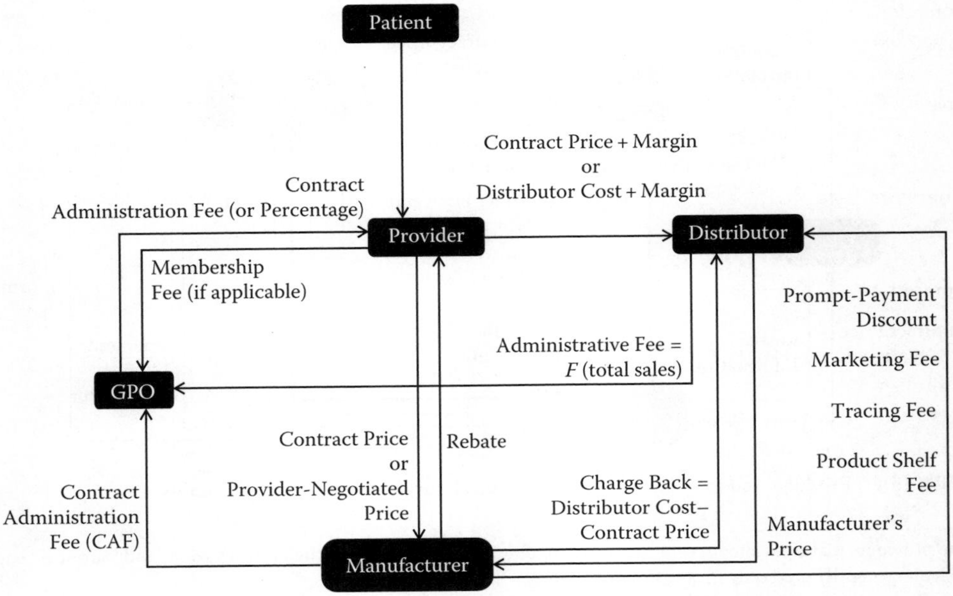

FIGURE 45.2 Dollar-flows in medical-surgical product supply chains.

TABLE 45.3 Dollar-Flows in Medical-Surgical Product Supply Chains

	From Manufacturers	From Distributors	From Providers	From GPOs
To manufacturers	—	Manufacturer's price	Contract price or Provider-negotiated price	—
To distributors	*Marketing fee* Tracing fee Product shelf fee Prompt-payment discount Charge-back = distributor cost − contract-price	—	Contract price + margin or Distributor cost + margin	—
To providers	Rebate	—	—	Contract administration fee (or percentage)
To GPOs	Contract administration fee (1%–3%)	Administrative fee = *F* (total sales)	Member fee (if applicable)	—

manufacturer's list price or a price the provider has negotiated with the manufacturer. The manufacturer may provide a rebate to the provider as an incentive to purchase its products.

Before detailing the dollar-flow involving distributors, it is important to understand that, in general, distributors operate on a "cost-plus" basis. The "cost" part of "cost-plus" is the cost of the product to the distributor; i.e., the price that the distributor pays the manufacturer for the product. The "plus" part is a percentage of the distributor's cost that the provider pays, depending on the services negotiated between the distributor and provider (e.g., delivery size, delivery frequency, and/or packaging). Burns (2002) describes these margins as being in the 1%–2% range. Others describe margins as large as 8%.*

Consider an item with a distributor's cost (i.e., manufacturer's price) of $50. If the provider purchases this item off contract, then the provider will pay the distributor $50 plus a margin. Now, suppose that the item has a GPO-negotiated price of $40—$10 less than the distributor's cost. In this case, the provider will pay the distributor $40 plus a margin. The distributor then "charges back" the difference, $10, to the manufacturer. Hence, Figure 45.2 displays a dollar-flow from the provider to the distributor as "contract price + margin" or as "distributor cost + margin." Figure 45.2 also displays the corresponding dollar-flow between the distributor and the manufacturer: the "manufacturer's price" (distributor's cost) going to the manufacturer and the "charge-back," if appropriate, going to the distributor.

In addition to charge-backs, distributors can avail themselves of prompt-payment discounts (estimated 1%–2%) from manufacturers. Distributors also charge manufacturers "tracing fees" for providing the information they provide to manufacturers about product sales. Distributors may also have negotiated marketing fees with manufacturers to feature their products in catalogs, sales presentations, etc.

The dollar-flows involving GPOs are as follows. Although GPOs negotiate with manufacturers on behalf of their members, they do not typically charge provider-members for this service. Instead, the manufacturer pays a "contract administration fee (CAF)" to the GPO, evidently in order to have its products on contract. CAFs range from 1% to 3% on the total contract value (price × volume) to the

* In some cases, the provider may pay the distributor no (i.e., a zero) margin; and, instead, pay a fixed annual fee-for-services to the distributor.

manufacturer.* In some instances, the CAF is paid by the manufacturer to the GPO at the beginning of the contract; in other instances, at the end of the contract. Some GPOs (e.g., Novation) pass CAF dollars back to their members; others pass back only a portion.† Finally, provider-members may pay a membership fee in order to belong to the GPO.‡

Finally, GPOs receive an "administrative fee" from the distributor in order to be authorized to sell to the GPO's provider-members under contract. This administrative fee is based on, among other things, total distributor sales to the GPO's provider-members (not only on-contract sales) and is in the 0.25%–0.5% range.

One consequence of on-contract vs. off-contract pricing, and the tiered nature of on-contract pricing, is that if the dollars involved in a given transaction are to flow correctly, then every organization in the chain must reconcile the information associated with that transaction. In particular: (1) the provider must verify that it is paying the price it is entitled to; (2) the distributor must charge the correct price and, if appropriate, charge back the correct amount to the manufacturer; (3) the manufacturer must verify the validity and accuracy of the charge-back, if appropriate; and (4) the GPO must verify the entire transaction.

Product-, Information-, and Dollar-Flow for Pharmaceutical Products

In this section, we describe the product-, information-, and dollar-flow for pharmaceutical products. In 2006, it was estimated that pharmaceutical purchases in the United States totaled $214 billion, 78% of the total spent for pharmaceuticals, devices, and medical-surgical supplies. We begin by describing the flows that involve providers (e.g., hospitals). Then we will describe the flows that involve retail/mail-order pharmacies.§

Product-Flow in the Provider Supply Chain

The product-flow and information-flow for pharmaceutical products in the provider supply chain are diagrammed in Figure 45.3. Product-flow is represented by heavy solid lines.

Most pharmaceutical products flow to providers through distributors. So-called specialty distributors are involved in the distribution of high-value, low-volume pharmaceuticals that may require special storage, handling, or delivery. Specialty pharmaceuticals target and treat specific complex conditions, such as cancer, multiple sclerosis, hepatitis C, and HIV/AIDS.

Information-Flow in the Provider Supply Chain

One very important characteristic distinguishes information-flow for pharmaceutical products from other healthcare products: the Food and Drug Administration (FDA) mandates the use of national

* Although such payments are generally regarded as illegal "kickbacks" under the Social Security Act (*Social Security Act 1988*), GPOs are permitted to charge CAFs under so-called "safe harbor" legislation. These CAFS are very controversial. (For example, see http://www.stopgpokickbacks.org/reports.asp.) According to Burns (2002, pp. 80–81), GPOs justify these fees as paying for services provided *to* the manufacturers in terms of maintaining or increasing market share, informing their provider-members about manufacturers' products, etc.

† According to Burns (2002), the portion of the CAF may depend on the provider-member's volume or level of compliance.

‡ According to Burns (2002, pp. 61–62), GPOs offer noncontract services to their members. "These include other cost reduction tools (for example, materials management, contract management, and operations consulting), programs to improve product standardization and reduce product utilization, programs to improve clinical operations (for example, benchmarking, clinical resource management, decision support tools, disease management, and process design), comparative data on supply-chain expenditures, technology management programs,..., insurance services, human resource management, education, marketing, ... and advocacy."

§ According to a 2008 study by Booz Allen Hamilton (conducted for the Healthcare Distribution Management Association), distributors distribute approximately 63% of pharmaceuticals, serving 130,000 pharmacy outlets (retail and provider).

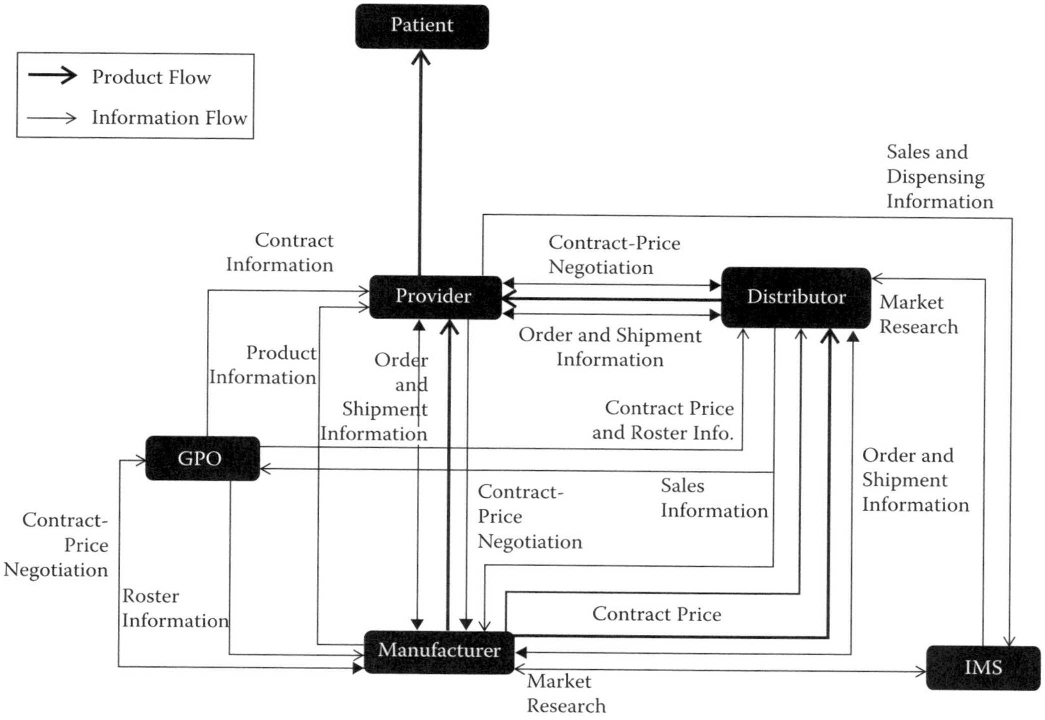

FIGURE 45.3 Product- and information-flows in provider pharmaceutical supply chains.

drug codes (NDCs) for all pharmaceutical products, branded or generic, as these products flow through their supply chains. This permits the tracking of individual batches of pharmaceuticals "up" the supply chain all the way to the manufacturer.* However, NDCs are not used for supply-chain management.

Order-information flows from the provider to the distributor (by phone, fax, Web-based catalog, etc.) or to the manufacturer. Distributors replenish their inventories by ordering from the manufacturer.†

Distributors are obligated to provide information (tracing) about on-contract product sales (e.g., by provider, sales territory) to the manufacturer and to the GPO. Distributors may also provide off-contract sales information to the GPO and/or the manufacturers. Depending on the information technology being used, this sales information might be detailed to specific SKUs and the specific units (i.e., departments) in the provider.

Distributors and providers, for a fee, often provide information about pharmaceutical sales and dispensing to an organization called IMS Health, Incorporated (IMS), which aggregates this information as market research and provides it (for a fee) to distributors and manufacturers.

Another set of information-flows is related to the role that GPOs play in pharmaceutical supply chains. As part of the process of negotiating prices with manufacturers on behalf of their provider-members, GPOs share their membership rosters with manufacturers. Contract-price information is exchanged between manufacturers and GPOs as new products are introduced, new prices are negotiated, etc. Both the manufacturer and the GPO inform the distributor about the contract price; i.e., what price should be

* Sales of controlled substances are routinely reported to the Drug Enforcement Administration (DEA).

† Branded pharmaceuticals are often marketed directly to providers and clinicians by manufacturer sales representatives.

paid for which product by which provider. The GPO communicates contract information (e.g., products, pricing) to its provider-members.

For noncontract items, the provider negotiates directly with the manufacturer and/or distributor.

Dollar-Flow in the Provider Supply Chain

The dollar-flows for pharmaceutical products in the provider supply chain are diagrammed in Figure 45.4. Table 45.4 describes these flows in tabular form.

These flows are similar to those involving medical-surgical products, but with a few important differences. First, there is the flow of dollars associated with IMS: fees paid by IMS to the distributors and providers in exchange for the information they provide; plus the fees paid by the manufacturers for the market research provided by the IMS. Second, there is a "product shelf fee" paid by the manufacturer to the distributor for stocking its products.

Without doubt, the most remarkable characteristic about the dollar-flow for pharmaceutical products involves the price the provider pays the distributor. As described above, medical-surgical products are typically sold on a "cost-plus" basis, where the "cost" is the price the distributor pays the manufacturer—in pharmaceuticals this is typically called the "wholesaler acquisition cost (WAC)—and the "plus" is the distributor's margin. However, for some pharmaceuticals, this margin is zero; i.e., the distributor charges the provider its cost. For other pharmaceuticals, this margin is negative; i.e., the distributor charges the provider less than its cost (i.e., WAC) for the product!

Here are some possible scenarios, all based on a manufacturer's price (WAC) of $100, and a GPO-negotiated price, if applicable, of $25. Note that in each of these scenarios, the distributor, at best, breaks even:

Contract Sale with 0% Margin

The provider-member pays the distributor $25; and the distributor charges back $75 (= $100 − 25) to the manufacturer. Nominally, the distributor earns a contribution to profit and overhead of $0.

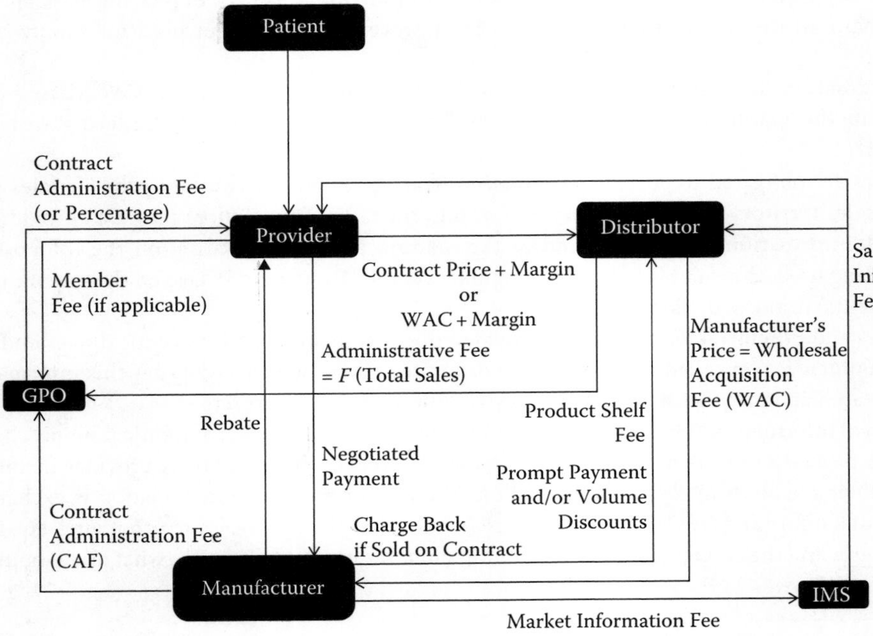

FIGURE 45.4 Dollar-flows in provider pharmaceutical supply chains.

TABLE 45.4 Dollar-Flows in Pharmaceutical Supply Chains

	From Manufacturers	From Distributors	From Retailer/ Mail-Order Business	From Providers	From PBMs	From GPOs (in Provider Supply Chains)	From IMS Health
To manufacturers	—	Wholesale acquisition cost (WAC)	Negotiated payment	Negotiated payment	—	—	—
To distributors	Product shelf fee (2%–7%) Prompt payment and/or volume discount Charge-back = WAC – contracted price	—	Negotiated payment	WAC + margin or contract-price + margin	—	—	Sales information fee
To retailer/ mail-order business	—	—	—	—	Dispensing fee	—	Sales information fee
To providers	Rebate	—	—	—	—	Contract administration fee (or %)	Sales information fee
To GPOs (in provider supply chains)	Contract administration fee (1%–3%)	Administration fee	—	Member fee	—	—	—
To IMS health	Market information fee	—	—	—	—	—	—

Contract Sale with –1.50% Margin

The provider-member pays the distributor \$24.63 = (\$25 – 0.015 × \$25); and the distributor charges back \$75 (= \$100 – 25) to the manufacturer. Nominally, the distributor earns a contribution to profit and overhead of –\$0.37 (i.e., a loss of \$0.37).

Off-Contract Sale with –1.5% Margin

The provider-member pays the distributor \$98.50 (= \$100 – 0.015 × \$100). Nominally, the distributor earns a contribution to profit and overhead of –\$1.50 (i.e., a loss of \$1.50).

How, then, do distributors earn positive contributions to profits and overhead from these transactions? First, through so-called fee-for-service arrangements, manufacturers pay distributors for distributing their products (such fees are estimated to be 1%–3% of the manufacturer's product dollar-flow through the distributor).* Second, through the management of working capital. Here is how: most manufacturers offer discounts (estimated 1%–2%) for payment within 20–30 days. For example, if a provider pays within 10 days, then the distributor has a 10- to 20-day float, which allows it to finance its inventory investment. In the scenarios above, note that a prompt-payment discount of 2% would yield a contribution to profit and an overhead of \$2, \$1.63, and \$0.50, respectively. Third, pharmaceutical

* Such fee-for-service (FFS) arrangements were one of the results of the general demise of "investment buying" (also known as "forward buying") by pharmaceutical distributors. This practice, which was widespread prior to 2002, worked as follows: Given the general upward trend in manufacturers' prices for name-brand pharmaceuticals during the 1990s and early 2000s, distributors developed elaborate systems to forecast *future* price increases. Given an anticipated price increase, distributors would buy large quantities of specific pharmaceuticals at the (then) current price and hold them in inventory. Once the price did increase, distributors were in a position to add this increase to their margins and fees, as described above. Indeed, depending on the size of the price increase, distributors were sometimes able to earn a profit even by charging a negative margin on the higher price.

distributors will sometimes take advantage of quantity discounts from the manufacturer. Fourth, distributors sometimes earn fees from manufacturers for increasing market share.*

Product-Flow in the Retail/Mail-Order Supply Chain

It is estimated that approximately 73% of all pharmaceuticals dispensed in the United States are dispensed through the retail/mail-order supply chain.

The product-flow and information-flow for pharmaceutical products in the retail/mail-order supply chain are diagrammed in Figure 45.5. Product-flow is represented by heavy solid lines. The product-flow is similar to those for provider pharmaceutical supply chains, the only exception being that many large pharmaceutical retailers/mail-order companies distribute their own products to their own outlets rather than have a pharmaceutical distributor distribute them.

Information-Flow in the Retail/Mail-Order Supply Chain

Although GPOs are not involved in retailer/mail-order supply chains for pharmaceuticals, PBMs typically are. In a sense, PBMs play the role of GPOs in these supply chains to the extent that they negotiate, on behalf of their third-party-payer clients, the products to be covered (i.e., the "formulary") in the benefits

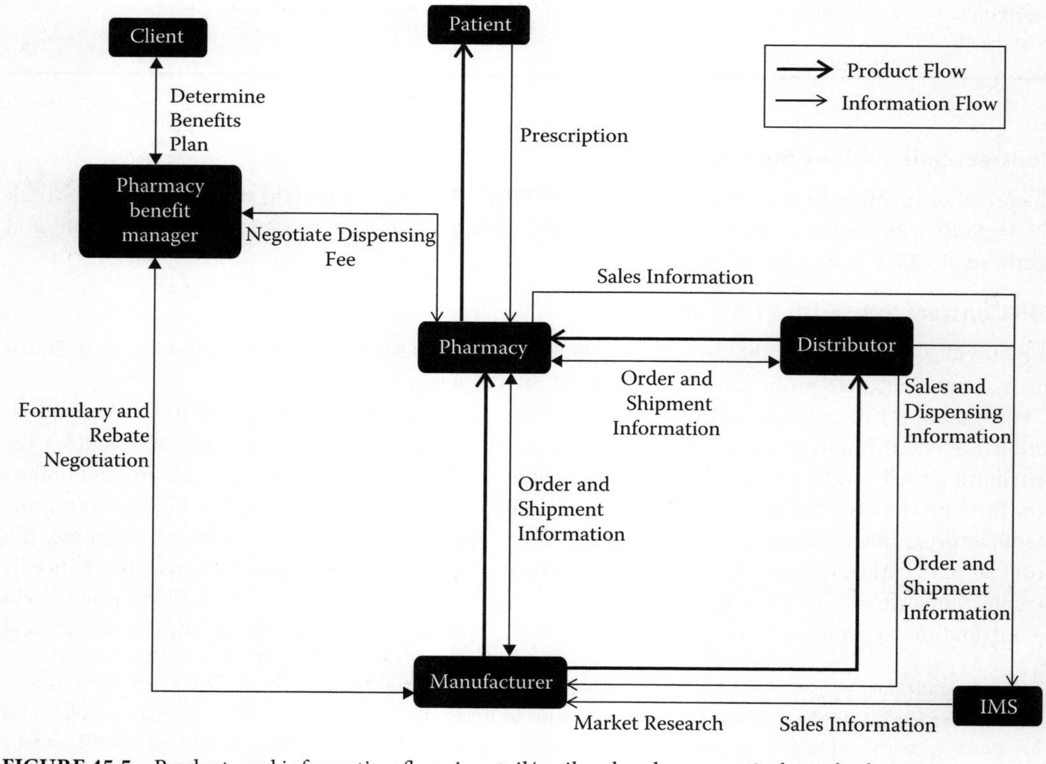

FIGURE 45.5 Product- and information-flows in retail/mail-order pharmaceutical supply chains.

* According to Burns (2002, p. 151), "The bulk of the distributors' gross margins came from manufacturers in the form of cash discounts for prompt payment for products received, manufacturer incentives to promote certain products and to move its own inventory and market share, and inventory profits based on both speculative and non-speculative buying."

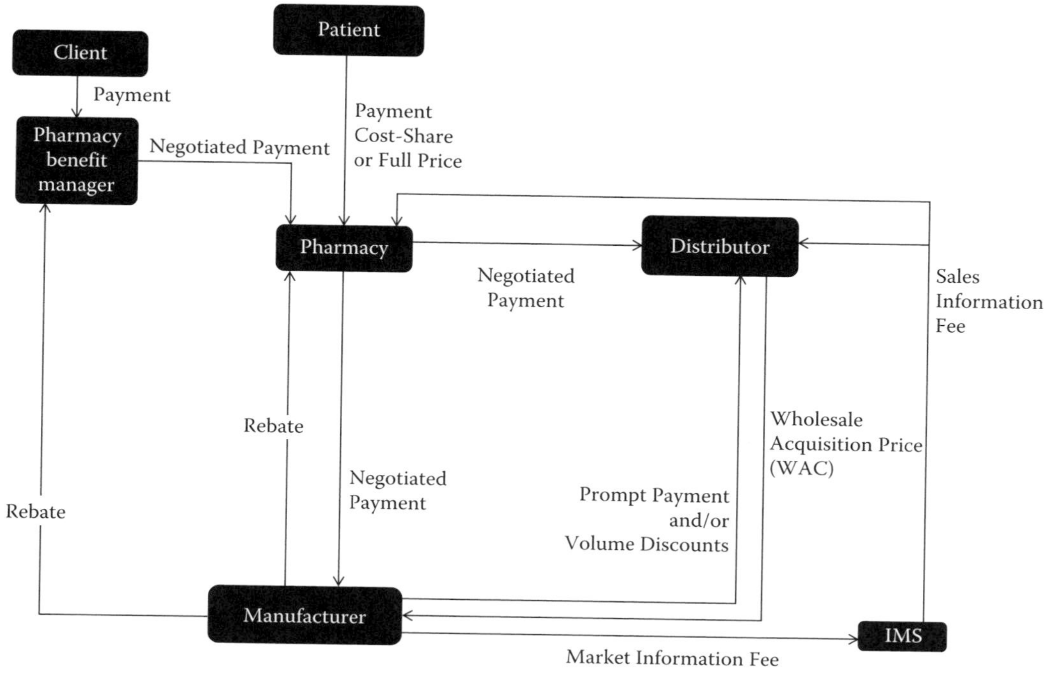

FIGURE 45.6 Dollar-flows in retail/mail-order pharmaceutical supply chains.

plan and the fees that the pharmacy will charge for dispensing pharmaceuticals to patients. Otherwise the information-flows in these chains are quite similar to those in provider pharmaceutical chains.

Dollar-Flow in the Retail/Mail-Order Supply Chain

The dollar-flow for pharmaceutical products in the retail/mail-order supply chain is diagrammed in Figure 45.6. Table 45.4 describes these flows in tabular form. These dollar-flows are similar to those for provider pharmaceutical supply chains, the only exception being those involving the PBMs. The PBMs pay their authorized retail/mail-order pharmacies for their clients' share of the pharmaceuticals' price plus a dispensing fee. PBMs are reimbursed for these fees by their clients, who also pay the PBM an administration fee.

Product-, Information-, and Dollar-Flow for Orthopedic Devices

Up to this point, for simplicity sake, our description of healthcare-product supply chains has ignored the role of the clinician, who, in most cases, is the interface between healthcare-product supply chains and patients. We have also ignored the fact that it is the clinician that prescribes the pharmaceuticals dispensed to patients (and, consequently, that branded pharmaceuticals are typically marketed by manufacturer's representatives directly to providers and clinicians).

However, we have chosen to include the surgeon in describing the supply chains for orthopedic devices in order to highlight the closeness of the relationship between the manufacturer and the surgeon.

Since the surgeon typically specifies the "make and model" of the device to be used in the patient, device manufacturers want surgeons to be knowledgeable about their products and how to use them. From the surgeon's perspective, this marketing/education process begins in medical school, and continues through their participation, as practicing surgeons, in manufacturer-sponsored workshops that

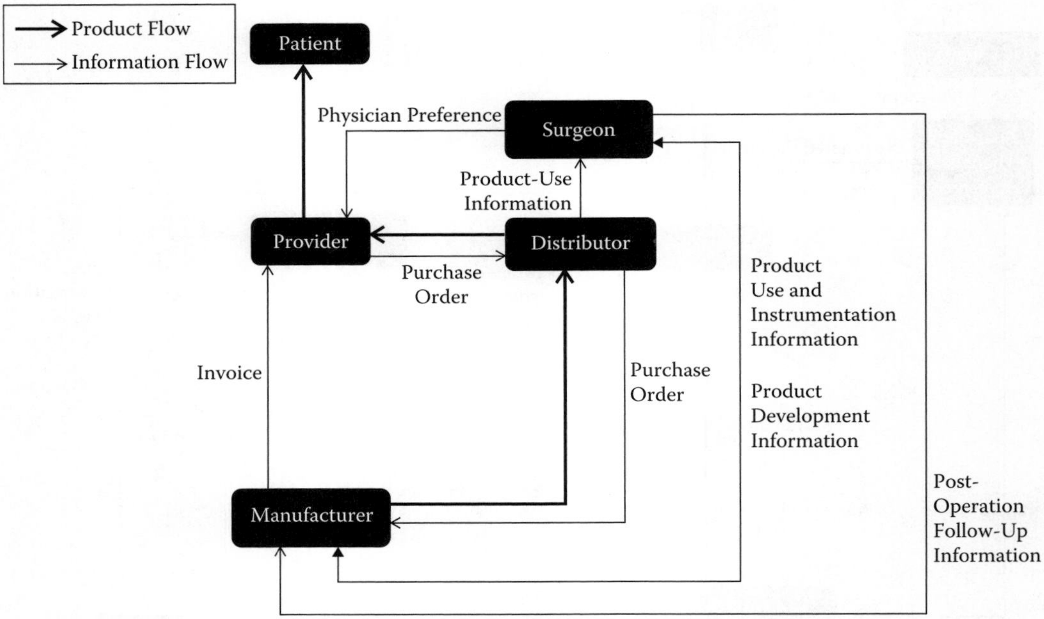

FIGURE 45.7 Product- and information-flows in orthopedic device supply chains.

feature the manufacturer's products. Manufacturers and their distributors also employ representatives with extensive product knowledge to call on surgeons. Sometimes these representatives are present during the surgeries, in order to provide product and process advice to the surgeon.

On the other hand, GPOs are not typically involved in the supply chains for orthopedic devices. To the extent they are, the corresponding product, information, and dollars among the organizations involved are similar to that for medical/surgical products.

Hence, GPOs are excluded and a surgeon is included in the product-flow and information-flow for orthopedic devices, diagrammed in Figure 45.7. Product-flow is represented by heavy solid lines.

Product-Flow

Another characteristic that distinguishes orthopedic-device supply chains from other healthcare-product supply chains is that device distributors typically represent only a single orthopedic manufacturer (e.g., Zimmer), although they operate as separate businesses—i.e., purchasing products from the manufacturer and selling to providers.

Despite the fact that orthopedic devices are fit to individual patients during surgery, the manufacturer produces them on a make-to-stock basis. Similarly, orthopedic distributors maintain inventories of devices. In some instances, the provider (e.g., hospital) also maintains an inventory of commonly used orthopedics and replenishes these inventories as they are used. It is reported that manufacturers'/distributors' representatives sometimes "vendor manage" these inventories for the provider. It is also reported that, when involved in a specific surgery, the manufacturer's/distributor's representative may bring with her/him a set of products or tools for possible use during that surgery.

Information-Flow

As described above, there is a great deal of information provided by manufacturers to surgeons regarding the development and use of their products. This information is supplemented by on-site information

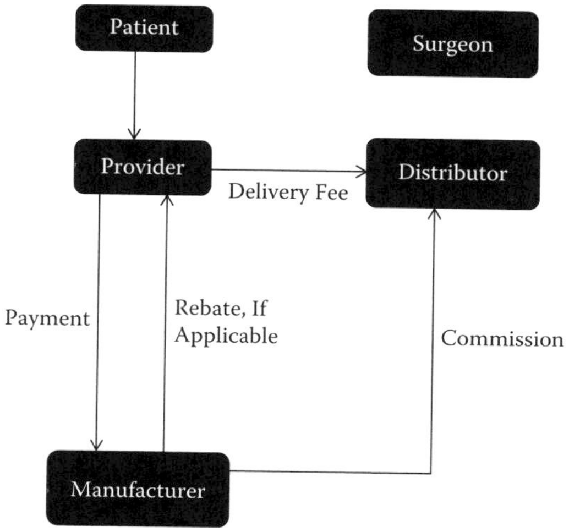

FIGURE 45.8 Dollar-flows in orthopedic device supply chains.

provided to the surgeon by the distributor. In addition, the surgeon provides post-operation information to the manufacturer regarding follow-up visits with the patient.

Purchase orders for devices specified by the surgeon are issued by the provider to the distributor, who forwards it to the manufacturer. Subsequently, the manufacturer invoices the provider for the item(s) purchased.

Dollar-Flow

The dollar-flow for orthopedic devices is diagrammed in Figure 45.8.

The provider pays the manufacturer for devices purchased and, if appropriate, receives a rebate from the manufacturer. The manufacturer pays a sales commission to the distributor. The provider may also pay a material loan and/or delivery fee to the distributor.

References

Burns, L. R., 2002. *The Health Care Value Chain*. San Francisco, CA: Jossey-Bass.

Burns, L. R. and J. A. Lee. 2008. Hospital purchasing alliances: Utilization, services, and performance, *Health Care Management Review*, 33(3):203–215.

Projections. 2006. U.S. Department of Health and Human Services, Centers for Medicare and Medicaid Services, Office of the Actuary, National Health Statistics Group, 2005 National Health Care Expenditure Data.

Schneller, E. S. 2009. The value of group purchasing—2009: Meeting the needs for strategic savings. *Health Care Advances, Inc.* San Francisco, CA: Jossey-Bass.

Design, Planning, Control, and Management of Healthcare Systems

IV.L Tracking and Information Systems

46 **Wireless Sensor Network** *James A.C. Patterson, Raza Ali, and Guang-Zhong Yang* **46**-1
Introduction • Wireless Sensor Networks • Body Sensor Networks: On-Board Processing • Trend and Behavior Analysis • Future of WSN in Healthcare • References

47 **Bar Coding in Medication Administration** *Ben-Tzion Karsh, Tosha B. Wetterneck, Richard J. Holden, A. Joy Rivera-Rodriguez, Hélène Faye, Matthew C. Scanlon, Pascale Carayon, and Samuel J. Alper* **47**-1
Introduction • BCMA Basics • BCMA Adoption • BCMA and Safety Outcomes • BCMA and Nursing Work • BCMA and Physician Administration • BCMA with Pediatric Patients • Conclusion • Acknowledgments • References

48 **Clinical Decision Support Systems** *Sze-jung Sandra Wu, Mark Lehto, and Yuehwern Yih* **48**-1
Introduction • Conclusions • References

49 Health Informatics: Systems and Design Considerations *Jose Antonio Valdez and Rupa Sheth Valdez* **49**-1
What Is Health Informatics? • Systems Context of Health Information Technologies • Designing Health Information Technologies • References

50 Privacy/Security/Personal Health Record Service *Jeff Donnell* **50**-1
Prevalence of Paper • Makeshift Solutions • Medical Consumerism • Enter the PHR • Paper and Privacy • Privacy of Electronic PHRs • HIPAA • Privacy Policy • ARRA and Privacy • PHRs and Privacy: Where to From Here?

46

Wireless Sensor Network

Introduction 46-1
Wireless Sensor Networks 46-3
Wireless Networking • Wireless Sensor Network Platforms
Body Sensor Networks: On-Board Processing 46-6
Context-Aware Sensing • Autonomic Sensing • Embedded Data Enhancement
Trend and Behavior Analysis 46-9
Activity Monitoring • Behavioral Analysis through Data Mining • Detecting Anomalies
Future of WSN in Healthcare 46-14
Clinical Uptake of Technology • Improved On-Node Processing • Miniaturization • Prediction • Data Standardization
References 46-15

James A.C. Patterson
Imperial College London

Raza Ali
Imperial College London

Guang-Zhong Yang
Imperial College London

Introduction

The average age of the population is increasing rapidly. Trends indicate that more than a third of the population of developed countries will be aged 60 or over by 2050 (World Population Ageing, 1950–2050, 2002). Older people require significantly greater healthcare resources, for both treatment and management of ailments. Thanks to modern medicine, a large number of diseases that used to be fatal are now treatable. However, many of these, such as diabetes and hypertension, will remain as chronic conditions that require continued management over the lifetime of the patient. This has resulted in a significant strain on healthcare systems. The financial burden of burgeoning healthcare needs has led to research into effective, low-cost alternatives to traditional medical practice, including pervasive healthcare enabled by body sensor networks (BSNs) (Yang, 2006).

In addition to lowering healthcare cost, providing care at home increases convenience and independence for patients and social careers. Avoiding frequent visits to healthcare facilities also reduces exposure to potential hospital infections. Postoperative recovery can be managed at home (Lo et al., 2007), reducing hospital stay after surgery. Many illnesses, for instance cardiac related, are associated with infrequent, yet potentially life-threatening episodes. Traditional assessment in a clinical laboratory-based environment has a low probability of catching transient events. The provision of continuous, pervasive sensing is set to transform our future of managing patients with chronic diseases. One important opportunity provided by such a sensing scheme is the early detection of disease through behavior profiling (Atallah et al., 2007). The onset or complication of a disease may be preceded by changes in patterns of behavior or activity. Changes in sleeping patterns, social activity, or eating, for example, can be due to gastroesophageal reflux, heart disease, and urinary tract infections. Changes in gait can indicate recovery from injury or exacerbation of it, or according to recent research, even neurological diseases such as dementia (Verghese et al., 2002).

TABLE 46.1 Clinical Requirements

Requirement	Approaches
Intuitive visualizations and user interfaces	Data abstraction, information-rich graphical user interfaces, decision support systems
High-resolution, context-rich data	Information utility directed sampling, incorporation of metadata, integration with medical systems
Privacy	Network encryption, bio-inspired immune systems, data anonymization, privacy preserving data mining
Disease-specific sensing	Sensing modalities and algorithms targeted to specific patient conditions, adaptive systems
Variable subject lifestyle	Sensing modalities and algorithms adaptive for different lifestyles and habits, robust sensors, on-board storage for storing data locally when out of network
Scalability	Distributed processing, on-board processing, autonomic sensing
Fault tolerance	Hardware and software failure recovery, feature redundancy, decoupled software components, autonomic sensing
Communication reliability	Local/on-board storage, autonomic sensing
Ergonomics and wearability	Miniaturization of hardware, contour-adaptive and unobtrusive devices, wireless communication

Nevertheless, pervasive sensing is still in its infancy. To be successful, it needs to meet several critical requirements both technically and clinically. These requirements are driven by the diverse stakeholders of this technology, which includes patients, clinicians, care-providers, researchers, and financial stakeholders. Some requirements, such as privacy, reliability, and fault tolerance, are crucial. Other requirements, such as intuitive visualizations and decision support systems, are needed if the system is to be adopted at a large-scale by care-providers. Table 46.1 lists some of the requirements that pervasive healthcare systems should aim to meet.

Addressing these requirements has led to the development of wireless BSN platforms (Yang, 2006), which is a subset of the wider field of wireless sensor networks (WSNs). BSN takes advantage of recent advances in low-power, low-cost wireless communications and embedded processors to implement miniaturized, ubiquitous healthcare monitoring systems. The general WSN is a distributed infrastructure of multiple autonomous sensor nodes which communicate with each other to create a pervasive monitoring system. A WSN node integrates a sensor, embedded processing, energy storage, and wireless communications into a single physical entity in order to perform both data acquisition and data distribution. To make the acquired data available outside of the sensor network, a combination of on-node embedded processing and wireless communications gives WSN many beneficial characteristics over traditional wired networks.

Foremost of these characteristics is the obsolescence of physical cabling. This can dramatically reduce the cost of deploying a sensor network infrastructure. Embedding a processor on each node provides robustness through autonomous interaction with the node's environment. By enabling WSN to detect if local communication channels or neighboring nodes fail and ensure that action is taken to compensate for these failures. Such action could be either rerouting the data paths of the wireless network or informing an observer, external to the network, where the faulty node is located. The range of applications that WSN can provide a solution for is continually expanding and with each new application comes a different set of challenges (Juang et al., 2002; Werner-Allen et al., 2005). However, combining wireless networking with sensors on its own will not provide a pervasive healthcare solution. Meeting clinical requirements will involve the combination of WSN hardware with novel solutions of how and where to process sensor data.

Wireless Sensor Networks

A BSN is a good illustration of the complexities involved in a WSN. There are three main types of sensor that can constitute a BSN: ambient sensors, wearable sensors, and implantable sensor. Also, each network node can be classified as being fixed or mobile (Figure 46.1).

Wireless Networking

At the very core of a pervasive monitoring system is the wireless network itself. Some of the key characteristics that drive the specification of a WSN platform are the number of sensor nodes, node location (e.g., wearable, implantable, ambient), node mobility (fixed, mobile), lifetime of the monitoring process (hours, days, weeks), the volume of data propagating through the network, and the reliability of the network. Derived from these functional specifications are more detailed technical specifications. For example, the location of a node may determine the maximum size of the node which in turn drives the amount of energy that can be stored. Combining the specification of energy storage with the lifetime requirement will specify the allowable power consumption of the node. Table 46.2 provides a list of sensor network characteristics from which a monitoring system can be specified.

Although a wireless network is not physically constrained by cables, it still needs some form of system architecture to determine how data are to be routed between sensor nodes. The arrangement of links between member nodes of a network is defined by a *topology*. As there are no cables to define the links between nodes, there is a lot of inherent flexibility in the choice of topology for wireless networks. While it is possible to use classical wired network topologies such as point-to-point, star, and ring for a WSN, they are designed for the requirements of a wired network. More adaptable topologies such as wireless mesh networks offer a more ad hoc solution to the requirements of WSN by defining a protocol to allow the network nodes to self-organize the network structure—even as the number and arrangement of nodes and links change throughout the lifetime of the network (Akyildiz et al., 2005).

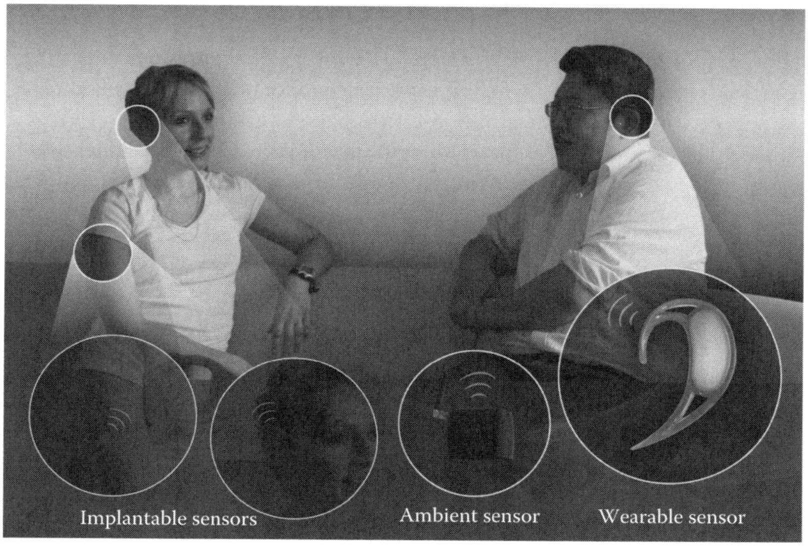

FIGURE 46.1 A BSN consisting of wearable, implantable, and ambient sensors for pervasive monitoring of a patient's health and lifestyle.

TABLE 46.2 Sensor Network Characteristics

Characteristic	Description	Challenges
Network scope	Size of the network based on geographical area and number of nodes associated with the network	Integrating low-power wireless personal area networks into wide-area networks to provide massive scope
Network capacity	Limit on the total amount of data that the network can handle in a given period of time	Minimizing the amount of raw data transferred across the network by performing data processing on-node
Network dynamics	How much the structure of the network changes over its lifetime as nodes move with respect to one another, join and leave the network	Finding a balance between flexibility and security where the access to sensor data cannot be compromised by node failure or malicious intruders
Node range	Maximum distance between nodes likely to be experienced	Reducing range lowers power consumption, but limits the network scope unless more nodes can be added
Node lifetime	Length of time a node must function properly without external intervention (for energy replenishment, repair, etc.)	Increasing lifetime predominantly means reducing power consumption. Introducing autonomy to nodes will provide robustness against failure
Node power source	Fixed external power source, battery powered or energy scavenging	Developing MEMS-based scavenging devices with power density to match battery- and fuel-based sources
Node data rate	Maximum amount of data that a node can transmit in a given period	Lowering the data rate with on-node processing will lead to reduced power consumption
Node conformity	If the node is to coexist and cooperate with other devices, it will have to conform to regulations and standards	Developing radio and communications standards specifically to meet clinical requirements
Node environment	Wearable and implantable devices have vastly differing requirements to differing geographical environments	Biocompatibility for implantable devices; increased temperature and humidity range, increased electromagnetic interference for wearable devices
Network security	What level of privacy is required for the data propagating through the network and how restricted is general access to the network	Encryption and authentication methods need to address both safety criticality of medical systems and low power consumption of embedded systems

The number of sensor nodes and the geographical area covered by a network determine the scale of a network. Consider a typical pervasive healthcare scenario where one or more healthcare professionals are required to remotely monitor the health of multiple patients from a single access point in a clinic. The scale of this network is potentially huge; it could have a radius of many miles and contain thousands of nodes. If each patient is to be monitored by multiple sensors, then it is less efficient for each sensor node to have to communicate over a direct connection to the clinician's monitoring terminal as would be the case for a star network topology. The communication range of each node would be too high to allow a low-power design methodology and the monitoring terminal would have to be shared by multiple healthcare professionals and manage an inconveniently large number of incoming physical connections (i.e., high fan-in). A more practical approach is to create a hierarchical structure where network nodes are classified by type and then tiered by their ability to communicate over a given range. This multi-tier architecture also leverages the rapid development in wireless mobile communication in recent years. For instance, wearable sensor nodes which are mobile and have the strictest constraints on power consumption populate the lowest tier of the hierarchy. Ambient sensor nodes, which can occupy fixed locations, afford larger power sources, and higher communication data rates, provide an intermediate tier on the hierarchy between the mobile sensor networks and an Internet Protocol (IP)-based network that can provide a gateway connection to the monitoring terminal using either a wide-area cellular network device, such as a 3G data modem, or to connect to a local WLAN-based Internet gateway (Konstantas and Herzog, 2003; Atallah et al., 2008) (Figure 46.2).

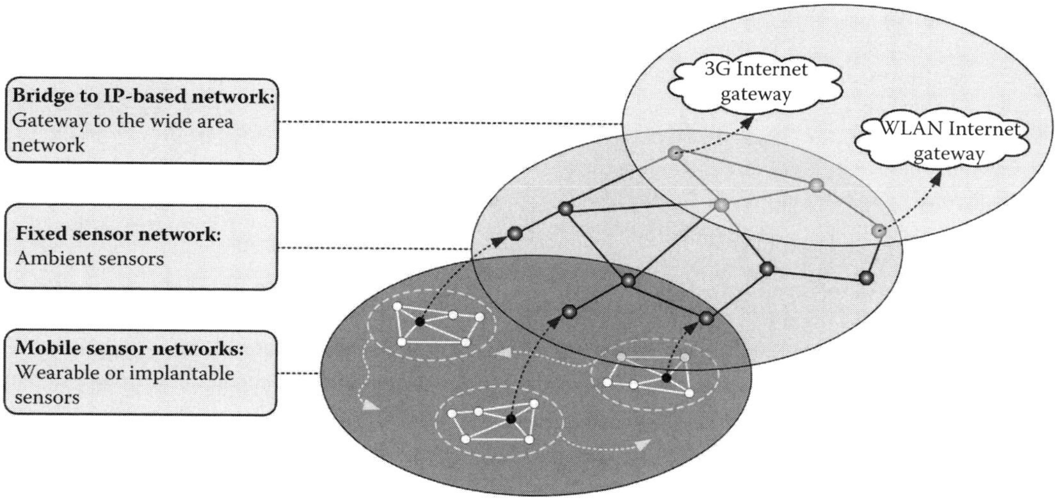

FIGURE 46.2 A multi-tier pervasive monitoring structure illustrating the key levels of abstraction in network node functionality.

Wireless Sensor Network Platforms

The development of a pervasive healthcare monitoring system, at the very least, requires sufficient electronic hardware to collect and condition the data from the sensor and to transmit the data into the wireless network. In reality, more data analysis and system control ability is required if the sensor node is to have any level of autonomy. Generally, this means the inclusion of a processor core and a wireless receiver on-node to allow two-way communications. Figure 46.3 illustrates the typical hardware system architecture required to implement a modern BSN node.

The autonomy of a sensor node relies on the ability to acquire data from the sensor, manage its power consumption, and maintain its connection to a wireless network. The quickest and most flexible method is to implement the processing and control algorithms in software—this requires the use of a microprocessor. Developed specifically for the requirements of low-power, low-cost embedded processing applications is the *microcontroller*, which integrates a processor core with *read only memory* (ROM) for storing programs and *random access memory* (RAM) for running those programs. In addition to memory, microcontrollers generally include peripheral interface circuitry such as digital counters and communication ports (e.g., UART, SPI, I^2C). Three of the most common families of microcontrollers available today are the PIC® family from Microchip®, the AVR® family from Atmel®, and the MSP430™ family from Texas Instruments. These have become a popular choice for both professional embedded circuit designers and hobbyists due to the wide variety of peripherals offered, comprehensive design support, and low cost. This type of device is suited to wearable sensors where power consumption and size are primary concerns.

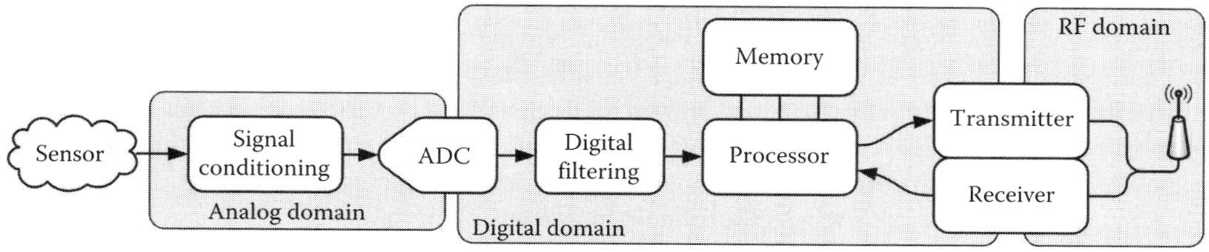

FIGURE 46.3 System architecture of a wireless sensor node.

For more data-intensive requirements, such as vision-based ambient sensors, where more processing power and memory is required, there are system-on-chip (SoC) solutions that incorporate much more powerful processor cores than microcontrollers (e.g., 32-bit data width compared to 8 or 16 bit), and the peripherals can perform more complex functions such as a USB interface or an Ethernet MAC. Example devices are the Marvell PXA family of application processors. This added functionality and performance does not leave much room for memory on-chip so external RAM and ROM is generally required for an application processor. These devices consume much more power than microcontrollers so are more suited to applications such as gateway nodes where it is possible to have a more substantial power source than is possible on a sensor node.

Rather than addressing all the difficulties of building bespoke wireless communications circuitry, most WSN platforms use a COTS digital radio transceiver. The semiconductor industry has produced a wide range of single-chip radio solutions. Low-level transceivers, such as the nRF24L01+ from Nordic Semiconductor®, only perform the radio modulation and data packet addressing on chip and higher functionality to be implemented in software by a separate microcontroller. This allows a designer flexibility in implementing a full radio communications solution, but comes at the cost of increased design effort. Alternatively, there are devices such as the BlueCore™ family of Bluetooth® chips from CSR and CC2480 ZigBee® processor from Texas Instruments which have the low-level radio frequency (RF) circuitry integrated with a simple processor core. The purpose of the processor core is to perform the software-intensive tasks of implementing the full communications protocol to leave only the user applications to be implemented on another chip.

A sensor outputs some form of electrical signal that is representative of a physical quantity that the system is trying to monitor. It is the task of the sensor interface to convert the electrical signal from the sensor into a form that is acceptable for either transmission into the wireless network or computational processing on the sensor node itself. Due to the digital nature of microcontrollers and the wireless communications used by almost all WSNs, it is essential that the signal from the sensor be digitized. Most physical phenomena are continuous in nature so the electrical signals generated by sensors tend to be analog, and an analog-to-digital converter (ADC) is required. Often microcontrollers have ADCs integrated as a peripheral device so no extra components are required for the sensor interface save for anti-aliasing filters.

Some sensors integrate ADCs into the device to provide a digital output. To keep the pin count of a sensor to a minimum, the digital signal can be serialized so a microcontroller can access the data with a serial port using the SPI or I^2C protocols. Another form of digitization is pulse width modulation (PWM) where a binary signal represents an analog signal by the percentage of time the signal is high (i.e., dutycycle). A microcontroller converts the signal by timing the dutycycle and calculating its percentage of the period. Analog Devices offer a microelectromechanical system (MEMS) based accelerometers with all three types of interface—the ADXL204, ADXL213, and ADIS16003, which are all two-axis accelerometers with analog, PWM, and SPI interfaces, respectively.

Body Sensor Networks: On-Board Processing

Traditional WSNs work on an *acquire-and-transmit* methodology where data captured continuously from a sensor are sent into the wireless network, with minimal processing being performed on the data beyond basic spectral noise reduction (i.e., averaging). Having a large accumulation of raw sensor data is fine for research purposes where it is required to test and validate new analytical techniques, but it is too costly, in terms of power consumption and robustness, for a clinically viable healthcare delivery solution. Moving the role of data processing from a PC to the sensor node itself can minimize the usage of the wireless data connection, allowing conservation of energy reserves and increased data integrity. BSNs aim to provide a healthcare-specific solution by addressing the issues of deciding how to interpret sensor data, if and how to react to sensed events, and how to actually implement the data processing on the sensor node.

Context-Aware Sensing

Context-awareness is the ability of a sensing system to observe how underlying trends affect an object. In the case of healthcare monitoring, these trends can indicate how the lifestyle of a patient is affecting their health or even how a course of treatment is affecting the patient's lifestyle. The raw data provided by a sensor, or a combination of sensors, might not directly present contextual information, although the data are influenced by the underlying context. As an example, an electrocardiogram (ECG or EKG) provides a measurement of heart rate, but to determine the fitness of the person requires knowing how their cardiac function is affected by physical activity. In this case, the sensor system is made context-aware by adding activity recognition (Seon-Woo and Mase, 2002). Activity recognition systems based on a range of motion sensors have received a significant amount of research interest and will be addressed in more detail later.

For BSNs, detecting underlying health trends is not the only purpose of context-aware sensing. Knowing how the ambient environment is affecting a measurement gives the sensor system the ability to compensate for the induced artifacts. One of the most studied environmental influences on sensors is temperature drift. Resistors and semiconductor devices can be particularly sensitive to temperature, although compensating for the drift is a well-understood process. However, the ubiquitous nature of BSNs means they will experience a much wider range of physical effects than just temperature drift. A sensor on a mobile patient will experience considerably more motion than a bed-bound patient, and the effect on a sensor can be illustrated with another heart rate measurement example. Photoplethysmography (PPG) can be used to measure heart rate by detecting how a pulse of blood through the capillaries modulates the optical transmission or reflection properties of the tissue that the PPG sensor is attached to. This technique works well on a stationary patient, but a moving patient introduces mechanical changes in the optical path which in turn induce *motion artifacts* into the photometric signal that reduce the ability of the sensor to detect heart rate.

Removing motion artifact from PPG measurements is a well-studied problem, and there are commercial systems such as the pulse-oximeters from Masimo (Graybeal and Petterson, 2004) that can address motion artifact, but it is designed specifically for the clinical environment—not for mobile patients. Commercially available pulse-oximeters tend to use *a priori* knowledge of how patient motion is likely to corrupt the PPG signal, but for a wearable PPG heart rate monitor context-aware sensing is a much more robust approach. Thus far, there are different approaches that rely on an extra measurement to compensate for motion artifact. For example, Asada et al. proposed using an accelerometer to measure the physical motion of a wearable PPG sensor and then using this extra information as an input to an adaptive filter that reduces the motion-induced corruption component of the signal (Asada et al., 2004).

Autonomic Sensing

The advantage of using the context-aware approach for correcting measurement corruptions is the robustness it provides by allowing the sensor to adapt to its environment. This is the first step in making the sensor node being fully self-sufficient or *autonomous*. Originating from the concept of *autonomic computing* (Kephart and Chess, 2003), *autonomic sensing* contrives to describe how a system containing a large number of sensor nodes can be managed by distributing the required control system intelligence throughout the nodes themselves rather than requiring a central, isolated administration controller. Each node should perform the tasks of management, configuration, optimization, healing, protection, adaptation, integration, and scaling (the so called *self-** properties) for themselves to make the sensing system autonomic (Yang, 2006).

In wireless sensors, preserving sensor energy reserves by minimizing the usage of power-hungry resources, such as radio communication, is an important goal for long-term operation. In the context of healthcare, the physiological state of the user can be used to adapt resource utilization. If the utility of information for patient states can be specified, the resource utilization of sensors can be adjusted according to the current state with a view to maximizing utility. This is the approach taken by Talukder et al. (2005). In this case, several sensors are used to monitor a patient's state, with known utility for specific states. Utilizing a genetic algorithm-based controller, the operation of sensors is adjusted in order to match the quality of information with the utility of the patient state. Here quality is measured in terms of both the sensing modality and the sampling rate. While one method relies on a centralized controller residing on the gateway (Talukder et al., 2005), the controller is shifted to the nodes themselves by Anand et al. (Panangadan et al., 2005), relying on a simpler Markov model to perform resource management. The controller is also shown to operate in more dynamic environments; the controller meets design imperatives (e.g., a minimum operating life) when the system model is not close to the real deployment conditions.

As noted earlier, an important requirement for pervasive sensing is fault tolerance. Dynamic operating conditions make it likely that some sensors may be faulty, out of range, or out of power. Data processing can explicitly be designed with a view to feature redundancy and minimization of communication. This is the approach taken by Thiemjarus and Yang (2007), who develop a multi-objective Bayesian framework for feature selection that can be used for robust distributed inferencing. Features are selected that optimize data redundancy and discriminative power and lower communication cost.

Inspiration for how to implement an autonomic system can be sought in nature, as in swarm intelligence. With swarm intelligence, relatively simple agents interact locally, but collective intelligence over a global scale emerges, allowing the system to perform complicated tasks. Wang et al. (2007) utilize the swarm intelligence framework for discovering and maintaining routing information in dynamic network settings. Another example of how the architecture of WSN is close to biological systems is security. Systems inspired from the *biological immune system* offer a useful multi-tier encapsulation of security requirements (Yang, 2006; Ko et al., 2008) that mimic the behavior of the auto-immune system, adapted to sensors design, and network communication.

Embedded Data Enhancement

In practice, rarely is the data acquired direct from a sensor a direct representation of the underlying event being monitored. For example, a PPG sensor outputs a period signal representative of the cardiac cycle, but to measure the heart rate requires an algorithm to determine the periodicity of that cycle. A software-based solution typically uses some form of peak detection algorithm in conjunction with a timer to measure the waveform's period. In this case, the algorithm is simple enough for even the most basic microcontroller to implement, but more mathematically intensive feature extraction methods will require a sensor node transmitting raw data over the wireless connection to a more powerful processor. This approach is unsuitable as a fundamental requirement of BSNs is to minimize the usage of such resources in order to maximize operating lifetime.

Performing the feature extraction on the sensor node is not solely for reducing the power consumption, but is essential for autonomy. A system that does not have to transmit sensor data for analysis will be far more responsive to external stimulus. In addition to improved response time, the node will be able to acquire and analyze useful data even if the node moves out of the communication range. Closing the control loop on-node means finding a solution to the opposing requirements of low power consumption and strong mathematical computational power. The problem lies with relying on the digital representations of data as is required by the memory storage and wireless communications components of a sensor node. To increase the computational power of a digital processor, it requires either more processing time to implement complex functions from combinations of more simple programs (e.g., calculating a logarithm using the Taylor's series) or using bespoke digital circuitry to perform the calculation (e.g., performing a multiplication with a binary multiplier circuit (Macsorley, 1961) as opposed to an accumulator loop in software). Both of these methods require additional transistors for the required extra program memory or custom circuitry respectively. Generally a balance is struck between the two methods, with the software solution being cheaper and the hardware method being faster. For autonomic sensing, neither solution is suitable as the inherent mathematical complexity in feature extraction would require too much memory and take too long to calculate if performed in software, and the extra circuitry required to perform it digitally in hardware would blow the budget on device power consumption and size.

Compared to digital electronics, analog circuitry is rich in mathematical properties. Addition and subtraction are implemented purely by Kirchhoff's current law, derived from the conservation of charge principle, where the sum of the currents flowing into a node must equal the sum of the currents flowing out of the node. Multiplication and division can be performed by converting linear signals into logarithmic signals using either bipolar transistors or CMOS transistors biased in the sub-threshold region. In the log domain, addition and subtraction are equivalent to multiplication and division in the linear domain. This translinear process is the basis of the Gilbert multiplier cell which only requires eight transistors to perform a full four-quadrant multiplication (Gilbert, 1968).

From the late 1980s, analog and mixed-signal artificial neural networks (ANNs) have received a considerable amount of interest and led to the development of a number of analog implementations such as the cellular neural network, self-organizing neural networks, and the SeeHear chip (Chua and Yang, 1988; Mann and Gilbert, 1989; Mead, 1989). These forms of ANNs have not yet found widespread use in commercial products due to their complexity in the design phase and relative specificity in feature extraction ability. To implement a useful mixed-signal ANN requires tens to hundreds of neuron which may require thousands of transistors (Lei et al., 2008). Modeling this kind of circuit with traditional Simulation Program with Integrated Circuit Emphasis (SPICE)-based simulators would take a very long time—even when using modern multicore processors. Contemporary analog behavioral modeling tools such VHDL-AMS and Verilog-AMS are more suited to this scale of system and should lead to reduced development times for mixed-signal ANNs (Michel and Herve, 2004).

Trend and Behavior Analysis

Information accumulated from continuous operation of the BSN enables long-term analysis. In the context of healthcare, this refers to understanding a person's routines, activities, and habits. Key indicators of well-being that can be inferred from sensor measurements include sleeping patterns, social interaction, gait, regular eating, and exercise. A noticeable change in any of these can indicate a health issue (Atallah et al., 2007; Katz et al., 1970). Furthermore, a person's lifestyle can be inferred from the extent of activities in said person's daily routine A recent study has shown that morbidly obese people have low activity levels for most of the day (Vanhecke et al., 2009).

There has been some use of monitoring through wearable or ambient sensors to encourage specific types of behavior. For instance, in the field of assisted living, elderly people are given advice on ways to improve their lifestyle on the basis of sensor information (Edwards et al., 2000; Maciuszek et al., 2005).

Smart home technology (Chan et al., 2008) relies on sensors (usually ambient) to provide intelligent environments that can be assistive to occupants, typically elderly occupants. The home may also facilitate the operation of devices in the house based on sensed information. The sensors utilized in these projects include temperature, water flow and utility usage sensors as well as pressure sensors on furniture, proximity sensors for tracking users' position in rooms, as well as devices for monitoring vital signs. Data from these sensors can be analyzed to observe patient behavior or to detect the occurrence of critical events such as falls.

Sensors that detect a user's activities are useful for behavior profiling, although physiological and location information can be used to provide additional context. Such sensors can be either body-worn or ambient. However, there are limitations of using ambient sensing alone for tracking user behavior. The analysis is complicated by the presence of other users in the sensed environment. Detailed records of changes in activity and physiological data are difficult to obtain with just ambient sensing.

In addition, wearable devices can track the user outside their home environments. Several studies have shown increased classification rates when ambient sensing is combined with wearable sensing (Pansiot et al., 2007).

In order to implement a system capable of analyzing trend and behavior requires the ability to detect and monitor activity, and the utilization of data mining and anomaly detection techniques with a view toward describing and predicting health.

Activity Monitoring

Activity monitoring has been an intensely researched area over the past decade (Lo et al., 2007; Atallah et al., 2007; Thiemjarus and Yang, 2007; Pansiot et al., 2007). In the context of studying behavior, it is important not only to detect the user's activity, but also to assess how this activity is being performed. For example, the gait of a user could be indicative of exacerbations in medical conditions. The activities performed can also characterize the extent to which a person is capable of living independently. The Katz activities of daily living (ADL) index is one such measure of the autonomy of a person (Katz et al., 1970).

In general, activity analysis can be divided into two broad tasks. The first is *activity detection*, which is the near-instantaneous detection of current user state based on a typically small time horizon. Subsequently, temporal aspects can be introduced, which is called *activity modeling*. To some extent, the distinction between the tasks can be seen on the basis of complexity. In the first case, "atomic" activities such as standing, sitting, walking etc. are detected. In the second, more complex activities that can be temporally composed of atomic activities are detected, for example, food preparation and eating. At this level, concurrent activities can be interleaved or pursued at the same time.

A first step in any system aiming to profile behavior over the long term is to detect atomic activities of users. This can range from providing specific information about the user's current activity, such as brushing teeth or reading, to abstracted, yet still medically relevant information such as the current intensity of activity. An example of this type of activity recognition is the work by Ravi et al. (2005), where the activities recognized include standing, walking, running, climbing upstairs and downstairs, sit-ups, vacuuming, and brushing teeth. Activities were detected using data collected from a triaxial accelerometer worn on the pelvic region. Four features are extracted from the data for each axis: mean, standard deviation, correlation, and energy. The authors compare the performance of different classifiers using these features.

While precise information about a user's activity provides valuable information for further mining, a pragmatic reason for avoiding this is the issue of user privacy. Lo et al. (2007) have developed a multivariate Gaussian Bayes classifier that produces an activity level from an ear worn accelerometer. The classifier defines activity in four values, the lowest of which indicates almost no movement (e.g., sleeping) and the highest indicates an activity involving vigorous movement (e.g., running). Quantitative measures of activity have been used in cardiorespiratory fitness studies (Vanhecke et al., 2009) and postoperative recovery (Lo et al., 2007). Low levels of activity have also been associated with type-II diabetes (Kriska et al., 2003).

A recent direction of research has been to analyze the transitions between activities. Joint diseases such as arthritis can impair the ability of patients to fluidly transition between activity states. More than two million people over 65 experience difficulty in rising from a chair. This difficulty has been associated with the likelihood of falls (Topper et al., 1993). A natural application therefore arises to detect disability based on this transition. A further application is compliance with physiotherapy guidelines on the optimal method of transitioning for such patients.

A decision-tree classifier is trained to discriminate between sit-to-stand strategies based on single and multiple sensors in Allin and Mihailidis (2008). A more general framework for transition detection and analysis is described in Tenenbaum et al. (2000). The raw sensor data are first segmented. Each consecutive pair of segments is then analyzed for transitions between them. This is performed by first embedding the data into a lower dimension manifold space.* The local neighborhoods of the manifold are represented in a graph, which is partitioned. The partitions represent principal activities. Segments that represent a transition between the partitions are identified based on the manifold geometry (Figure 46.4).

It is worth noting that most of the existing work on activity recognition is limited to detecting atomic activities. Sequences of atomic activities can be temporally composed into more complex activities through generative models such as hidden Markov model (HMM) (Olivier et al., 2005). In addition to their modeling power, HMMs amortize the computation cost and can be trained offline and deployed online with relatively small computation cost. The HMM shown in Figure 46.5a contains two layers: an observable and a hidden layer of states. The hidden states are governed by a Markov model—a model where future behavior depends only on the present state. Each observable state is related to a hidden state via an observation probability. In Figure 46.5a, A1 can represent a simple activity, such as preparing breakfast. The hidden states, shown as circles, indicate separate stages that comprise preparing

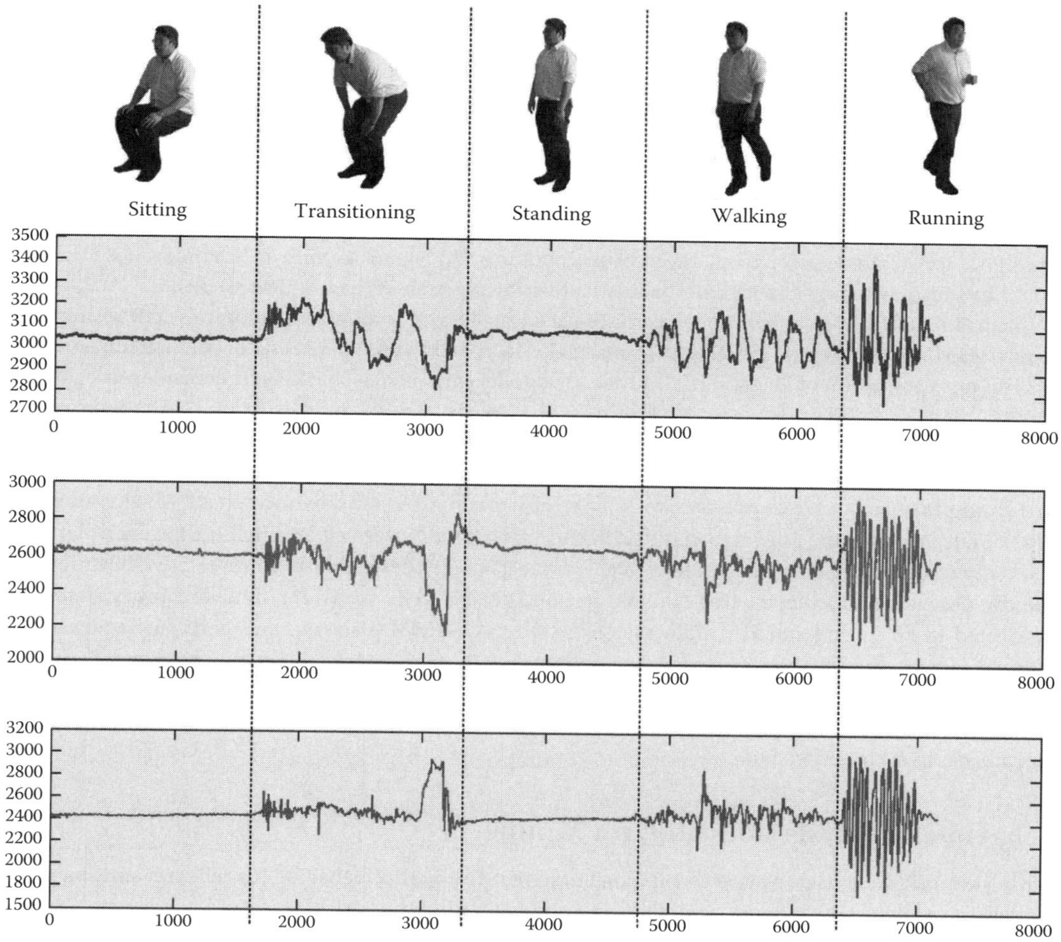

FIGURE 46.4 Transient activity detection, changes in dynamic behavior, such as sitting to standing, could indicate underlying health issues such as arthritis.

* Manifold methods, such as IsoMap (Tenenbaum et al., 2000), are nonlinear dimensionality reduction techniques that preserve the geometric properties of the data

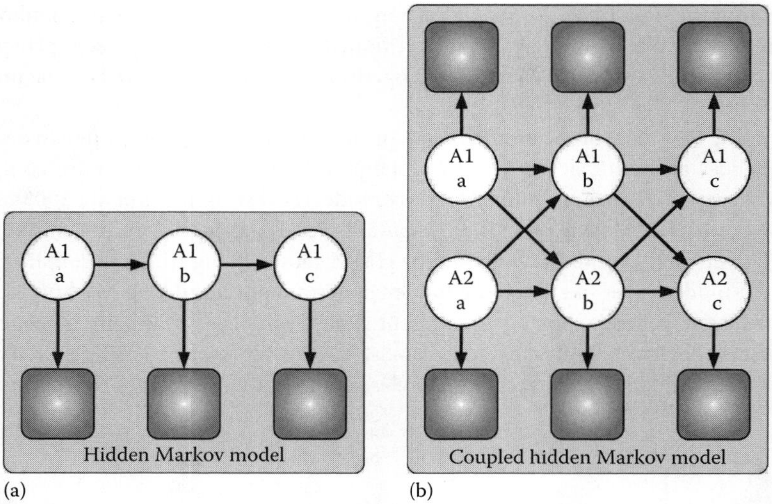

FIGURE 46.5 HMMs used in activity recognition: (a) illustrates a simple activity, such as preparing breakfast, where the circles represent the constituent tasks involved in the overall process and shaded boxes represent observations made by sensors. For more complex activities, a coupled HMM (b) allows a collection of HMMs to represent multiple interleaving activities.

breakfast, for example, preparing ingredients, cooking food, and serving it. Example observations would be sensor readings that can probabilistically indicate each of these hidden states.

Extensions of HMMs allow modeling of more complex and interleaving activities. For example, a coupled HMM (Brand et al., 1997), shown in Figure 46.5b, allows the modeling of concurrent activities by utilizing a collection of HMMs. In this case, the model can "switch" between independently evolving Markov models. Another extension of HMMs is that of hierarchical models. Hierarchical approaches for modeling activity and behavior mirror research in the field of ethology (the biological study of behavior) where hierarchy has been shown to be underlying certain kinds of behavior (Dawkins, 1976). One example of such an extension is work is the abstract hidden Markov model (AHMM) (Bui et al., 2002). Plan recognition is the artificial intelligence problem of inferring an intelligent agent's plans—a hierarchy of actions that allow an agent to carry out its goal. These actions however are deterministic, and the observations are error free. This limitation is resolved by the AHMM, where policy states are connected to an underlying HMM. A system based on AHMM discriminates between sequences of actions, such as different strategies of movement in an office space. Based on this, the user is classified as having a particular "plan" based on a predefined plan library. AHMM offers a powerful model for defining how low level activities compose into higher level plans and allows the inference of the goals of subjects based on their behavior.

Behavioral Analysis through Data Mining

With the emergence of pervasive sensing technologies, the goal of behavior modeling is shifting from modeling and detecting individual activities to understanding the typical structure of a person's activities. One instance of this is capturing daily routines. Living beings have *circadian rhythms* (Gachon et al., 2004), 24-hour cycles in their behavioral, biochemical, and physiological processes. Healthy people have characteristic circadian rhythms, deviations from which can indicate a change in the state of health.

Behavior is manifested over a period of time, and therefore methods designed to analyze large datasets, such as those developed in the field of data mining, can be utilized. Frequent pattern mining is one such problem in data mining, related to searching for frequently repeating patterns in a database.

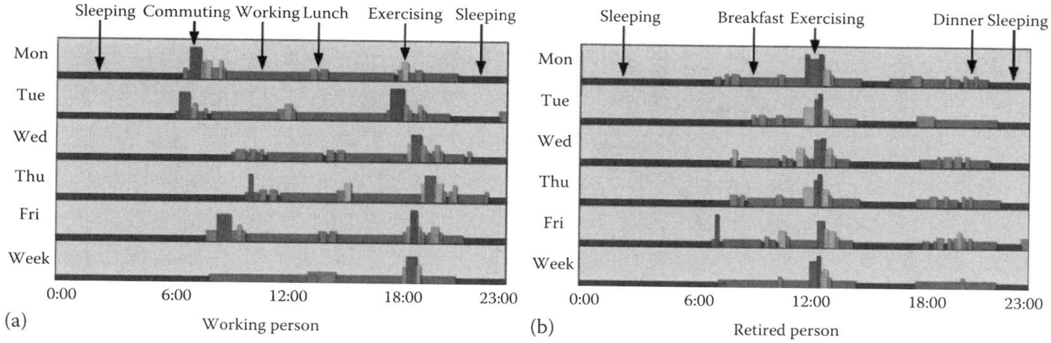

FIGURE 46.6 Routine trees used for visualizing the activity patterns of a user. Presented here are simulated daily routines of two different users: (a) an office worker and (b) a retired person. The height of each bar is proportional to the intensity of an activity, making it easy to interpret a user's activity profile without any specialist data analysis training.

A pattern is considered to be frequent if its occurrence in the database (called support) is above a user-specified threshold. Lühr et al. (2007) use an extension of frequent pattern mining in a smart home to model temporal relationships in activities. Data are obtained from activations on object sensors. Associations between these activations are mined over the long term, and the extended mining algorithm allows these associations to span database transactions. An example of these approaches can be learning typical paths taken by users in moving between rooms or the sequence of objects activated during a typical kitchen task.

An effort to associate patterns of activity with time has been taken in Ali et al. (2008), where a data structure, called *routine tree*, is constructed to represent a 24-hour period of activity data. Activity data is progressively mined at finer resolutions in order to obtain a compact, multiresolution tree data structure. The frequent pattern mining algorithm Closet+ is used; the patterns generated are detected with the time period, which is a node in the tree. Figure 46.6 shows visualizations generated from the leaves of the pattern tree (information at the highest resolution), which provided a high-level picture of a person's day. Alternatively, the whole tree can be visualized, showing a temporal hierarchy of activity patterns with different degrees of specificity. The visualizations are geared to be easily understandable for nonspecialists in data analysis, such as healthcare professionals. Figure 46.6 shows profiles of the activity patterns during a day of two individuals, the first an office-going user and the second a retired person with scheduled exercise visits. Shorter bars indicate lower intensity activity (e.g., sleep or no activity), and conversely taller bars indicate activities involving more movement (e.g., exercise). Activity patterns are plotted against a time-grid. Not only is the general structure of the day apparent from this, but important health indicators can be analyzed. For instance, the first individual routinely exercises in the evening and is active throughout the day. On the other hand, there is little activity in the retired person's routine aside from the scheduled activity, and much of the day is spent resting. This indicates the importance of the scheduled exercises to this user: in their absence, the user may lead a completely sedentary, unhealthy lifestyle as some individuals have been shown to be prone to (Vanhecke et al., 2009).

Detecting Anomalies

Anomaly detection algorithms seek to find deviation from normal behavior in a given dataset. It involves detecting meaningful change in the activities, transitional activities, or routines of the user. The variable nature of human activity and behavior makes this is a challenging area of research.

The movement of a user from room to room can be represented as a sequence of symbols on a temporal grid. Two such activity grids are shown in Figure 46.7 to illustrate different behaviors. Figure 46.7a shows a user spending most of their time in the living room and kitchen while Figure 46.7b shows a user

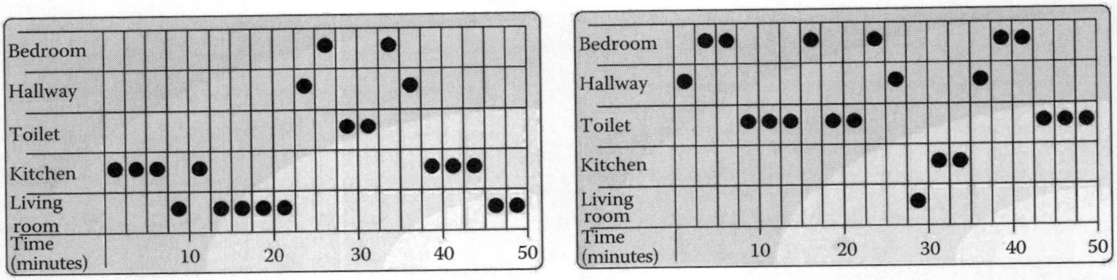

(a) (b)

FIGURE 46.7 Intuitive activity grids used to visualize a user's overall behavior pattern in a home environment. These two simulated activity grids illustrate contrasting behavioral patterns: (a) the user spends most time in the living room and (b) more time is spent in the bedroom and toilet indicating anomalous behavior.

spending most of their time in either the bedroom or toilet which may be indicative of a health issue. For each sequence, an HMM is trained on a selected reference sequence from the dataset. These trained HMMs can then be used to analyze new sequences based on the distance of the given sequence to the trained models. Sequences with large distances can be identified as anomalous.

Li and Parker (2008) utilize a Fuzzy-ART (adaptive resonance theory) neural network supplemented with a Markov model to detect abnormal events generated by ambient sensors. The neural network categorizes raw sensor data, with each category representing a state in the Markov model which then learns the state transitions during normal behavior. Detection of anomalous behavior is based on state occupancy time by recording the average time spent in each state during normal behavior.

One such approach is a behavior profiling system for elderly patients residing in a smart home (Mori et al., 2008). The smart home is equipped with ambient pyroelectric (i.e., location) sensors tracking the time a patient spends in each room. Behavior is tracked by maintaining a Gaussian mixture model (GMM) of room occupancy duration at different time periods. Changes are detected at two scales. The first is at the level of "local anomaly" where an outlier detection algorithm is used to detect behaviors with unlikely timing or duration. For example, an inordinate time spent in the bedroom would be classified as an anomaly. The second is a "global anomaly" where changes in the model are tracked over longer time periods. Daily differences in behavior are computed and an anomaly is flagged if a sudden change in 1 day exceeds a threshold after discounting for seasonal variations.

One of the key problems in anomaly detection is to determine when it is actually likely to indicate the onset of an adverse event as opposed to the normal variation in behavior. This relates to the concept of *Interestingness*, i.e., the importance of discovered knowledge to the application at hand. Ohsaki et al. (2007) consider this with respect to the analysis of medical data. Incorporating interestingness into the capabilities of BSN can ensure the medical relevancy of any anomalies detected.

Future of WSN in Healthcare

Clinical Uptake of Technology

As pervasive systems move from research laboratories into people's homes and from toy problems to addressing real healthcare concerns, it is very clear that there is a wide scope and range of challenges that need to be met. Healthcare systems are critical for the well-being of their users; failure in this domain comes at a very high cost, which is a significant reason for why the adoption of this technology has been with caution and deliberation. To take BSN-based healthcare monitoring solutions to commercial reality will require investment of both time and money in clinical trials to prove to regulatory boards the validity of pervasive healthcare devices and its clear patient management advantages.

Improved On-Node Processing

A major hurdle to overcome is finding a way of embedding processing power capable of providing context-awareness without compromising power consumption. Digital processors have always been preferred to analog computational methods as they can be reprogrammable and are not constrained by circuit noise in the same way that analog circuits are despite the power and silicon area overheads required to implement mathematics in digital circuitry. Bio-inspired circuitry such as analog ANNs has huge computational potential, but will require significant research and development effort to transform it into a clinically viable solution.

Miniaturization

Current BSN development platforms are still too large to be truly unobtrusive as a wearable or implantable sensor device due to their multichip, PCB-based construction. Modern packaging techniques, such as system-in-package (SiP) (Wei, 2005) and three-dimensional integrated circuits (3D-IC) (Schaper, 2008), take advantage of the third dimension to drastically increase the amount of silicon that can fit onto a given area of circuit board. It is these modern IC packaging techniques that offer the best opportunities in reducing the physical outline of sensor nodes for minimal intrusion to the sensing environment while increasing the amount of on-node processing that can be performed.

Prediction

With an adequate framework for capturing behavior and enhanced metadata, it is possible to predict likely states of the user and potentially identify at risk patients early based on their current behavior. As yet, there has been relatively little research in predicting future health states based on behavior, especially in the context of pervasive sensing. Recent research (Nor et al., 2008) by the (World Health Organization) WHO provides a framework for finding patterns of health-related events. The framework enables the association of key medical events, such as the prescription of a new medicine, with likely future events.

Data Standardization

One promising technology to assist with the metadata requirement is electronic medical record (EMR) systems. Increasingly medical records are computerized. Integrating pervasive healthcare systems with EMR systems could provide a wealth of metadata to supplement sensor data, which can be used by behavior profiling and data mining algorithms. Another technology worth exploring is the field of medical ontologies, such as Unified Medical Language System (UMLS) and SNOMED (http://www.nlm.nih.gov/research/umls/Snomed/snomedmain.html). As pervasive systems discover deeper medical information, capturing that and sharing with the medical community in a standardized format will be important.

References

Akyildiz, I.F., X. Wang, and W. Wang. 2005. Wireless mesh networks: A survey. *Computer Networks* 47(4):445–487.

Ali, R. et al. 2008. Pattern mining for routine behaviour discovery in pervasive healthcare environments. In *5th International Conference on Information Technology and Application in Biomedicine* (ITAB), pp. 241–244, Schenzen, China.

Ali, R. et al. 2009. Transitional activity recognition with manifold embedding. In *6th International Workshop on Wearable and Implantable Body Sensor Networks* (BSN 2009), pp. 98–102, Berkeley, CA.

Allin, S. and A. Mihailidis. 2008. Sit to stand detection and analysis. In *AI in eldercare: New solutions to old problems. Papers from the AAAI Fall Symposium*, AAAI, Arlington, VA.

Analog Devices, Inc. iMEMS® Accelerometers. Norwood, MA, Available from: http://www.analog.com/en/mems-and-sensors/imems-accelerometers/products/index.html

Asada, H.H., J. Hong-Hui, and P. Gibbs. 2004. Active noise cancellation using MEMS accelerometers for motion-tolerant wearable bio-sensors. In *26th Annual International Conference of the IEEE Engineering in Medicine and Biology Society, 2004* (IEMBS '04), pp. 2157–2160, San Francisco, CA.

Atallah, L. et al. 2007. Behaviour profiling with ambient and wearable sensing. In *4th International Workshop on Wearable and Implantable Body Sensor Networks*, pp. 133–138, Aachen, Germany.

Atallah, L. et al. 2008. Wirelessly accessible sensor populations (WASP) for elderly care monitoring. In *Second International Conference on Pervasive Computing Technologies for Healthcare. PervasiveHealth 2008*, Tampere, Finland.

Atmel Corporation. 8bit AVR microcontrollers. San Jose, CA, Available from: http://www.atmel.com/dyn/resources/prod_documents/doc2467.pdf

Brand, M., N. Oliver, and A. Pentland. 1997. Coupled hidden Markov models for complex action recognition. In *Proceedings of the 1997 IEEE Computer Society Conference on Computer Vision and Pattern Recognition*, p. 994, San Juan, PR.

Bui, H., S. Venkatesh, and G. West. 2002. Policy recognition in the abstract hidden Markov models. *Journal of Artificial Intelligence Research* 17:451–459.

Chan, M. et al. 2008. A review of smart homes-Present state and future challenges. *Computer Methods and Programs in Biomedicine* 91(1):55–81.

Chua, L.O. and L. Yang. 1988. Cellular neural networks: Theory. *Circuits and Systems, IEEE Transactions* 35(10):1257–1272.

CSR. Single-chip Bluetooth®: An overview of BlueCore design options. Cambridge, U.K., Available from: http://www.csr.com/products/bcrange.htm

Dawkins, R. 1976. Hierarchical organization: A candidate principle for ethology. In *Growing Points in Ethology*, P.G. Bateson and R.A. Hinde (eds.), Cambridge, U.K.: Cambridge University Press.

Edwards, N. et al. 2000. Life-style monitoring for supported independence. *BT Technology Journal* 18(1):64–65.

Gachon, F. et al. 2004. The mammalian circadian timing system: From gene expression to physiology. *Chromosoma* 113(3):103–112.

Gilbert, B. 1968. A precise four-quadrant multiplier with subnanosecond response. *Solid-State Circuits, IEEE Journal* 3(4):365–373.

Graybeal, J.M. and M.T. Petterson. 2004. Adaptive filtering and alternative calculations revolutionizes pulse oximetry sensitivity and specificity during motion and low perfusion. In *26th Annual International Conference of the IEEE Engineering in Medicine and Biology Society, 2004* (IEMBS '04), pp. 5363–5366, San Francisco, CA.

Juang, P. et al. 2002. Energy-efficient computing for wildlife tracking: Design tradeoffs and early experiences with ZebraNet. *SIGARCH Computer Architecture News* 30(5):96–107.

Katz, S. et al. 1970. Progress in development of the index of ADL. *Gerontologist* 10(1):20–30.

Kephart, J.O. and D.M. Chess. 2003. The vision of autonomic computing. *Computer* 36(1):41–50.

Ko, A., H. Lau, and N. Lee. 2008. AIS based distributed wireless sensor network for mobile search and rescue robot tracking. In *Proceedings of the 7th International Conference on Artificial Immune Systems*, pp. 399–411, Phuket, Thailand.

Konstantas, D. and R. Herzog. 2003. Continuous monitoring of vital constants for mobile users: The MobiHealth approach. In *Proceedings of the 25th Annual International Conference of the IEEE Engineering in Medicine and Biology Society*, Cancun, Mexico.

Kriska, A.M. et al. 2003. Physical activity, obesity, and the incidence of type 2 diabetes in a high-risk population. *American Journal of Epidemiology* 158(7):669–675.

Lei, W. et al. 2008. Toward a mixed-signal reconfigurable ASIC for real-time activity recognition. In *5th International Summer School and Symposium Medical Devices and Biosensors*, ISSS-MDBS 2008, pp. 227–230, Hong Kong.

Li, Y.Y. and L.E. Parker. 2008. Detecting and monitoring time-related abnormal events using a wireless sensor network and mobile robot. In *International Conference on Intelligent Robots and Systems* (IROS), pp. 3292–3298, Nice, France.

Lo, B. et al. 2007. Real-time pervasive monitoring for postoperative care. In *4th International Workshop on Wearable and Implantable Body Sensor Networks*, pp. 122–127, Aachen, Germany.

Lühr, S., G. West, and S. Venkatesh. 2007. Recognition of emergent human behaviour in a smart home: A data mining approach. *Pervasive and Mobile Computing* 3(2):95–116.

Maciuszek, D., J. Aberg, and N. Shahmehri. 2005. What help do older people need?: Constructing a functional design space of electronic assistive technology applications. In *Proceedings of the 7th International ACM SIGACCESS Conference on Computers and Accessibility*, pp. 4–11, Baltimore, MD.

Macsorley, O.L. 1961. High-speed arithmetic in binary computers. *Proceedings of the IRE* 49(1):67–91.

Mann, J.R. and S. Gilbert. 1989. An analog self-organizing neural network chip. In *Advances in Neural Information Processing Systems*, pp. 739–747. San Francisco, CA: Morgan Kaufmann Publishers Inc.

Marvell Semiconductor, Inc. Marvell PXA applications processor family. Santa Clara, CA, Available from: http://www.marvell.com/products/cellular/applications.jsp

Mead, C. 1989. *Analog VLSI and Neural Systems*, p. 371. Boston, MA: Addison-Wesley Longman Publishing Co., Inc.

Michel, J. and Y. Herve. 2004. VHDL-AMS behavioral model of an analog neural networks based on a fully parallel weight perturbation algorithm using incremental on-chip learning. In *IEEE International Symposium on Industrial Electronics*, 2004, Ajaccio, France.

Microchip Technology, Inc. PICmicro microcontrollers from microchip. Chandler, AZ, Available from: http://www.microchip.com/stellent/idcplg?IdcService=SS_GET_PAGE&nodeId=74

Mori, T. et al. 2008. Anomaly detection algorithm based on life pattern extraction from accumulated sensor data. In *International Conference on Intelligent Robots and Systems*, pp. 2545–2552, Nice, France.

Nor, G.N. et al. 2008. Temporal pattern discovery for trends and transient effects: Its application to patient records. In *Proceeding of the 14th ACM SIGKDD International Conference on Knowledge Discovery and Data Mining*, pp. 963–971, Las Vegas, NV.

Nordic Semiconductor, Inc. nRF24L01+ datasheet. Sunnyvale, CA, Available from: http://www.nordicsemi.com/files/Prod_brief_RFSilicon_nRF24L01p.pdf

Ohsaki, M. et al. 2007. Evaluation of rule interestingness measures in medical knowledge discovery in databases. *Artificial Intelligence in Medicine* 41(3):177–196.

Olivier, C., M. Eric, and R. Tobias. 2005. *Inference in Hidden Markov Models* (*Springer Series in Statistics*). New York: Springer-Verlag Inc.

Panangadan, A., M. Ali, and A. Talukder. 2005. Markov decision processes for control of a sensor network-based health monitoring system. In *Proceedings of the Seventeenth Conference on Innovative Applications of Artificial Intelligence*, pp. 1529–1534, Menlo Park, CA.

Pansiot, J. et al. 2007. Ambient and wearable sensor fusion for activity recognition in healthcare monitoring systems. In *4th International Workshop on Wearable and Implantable Body Sensor Networks* (BSN 2007), pp. 208–212, Aachen, Germany.

Ravi, N. et al. 2005. Activity recognition from accelerometer data. In *Twentieth National Conference on Artificial Intelligence*, Pittsburgh, PA.

Schaper, L.W. 2008. 3D-SiP: The latest miniaturization technology. In *IEEE 9th VLSI Packaging Workshop of Japan, 2008*, VPWJ 2008, pp. 3–6, Kyoto.

Seon-Woo, L. and K. Mase. 2002. Activity and location recognition using wearable sensors. *Pervasive Computing, IEEE* 1(3):24–32.

Talukder, A. et al. Predictive controller for heterogeneous sensor network operation in dynamic environments. In *Proceedings of the IEEE/RSJ International Conference on Intelligent Robots and Systems, 2005* (IROS 2005), pp. 1710–1716, Las Vegas, NV.

Tenenbaum, J.B., V.D. Silva, and J.C. Langford. 2000. A global geometric framework for nonlinear dimensionality reduction. *Science* 290: 2319–2323.

Texas Instruments, Inc. CC2480 network processor. Dallas, TX, Available from: http://www.ti.com/corp/docs/landing/cc2480/index.htm

Texas Instruments, Inc. Getting started with MSP430. Dallas, TX, Available from: http://focus.ti.com/mcu/docs/mcugettingstarteddetail.tsp?sectionId=97&tabId=1511&familyId=342

Thiemjarus, S. and G.Z. Yang. 2007. An autonomic sensing framework for body sensor networks. In *Proceedings of the ICST 2nd International Conference on Body Area Networks*, Florence, Italy, Institute for Computer Sciences, Social-Informatics and Telecommunications Engineering (ICST).

Topper, A.K., B.E. Maki, and P.J. Holliday. 1993. Are activity-based assessments of balance and gait in the elderly predictive of risk of falling and/or type of fall? *Journal of the American Geriatrics Society* 41(5):479–487.

Vanhecke, T.E. et al. 2009. Cardiorespiratory fitness and sedentary lifestyle in the morbidly obese. *Clinical Cardiology* 32(3):121–124.

Verghese, J. et al. 2002. Abnormality of gait as a predictor of non-Alzheimer's dementia. *New England Journal of Medicine* 347:1761–1768.

Wang, J. et al. 2007. A swarm intelligence inspired autonomic routing scenario in ubiquitous sensor networks. In *Proceedings of the 2007 International Conference on Multimedia and Ubiquitous Engineering*, IEEE Computer Society, Seoul, Korea.

Wei, K. 2005. System in package (SiP) technology applications. In *Sixth International Conference on Electronic Packaging Technology*, pp. 61–66, Shenzhen, China.

Werner-Allen, G. et al. 2005. Monitoring volcanic eruptions with a wireless sensor network. In *Proceedings of the Second European Workshop on Wireless Sensor Networks*, Istanbul, Turkey.

World Population Ageing: 1950–2050. 2002, United Nations Department of Economic and Social Affairs—Population Division. New York.

Yang, G.Z. (ed.) 2006. *Body Sensor Networks*, London: Springer-Verlag.

47

Bar Coding in Medication Administration

Ben-Tzion Karsh
University of Wisconsin–Madison

Tosha B. Wetterneck
University of Wisconsin–Madison

Richard J. Holden
University of Wisconsin–Madison

A. Joy Rivera-Rodriguez
University of Wisconsin–Madison

Hélène Faye
Institut de Radioprotection et de Sûreté Nucléaire

Matthew C. Scanlon
Medical College of Wisconsin

Pascale Carayon
University of Wisconsin–Madison

Samuel J. Alper
Exponent

Introduction 47-1
BCMA Basics 47-2
BCMA Adoption 47-4
BCMA and Safety Outcomes 47-5
BCMA and Nursing Work 47-6
Time on Task and Perceptions of Medication Administration • BCMA Problems and Problem Solving • BCMA and Interruptions • BCMA Workarounds and Violations
BCMA and Physician Administration 47-9
BCMA with Pediatric Patients 47-10
Conclusion 47-10
Acknowledgments 47-11
References 47-11

Introduction

Research applying human factors and safety engineering to patient safety dates back to at least 1960 (Chapanis and Safren 1960, Safren and Chapanis 1960) to a study on hospital medication errors by one of the founders of human factors engineering (Chapanis). The authors concluded, among other things, that a variety of risks existed in the medication process including hard-to-read decimal places in drug orders, use of abbreviations, poor handwriting, difficult drug labels, poor arrangement of drugs in the pharmacy, and distractions. Recently, especially in hospital settings, many of those risk factors, and resultant medical errors, are receiving renewed attention (Institute of Medicine 2000, 2001, 2007).

Among medical errors, it is estimated that about 19% are medication errors (Leape et al. 1991), of which 40% are believed to occur in the administration and dispensing phases (Bates et al. 1995). In hospitals, the medication administration stage accounts for 26%–32% of adult patient medication errors (Bates et al. 1995, Kopp et al. 2006) and 4%–60% of pediatric patient medication errors (Walsh et al. 2005). More recently, an Institute of Medicine (IOM) report indicated that hospitalized patients experience one medication administration error per day (Institute of Medicine 2007), where an error can be an omitted drug, wrong drug, unauthorized drug, wrong dose, extra dose, wrong route, wrong form, wrong technique, or wrong time (Barker et al. 1982, 2002). Errors in the administration stage are especially concerning because they are far less likely to be intercepted and far more likely to reach patients than errors in any preceding stage (Bates et al. 1995, Leape et al. 1995, Kopp et al. 2006, Shane 2009).

The reasons for such high rates of errors in medication administration is that administration requires many complex steps, each that can fail (Shane 2009), and takes up approximately 25% of all nursing time (Keohane et al. 2008). Well known is that to safely administer medications, clinicians, typically nurses, must perform visual inspection to match medication name, dose, route, time, form, and sometimes rate to the right patient. But nurses must also engage in a variety of other cognitive activities during medication administration such as communicating with pharmacists and physicians, determining appropriate times for PRN (as needed) medications, evaluating patients, teaching patients and family members about diagnoses and treatments, monitoring for medication side effects, and anticipating or detecting problems (Eisenhauer et al. 2007). They might also have to prepare the medication. Administrations can take place dozens of times per shift, potentially with several different patients per nurse (depending on the acuity of the unit or patients), all in highly dynamic and interruption-filled environments. The presence of pharmacists on the unit, how medications are dispensed from the pharmacy, and the way drugs are delivered to the units may also affect the complexity of administration. Drugs may be delivered to special medication rooms on each unit, to controlled access cabinets that dispense medications, directly to nurses, to locked boxes in patient rooms, etc. Some of these practices vary by country, within countries, and in some cases, even within hospitals. Because of these facts, medication administration is highly complex and its safety is a high priority.

The most recommended technology for controlling medication administration errors is bar coded medication administration (BCMA) (Bates 2000, Wald and Shojania 2001, Bates and Gawande 2003, Institute of Medicine 2007, Cescon and Etchells 2008), alternatively referred to as bar code point of care (BPOC) medication systems. The idea of using bar codes for medications dates back to at least 1985, when some urged their adoption in hospital pharmacies for quality assurance, inventory control, and tracking of expired stock (Hokanson et al. 1985, Nold and Williams 1985). Since then, bar codes have been used in hospitals for many purposes including lab specimen management (Tilzer and Jones 1988, Willard and Shanholtzer 1995, Yu et al. 2008), identifying transfusion products (Turner et al. 2003, LaRocco and Brient 2008), tracking surgical tools and sponges during surgery (Berger and Sanders 2008, Gamble 2008), patient identification (Renner et al. 1993, Howanitz et al. 2002, Lanoue and Still 2008), and for tracking investigational drugs (Sweet et al. 2008). This chapter focuses only on the use of bar codes for medication administration, describes their use, and discusses evidence of their efficacy.

BCMA Basics

BCMA systems, if designed and implemented appropriately, are meant to help ensure the five "rights" of medication administration: right medication, right patient, right dose, right route, right time (Neuenschwander et al. 2003, Cummings et al. 2005), and ensure complete and accurate documentation of the administration process (McRoberts 2005). BCMA systems also address the first Joint Commission National Patient Safety Goal of 2009—improve the accuracy of patient identification (Neuenschwander 2009). To be effective in guarding against administration errors, BCMA systems at minimum require machine readable bar code labels that uniquely identify all medications, nursing staff, and patients (Cummings et al. 2005). This seemingly simple requirement is in fact complicated by the size and shape of medication packages and patients (consider infants, for example), as well as the environments of use. The environment can subject bar codes to soaps, alcohol, water, blood, different kinds of lighting, high humidity, radiation, sterilization, human waste products, heat and cold (Murphy 2007, Hagland 2009). Therefore, the symbology (bar code format), printer, and media upon which the bar codes are printed need careful consideration. BCMA systems may rely on linear, composite, or two-dimensional symbologies (Neuenschwander et al. 2003, Cummings 2005); however, two-dimensional symbology is likely to see increased use because it can store more information in less space, making it more flexible (Lanoue and Still 2008).

Machine-readable bar codes are necessary, but not sufficient for BCMA systems to lead to safe administration. In addition, the medication order must be correct, the BCMA software must be easy to use, useful, and fit into the complex and variable conditions of work, the scanners must be available and working, the alerts and/or warnings must be working and useful, and the nurse must actively perform all the necessary scans (Karsh 2005). As will be discussed, these other conditions for success are not always met.

BCMA systems are typically integrated with an electronic medication administration record (eMAR, 86% of BCMA systems) and electronic nurse documentation (91% of BCMA systems) (Pedersen and Gumpper 2008). The eMAR is an electronic version of the paper MAR, and contains, for each patient, the names of medications to be administered, dose, route, time and/or schedule, and the form of the medication. eMARs can be used with or without BCMA systems. Currently, standard infusion pumps do not interface with BCMA systems and only 3% of hospitals with smart infusion pumps have them interfaced with eMARs (Pedersen and Gumpper 2008).

Supporting an effective BCMA system requires significant capital expenditures. One estimate suggests initial capital costs can range from $1 million to $10 million considering all infrastructure, staffing, hardware, software, and training costs (Cummings 2005). Ideally, medications would be bar code–labeled by drug manufacturers at the unit dose level (American Hospital Association, Health Research and Education Trust, and Institute for Safe Medication Practice 2002); however, this is not currently a reality and was not required in the 2004 U.S. Food and Drug Administration (FDA) bar code regulation (Food and Drug Administration 2004). Therefore, hospital pharmacies must implement medication repackaging centers, or outsource repackaging processes, for repackaging medications at the unit of use and affixing the new packaging with the appropriate bar code (Ragan et al. 2005, Poon et al. 2006, Pedersen and Gumpper 2008). Unless repackaging is outsourced, this will require software, hardware, and processes for printing high volumes of bar code labels. Current estimates are that nearly 40% of doses require repackaging for use with BCMA systems, so hospitals with BCMA may need to dedicate staff just for repackaging medications (Pedersen and Gumpper 2008). About 40% of pharmacy directors that have repackaging centers report that repackaging, while necessary, took more time and money than they initially anticipated. To support BCMA system use, hospitals also require wristband printers for every unit, wireless communication networks, information technology infrastructure to link BCMA software to other software systems, and new processes and procedures. Then there is the BCMA hardware itself.

BCMA hardware generally comes in two varieties: (1) wireless, handheld devices that both read bar codes and have a screen that displays the eMAR, or (2) a handheld scanner that is tethered to a wireless computer-on-wheels (COW) that displays the eMAR and allows access to other relevant software. Alternatively, a tethered scanner can be attached to a fixed computer station in the patient room. The different types of hardware provide different trade-offs. The handheld wireless system is highly portable, assuming ubiquitous wireless connectivity, and not constrained by the length of the tether. But the handheld screen may be too small to display all relevant medication data on one screen and thus may require considerable manipulation (scrolling or tapping with a stylus) to access data. The tethered version permits full-screen viewing of much more data because larger monitors or laptops can be used with the wheeled cart. However, the tether may make scanning patient ID bands difficult depending on tether length, COW size, and room configuration. Also, because the tethered scanner does not itself have a screen, the user of the device may not be able to see the relevant data at the point of scanning (Koppel et al. 2008). Typically, there should be one scanner available per nurse.

Regardless of the hardware configuration, BCMA use typically follows a common protocol (Larrabee and Brown 2003, Neuenschwander et al. 2003, Cummings 2005, McRoberts 2005, Carayon et al. 2007).

Users, typically nurses, but possibly others who administer medications (e.g., respiratory therapists, anesthesiologists) scan their own ID badges to access the eMAR or otherwise log into the system. Next, the user will acquire the necessary medications, compare the labels on the medications to the data in the eMAR and scan the medication bar codes. There are variations in this typical protocol, such as having nurses obtain the medication, bring it to the patient's room, and then, in order, scan his or her ID badge, the patient ID band, and then the medication (Lawton and Shields 2005, Paoletti et al. 2007). Whichever protocol is followed, if there is a mismatch between the medications scanned and those currently active in the eMAR, audible and/or visual alerts are triggered. In such cases, users need to determine if they need to take corrective action (Koppel et al. 2008). In some cases an alert might indicate the user was scanning the wrong medication, in which case the user would find and scan the correct medication. In other cases, the alert might be triggered by having the wrong bar code on the right medication, by giving the medication earlier than the scheduled administration time, or by having a medication formulation that is not consistent with what was in the eMAR even though the dose is correct (e.g., the software was expecting two 5 mg tablets, but the pharmacy sent one 10 mg tablet). In these cases, users can override such alerts and document the reason.

The users should next scan the patients ID band. ID bands are most commonly found on patient's wrists, but might be found on ankles, especially when patients are small children. ID bands might also be found in locations external to the patient, such as when premature infants are in isolettes. Isolettes complicate having the ID band directly on the patient (Karsh and Scanlon 2005). As when scanning the medications, scanning the patient ID can result in an alert, which may require corrective action or an override with documentation. Every alert, override, and medication administration is logged in a central database (Larrabee and Brown 2003, Koppel et al. 2008). If the five rights have been confirmed, the user may administer the medication and document the administration. High-risk medications require double checks by a second clinician and in some hospitals these visual double checks are documented in the eMAR as well. Documentation is typically automated with BCMA systems; after scanning the patient's ID band, the system allows the nurse to easily document that the medication was given, noting the date, time and administering user. Sometimes the user must confirm administration manually in the system. Documentation is used for quality assurance, regulatory purposes, analysis, and billing.

BCMA systems can range considerably in their level of functionality (Grotting et al. 2002). Basic systems confirm the five rights of administration and also provide an eMAR; intermediate system additionally provide drug references, formulary information and nursing workflow tools; advanced systems add maximum daily dose warnings, look-alike and sound-alike warnings, high risk warnings, clinical reminders, near miss reporting and/or order reconciliation (Bridge Medical Inc. 2001). Depending on the level of functionality, the design of the software, and the implementation of the system, BCMA systems cannot only decrease medication errors and rework, but also increase documentation accuracy and speed (Neuenschwander et al. 2003) as well as improve inventory control and billing accuracy (American Hospital Association, Health Research and Education Trust, and Institute for Safe Medication Practice 2002).

BCMA Adoption

Clearly, BCMA systems have great appeal for reducing administration errors and this is reflected in recent adoption trends. In 2002, only 1.5% of hospitals in the United States used BCMA systems for medication administration (Pedersen et al. 2003), but at that time it was anticipated that the number of adopters may grow because the U.S. FDA planned to mandate that drug manufacturers put bar codes on medications by April 2006 (Food and Drug Administration 2004). In fact, adoption among U.S. hospitals grew to 24% in 2007, with 70% of non-adopters planning to implement BCMA in the future (Pedersen and Gumpper 2008). Despite the FDA mandate, there are still reports that not all medications are appropriately bar coded (Hook et al. 2008). The 24% adoption figure included 100% of U.S. Veterans Hospitals using BCMA (Pedersen and Gumpper 2008). The U.S. Veterans Health Administration hospitals have invested significant national resources into BCMA, are the source of many publications about BCMA, and have been using BCMA since 1999 (Patterson et al. 2004, Schneider et al. 2008).

BCMA and Safety Outcomes

There are many case studies published about BCMA implementations (Bridge Medical Inc. 2001, Coyle and Heinen 2002, Grotting et al. 2002, Johnson et al. 2002, Sublett 2002, Larrabee and Brown 2003, Carlson 2004, Kester 2004, Traynor 2004, Swenson 2007, Foote and Coleman 2008, Gee 2009, Hagland 2009), of which many claim that BCMA improved safety (Puckett 1995, Coyle and Heinen 2002, Johnson et al. 2002, Foote and Coleman 2008). For example, one report stated that a U.S. Veterans Hospital had no known medication administration errors following BCMA implementation and that BCMA prevented 549,000 errors (Johnson et al. 2002). Another reported an 80% reduction in medication errors just during BCMA pilot testing (Foote and Coleman 2008).

However, through 2002, there was very little scientific study of BCMA (Shojania et al. 2001). In fact, one systematic review of research published between 1982 and 2002 found no scientific publications on the impact of bar coding on administration outcomes (e.g., errors) or patient outcomes (e.g., patient harm) (Oren et al. 2003). The authors did identify seven studies that reported the impact of bar codes on a number of pharmacy outcomes, data entry errors, and patient accountability for charges. Between 2002 and 2009, the picture was similar with few scientific studies of the impact of BCMA on administration or patient outcomes.* Several studies have been published, though, on the impact of BCMA on nursing work.

Among the studies assessing the impact of BCMA on administration or patient outcomes, one found that BCMA did not reduce medication errors in one test unit, but in a second test unit reduced them by 36% when wrong time and wrong technique errors were counted, and by 54% when those errors were not counted (Paoletti et al. 2007). The post-implementation administration error rate in the second unit was 10% if counting wrong time and wrong technique errors or 2.9% if not counting them. Bar code scanning compliance at the hospital remained at about 90% 18 months post-implementation. Another study found that during 1 year at a four-hospital system using BCMA there were 23,828 BCMA alerts of drug or patient mismatches (Koppel et al. 2008). These alerts appeared to prompt users to change their action by changing the medication or administering the medication to the correct patien. In a study of a small hospital that implemented BCMA, the system detected and averted 27 potential administration errors during the 9 month study period (Lawton and Shields 2005). Also, an analysis of BCMA-related reports to MEDMARX, a national database of voluntarily reported medication errors, submitted from January 1, 2000 to December 31, 2005, found 70 reports of BCMA preventing errors. Among those, 51 were dispensing errors caught during administration by the nurse using BCMA. The remaining 19 errors that were caught by the BCMA system either related to attempts to administer medications too early or attempts to administer medications for which there were no orders (Cochran et al. 2007).

Perhaps the strongest data to support the positive impact of BCMA on safety comes from a study in which a panel of six healthcare providers reviewed medication administration error scenarios generated from BCMA error logs at six community hospitals (Sakowski et al. 2008). They found that only 1% of errors caught by BCMA were rated as having the potential for severe or life-threatening adverse events, 9% were thought to have the potential to produce moderate adverse effects, and 91% were judged capable of producing minimal or no effects. However, importantly, the authors pointed out that extrapolating the findings to the 18 million doses administered by the six hospitals since BCMA was implemented translated to 17,000 errors that were prevented that could have produced moderate to severe consequences. Taken together, it appears that evidence about the impact of BCMA on safety is positive; BCMA implementation leads to decreased administration errors reaching the patient. At the same time, as described below, there is evidence that the path to safety is not straight forward.

* While this chapter was in press, a large scientific study of BCMA was published (Poon et al. 2010). The study found substantial reductions in administration errors post BCMA implementation, though errors continued to occur.

Instead, there are fundamental changes to nursing work that may mediate the relationship between BCMA and patient safety.

BCMA and Nursing Work

Slightly more studies have been published identifying how BCMA affects nursing work, compared to how it impacts administration errors or patient outcomes, though the numbers are still very small. These are important studies because they demonstrate that information technologies do *not* produce safety in and of themselves; rather, outcomes such as safety depend on the information technology design (e.g., do they support the physical and cognitive work required?), implementation (e.g., were end users involved? was training adequate?) and integration with workflow and the clinical contexts of use (Patterson et al. 2002, Karsh 2004, Karsh and Holden 2006, Koppel et al. 2008, Sakowski et al. 2008, Holden and Karsh 2009). These studies have been grouped into those that examined the relationship of BCMA to (1) time on task and perceptions of medication administration, (2) problems and problem-solving, (3) interruptions, and (4) workarounds and violations. Those four types of studies are highly related and the distinctions may be somewhat artificial; for example, interruptions are types of problems, and workarounds may be responses to problems.

Time on Task and Perceptions of Medication Administration

The percent of time nurses spend in different nursing activities may change after BCMA is implemented. One study found that the proportion of time nurses spent on medication administration activities did not significantly change overall (pre-BCMA: 26.9%, post-BCMA: 24.9%), but time spent on specific tasks did (Poon et al. 2008). The percent of time spent on information retrieval (e.g., looking up drug information), verifying patient ID, and waiting (e.g., for the computer to operate) increased, while the percent of time spent managing orders and delivering medications decreased. Also, post-BCMA, the percent of time that nurses spent communicating with patients or patients' families decreased. On the positive side, time spent on inefficient activities decreased post-BCMA, mostly due to less travel and less searching for records. Interestingly, the percent of time spent documenting medication administration did not change even though the BCMA system automatically documented when a nurse scanned his or her badge post administration. At the same institution, nurse satisfaction with medication administration efficacy, safety, and access to information and medications significantly improved post-BCMA implementation (Hurley et al. 2007).

Another study assessing nurse self-reports about BCMA systems found more conflicting results (Holden et al. 2008b). In the study, nurses rated medication administration processes—matching the medication to the MAR, checking patient ID, documenting administration, and the overall administration process—on seven dimensions. Those dimensions were usefulness, accuracy, likelihood of an error occurring, likelihood that an error would be detected before leading to harm, consistency, time efficiency, and ease of performance. There was little change in nurse perceptions of the matching medications to the MAR process, other than improved perceptions that errors could be detected post-BCMA. ID checking and documentation processes were more affected. Nurses reported more positive perceptions of the usefulness, accuracy, consistency and time efficiency of checking patient ID, and nurses perceived a lower likelihood of error during this step post-BCMA. For documentation, there were improved perceptions that errors could be detected post-BCMA, but documentation was perceived to be more difficult and less time efficient post-BCMA.

BCMA Problems and Problem Solving

One of the first studies to thoroughly document BCMA problems was done at a U.S. VA hospital (Patterson et al. 2002). Five "negative side effects" of BCMA implementation were discovered. The first was nurse confusion over automated removal of medications by BCMA. Such automation surprises are problematic in other forms of automation (Sarter et al. 1997) and degrade performance. Other studies of BCMA have also documented automation surprises (e.g., loss of wireless connectivity, the device timing out the user, or screens being out of alignment preventing the user from being able to scroll through screens), a few of which resulted in unsafe administration sequences and even a nurse discontinuing the process without completing it due to frustration (Carayon et al. 2007). The second side effect was degraded coordination between nurses and physicians, presumably because physicians no longer knew how to access medication administration information and because BCMA restricted the window of medication-related information that could be viewed. Third, nurses were found having to drop activities or work around BCMA activities they felt were inefficient (e.g., having to scan an ID band multiple times before it registered) to reduce workload during busy periods. Fourth, nurses increased prioritization of monitored activities during goal conflicts; because nurses knew administration times were now easily monitored by supervisors, time accuracy became more important than other tasks that could not be monitored as easily. Finally, BCMA led to decreased ability to deviate from routine sequences, which might be necessary in some cases.

The aforementioned analysis of BCMA-related reports to MEDMARX also found BCMA problems. There were 445 reports of BCMA systems contributing to errors (Cochran et al. 2007). The most commonly reported errors were due to wrong bar codes on the medication package, missing bar codes, and inability to scan bar codes. However, among all 445 reports only one was thought to be potentially harmful to a patient.

BCMA systems appear to alter both the problems encountered and the strategies applied by nurses during medication administration (Vogelsmeier et al. 2008). Holden et al. (2008a) described situations where BCMA created new problems and required new problem-solving strategies. In one case, medication administration was delayed despite the nurse having the correct dose for the patient. The problem was that the BCMA software expected one 20 mg dose, but pharmacy dispensed two 10 mg doses. Pre-BCMA, nurses commonly made, and then documented, reasonable substitutions such as this. That strategy was blocked post-BCMA, as only a 20 mg dose could be accepted by the system. To speed up administration, a pharmacist improvised an effective, if inelegant, solution involving the entry of two new 10 mg dose orders. BCMA systems can also provide new solutions to problems that existed pre-BCMA. For example, nurses still have to keep track of which medications to administer, when to do so, and when previous doses of the medication were administered. BCMA provides a solution because nurses can access, sort, or print a list of medications, scheduled administration times, and records of when medications were scanned in the past. There are also cases where preexisting problems within medication administration are not solved with BCMA. BCMA systems do not ensure that a second nurse is available to witness the preparation of high-risk medications. Nurses cannot typically use BCMA in order to determine infusion rates, how to dilute a medication, or whether two medications are compatible (though some systems could provide compatibility checks). Also, wrong route errors continue to occur as BCMA only double-checks the form of the medication (e.g., tablet, suspension, intravenous [IV] injection) against the medication order but does not ensure that the nurses administers the medication via the correct route to the patient.

BCMA and Interruptions

BCMA problems can interrupt the flow of nurses' work. Interruptions were already inherent to healthcare work before BCMA was introduced, as studies have shown that no matter the healthcare setting or technologies used, clinicians experience interruptions that disrupt them throughout their day and interfere with their already demanding workload (Shvartzman and Antonovsky 1992, Flynn et al. 1999, Potter et al. 2005, Wiegmann et al. 2007). Interruptions can come from a variety of different sources, such as phone calls, pages, other colleague requests, patients, patients' families, alarms and equipment failure. When clinicians are interrupted, their attention is shifted away from the primary task to the interrupting task (Potter et al. 2005). This shift in attention can be detrimental to the primary task at hand.

BCMA systems can provide helpful interruptions, help nurses to recover from interruptions, and can contribute to unwanted interruptions. BCMA systems interrupt nurses by alarming when a medication or patient is scanned and there is a mismatch. Although this may stop the nurse's workflow, the alarm usually alerts the nurse that something is wrong (e.g., one or more of the five rights are not met). Nurses may welcome these types of interruptions, as long as the alarms are meaningful, because they help prevent medication errors.

BCMA systems can also help nurses recover from interruptions during medication administration. For example, nurses are often interrupted while doing patient documentation. If a nurse is interrupted while documenting the time he/she administered a medication, and forgets to resume documenting or forgets the administration time, the BCMA system can be accessed to see when and what medication was last scanned. As another example, if a nurse is interrupted while administering multiple medications to a patient, the nurse might forget which medications were administered and which were not. The nurse can check the BCMA system for that information.

Other interruptions caused by BCMA may negatively impact nurse performance. These interruptions are often related to hardware or software problems (Carayon et al. 2007, Koppel et al. 2008, Patterson et al. 2002), such as when a nurse is trying to scan a patient and the tethered scanner does not reach the patient. This interrupts the nurse's workflow and he or she must work around the obstacle to finish the task. A nurse must stop his or her primary task and deal with the malfunctions before continuing. Additionally, these malfunctions may cause nurses to interrupt each other to ask for help in fixing such situations.

BCMA Workarounds and Violations

Violations and workarounds related to BCMA systems are receiving growing attention, as they are in other industries (Alper and Karsh 2009). Some of the earlier workarounds reported by Patterson et al. (2002) have been substantiated by others. For example, van Onzenoort et al. (2008) found that bar code scanning was only performed in 55% of administrations that should have been scanned. The top reasons for not scanning were difficulties scanning the bar codes on medication labels, lack of awareness of bar codes on medication labels, delays in response from the BCMA systems, shortage of time, and administration of a medication before the order.

In a similar study (Carayon et al. 2007), 63 observations of nurses administering medications revealed 18 different process sequences for the prescribed 8–9-step process of medication administration. The two sequences consistent with policy occurred 39% of the time. The most common deviation from procedure was documenting medication administration in the BCMA before administering the medication. This could represent a major safety problem if a full dose was documented as administered, but the medication was not actually administered (e.g., because patient was asleep) or only a partial dose was administered.

Four of the sequences in Carayon et al. (2007) were deemed unsafe because a medication or patient ID band was not scanned or administration was not documented. In fact, 34% of the observations had at least one medication administered without bar code verification due to the bar code not being in the medication database, a lack of a bar code on the medication, a non-scannable bar code (e.g., crinkled, ripped), the medication dose size differing from the ordered dose, and the lack of an order for the medication in the computer. Other witnessed unsafe acts during medication administration included the scanning of patient ID bands that were not physically on the patient and giving a different dose of medication other than what was ordered despite a BCMA alert for wrong medication dose. During brief interviews after the observations, nurses were asked about their views (positive and negative) of the BCMA system, providing insight into procedural violations. Nurses stated that it was easier and faster to rely on the BCMA system to alarm indicating the wrong medication, dose, time or patient rather than to visually check the medication label or patient ID. Nurses also stated it was much easier and faster to document administration immediately after scanning the patient ID band rather than after administering the medications. This was especially true when the administration was expected to take more than a few minutes because the device would time out in the interim, requiring the nurse to log back into the system in order to document the administration.

Data from five hospitals that used BCMA were used for the first study designed to systematically assess the nature, causes, and consequences of BCMA workarounds (Koppel et al. 2008). Fifteen types of workarounds were identified. These were grouped into omissions of process steps (e.g., failure to scan medication or patient ID bar codes, failure to review BCMA system computer screens or alerts), steps out of sequence (e.g., documenting medications as administered before actually administering the medication or observing patient ingestion, or administering medications and documenting it much later), and unauthorized steps such as disabling audio alarms. The study also found that nurses overrode BCMA-alerts for 4.2% of patients charted and for 10.3% of medications charted, a phenomenon reported by others as well (Sakowski et al. 2008).

Importantly, there were also 31 different causes of workarounds identified. These were categorized into (1) technology-related causes such as failing batteries of handheld scanners or linked computers, difficult-to-read or navigate screens, alert beeps that sound like confirmation beeps; (2) task-related causes that were related to BCMA steps that were perceived as slowing performance; (3) organizational causes such as patients or medications without bar codes (due to organizational or workflow flaws), and pharmacies sending only partial doses; (4) patient-related causes such as patients refusing medications, vomiting medications, sleeping, or in contact isolation; and (5) environmental causes such as hospital areas that lack wireless BCMA connectivity (operating rooms, labs), and doorways and patient-room configurations that hinder bedside access of BCMA systems that use COWs.

The studies documenting workarounds or violations of BCMA use protocols do not blame the nurses. Rather, the data show that poor system design, implementation, and integration into workflow create new problems; this has been documented with others types of health information technology as well (Berg et al. 1998, Berg and Goorman 1999, Karsh 2004, Gosbee and Gosbee 2005, Wears and Berg 2005, Aarts and Berg 2006, Karsh et al. 2006, Schiff 2006, Wears et al. 2006, Harrison et al. 2007). The data also suggest that some of the workarounds are reasonable in certain circumstances. Workarounds perceived as necessary by the user for patient care, efficiency (Kobayashi et al. 2005), or safety (Reason et al. 1998) may be beneficial, neutral, or dangerous for patients' safety (Kobayashi et al. 2005, Koppel et al. 2008). Some workarounds are trade-offs made when confronted by competing goals, for example, providing urgently needed medications without taking the time to scan patient or medication (Patterson et al. 2002, Alper et al. 2008b, Koppel et al. 2008). Also interesting is that the workarounds identified were neither rare nor secret (Koppel et al. 2008). They were known to staff; some may have been accepted as the norm. Only one study appears to have quantitatively examined the extent of violations or workarounds during medication administration before and after BCMA implementation (Alper et al. 2008a). Nurses' self-reported violations did not change for the process step of matching medications to the MAR, but decreased for checking patient ID, and increased for documentation after BCMA implementation. These changes could be expected as the BCMA scanner promotes patient ID checking, but the design of the BCMA may also lead to documenting administration before the medication is administered (Carayon et al. 2007).

BCMA and Physician Administration

While nearly every publication about BCMA focuses on nurse users, physicians, such as anesthesiologists also administer medications and could benefit from BCMA. During surgery, an anesthesiologist, may order, dispense, prepare, and administer his or her own medications for the patient. In one study, a BCMA system designed to help identify anesthetic drugs and improve billing capture increased the quantity of drugs documented per case by 22% and drug revenue capture per case by 19% (Nolen and

Rodes 2008). Also, total time required by operating room staff to process drug-related data was reduced by 8 minutes per case.

BCMA with Pediatric Patients

There are important differences in the medication ordering, dispensing, and administration processes for adult versus pediatric patients (Marino et al. 2000, Kaushal et al. 2001, Scanlon et al. 2006). Issues related to the size of pediatric patients, the ability of clinicians and pediatric patients to communicate, and the unique pediatric care environments complicate BCMA use with children (Karsh and Scanlon 2005). To fit an ID band with a readable bar code label onto an infant is a challenge because small wrists lead to bar code label size and curvature problems, particularly for the larger, one-dimensional symbologies. Patient ID location and skin vulnerability problems also exist. Again, because of their small size, ID bands on children are not necessarily located on the wrist, but might be on the ankle or an IV access pole.

Because ID bands may not be in a consistent location, and because pediatric patients may not be able to communicate to the nurse about where the ID band is, or make it accessible to the nurse for scanning, nurses may have to hunt for the patient ID bands, which adds to their work time. Also, because children are smaller than most adults, there is a problem of competing real estate; the small space on a child's wrist or ankle that is needed for an ID band is also needed for IV access. This real estate shortage can lead to a number of different problems. First, as IVs are added or moved, it is likely that wristbands will either be moved or removed completely. Second, clinicians often secure IV lines with an abundance of tape or gauze, which may cover the ID bands.

Certain pediatric environments of care, such as the neonatal intensive care units (NICUs), present additional challenges. Neonates may be located inside of isolettes for thermal control, requiring special considerations for bar codes (Hagland 2009) and scanning devices. If identification bands are secured around NICU patients' wrists or ankles, a nurse would have to potentially place a scanning device inside of an isolette to accurately identify the patient. This makes infection control and contamination from the device an important issues to deal with. Even if a scanner can be safely inserted into an isolette, the skin of neonates is easily injured, requiring that identification bands be made out of material that is benign enough to not damage neonate skin. As a result, one "solution" to the challenge of the use of bar codes with neonates is to place the wristband outside of the isolette on IV tubing that is connected to the patient or attached to the isolette itself. Those problems are but the tip of the iceberg. Fortunately, there is some evidence that BCMA systems can be implemented in pediatric inpatient units for improved medication administration safety (Morriss et al. 2009).

Conclusion

The growing number of case studies, reports (American Hospital Association, Health Research and Education Trust, and Institute for Safe Medication Practice 2002, Grotting et al. 2002, Cummings 2005, Hook et al. 2008), and peer-reviewed publications (Patterson et al. 2002, Karsh 2005, Karsh and Scanlon 2005, Barber et al. 2007, Carayon et al. 2007, Koppel et al. 2008) make it clear that BCMA has significant potential to improve medication administration safety, but that there are also design and implementation challenges. BCMA design issues are often not identified until BCMA has been implemented (Koppel et al. 2008); this speaks to the need to improve the methodologies used to design and pilot test BCMA, such as human-centered design and usability evaluation with realistic scenarios and realistic simulated environments. Even if design and ergonomics principles were systematically applied to the design of BCMA technologies, there may still be problems after BCMA implementation (Carayon et al. 2007). Therefore, a process for continuous optimization and evaluation post-BCMA implementation is necessary (Harrison et al. 2007, Koppel et al. 2008).

BCMA systems fundamentally change nursing work, and cause significant changes in other processes in the healthcare organization, in particular pharmacy processes and physician monitoring. Because of that, practical and evidence-based information technology implementation practices related to champions, fairness, culture, workload, policies, end user involvement, training, technical support, management commitment, simulation, and pilot testing must all be followed (Mahmood et al. 2000, Frambach and Schillewaert 2002, Venkatesh et al. 2003, Karsh and Holden 2006, Holden and Karsh 2009). These implementation principles are likely to contribute to the early identification of issues and quick problem solving before patients are harmed.

Technology such as radio frequency identification (RFID) may someday replace bar codes for medication administration, but cost has prevented widespread RFID use for medication applications (Cescon and Etchells 2008). Some are designing medication administrations systems using both bar codes and RFID (Sun et al. 2008); and RFID technology is being used in hospitals for other applications (Inglesby 2006). But, for the foreseeable future, BCMA systems will be the technologies of choice for improving with medication administration safety.

Acknowledgments

This publication was supported by grants 1R01LM008923 from the National Institutes of Health (to Karsh), 1 R01 HS013610 from the Agency for Healthcare Research and Quality (to Karsh), 1R01 HS015274 from the Agency for Healthcare Research and Quality (to Carayon), 61148 from the Robert Wood Johnson Foundation (to Carayon and Karsh), and 1UL1RR025011 from the Clinical & Translational Science Award (CTSA) program of the National Center for Research Resources National Institutes of Health.

References

Aarts, J. and M. Berg. 2006. Same systems, different outcomes—Comparing the implementation of computerized physician order entry in two Dutch hospitals. *Methods of Information in Medicine* 45(1):53–61.

Alper, S. J., R. J. Holden, M. C. Scanlon, N. Patel, K. Murkowski, T. M. Shalaby, and B. Karsh. 2008a. Violation prevalence after introduction of a bar coded medication administration system. Paper read at *2nd International Conference on Healthcare Systems Ergonomics and Patient Safety*, Strasbourg, France.

Alper, S. and B. Karsh. 2009. A systematic review of the causes of safety violations in industry. *Accident Analysis and Prevention* 41(4):739–754.

Alper, S. J., M. C. Scanlon, K. Murkowski, N. Patel, R. Kaushal, and B. Karsh. 2008b. Routine and situational violations during medication administration. Paper read at *9th International Symposium on Human Factors in Organizational Design and Management*, Guarujá, São Paulo, Brazil.

American Hospital Association, Health Research and Education Trust, and Institute for Safe Medication Practice. 2002. *Assessing Bedside Bar-Coding Readiness*. Available from http://www.medpathways.info/medpathways/tools/tools.html (retrieved October 21, 2010).

Barber, N., T. Cornford, and E. Klecun. 2007. Qualitative evaluation of an electronic prescribing and administration system. *Quality & Safety in Health Care* 16(4):271–278.

Barker, K. N., E. A. Flynn, G. A. Pepper, D. W. Bates, and R. L. Mikeal. 2002. Medication errors observed in 36 health care facilities. *Archives of Internal Medicine* 162(16):1897–1903.

Barker, K. N., R. L. Mikeal, R. E. Pearson, N. A. Illig, and M. L. Morse. 1982. Medication errors in nursing-homes and small hospitals. *American Journal of Hospital Pharmacy* 39(6):987–991.

Bates, D. W. 2000. Using information technology to reduce rates of medication errors in hospitals. *British Medical Journal* 320:780–791.

Bates, D. W., D. J. Cullen, N. Laird, L. A. Petersen, S. D. Small, D. Servi, G. Laffel, B. J. Sweitzer, B. F. Shea, R. Hallisey, M. Vandervliet, R. Nemeskal, and L. L. Leape. 1995. Incidence of adverse drug events and potential adverse drug events—Implications for prevention. *JAMA—Journal of the American Medical Association* 274(1):29–34.

Bates, D. W. and A. A. Gawande. 2003. Patient safety: Improving safety with information technology. *New England Journal of Medicine* 348(25):2526–2534.

Berg, M. and E. Goorman. 1999. The contextual nature of medical information. *International Journal of Medical Informatics* 56(1–3):51–60.

Berg, M., C. Langenberg, I. vd Berg, and J. Kwakkernaat. 1998. Considerations for sociotechnical design: Experiences with an electronic patient record in a clinical context. *International Journal of Medical Informatics* 52:1–3.

Berger, P. S. and G. Sanders. 2009. *Objects Retained During Surgery: Human Diligence Meets Systems Solutions*. Patient Safety and Quality Healthcare 2008. Available from http://www.psqh.com/sepoct08/objects.html (retrieved March 1, 2009).

Bridge Medical Inc. 2001. *The Effect of Bar-Code Enabled Point of Care Technology on Medication Administration Errors*, San Diego, CA.

Carayon, P., T. B. Wetterneck, A. S. Hundt, M. Ozkaynak, J. Desilvey, B. Ludwig, P. Ram, and S. S. Rough. 2007. Evaluation of nurse interaction with bar code medication administration technology in the work environment. *Journal of Patient Safety* 3(1):34–42.

Carlson, R. 2004. Setting safe standards. Homegrown bar coding medication administration system helps VA hospitals minimize mistakes at the point of care. *Health Management Technology* 25(4):30–33.

Cescon, D. W. and E. Etchells. 2008. Barcoded medication administration—A last line of defense. *JAMA—Journal of the American Medical Association* 299(18):2200–2202.

Chapanis, A. and M. Safren. 1960. Of misses and medicines. *Journal of Chronic Diseases* 12(4):403–408.

Cochran, G. L., K. J. Jones, J. Brockman, A. Skinner, and R. W. Hicks. 2007. Errors prevented by and associated with bar-coded medication administration systems. *Joint Commission Journal on Quality and Patient Safety* 33:293–301.

Coyle, G. A. and M. Heinen. 2002. Scan your way to a comprehensive electronic medical record. Augment medication administration accuracy and increase documentation efficiency with bar coding technology. *Nursing Management* 33(12):56, 58–59.

Cummings, J. P. 2005. *UHC Technology Report: Bar-Coded Medication Administration*. Oak Brook, IL: University HealthSystem Consortium.

Cummings, J., P. Bush, D. Smith, and K. Matuszewski. 2005. Bar-coding medication administration overview and consensus recommendations. *American Journal of Health-System Pharmacy* 62:2626–2629.

Eisenhauer, L. A., A. C. Hurley, and N. Dolan. 2007. Nurses' reported thinking during medication administration. *Journal of Nursing Scholarship* 39(1):82–87.

Flynn, E. A., K. N. Barker, J. T. Gibson, R. E. Pearson, B. A. Berger, and L. A. Smith. 1999. Impact of interruptions and distractions on dispensing errors in an ambulatory care pharmacy. *American Journal of Health-System Pharmacy* 56(13):1319–1325.

Food and Drug Administration. 2004. *Bar Code Label Requirement for Human Drug Products and Biological Products (21 CFR Parts 201, 606, and 610)*. Available from http://www.fda.gov/cber/rules/barcodelabel.htm (retrieved February 20, 2005).

Foote, S. O. and J. R. Coleman. 2008. Medication administration: The implementation process of bar-coding for medication administration to enhance medication safety. *Nursing Economics* 26(3):207–210.

Frambach, R. T. and N. Schillewaert. 2002. Organizational innovation adoption—A multi-level framework of determinants and opportunities for future research. *Journal of Business Research* 55(2):163–176.

Gamble, K. H. 2009. *No Sponge Left Behind*. Healthcare Informatics 2008. Available from http://healthcare-informatics.com (retrieved February 2, 2009).

Gee, T. 2009. *Barcoding: Implementation Challenges*. Patient Safety and Quality Healthcare 2009. Available from http://www.psqh.com/marapr09/barcoding.html (retrieved April 24, 2009).

Gosbee, J. W. and L. L. Gosbee. 2005. *Using Human Factors Engineering to Improve Patient Safety*. Oak Brook, IL: Joint Commission Resources.

Grotting, J. B., M. Yang, J. Kelly, M. M. Brown, and B. Trohimovich. 2002. *The Effect of Barcode-Enabled Point-of-Care Technology on Patient Safety*. San Diego, CA: Bridge Medical, Inc.

Hagland, M. 2009. *A Model of Innovation*. Healthcare Informatics 2009. Available from http://healthcare-informatics.com (retrieved April 24, 2009).

Harrison, M., R. Koppel, and S. Bar-Lev. 2007. Unintended consequences of information technologies in health care—An interactive sociotechnical analysis. *Journal of the American Medical Informatics Association* 14(5):542–549.

Hokanson, J. A., M. R. Keith, B. G. Guernsey, R. R. Grudzien, W. H. Doutre, D. J. Luttman, and M. C. Trachtenberg. 1985. Potential use of bar codes to implement automated dispensing quality assurance programs. *Hospital Pharmacy* 20(5):327–329, 333, 337.

Holden, R. J., S. J. Alper, M. C. Scanlon, K. Murkowski, A. J. Rivera, and B. Karsh. 2008a. Challenges and problem-solving strategies during medication management: A study of a pediatric hospital before and after bar-coding. Paper read at *Proceedings of the 2nd International Conference on Healthcare Systems Ergonomics and Patient Safety*, Strasbourg, France.

Holden, R. J. and B. T. Karsh. 2009. A theoretical model of health information technology usage behaviour with implications for patient safety. *Behaviour & Information Technology* 28(1):21–38.

Holden, R. J., M. C. Scanlon, R. L. Brown, and B. Karsh. 2008b. What is IT? New conceptualizations and measures of pediatric nurses' acceptance of bar-coded medication administration information technology. *Proceedings of the 52nd Annual Meeting of the Human Factors and Ergonomics Society*, New York City, pp. 768–772.

Hook, J., J. Pearlstein, and C. Cusack. 2008. *Using Barcode Medication Administration to Improve Quality and Safety: Findings from the AHRQ Health IT Portfolio*. Rockville, MD: Agency for Healthcare Research and Quality.

Howanitz, P. J., S. W. Renner, and M. K. Walsh. 2002. Continuous wristband monitoring over 2 years decreases identification errors—A college of American pathologists Q-tracks study. *Archives of Pathology & Laboratory Medicine* 126(7):809–815.

Hurley, A. C., A. Bane, S. Fotakis, M. E. Duffy, A. Sevigny, E. G. Poon, and T. K. Gandhi. 2007. Nurse's satisfaction with medication administration point-of-care technology. *Journal of Nursing Administration* 37(7/8):343–349.

Inglesby, T. 2009. *Ready for Prime Time?* Patient Safety and Quality Healthcare 2006. Available from http://www.psqh.com/mayjun06/rfid.html (retrieved April 24, 2009).

Institute of Medicine, ed. 2000. *To Err Is Human: Building a Safer Health System*. Washington, DC: National Academy Press.

Institute of Medicine, ed. 2001. *Crossing the Quality Chasm: A New Health System for the 21st Century*. Washington, DC: National Academy Press.

Institute of Medicine. 2007. *Preventing Medication Errors*. Washington, DC: National Academy Press.

Johnson, C. L., R. A. Carlson, C. L. Tucker, and C. Willette. 2002. Using BCMA software to improve patient safety in Veterans Administration Medical Centers. *Journal of Healthcare Information Management* 16(1):46–51.

Karsh, B. 2004. Beyond usability for patient safety: Designing effective technology implementation systems. *Quality and Safety in Healthcare* 13(5):388–394.

Karsh, B. 2005. A conceptual framework for understanding the safety implications of bar code enabled point of care (BPOC) systems. *Proceedings of the 11th International Conference on Human–Computer Interaction*, Las Vegas, Nevada.

Karsh, B., K. H. Escoto, J. W. Beasley, and R. J. Holden. 2006. Toward a theoretical approach to medical error reporting system research and design. *Applied Ergonomics* 37(3):283–295.

Karsh, B. and R. Holden. 2006. New technology implementation in health care. In *Handbook of Human Factors and Ergonomics in Patient Safety*, ed. P. Carayon. Mahwah, NJ: Lawrence Erlbaum Associates.

Karsh, B. and M. Scanlon. 2005. Using bar code technology for medication administration: Special human factors considerations for pediatric populations. *Proceedings of the International Conference on Healthcare Systems Ergonomics and Patient Safety*, pp. 135–138, Florence, Italy.

Kaushal, R., D. W. Bates, C. Landrigan, K. J. McKenna, M. D. Clapp, F. Federico, and D. A. Goldmann. 2001. Medication errors and adverse drug events in pediatric inpatients. *JAMA—Journal of the American Medical Association* 285(16):2114–2120.

Keohane, C. A., A. D. Bane, E. Featherstone, J. Hayes, S. Woolf, A. Hurley, D. W. Bates, T. K. Gandhi, and E. G. Poon. 2008. Quantifying nursing workflow in medication administration. *Journal of Nursing Administration* 38(1):19–26.

Kester, M. 2004. Bar coding at the bedside. New England hospital implements an automated point-of-care medication administration system to reduce medication errors and their associated complications. *Health Management Technology* 25(5):42–44.

Kobayashi, M., S. R. Fussell, Y. Xiao, and F. J. Seagull. 2005. Work coordination, workflow, and workarounds in a medical context. Paper read at *CHI '05: Conference on Human Factors in Computing Systems*, Portland, OR.

Kopp, B. J., B. L. Erstad, M. E. Allen, A. A. Theodorou, and G. Priestley. 2006. Medication errors and adverse drug events in an intensive care unit: Direct observation approach for detection. *Critical Care Medicine* 34:415–425.

Koppel, R., T. Wetterneck, J. L. Telles, and B. T. Karsh. 2008. Workarounds to barcode medication administration systems: Their occurrences, causes, and threats to patient safety. *Journal of the American Medical Informatics Association* 15(4):408–423.

Lanoue, E. and C. J. Still. 2009. *Patient Identification: Producing a Better Barcoded Wristband*. Patient Safety and Quality Healthcare 2008. Available from http://www.psqh.com/mayjun08/identification.html (retrieved March 1, 2009).

LaRocco, M. and K. Brient. 2009. *An Interdisciplinary Approach to Safer Blood Transfusion*. Patient Safety and Quality Healthcare 2008. Available from http://www.psqh.com/marapr08/transfusion.html (retrieved April 24 2009).

Larrabee, S. and M. M. Brown. 2003. Recognizing the institutional benefits of bar-code point-of-care technology. *Joint Commission Journal on Quality & Safety* 29(7):345–353.

Lawton, G. and A. Shields. 2005. Bar-code verification of medication administration in a small hospital. *American Journal of Health-System Pharmacy* 62(22):2413–2415.

Leape, L. L., D. W. Bates, D. J. Cullen, J. Cooper, H. J. Demonaco, T. Gallivan, R. Hallisey, J. Ives, N. Laird, G. Laffel, R. Nemeskal, L. A. Petersen, K. Porter, D. Servi, B. F. Shea, S. D. Small, B. J. Sweitzer, B. T. Thompson, and M. Vander Vliet. 1995. Systems analysis of adverse drug events. *Journal of the American Medical Association* 274(1):35–43.

Leape, L. L., T. A. Brennan, N. Laird, A. G. Lawthers, A. R. Localio, B. A. Barnes, L. Hebert, J. P. Newhouse, P. C. Weiler, and H. Hiatt. 1991. The nature of adverse events in hospitalized-patients—Results of the Harvard Medical Practice Study II. *New England Journal of Medicine* 324(6):377–384.

Mahmood, M. A., J. M. Burn, L. A. Gemoets, and C. Jacquez. 2000. Variables affecting information technology end-user satisfaction: A meta-analysis of the empirical literature. *International Journal of Human–Computer Studies* 52(4):751–771.

Marino, B. L., K. Reinhardt, W. J. Eichelberger, and R. Steingard. 2000. Prevalence of errors in a pediatric hospital medication system: Implications for error proofing. *Outcomes Management for Nursing Practice* 4(3):129–135.

McRoberts, S. 2005. The use of bar code technology in medication administration. *Clinical Nurse Specialist* 19(2):55–56.

Morriss, F. H., P. W. Abramowitz, S. P. Nelson, G. Milavetz, S. L. Michael, S. N. Gordon, J. F. Pendergast, and E. F. Cook. 2009. Effectiveness of a barcode medication administration system in reducing preventable adverse drug events in a neonatal intensive care unit: A prospective cohort study. *Journal of Pediatrics* 154(3):363–368.

Murphy, D. 2009. *Barcode Basics: Why Printing, Symbology, and Media Choices Matter*. Patient Safety and Quality Healthcare 2007. Available from http://www.psqh.com/julaug07/barcode.html (retrieved March 1, 2009).

Neuenschwander, M. 2009. *National Patient Safety Goals and Barcoding*. Patient Safety and Quality Healthcare 2009. Available from http://www.psqh.com/marapr09/technology.html (retrieved April 20, 2009).

Neuenschwander, M., M. R. Cohen, A. J. Vaida, J. A. Patchett, J. Kelly, and B. Trohimovich. 2003. Practical guide to bar coding for patient medication safety. *American Journal of Health-System Pharmacy* 60(8):768–779.

Nold, E. G. and T. C. Williams. 1985. Bar codes and their potential applications in hospital pharmacy. *American Journal of Hospital Pharmacy* 42(12):2722–2732.

Nolen, A. L. and W. D. Rodes. 2008. Bar-code medication administration system for anesthetics: Effects on documentation and billing. *American Journal of Health-System Pharmacy* 65(7):655–659.

Oren, E., E. R. Shaffer, and B. J. Guglielmo. 2003. Impact of emerging technologies on medication errors and adverse drug events. *American Journal of Health-System Pharmacy* 60(14):1447–1458.

Paoletti, R. D., T. M. Suess, M. G. Lesko, A. A. Feroli, J. A. Kennel, J. M. Mahler, and T. Sauders. 2007. Using bar-code technology and medication observation methodology for safer medication administration. *American Journal of Health-System Pharmacy* 64(5):536–543.

Patterson, E. S., R. I. Cook, and M. L. Render. 2002. Improving patient safety by identifying side effects from introducing bar coding in medication administration. *Journal of the American Medical Informatics Association* 9(5):540–553.

Patterson, E. S., M. L. Rogers, and M. L. Render. 2004. Fifteen best practice recommendations for bar-code medication administration in the Veterans Health Administration. *Joint Commission Journal on Quality & Safety* 30(7):355–365.

Pedersen, C. A. and K. F. Gumpper. 2008. ASHP national survey on informatics: Assessment of the adoption and use of pharmacy informatics in US hospitals-2007. *American Journal of Health-System Pharmacy* 65(23):2244–2264.

Pedersen, C. A., P. J. Schneider, and D. J. Scheckelhoff. 2003. ASHP national survey of pharmacy practice in hospital settings: Dispensing and administration—2002. *American Journal of Health-System Pharmacy* 60(1):52–68.

Poon, E. G., J. L. Cina, W. Churchill, N. Patel, E. Featherstone, J. M. Rothschild, C. A. Keohane, A. D. Whittemore, D. W. Bates, and T. K. Gandhi. 2006. Medication dispensing errors and potential adverse drug events before and after implementing bar code technology in the pharmacy. *Annals of Internal Medicine* 145(6):426–434.

Poon, E. G., C. A. Keohane, A. Bane, E. Featherstone, B. S. Hays, A. Dervan, S. Woolf, J. Hayes, L. P. Newmark, and T. K. Gandhi. 2008. Impact of barcode medication administration technology on how nurses spend their time providing patient care. *Journal of Nursing Administration* 38(12):541–549.

Poon, E. G., C. A. Keohane, C. S. Yoon, M. Ditmore, A. Bane, O. Levtzion-Korach, T. Moniz, J. M. Rothschild, A. B. Kachalia, J. Hayes, W. W. Churchill, S. Lipsitz, A. D. Whittemore, D. W. Bates, T. K. and Gandhi. 2010. Effect of bar-code technology on the safety of medication administration. *New England Journal of Medicine* 362:1698–1707.

Potter, P., L. Wolf, S. Boxerman, D. Grayson, J. Sledge, C. Dunagan, and B. Evanoff. 2005. Understanding the cognitive work of nursing in the acute care environment. *Journal of Nursing Administration* 35(7–8):327–335.

Puckett, F. 1995. Medication-management component of a point-of-care information system. *American Journal of Health-System Pharmacy* 51:1305–1309.

Ragan, R., J. Bond, K. Major, T. Kingsford, L. Eidem, and J. C. Garrelts. 2005. Improved control of medication use with an integrated bar-code-packaging and distribution system. *American Journal of Health-System Pharmacy* 62(10):1075–1079.

Reason, J., D. Parker, and R. Lawton. 1998. Organizational controls and safety: The varieties of rule- related behaviour. *Journal of Occupational and Organizational Psychology* 71:289–304.

Renner, S. W., P. J. Howanitz, and P. Bachner. 1993. Wristband identification error reporting in 712 hospitals—A College-of-American-Pathologists Q-probes study of quality issues in transfusion practice. *Archives of Pathology & Laboratory Medicine* 117(6):573–577.

Safren, M. and A. Chapanis. 1960. A critical incident study of hospital medication errors. *Hospitals* 34:53–68.

Sakowski, J., J. M. Newman, and K. Dozier. 2008. Severity of medication administration errors detected by a bar-code medication administration system. *American Journal of Health-System Pharmacy* 65(17):1661–1666.

Sarter, N. B., D. D. Woods, and C. E. Billings. 1997. Automation surprises. In *Handbook of Human Factors and Ergonomics*, ed. G. Salvendy. New York: Wiley.

Scanlon, M. C., B. Karsh, and E. Densmore. 2006. Human factors and pediatric patient safety. *Pediatric Clinics of North America* 53:1105–1119.

Schiff, G., ed. 2006. *Getting Results: Reliably Communicating and Acting on Critical Test Results.* Oak Brook, IL: Joint Commission Resources.

Schneider, R., J. Bagby, and R. Carlson. 2008. Bar-code medication administration: A systems perspective. *American Journal of Health-System Pharmacy* 65(23):2216–2219.

Shane, R. 2009. Current status of administration of medicines. *American Journal of Health-System Pharmacy* 66(Suppl 3):S42–S48.

Shojania, K. G., B. Duncan, K. McDonald, and R. M. Watcher. 2001. Making healthcare safer: A critical analysis of patient safety practices. Rockville, MD: Agency for Healthcare Research and Quality. Evidence Report/Technology Assessment No. 43; AHRQ publication 01-E058.

Shvartzman, P. and A. Antonovsky. 1992. The interrupted consultation. *Family Practice* 9(2):219–221.

Sublett, P. 2002. Technology's impact on reducing medication errors. At Danville Regional Medical Center, not a single medication is administered without the benefit of bar code verification technology. *Health Management Technology* 23(11):24–26.

Sun, P. R., B. H. Wang, and F. Wu. 2008. A new method to guard inpatient medication safety by the implementation of RFID. *Journal of Medical Systems* 32(4):327–332.

Sweet, B. V., H. R. Tamer, R. Siden, S. R. McCreadie, M. E. McGregory, T. Benner, and R. M. Tankanow. 2008. Improving investigational drug service operations through development of an innovative computer system. *American Journal of Health-System Pharmacy* 65(10):969–973.

Swenson, D. 2009. *Point-of-Care Medication Error Prevention*. Patient Safety and Quality Healthcare 2007. Available from http://www.psqh.com/mayjun07/pointofcare.html (retrieved April 24, 2009).

Tilzer, L. L. and R. W. Jones. 1988. Use of bar code labels on collection tubes for specimen management in the clinical laboratory. *Archives of Pathology & Laboratory Medicine* 112(12):1200–1202.

Traynor, K. 2004. Details matter in bedside bar-code scanning. *American Journal of Health-System Pharmacy* 61(19):1987–1988.

Turner, C. L., A. C. Casbard, and M. F. Murphy. 2003. Barcode technology: Its role in increasing the safety of blood transfusion. *Transfusion* 43(9):1200–1209.

van Onzenoort, H. A., A. van de Plas, A. G. Kessels, N. M. Veldhorst-Janssen, P. H. M. van der Kuy, and C. Neef. 2008. Factors influencing bar-code verification by nurses during medication administration in a Dutch hospital. *American Journal of Health-System Pharmacy* 65(7):644–648.

Venkatesh, V., M. G. Morris, G. B. Davis, and F. D. Davis. 2003. User acceptance of information technology: Toward a unified view. *Mis Quarterly* 27(3):425–478.

Vogelsmeier, A. A., J. R. B. Halbesleben, and J. R. Scott-Cawiezzel. 2008. Technology implementation and workarounds in the nursing home. *Journal of the American Medical Informatics Association* 15:114–119.

Wald, H., and K. G. Shojania. 2001. Prevention of misidentifications. In *Making Health Care Safer: A Critical Analysis of Patient Safety Practices*, eds. K. G. Shojania, B. W. Duncan, K. M. McDonald, and R. M. Wachter. Rockville, MD: Agency for Healthcare Research and Quality.

Walsh, K. E., R. Kaushal, and J. B. Chessare. 2005. How to avoid paediatric medication errors: A user's guide to the literature. *Archives of Disease in Childhood* 90(7):698–702.

Wears, R. L. and M. Berg. 2005. Computer technology and clinical work: Still waiting for Godot. *JAMA—Journal of the American Medical Association* 293(10):1261–1263.

Wears, R. L., R. I. Cook, and S. J. Perry. 2006. Automation, interaction, complexity, and failure: A case study. *Reliability Engineering & System Safety* 91(12):1494–1501.

Wiegmann, D. A., A. W. ElBardissi, J. A. Dearani, R. C. Daly, and T. M. Sundt. 2007. Disruptions in surgical flow and their relationship to surgical errors: An exploratory investigation. *Surgery* 142(5):658–665.

Willard, K. E. and C. J. Shanholtzer. 1995. User-interface reengineering—Innovative applications of bar coding in a clinical microbiology laboratory. *Archives of Pathology & Laboratory Medicine* 119(8):706–712.

Yu, L., M. S. Alminski, and U. J. Balis. 2008. Just-in-time surgical pathology specimen workflow with comprehensive barcode tracking and lean/six sigma software design as a prototypic next generation laboratory information system for comprehensive error reduction. Paper read at *97th Annual Meeting of the United-States-and-Canadian-Academy-of-Pathology*, March 4, Denver, CO.

48

Clinical Decision Support Systems

Sze-jung Sandra Wu
JP Morgan Chase

Mark Lehto
Purdue University

Yuehwern Yih
Purdue University

Introduction 48-1
Systems for Diagnosis • Reminders for Preventive Care and Disease Management • Systems for Drug Dosing and Prescribing • Effects of CDSS: Outcome Measures • Issues Associated with CDSS Implementation Success • Roadmap to a Successful CDSS • Workflow Integration • User-Centered Approach for System Design
Conclusions 48-10
References 48-10

Introduction

Decision support in the clinical setting has been defined as "advice and guidance offered by information and communication technology to aid the problem-solving and decision making of healthcare providers" (Greenes, 2007). Clinical decision support systems (CDSSs) are health information systems that utilize patient data and clinical knowledge to generate patient-specific information at the place and time decisions are made. The type of clinical knowledge incorporated in a computerized clinical knowledge base might include guidelines, research literature, or outcome-based knowledge, or even knowledge developed by a machine-learning tool that allows computers to learn from past experiences. CDSSs have been implemented as stand-alone systems or add-ons to local electronic medical record (EMR) systems that augment the use of EMR and improve quality of healthcare.

CDSSs provide support and address clinical needs at various stages of the patient care process, ranging from monitoring, preventive care, evaluation, diagnosis, treatment, to follow-up. The characteristics of CDSSs can be generalized into four categories by functionality, including systems for diagnosis, reminders for prevention, systems for disease management, and systems for drug dosing and prescribing (Garg et al., 2005). Because of the need for system integration and the need to provide recommendations at the point of care, clinical reminder systems have gradually extended in scope to include disease management items (Sequist et al., 2005). The following section will introduce each of these types of CDSSs.

Systems for Diagnosis

A diagnostic CDSS provides suggestions for possible diagnoses that match a patient's signs and symptoms. Its knowledge representation derives from an expert knowledge base developed using artificial intelligence approaches (Uzuner et al., 2009), such as artificial neural networks (Zhang and Szolovits, 2008) and case-based reasoning (Fritsche et al., 2002), or statistical algorithms, such as Markov model or logistic classifier (Gellerstedt et al., 2006). Given a patient symptom description entered through a structured data entry interface, a diagnostic CDSS typically provides diagnostic suggestions by generating a rank-ordered list of likely diagnoses, each with estimated probability, or relationships between clinical findings and disease expressed on heuristic scales. A diagnostic CDSS can also provide comparisons and contrasts of paired diseases to help clinicians refine their diagnoses (Friedman et al., 1999), or continuously monitor patient data to detect lift-threatening conditions in critical care (Chen et al., 2008; Zhang and Szolovits, 2008).

Other diagnostic CDSSs utilize free-text patient medical records, including narrative medical reports, triage chief complaints, and discharge summaries, to generate diagnostic recommendations. These free-text data entries contain valuable information that may be evident in text but not indexed in a structured database, such as negative symptom narratives. However, most clinical narratives are in the form of fragmented free text (e.g., abbreviating "smok," "tobac" for "smoking"), which poses a challenge for the development of diagnostic CDSSs. Accurately extracting and analyzing data from free-text records requires lexically and semantically profiling the diseases and their associated symptoms and treatments, along with dictionary look-up and other rule-based or machine-learning methods (Yang et al., 2009).

Reminders for Preventive Care and Disease Management

A computerized clinical reminder (CCR) system provides patient-specific recommendations. The scope of the recommendations includes a broad range of clinical activities, such as alerts about at-risk status, and reminders for appropriate screening, assessment, or treatment. CCRs can be integrated with information management services that improve workflow and increase chance for success in implementation. More specifically, in addition to providing recommendations, a CCR system can be equipped with the functionality to document relevant findings, provide explanations and literature citations, record, store, and identify data, generate outputs, calculate patient data to trigger rules, capture data to generate aggregated reports, and provide an interface to other components of EMR systems (Shiffman et al., 1999).

Systems for Drug Dosing and Prescribing

A dosing and prescribing CDSS (DP-CDSS) system provides decision support to a prescriber (usually a physician) or pharmacist when they are writing or filling a prescription. Support ranges from checking for drug allergies, drug–drug interactions, and basic dosing guidelines, to consideration of patient-specific diagnoses and history to provide drug recommendations or drug–disease interactions (Steele et al., 2005; Kuperman et al., 2007). A computerized physician order entry (CPOE) system integrated with a DP-CDSS can facilitate documentation and potentially reduce possible prescribing errors and adverse drug events (ADE) (Bates et al., 1998; Wolfstadt et al., 2008), which is one of the significant causes of hospitalized patient morbidity and mortality (Knight et al., 2005). Integration also provides other benefits, such as linking to algorithms to select cost-effective medications, and to reduce under-prescribing, overprescribing, and incorrect drug choices (Koppel et al., 2005).

Effects of CDSS: Outcome Measures

Impacts of CDSS on clinical performance have been shown in a large number of studies. A series of systematic reviews or meta-analysis demonstrate that CDSSs have great potential to improve clinician performance (Johnston et al., 1994; Shea et al., 1996; Hunt et al., 1998; Kaplan, 2001), decision quality (Sintchenko et al., 2004) and quality of care (Gorton et al., 1995; Shea et al., 1996; Calabrisi et al., 2002; Gandhi et al., 2003; Kralj et al., 2003; Sequist et al., 2005). However, the impact on patient outcomes remains understudied and, when studied, inconsistent results have been found (Hunt et al., 1998; Garg et al., 2005).

Mixed results have also been found for the impact of CDSSs on medication safety (Gandhi et al., 2003; Steele et al., 2005); costs (Tierney et al., 2003; McMullin et al., 2004); (organizational) efficiency (Tierney et al., 1993; Bates et al., 1999); adherence to guidelines and other standards (Walton et al., 1997; Tierney et al., 2005); time (Tierney et al., 1993; Overhage et al., 2001; Poissant et al., 2005; Pizziferri et al., 2005); and satisfaction, usage, and usability (Eslami et al., 2007). A diagnostic CDSS may also be evaluated based upon the consistency and accuracy of its classification of disease. It is worth mentioning that many of the studies used the designs based on observational studies or controlled trials that controlled the exposure to intervention. Other approaches for Health IT evaluation that have been commonly achieved in aviation, military, and consumer software industry, such as simulation, usability testing, or cognitive studies were rarely found in the healthcare literature.

Issues Associated with CDSS Implementation Success

CDSS Implementation Barriers

As with any other technology, CDSSs may introduce adverse consequences. For example, a CDSS for diagnostic management of young children with fever was successful regarding compliance and adherence to CDSS recommendations, but had unexpected effects on patient outcome in terms of ED length of stay and number of laboratory tests (Roukema et al., 2008). In another study, an unexpected increase in patient mortality rate from 2.80% to 6.57% has been observed after a commercially sold CPOE implementation, despite its evident reduction in medication error rates (Han et al., 2005). These examples showed that under certain circumstances, a CDSS may actually foster unintended adverse consequences.

Campbell et al. identified 245 and more unintended adverse consequences of CPOE and sorted these consequences into nine major categories, including more work, workflow, system demands, paper persistence, communication, emotions, new errors, and dependence on the technology (Campbell et al., 2006). A follow-up of their study showed that these adverse consequences had occurred in all of the 176 studying hospitals in the United States, and were ranked as moderately to very important by at least 72% of respondents (Ash et al., 2007). These adverse consequences often account for the reason why clinicians do not access or choose to ignore CDSS recommendations.

The adverse consequences are just one of the significant barriers to the implementation of CDSSs. Some of the many barriers to physician guideline adherence include providers' lack of familiarity with CDSSs, outcome expectancies, and guideline-, patient- and environmental-related issues (Cabana et al., 1999). Many of these barriers are also present for more conventional paper-based guidelines, and some of them can be overcome by changes in CDSSs, such as including features such as real-time support. Other barriers, including inadequate technology integration with workflow practices and poor user-interface design, may require significant changes in the design of CDSSs.

Barriers to the implementation of CDSSs have been classified into three categories: (1) organizational factors, (2) technical factors, and (3) human factors (Trivedi et al., 2002). Organizational factors are related to the culture and climate of the organization, such as its readiness and ability to change, and the management strategies and supports required to incorporate CDSS into practice. Providing adequate training and education throughout the implementation process is one of the critical organizational strategies to reduce providers' resistance to new software (Patterson et al., 2004; Varonen et al., 2008). Not only providers should be educated to use the software to a level of efficiency. Patient education combined with patient-specific recommendations to providers has been shown to be superior to provider education alone (Roumie et al., 2006). Other organizational issues include the administration benefiting more than provider from CDSS use (Patterson et al., 2005), communication between primary and secondary care (Hayrinen et al., 2008), clear incentive for users to use CDSS (Mollon et al., 2009), and involving local users in development process (Kawamoto et al., 2005; Mollon et al., 2009).

Technical factors reduce the functionality of the CDSS, and often involve software issues related to data standards, compatibility, transportability, usability, flexibility, reliability, and integration with other clinical programs (Patterson et al., 2004, 2005; Varonen et al., 2008; Mollon et al., 2009). These issues are generally encountered at the implementation stage of a CDSS and directly affect users' acceptance.

Effects on acceptance are closely related to response time and efficiency. If any of the technical deficiencies delay or interfere with providers' daily work, the consequent frustration and loss of confidence in the system will result in low acceptance and use of the CDSSs.

Unlike the technical issues that often emerge at the later stages of CDSS implementation, human-factors-related issues often arise in the design, planning, and development stages of CDSSs. One frequently mentioned human factors issue in the literature is provider–patient interaction (Patterson et al., 2004; Hayrinen et al., 2008; Varonen et al., 2008), which was reported to be influenced by the level of user IT literacy (Patel et al., 2000).

Increased workflow and time to use a CDSS are the most frequently identified human factors issues impeding CDSS implementation. Graham et al. conducted a cross-sectional survey of randomly selected physicians, and only 27% of 270 physicians felt that the CDSSs would save time (Graham et al., 2007). Another systematic literature review found that use of a CPOE significantly increased total prescribing time in most of the cases (Eslami et al., 2007). In addition, the issue of inapplicable recommendations, fatigue, and information overload is problematic with many CDSSs. Other human factors barriers include threats to clinician's autonomy (Varonen et al., 2008), resistance toward change (Varonen et al., 2008), extra work load (Patterson et al., 2004; Saleem et al., 2005; Varonen et al., 2008), time to remove inapplicable recommendations (Patterson et al., 2004; Saleem et al., 2005), false alarms (Patterson et al., 2004; Saleem et al., 2005), and lack of coordination between nurses and providers (Patterson et al., 2005; Saleem et al., 2005).

The aforementioned organizational, technical, and human-factors-related barriers are a major reason why CDSSs are still not in widespread use. Even though these factors may not be generalizable to all systems because of the different settings and constraints in each study, they provide diverse diagnoses of potential problems that can be avoided through vigorous design, planning, and development of CDSSs.

Roadmap to a Successful CDSS

As of 2000, the failure rate of clinical information systems implementation was reported to be greater than 50% (Kaplan, 2001). The many studies conducted tend to focus on identifying barriers rather than explaining why some CDSSs succeed. A notable exception is the study conducted by Kawamoto et al., which evaluated 15 features of CDSSs and found the following four features to be significantly correlated with system success, including (1) providing decision support automatically as part of clinician workflow, (2) delivering decision support at the time and location of decision making, (3) providing actionable recommendations, and (4) using a computer to generate the decision support (Kawamoto et al., 2005). Other studies of factors contributing to the success of CDSSs include the work of Rousseau et al., who concluded from semi-structured interviews of system users that improving relevance and accuracy of messages, ease of use of the system, and timing of the triggered guideline are critical for the success of CDSS implementation (Rousseau et al., 2003). In addition, clinicians' positive perception of CDSS usefulness is found to be crucial to foster their adoption of a CDSS (Pare et al., 2006). An overall conclusion is that workflow considerations and system usability are among the most important challenges in CDSS implementation. It is believed that most of the barriers can be overcome by integrating workflow and systematically developing and applying human-centered design, implementation, and evaluation methods to point-of-care CDSSs (Sittig et al., 2006).

Workflow Integration

The capability and degree for a CDSS to fit into the clinical workflow is shown to be critical for effective care coordination (Bates et al., 2003; Zai et al., 2008). For example, when a CPOE system is not electronically linked to pharmacy systems, pharmacists must manually reenter orders into the pharmacy system. However, as a national survey in 2001 shows, 25.7% of surveyed hospitals still required reentry of medication orders, which can possibly result in mistranscription of medication errors (Pedersen et al.,

2001). A proper designed CDSS should take advantage of structured data entry and maximize its reuse throughout the application.

When implementing a new CDSS, the sequence of work flow is often required to be changed to optimize healthcare delivery and efficiency. The altered workflow has different effects on different jobs and people (Ash et al., 2007). These changes of workflow are usually implemented either prior to or during the adoption of a CDSS. Changes in workflow that will be required to implement the CDSS and their potential impact must be carefully assessed in the planning and design phase of software development process to ensure success.

Workflow integration is not limited to "physical" workflow in the context of CDSS. A CDSS also needs to be nonintrusive to clinicians' "mental," or "cognitive" workflow. For instance, clinical reminders that are inapplicable or not provided "just-in-time" at the point of care may cause frustration or even "alert fatigue." In order to increase its utilization rate, a CDSS has to be less disruptive to the users' daily chores and workflow, and designed in a way that users can choose on demand (Rosenbloom et al., 2005).

Human-centered approaches have recently been applied in the domain of clinical workflow investigation to address these and other related issues. For example, Weir et al. used cognitive task analysis to identify the common components across tasks when using a CPOE system (Weir et al., 2007). Their study revealed that nearly half of the identified task components were not fully supported by the available CPOE technology. Clinicians thus had to spend extra efforts in retrieving relevant data, ensuring accuracy, and prioritizing information, in order to adapt to the CDSS. The disintegration of workflow had adversely imposed additional cognitive workload on the clinicians. Jalloh et al. prioritized clinical orders in their CPOE system by clinicians' search preference and the frequency of orders, and found significant reduction of orderable selection time (Jalloh and Waitman, 2006). These studies show that a good CDSS should assess the clinical and cognitive workflow early in the planning phase of CDSS development, with the aid of user-centered approaches to achieve this goal.

User-Centered Approach for System Design

A user-centered approach for system design by definition incorporates the need and preferences of the users throughout a system's development. User-centered techniques have been commonly practiced in industries such as aviation, automobiles, and consumer electronics. However, they are not currently widely used in the design and development of CDSSs. Often, this only involves conducting a user satisfaction survey in the evaluation stage after a CDSS has been implemented or after problems have been encountered.

A more complete user-centered approach will include a user needs assessment and analysis, followed by application of user interface design guidelines, rapid prototyping, and testing, prior to application release. Testing using a quick mock-up or prototype can provide an efficient and effective way to solicit users' feedback in order to understand users' needs, identify problems, and to collect expected outcomes before a new design is completely implemented. This allows time for system adjustment, and most importantly prevents unintended adverse consequences.

User-centered CDSS design is the protocol to improving the usability of a CDSS. Usability is not limited to the hardware and software that compose the computer systems. From the user's point of view, usability of an interface must be judged in the context of use, which also includes activity associated with the use of help systems, training, and other associated operating procedures required to complete the task.

Incorporating user-centered approaches into CDSS design and implementation processes can potentially overcome many of the aforementioned technical and human-factors-related barriers. One conspicuous example is designing a user-centered human–computer interface of CDSSs, which has been one of the most important challenges in clinical decision support (Sittig et al., 2008). A user-centered CDSS interface should support, rather than impede, clinical workflows, to provide clear, concise, and actionable warnings and advice (Bates et al., 2003; Ash et al., 2004; Kuperman et al., 2007). The alerts or reminders should display sufficient information so that clinicians understand the rationale for the interruption. To accomplish this type of advanced CDSSs, it presents a great human factors challenge, and requires user interface capabilities that are often lacking in most CDSS design and development.

The case study in the following section provides an example demonstrating how user-centered techniques can be employed to improve the interface of a CDSS and further affect users' clinical decisions. The methodology used in the study is typical in project design lifecycle management, including needs assessment, application of user interface design guidelines, rapid prototyping, and evaluation.

Gearing up for Better Performance: A Case Study

VA'S COMPUTERIZED PATIENT RECORD SYSTEM AND COMPUTERIZED CLINICAL REMINDERS

The Veterans Health Information Systems and Technology Architecture (VistA) is a health information system implemented by the U.S. Department of Veterans Affairs (VA) in VA's over 1000 healthcare facilities. Its graphical user interface, the computerized patient record system (CPRS), integrates an EMR database with numerous decision support modules to allow healthcare providers to review and update patients' records (Figure 48.1). A point-and-click CPOE system allows providers to place orders, including medications, laboratory tests, and special procedures. An order checking system enables the CPOE system to alert clinicians when potential problems are found.

In addition to providing a CPOE, other decision support in CPRS includes critical alerts for abnormal lab results or crisis notes, a remote date viewer to access information from other VA facilities, and the CCR system. The CCR system is an automated system that provides reminders based on evidence-based clinical guidelines, and is intended to reduce providers' workload and their reliance on memory. The CCR system in the VA is both context and time sensitive.

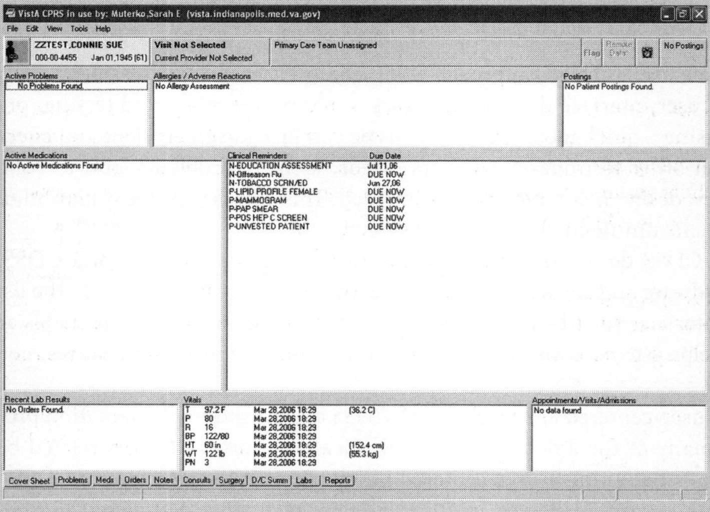

FIGURE 48.1 The VA's CPRS.

It recognizes the patients' specific diagnosis and the time elapsed since the last reminder was provided. The VA's CCR system also provides standardized screening protocols in its dialog boxes and automatically generated documentation.

Recent studies have reported that CCRs have been underused by clinicians, resulting in missed opportunities for provision of preventive care (Schellhase et al., 2003). Moreover, adherence to individual CCRs has been found to be variable (Agrawal and Mayo-Smith, 2004). A prior investigation by Wu et al. shed light on several important factors associated with CCR adherence. One finding was that the perceived clinical importance of particular reminders was related to the likeliness of adherence with them. Moreover, physicians' projected resolution time was found to be inversely correlated to their adherence rate (Wu et al., 2007). This finding implies that a CCR perceived as taking longer to resolve is more likely to be deferred. One explanation comes from time restriction and work load, which often forces primary care providers to choose among multiple problems and tasks during a given visit. Another possible explanation is that the "black-box" design of some VA CCRs fails to provide conspicuous reasons why a CCR is triggered. Consequently, it is important to develop a CCR system that facilitates the retrieval of relevant data by prioritizing information, and providing it at the time it is needed in the patient care process (Weir et al., 2007).

To address these issues, we designed a new CCR system to assist clinicians in achieving more effective prioritization decisions. The design modifications included a knowledge-based risk factor repository, a role-based filter, and a prioritization mechanism, as will be elaborated in the following section. The performance of the original and new CCR designs were prototyped and tested in a study involving primary care physicians in a controlled human–computer interaction (HCI) lab.

PROTOTYPING AND TESTING OF THE NEW CCR DESIGN

A web-based prototype was developed as a mock-up of the current VA CPRS system (Figure 48.2). This web-based CPRS simulation provided a platform for studying use of CRPS in simulated

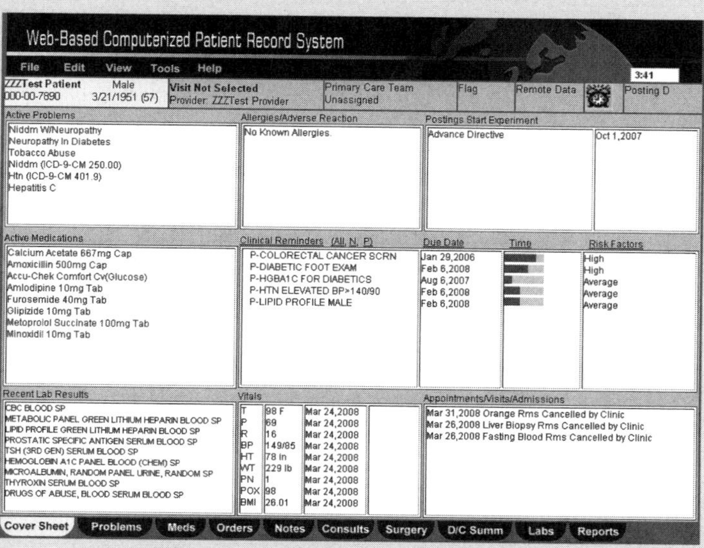

FIGURE 48.2 The CPRS prototype with the new design of CCR system (simulated data).

clinic settings. Two different designs of the web-based CPRS were developed. Design A, representing the original design, has the interface built upon the current VA CPRS system. In design B, numerous design modifications were implemented. Three major design features were added to the modified design in order to assist providers in prioritizing CCRs, as expanded upon below.

Risk Factor Repository

We designed a risk factor repository that connected to patient's EHR to populate a systematic review of patient's risk factors (i.e., problem list, laboratory results, other diagnostic tests), past encounter summary, and pending exams. This tool automatically summarized risk factor assessment through a knowledge base in order to facilitate early detection of a disease or other preventive services. The interface for the risk factor repository was programmed using JavaScript to include an expandable tree feature to facilitate navigation. This repository was connected to the CPRS database and accessible as a pop-up window with a single click on the corresponding CCR (Figure 48.3). The intent was to make it easy for clinicians to quickly retrieve desired information without having to manually browse through various locations for patient information.

Prioritization Mechanism

The second feature added to the prototype CCR system was a prioritization mechanism that enabled users to prioritize the clinical reminders according to several CCR attributes, including CCR due date, estimated resolution time, and risk factors. Due date information enabled clinicians to easily tell how long a CCR was past due. Resolution time estimated how long it would take to resolve a CCR, including the time needed to both address the issue and document the resolution. A "risk" score of "average" or "high" was also assigned to represent a person's chances of developing a disease. This risk score was triggered by the same knowledge base that powered the risk factor repository. The prioritization mechanism facilitates providers' decision process and assists them in recognizing important reminder recommendations by their own criteria.

Role-Based Filter

The third design feature, the role-based filter, was designed to optionally display the CCRs to be addressed by nurses (N), physicians (P), or both, as designated by the users. The role-based filter was designed as a system intervention to prioritize who should best receive the reminder in order to reduce information overload and improve the use of the CCR system.

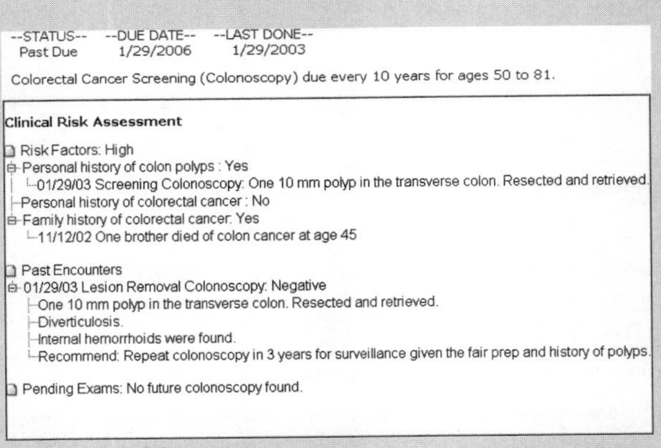

FIGURE 48.3 The risk factor repository for colorectal cancer screening.

EXPERIMENTAL PROCEDURE

Sixteen VA physicians were recruited opportunistically to participate in the experimental study. The first participant's data was later discarded because the simulated patient history was modified following the first experiment. The experiment was conducted in a HCI laboratory to provide a controlled, closed setting to simulate physicians using a workstation in an exam room.

The experiment started with a structured exploration session that acquainted the subjects with the CPRS prototype with the original CCR design (design A) and simulated patient data. The base case scenario was a 55-year-old male smoker with 4-year history of type II diabetes, and other active problems, including hypertension, tobacco abuse, and neuropathy in diabetes. The participants further used an interactive simulator programmed with JavaScript to simulate the procedure of a typical patient encounter in an exam room. The simulator provided real-time interactive feedback pertaining to patient symptoms, examination and checkup results as the participants walked through a simulated physical exam.

Near the end of the simulated patient encounter, the participants were asked to prioritize the five remaining CCRs in a ranked order and explain their decisions. These clinical reminders were diabetic foot exam, hemoglobin A1c, colorectal cancer screening, hypertension, and LIPID profile.

In the second half of the experiment, the subjects were introduced to the new CCR design (design B) and its new features. After the subjects walked through each feature in the new design, they were then asked the same questions to prioritize the same CCRs, assuming they were seeing the same patient. Finally, the interview concluded by a web-based survey for the subject to rate the usefulness of each design feature on a five-point Likert scale.

STUDY RESULTS

This study investigated how physicians prioritized CCRs under time pressure given both the original and new designs (Table 48.1). With the original design, participants on average prioritized the reminders in the following ranked order: hypertension (mean = 1.69, s.d. = 0.85), hemoglobin A1c (mean = 1.93, s.d. = 1.10), LIPID profile (mean = 2.67, s.d. = 1.35), diabetic foot exam (mean = 3.47, s.d. = 1.46), and colorectal cancer screening (mean = 3.53, s.d. = 1.51). For the new design, 12 out of the 15 subjects modified their prioritization decisions. The average priority of the reminders when using the new system was: colorectal cancer screening (mean = 1.87, s.d. = 1.51), hemoglobin A1c (mean = 2.53, s.d. = 1.19), hypertension (mean = 2.62, s.d. = 0.96), diabetic foot exam (mean = 2.62, s.d. = 0.96), and lipid profile (mean = 3.27, s.d. = 1.33). This result showed that the new design changed physician's prioritization decision substantially. The new design impacted 12 (80%) out of 15 subjects and 33 (44%) out of a total of 75 prioritization decisions. The proposed design features were also rated useful or very useful by the participants.

Figure 48.4a and b demonstrates the relationship between resolution time and CCR priority for the original and the new design, respectively. As indicated in Figure 48.4a, a positive

TABLE 48.1 Priority Order Elicited from Each Participant with Original Design (on the Left) and Modified Design (on the Right)

	With Original Design					With Modified Design				
Priority	CRC	D.Foot	HTN	HgbA1c	LIPID	CRC	D.Foot	HTN	HgbA1c	LIPID
Mean	3.53	3.47	1.69	1.923	2.67	1.87	2.73	2.62	2.53	3.27
s.d.	1.51	1.46	0.85	1.10	1.35	1.51	1.53	0.96	1.19	1.33

Note: CRC, colorectal cancer screening; D.Foot, diabetic foot exam; HTN, hypertension screening; HgbA1c, hemoglobin A1c test; LIPID, lipid profile.

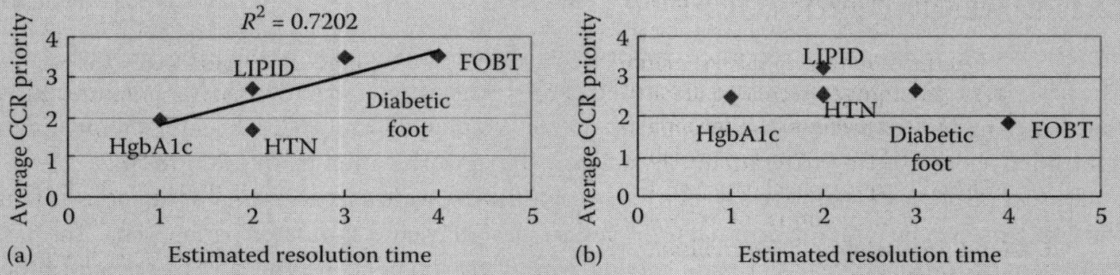

FIGURE 48.4 Average CCR priority versus estimated resolution time in the (a) original design and (b) the modified design. (*Note*: Lower numerical value in *Y* axis stands for higher priority.)

linear correlation between CCR resolution time and priority was found in the original design (R^2 = 0.7202), when, in fact, no resolution time information was provided to the participants. The results also showed that clinicians consider CCR resolution time during a patient encounter, subconsciously or not, and factored the time into their prioritization decisions. This result is consistent with our prior study, where a CCR perceived easier to resolve would be more likely to be resolved (Wu et al., 2007).

Intriguingly, the correlation between resolution time and priority was much lower when the subjects used the new design (R^2 = 0.3101) (see Figure 48.4b). This result supports the conclusion that the new design caused a shift in physician decision making for the simulated patient's scenario, in which resolution time was no longer a dominant decision criterion.

Conclusions

CDSSs provide clinicians, staffs, and patients with patient-specific information at the place and time decisions are to be made. Evidences have shown that CDSSs can improve practitioner performance, especially in increasing adherence to guidelines and other standards. However, research has shown mixed results where, in some cases, the benefits have not been demonstrated to their expected degree. Significant barriers remain, such as unintended adverse consequences after CDSS implementation, and the organizational, technical, and human factors. Several solutions have been proposed, including workflow integration and user-centered design to overcome human–machine interface flaws. The feasibility of successfully removing some of these barriers was illustrated by the case study given in this chapter.

This case study demonstrated that a user-centered redesign of the VA's CCR system changed the way providers incorporated CCR information to achieve a clinical decision. This reaffirmed the need for a user-centered system that is able to align the system's information flow with physician's workflow to facilitate retrieving desired information at the right place and right time. The proposed design features and usability testing approach can be beneficial to the audience who are in the planning and design phase for implementing clinical information systems, as well as those who are adding heuristic modules to their preexisting CCR system.

References

Agrawal, A. and M.F. Mayo-Smith. 2004. Adherence to computerized clinical reminders in large healthcare delivery network. *Medinfo* 11:111–114.

Ash, J.S., M. Berg, and E. Coiera. 2004. Some unintended consequences of information technology in health care: The nature of patient care information system-related errors. *J Am Med Inform Assoc* 11(2):104–112.

Ash, J.S. et al. 2007. The extent and importance of unintended consequences related to computerized provider order entry. *J Am Med Inform Assoc* 14(4):415–423.

Bates, D.W. et al. 1998. Effect of computerized physician order entry and a team intervention on prevention of serious medication errors. *JAMA* 280(15):1311–1316.

Bates, D.W. et al. 1999. A randomized trial of a computer-based intervention to reduce utilization of redundant laboratory tests. *Am J Med* 106(2):144–150.

Bates, D.W. et al. 2003. Ten commandments for effective clinical decision support: Making the practice of evidence-based medicine a reality. *J Am Med Inform Assoc* 10(6):523–530.

Cabana, M.D. et al. 1999. Why don't physicians follow clinical practice guidelines? A framework for improvement. *JAMA* 282(15):1458–1465.

Calabrisi, R.R., T. Czarnecki, and C. Blank. 2002. The impact of clinical reminders and alerts on health screenings. The VA Pittsburgh Healthcare System achieves notable results by enhancing an automated clinical reminder system within its CPR—And has the data to prove it. *Health Manag Technol* 23(12):32–34.

Campbell, E.M. et al. 2006. Types of unintended consequences related to computerized provider order entry. *J Am Med Inform Assoc* 13(5):547–556.

Chen, L. et al. 2008. Decision tool for the early diagnosis of trauma patient hypovolemia. *J Biomed Inform* 41(3):469–478.

Eslami, S., A. Abu-Hanna, and N.F. de Keizer. 2007. Evaluation of outpatient computerized physician medication order entry systems: A systematic review. *J Am Med Inform Assoc* 14(4):400–406.

Friedman, C.P. et al. 1999. Enhancement of clinicians' diagnostic reasoning by computer-based consultation: A multisite study of 2 systems. *JAMA* 282(19):1851–1856.

Fritsche, L. et al. 2002. Recognition of critical situations from time series of laboratory results by case-based reasoning. *J Am Med Inform Assoc* 9(5):520–528.

Gandhi, T.K. et al. 2003. Adverse drug events in ambulatory care. *N Engl J Med* 348(16):1556–1564.

Garg, A.X. et al. 2005. Effects of computerized clinical decision support systems on practitioner performance and patient outcomes: A systematic review. *JAMA* 293(10):1223–1238.

Gellerstedt, M., A. Bang, and J. Herlitz. 2006. Could a computer-based system including a prevalence function support emergency medical systems and improve the allocation of life support level? *Eur J Emerg Med* 13(5):290–294.

Gorton, T.A. et al. 1995. Primary care physicians' response to dissemination of practice guidelines. *Arch Fam Med* 4(2):135–142.

Graham, I.D. et al. 2007. Physicians' intentions and use of three patient decision aids. *BMC Med Inform Decis Making* 7:20.

Greenes, R. (Ed.). 2007. *Clinical Decision Support: The Road Ahead*, Elsevier, Academic Press: Burlington, MA.

Han, Y.Y. et al. 2005. Unexpected increased mortality after implementation of a commercially sold computerized physician order entry system. *Pediatrics* 116(6):1506–1512.

Hayrinen, K., K. Saranto, and P. Nykanen. 2008. Definition, structure, content, use and impacts of electronic health records: A review of the research literature. *Int J Med Inform* 77(5):291–304.

Hunt, D.L. et al. 1998. Effects of computer-based clinical decision support systems on physician performance and patient outcomes: A systematic review. *JAMA* 280(15):1339–1346.

Jalloh, O.B. and L.R. Waitman. 2006. Improving computerized provider order entry (CPOE) usability by data mining users' queries from access logs. *AMIA Annu Symp Proc* 379–383.

Johnston, M.E. et al. 1994. Effects of computer-based clinical decision support systems on clinician performance and patient outcome. A critical appraisal of research. *Ann Intern Med* 120(2):135–142.

Kaplan, B. 2001. Evaluating informatics applications—Clinical decision support systems literature review. *Int J Med Inform* 64(1):15–37.

Kawamoto, K. et al. 2005. Improving clinical practice using clinical decision support systems: A systematic review of trials to identify features critical to success. *BMJ* 330(7494):765–768.

Knight, A.M. et al. 2005. The effect of computerized provider order entry on medical student clerkship experiences. *J Am Med Inform Assoc* 12(5):554–560.

Koppel, R. et al. 2005. Role of computerized physician order entry systems in facilitating medication errors. *JAMA* 293(10):1197–1203.

Kralj, B. et al. 2003. The impact of computerized clinical reminders on physician prescribing behavior: Evidence from community oncology practice. *Am J Med Qual* 18(5):197–203.

Kuperman, G.J. et al. 2007. Medication-related clinical decision support in computerized provider order entry systems: A review. *J Am Med Inform Assoc* 14(1):29–40.

McMullin, S.T. et al. 2004. Impact of an evidence-based computerized decision support system on primary care prescription costs. *Ann Fam Med* 2(5):494–498.

Mollon, B. et al. 2009. Features predicting the success of computerized decision support for prescribing: A systematic review of randomized controlled trials. *BMC Med Inform Decis Making* 9:11.

Overhage, J.M. et al. 2001. Controlled trial of direct physician order entry: Effects on physicians' time utilization in ambulatory primary care internal medicine practices. *J Am Med Inform Assoc* 8(4):361–371.

Pare, G., C. Sicotte, and H. Jacques. 2006. The effects of creating psychological ownership on physicians' acceptance of clinical information systems. *J Am Med Inform Assoc* 13(2):197–205.

Patel, V.L. et al. 2000. Impact of a computer-based patient record system on data collection, knowledge organization, and reasoning. *J Am Med Inform Assoc* 7(6):569–585.

Patterson, E.S. et al. 2004. Human factors barriers to the effective use of ten HIV clinical reminders. *J Am Med Inform Assoc* 11(1):50–59.

Patterson, E.S. et al. 2005. Identifying barriers to the effective use of clinical reminders: Bootstrapping multiple methods. *J Biomed Inform* 38(3):189–199.

Pedersen, C.A., P.J. Schneider, and J.P. Santell. 2001. ASHP national survey of pharmacy practice in hospital settings: Prescribing and transcribing-2001. *Am J Health Syst Pharm* 58(23):2251–2266.

Pizziferri, L. et al. 2005. Primary care physician time utilization before and after implementation of an electronic health record: A time-motion study. *J Biomed Inform* 38(3):176–188.

Poissant, L. et al. 2005. The impact of electronic health records on time efficiency of physicians and nurses: A systematic review. *J Am Med Inform Assoc* 12(5):505–516.

Rosenbloom, S.T. et al. 2005. Effect of CPOE user interface design on user-initiated access to educational and patient information during clinical care. *J Am Med Inform Assoc* 12(4):458–473.

Roukema, J. et al. 2008. Randomized trial of a clinical decision support system: Impact on the management of children with fever without apparent source. *J Am Med Inform Assoc* 2008 15(1):107–113.

Roumie, C.L. et al. 2006. Improving blood pressure control through provider education, provider alerts, and patient education: A cluster randomized trial. *Ann Intern Med* 145(3):165–175.

Rousseau, N. et al. 2003. Practice based, longitudinal, qualitative interview study of computerised evidence based guidelines in primary care. *BMJ* 326(7384):314–318.

Saleem, J.J. et al. 2005. Exploring barriers and facilitators to the use of computerized clinical reminders. *J Am Med Inform Assoc* 12(4):438–447.

Schellhase, K.G., T.D. Koepsell, and T.E. Norris. 2003. Providers' reactions to an automated health maintenance reminder system incorporated into the patient's electronic medical record. *Am Board Fam Pract* 16:312–317.

Sequist, T.D. et al. 2005. A randomized trial of electronic clinical reminders to improve quality of care for diabetes and coronary artery disease. *J Am Med Inform Assoc* 12(4):431–437.

Shea, S., W. DuMouchel, and L. Bahamonde. 1996. A meta-analysis of 16 randomized controlled trials to evaluate computer-based clinical reminder systems for preventive care in the ambulatory setting. *J Am Med Inform Assoc* 3(6):399–409.

Shiffman, R.N. et al. 1999. Computer-based guideline implementation systems: A systematic review of functionality and effectiveness. *J Am Med Inform Assoc* 6(2):104–114.

Sintchenko, V. et al. 2004. Comparative impact of guidelines, clinical data, and decision support on prescribing decisions: An interactive web experiment with simulated cases. *J Am Med Inform Assoc* 11(1):71–77.

Sittig, D.F. et al. 2006. Lessons from "Unexpected increased mortality after implementation of a commercially sold computerized physician order entry system." *Pediatrics* 118(2):797–801.

Sittig, D.F. et al. 2008. Grand challenges in clinical decision support. *J Biomed Inform* 41(2):387–392.

Steele, A.W. et al. 2005. The effect of automated alerts on provider ordering behavior in an outpatient setting. *PLoS Med* 2(9):255.

Tierney, W.M. et al. 1993. Physician inpatient order writing on microcomputer workstations. Effects on resource utilization. *JAMA* 269(3):379–383.

Tierney, W.M. et al. 2003. Effects of computerized guidelines for managing heart disease in primary care: A randomized, controlled trial. *J Gen Intern Med* 18(12):967–976.

Tierney, W.M. et al. 2005. Can computer-generated evidence-based care suggestions enhance evidence-based management of asthma and chronic obstructive pulmonary disease? A randomized, controlled trial. *Health Serv Res* 40(2):477–497.

Trivedi, M.H. et al. 2002. Development and implementation of computerized clinical guidelines: Barriers and solutions. *Methods Inform Med* 41(5):435–442.

Uzuner, O., X. Zhang, and T. Sibanda. 2009. Machine learning and rule-based approaches to assertion classification. *J Am Med Inform Assoc* 16(1):109–115.

Varonen, H., T. Kortteisto, and M. Kaila. 2008. What may help or hinder the implementation of computerized decision support systems (CDSSs): A focus group study with physicians. *Fam Pract* 25(3):162–167.

Walton, R.T. et al. 1997. Evaluation of computer support for prescribing (CAPSULE) using simulated cases. *BMJ* 315(7111):791–795.

Weir, C.R. et al. 2007. A cognitive task analysis of information management strategies in a computerized provider order entry environment. *J Am Med Inform Assoc* 14(1):65–75.

Wolfstadt, J.I. et al. 2008. The effect of computerized physician order entry with clinical decision support on the rates of adverse drug events: A systematic review. *J Gen Intern Med* 23(4):451–458.

Wu, S.J. et al. 2007. Relationship of estimated resolution time and computerized clinical reminder adherence. *AMIA Annu Symp Proc* 334–338.

Yang, H. et al. 2009. A text mining approach to the prediction of disease status from clinical discharge summaries. *J Am Med Inform Assoc* 16(4):596–600.

Zai, A.H. et al. 2008. Lessons from implementing a combined workflow-informatics system for diabetes management. *J Am Med Inform Assoc* 15(4):524–533.

Zhang, Y. and P. Szolovits. 2008. Patient-specific learning in real time for adaptive monitoring in critical care. *J Biomed Inform* 41(3):452–460.

49

Health Informatics: Systems and Design Considerations

Jose Antonio Valdez
University of Wisconsin Hospital and Clinics

Rupa Sheth Valdez
University of Wisconsin–Madison

What Is Health Informatics? 49-1
Systems Context of Health Information Technologies 49-2
Cybernetics • Macroergonomics • Behavior Change and Social Networks • Systems Life Cycle
Designing Health Information Technologies 49-4
Defining User Needs • Design Heuristics • Deployment Issues
References 49-7

What Is Health Informatics?

The field of health informatics, also referred to as medical informatics, lies at the intersection of multiple disciplines including the health sciences, computer science, information science, and management and decision science. By combining knowledge from these diverse disciplines, health informaticians work to improve the acquisition, storage, and use of information. Health information technologies (HITs) have been implemented across the healthcare sector to advance cognate domains as medical decision making, healthcare delivery, health and health information management, and health education.

Multiple subdisciplines, named for the intended user of the developed technology, are contained within the field of health informatics. Although no definitive taxonomy exists, cited subdisciplines include bioinformatics, clinical informatics, consumer health informatics, dental informatics, imaging informatics, nursing informatics, pharmacoinformatics, and public health informatics (Shortliffe and Blois, 2001; Hersh, 2002; American Medical Informatics Association, 2008). As reflected in the titles of these subdisciplines, HITs are used by health practitioners, patients, and policy makers in clinical, home, and community settings.

Successful design, development, and deployment of HITs involves addressing both micro-level factors such as the terminologies used and macro-level factors like how the technology will be integrated into existing workflow. Multiple systems approaches exist to facilitate the design of HITs. These approaches highlight the macro- and micro-level factors that must be simultaneously considered to create technology that may be effectively implemented and sustained. These systems perspectives are relevant regardless of the intended type, location, and user of the HIT.

Systems Context of Health Information Technologies

A *system* can be defined as a set of interacting elements that form an integrated, often complex, whole. In the design, development, and deployment of HITs, several systems perspectives become relevant.

Cybernetics

Cybernetics is the scientific study of communication and control processes in biological and artificial systems (Wiener, 1948). Figure 49.1 shows the components of a typical cybernetic system. *Inputs* go through a *conversion process* from which desired *outputs* emerge. Outputs are then monitored through a *sensor* that compares it with *standards*. *Error signals* are then sent to a *control* unit that undertakes corrective action on the inputs and/or conversion processes. All of these elements are influenced by the *environment* in which the system is operating.

This model becomes immediately relevant in the context of building HITs in several ways. First, there is the teleological issue: what is the *purpose* of the system? Complex systems often suffer from "featuritis"—additional functionality that users do not necessarily need or want—due to poor definition and anticipation of user requirements, or what problem needs to be solved. This often stems from decision makers having an innate bias to adopt new technologies, regardless of whether or not they have been proven to be superior over existing ones.

Second, a good system requires the existence of an effective and efficient *feedback and control loop*—a sensor/monitor function, clearly defined standards, the timely transmission of error signals to the control unit, and the subsequent execution of corrective action. Deliberate consideration of these elements at the design stage goes a long way toward ensuring that system goals are met.

Third, this perspective also implies that one examines and monitors how *structure or environment* influences processes and behavior, which in turn influences events and system outcomes. Variables such as organizational structure and priorities, industry demand patterns and supply constraints, regulatory requirements, sociocultural norms, and technological advancements, exert pressure on these system

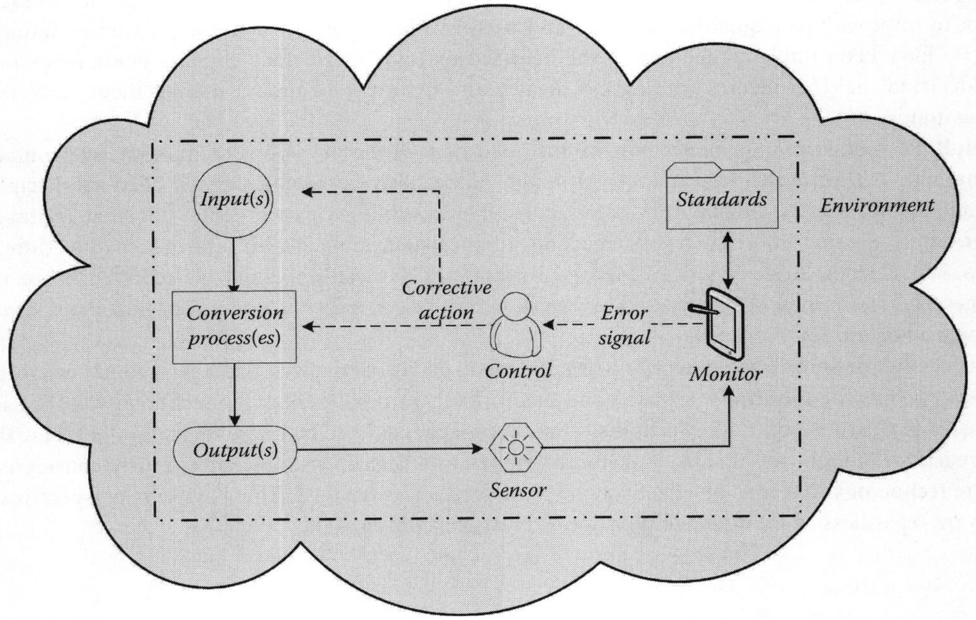

FIGURE 49.1 Components of a typical cybernetic system.

elements. Some effects may be drastic and immediate, while others can be largely unseen as changes occur slowly over time.

Macroergonomics

Macroergonomics conceptualizes HIT as one element of a total work system. The role of the designer is to create the proper fit between the multiple elements of the work system and the HIT being developed. Multiple models of the work system exist; the primary difference between these models is the scope. Smith and Carayon-Sainfort (1989) propose a model that constrains the work systems to elements contained within a single institution. In this model, the work system elements are the tasks, individuals, tools and technologies, physical and organizational environments. More recent models of the work system have expanded this definition to include the legal and regulatory environment in which an institution operates (Rasmussen, 2000) and the sociocultural context in which the legal and regulatory environment and institution are embedded (Moray, 2000; Wilson, 2000). Common to all models, however, is the philosophy that a technology is embedded within a larger work system and that changes in any work system element affect other system elements.

Interactions that may occur between the HIT and other elements of the work system must, therefore, be considered during the design process. A balance should be achieved between elements of the system, and one system element may be enhanced to compensate for a deficiency in another system element (Smith and Carayon-Saintfort, 1989). For example, dim lighting in a workspace may be balanced by bright lighting on the screen of a computer technology. When more macro-level elements such as the legal and regulatory environments or sociocultural context are conceptualized as part of the work system, designers should begin by understanding and designing for interactions between the HIT and the macro-level elements (Hendrick and Kleiner, 2002), and then progressively working toward understanding and designing for interactions between the HIT and more micro-level elements. For example, the sociocultural practices of the patient population and the standards advanced by legal and regulatory bodies like the Joint Commission (an independent, non-profit organization that accredits and certifies healthcare organizations in the United States) should inform the design of the organization's policies and procedures.

Behavior Change and Social Networks

What makes the domain of healthcare intrinsically difficult to manage is the fact that it can be simultaneously conceptualized as a machine, an organism, and as a social system (Ackoff, 1994). We can view users of HITs as being organismic systems in and of themselves, with individual learning styles, preferences, values, motivations, expectations—each one exerting influence over the other, as well as the environment in which they are embedded. It is therefore necessary to consider an *individual's readiness for and propensity to change*, given the natural tension that comes with adopting a new HIT.

The stages of change model (Prochaska et al., 1992), while initially developed within the field of addiction treatment, can prove useful in understanding the change process and the difficulties associated with changing people's habits and rituals. In this model, people undergoing behavior change are posited to go through distinct, sequential stages: (1) pre-contemplation (the individual does not recognize the need for change, or is not actively pursuing it); (2) contemplation (the individual is considering changing his/her behavior); (3) preparation (the individual is taking steps preparing for the change); (4) action (the individual has initiated the change); and (5) maintenance (the individual is sustaining new behaviors). Often, people relapse back to the status quo prior to the change, and the process begins anew. Knowledge that most people go through this progressive spiral of behavior change can be leveraged to make pilot testing and/or deployment efforts of HITs more successful. Forcing individuals to accept new technologies without regard to their degree of readiness can lead to protracted implementation difficulties.

As individuals interact and aggregate into groups, organizations, and populations, it is also important to consider how HITs *spread* throughout social networks. In this vein, Rogers' work (2003) on diffusion theory provides guidance on how to improve the rate of adoption of HITs. Perceptions of the relative advantage of the new HIT as well as the strength of interpersonal network channels lie at the heart of the diffusion process. Additionally, models and methods of social network analysis (Wasserman and Faust, 2004) allow measurement of network characteristics (e.g., network density, degree of centralization, clustering tendencies) and the identification of opinion leaders and effective change agents, which can likewise be leveraged to smooth out the technology adoption process.

Systems Life Cycle

Every system evolves through time, and follows the sequential steps of conception, design, creation, transition (to use), utilization, and eventually, senility and replacement. The notion of a systems life cycle (Blanchard and Fabrycky, 2005) is important in the context of building HITs, given the pace with which modern HITs evolve vis-à-vis constantly changing user needs and expectations. Even as HITs get diffused within organizations and populations, new technologies are being developed, waiting for their turn in the technology adoption process.

As HITs transition to widespread use, issues of scalability, robustness, and adaptivity become relevant, constant monitoring of system performance is therefore required in order to ensure that new technologies consistently meet users' needs. At a certain point in the system life cycle, the cost-effectiveness of maintaining existing HITs will be less than optimal when compared to new HITs. New HITs may be more cost effective because they increase efficiency, reduce medical errors, or increase quality of care. Upon deciding to replace an existing HIT, careful consideration must be given to the environmental impact of materials and equipment when it comes time for disposal and replacement.

In summary, the term "system" can be defined in multiple ways and each provides a unique framework for elucidating design requirements as well as in guiding deployment activities. Adopting a systems approach then implies taking different perspectives (cybernetic, macroergonomic, social, and temporal) and factoring in critical elements (environmental impact, feedback loops, standards, workload balance, individual behavior change, network diffusion, and system life cycles) in order to build and use effective HITs.

Designing Health Information Technologies

Suppose we are asked to explore the potential of using a computerized physician order entry system (CPOE)—technology that allows doctors to enter orders through the computer instead of traditional handwriting. Where do we begin and what are the salient points of systems design?

Developers of new HITs have a tacit assumption that the quality of care will be improved; yet, it is not prudent to base the decision to adopt new technologies on this alone. Neither is it conscientious to embrace new HITs just because they are in vogue—i.e., everyone else is doing it, and therefore we should, too. A thorough understanding of potential benefits provided by CPOE, weighed against the costs and risks involved, should serve as the primary backdrop for decision making. Benefit–cost analysis should also be informed by *actual* experiences of organizations that have adopted the technology, as well as any systematic reviews published on the subject (Kaushal et al., 2003; Kuperman and Gibson, 2003).

Defining User Needs

It is important to define clear system goals at the outset, which are predicated on an exhaustive assessment of user needs for all key stakeholders. An enterprise-wide CPOE system can have several components—i.e., lab, radiology, pharmacy—making the task of needs assessment arduous and complex. To this end, visualization techniques from process engineering (e.g., process flowcharts, cross-functional (swimlane) diagrams, value-stream maps) could be used as the first step in eliciting specific user requirements; these diagrams also provide a practical design guide to how CPOE can be integrated into the workflow.

In practical terms, creating collaborative, high-level value-stream maps (Lummus et al., 2006) with representatives from each of the key functions involved provides a common bird's eye view for system users. Development of a "present state" value-stream map enables the identification of areas of waste in the current process; a "future state" map can then be created to show how the system *should* be, taking into account the CPOE technology to be adopted. Cross-functional flowcharts can be developed for each process identified in the value-stream maps created to provide further depth and detail for identified workflows.

Gathering data for user needs assessment in general can essentially be classified into three categories: interaction, observation, and personal experience (Figure 49.2). The most common method applied is user *interaction*: *asking* users what they need or want. This can be done through a variety of methods—i.e., surveys, interviews, focus groups—with the objective of identifying the range of user needs, their relative importance, and the variations that exist within and among groups. These basic knowledge elicitation techniques have been adapted and combined into stylized methods (e.g., the critical incident technique, cognitive "walkthroughs") or more rigorous analytical approaches (e.g., cognitive task analysis, failure mode, and effects analysis), which can be effectively used for CPOE needs assessment.

More often than not, however, what people say they do is different from what they *actually* do. This is the reason why user *observation* is necessary to corroborate data derived through user interaction. *Shadowing* users as they go through work tasks is one of the most effective means of defining user requirements for CPOE-supported systems. Classic *time-and-motion studies* could also be used to get a sense of overall workflow throughput, as well as potential resource bottlenecks. When possible, *data mining of electronic tracking data* (e.g., phone logs, pager data, database use statistics) should also be conducted to better understand system performance and integration issues.

Last, personal *experience* can be the most powerful way to understand what users need. Role-playing can provide insight into what system users actually experience, as it simulates the CPOE decision-making environment in real time. Participant observation, a staple of ethnographic methods, can provide a sense of the impact on user affect and cognition—variables that may be hard to capture through user interaction or traditional observation.

Each of these approaches—interaction, observation, and personal experience—affords unique advantages as well as its own share of shortcomings. Employing elements of all three approaches in the user needs assessment phase allows one to *triangulate* on what the system requires, as well as anticipate potential sources of error.

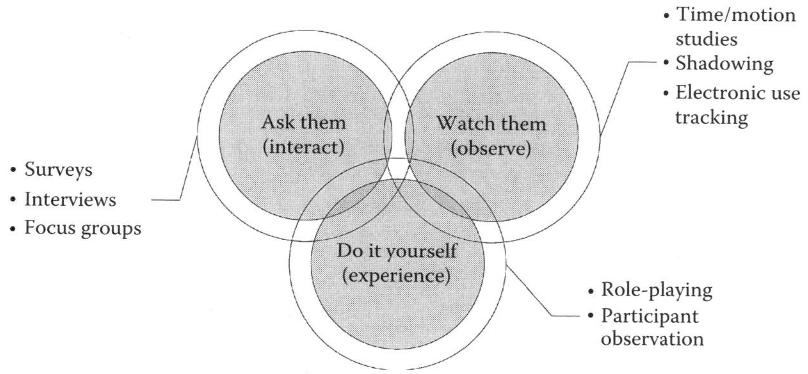

FIGURE 49.2 User needs triangulation.

Functionality	Technical Advantage	Emotional Impact	Cultural Acceptability
Is it **safe?**	Is it **fast?**	Does it have good **aesthetics?**	Is it within social **norms?**
Is it **reliable?**	Is it **easy to learn?**	Are users given a **choice?**	Does it have **currency?**
Does it provide good **feedback?**	Is it **error-forgiving?**	Does it **engage** or **entertain?**	Does it have **credibility?**
Is it **easy to use?**	Is it **standardized?**	Does it **anticipate** user needs?	Is it culturally **inclusive?**

FIGURE 49.3 Design heuristics.

Design Heuristics

Specific design components needed to build HITs will, in part, be dictated by the nature of the technology being built (i.e., data storage and retrieval, communication, decision support, education, etc.). There are, however, overall design heuristics that can be followed regardless of the specific type of technology under consideration. We can classify these heuristics into four domains: functionality, technical advantage, emotional impact, and cultural acceptability (Figure 49.3).

The first consideration in designing HITs is that of functionality (i.e., does it do what it's supposed to do) given the requirements elicited in the user needs assessment phase. Safety is of utmost concern in this domain—the CPOE system must do no harm to the ultimate beneficiary, the patient. This encompasses not only reducing potential medication errors (Koppel et al., 2005), but also threats to patient privacy and confidentiality of health-related privacy rules (http://www.hhs.gov/ocr/privacy/). Basic functionality also implies overall system reliability, providing good man–machine feedback, as well as fundamental ease of use to prevent user confusion.

Once functionality has been determined, elements of *technical efficiency* need to be evaluated. *Speed of response* needs to be considered early as it has a direct impact on overall system efficiency. With any CPOE set up, how users *learn* and how user *errors* are minimized also have to be addressed substantially in order to reduce user frustration—a good system has high learnability and should be as "error-forgiving" to the average user as possible. Last, any CPOE system adopted should aim for compliance with *standards* for interoperability of HITs (Health Level Seven: http://www.hl7.org) to facilitate future expansion and integration with other systems.

Emotional impact and *cultural acceptability* should also be considered in the design and evaluation of a CPOE system. Aesthetic considerations, degree of user personalization or tailoring, level of user engagement, and the ability to anticipate user needs all affect the emotional impact of CPOE on users, thus facilitating easier technology adoption and diffusion throughout the network. Finally, accommodating cultural nuances of patient populations being served will increasingly become more relevant given demographic trends in healthcare delivery.

Deployment Issues

When designing a CPOE system, careful attention must be paid to how the technology will interface with other aspects of the existing work system. At the institutional level, consideration must be given to interaction between the technology and the organization's policies and procedures, the physical environment, the physicians and other clinical users of the system, the tasks that must be executed, and other existing technologies in use in the work system. Designing for these interactions in advance can decrease the likelihood of unintended consequences of CPOE implementation (Campbell et al., 2006)

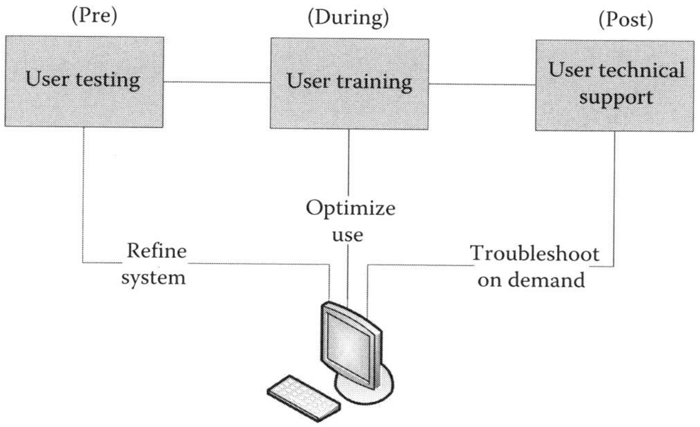

FIGURE 49.4 System deployment considerations.

such as poor interoperability between technologies, suboptimal human–computer interaction, conflicting role definitions, and inefficient workflows. For example, informal or formal organizational policies and the rules embedded in the CPOE technology may advance different expectations as to who enters orders into the system. Similarly, attention to interactions between macro-level factors such as cultural considerations must also be attended to in advance. If a clinic's patient population takes traditional herbal remedies, these should, for example be added into the system to ensure that no interacting medications are prescribed (Figure 49.4).

The adoption of any new HIT will always be disruptive by nature. Significant organizational effort and resources should be given to user testing, user training, and user technical support/troubleshooting—before, during, and after the CPOE system goes "live."

References

Ackoff, R. L. 1994. Systems thinking and thinking systems. *System Dynamics Review* 10(2–3): 175–188.

American Medical Informatics Association. 2008. http://www.amia.org/mbrcenter/wg

Blanchard, B. S. and W. J. Fabrycky. 2005. *Systems Engineering and Analysis*, 4th edn. Lebanon, IN: Prentice-Hall.

Campbell, E. M., D. F. Sittig, J. S. Ash, K. P. Guappone, and R. H. Dykstra. 2006. Types of unintended consequences related to computerized provider order entry. *Journal of the American Medical Informatics Association* 13(5):547–556.

Hendrick, H. W. and B. M. Kleiner. 2002. *Macroergonomics: Theory, Methods, and Applications*. Mahwah, NJ: Lawrence Erlbaum Associates.

Hersh, W. R. 2002. Medical informatics: Improving health care through information. *Journal of the American Medical Association* 288:1955.

Kaushal, R., K. G. Shojania, and D. W. Bates. 2003. Effects of computerized physician order entry and clinical decision support systems on medication safety: A systematic review. *Archives of Internal Medicine* 163:1409–1416.

Koppel, R., J. P. Metlay, A. Cohen et al. 2005. Role of computerized physician order entry systems in facilitating medication errors. *JAMA* 293(10):1197–1203.

Kuperman, G. J. and R. F Gibson. 2003. Computer physician order entry: Benefits, costs, and issues. *Annals of Internal Medicine* 139:31–39.

Lummus, R. R., R. J. Vokurka, and B. Rodeghiero. 2006. Improving quality through value stream mapping: A case study of a physician's clinic. *Total Quality Management* 17(8):1063–1075.

Moray, N. 2000. Culture, politics, and ergonomics. *Ergonomics* 43(7):858–868.

Prochaska, J. O., C. C. DiClemente, and J. C. Norcross. 1992. In search of how people change—Applications to addictive behaviors. *American Psychologist* 47(9):1102–1114.

Rasmussen, J. 2000. Human factors in a dynamic information society: Where are we heading. *Ergonomics* 43(7):869–879.

Rogers, E. M. 2003. *Diffusion of Innovations*, 5th edn. New York: Free Press.

Shortliffe E. H. and M. S. Blois. 2001. The computer meets medicine and biology: Emergence of a discipline. In *Medical Informatics: Computer Applications in Health Care and Biomedicine*, vol. 3, E. H. Shortliffe and L. E. Perreault (eds.), New York: Springer-Verlag.

Smith, M. J. and P. Carayon-Sainfort. 1989. A balance theory of job design for stress reduction. *International Journal of Industrial Ergonomics* 4:67–69.

Wasserman, S. and K. Faust. 2004. *Social Network Analysis: Methods and Applications*. Cambridge, U.K.: Cambridge University Press.

Wiener, N. 1948. *Cybernetics: OR Control and Communication in the Animal and the Machine*. Paris, France: Librairie Hermann & Cie/Cambridge, MA: MIT Press.

Wilson, J. R. 2000. Fundamentals of ergonomics in theory and practice. *Applied Ergonomics* 31:557–567.

50

Privacy/Security/Personal Health Record Service

Prevalence of Paper 50-1
Makeshift Solutions 50-1
Medical Consumerism 50-2
Enter the PHR 50-2
PHR History • PHR Product Models • PHR Challenges
Paper and Privacy 50-6
Privacy of Electronic PHRs 50-6
HIPAA 50-6
Privacy Policy 50-7
ARRA and Privacy 50-8
PHRs and Privacy: Where to From Here? 50-11

Jeff Donnell
NoMoreClipboard.com

Prevalence of Paper

As this chapter is written, most physician practices still capture patient health information on paper. As patients enter a physician office for a visit, a clipboard full of registration forms along with a pen is placed in their hands by the receptionist. Patients then struggle to complete those forms, trying to recall the names and proper spellings of medications, when they had their last tetanus shot, what year they had hernia surgery, and the phone number for their primary care physician.

Patients report frustration and aggravation, and wonder why in this day and age they are forced to participate in this antiquated approach to data collection. Worse yet, when these same patients are referred to another specialist, they must answer the same questions in the same outmoded fashion.

Paper registration forms are no picnic for medical professionals. Not only do paper forms start a clinical visit off on the wrong foot in terms of patient satisfaction, the practice generally receives forms that are illegible, incomplete, and inaccurate.

This outdated method of information sharing contributes to ineffective communication, poor care coordination, duplicated services, medical errors, and unnecessary costs.

Makeshift Solutions

Consumers, especially those managing chronic conditions, taking care of aging or infirm relatives, or overseeing the health and wellness of a family, often resort to makeshift methods of health information management. File folders, bankers boxes, and home-grown spreadsheets are used to compile and organize family health information.

Many physician practices have begun to employ technology to improve information gathering. This may be as simple as placing forms on a practice Web site, where they can be downloaded and completed at home prior to a visit. Other practices enable patients to complete registration forms online. Forward thinking practices offer patient portals, enabling their patients to register, request appointments, request medication refills, ask questions, and pay medical bills online.

While physician use of technology solutions is an encouraging sign, most of these solutions are tethered to the sponsoring practice. A patient can register online prior to visiting a sponsoring practice, but when they go elsewhere they again must answer the same questions.

Medical Consumerism

Employees were once passive consumers of often-generous health plan benefits, paid largely by their employers. These workers are now being asked to engage with their physicians and other medical professionals to adopt healthier lifestyles and to actively manage the more expensive and confusing benefits associated with a leaner health plan, health savings account, or other alternative insurance program.

As the cost burdens shift, consumers have financial incentives to use the Internet to learn about medical conditions, evaluate physician practices, and manage family health and wellness. Patients are now engaged in self-diagnosis and often self-treatment. When individuals are diagnosed or experience symptoms of an illness, they commonly go online, enter the appropriate keywords in a search engine, and for better or worse immerse themselves in a multitude of health-information Web sites. When Google launched its Google Health consumer platform, company executives acknowledged that the product concept began to take shape when the company realized that a significant percentage of its search activity was related to health.

Enter the PHR

The term personal health record (PHR) offers an alternative approach to managing patient health information. PHR definitions vary. The Healthcare Information and Management Systems Society (HIMSS) states that

> "An electronic Personal Health Record ("ePHR") is a universally accessible, layperson comprehensible, lifelong tool for managing relevant health information, promoting health maintenance and assisting with chronic disease management via an interactive, common set of electronic health information and e-health tools. The ePHR is controlled, managed and shared by the individual or his or her legal proxy(s) and must be secure to protect the privacy and confidentiality of the health information it contains. It is not a legal record unless so defined and is subject to various legal limitations."

The American Health Information Management Association (AHIMA) employs a simpler definition and describes a PHR as "A collection of important information that you maintain about your health or the health of someone you're caring for, such as a parent or a child, which you actively maintain and update."

In practical terms, a PHR is a tool that helps consumers compile, organize, manage, and share health information, and a repository of the record is critical to its versatility. Recent trends in the PHR space have records managed through the use of a software platform that enables the patient to engage digitally with physicians, clinics, and hospitals.

PHR History

The useful genesis of PHRs dates from the Massachusetts Institute of Technology publication of "Guardian Angel—Patient-Centered Health Information Systems" (Szlovits, Doyle, Long) in 1994. They envisioned interoperability *through the patient* in the form of a life-long, electronic record that might be broadly used for personal health and wellness. Their prophetic proposed mission included data collection, monitoring disease and treatment progress, providing patient information, customization of therapy, "sanity checks" on diagnosis and therapy, appointment scheduling, physician communication, interfacing with information systems, and social networking. "We believe," they said, "that comprehensive information can greatly improve the quality of medical decision making, reduce errors in healthcare, and allow people to make better personal decisions…."

PHR models tethered to a treating hospital system such "Ping" in the United Kingdom and Indivo at Harvard University followed. Scores of PHRs were developed over the next decade, ranging from paper-based binders to glorified electronic spreadsheets to web-based applications. Many of these early PHRs were stand-alone applications developed for a narrow purpose such as emergency access to health information. The founders of those organizations were often motivated by the injury of a loved one in an accident and the subsequent lack of health information available to emergency room physicians. These "in case of emergency" PHRs were designed to provide first responders with critical information such as medication lists, allergies, and the presence of serious conditions such as diabetes. In the quest to make this information available, the need to protect patient privacy was often overlooked.

Other early PHR models were focused on the consumer market, with the expectation that consumers would rush to adopt PHRs just as they rapidly embraced the use of search engines to search for health information. The early experience at PHR vendor NoMoreClipboard.com was typical—the product was launched with a direct-to-consumer marketing strategy, and the organization quickly learned that most consumers were not yet at the point where they understood the PHR concept, let alone the value in creating and using a PHR account.

More recently, Google Health and Microsoft HealthVault have entered the PHR space with their own consumer health offerings. The presence of Google and Microsoft in the market is expected to help build the PHR category, as their brand strength and consumer footprints can contribute mightily to consumer awareness of PHRs and their potential benefits.

Sponsored Model: Part One

Recognizing that consumer adoption of PHRs was anemic at best, many PHR vendors shifted to a sponsored model of distribution, where an organization sponsors the PHR on behalf of a patient population. Several health plans began offering PHR solutions to their members, often enabling the member to populate the PHR with claims data. Most of these solutions were tethered—meaning that the member can access and use the PHR for only as long as they are covered by the sponsoring health plan, and they lose access to their PHR data if they go elsewhere for health insurance. In general, consumer adoption of health plan–sponsored solutions has been weak, likely based on consumer distrust about how PHR information might be used in insurance coverage decisions.

Progressive employers concerned about rapidly escalating healthcare costs also began to investigate the role PHR solutions might play in engaging employees and their families in managing health and wellness. Most notable was the formation of Dossia, a consortium of large U.S. corporations who joined forces to create an employer-sponsored PHR. Organizations including AT&T, BP America, Intel, Pitney-Bowes, and Wal-Mart launched this effort with much fanfare in 2006, with the stated mission "To empower people and their doctors to be active partners for health by providing secure, convenient access to lifelong health information." After a slow start based largely on a falling out and ensuing legal battle with their original technology partner, Dossia was made available to Wal-Mart employees in 2009.

In general, consumer adoption of an employer-sponsored PHR requires a culture of trust between the employer and its employees. Employees are understandably concerned that unscrupulous employers might try to use health information to make decisions about hiring, promotions, and continued employment. Where the employer-sponsored model has been accepted, the workplace culture is such that employees feel confident that personal health information will remain private and secure and will not be available to supervisors or others in the organization. Often, corporations elect to keep worker health records "outside the firewall" and clearly separate from personnel records. A portable PHR tool is ideal for corporations interested in giving employees ownership and control of their health information.

Sponsored Model: Part Two

While health plan- and employer-sponsored PHR models have had limited success thus far, sponsorships by hospitals, health systems, and physician practices appear to be more effective. At NoMoreClipboard, our surveys indicate that physician recommendation is the top reason for consumer creation of a PHR account—indicating that when physicians prompt their patients to use a PHR, those patients are likely to comply.

Much of the success with hospital- and physician-sponsored models can be attributed to context. A significant portion of today's patient population is used to conducting business online, and using an electronic PHR tool to communicate with a healthcare provider is a logical pursuit. In addition, there is generally an existing or at least implied trust relationship between a patient and a healthcare provider. Patients are accustomed to sharing sensitive health information with physicians or other medical professionals, and doing so electronically is simply a different means to move the data.

PHR sponsorships by participants in the medical community are expected to expand rapidly with the availability of the American Recovery and Reinvestment Act of 2009 (ARRA) incentive funding. This legislation makes approximately $20 billion available to physicians and hospitals for the implementation and meaningful use of certified electronic health record (EHR) solutions. As of this writing, proposed meaningful use criteria include requirements for engaging patients and their families in their healthcare. Patient engagement criteria require providers to:

- Send reminders to patients per patient preference for preventive/follow-up care, measured by sending reminders to at least 50% of all unique patients seen by the eligible physician (EP) that are 50 or over.
- Provide patients with an electronic copy of their health information (including diagnostic test results, problem list, medication lists, and allergies) upon request, providing electronic copies to at least 80% of all patients who request an electronic copy of their health information within 48 hours.
- Provide patients with timely electronic access to their health information (including lab results, problem list, medication lists, and allergies) within 96 hours of the information being available to the EP. At least 10% of all unique patients seen by the EP should be provided with timely access to their health information.
- Provide clinical summaries for patients for each office visit, with clinical summaries provided for at least 80% of all office visits.
- Provide patients with an electronic copy of their discharge instructions and procedures at time of discharge, upon request, providing this information to at least 80% of all patients who are discharged from an eligible hospital and who request an electronic copy.

These requirements are expected to phase in by 2011, and by 2013 it appears that qualifying physicians and hospitals will have to offer patients a PHR. ARRA incentives are expected to drive widespread EHR and PHR adoption and facilitate the flow of electronic information between patients and their healthcare providers. This likelihood is increased by financial penalties to be levied against providers who fail to adopt a qualified EHR system after 5 years.

PHR Product Models

A number of different PHR models exist today. One is a tethered or connected model. A tethered PHR is offered by a sponsoring organization such as a health plan or health system and enables sponsored patients to access electronic health information that exists within the sponsoring organization. As an example, the Cleveland Clinic offers its patients a PHR that provides a view of selected information that exists within the EHR system used by this health system. While tethered systems generally offer the benefit of a patient record that is populated with existing electronic data, they usually lack portability. When patients go elsewhere for treatment, they are unable to take their tethered data with them—the

PHR only "works" when care is sought from the sponsor. In addition, tethered systems do not enable patients to populate the PHR with data from outside the sponsoring organization.

An un-tethered or stand-alone PHR provides more flexibility—the patient has a PHR that is portable and can be used with any healthcare provider or health plan in virtually any location. These PHRs may be offered in a direct-to-consumer model, or they may be offered by a sponsoring entity that chooses not to tether the PHR exclusively to their organization. In some cases, these PHRs must be populated by patient self-entry. In other cases, the PHR may be populated with data from a sponsoring organization or from other external data sources.

Another emerging model is often referred to as a PHR platform (sometimes referred to as a consumer health platform). Google Health and Microsoft HealthVault fall into this category. PHR platforms include elements of a PHR and also serve as an aggregation point for consumer health information from a variety of sources—healthcare providers, pharmacies, remote monitoring devices, health plans, and other health management products and services. Google and Microsoft have both created partner communities, integrating their consumer health platforms with product and services from other organizations in the healthcare space.

PHR Challenges

Significant consumer adoption and use of PHRs has the potential to generate myriad benefits, especially as those consumers become able to share information electronically with their healthcare providers with relative ease. A PHR, properly deployed and utilized, should enable consumers to create a complete health record that can be shared with everyone involved in their care. As care providers receive more complete and accurate information, including data from other care providers, coordination of care can improve. A current medication list along with all known allergies will reduce medical errors. A complete picture of recent lab results or medical images should reduce service duplication. As consumers and healthcare providers begin to share electronic health information as a matter of course, it stands to reason that costs can be reduced and clinical outcomes improved.

While the value of PHRs is evident, concerns about the privacy and security of health information is a legitimate cause for concern. This concern begins with the nature of the information contained in a PHR. To be considered complete, a PHR should contain demographic information, medications, allergies, immunizations, current and past medical conditions, a procedure history, family history, and social history. PHRs that are considered robust often contain more than this basic information, including health measures such as blood pressure or blood glucose readings, lab results, medical images, legal documents, copies of past medical records, personal health journal entries, and care plans provided by health professionals.

The abundance of this information contributes materially to the realization of the value of a PHR described above. The presence of this same material, ironically, is what fuels privacy fears. Consumers, privacy advocates, and policy makers are understandably concerned about the potential for nefarious use of personal health information. In the wrong hands, PHR data could be used for identity theft, to deny employment or health plan coverage, or to simply spread embarrassing information. Most individuals lack the celebrity status that might tempt a hospital or physician practice employee to sneak a peek at medical records in search of tabloid fodder. However, average Joes and Janes still harbor concern over the possible exposure of a bout with depression, past treatment for a sexually transmitted disease, or a family history of a genetic disorder.

The model for sharing PHR information employed by many PHR vendors also contributes to privacy and security concerns. For example, many PHRs enable consumers to carry a complete PHR around with them on a USB device. From a privacy point of view, individuals who get their hands on one of these USB devices may be able to access the information contained therein. In terms of security, many healthcare providers are wary of plugging this type of media into their office computers for fear of introducing a virus onto their networks. In fact, many health systems have strict policies which restrict the use of outside media such as USB devices or CDs.

Paper and Privacy

While apprehension over sharing electronic health information is justifiable, the prevalent methodology for sharing health information has serious drawbacks. At the time of this writing, approximately 80% of physician practices still utilize paper charts. The management of those charts is a major challenge for the medical profession. It is not uncommon for these charts to be lost or misplaced—often within the four walls of the practice. Those same charts may travel—perhaps with a physician or other practice employee seeing a patient at a remote location. Information from those charts may be copied and mailed, faxed or hand delivered to another physician. While most practices do their best to restrict access to charts, gaining access to chart contents would be a simple matter for an unscrupulous employee. Worse yet, with the absence of electronic tracking and audit trails found in most electronic record systems, determining who gained access to a paper record is virtually impossible.

Privacy of Electronic PHRs

It is when patient health information becomes electronic that privacy concerns escalate, and a model for the life cycle of those concerns can be found in the financial industry. When automatic teller machines were initially introduced, the prevailing consumer refrain was "I will never use one of those things." Today, ATM use is as routine as brushing one's teeth. Early reactions to online banking were equally negative, and now paying bills over the Internet is making the mailing of checks obsolete. While electronic commerce is commonplace, it is not without its risks. Without the proper privacy protection and security measures, financial information can fall into the wrong hands—often with dire consequences.

PHRs will likely follow a similar path to everyday use, and concerns about privacy and security will persist. However, the lessons learned from credit cards and ATM machines are instructive, and much attention is being paid to protecting consumers from the inappropriate use of their health information.

HIPAA

The Health Information Portability and Accountability Act (HIPAA) is the primary law which applies to the privacy and security of health information. HIPAA is applied to covered entities including healthcare providers, health plans, and healthcare clearinghouses. HIPAA rules apply indirectly to business associates, which are entities that assist covered entities in performing treatment, payment, or operations functions. HIPAA mandates that covered entities have business associate agreements in place with business associates so that the associates are contractually bound to comply with the HIPAA regulations that apply to the business function that is being performed.

If a covered entity hosts a PHR application, HIPAA rules apply to that covered entity. HIPAA regulations do not apply directly to a PHR vendor that hosts a PHR application, as that PHR vendor is not a covered entity. When a PHR vendor hosts a PHR on behalf of a covered entity, a business associate agreement should be in place to ensure that the PHR vendor adheres to HIPAA rules.

HIPAA does extend to PHR security. Covered entities must have a security officer to comply with HIPAA, which would likely apply to a tethered PHR model. For non-tethered PHRs, the host, supplier, and consumer would have varying security roles. Consumers would assume responsibility for setting their usernames, passwords, and other access credentials. The host of the PHR would be responsible for assessing security threats, identity authentication, and authorization for providing and accessing data, and the supplier would be responsible for designing and operating a secure technical architecture. In many cases, the host and supplier or vendor would be one and the same.

Privacy Policy

A number of organizations are actively working to protect the privacy and security of patient health information, including this information in the context of a PHR. One of the most respected is the Markle Foundation. Markle's Connecting for Health Initiative brings together leading government, industry, and healthcare experts to accelerate the development of a health-sharing environment to improve the quality and cost-effectiveness of healthcare. Markle's Center for Democracy and Technology promotes privacy and security policies to protect health data through its Health Privacy Project.

In a survey released by the Markle Foundation, consumers cited privacy concerns as a significant PHR adoption barrier. Of those surveyed who indicated they were not interested in having a PHR, 57% cited privacy concerns as their number one reason for avoiding a PHR. This same study found that 24% of the public have high concerns regarding health privacy, and roughly 50% have moderate concerns. While privacy concerns are formidable, Markle research also indicates strong consumer interest in having access to their electronic health information.

With the context, Markle Connecting for Health released the Common Framework for Networked Personal Health Information in 2008. This framework, developed with input from technology companies, healthcare providers, health insurers, and consumer and privacy organizations, outlines consumer access and privacy practices for PHRs and other web-based health information services. The framework includes specific technology and policy approaches for consumers to access health services, obtain and control copies of health information about them, authorize the sharing of their information with others, and sound privacy and security practices.

Perhaps the most vocal proponent of patient privacy is the advocacy group PatientPrivacyRights (PPR). In 2009, PPR published a PHR Privacy Report card that graded leading PHR vendors on several criteria. These criteria include

Privacy Policy/Notice

- Location: Privacy Policy must be easy to find and accessible from the organization's home page. Should be unavoidable and accessible on any page that collects information.
- Readability: Privacy Policy must be clear, easy to understand, and at a low reading level.
- Transparency: Privacy Policy is comprehensive; individuals should not have to read multiple policies to understand how their information can be used.

Patient Control/Choice

- Consent for Identifiable Data: No information is shared or collected without explicit, informed consent. Privacy Policy states how information will be shared and ideally, how it will NOT be shared.
- "De-Identified Data": No de-identified or aggregate data should be used without explicit, informed individual consent.
- Segmentation: Patients can segment/hide sensitive information.

Access/Participation

- Patients can easily find out who has accessed or used their information.
- Patients must be able to promptly and permanently remove themselves and their health information from the system upon request.

Integrity/Security

- Patients can expect their data to be secure. Data should only be stored in the United States and use authentication that goes beyond username and password login.

Customer Service/Enforcement

- Patients can easily report concerns and get answers.

Of course, the federal government is quite involved in shaping policy. For example, in 2008, the Department of Health and Human Services began a multiphase research project to develop a model for presenting easy-to-understand information about PHRs to consumers. The project purpose is to develop a "plain language" model PHR fact sheet that will enable consumers to clearly understand and compare privacy policies across PHRs. The final product is envisioned to be a template for a web-based PHR fact sheet for vendors to use to deliver complex PHR privacy and security information simply and clearly so that consumers can make informed decisions, similar to the nutrition label that provides a format for consumers to quickly learn nutritional information about a food or the financial services industry model privacy notice that dictates how the financial institutions inform consumers about financial privacy information practices.

ARRA and Privacy

The work of organizations like Markle and PPR has clearly influenced legislative policy, as is evidenced in privacy and security language that is part of ARRA legislation. Under ARRA, the Department of Health and Human Services was directed to develop regulations or guidance related to privacy, including

- HIPAA security and privacy rules extended to business associates of HIPAA covered entities.
- New provisions for notification to consumers of information breaches.
- Limitations on sales of protected health information (PHI).
- New guidance on "minimum necessary."
- Guidance on implementation specification to de-identify PHI.
- Individual right to access personal information in an electronic format.
- Annual guidance on the most effective technical safeguards for carrying out the HIPAA Security Rule.
- Recommendations on technologies that protect the privacy of health information and promote security.
- Restrictions on use of PHI for marketing.
- Requirement for consumer access to an accounting of full disclosures of information contained in EHRs.

An example of the regulations that resulted from this direction to United States Department of Health and Human Services (HHS) became effective in September of 2009. PHRs are now subject to a Security Breach Notification Rule administered and enforced by the Federal Trade Commission. This rule strives to extend HIPAA-like protections to PHI contained in PHR systems managed and maintained by organizations that are not subject to the HIPAA "covered entity" provisions.

To comply with the FTC PHI protections, PHR vendors must do the following:

- Quickly and comprehensively recognize when unsecured PHI that is contained in PHR systems has been "acquired without authorization."
- Provide notification to the individuals (who are citizens or residents of the United States) whose PHI has been acquired without authorization notice of the breach within 60 days of discovery.
- In the event a PHR is offered through a sponsoring entity, the PHR also has an obligation to provide notice to the sponsoring organization.
- The notice must be
  - Written
  - Delivered via first class mail to the last known address (or via e-mail if the individual agrees; or to next-of-kin if individual is deceased)
  - Provided to the FTC within 10 days if 500 or more individuals are affected, or annually via log if less than 500 individuals are affected in any given breach

- Provided to the local media for publication if 500 or more individuals in the same state or jurisdiction are affected
- In plain language and include a brief description of what happened, the date of the breach, a description of the types of PHI involved, steps recommended to protect parties affected, what we are doing to mitigate the negative effect, contact procedures (an 800 number, e-mail address, Web site, and postal address are all highly recommended) for questions or additional information

Privacy Case: Indiana University

In late 2008, the Indiana University Health Center (IUHC) at IU's main Bloomington, IN, campus began working on a PHR solution to facilitate improved communication with the student population. Working with PHR vendor NoMoreClipboard, a patient portal sponsored by the university was developed.

Originally, this initiative was designed to integrate with OneStart, a central portal where students can conduct university business—registering for classes, accessing grades, and paying tuition. The intent was to employ a single sign-on approach, such that OneStart credentials would be used to access the student PHR account. However, the team working on the project realized during the implementation process that single sign-on posed a privacy challenge, as a significant percentage of the student population shared their OneStart credentials with parents or other family members so they could also view grades or pay bursar bills. While these students are perfectly happy to have their parents use OneStart to pay their tuition, they may not want those parents to know why they had to visit the student health center.

While many university students are not hesitant to post intimate photos or other potentially damaging information on social networking sites such as Facebook, the IU PHR team was sensitive to its role in helping educate its student population on the importance of protecting private health information.

IU elected to use OneStart as the site for creating and accessing a PHR account, using OneStart credentials to verify student status. When students elect to create an account, they are linked to a landing page outside the OneStart environment where they encounter a message about the importance of protecting personal health information, including the fact that the student may not want family members to have access to their PHR account. Students are urged to create a unique username and password to access the PHR—one that is different from their OneStart credentials.

While this approach encourages students to manage yet another set of access credentials, it also reminds students of the private nature of their health information. This added burden has not deterred student adoption. Forty percent of the incoming freshman class voluntarily created a PHR account prior to arriving on campus in the fall of 2009, and more than half of those students have used their PHR accounts to share data with the student health center as of this writing. These best-in-class adoption figures give us a glimpse of the future of PHRs, as today's student population expects to conduct business online and scoff at the notion of filling out paper registration forms. "Our students are extremely web-savvy and we wanted incoming students to realize the benefit of managing their health information securely online. We want the adoption of a PHR to be seen as a normal part of the college registration process," says Pete Grogg, associate director at the IUHC.

Privacy Case: Centers for Medicare and Medicaid Services

At the other end of the spectrum from IU is a PHR pilot conducted by Center for Medicare and Medicaid Services (CMS) in Arizona and Utah. This pilot was designed to enable Medicare beneficiaries in those states to create a PHR account and populate it with Medicare claims data.

This pilot requires Medicare patients to create a PHR account with one of a handful of PHR vendors, and to then opt-in with a CMS claims processing entity to import claims data. To ensure that beneficiaries only have access to their claims data, they must provide information unique to themselves, including their name, Medicare ID number, and date of birth. This enables an electronic connection between the Medicare claims processing entity and the patient PHR account. In addition, participating beneficiaries can opt-out of the program at any point in time.

For Medicare beneficiaries considering pilot participation, questions about the privacy and security of their health information are common. While this population often stands to benefit tremendously from having access to a complete and accurate health record, they are generally careful about sharing personal information and suspicious about the idea of placing their health data "in the cloud."

Privacy Case: NoMoreClipboard

PHR vendor NoMoreClipboard has carefully followed PHR privacy and security developments. Like other PHR vendors, NoMoreClipboard has addressed privacy and security concerns in its product offering, underlying architecture, and service delivery. The company is particularly careful, given their Software as a Service approach to managing information.

Examples of actions taken relative to privacy and security include

- Development and implementation of a consent module in the application that enables consumers to grant (or revoke) PHR access to family members, physicians, or others involved in their care. This access includes different levels ranging from read-only to full administrative rights.
- Storing patient data in a secure data center based in the United States. Access to the data center environment is highly restricted, and the data center has back-up power, including uninterruptible power supply systems and an on-site natural gas–fired generator.
- Patients are in complete control—they determine their own username, password, and security settings. Patients determine what information goes in their PHR, what is excluded, and who that information can be shared with.

As a result of these and other actions, NoMoreClipboard was awarded an "A" grade by PPR when they issued their PHR Privacy Report Card in late 2009.

PHRs and Privacy: Where to From Here?

Significant adoption of PHR technology is generally viewed as a when, not if proposition. The presence of tens of billions of dollars of stimulus funds earmarked to stimulate EHR adoption all but guarantees the spread of PHRs, and consumer awareness and education efforts will answer questions, address obstacles, and convey value propositions. Attention to PHR privacy and security already has momentum, and concerns about consumer protection are actually ahead of consumer understanding at this juncture. These consumer protection efforts—including advocacy, policy, and legislation—will no doubt continue to gather momentum. As privacy protection and consumer adoption converge, Americans will no doubt benefit from robust PHR products that are engineered to keep health information private and secure and are offered by organizations that are governed by strict regulations that mandate strong protection.

Index

A

Accountable care organization, 1-13–1-14
Acute care system, 32-4
Acute psychiatric symptoms, 42-4
Acute to chronic care, 8-3, 8-9
Adaptive treatment planning (ATP), 15-9–15-10
Adverse drug events (ADEs), 12-4
Agent-based modeling (ABM), 14-11–14-12
Ambulatory-care systems, 32-5
American hospital association's (AHA), 33-2
American Recovery and Reinvestment Act (ARRA)
  Indiana University, 50-9
  medicare and medicaid service centers, 50-10
  NoMoreClipboard, 50-10
Americans for Relief and Recovery Act, 5-1
Americans with Disabilities Act (ADA), 21-5
Anesthesia group management and strategies
  autonomy, 36-5
  change and transitions, 36-6
  closed staffs and exclusive contracts, evolution, 36-4
  cultural differences, 36-3
  culture and strategy alignment, 36-8–36-9
  history, 36-2–36-3
  leadership
    communication, 36-11
    essence, 36-9
    organizational change factors, 36-10, 36-11
    psychological contract advantage, 36-9
  macro-level transition models
    classification, 36-6
    impact, 36-6–36-8
  market determination, 36-6
  physician practice management companies, 36-4–36-5
  trade union, definition, 36-11
Anthrax drills, 41-17–41-18
Anti-cervical cancer vaccines, 27-5
Antiretroviral therapy (ART), 25-3
Appropriations, 3-9–3-10
A3 problem solving, 22-10–22-11
Asian flu, 40-5
Aspirin, 31-9
Assisted living facilities, 6-5–6-6; *see also* Long-term care
Association rules, 24-9–24-11
Attributional rule-based models
  AQ programs, 19-6
  attributional rules, 19-5–19-6
  data preparation guidelines, learning rules, 19-6–19-7
Autonomy, 1-3–1-4
Avian flu, 41-5

B

Balanced healthcare, 1-9
Bar coded medication administration (BCMA)
  adoption, 47-4–47-5
  capital expenditures, 47-3
  eMAR, 47-4
  ergonomics principles, 47-10
  hardware, 47-3
  high-risk medications, 47-4
  ID bands, 47-4
  machine-readable bar codes, 47-3
  medical errors, 47-1–47-2
  medication repackaging centers, 47-3
  nursing work
    interruptions, 47-7–47-8
    negative side effects, 47-6–47-7
    problem-solving strategies, 47-7
    time on task and perceptions, 47-6
    workarounds and violations, 47-8–47-9
  patient safety, 47-1
  pediatric patients, 47-10
  physician administration, 47-9–47-10
  safety outcomes, 47-5–47-6
  symbology, 47-3
Barriers, 2-4–2-5
Bayesian inference, 18-6–18-7
BCMA, *see* Bar coded medication administration
Bed planning, 34-2–34-3
Benefit–risk analyses, 31-9
Biosurveillance, 24-9

Blue Cross Blue Shield Plans, 7-5
Body sensor networks
  autonomic sensing, 46-7–46-8
  context-aware sensing, 46-7
  embedded data enhancement, 46-8–46-9
Brachytherapy treatment planning, 15-6–15-7
Branch and bound algorithm, 15-12–15-14

C

Capacity planning
  operating rooms
    aggregate planning process, 34-1
    bed planning, 34-2–34-3
    definition, 34-2
    healthcare, 34-2
    operational planning (*see* Operational capacity planning)
    tactical planning (*see* Tactical capacity planning)
  panel management, primary care, 10-6
Capillary electrophoresis (CE) method, 27-15
Cardiovascular disease (CVD), 43-2
Care episode, 8-5–8-6, 8-11
Catering, 44-6–44-7
Causal risk analysis
  breast cancer, 26-1
  cardiac events, 26-2
  causal *vs.* noncausal analysis, 26-8–26-9
  cause, 26-3–26-4
  history, 26-2–26-3
  multiple causes modeling
    causal diagrams, 26-5
    probability networks, 26-5–26-7
    simultaneous equations, 26-7–26-8
  patient safety, 26-2
  risk factors, 26-1
  structure, 26-1, 26-2
CCR, *see* Computerized clinical reminders
CDSS, *see* Clinical decision support systems
Centers for Medicare and Medicaid Services (CMS), 4-2
Central Sterile Supply Department (CSSD), 38-3
Cervarix, 27-1
Chemoprophylaxis, 25-7
Chronic disease self-management program (CDSMP), 43-6
Classification and regression trees (CART), 10-3
Clinical decision support systems (CDSS)
  barriers implementation, 48-3–48-4
  CCR (*see* Computerized clinical reminders)
  CPRS, 48-6–48-7
  definition, 48-1
  diagnosis system, 48-1–48-2
  drug dosing and prescribing, 48-2
  effects of, 48-2–48-3
  electronic medical record (EMR) systems, 48-1
  experimental procedure, 48-9
  information retrieval, 48-10
  preventive care and disease management, 48-2
  resolution time *vs.* CCR priority, 48-9, 48-10
  roadmap, 48-4
  user-centered approach, 48-5–48-6
  workflow integration, 48-4–48-5
Commercial Health Insurers, 7-5
Communication, 2-5–2-6
Communities of practice (CoP)
  community element, 13-9
  context, 13-10
  definition, 13-8
  evidence, 13-9–13-10
  facilitation, 13-10
Community-based outpatient clinics (CBOC), 3-9
Computerized clinical reminders (CCR)
  black-box design, 48-7
  prototyping and testing
    CPRS prototype, 48-7
    prioritization mechanism, 48-8
    risk factor repository, 48-8
    role-based filter, 48-8
  standardized screening protocols, 48-6
Computerized patient record system (CPRS), 3-11, 48-6–48-7
Computerized physician/provider order entry (CPOE), 49-4
  adverse drug events quantitation, 12-4–12-5
  ICU, 12-10–12-11
  vs. manual system, 12-5
Computer simulation
  agent-based modeling, 14-11–14-12
  discrete-event simulation, 14-8–14-9
  experimentation and optimization, 14-12–14-13
  healthcare
    doctor arrivals, 14-2
    nurses, emergency department, 14-2
    outpatient surgery center, 14-2
    simulation model construction, 14-2–14-3
  health system
    capacity analysis, 14-3
    emergency department, 14-3–14-4
    probabilistic sensitivity analysis, 14-4
  models
    data, 14-6–14-7
    validation, 14-4–14-5
  Monte Carlo simulation, 14-8
  object-oriented simulation, 14-9–14-10
  systems dynamics model, 14-10–14-11
  technology, 14-7
Congestive heart failure (CHF), 29-11
Consumer-health ecosystem, 1-11–1-12
Continuing Care Retirement Communities (CCRC), 6-7
Continuous drug infusion delivery, 12-4–12-5
Contract care, 3-10

Cookbook medicine, 1-4
CoP, *see* Communities of practice
Cost–benefit analysis, 28-5
Cryptosporidium, 28-7
Cybernetics, 49-2–49-3

D

Data mining, 46-12–46-13
    application, 24-1
    clinical and health-related information, 24-1
    clinical biochemical analysis, 24-3
    data exploration
        disadvantage, 24-6
        histogram, arterial oxygen pressure, 24-4–24-5, 24-6
        minimal mean blood pressure *vs.* minimal systolic blood pressure, 24-6, 24-7
        Pearson's correlation coefficient, definition, 24-6
        summary statistics, 24-4, 24-5
    decision tree, 24-2
    definition, 24-1
    descriptive data
        association rules, 24-9–24-11
        biosurveillance application, 24-9
        hierarchical clustering algorithms, 24-8
        k-means clustering algorithm, 24-8
        market basket analysis, 24-9
        PCA, 24-7
    emergency cases, 24-3
    knowledge representation, 24-4
    predictive data
        Bayesian network, 24-14
        black box models, 24-14
        cardiovascular failure, 24-13
        decision boundary, 24-12
        decision tree, 24-13
        discriminant analysis, 24-11–24-12
        linear discriminant analysis, 24-12
        multilayer perceptron, 24-14
        naive Bayesian classifier, 24-12
        overfitting phenomenon, 24-14
        patient-specific information, 24-10–24-11
        recursive partitioning method, 24-12
        regression and classification, 24-10
        validation set, 24-11
    risks, 24-3
    software, 24-15
    temporal sequence data analysis, 24-4
Decision analysis
    advantages, 19-1
    alternatives, 19-7–19-8
    automated methods, decision making, 19-2
    classification/prediction models, 19-8
    medication outcomes evaluation, 19-8–19-9
    models
        attributional rule-based models, 19-5–19-7
        cause and effect, Vioxx, 19-5
        if-then rules, 19-5
    process
        alternatives, 19-2–19-3
        data sources selection, 19-3
        goal, 19-2
        models for alternatives, 19-3–19-4
        perspectives, 19-3
        predictions/evaluation, alternatives, 19-4
        recommendation, 19-4
        sensitivity analysis, 19-4
Decision making, 1-3, 20-3
Decision support system, 41-32–41-33; *see also* Clinical decision support systems
Decision tree, 24-2, 24-13
Decontamination service
    cleaning
        definition, 38-2
        manual cleaning, 38-6
        thermal washer disinfectors, 38-6
        ultrasonic cleaners, 38-6
    conditions, 38-3
    CSSD, 38-3
    definition, 38-2
    degree of specialization, 38-3
    disinfection, 38-2–38-3, 38-6–38-7
    endoscope washer disinfectors (EWD), 38-4
    infection prevention and control, 38-1
    instrument life cycle, 38-4–38-5
    monitoring, 38-10–38-11
    procedures, 38-1
    sterilization
        choice of sterilizing process, 38-10
        definition, 38-3
        dry heat sterilizers, 38-9
        kinetics, 38-7
        low-temperature sterilizers, 38-9–38-10
        steam, properties, 38-7–38-8
        steam sterilization cycle, 38-8–38-9
Demand management, 32-6
Demographics and demand
    diversity, care system, 1-7–1-8
    growth and aging, care system, 1-7–1-8
    implications, care delivery, 1-8
    prevention and wellness services, 1-9
Discrete-event simulation, 14-8–14-9
Disease-propagation analysis
    differential equation systems, 41-13
    n-server system, 41-15
    prophylaxic vaccination, 41-16
    SEPAIR model, 41-13–41-14
    triage accuracy *vs.* symptomatic proportion, 41-15
DNA-based vaccines, 27-5
Doctor of Nursing Practice (DNP), 5-2
    advanced practice nursing, 5-7–5-8
    educational models, 5-7

evidence-based practice, 5-8–5-9
healthcare dilemmas, 5-8
program design, 5-7
Drug approval process, 31-2–31-3
Drug prescription, 12-5

E

EBP, *see* Evidence-based practice
Economic order quantity (EOQ), 20-2–20-3
Electronic medication administration record (eMAR), 47-4
Electronic patient tracking systems, 32-12
Electronic personal health record; *see also* Personal health record
definition, 50-2
privacy, 50-6
Emergency communication
emergency response system model, 41-24
multi-organizational radio interoperability issue, 41-24
radio networks, 41-21, 41-22–41-23
tabletop exercises, 41-20
telephony networks, 41-21
Emergency department crowding
administrative and policy response, 32-14–32-15
ambulance diversion, 32-3
bed capacity, 37-1
conceptual framework
access block phenomenon, 32-8
acute care system, 32-4
ambulatory-care systems, 32-5
clinical decision units, 32-10
demand management, 32-6
diagnostic testing and treatment, 32-7
emergency admissions, 32-9
EMTALA, 32-6
financial incentives, 32-9
follow-up care, 32-8
healthcare safety net, 32-5
input–throughput–output model, 32-4, 32-5
low-acuity patients, 32-6
operational processes, 32-7
operational strategies, 32-10
primary care, 32-6
queuing theory and discrete event simulation, 32-8
triage, definition, 32-8
unscheduled urgent care, 32-5
definitions, 32-4
downstream effects, 32-3
epidemiology, 32-2–32-3
history, 32-1–32-2
measurement
electronic patient tracking systems, 32-12
emergency department work index, 32-13–32-14
multiple different scoring systems, 32-12
National Emergency Department Overcrowding Study (NEDOCS), 32-14
potential measures, 32-11
scoring, 32-12
patient care, 32-3
supply and demand relationships, 32-3
Emergency department, healthcare leader's perspective
demand–capacity divergence, symptoms, 33-2
diagnostic imaging, 33-6–33-7
diagnostic procedure area, 33-5–33-6
disease control center, 33-1
housekeeping room turnover, 33-11–33-12
inpatient capacity bottleneck, 33-10
inpatient pull system, 33-10, 33-11
intradepartmental flow bottleneck, 33-6
laboratory services, 33-7–33-9
mini-registration and mobile bedside registration, 33-3–33-4
patient reception bottleneck, 33-2–33-3
primary care, 33-1
sustainment strategy
control and monitoring mechanisms, 33-15
thumb rule, 33-17
tracking mechanism, 33-17
team-based approach, 33-9–33-10
throughput, 33-2
4-tier high census alert strategy
functional chaos, 33-12
initiating mechanisms, 33-14
key action strategies, 33-14
normalcy state, 33-14
proactive demand management, 33-15, 33-16–33-17
revolving door theory, 33-14
transformation, 33-18–33-19
triage, 33-4
Emergency department work index (EDWIN), 32-13–32-14
Emergency Medical Treatment and Active Labor Act (EMTALA), 32-6
Emergency planning model, pandemics, *see* Pandemics emergency planning model
Employer-sponsored healthcare insurance
coverage, 7-3–7-4
distribution, 7-5
Endoscope washer disinfectors (EWD), 38-4
Engineering and health delivery system
barriers to cooperation, 2-4–2-5
challenges, 2-3–2-4
definition, 2-1
healthcare quality, 2-1–2-2
long-term opportunities
engineering and management students, 2-7
health professional educators, 2-7
information and communication, 2-5–2-6
multidisciplinary centers, 2-6–2-7

short-term projects, 2-5
tools, 2-2–2-3
Erlang delay model, *see* M/M/s model
Evidence-based practice (EBP)
definition, 13-1
implementation, 13-1–13-3
complexity, heathcare system, 13-2–13-3
healthcare quality, effectiveness, and outcomes, 13-1–13-2
innovation implementation, 13-2
PARiHS framework, 13-3
social capital theory
communities of practice, 13-8–13-10
forms, 13-3
PARiHS framework, 13-3–13-5
social network analysis, 13-5–13-8
Explicit services, 8-5
External peer review program (EPRP), 9-7

F

Facility planning and design
assessment, 21-2
capital building project, 21-1
facility design process, 21-3, 21-5
master facility plan deliverables, 21-3, 21-4
mission and strategic vision, 21-1
new design and construction project, 21-3
physical plant, 21-2
site selection and evaluation, 21-2–21-3
stakeholders, 21-1
strategic planning phase, 21-1–21-2
Williamson Medical Center (WMC)
growth and reputation, 21-5–21-6
master facility plan recommendations, 21-8
project phasing plan, 21-8–21-12
site evaluation, 21-7–21-8
team initiates feasibility phase, 21-6
value of planning, 21-12–21-13
Faculty practice model; *see also* Nurse-managed clinics
categories, 5-1
University of Texas-Houston, 5-2
Failure modes and effects analysis (FMEA), 12-2
continuous drug infusion delivery, 12-4–12-5
drug prescribing process, 12-5
intravenous (IV) medication administration, 12-7–12-10
limitations, 12-3
performance, 12-3
Failure modes, effects, and criticality analysis (FMECA), 12-5
Family caregiver
burden, 6-2
caregiving activity, 6-1–6-2
involvement, 6-4–6-5
norms and duration, 6-2
prevalence, 6-1
Family Medical Leave Act (FMLA), 4-3
Fixed capacity analysis, queueing theory
benefits of flexibility, 16-13–16-14
delay standard, 16-11–16-12
demand prediction, 16-12–16-13
M/M/s model, 16-9
target occupancy levels, 16-9–16-11
Flexible capacity analysis, queueing theory
data collection and model choices, 16-14–16-15
delay standard and queueing results, 16-15
model construct, 16-15
Food safety and security, 44-10; *see also* Healthcare foodservice
Fragmentation, healthcare services, 8-2–8-3, 8-8–8-9

G

GAO, *see* Government accountability office
Gardasil, 27-5
Genetic algorithm (GA), 15-15
Good manufacturing practice (GMP), 20-8
Government accountability office (GAO), 41-7–41-8
Group purchasing organizations (GPO), 45-3–45-4

H

Healthcare foodservice
acute care, 44-1
cafés, 44-9
catering, 44-6–44-7
current trends, 44-3
emergency, disaster preparedness, 44-10–44-11
food safety and security, 44-10
hospices, 44-2
hospital system, 44-2
layout and design, 44-7
long-term care, 44-2
management
patient/resident feeding, 44-4–44-5
self-operated *vs.* contracted, 44-3–44-4
nutrition therapy, 44-5–44-6
offices, 44-9
patient feeding, 44-8
patient service centers, 44-10
production, 44-8
receiving and storage, 44-7–44-8
retail operations, 44-6
Healthcare insurance
employer-sponsored insurance, 7-3–7-4
healthcare financing, 7-2–7-3
private healthcare insurance, 7-5
products, 7-5–7-6
regulation, 7-6
reimbursement system
capitation, 7-7
diagnostic-related groups (DRGs), 7-6–7-7
fee-for-service, 7-6
pay for performance, 7-7

third-party payers
characteristics, 7-1–7-2
issues, 7-4
Healthcare simulation, *see* Computer simulation
Health informatics
behavior change and social networks, 49-3–49-4
cybernetics, 49-2–49-3
design
CPOE technology, 49-4
deployment issues, 49-6–49-7
heuristics, 49-6
user definition, 49-4–49-5
life cycle, 49-4
macroergonomics, 49-3
macro-level factors, 49-1
micro-level factors, 49-1
Health Information Portability and Accountability Act (HIPAA), 50-6
Health information technologies (HIT), *see* Health informatics
Health Maintenance Organizations (HMOs), 7-5
Health professional educators, 2-7
Healy Murphy Alternative High School and Day Care Center, 5-6
Heathcare information and communications, 8-3, 8-9–8-10
Hepatitis B vaccines, 27-4, 28-2
HIV prevention strategies
biomedical approaches, 25-3
economic evaluation techniques, 25-1–25-2
epidemic, 25-2–25-3
mathematical modeling, 25-11
popular opinion leader intervention
behavioral intervention, 25-9
Bernoulli process model, 25-9
description, 25-8
intervention costs, 25-9
postexposure prophylaxis (PEP), 25-3
PrEP (*see* Preexposure prophylaxis)
Home-based monitoring, 1-6, 29-11
Hong Kong flu, 40-5
Horizontal integration model, 5-2
Hospices, 44-2
Hospital-based clinics, 4-3
Hospital bed turnaround
cleaning procedures, 37-3
definition, 37-1, 37-3
high-level flow diagram, 37-3, 37-5
staffing roles, 37-4
Housekeeping room turnover, 33-11–33-12
Human papilloma virus (HPV), 27-1
Hurricane Katrina, 41-5

I

Incident management system, 41-7
Incremental cost-effectiveness ratio (ICER), 25-6
Indian Health Service, 7-3
Information, 2-5–2-6
Inpatient Evaluation Center (IPEC), 9-7
Inpatient pull system, 33-10, 33-11
Insurance, healthcare, *see* Healthcare insurance
Integrated and/or coordinated care, 4-7
Integrated care organization, 1-2
Integrated healthcare delivery model
barriers, healthcare services
acute to chronic care, 8-3
complexity, 8-2
fragmentation, 8-2–8-3
information and communications technology, 8-3
linking system, 8-3
care cycles, 8-6–8-7
care episode, 8-5–8-6
explicit services, 8-5
outcomes, 8-7
population extension, 8-7–8-8
provider levels, 8-4–8-5
research opportunities
acute to chronic care, 8-9
complexity, 8-8
fragmentation, 8-8–8-9
healthcare system, 8-10–8-11
individual in, 8-10
information and communications technology, 8-9–8-10
multidimensional metrics, 8-10
system support, 8-7
Intensity modulated radiation therapy (IMRT), 15-4–15-5
Interactive medicine
asynchronous technologies, 29-2
barriers and nonbelievers, 29-7–29-8
CHF patients, home monitoring, 29-11
chronic disease management, 29-4–29-5
definition, 29-1–29-2
diagnosis and treatment
dentistry, 29-4
pathology, 29-3
pediatrics, 29-4
store-and-forward technology, 29-2
teledermatology, 29-3
telehospice, 29-4
telepsychiatry, 29-3
teleradiology, 29-2
education and training, 29-8
e-health, 29-9
health Web site, 29-9
information retrieval, 29-2
isolated medicine, 29-5–29-7
synchronous technology, 29-2
telehospice, 29-10–29-11
TeleKid Care, 29-9–29-10
Intervention/allocation scheduling, 23-12

Intravenous (IV) medication administration, 12-7–12-10
Inventory management system
  decision-making process, 20-3
  design, 20-2
  Dutch Hospital
    overall performance objectives, 20-9–20-10
    planning and control, 20-8–20-9
    reasons for failure, 20-9
    redesign process, 20-10
    strengths and weakness, 20-8
  economic order quantity, 20-2–20-3
  framework
    information system, 20-6–20-7
    internal and external performance objectives, 20-4–20-5
    inventory planning and control, 20-6
    management concept, 20-4
    organizational embedding, 20-7–20-8
    organizational issues, 20-3–20-4
    physical infrastructure, 20-5–20-6
  healthcare setting, 20-1–20-2
  qualitative approach, 20-3
Inventory planning and control, 20-6
Irritable bowel syndrome (IBS), 43-3
Isolated medicine, 29-5–29-7

K

Key (process) performance indicators (KPI), 9-3, 9-9, 9-11
Knowledge representation, 24-4

L

Lean, heathcare
  analysis
    causes of operational problems, 11-8–11-10
    problems with implementation, 11-10–11-12
  discussion, 11-1–11-2
  doctors' orders, 11-9–11-10
  GDP, 11-1
  Great Britain's National Health Service, 11-6
  historical perspective, 11-4–11-5
  infusion suite, 11-8–11-9
  Intermountain Healthcare in Salt Lake City, 11-6
  kaizen event, 11-3–11-4
  Lean tools, 11-2–11-3
  principles, 11-2
  quality problems, 11-7
  radio frequency identification, 11-6
  Six Sigma technology, 11-4, 11-6–11-7
  VSM, 11-3
  waste, 11-3
Linear discriminant analysis, 24-12
Linear programming (LP)
  formulation, 15-3
  IMRT fluence map optimization, 15-4–15-5
  representation, 15-4
Liver transplantation decision models, 17-14–17-15
Long-term care
  assisted living facilities, 6-5–6-6
  culture
    autonomy, 6-7
    CCRC, 6-7
    health and the appearance of being healthy, 6-7–6-8
    meal time to residents, 6-8
    stigmatization widows and widowers, 6-8–6-9
  definition, 6-1
  family caregiver
    burden, 6-2
    caregiving activity, 6-1–6-2
    involvement, 6-4–6-5
    norms and duration, 6-2
    prevalence, 6-1
  financing, 6-6
  nursing homes
    vs. acute care settings, 6-4
    decision, 6-2–6-3
    physical care, 6-3–6-4
    quality of care, 6-3
    staff turnover, 6-4

M

Machine learning; *see also* Decision analysis
  alternative choice, 19-4
  AQ programs, 19-6–19-7
  decision making, 19-2
  medication outcomes, 19-8–19-9
Macroergonomics, 49-3
Maricopa County mental health system, 42-15
Market basket analysis, 24-9
Markov decision process (MDP)
  challenges and future research, 17-14
  clinical decision making, 17-14–17-15
  clinical healthcare applications, 17-9–17-10
  healthcare management, 17-10–17-13
  operational healthcare applications, 17-8–17-9
  theory
    actions and action sets, 17-2–17-3
    continuous time models, 17-7
    decision epochs, 17-2
    finite horizon MDP, 17-4–17-5
    infinite horizon models, 17-5–17-7
    limitations, 17-7
    reward/cost functions, 17-3
    states and state spaces, 17-2
    transition probabilities, 17-3
Marvell PXA family, application processors, 46-6

Master facility plan
  deliverables, 21-3, 21-4
  recommendations, 21-8
Master surgery scheduling, 23-10–23-11
  block scheduling strategy, 35-2
  definition, 35-2
  nurse scheduling, 35-6–35-7
  open scheduling strategy, 35-2
  optimization, 35-5–35-6
  visualization, 35-3–35-5
MDP, *see* Markov decision process
Medicaid, 7-2
Medical consumerism, 50-2
Medical expenses, 1-1–1-2
Medical informatics, *see* Health informatics
Medical science growth
  advances, 1-6–1-7
  biological science, 1-5
  home-based monitoring, 1-6
  population science, 1-6
  social science, 1-6
  wireless-based tools, 1-6
Medical surge
  capacity and capability, 41-2
  capacity components
    care personnel and staff, 41-5–41-6
    decision-making process, 41-5
    disposition classification, 41-5
    equipment, supplies, 41-6–41-7
    facility, 41-6
    incident management system, 41-7
    multidimensional aspects, 41-4
  definitions, 41-2, 41-3
  GAO, 41-7–41-8
  international collaboration, 41-8
  medical system resiliency, 41-2
  patterns, 41-3–41-4
  surge-in-place solutions, 41-2
Medical-surgical products
  definition, 45-5
  dollar-flow, 45-6–45-8
  information flow, 45-6
  product-flow, 45-5–45-6
Medical system resiliency, 41-2
Medicare, 1-1, 7-2
Mental health allocation and planning simulation model
  Arnold v. Sarn service capacity plan
    annual service system costs, 42-12, 42-14
    background, 42-10
    functional level distribution estimation, 42-10–42-11
    rehabilitation costs, 42-12
    service definitions, 42-11
    service package costs, 42-12, 42-14
    service unit cost estimation, 42-11–42-13
    transition probabilities estimation, 42-12
  criminal justice, 42-16–42-17
  expenditures distribution, 42-14, 42-15
  frictionless system, 42-16
  human services research institute
    acute psychiatric symptoms, 42-4
    conceptual framework, 42-3
    delivery of services, 42-3
    functional level groups, 42-5–42-6
    level of functioning, 42-3
    mathematical formulation, 42-4–42-5
    outcome estimation, 42-8–42-9
    planning service packages, 42-6–42-8
    unit costs and revenues, 42-8
    Web-based implementation, 42-9–42-10
  Maricopa County mental health system, 42-15
  operations research models, 42-1–42-3
  Quebec planning, 42-17
  remedial strategic plans, 42-15
Meta-heuristic approach, 15-14–15-15
Methicillin-resistant *Staphylococcus aureus* (MRSA), 13-5–13-6
M/G/1 and G/G/s models, 16-8
Microcontrollers, 46-5
Military Health System, 7-3
Mixed integer programming (MIP), 15-5–15-7
M/M/s model
  advantage, 16-6
  average delay, 16-6
  construction, 16-15
  finite capacity models, 16-7–16-8
  obstetrics unit, 16-9
  performance constraint, 16-7
  priority models, 16-7
  probability of delay, 16-12
  target occupancy levels, 16-9, 16-10
Model for end-stage liver disease (MELD)
  encephalopathy and ascites, 30-6
  formulaic scoring system, 30-6
  liver allocation policy, 30-6
  policy compliance and patient safety, 30-7–30-8
Monte Carlo simulation, 14-8
Multi-criteria optimization, *see* Multi-objective optimization
Multidisciplinary centers, 2-6–2-7
Multilayer perceptron, 24-14
Multi-objective optimization (MOO)
  medical resource planning and management, 15-11
  nurse scheduling, 15-10–15-11
  representation, 15-10
  solution strategies, 15-10
Multi-priority patient scheduling, 17-10–17-13

N

Naive Bayesian classifier, 24-12
National drug codes (NDC), 45-8–45-9
National Healthcare Expenditure, 7-3

National Institutes of Health (NIH), 1-5
Natural language processing (NLP), 9-10
Neonatal Intensive Care Units (NICU), 47-10
Nonhomogeneous Poisson arrival process (NHPP), 14-7
Nonlinear programming (NLP), 15-7–15-8
North Central Nursing Clinics (NCNC), 5-1, 5-3–5-4
Nurse-managed clinics
  challenges, 5-7
  consultation, 5-4–5-5
  direct practice, 5-2
  DNP development, 5-7–5-9
  indirect care contracts, 5-4
  models, 5-1–5-2
  North Central Nursing Clinics, 5-3–5-4
  payment models, 5-5
  program costs, 5-3
  survival, 5-1
  UT Nursing Clinical Enterprise, 5-5–5-7
Nurse rostering
  constraint programming, 23-4
  constraints and objectives, 23-2
  heuristic approach, 23-4–22-5
  mathematical programming, 23-3–23-4
  optimization methods, 23-3
  research and development of technologies and methodologies, 23-2
  VNS approach, IP model
    constraints, 23-6–23-9
    decision variables, 23-5
    heuristic shift ordering, 23-8
    hybrid method, 23-8, 23-9
    parameters, 23-5
Nursing homes
  vs. acute care settings, 6-4
  decision, 6-2–6-3
  physical care, 6-3–6-4
  quality of care, 6-3
  staff turnover, 6-4
Nursing medication management process, 12-11–12-12
Nutrition therapy, 44-5–44-6

O

Object-oriented simulation (OOS), 14-9–14-10
Office-based clinics, 4-2–4-3
On-board processing, *see* Body sensor networks
Online analytical processing (OLAP) systems, 9-10–9-11
Ontologies, 46-15
Open access, primary care, 10-2–10-3
Operating room turnover
  ambulatory surgery centers, 37-5
  circulator, 37-2
  cleaning tasks, 37-6
  definition, 37-1, 37-2
  high-level flow diagram, 37-3, 37-4
  housekeeping personnel, 37-2
  registered nurse (RN) or surgical technologist, 37-2
  scrub person roles, 37-6
Operational business intelligence (OBI), 9-10–9-11
Operational capacity planning
  advance and allocation scheduling, 34-3
  booking control, 34-4
  case duration estimation, 34-8–34-9
  case sequencing, 34-6–34-8
  external resource scheduling, 34-4
  patient flow optimizing, 34-9–34-10
Operational healthcare, 17-8–17-9
Operational surgery scheduling, 23-11–23-13
Optimization techniques
  application, 15-2–15-3
  categories, 15-2
  computer simulation, 14-12–14-13
  concept, 15-1
  implementation, 15-1–15-2
  mathematical models
    linear programming, 15-3–15-5
    mixed integer programming, 15-5–15-7
    multi-objective optimization, 15-10–15-11
    nonlinear programming, 15-7–15-8
    stochastic programming, 15-8–15-10
  solution algorithms
    meta-heuristic approach, 15-14–15-15
    traditional solution algorithms, 15-12–15-14
Organizational embedding, 20-7–20-8
Organ procurement and transplantation network (OPTN)
  bylaws and policies, 30-4–30-5
  membership and representation, 30-3–30-4
  policy development process, 30-5–30-6
  roles and scientific registry, 30-3
Orthopedic devices
  dollar-flow, 45-15
  information-flow, 45-14–45-15
  manufacturer, surgeon relationship, 45-13
  product-flow, 45-14
Outpatient clinics
  care coordination, 4-7–4-8
  medical home, 4-7
  practice expenses and overhead, 4-3–4-4
  primary care shortage, 4-8
  quality, 4-5–4-7
  revenue and payment for services, 4-4–4-5
  size and scope, 4-1–4-2
  structure, 4-2–4-3

P

Pandemics emergency planning model
  epidemiology, 40-2
  health- and logistics-related tasks, 40-14
  hospital plan, 40-11–40-12
  hospital staffing strategies, 40-8–40-9
  incident command selection, 40-8

influenza, 40-5–40-6
military application, 40-1
military tactics
CDC surveillance system, 40-4
infodemiology and infoveillance, 40-3
minimal intervention, 40-4
office of surgeon general (OSG), 40-3
primary and secondary prevention method, 40-5
principles, 40-3
prophylaxes *vs.* treatment, 40-4
swine flu, 40-3
past history, 40-2
planning benefits, 40-2
prevention, 40-6
individual strategies, 40-8
national strategy, 40-8
strategic planning
development and implementation, 40-9–40-11
planning constraints, 40-6–40-7
situational uncertainties, 40-7
and tactics, 40-14–40-15
TTX
areas for improvement, evaluators, 40-13–40-14
survey, 40-13
Panel design genetic algorithm (PDGA), 10-7–10-8; *see also* Primary care
PARiHS framework
implementation, 13-3
social capital
contextual factor, 13-4
elements, 13-5
evidence, 13-4
facilitation, 13-4–13-5
Patient care cycles, 8-6–8-7, 8-11
Patient-Centered Medical Home (PC-MH), 4-7, 10-8–10-9
Patient-physician continuity, 10-2–10-3
Patient/resident feeding
acute-care patients, 44-4
design, 44-8
hospice care, 44-5
long-term care, 44-4–44-5
Patient safety, 37-6; *see also* Proactive risk assessment
goals of safety engineering, 12-2
paradigms, 12-1–12-2
Patient scheduling
offline sequencing step, 35-9–35-10
taxonomy, 35-8
Patient service centers/call centers, 44-10
Pay-for-performance (P4P), 4-5–4-6
Pearson's correlation coefficient, definition, 24-6
Pediatric end-stage liver disease (PELD) model, 30-7
Performance measurement, healthcare organizations
barriers
aggregation, 9-8–9-9
clinical guidelines, 9-7–9-8
data analysis, 9-8
individual measures effectiveness, 9-8
challenges, 9-3
design principles, 9-5, 9-6
diabetes outcomes, 9-4
Donabedian model, 9-4–9-5
healthcare measurement system, 9-5–9-6
natural language processing, 9-10
operational business intelligence, 9-10–9-11
proliferation, 9-8
rationale
comparison and competition, 9-2–9-3
discussions and decision making, 9-3
goals, 9-1–9-2
performance measurement-driven behavior, 9-2
vertical and horizontal integration, 9-5
veterans health administration, 9-6–9-7
Personal health record (PHR)
definition, 50-2
electronic health information, 50-5
health information managing tool, 50-2
health information on paper, 50-1
history, 50-2–50-4
makeshift solutions, 50-1–50-2
medical consumerism, 50-2
privacy
ARRA, 50-8–50-10
ePHR, 50-6
HIPAA, 50-6
paper record, 50-6
policy, 50-7–50-8
product models, 50-4–50-5
security, health information, 50-5
Personalized medicine, 1-12–1-13
Pervasive healthcare, 46-4
Pharmaceutical products
provider supply chain
dollar-flow, 45-10–45-12
information-flow, 45-8–45-10
product-flow, 45-8
retail/mail-order supply chain
dollar-flow, 45-13
information-flow, 45-12–45-13
product-flow, 45-12
Pharmacoeconomics and drug development process
aspirin, 31-9
cardiovascular event prevention, 31-9
cost control, 31-1
decision-analytic modeling, 31-1, 31-6
drug approval process, 31-2–31-3
economic modeling, 31-2
guidelines, 31-3–31-5
incremental cost, 31-10
ischemic *vs.* hemorrhagic stroke, 31-9
model analyses
benefit–risk analyses, 31-9
budget impact analyses, 31-7

clinical planning, 31-8
cost-effectiveness analyses, 31-5–31-7
hypertensive agents, 31-5
threshold analyses, 31-7–31-8
valuation modeling, 31-10
pharmacotherapy, 31-2
statins, 31-9
Pharmacy benefits managers (PBM), 45-4
PHR, *see* Personal health record
Physician culture
autonomy, 1-3–1-4
intuition *vs.* prediction, 1-4–1-5
physician exceptionalism, 1-4
Physician explained variation (PEV), 18-7–18-8, 18-10–18-11
Physician Quality Reporting Initiative (PQRI), 4-6
Pigouvian welfare model, 28-5
Points of dispensing (POD), 41-11–41-13
Poisson process
arrival and demand process, 16-5–16-6
assumption, 16-4–16-5
properties, 16-5
Post-Anesthesia Recovery Unit (PACU), 14-4, 14-12
Postexposure prophylaxis (PEP), 25-3
Preemptive and non-preemptive model, 16-7
Preexposure prophylaxis
chemoprophylaxis, 25-7
compartmental models, 25-5
description, 25-4–25-5
economic and disease modeling, 25-5
economic evaluation, 25-5
incremental cost-effectiveness ratio (ICER), 25-6
quality-adjusted life year (QALY), 25-6–25-7
sensitivity analysis, 25-7
tenofovir plus emtricitabine, 25-5
treatment cost estimation, 25-6
Preventive care, economic implications
cost-effectiveness evaluation
anti-tobacco programs, 28-4
cost-benefit analysis, 28-5
cost-utility analysis, 28-5
welfare-enhancing income transfer effect, 28-6
welfare-maximizing preventive interventions, 28-5
definition, prevention, 28-3
disease management programs, 28-1
environmental risk regulation, 28-2
incentives, 28-3–28-4
medicine, 28-1
morbidity and mortality rates, 28-2
primary prevention
air quality, 28-7–28-8
drinking water quality, 28-7
physical activity promotion, 28-8
vaccinations, 28-6–28-7
rehabilitation, 28-10–28-11
secondary prevention
breast cancer, 28-9–28-10
colorectal cancer, 28-9
tertiary prevention, 28-10
Primary care, 32-6
appointment scheduling, 10-2
benefits, 10-1
emerging trends
patient-centered medical home, 10-8–10-9
team care, 10-8
open access adoption, 10-2–10-3
panel management
capacity planning, 10-6
definition, 10-2
genetic algorithm, 10-7–10-8
histogram, weekly appointments, 10-5
optimization problem, 10-6–10-7
patient classification, 10-3–10-5
patient-physician continuity, 10-2–10-3
timely access to care, 10-1–10-2
Primary care internal medicine (PCIM), 10-2
Principal component analysis (PCA), 24-7
Private healthcare insurance
regulation, 7-6
state-licensed/self-funded insurance, 7-5
top companies, 7-2
Proactive risk assessment; *see also* Patient safety
adverse drug events, 12-4
continuous drug infusion delivery, 12-4–12-5
CPOE/EHR, ICUs, 12-10–12-11
diversity, 12-2–12-3
drug prescribing process, 12-5
for health hazards, 12-2
intravenous (IV) medication administration, 12-7–12-10
nursing medication management process, 12-11–12-12
organizational learning and sensemaking, 12-3
practical considerations
advice for conducting, 12-5–12-6
selection process, 12-6, 12-7
process analysis, 12-4
thoracic organ transplantation process, 12-4
Probability networks
arthritis pain, 26-6
Bayesian probability network, 26-5
cyclic causal diagram, 26-5
mortality causes, 26-6
structures, 26-6
Process-interaction approach, 14-9
Process mapping, 14-9
Product supply chains
organizations
distributors, 45-2–45-3
GPO, 45-3–45-4
major players, 45-1, 45-2

manufacturer, 45-2
PBM, 45-3–45-4
provider, 45-2
purchase products, 45-4–45-5
Profiling/report cards, 18-1, 18-3
Prophylaxis
vs. treatment, 40-4
vaccination, 41-16
Provider supply chain
dollar-flow, 45-10–45-12
information-flow, 45-8–45-10, 45-9
product-flow, 45-8
Psychosocial distress
assessment, 43-5–43-6
barriers, 43-9–43-10
baseline depressive symptoms, 43-8
caregiving and healthcare delivery, 43-3–43-4
definitions, 43-1–43-2
disease outcomes, 43-2–43-3
interventions, 43-6–43-7, 43-10
peer-led self-management program, 43-8–43-9
professional caregivers, 43-11
quality-of-life issues, 43-11
racial concordance, 43-8
research challenges, 43-10–43-11
risk factors, 43-4–43-5
rural *vs.* urban residents, 43-9
spirituality, 43-7–43-8
Public health and medical preparedness
catastrophic health event, 41-1
challenges, 41-33–41-34
communication system
facilitation programs, 41-24
organizational factors, 41-24, 41-26
physical infrastructure (*see* Emergency communication)
robust communication infrastructure, 41-20
sociological factors, 41-26
two-way communication lines, 41-20
decision support systems, 41-32–41-33
emergency evacuation
affecting factors, 41-27
behavior, 41-29–41-30
definition, 41-26
hospital, 41-27–41-29
epidemiology and disease propagation models, 41-31
hybrid fuzzy clustering-optimization approach, 41-31
MASSVAC 4.0 software tool, 41-31
medical surge (*see* Medical surge)
New York City-RAND Institute (NYCRI), 41-30
planning, 41-2
population protection
anthrax drills, 41-17–41-18
communication and public information, 41-16–41-17
department of health and human services, 41-9
disease-propagation analysis (*see* Disease-propagation analysis)
dispensing mode, 41-10–41-11
large-scale disaster relief efforts, 41-19–41-20
mass dispensing operations, 41-9
multilayer protection, 41-18
POD layout design, 41-13
POD placement, 41-11–41-12
points of dispensing (POD) placement, 41-11–41-12
public-health emergencies, 41-8
resource allocation, 41-12–41-13
smallpox vaccine, 41-9
supply chain management, 41-16
trauma resource allocation model, 41-30

Q

Quality-adjusted life year (QALY), 17-10, 25-6–25-7
Quality control
healthcare, 2-1–2-2
hospital clinical laboratories
accuracy and precision, 39-5–39-6
blood and urine testing services, 39-1
blood collection flow diagram, 39-3, 39-6
error budget, 39-4
performance limits, 39-4
quality control management systems, 39-1
system analysis and flowcharting, 39-2–39-4
turnaround time (TAT) expectation, 39-6
management systems, 39-1
Quality-of-life, 43-11
Quebec planning, 42-17
Queueing theory and modeling
basic principles
delays, utilization, and system size, 16-3–16-4
M/G/1 and G/G/s models, 16-8
M/M/s model, 16-6–16-8
Poisson process, 16-4–16-6
fixed capacity analysis
benefits of flexibility, 16-13–16-14
delay standard, 16-11–16-12
demand prediction, 16-12–16-13
M/M/s model, 16-9
target occupancy levels, 16-9–16-11
flexible capacity analysis
data collection and model choices, 16-14–16-15
delay standard and queueing results, 16-15
model construct, 16-15
healthcare, 16-1–16-2
opportunities and challenges, 16-16–16-17
queueing fundamentals, 16-2–16-3

R

Radio frequency identification (RFID), 47-11
Radiotherapy treatment planning, 15-8
Recursive partitioning method, 24-12
Relative value units (RVUs), 4-5
Resource allocation, 41-12–41-13
Retail/mail-order supply chain
 dollar-flow, 45-13
 information-flow, 45-12–45-13
 product-flow, 45-12
Reverse genetics, 27-12
Reward/cost functions, 17-3
RNA-based vaccines, 27-5
Rofecoxib, *see* Vioxx
Run and control charts, 18-2
Rural physicians, 4-2

S

SARS, 41-5
Scheduling and sequencing
 common scenarios, 23-1
 disadvantages, manual schedules, 23-1
 nurse rostering
  constraint programming, 23-4
  constraints and objectives, 23-2
  heuristic approach, 23-4–22-5
  mathematical programming, 23-3–23-4
  optimization methods, 23-3
  research and development, technologies and methodologies, 23-2
  VNS approach, 23-5–23-9
 surgery scheduling
  master surgery schedule, 23-10–23-11
  operating room management, 23-9
  operational surgery scheduling, 23-11–23-13
  patient mix planning, 23-9
Scientific registry of transplant recipients (SRTR), 30-1
Self-Funded Employer Health Benefit Plans, 7-5
Self-operated *vs.* contracted foodservice, 44-3–44-4
Sequential decision problems (SDPs), 17-2
Sick care delivery system, 1-6, 1-10–1-11
Sickness syndrome, 43-2
Simplex method, 15-12
Simulated annealing (SA), 15-15
Smallpox vaccine, 41-9
Smart home technology, 46-9
Social capital theory
 communities of practice, 13-8–13-10
 PARiHS framework
  contextual factor, 13-4
  elements, 13-5
  evidence, 13-4
  facilitation, 13-4–13-5
 social network analysis (SNA)
  context, 13-7–13-8
  evidence, 13-7
  facilitation, 13-8
  methicillin-resistant *Staphylococcus aureus,* 13-5–13-6
  network density, 13-6–13-7
Spanish flu, 40-5
Spirituality, 43-7–43-8
State Children's Health Insurance Program (SCHIP), 7-2–7-3
State-Licensed Insurance Companies/ Organizations, 7-5
Statins, 31-9
Statistical analysis and modeling
 Bayesian inference, 18-6–18-7
 challenges, 18-4
 classical statistical approach, provider profiling
  ordinary least squares regression, 18-4–18-5
  random effects approach, 18-5
 multi-institutional analysis, 18-2
 numerical property of outcomes, 18-3–18-4
 pharmacy expenditures, health maintenance, organization
  disease types and medication prescription, 18-9–18-10
  PEV and APEV estimation, 18-10–18-11
  physician performance index, 18-11–18-12
  ranking, physician, 18-12–18-13
  statistical inference, 18-9
  two-part hierarchical model estimation, 18-9–18-10
  unit of analysis, 18-9
 physician explained variation (PEV), 18-7–18-8
 profiling/report cards, 18-1, 18-3
 risk adjustment, 18-3
 statistical inference, 18-1
 statistical process control, graphical time series, 18-2–18-3
 statistical testing, 18-1–18-2
 two-part hierarchical model, 18-5–18-6
Sterilization, 38-7–38-10
 choice of sterilizing process, 38-10
 definition, 38-3
 dry heat sterilizers, 38-9
 kinetics, 38-7
 low-temperature sterilizers, 38-9–38-10
 steam, properties, 38-7–38-8
 steam sterilization cycle, 38-8–38-9
Stochastic programming (SP)
 adaptive treatment planning, 15-9–15-10
 fuzzy optimization, 15-8–15-9
Strategic facility planning, 21-1–21-2
Strategic national stockpile (SNS) program, 41-6
Subject-matter experts (SMEs), 14-5
Supply chain management, 41-16

Surgery scheduling
advance scheduling and allocation scheduling, 35-2
case mix planning, 35-2
managerial aspect, 35-1
master surgery schedule, 23-10–23-11
master surgery scheduling
block scheduling strategy, 35-2
definition, 35-2
nurse scheduling, 35-6–35-7
open scheduling strategy, 35-2
optimization, 35-5–35-6
visualization, 35-3–35-5
operating room management, 23-9
operational surgery scheduling
intervention/allocation scheduling, 23-12
intervention assignment, 23-11–23-12
variations, 23-13
patient mix planning, 23-9
patient scheduling
offline sequencing step, 35-9–35-10
taxonomy, 35-8
Swine flu, 28-6, 40-3
System-on-chip (SoC), 46-6
Systems dynamics, 14-10–14-11
System support, 8-7, 8-11

T

Tabletop exercises (TTX)
areas for improvement, evaluators, 40-13–40-14
community involvement, 40-13
pandemic preparation, 40-14
physical infrastructure, emergency communication, 41-20
survey, 40-13
Tactical capacity planning
advance and allocation scheduling, 34-3
block and nonblock system, 34-3–34-4
booking control, 34-4
external resource scheduling, 34-4
time allocation, 34-4–34-6
Task analysis
continuous work flow, 22-7–22-8
future state plan, 22-8
personal worksheet, medical administration, 22-7, 22-9
time and activity study, 22-7, 22-8
Team care, 10-8
Telehospice, 29-10–29-11
TeleKid Care, 29-9–29-10
Tenofovir plus emtricitabine, 25-5
Thermal washer disinfectors, 38-6
Thoracic organ transplantation, 12-4
Toyota Production System (TPS), 22-2
Trade union, 36-11
Transition probabilities, 17-3
Transjugular intrahepatic portosystemic shunt (TIPS) procedures, 30-6
Triage, 33-4
Turnaround time (TAT), 39-6
Two-part hierarchical model, 18-5–18-6

U

Ultrasonic cleaners, 38-6
Unit cost estimation, 42-11–42-13
United Network for Organ Sharing (UNOS), 30-1
United States Environmental Protection Agency (USEPA), 28-2
University of Texas
Houston School of Nursing, 5-2
Nursing Clinical Enterprise, 5-5–5-7
U.S organ transplant network
data collection and analysis, 30-12–30-13
federal legislation and regulation, 30-2
heart allocation policy, 30-13–30-14
history, 30-1–30-2
MELD (*see* Model for end-stage liver disease)
OPTN (*see* Organ procurement and transplantation network)
organ placement activities
host OPO, 30-9
medical judgment, 30-9
UNet^{sm} and DonorNet®, 30-9–30-10
UNOS organ center, 30-10–30-11
organ wastage prevention, 30-11
transplant community, 30-11

V

Vaccinations, 28-6–28-7
Vaccines
applications, 27-1–27-2
cell culture-derived vaccines
avian fibroblasts, 27-11
bacterial cells, 27-8–27-9
Chinese hamster ovary cells, 27-11
host systems and current applications, 27-7
human embryonic kidney-293 cells, 27-10
insect cells, 27-9
Madin-Darby bovine kidney cells, 27-10
Madin-Darby canine kidney cells, 27-10
mammalian cells and transfection, 27-10–27-12
MRC-5 cells, 27-10–27-11
PER.C6 cells, 27-11
plant cells, 27-7–27-8
reverse genetics, 27-12
vero cells, 27-10
yeast cells, 27-9
cervical cancer prevention, 27-1
evolution, 27-2

market, 27-1–27-2
production system
eggs, 27-5
non-plant cells, 27-6–27-7
plants, 27-5–27-6
product purification
antigens, 27-13–27-14
downstream processing, 27-13
egg-based viral vaccines, 27-13
flow diagram, 27-13
planning and scheduling, 27-15
product quality assessment, 27-15
quality control, 27-14–27-15
whole virus vaccines, 27-13
smallpox, 41-9
types
anti-cervical cancer vaccines, 27-5
component, 27-4
DNA-based vaccines, 27-5
hepatitis B vaccines, 27-4
RNA-based vaccines, 27-5
whole organism, 27-3–27-4
VA healthcare delivery system
computerized patient record system, 3-11
healthcare budget and financing mechanisms
appropriations, 3-9–3-10
fee basis and contract care, 3-10
medical care cost recovery, 3-10
veterans equitable resource allocation system, 3-10
healthcare settings
Iraq and Afghanistan freedom veterans, 3-15–3-16
mental health and/or substance abuse, 3-14
spinal cord injuries, 3-14–3-15
women veterans, 3-15
healthcare utilization, 3-12
health status of users, 3-11–3-12
historical evolution, 3-1–3-3
leadership and organizational structure
community-based outpatient clinics, 3-9
medical centers, 3-8–3-9
veterans health administration, 3-6–3-7
veterans integrated service networks, 3-7–3-8
mission and goals
contingency support and emergency management, 3-6
education and training mission, 3-5
healthcare-related research, 3-5–3-6
medical care mission, 3-5
patient care service
eligibility, 3-4–3-5
scope, 3-11
quality of care
national VA patient safety registry, 3-13
performance measurement system, 3-13
research–clinical partnerships, 3-14
quality transformation, 3-3–3-4
Value stream map (VSM)
activities and order, work flow, 22-3–22-4
vs. conventional process maps, 22-5–22-6
lean, 11-2, 11-3
policy deployment, 22-5
process box, 22-4–22-5
time and motion study, 22-5
unhappy patient, 22-4
Vertical integration model, 5-2
Veterans equitable resource allocation (VERA) system, 3-10
Veterans health administration (VHA), 7-3, 9-6–9-7, 44-2
Veterans integrated service networks (VISNs), 3-7–3-8
Vioxx; *see also* Causal risk analysis
arthritis, 26-2
and aspirin, 26-4
cause and effect, 19-5, 26-3
decision analysis, withdrawal, 19-3
medication outcome evaluation, 19-8–19-9
rule based models, 19-5–19-7
side effects, 26-5, 26-6
treatment, 26-2
VSM, *see* Value stream map

W

Wearable/ambient sensor monitoring, 46-9
Whole organism vaccines, 27-3–27-4
Wilcoxon rank sum test, 24-6
Williamson Medical Center (WMC)
growth and reputation, 21-5–21-6
master facility plan recommendations, 21-8
project phasing plan, 21-8–21-12
site evaluation, 21-7–21-8
team initiates feasibility phase, 21-6
value of planning, 21-12–21-13
Wireless-based tools, 1-6
Wireless sensor networks
ambient sensor nodes, 46-4
behavior analysis
activity monitoring, 46-10–46-12
anomaly detection, 46-13–46-14
data mining, 46-12–46-13
smart home technology, 46-9
wearable/ambient sensor monitoring, 46-9
body sensor networks
autonomic sensing, 46-7–46-8
context-aware sensing, 46-7
embedded data enhancement, 46-8–46-9
characteristics, 46-3, 46-4
clinical requirements, 46-2
clinical uptake, 46-14
data standardization, 46-15

healthcare monitoring systems, 46-2
microcontrollers, 46-5
miniaturization, 46-15
node classification, 46-3
on-node processing, 46-15
pervasive healthcare scenario, 46-4
postoperative recovery, 46-1
prediction, 46-15
SoC solutions, 46-6
SPI/I^{2}C protocols, 46-6
system architecture, 46-5
topology, 46-3

Work design; *see also* Task analysis
continuous work flow, 22-3
current state to future state, 20-6–20-7
future state plan, 22-9–22-11
ideal approach, 22-2
inconsistency, 22-1, 22-2
interruptions in work, 22-3
organization functions, 22-1
random and standard work, 22-2
task analysis, 22-7–22-9
validation, work revisions, 22-6
VSM (*see* Value stream map)